Gerontology

Gerontology

Changes, Challenges, and Solutions

Volume 2: Health and Wellbeing

Madonna Harrington Meyer and
Elizabeth A. Daniele, Editors

PRAEGER™

An Imprint of ABC-CLIO, LLC
Santa Barbara, California • Denver, Colorado

Library of Congress Cataloging-in-Publication Data

Names: Harrington Meyer, Madonna, 1959– , editor. | Daniele, Elizabeth A., editor
Title: Gerontology : changes, challenges, and solutions / Madonna Harrington Meyer, Elizabeth A. Daniele, editors.
Description: Santa Barbara, California : Praeger, 2016. | Includes bibliographical references and index.
Identifiers: LCCN 2015039168 | ISBN 9781440834264 (set) | ISBN: 978-1-4408-4491-1 (vol. 1) | ISBN: 978-1-4408-4492-8 (vol. 2) | ISBN: 978-1-4408-3427-1 (set : ebook)
Subjects: | MESH: Aging. | Geriatrics. | Aged.
Classification: LCC RC952.55 | NLM WT 100 | DDC 618.97—dc23
LC record available at http://lccn.loc.gov/2015039168

ISBN: 978-1-4408-3426-4 (set)
978-1-4408-4491-1 (vol 1)
978-1-4408-4492-8 (vol 2)
EISBN: 978-1-4408-3427-1

20 19 18 17 16 1 2 3 4 5

This book is also available on the World Wide Web as an eBook.
Visit www.abc-clio.com for details.

Praeger
An Imprint of ABC-CLIO, LLC

ABC-CLIO, LLC
130 Cremona Drive, P.O. Box 1911
Santa Barbara, California 93116-1911

This book is printed on acid-free paper ∞

Manufactured in the United States of America

To my family,
my greatest joy
M.H.M.

To my family,
my first teachers and greatest support
E.A.D.

Contents

Introduction

Madonna Harrington Meyer

Volume 2: Health and Wellbeing

As socioeconomic disparities grow in the United States, so do health disparities. Volume 2 focuses on causes and consequences of growing inequalities in health and well-being. The health and wellness of older people is tremendously diverse. By the time they reach age 65, millions of older Americans have enjoyed decades of cumulative advantage and report good health and abundant resources with which to protect their health. But millions of others have faced decades of cumulative disadvantage and report poor health and insufficient resources with which to protect their health (Ferraro, Shippee, & Schafer, 2009; Avendano & Kawachi, 2014). While some fight hard against age-related health and disability problems, others are overwhelmed by both the physical and economic consequences.

These differences become apparent in a comparison of Harriette and Bennie. In May of 2015, Syracuse University Alumni Harriette Thompson of Charlotte, North Carolina, completed her 16th Rock 'n' Roll Marathon in San Diego in less than 7½ hours. At age 92, she became the oldest woman to finish a marathon (Associated Press, 2015). It wasn't easy. Harriette is a cancer survivor who had, just months earlier, buried her husband and struggled with a staph infection in her leg. But the classically trained pianist, who studied at the New England Conservatory and performed at Carnegie Hall three times, told reporters that she mentally played piano pieces as she ran more than 26 miles. Perhaps most surprising? When she ran her very first marathon, she was already in her seventies (Associated Press, 2015). During her runs, she raises money for cancer research. Additionally, she told reporters, running has helped to keep her healthy. "I don't think I'd be living today if I didn't do this running."

In stark contrast, 53-year-old Bennie is struggling to walk any distance at all. I interviewed Bennie, a white, married, mother of three and grandmother of three, for my book, *Grandmothers at Work: Juggling Families and*

Jobs (Harrington Meyer, 2014). She told me that her husband no longer works due to a series of health problems and disabilities. "My husband is disabled. He has a bad back from working years as a mechanic. He is only 47, and he has been disabled for three years. Just two weeks ago he had a heart attack, and had two stents put in. And he is borderline diabetic and has a hernia." Bennie completed high school and works full time as a lab technician. "Now I have the only job, I have the only income." But health problems have also interfered with Bennie's mobility. "I have just spent three months recovering from my second knee replacement." Her salary—and his disability benefits—provide them with a household income of just $40,000. Though they find a great deal of joy caring for their grandchildren, they are foregoing plans to travel or move to a quieter neighborhood. "We are much more financially strapped and have many more physical problems than we ever thought. It has been rough, had a hard life," she explained. "I thought we would be working, travelling, spending on the grandkids, not struggling with health and money."

As the U.S. population ages, and we reach record numbers and proportions of older Americans, how healthy will we be? The answer is not simple. For every article tracing improvements in life expectancy or decreases in cancer rates, there are articles predicting longer but sicker older ages (Siegel, Miller, & Jemal, 2015; Avendano & Kawachi, 2014). Will we see more like Harriette or more like Bennie? Surely we will see more of both. Scholars expect to see growing diversity in health and well-being and, as the chapters in this volume suggest, our old-age health will be shaped by macrolevel factors including economic inequality, social policies, and health-care policies, as well as microlevel factors including our own health behaviors.

Overview of Chapters

With each generation, higher proportions of Americans are completing higher levels of education. That said, access to, and quality of, education continues to vary significantly by race, ethnicity, and socioeconomic status. Moreover, we are not keeping pace with our European neighbors. In Chapter 1, Elizabeth Daniele examines trends in, and impacts of, educational attainment across the life course. She demonstrates the powerful impact of education on health and well-being across the life course. She then focuses on lifelong learning for older adults, assessing the importance of adult education, various types of learning, best practices for older learners, and the increasingly important role of technology. She concludes with thoughts about the future of education for all ages.

Many artists produce some of their most creative works after serious health problems and when they are well into old age (Dormandy, 2000). Georgia O'Keefe was still painting when she was nearly blind and 96 years old. Creativity and wisdom are a highly valued part of human existence throughout the life course. In Chapter 2, Monika Ardelt and Carolyn Adams-Price review how researchers define and measure creativity and wisdom. They explore similarities and differences related to age and personality and then describe the benefits in later life. They reveal that both creativity and wisdom improve well-being in old age, particularly during difficult times.

How important is it to volunteer? Or go to church? Both have significant positive impacts on health and well-being, and it turns out that those who do one are more likely to do the other. Though religious preferences and attachments may change over the life course, generally those who attend church during childhood are more likely to attend, and volunteer, at older ages. In Chapter 3, Fengyan Tang explores the links between volunteering and religion by analyzing the four dimensions in religion: religiosity, religious identity, religious socialization, and religious social networks. Tang explores how the links between volunteering, religion, and the four dimensions influence health and well-being, paying careful attention to how those links vary by age, gender, race, and socioeconomic status. Ultimately, most research suggests that those who volunteer and are religious have longer, healthier, more satisfying lives (McDougle, Handy, Konracth, & Walk, 2014; Li & Ferraro, 2006).

Since the 1800s, the human lifespan has increased worldwide. Dramatic increases have caused us to ponder, what are the limits? In Chapter 4, Donna Holmes demonstrates how the answers to that question integrate evolutionary, demographic, physiological, cellular, and molecular approaches. Currently scientists are focusing their studies on cell-signaling pathways involved in energy metabolism, the accumulation of cellular damage, and physiological dysregulation. She notes the extent to which morbidity and mortality vary by gender, particularly with regard to cardiovascular disease and various forms of disability, providing important insights into the evolving human lifespan. But of course lifespan depends on more than biological factors; a wide variety of cultural factors also shape these trends.

Americans are living longer but how healthy are those added years? The answers to this question are complex. Gerontologists have long said that men have higher mortality rates and women have higher morbidity rates, meaning that women live longer, but sicker, lives. In Chapter 5, Anna Zajacova and Vicki Johnson-Lawrence explore new and conflicting trends in morbidity and mortality among our aging populations. They focus on fundamental causes of health disparities and contextualize health behaviors as risk factors for morbidity and mortality. In examining the leading causes of morbidity and mortality, they pay close attention to the disparities by socioeconomic status, gender, and race/ethnicity. Ultimately, they demonstrate how a complete understanding of morbidity and mortality is critical to individuals, their families, and our national economic and health-care policies.

Mental and cognitive health are complex matters. The risk of mental health problems such as depression are highest at younger ages, the risk of cognitive disorders such as dementia are highest at older ages, and the risk of both are higher for those who have additional medical conditions. In Chapter 6, Donna McAlpine and Taeho Greg Rhee examine social and life-course characteristics that help explain class and race differences in risk factors, costs, burdens, and consequences of cognitive and other mental health disorders in later life. They emphasize the degree to which cognitive disorders, particularly when they coexist with other mental disorders, create significant burdens for individuals, their families, and our society.

Experts estimate that care provided by family and friends comprised well over one-half of all long-term care costs for the elderly in the United States (Congressional Budget Office, 2013). In fact most of us will, at some point in our lives, be both the provider, and the recipient, of informal care. In Chapter 7, Eliza Pavalko and Joseph Wolfe examine who provides care, how it has changed over time, and how it varies by gender, race, ethnicity, and socioeconomic status. They review the health and economic consequences of providing care and explore the ways people balance unpaid care work with employment. They conclude by discussing workplace and national policies that help—and hinder—care workers balance competing demands.

Elder abuse is one of the darkest secrets of old age. As many as 10 percent of those aged 60 and older living in the community, and an even higher percent of those living in nursing homes and assisted living facilities, have experienced some form of abuse in the past year (Acierno et al., 2010). Rates may be even higher given that many are too fearful, or too embarrassed, to report abuse. In Chapter 8, Joah Williams, Melba Hernandez-Tejada, Emily Fanguy, and Ron Acierno review the types of abuse and neglect, including psychological, physical, sexual, and financial. They assess the risk and protective factors associated with elder abuse, screening and assessment strategies, and elder abuse policy issues. Most important, they highlight preventive interventions, such as maintaining social connection and educating proximal bystanders about intervening.

If you ask Americans whether they would like to someday move to a nursing home, few will say yes. Indeed, though the proportion of older Americans is rising steadily, the proportion moving into nursing homes is shrinking steadily. In Chapter 9, Stephanie W. Burge explores what is behind this trend. She discusses functional health and cognitive status of those in nursing homes and in residential care facilities, the factors that determine nursing home placement, and barriers to nursing home access for minority elders. She concludes by analyzing recent changes in nursing home culture and the impact on residents and their families.

We know that we should plan ahead for our own deaths, but there is little about U.S. tradition or health practices that encourages us to do so. In Chapter 10, Megumi Inoue, Sara Keary, and Sara Moorman discuss death and dying, perceptions of good and bad deaths, and the much overlooked capacity to plan death. Though most wish to die at home, without pain or anguish, and in the company of loved ones, medical technology sustains many for longer than they and their families may wish. The authors review the alternatives, including advance care planning, hospice, euthanasia, physician-assisted suicide, and palliative sedation. Whether death comes quickly from an accident or acute illness, or slowly from a long-term chronic condition, the quality of the experience for us, and our families, can be much improved with forethought.

One of the most difficult challenges of old age is saying good-bye to all of those who pass before you. Bereavement and grief become increasingly commonplace as we age. But as Deborah Carr shows in Chapter 11, the intensity of grief varies based on characteristics of the survivor, the decedent, and circumstances surrounding the death. Carr provides a historical overview of death in the United States, describes the types of grief reactions, and summarizes the distinctive characteristics of spouse, partner, sibling, parent, and child loss. She concludes with recommendations for future research.

Resources for those who want to work with, or learn more about, older Americans are plentiful. The appendices provide links for a variety of such resources. In Appendix A, Elizabeth Daniele provides an annotated list of several of the many federal, state, and local organizations that represent the interests of aging Americans. Far from exhaustive, the list provides links to numerous important and diverse organizations that research, serve, and lobby for our aging population. In Appendix B, Elizabeth Daniele provides summaries of several documentaries on older persons. Such documentaries are multiplying, and her list describes only some of the recent films that highlight variation in the old-age experience by gender, class, race, and ethnicity. These films are useful for older persons and their families, scholars and their students, and policy makers and their constituents.

Together the chapters in this volume reveal the structural, and the individual, factors that shape health and well-being at older ages. They show sweeping trends and stark inequalities. They also demonstrate what we, as a society and as individuals, might do to reduce disparities in health and well-being for generations to come.

References

Acierno, R., Hernandez, M. A., Amstadter, A. B., Resnick, H. S., Steve, K., Muzzy, W., & Kilpatrick, D. G. (2010). Prevalence and correlates of emotional, physical, sexual, and financial abuse and potential neglect in the United States: The National Elder Mistreatment Study. *American Journal of Public Health, 100*, 292–297.

Associated Press. 2015. *92 year old becomes oldest woman to finish marathon. May 31, 2015.* http://www.nytimes.com/aponline/2015/05/31/us/ap-ath-marathon-record.html?_r=0

Avendano, M., & Kawachi, I. (2014). Why do Americans have shorter life expectancy and worse health than people in other high-income countries? *Annual Review of Public Health, 35*, 307.

Congressional Budget Office (2013). *Rising demand for long-term services and supports for elderly people*. Washington, DC.

Dormandy, T. (2000). *Old masters: Great artists in old age*. New York: Hambledon Press.

Harrington Meyer, M. (2014). *Grandmothers at work: Juggling families and jobs*. New York, NY: NYU Press.

Li, Y., & Ferraro, K. F. (2006). Volunteering in middle and later life: Is health a benefit, barrier or both? *Social Forces, 85*, 497–519.

McDougle, L., Handy, F., Konrath, S., & Walk, M. (2014). Health outcomes and volunteering: The moderating role of religiosity. *Social Indicator Research, 117*, 337–351.

Siegel, R. L., Miller, K. D., & Jemal, A. (2015). Cancer statistics, 2015. *CA: A Cancer Journal for Clinicians, 65*(1), 5–29.

CHAPTER ONE

Education across the Life Course

Elizabeth A. Daniele

While the United States has become a more educated society over time, persistent gaps in educational attainment remain. This chapter reviews educational trends at the secondary and tertiary levels, while highlighting disparities by age, race and ethnicity, gender, and socioeconomic status. The chapter then explores the impacts of education on earnings and economic well-being, unemployment, and health at the individual and societal levels. Finally, the chapter focuses on adult education and lifelong learning, exploring the reasons to educate adults, the types of learning encompassed by adult education, best practices for educating older adults, and the increasing importance of technology in the information age. I conclude with some thoughts about the future of education in the United States.

Trends in Education

For the past 50 years, each cohort has had higher educational attainment than the one that preceded it. According to the Profile of Older Americans (AoA, 2013), in 1970 only 28 percent of Americans aged 65 or older had completed high school, whereas by 2013 the percentage of older Americans who had completed high school was 83 percent. Among adults aged 25 to 29 in 2013, 90 percent had a high school diploma or an equivalent certification (Kena et al., 2014).

Similarly, college-degree-attainment trends have generally been increasing since the middle of the 20th century—except during the 1980s, when the proportion of adults aged 25 to 34 with bachelor's degrees consistently hovered around 24 percent (Baum, Ma, & Payea, 2010; Mettler, 2014). In 1947, only 6 percent among those aged 25 to 29 had bachelor's degrees, compared to 24 percent in 1977 (Mettler, 2014). Compared to 1940 when only 1 in 20 Americans had a bachelor's degree, by 1977 1 in 4 Americans had a four-year college education (Mettler, 2014). The proportion of adults between 25 and 34 years old with bachelor's degrees increased by an average of 2 percent per year throughout the 1990s; between 2000 and 2009, the rate of increase for 25- to 34-year-old adults with four-year degrees was about 1 percent per year (Baum, Ma, & Payea, 2010).

Because more Americans have pursued and completed bachelor's degrees, the younger cohorts of adults are more educated than their predecessors. In 2013, approximately 25 percent of adults, aged 65 and over, had a bachelor's degree or higher (AoA, 2013) compared to 34 percent of young adults aged 25 to 29 (Kena et al., 2014). For adults aged 65 and older in 2000, only 4 percent had a graduate or professional degree (National Center for Higher Education Management Systems, 2015). Among 25- to 29-year-olds in 2013, approximately 7 percent had already completed a master's degree or higher despite their young age (NCES, 2013). As these young adults continue to age, we will see a more highly educated population of older adults in the next 30 years.

But when compared to other nations, U.S. higher education enrollment lags far behind. As Mettler (2014) cautions, despite the upward trajectory in postsecondary education completion rates, the United States is losing ground to other nations. Based on the percentage of 25- to 34-year-olds with higher education in 2012, the United States ranked 14th in the world (Organization for Economic Cooperation and Development [OECD], 2012). Other nations are increasing their proportions of citizens with tertiary educational attainment at faster rates than the United States. In 2012, about 26 percent of 20- to 29-year-olds in the United States were enrolled in education compared to 43 percent in Denmark (OECD, 2014). Further, because higher education systems are dependent upon well-educated elementary- and secondary-level students, it is worth noting that the United States spends above average on each pupil, but yields average or below average results as compared to other nations in the OECD. The Programme for International Student Assessment, or PISA, is a test given to 15-year-olds in 65 countries and used as a tool to compare student skill in different subject areas across national borders. Out of 34 OECD nations, the U.S. students ranked 27th on mathematics; U.S. scores were closer to average performance on reading and science despite the fact that the United States ranks 5th on spending per student (OECD-PISA, 2012).

Though education rates are rising, they are not rising for all in the United States. Whites and Asians continue to be more educated than African Americans and Latinos (the terms Latino and Hispanic are used interchangeably throughout). As shown in Figure 1.1, among older Americans in 2012, non-Hispanic whites were the group most likely to have completed high school. Nearly 87 percent of older whites compared to 76 percent of older Asians, 71 percent of older African Americans, and 60 percent of older Native Americans had completed high school (AoA, 2013). Only 51 percent of older adult Hispanic Americans had completed high school in 2012 (AoA, 2013). Among the 25- to 29-year-old U.S. population in 2014, the percentages of those with a high school diploma or an equivalent certification were 96 percent for whites, 92 percent for blacks, and 75 percent for Hispanics (NCES, 2014b). Hispanics increased high school attainment by 17 percentage points since 1990 when the rate was 58 percent of Hispanics in this age range having high school certifications; most of this educational progress occurred after 2005 (NCES, n.d.). These educational attainment rates reflect considerable reductions of gaps between whites and blacks, and whites and Hispanics from two decades prior. High school completion rates for Asians/Pacific Islanders between 1990 and 2014 increased from 92 percent to 97 percent (NCES, 2014b).

Postsecondary educational levels also reflect persistent inequality. As shown in Figure 1.1, among young adults aged 25 to 29 years in 2013, attainment of a bachelor's degree or higher for whites was almost double that

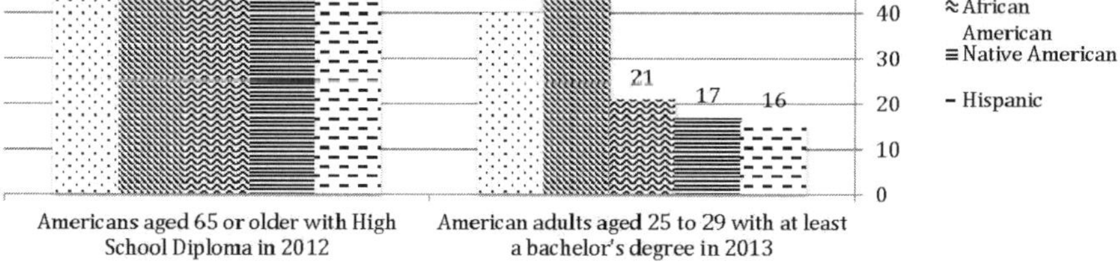

Figure 1.1 Percentage of U.S. population with completed degree by age and race. (Administration on Aging [2013]. A Profile of Older Americans: 2013. Retrieved from http://www.aoa.acl.gov/Aging_Statistics/Profile/2013/docs/2013_Profile.pdf. National Center for Education Statistics. (2013). Table 104.20. Retrieved from https://nces.ed.gov/programs/digest/d13/tables/dt13_104.20.asp/)

of African Americans, 40 percent compared to 21 percent (NCES, 2013). Attainment of at least a bachelor's degree for Hispanic young adults was 16 percent whereas for Asian/Pacific Islanders it was 58 percent (NCES, 2013). When disaggregated, these data reflect a graduation rate for Asians more than double that of Pacific Islanders, who comprise such a numerically small population that it is difficult to get accurate statistics (NCES, 2013). American Indian/Alaskan Native young adult college attainment rates were at 17 percent in 2013 while 30 percent of those identifying as two or more races had a bachelor's degree or higher that year (NCES, 2013). Between 1991 and 2011, there was a 67 percent increase in the number of doctorates conferred upon African Americans, but they still earned only 6 percent of all doctorates in 2011 (National Science Foundation, 2012). Similarly, in that same 20-year timespan Latinos more than doubled their proportion of doctorates to 6 percent, but these groups are still underrepresented at all levels of higher education (National Science Foundation, 2012).

Throughout U.S. history, federal and state government legislation as well as individual college and university policies enabled some segments of the population to become better educated than others. White males dominated postsecondary education since the first higher educational institution was founded in 1636 (see Beckert et al., 2011 for Harvard's connections with slavery). This practice of providing more education to a white male demographic was supported and reinforced by legal segregation, exclusion of racial and ethnic minorities from most institutions of higher education, and de facto practices of institutional discrimination (Thelin, 2004; Wallenstein, 2008). It seems likely that the nation's history of exclusion is reflected in persistent racial gaps in education.

Presently there are some programs in place to improve the enrollment and retention rates for underrepresented minorities. The federal definition pertaining to underrepresented minorities in education includes African Americans, Native Americans, Pacific Islanders, Alaskan Natives, and Hispanics/Latinos (U.S. Government Printing Office, 2011); international students are not underrepresented minorities (National Academies Press, 2011). These demographics are underrepresented in higher education insofar as they enroll in postsecondary education at rates below parity with their representation in the general population. In some cases, there are opportunities for underrepresented minorities to apply for programs to increase minority participation in higher education. Some federally funded TRiO programs, for example, like the Ronald E. McNair Postbaccalaureate Achievement Program, serve primarily low-income and first-generation students who are interested in pursuing graduate education, but also underrepresented minorities (http://www2.ed.gov/programs/triomcnair/eligibility.html).

How will the future look? As the nation moves toward the majority-minority population composition predicted for 2050 (Passel & Cohn, 2008), it will be ever more important to incorporate all segments of the American populace into the higher educational system and adjust the college and university structure to serve increasingly diverse student populations, faculty, and staff. Without such efforts, it is not clear that greater proportion of people of color in the general population will lead to a correspondingly greater presence in higher education.

Traditionally women's educational attainment lagged behind men's, but now women are ahead of men at every level. Women were typically excluded from formal higher education until the 1840s (American Association of University Women in St. Lawrence County, n.d.), which contributed to the construction of women's colleges toward the end of the 19th century. Much of higher education remained single-sex until the late 1960s and early 1970s. In 1972, the creation of Pell grants for low-income students and passage of Title IX—mandating that institutions receiving federal funds treat individuals equitably regardless of sex—both opened doors for lower-income students to access higher education and for women to take advantage of student loans and work-study (Mettler, 2014). Due to such legislation and increasingly widespread feminist sentiments, trends in higher education attainment shifted from postsecondary education being male dominated to being increasingly female dominated (DiPrete & Buchmann, 2013).

In recent years, women are consistently achieving higher educational attainment than men—a trend that holds across various demographics. Kim and Joo (2013) used longitudinal data to show that between 1960 and 1990 women became more likely to obtain general educational development (GED) credentials and pursue postsecondary education than men. Zhang (2010) found that female GED holders were substantially more likely to participate in postsecondary education than male GED holders. As Figure 1.2 shows, women have been more likely to earn degrees than men at almost every level of education since 2000 (NCES, n.d.). Between 2000 and 2010, females earned between 60 percent and 62 percent of associate's degrees, as well as 58 percent of bachelor's degrees conferred to U.S. residents during those years (NCES, 2012). Women between the ages of 25 and 29 in 2009 pursued and completed bachelor's degrees at rates higher than men within white, black, and Latino demographics (Baum, Ma, & Payea, 2010). In 2014, females in the 25- to 29-year-old age range were 6 percentage points higher than males for educational attainment of a bachelor's degree or higher (NCES, n.d.).

This trend of females surpassing males in educational attainment is true at the highest levels of education as well. The postgraduate trend

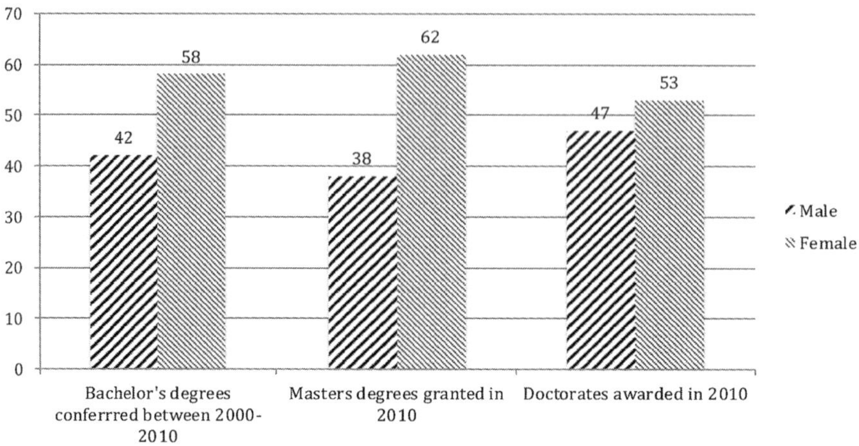

Figure 1.2 Percentage of U.S. population who attained degree by gender. (National Center for Education Statistics [2012]. Degrees conferred by sex and race. Retrieved from http://nces.ed.gov/FastFacts/display.asp?id=72/)

for women between 2000 and 2010 indicates an increased participation, with women earning 62 percent of master's degrees awarded in 2010 and 53 percent of doctorates that year (NCES, 2012). In 2013, 9 percent of women had completed a master's degree or higher whereas only 6 percent of males had (NCES, n.d.). Barriers remain, among them the equal representation and full incorporation of women into faculty positions in Science, Technology, Engineering, and Math (STEM) fields at research universities (National Academies Press, 2011).

Thus far, I have focused on education attainment, but it is important to also examine differences in quality of education. Because students throughout the United States are generally required to go to neighborhood schools, those with higher incomes, greater wealth, and comparatively more power continue to tend to have significantly better schools than those with fewer resources. Nationwide the poverty rate for the United States was 15 percent in 2013 (Kaiser Family Foundation, 2015), but that same year more than half of the public school students were low income (Jordan, 2015). Poor and low-income students are likely to attend schools where poverty is concentrated, known by the federal government as high-poverty schools, and also sometimes known as Title I schools, in which 76 percent to 100 percent of students are eligible for free or reduced price lunch, or FRPL (Aud et al., 2010). In recent years, high-poverty schools produced fewer graduates than they used to; in 2008 the graduation rate of 68 percent for high-poverty schools was 18 percentage points lower than the 1999–2000 high-poverty schools graduation rate of 86 percent

(Aud et al., 2010). As compared to low-poverty schools, where up to 25 percent of students are eligible for FRPL, between 2000 and 2009, high-poverty schools consistently averaged lower scores on fourth and eighth grade tests of reading, mathematics, and music and visual arts (Aud et al., 2010). High-poverty high schools consistently produce significantly fewer graduates than low-poverty high schools. In 2007–2008, only 68 percent of 12th graders in high poverty schools graduated while 91 percent of 12th grade students from low-poverty schools received diplomas that year (Aud et al., 2010). Reports on the tests and surveys of PISA indicate that socioeconomic disadvantage has a greater impact on the scores of American students than it does on the score differentials of students of different socioeconomic statuses in other nations (OECD-PISA, 2012).

There is increasing racial and ethnic wealth inequality (Kochhar & Fry, 2014; Pfeffer, Danzinger, & Schoeni, 2013), which may interact with other social identities like gender. In both rural and urban areas, high-poverty schools were disproportionately attended by African American and Latino students (Aud et al., 2010; Jordan, 2015). In addition to financial resources, other types of capital may be important for student success as well. A study by Perna and Titus (2005) suggested that lower rates of enrollment for African Americans and Hispanics as compared to whites may be due to the fact that their schools have fewer resources regardless of the cultural, social, and economic capital possessed by a given individual.

Low-income students and students from districts with highly concentrated poverty show lower rates of immediate college enrollment, college persistence, and college graduation. In 2007–2008, high-poverty high schools had an average rate of 28 percent of students going to a four-year college or university the autumn following high school graduation; among high school graduates from low-poverty schools, the rate was 52 percent (Aud et al., 2010). College-continuation rates by family income quartile in 2012 revealed a 37 percentage point gap between top and bottom quartiles; while 82 percent of 18- to 24-year-olds from the top family income quartile went to college, only 45 percent of those from families in the bottom income quartile did so (Pell Institute, 2015). In 2013, bachelor's degree attainment rates were 66 percentage points lower for students from low-income families than for students from high-income families such that students from high-income families were eight times more likely to graduate with a bachelor's degree by age 24 than those from low-income families (Pell Institute, 2015).

Not only have low-income students been less likely to go to college and persist to graduation, but first-generation students also show similar struggles. Parental education level and family income are among the strongest predictors of college enrollment and success. Children of college-educated parents have been more likely to go to college themselves (Robert Wood Johnson Foundation [RWJF], 2013), which implies a unique struggle for those who are first-generation college students, namely individuals whose parents did not attend or complete college. In 2008, the immediate college enrollment rate for students whose parents had a bachelor's degree or higher was 82 percent whereas it was 54 percent for those whose parents' highest educational attainment was high school or less (Aud et al., 2010).

The cost of education has risen dramatically, leading to increased accrual of debts to pay for postsecondary education. In 1972, the federally funded Pell grant program opened the doors of higher education for more low-income students (Mettler, 2014). Since that time, the cost of college has increased tremendously, and more Americans have taken out loans to fund their education (Ratcliffe & McKernan, 2013). In 2010, outstanding student loans totaled $1 trillion worth of debt (Ratcliffe & McKernan, 2013), and this debt burden is disproportionately concentrated in the bottom-income quintile (Fry, 2012). Though fewer than 5 percent of households headed by Americans aged 65 and older had outstanding student debt in 2010, 19 percent of all American households had outstanding student debt at that time (Fry, 2012). The disparity between low levels of debt for older Americans and higher levels of debt among younger populations likely reflects the fact that college education is more expensive now than when older adults were traditional college-going age (see College Board, 2013).

In addition to evidence that cost of higher education is already a deterrent or prohibitive for many Americans, as time goes on there is some concern whether it will become increasingly difficult for middle-income Americans to afford higher education. Astin and Oseguera (2004) found that there is significant inequity of access to highly selective postsecondary educational institutions, which increased over time. With the proportion of high-income students growing while the lowest income students remained at a steady proportion, middle-income students were increasingly underrepresented.

While approximately one-third of younger adults in the United States have bachelor's degrees, many American adults remain undereducated. In 2013, slightly more than 45 percent of all Americans aged 25 years or older, which is nearly half the total adult population in the United States, had either not finished high school or had not pursued any education beyond the secondary level (RWJF, 2013). In 2000 more than 39 million adults over age 16 lacked a high school credential and were not enrolled in any educational program (American Council on Education, 2011). Though 2013 represented the lowest U.S. high school dropout rates ever recorded (Fry, 2014), that year there were over 2 million 18- to 24-year-olds who neither had completed high school nor were enrolled in school. In 2007, the percentage of high school status dropouts, those 16- to 24-year-olds who are not enrolled in school and do not have a high school degree, was at 9 percent overall and 21 percent for Hispanics, which was more than double the dropout rate of any of the other groups (Aud, Fox, & KewelRamani, 2010). More recently, dropout rate levels were lower due largely to the fact that Latino and black youth were persisting to finish high school at higher rates than in years prior. Though Hispanics still had the highest dropout rate among any racial or ethnic group in 2013, at 14 percent, their high school completion and college-going rates had increased even as the youth population had grown considerably (Fry, 2014).

The GED is a "uniquely American education credential" (Tyler, 2005, p. 46) available to individuals who did not complete high school following a proscribed course of study. The history of the GED is tied to the U.S. military, but today people of many demographic characteristics take the GED subtests on writing, reading, social studies, mathematics, and science. Army leaders created the GED in the early 1940s to demonstrate that vets who left high school for military service were cognitively on par with high school graduates (Boesel, Alsalam, & Smith, 1998; Tyler, 2005). By 1959, more of the 56,500 GED test takers were civilians than armed forces affiliates (Boesel, Alsalam, & Smith, 1998; GED Testing, 2014). In the mid-1960s, high school dropout rates shot up, and there was tremendous growth in GED testing such that by 1970, 331,500 people took the GED and a decade later 816,000 completed at least one subsection (GED Testing, 2014; Tyler, 2005). In 2013, 743,000 people took the GED exam and three-quarters of them passed, which brings the total number of people who have passed the GED close to 20 million (GED Testing, 2014). Over 46,000 took the Spanish version of the exam in 2013 and 1,000 people took the French language version (GED Testing, 2014). Whites comprised 43 percent of test takers, but of the 50 percent who passed, Hispanics were 25 percent of takers and 23 percent of passers, African Americans were 27 percent of test takers and 22 percent of test passers; American Indian/Alaskan Natives as well as Asians each represented 2 percent of test takers and passers (GED Testing, 2014).

Noncompletion of high school may occur for any number of reasons, but regardless of cause to pursue a GED, many postsecondary educational institutions plus most employers accept this credential as representing educational equivalency to a high school diploma (American Council on Education, 2009). Since its inception, there have been four versions of the GED exam; the 2002 series GED test concluded in 2013 and comprised five parts that took just under 8 hours to complete (GED Testing Service,

2014; Tyler, 2005). It may be thought of as an alternative pathway or second chance for individuals who wish to pursue their educational aspirations. Data suggest, however, that in comparison to those who graduate high school, those with GEDs do not earn as much in wages or income and do not enroll in, or complete postsecondary education at the same rate; nor do GED-credentialed individuals obtain employment at the same rates as high school graduates (Cameron & Heckman, 1993; Chapman, Laird, Ifill, & KewelRamani, 2011). Tyler (2002) poignantly pointed out that "earning a GED is not a path out of poverty" (p. 4).

Today the GED remains pertinent as a field of study because it raises and addresses questions about how the nation plans to handle its least-educated citizens who have not obtained a high school diploma or equivalent credential. Among the most pressing of these questions is whether to direct public funds toward supporting individuals to pass the GED. Some studies challenge the value of the GED (Tyler & Lofstrom, 2010; Tyler, Murnane, & Willett, 2000) while others suggest the primary benefit of the GED seems to be the potential to pursue postsecondary degrees and reap subsequent benefits of those more advanced credentials (Boesel, Alsalam, & Smith, 1998; Murnane, Willett, & Boudett, 1999). Work by Kim and Joo (2013) indicates that from the 1960s to the 1990s, high-school dropouts from all racial or ethnic groups have become more likely to obtain a GED, but over these generations only white and African Americans have become more likely to pursue postsecondary education; probability for Hispanics to do so has not changed over time. It is also important to query how the GED differentially impacts incarcerated versus nonimprisoned individuals. Tyler (2002) suggested that earning the degree while incarcerated limited the positive effects associated with the credential.

Worldwide, and in the United States, there is a rising bar of expected minimum education, but not all are reaching that bar. Given the patterns of differential educational attainment that exist along racial and gender differences as well by varying socioeconomic status and parental education, it is important to note that despite improvements in education overall, there is no guarantee of continued educational advancement for the United States overall. The following section explores the effects of education on individuals and also at the societal level.

Impacts of Education

The positive effects of education are myriad and accrue to both the educated individuals and the society in which they live. Those with more education tend to have better fiscal, employment, and health outcomes over the life course.

Higher levels of education are generally associated with better economic standing over the life course. The relationship between socioeconomic status and college can be thought of as mutually reinforcing: "Poverty of education is a principal factor responsible for income poverty; and income poverty, in turn, does not allow the people to overcome poverty of education" (Tilak, 2002, p. 198). In the aggregate, the more postsecondary education individuals accrue, the better their earnings are. Also, because those with postsecondary education are generally in higher-paid positions, they usually contribute to the tax base at higher rates (Baum, Ma, & Payea, 2013). According to a report from the Robert Wood Johnson Foundation (2013), college graduates earned nearly double what high school graduates earned over the course of their lives. Those with a professional degree earned $3.2 million more over the course of their working lives compared to those with a maximum educational attainment of eighth grade education (Julian, 2012). One exception to the rule of economic return on education is that as compared to high school dropouts, high school graduates do not have many benefits in terms of earnings and wealth benefits (Bernstein, 2007). Recently the Pew Research Center (2014b) suggested the benefits of education in the United States showed "the dramatic decline in the value of a high school education" (p. 7) and corresponding "growing economic return to a college degree" (p. 8). Though since 2000, wages of college graduates and benefits like health insurance coverage from one's employer fell (Mishel, Gould, & Bivens, 2015), there is also evidence that pursuing postsecondary education was worth the investment: "the typical bachelor's degree recipient," for example, "can expect to earn about 66% more during a 40-year working life than the typical high-school graduate earns over the same period" (Baum, Ma, & Payea, 2010, p. 12). More education leads to higher likelihood of full-time work and greater fulfillment from work (Ross & Wu, 1995), but even among those with parity of educational attainment, there are different levels of earnings. There is greater return on educational investment for males of almost any race when compared with women, and for whites and Asians when compared with blacks and Hispanics (Ashton, 2014; Pew Research Center, 2014a).

Those with lower levels of education are more likely to suffer from higher unemployment rates and have a greater likelihood of living in poverty. In both good and bad economic times, those with lower levels of educational attainment were hit harder by unemployment than those with more education (Hoynes, Miller, & Schaller, 2012). Unemployment rates were usually lower for those with high school education than dropouts and were lower for those with tertiary education than secondary (Chapman, Laird, & KewalRamani, 2011; Stanford Center on Poverty and Inequality,

2014). In 2014, the poverty rates for Americans aged 25- to 64-years were 4 percent for those with college degrees, 11 percent for those with some college, 16 percent for those with only high school, and 34 percent for those with less than high school education (Stanford Center on Poverty and Inequality, 2014).

Individuals with more education are more likely to get benefits from employers such as private pensions and health insurance through their job. College-educated workers are more likely to be offered employer-provided pension plans than those with lower levels of education, and likelihood of employee participation increases as education level increases such that those with advanced degrees are most likely to participate in such plans (Baum, Ma, & Payea, 2013). Individuals with more advanced levels of tertiary education are more likely to have employer-provided health insurance regardless of status as a full-time or part-time employee. In 2008, only 50 percent of high school graduates had employer-provided health insurance whereas 68 percent of those with a bachelor's degree or higher who were working at least half time in the private sector had this benefit; this 18 percentage point gap in coverage between those with secondary and tertiary education grew from a 10 percentage point difference in 1979 (College Board, n.d.). In 2011, 73 percent of full-time, year-round workers over age 25 who had advanced degrees had employer-provided health insurance; among part-time workers in 2011, 39 percent of those with a bachelor's degree and 48 percent of those with an advanced degree had this benefit (Baum, Ma, & Payea, 2013). That same year 30 percent of all adults over age 17 had government-sponsored health-care plans, which included 36 percent of high school graduates and 20 percent of those with a four-year degree or higher (Baum, Ma, & Payea, 2013).

Higher levels of education are consistently associated with better health outcomes. Higher education indicates lower likelihood of working in the most dangerous jobs, fewer health-risking behaviors such as smoking and alcohol use, and greater use of health services (Cutler & Llevras-Muney, 2006; Feinstein et al., 2006). Even among individuals with similar health-care coverage, those with higher levels of education exhibit better health outcomes (see Klein, 2014). Those with college degrees have better health outcomes compared to those without high school diplomas along metrics of increased longevity—living five or more years longer; overall higher reports of healthy behaviors like not smoking; and lower likelihood to have or die from common diseases, like heart disease or diabetes (RWJF, 2013). According to Feinstein et al. (2006, p. 187), health services utilization can be preventative, for example, by having regular physical examinations; or responsive when one seeks medical attention in situations of pain, ailment, or injury; and can also happen in the context of management of conditions that require ongoing treatment. There are also benefits such as the fact that higher levels of education are associated with greater likelihood of receiving retirement benefits and health insurance from the employer (Baum, Ma, & Payea, 2010; RWJF, 2013). Finally, well-educated citizens tend to produce to better educated future generations because children of college-educated parents are more likely to pursue and obtain bachelor's degrees. RWJF (2013) suggested that higher earnings associated with advanced education produce greater access to healthy foods and safer home environments in addition to noting that college-educated women demonstrated lower infant mortality rates as compared to those who never graduated high school. A consequence of well-educated society can be reduced public expenditure on public health and medical care.

Older Adult Learning and Geragogy

Though we tend to emphasize education for children, education for adults generally, and older adults specifically, can be beneficial as well. Adult learning can be defined as the acquisition of skills, knowledge, and abilities during the course of adult life. Learning among older adults takes a variety of forms. Adult learning encompasses formal education like earning credentials and certifications, as well as vocational trainings, or leisure-based educational enrichment, and learning health-related information for self-care. This section details the what, how, and why of older adult education.

Defining Education and Learning

Older adult education may be formal, nonformal, or informal to use the language of Jarvis (as cited in Findsen, 2006). These frameworks correspond to notions of education, training, and learning. Education denotes a formal process that occurs at officially recognized institutions; education is schooling replete with formal and sequential paths to earning a credential. Nonformal learning among older adults is any form of structured and organized learning that occurs outside formal educational institutions. An example would be training, which implies absorbing new information in order to achieve professional or vocational success. As a type of learning with the aim of acquiring a set of skills usually tied to employer initiatives or individual aims to maximize employment outcomes such as earning capacity, training is usually formalized, likely comprises in-person or web-based instruction, and increasingly relevant as seniors are working longer (Liu, Courtenay, & Valentine, 2011). Other examples of nonformal learning include seniors enrolled in art or music classes at a local museum or senior center.

While few adults pursue formal education, many are engaged in the pursuit of knowledge, skills, and abilities or the informal learning that enhances life. In contrast to education, which tends to be regulated by policies and receives recognition from the public, learning is a personal endeavor that can be ongoing and private (Jarvis in Preece, 2009). The seemingly semantic distinction between education and learning belies an ongoing debate over choice of language in the field of adult education (see Hager, 2011). To stress the ongoing nature of learning, the term lifelong learning evolved in the 1970s. The European Commission (2001) defines lifelong learning (LLL) as "all learning activity undertaken throughout life with the aim of improving knowledge, skills and competences within a personal, civic, social and/or employment-related perspective" (p. 9). This expansive definition is inclusive of the fact that one cannot learn during formal schooling in early life, every aspect of what they will need for rewarding employment over the life course (London, 2011). As Cross (1981) famously highlighted, learning is necessary for everyone who wishes to survive in the modern age.

Adult learning can be understood as an extension of education that occurred in earlier phases of life, but it may also be considered a different type of learning that requires altogether different modes and philosophies of teaching. Like most nations, the United States generally follows an age-differentiated (Riley & Riley, 2000, p. 267) model of life that designates early life or youth as the time for education, assigns midlife as the time for work, and expects later life stages to be filled with leisure. This model has become highly normalized as the schooling-employment-retirement trajectory. Adult education challenges this model by inserting formal learning later in life.

Educating Adults

Pedagogy is the method for instructing children, so andragogy has been proposed as a means of teaching adults; geragogy is a method for educating older adults. According to Schuetz (1982), "geragogy emphasizes the guided learning of persons in old age" (p. 339). This concept recognizes older adults as a distinctive learning population that merits unique teaching methods. McClusky (cited in Hiemstra, 1998) proposed that older learners must have five needs met: coping needs, expressive needs, contributive needs, influence needs, and transcendence needs. These needs cover the ability to be minimally literate and self-sufficient, be involved in activities, help others, improve quality of life, and to rise above limitations associated with one's age (Hiemstra, 1998). There is some debate over whether working with older populations necessitates different methods of teaching (see Tam, 2014). Accompanying questions over how to best teach for particular results are concerns over what older learners need to learn. Ansello (2011) highlights older adults' need for wisdom more than facts or figures. With so much data readily available in the information age, he suggests that it may be useful to turn toward "reflections on what we are, who we have been, what it means to 'be'" (p. 210), which can be explored, for example, through study of literary and visual arts that inspire the soul, heart, and mind. Ansello (2011) astutely suggests that wisdom may include more ethereal ways of knowing that do not fit categorically into typical classifications of substantial knowledge such as tying a shoelace or doing an algebra problem.

Older adults have different cognitive abilities and physical abilities than younger learners. According to Van Gerven, Paas, Van Merrienboer, and Schmidt (2000) cognitive aging occurs on three levels: "(1) working-memory capacity decreases, (2) processing speed goes down, and (3) there is a reduced ability to distinguish relevant from irrelevant information" (p. 507). These authors propose using Cognitive Load Theory to modify instructions to enable older learners to grasp otherwise overly complicated new skills. By providing less extraneous information and reducing the cognitive load on the learner, individuals can learn more complicated skills. The authors suggest that a diagram and caption, for example, is unnecessary separation of two pieces of information that can be integrated and unified into a single depiction, thereby focusing rather than splitting the attention of the viewer. Jeske and Roßnagel (2015) propose a *contextual view* suggesting that cognitive decline is neither linear nor inevitable; they argue that training and development among older adults can continue and flourish in supportive work climates that encourage learning among older workers.

Nonformal learning programs can be found in the United States and many European nations as well—some of the more established examples from the United States are Elderhostel's Road Scholar program, and Osher Foundation's Lifelong Learning Institutes. Elderhostel is an organization started in 1975 at colleges in New Hampshire designed as a living and learning educational model. Since the 1980s, Elderhostel has offered international experiential learning that combines study and travel for middle-aged to older adults (http://www.roadscholar.org/about/history.asp). In 2010, Elderhostel renamed their travel component Road Scholar, and presently they offer travel-and-learn programs in 150 countries on all 7 continents (http://www.roadscholar.org/default.asp). Research on Elderhostel program participants by Ahn and Janke (2011) indicates that those who enroll in the Road Scholar program are interested in physical benefits as well as maintaining their sharpness through mental stimulation. Osher Lifelong Learning Institute's Programs, which have existed since 2001, occur on college campuses throughout the United States and offer noncredit courses for adults aged 50 or above. These programs feature recreational learning, which is noncredit and does not lead toward a formal educational credential. Indeed their website advertises the programs as for those "who are interested in learning for the joy of learning" (http://www.osherfoundation.org/index.php?programs). Participation in noncredit programs such as Elderhostel and Osher Institutes tends to be dominated by those with higher socioeconomic status backgrounds though both programs offer scholarship opportunities.

In addition to nonformal learning for fulfillment, vocational learning is also important for older adults who continue working in an increasingly knowledge-based economy that almost always requires mastery of at least some technology—frequently computer-based skill sets for individual workers. Trainings may occur in the workplace or be mandated and contracted out by the employer. As the population around the world ages and technology continues to develop, these trends of aging and rapidly developing technology will have significant impact on economic development (Huber & Watson, 2014). In the postindustrial labor market that has emerged since 1970, there is an increasingly bifurcated economy with professional and technical occupations at the top, semi-skilled jobs at the bottom, and a shrinking pool of lower white collar jobs in the middle (see Portes & Rumbaut, 2014). The Information Age features greater economic disparity that often falls along lines of education; those who have degrees are more likely to find jobs that are well paid and feature benefits.

Health-related education is another important arena of nonformal education of older adults that happens outside the realm of schooling but can have important impacts. This type of education includes patient release instructions or giving clear instruction to seniors on using new medications. Successful health-related education includes teaching older African Americans about diabetes, high blood pressure through storytelling (Bertera 2014), and about fall prevention (Gitlin et al., 2008; Hill et al., 2011: Perry et al., 2012). Educating communities that have traditionally not been targeted or included does pose challenges that are not guaranteed to disappear as our society becomes more diverse. Work by Dentato et al. (2014) indicates that older adults who are LGBT often avoid seeking care because they mistrust health and mental health-care professionals due to past experiences with denial of services or discrimination based on their sexual orientation. This illustrates a two-fold need for adult education insofar as there is need to educate an isolated population of older LGBT adults, and because it prompts us to think about how we educate caregiving professionals who will be encountering an ever-more diverse older adult population.

There is much to be resolved in terms of logistics of educating an adult population. The formal American education system has not been particularly concerned with the need to provide service for adults and older adults even though adults are an increasing component of the student population—particularly at community colleges (Lane, Michelau, & Palmer, 2012). Yet Many of the practices that benefit older adults may also benefit other types of students. Persistence rates for older adult and first-generation college students, for example, can generally be improved by attention to academic advising and counseling, flexibility in scheduling options, academic assistance services, financial support, and resources that promote and assist students with balancing multiple responsibilities (Cummins, 2014). Because outreach programs with a particular target population and student-centered advising will differ based on the individuals served, it is important to take into consideration the unique facets of adult and older adult learners.

Why Educate Adults?

The primary reasons to educate adults fall into categories of economic, social/citizenship, and individual well-being. Adult education offers the opportunity to teach nontraditionally aged students skills for economic productivity in a knowledge-based economy. This is in accord with the human capital model of education, which states that individuals accumulate skills for increased competitiveness on the market. As the population becomes more educated overall, it requires a higher minimum level of education for sustainable employment. With the advent of digital communication and the computer age, for example, there is increased need to constantly update one's skill set in order to keep current and stay relevant in the job market. The other framework or model for education has more to do with the fact that education accrues benefits to the broader society as well as the individual. Well-educated persons are more likely to be actively engaged citizens who vote and volunteer at higher rates than those with lower levels of education; thus, ramifications of education as a social good, such as a politically engaged and civically active populace as well lower public expenditures, will accumulate at a higher rate in societies that nurture LLL (Baum, Ma, & Payea, 2013). Finally, we must remember the health and well-being that individuals garner from LLL (Weinstein, 2004). In addition to health benefits such as maintaining mental sharpness in older adults, for many there is genuine thrill in learning. Regardless of whether one chooses immersion in government-run or government-overseen institutional settings, which could be readily identified as supporting education for older adults, we would be remiss to reject out of hand the possibilities for LLL. There should be some attention to the benefits of some formal structuring for those who seek or appreciate such a format.

Education promotes both tangible and intrinsic benefits that accrue at individual and societal levels, but the efforts to promote educating adults have been too few and far between. A pronouncement from the World Conference on Education for All in 1990 stated, "basic education is more than an end in itself. It is the foundation for lifelong learning and human development on which countries may build, systematically, further levels and types of education and training" (UNESCO 1990:3–4 as quoted in Preece, 2009: 11). If we accept the idea that learning begets learning, we must foster initiatives across all age sectors of our society so that individuals can remain economically competitive, accrue social benefits for the greater good, and remain physically healthy.

Role of Technology in the Information Age

It is common for older adults to seek training regarding technology. Though only about half of American adults aged 65 and older reported using the Internet or e-mail in 2012, this figure represents progress since August of 2008 when only 38 percent of the same demographic reported going online, or in 2011 when 41 percent of seniors reported being online at least occasionally (Pew Internet and American Life Project, 2012). Huber and Watson (2014) insightfully claim that "designers are inclined toward the new and cool, creating a rapidly moving target of web-based interfaces that requires constant relearning," and hence, "the digital divide must be crossed not once, but many times" (p. 19). Wide ranges of trainings cover a broad swath of topics to help older adults constantly cross the digital divide. One can find, for example, private corporations offering workshops that train customers on how to use their new cell phone or other devices (Verizon Wireless, n.d.). According to the Pew Internet and American Life Project (2012), once older adults "are given the tools and training needed to start using the internet, they become fervent users of the technology" (n.p.). Many consider basic literacy in the contemporary age as including ability to manipulate computers and search the Internet.

It has become somewhat common for community colleges to offer programs teaching computer skills. Some such courses attract significant numbers of adult learners in no small part because most occupations require some ability to use computers. Familiarity with technology can be a barrier for older adults—especially those reentering the workforce who find they are seeking work in a different type of economy. Many turn to community colleges to learn new skills that both increase employability and exhibit willingness to learn: "recent education, especially in the use of technology, is important to potential employers; it demonstrates that the potential employee is teachable" (Cummins, 2014, p. 347). This type of learning allows older workers to maximize their employability, which harkens to the human capital model discussed above.

Learning about technology is not limited to vocational training, but can also be nonformal enrichment learning as well. Russell (2008) reports that older adults learning about computers have a unique perspective on time that is informed by the facts that they have more time available following retirement, and that they have a limited amount of time left to live. As such, time becomes valuable to the participant-learners because it is clearly finite. Russell (2008: 221) summarizes that the later-life learners she studied "want continuity, inclusion, and integrity in their relations with others and prefer autonomy to dependence... . Participants found ways of authenticating the self in learning." There is a valuable takeaway from Russell's eloquent phrasing, which captures the fact that many individuals can *authenticate the self* through learning, which is certainly one of the more lofty goals of LLL as it pertains to acquisition of any skill, ability or knowledge—ranging from using a new mobile device to learning to play an instrument or gaining a credential. There may also be intrinsic benefits to connecting through media that enable older adults to reconnect with friends or family members who use technology like e-mail, texting, and social networking sites.

Discussion

The dilemmas of financing older adult education, advocating for it, and providing instruction for adults and older adults have proven significant. In the foreword of Weinstock's (1978) *The Graying of the Campus*, she suggested, "with 'the graying of America,' educators will face an entirely new series of financial, political, and curricular problems" (p. 6). Moving forward, the questions of convincing the public of the need for a "learning society" (London, 2011, p. 5) will continue to plague efforts to remain competitive. Moreover, the persistent racial and socioeconomic inequality of the American educational system—from the elementary through postsecondary levels—indicates that the United States must travel a difficult path before reclaiming its status as the most college-educated nation in the world. Because younger American adults aged 25 to 34 are currently not educated at the same rates as those of other OECD nations and the college-going rates among the youngest adults aged 18 to 24 are not spiking,

Americans will see a persistent educational lag in the coming decades. This fact creates a pressing need to educate midlife and older adults if we wish to close the education gap with economic competitors on the global scale. We must adamantly resist the idea of "lifelong learning as serious leisure" (Jones & Symon, 2001, p. 269).

Despite the fact that the United States lags behind other nations, there is also the quandary of how to continue education for advanced credentials among a population that has more bachelor's degrees than any previous generation in this country. Infinite educational growth is impossible, but more learning among adults of all ages promises better nationwide fiscal well-being and health. Moreover, given the inequitable access to good education across many sectors of American society, providing more opportunities for learning to more people is a matter of social justice. There are questions as to what type of learning is necessary, how to motivate older learners to pursue such initiatives, as well as how to most effectively provide, fund, and legislatively support formal and informal learning programs. There are still questions about adult-learner motivations in general, and specifically how those may differ over time due to cohort effects. We know that World War II veterans went to college at much higher rates than their parents due to legislation, namely the first GI Bill. The impact of the 9/11 GI Bill on veterans and their families is not yet clear. Answers may be found in pursuit of the learning society, but our nation is largely distracted by extant, and very serious, problems in K-12 education. These problems of youth- and adult-oriented education are likely not as separate as they appear, but it will take "transformative learners [who] have the skills to confront and create frame-breaking change" (London, 2011, p. 4) if we are to accrue, as a nation, the benefits of widespread education and the justice of broad educational access.

References

Ahn, Y., & Janke, M. C. (2011). Motivations and benefits of the travel experiences of older adults. *Educational Gerontology, 37*, 653–673. doi: 10.1080/03601271003716010

American Council on Education (July 2009). *2008 GED testing program statistical report*. Retrieved from http://www.gedtestingservice.com/uploads/files/9d42c6660ec6184f73f466f2c53ef279.5MB%29

American Council on Education (2011). *2010 GED testing program statistical report*. Retrieved from http://www.gedtestingservice.com/uploads/files/3ba1916d8a9c6f7682f51216b9f10ff7.3MB/

American Association of University Women in St. Lawrence County (n.d.). Retrieved from http://www.northnet.org/stlawrenceaauw/college.htm

Ansello, E. F. (2011). Marginal gerontology and the curriculum palette. *Gerontology & Geriatrics Education, 32*, 199–214. doi: 10.1080/02701960.2011.583962

AoA/Administration on Aging (2013). *A profile of older Americans: 2013*. Retrieved from http://www.aoa.acl.gov/Aging_Statistics/Profile/2013/docs/2013_Profile.pdf

Ashton, D. (2014, June 10). Does race or gender matter more to your paycheck? *Harvard Business Review*. Retrieved from https://hbr.org/2014/06/does-race-or-gender-matter-more-to-your-paycheck/

Astin, A. W., & Oseguera, L. (2004). The declining "equity" of American higher education. *The Review of Higher Education, 27*(3), 321-341.

Aud, S., Fox, M. A., & KewelRamani, A. (2010). *Status and trends in the education of racial and ethnic groups* (NCES 2010-106). US Department of Education, National Center for Education Statistics. Washington, DC: US Government Printing Office.

Aud, S., Hussar, W., Planty, M., Snyder, T., Bianco, K., Fox, M., Frohlich, L., Kemp, J., & Drake, L. (2010). *The condition of education 2010* (NCES 2010-028). National Center for Education Statistics, Institute of Education Sciences, US Department of Education. Washington, DC. Retrieved from http://nces.ed.gov/pubs2010/2010028.pdf

Baum, S., Ma, J., & Payea, K. (2010). *Education pays 2010: The benefits of higher education for individuals and society*. College Board. Retrieved from https://trends.collegeboard.org/sites/default/files/education-pays-2010-full-report.pdf

Baum, S., Ma, J., & Payea, K. (2013). *Education pays 2013: The benefits of higher education for individuals and society*. College Board. Retrieved from https://trends.collegeboard.org/sites/default/files/education-pays-2013-full-report.pdf

Beckert, S., Stevens, K., et al. (2011). *Harvard and slavery: Seeking a forgotten history*. Retrieved from http://www.harvardandslavery.com/wp-content/uploads/2011/11/Harvard-Slavery-Book-111110.pdf

Bernstein, J. (2007, April 22). Is education the cure for poverty? *The American Prospect*. Retrieved from http://prospect.org/article/education-cure-poverty

Bertera, E. M. (2014). Storytelling slide shows to improve diabetes and high blood pressure knowledge and self-efficacy: Three-year results among community dwelling older African Americans. *Educational Gerontology, 40*(11), 785–800. doi: 10.1080/03601277.2014.894381

Boesel, D., Alsalam, N., & Smith, T. M. (1998). *Educational and labor market performance of GED recipients: Research synthesis. Executive summary* (NLE-98-2033). Washington, DC: National Library of Education. Retrieved from http://files.eric.ed.gov/fulltext/ED418239.pdf

Cameron, S. V., & Heckman, J. J. (1993). The nonequivalence of high school equivalents. *Journal of Labor Economics, 11*(1), 1–47.

Chapman, C., Laird, J., Ifill, N., & KewelRamani, A. (2011). *Trends in high school dropout and completion rates in the United States: 1972–2009* (NCES 2012-006). US Department of Education. Washington, DC: National Center for Education Statistics. Retrieved from http://nces.ed.gov/pubsearch/pubsinfo.asp?pubid=2012006

College Board (n.d.). *Health insurance coverage by education level, 1979–2008.* Retrieved from http://trends.collegeboard.org/education-pays/figures-tables/health-insurance-coverage-education-level-1979-2008

College Board (2013). *Trends in college pricing 2013.* Retrieved from http://trends.collegeboard.org/sites/default/files/college-pricing-2013-full-report.pdf

Cross, P.K. (1981). *Adults as learners: Increasing participation and facilitating learning.* San Francisco, CA: Jossey-Bass.

Cummins, P.A. (2014). Effective strategies for educating older workers at community colleges. *Educational Gerontology, 40*(5), 338–352. doi: 10.1080/03601277.2013.802193

Cutler, D.M., & Lleras-Muney, A. (2006). *Education and health: Evaluating theories and evidence* (working paper 12352). Cambridge, MA: National Bureau of Economic Research. Retrieved from http://www.nber.org/papers/w12352.pdf

Dentato, M.P., Orwat J., Spira M., & Walker, B. (2014). Examining cohort differences and resilience among the aging LGBT community: Implications for education and practice among an expansively diverse population. *Journal of Human Behavior in the Social Environment, 24*(3), 316–328. doi: 10.1080/10911359.2013.831009

DiPrete, T.A., & Buchmann, C. (2013). *The rise of women: The growing gender gap in education and what it means for American schools.* New York: Russell Sage Foundation.

European Commission (2001). *Making a European area of lifelong learning a reality.* Brussels: European Commission. Retrieved from http://eur-lex.europa.eu/legal-content/EN/TXT/PDF/?uri=CELEX:52001DC0678&qid=1424849728990&from=EN

Feinstein, L., Sabates R., Anderson, T.M., Sorhaindo, A., & Hammond, C. (2006). What are the effects of education on health? *Measuring the effects of education and civic engagement: Proceedings of the Copenhagen Symposium.* Retrieved from http://www.oecd.org/edu/innovation-education/37425753.pdf

Findsen, B. (2006). Social institutions as sites of learning for older adults: Differential opportunities. *Journal of Transformative Education, 4,* 65–81. doi: 10.1177/1541344605282429

Fry, R. (2012, September 26). *A record one-in-five households now owe student loan debt.* Pew Research Center Social and Demographic Trends. Washington, DC. Retrieved from http://www.pewsocialtrends.org/files/2012/09/09-26-12-Student_Debt.pdf

Fry, R. (2014, October 2). *US high school dropout rate reaches record low, driven by improvements among Hispanics, blacks.* Pew Research Center. Washington, DC. Retrieved from http://www.pewresearch.org/fact-tank/2014/10/02/u-s-high-school-dropout-rate-reaches-record-low-driven-by-improvements-among-hispanics-blacks/

GED Testing Service (2014). *Annual statistical report on the GED test: The close of the 2002 series GED test.* Retrieved from http://www.gedtestingservice.com/uploads/files/5b49fc887db0c075da20a68b17d313cd.pdf

Gitlin, L.N., Winter, L., Dennis, M.P., & Hauck, W.W. (2008). Variation in response to a home intervention to support daily function by age, race, sex, and education. *The Journals of Gerontology, Series A: Medical Sciences, 63A*(7), 745–750.

Hager, P.J. (2011). Concepts and definitions of lifelong learning. In M. London (Ed.), *The Oxford handbook of lifelong learning* (pp. 12–25). New York: Oxford University Press.

Hiemstra, R. (1998). From whence have we come? The first twenty-five years of educational gerontology. *New Directions for Adult and Continuing Education, 77*, 5–14.

Hill, A., et al. (2011). Evaluation of the sustained effect of inpatient falls prevention education and predictors of falls after hospital discharge—Follow-up to a randomized controlled trial. *The Journals of Gerontology, Series A: Medical Sciences, 66A*(9), 1001–1012. doi: 10.1093/gerona/glr085

Hoynes, H., Miller, D.L., & Schaller, J. (2012). Who suffers during recessions? *The Journal of Economic Perspectives, 26*(3), 27–47.

Huber, L., & Watson, C. (2014). Technology: Education and training needs of older adults. *Educational Gerontology, 40*(1), 16–25. doi: 10.1080/03601277.2013.768064

Jeske, D., & Roßnagel, C.S. (2015). Learning capability and performance in later working life: Towards a contextual view. *Education + Training, 57*(4), 378–391.

Jones, I., & Symon, G. (2001). Lifelong learning as serious leisure: Policy, practice and potential. *Leisure Studies, 20*(4), 269–283. doi: 10.1080/02614360110098676

Jordan, R. (2015, May 13). *A closer look at income and race concentration in public schools. Urban Institute*. Retrieved from http://www.urban.org/features/closer-look-income-and-race-concentration-public-schools

Julian, T. (2012, October). *Work-life earnings by field of degree and occupation for people with a bachelor's degree: 2011* (ACSBR/11-04). American Community Survey Briefs.

Kaiser Family Foundation (2015). *State health facts: Poverty rate by race/ethnicity*. Retrieved from http://kff.org/other/state-indicator/poverty-rate-by-raceethnicity/

Kena, G., Aud, S., Johnson, F., Wang, X., Zhang, J., Rathbun, A., Wilkinson-Flicker, S., & Kristapovich, P. (2014). *The condition of education 2014* (NCES 2014-083). U.S. Department of Education, National Center for Education Statistics. Washington, DC. Retrieved from http://nces.ed.gov/pubsearch

Kim, J., & Joo, M. (2013). Trend in U.S.-born dropouts' GED and postsecondary degree acquisition: Differences by gender and race/ethnicity. *Journal of the Society for Social Work and Research, 4*(3), 171–181.

Klein, R. (2014, September 26). This is how your education level impacts your health. *The Huffington Post*. Retrieved from http://www.huffingtonpost.com/2014/09/26/education-impacts-health-data_n_5871290.html

Kochhar, R., & Fry, R. (2014, December 12). *Wealth inequality has widened along racial, ethnic lines since end of Great Recession*. Pew Research Center. Retrieved from http://www.pewresearch.org/fact-tank/2014/12/12/racial-wealth-gaps-great-recession/

Lane, P., Michelau, D.K., & Palmer, I. (2012). *Going the distance in adult college completion: Lessons from the non-traditional no more project*. Western Interstate Commission for Higher Education. Retrieved from http://www.wiche.edu/pub/15637

Liu, S., Courtenay B. C., & Valentine, T. (2011). Managing older worker training: A literature review and conceptual framework. *Educational Gerontology 37*(12), 1040-1062. doi: 10.1080/03601277.2010.500576

London, M. (2011). *The Oxford handbook of lifelong learning*. New York: Oxford University Press.

Mettler, S. (2014). *Degrees of inequality: How the politics of higher education sabotaged the American Dream*. New York: Basic Books.

Mishel, L., Gould, E., & Bivens, J. (2015.) *Wage stagnation in nine charts*. Policy Institute. Retrieved from http://www.epi.org/publication/charting-wage-stagnation/

Murnane, R. J., Willett, J. B., & Boudett, K. P. (1999). Do male dropouts benefit from obtaining a GED, postsecondary education, and training? *Evaluation Review 23*(5), 475-503.

National Academies Press (2011). *Expanding underrepresented minority participation*. Washington, DC: National Academies Press. Retrieved from https://grants.nih.gov/training/minority_participation.pdf

National Center for Higher Education Management Systems (2015). *Educational attainment by degree level and age group (decennial census)*. Retrieved from http://www.higheredinfo.org/dbrowser/index.php?submeasure=221&year=1990&level=nation&mode=map&state=0

National Science Foundation. (2012, December). *Doctorate recipients from U.S. universities: 2011* (NSF 13-301). National Center for Science and Engineering Statistics Directorate Social, Behavioral and Economic Sciences.

NCES/National Center for Education Statistics (2012). *Degrees conferred by sex and race*. Retrieved from http://nces.ed.gov/FastFacts/display.asp?id=72

NCES/National Center for Education Statistics (2013). *Table 104.20: Percentage of persons 25 to 29 years old with selected levels of educational attainment, by race/ethnicity and sex: Selected years, 1920 through 2013*. Retrieved from https://nces.ed.gov/programs/digest/d13/tables/dt13_104.20.asp

NCES/National Center for Education Statistics (2014a). *Condition of education 2014*. Retrieved from http://nces.ed.gov/pubsearch/pubsinfo.asp?pubid=2014083

NCES/National Center for Education Statistics (2014b). *Table 104.20: Percentage of persons 25 to 29 years old with selected levels of educational attainment, by race/ethnicity and sex: Selected years, 1920 through 2014*. Retrieved from https://nces.ed.gov/programs/digest/d14/tables/dt14_104.20.asp

NCES/National Center for Education Statistics (n.d.). *Educational attainment*. Retrieved from https://nces.ed.gov/fastfacts/display.asp?id=27

OECD (2012). *Education at a glance: OECD indicators 2012: United States*. Retrieved from http://www.oecd.org/unitedstates/CN%20-%20United%20States.pdf

OECD (2014). *Education at a glance 2014: Highlights, OECD publishing*. Retrieved from http://dx.doi.org/10.1787/eag_highlights-2014-en

OECD-PISA (2012). *Country note: Programme for International Student Assessment (PISA) Results from PISA 2012: United States*. Retrieved from http://www.oecd.org/unitedstates/PISA-2012-results-US.pdf

Passel, J. S., & Cohn, D. (2008). *U.S. Population projections: 2005–2050*. Retrieved from http://www.pewhispanic.org/2008/02/11/us-population-projections-2005-2050/

Pell Institute (2015). *Indicators of higher education equity in the United States: 45 year trend report*. The Pell Institute for the Study of Opportunity in Higher Education and The University of Pennsylvania Alliance for Higher Education and Democrat (PennAHEAD). Retrieved from http://www.pellinstitute.org/downloads/publications-Indicators_of_Higher_Education_Equity_in_the_US_45_Year_Trend_Report.pdf

Perna, L. W., & Titus, M. A. (2005). The relationship between parental involvement as social capital and college enrollment: An examination of racial/ethnic group differences. *The Journal of Higher Education, 76*(5), 485–518.

Perry, L., et al. (2012). Completion and return of fall diaries varies with participants' level of education, first language, and baseline fall risk. *The Journals of Gerontology, Series A: Medical Sciences, 67A*(2), 210–214. doi: 10.1093/gerona/glr175

Pew Internet and American Life Project (2012). *Older adults and Internet use*. Retrieved from http://pewinternet.org/Reports/2012/Older-adults-and-internet-use.aspx

Pew Research Center (2014a). *There's more to the story of the shrinking pay gap*. Retrieved from http://www.pewsocialtrends.org/2014/01/09/theres-more-to-the-story-of-the-shrinking-pay-gap/

Pew Research Center (2014b). *The rising cost of not going to college*. Retrieved from http://www.pewsocialtrends.org/files/2014/02/SDT-higher-ed-FINAL-02-11-2014.pdf

Pfeffer, F. T., Danzinger, S., & Schoeni, R. F. (2013). *Wealth disparities before and after the great recession*. Retrieved from https://www.russellsage.org/sites/all/files/PfefferDanzigerSchoeni_InterimReport_2013.pdf

Portes, A., & Rumbaut, R. G. (2014). *Immigrant America*. Oakland: University of California Press.

Preece, J. (2009). *Lifelong learning and development: A southern perspective*. London: Continuum.

Ratcliffe, C., & McKernan, S. (2013). *Forever in your debt: Who has student loan debt, and who's worried?* The Urban Institute. Retrieved from http://www.urban.org/research/publication/forever-your-debt-who-has-student-loan-debt-and-whos-worried

Riley, M. W., & Riley, J. W., Jr. (2000). Age integration: Conceptual and historical background. *The Gerontologist, 40*(3), 266–270.

Ross, C. E., & Wu, C. (1995). The links between education and health. *American Sociological Association 60*(5), 719–745.

Russell, H. (2008). Later life: A time to learn. *Educational Gerontology, 34*(3), 206–224. doi: 10.1080/03601270701835981

RWJF/Robert Wood Johnson Foundation (2013). *Why does education matter so much to health?* Health policy snapshot: Public health and prevention, Issue brief, March 2013. Retrieved from http://www.rwjf.org/content/dam/farm/reports/issue_briefs/2012/rwjf403347

Schuetz, J. (1982). Geragogy: Instructional programs for elders. *Communication Education 31*, 339-347.

Stanford Center on Poverty and Inequality (2014). *State of the union: The poverty and inequality report*. Stanford, CA: Center on Poverty and Inequality. Retrieved from http://web.stanford.edu/group/scspi/sotu/SOTU_2014_CPI.pdf

Tam, M. (2014). A distinctive theory of teaching and learning for older learners: Why and why not? *International Journal of Lifelong Education, 33*(6), 811–820, doi: 10.1080/02601370.2014.972998

Thelin, J. R. (2004). *A history of American higher education*. Baltimore, MD: The Johns Hopkins University Press.

Tilak, J. B. G. (2002). Education and poverty. *Journal of Human Development: A Multi-Disciplinary Journal for People-Centered Development, 3*(2), 191–207. doi: 10.1080/14649880220147301

Tyler, J. H. (2002). So you want a GED? *Estimating the impact of the GED on the earnings of dropouts who seek the credential*. Boston, MA: National Center for the Study of Adult Learning and Literacy.

Tyler, J. H. (2005). The general educational development (GED) credential: History, current research, and directions for policy and practice. In *Review of adult learning and literacy* (Vol. 5, pp. 45–84). Retrieved from http://www.ncsall.net/index.html@id=778.html

Tyler, J., & Lofstrom, M. (2010). Is the GED an effective route to postsecondary education for school dropouts? *Economics of Education Review, 29*, 813–825.

Tyler, J. H., Murnane, R. J., & Willett, J. B. (2000). Estimating the labor market signaling value of the GED. *NCSALL*. Retrieved from http://www.ncsall.net/?id=667

U.S. Government Printing Office (2011). *Definitions*. Retrieved from http://www.gpo.gov/fdsys/pkg/USCODE-2011-title20/html/USCODE-2011-title20-chap28-subchapIII-partE-subpart3-sec1067k.htm

Van Gerven, W. M., Paas, F. G. W. C., Van Merrienboer, J. J. G., & Schmidt, H. G. (2000). Cognitive load theory and the acquisition of complex cognitive skills in the elderly: Towards an integrative framework. *Educational Gerontology 26*(6), 503-521. doi: 10.1080/03601270050133874

Verizon Wireless (n.d.). *Workshops*. Retrieved from https://www.verizonwireless.com/vzw/storelocator/workshop/workshop-landing.jsp

Wallenstein, P. (2008). (Ed.). *Higher education and the Civil Rights Movement: White supremacy, black southerners, and college campuses*. Gainesville: University Press of Florida.

Weinstein, L. B. (2004). Lifelong learning benefits older adults. *Activities, Adaptation and Aging, 28*(4), 1–12. doi: 10.1300/J016v28n04_01

Weinstock, R. (1978). *The graying of campus*. New York, NY: Educational Facilities Laboratories.

Zhang, J. (2010). *From GED credential to college: Patterns of participation in postsecondary education programs*. Retrieved from GED Testing Service website http://www.gedtestingservice.com/uploads/files/e28d9ff32e78d2de273b67c09a03d48d.pdf

CHAPTER TWO

Creativity and Wisdom across the Life Course

Monika Ardelt and Carolyn E. Adams-Price[1]

Creativity and wisdom are both considered desirable qualities. Creative people are exceptional due to their ability to create something new, depict reality in a new light, and transcend conceptual boundaries (Mumford, 2003), whereas wise individuals are deemed exceptional, because wisdom represents the apex of human development (Baltes & Staudinger, 2000; Erikson, 1963; Staudinger & Kessler, 2008). In this chapter, we explore the similarities and differences between creativity and wisdom, how they might develop across the life course, and how they might benefit people, particularly during the later years of life.

Definition and Measurement

Creativity and wisdom are concepts that are not easy to define and measure. Hence, before we can discuss how creativity and wisdom develop across the life course and their potential benefits, we first need to determine what creativity and wisdom are and how researchers try to study those elusive concepts.

Definition and Measurement of Creativity

Although the contemporary study of creativity started around 1950 (Hennessey & Amabile, 2010), creativity researchers do not always agree on the proper way to study creativity. Some researchers take an eminent creators or *Big-C* creativity approach, studying individuals from the past or present who are generally thought to be highly creative. These researchers might analyze creative products or the personality of exceptionally creative renowned individuals (Simonton, 1994). Other researchers study everyday creativity or *little-c* creativity, which consists of creative solutions to everyday problems and less prominent creative achievements (Richards, 2007).

The creativity of products is typically assessed through the Consensual Assessment Technique (Amabile, 1982), which asks independent judges who are familiar with the domain to rate creative products on several dimensions appropriate to the specific domain, such as creativity, novelty, and originality. The Lifetime Creativity Scales can be used to assess everyday creativity of individuals, based on independent ratings of the quantity and quality of individuals' lifetime creativity at work and as part of leisure activities (Richards et al., 1988).

To measure the creativity of individuals, Gough (1979) developed a 30-item Creative Personality Scale based on items from the Adjective Check List (ACL). In addition to creative personality items, this scale includes items that measure cognition, reflection, self-confidence, unconventionality, resilience, humor, self-expression, and egotism. Nassif and Quevillon (2008) selected items from the Minnesota Multiphasic Personality Indicator, 2nd edition (MMPI-2) to create a 31-item creativity (C) scale that assesses creativity as a combination of creative tendencies, caring, and extraversion.

One of the biggest subtopics in creativity research over the past 40 or 50 years is research on cognitive processes that are thought to be involved in creativity, such as the ability to come up with unique and valuable ideas, products, or problem solutions (Hennessey & Amabile, 2010; Mumford, 2003). Much of that research is on divergent thinking, defined as the ability to generate many ideas, including ideas that are unique and those that are useful. The most widely used test in this area is the Torrance Test of Creative Thinking (TTCT), which consists of several subtests, including the Unusual Uses Test that requires participants to invent as many uses as possible for a common object, such as a brick or paper clip, or the Consequences Test that asks participants to think about all possible consequences to impossible events, such as the ability to become invisible (Torrance, 1962). Divergent thinking is relatively easy to test and is typically found to be independent of performance on intelligence tests, which test the ability to generate the *one right answer*. Yet, divergent thinking does not tend to correlate with performance on creative tasks in the arts and sciences, nor does it predict future performance (Zeng, Proctor, & Salvendy, 2011). Thus, it might not be very useful as a measure of creativity.

Other researchers believe that in addition to cognitive abilities, creativity also requires certain personality qualities and an intrinsic motivation to pursue creative activities. For example, Amabile's (1983) componential framework of creativity conceptualizes creativity as a combination of domain-relevant skills, consisting of knowledge, talent, and technical skills, creativity-relevant skills, such as cognitive style, work style, and the ability to generate novel ideas, and intrinsic motivation and attitude. A third group of creativity researchers study the benefits of participating in creative activities, especially in later life and among nonfamous creators. These different approaches make very different judgments about creativity across the life course.

It should also be noted that creative acts occur in a cultural context. Hence, creative acts can be considered a function of the person, the creative materials, and the sociocultural context (Tanggaard, 2013). The materials available and the conventions of their social context play a large role in determining the value of a creative product. Thus, different cultures might value different creative products or value products for different reasons or features.

Kharkhurin (2014) compared typical Western definitions of creativity with Eastern definitions. He found that definitions of creativity from the East tend to incorporate the concepts of esthetics and authenticity. Esthetics is defined as beauty, elegance, and the embodiment of truth or deeper meaning. Authenticity is defined as honest self-expression and the incorporation of personal values into a creative piece. Kharkhurin (2014) suggested that the inclusion of esthetics and authenticity into the definition of creativity, while retaining novelty and utility as components, expands creativity beyond the classic fine arts and sciences.

One type of creative activity that has not been examined much in the literature is the creation of traditional crafts. Crafts are sometimes considered less than creative because they are often not high on novelty. However, they are likely to be high on authenticity and esthetics, especially cultural meaning. Glaveanu (2013) argued strongly that craft products are creative products worthy of study. Like other creative products, high-quality craft products are produced by individuals who have been working a long time to develop their skills and who are well-versed in the conventions of their craft to produce products high in esthetics and authenticity. Moreover, producing traditional crafts might be one of the best ways that people can participate in the continuity of their culture (Glaveanu, 2013).

Definition and Measurement of Wisdom

Contemporary empirical research on wisdom is even newer than creativity research. Starting in the 1980s, several teams of researchers attempted to define wisdom by pursuing either implicit or explicit approaches. The first approach asks lay persons of different ages to describe or rate characteristics of wisdom or wise persons. Implicit wisdom theories tend to describe wisdom as a combination of cognitive ability, insight, reflective attitude, concern for others, and real-world skills (Bluck & Glück, 2005). Yet, research has also shown that some people perceive wisdom primarily as a cognitive/reflective construct, whereas others hold an integrative view, which gives equal weight to cognitive, reflective, and compassionate characteristics (Glück & Bluck, 2011). Implicit wisdom theories of the East appear to emphasize benevolent and other-centered elements even more than Western implicit theories (Takahashi & Overton, 2005). For example, Yang (2001) found that Taiwanese Chinese adults characterized wisdom as a combination of real-life competencies, knowledge, openness, profundity, modesty, unobtrusiveness, benevolence, and compassion.

In contrast to implicit wisdom theories, explicit wisdom theories were developed by researchers based on a review of the wisdom literature rather than people's conception of wisdom. Some explicit wisdom theories refer to the products of wisdom or the general wisdom of knowledge and texts, similar to the products of creativity, whereas others describe the characteristics of wise individuals. Unlike implicit wisdom theories, explicit wisdom theories show less overlap and range from purely cognitive/reflective conceptions of wisdom to noncognitive wisdom definitions.

The most prominent explicit theory of general wisdom is the Berlin Wisdom Paradigm, which conceptualizes wisdom as expertise and knowledge in the fundamental pragmatics of life, including life planning, life management, and life review, and in the meaning and conduct of life (Baltes & Smith, 2008; Baltes & Staudinger, 2000). General wisdom-related knowledge is assessed by asking participants to address ill-structured hypothetical life problems, such as "A 15-year-old girl wants to get married right away. What should one/she consider and do?" The transcribed responses are then rated by independent judges according to rich factual knowledge and rich procedural knowledge about the fundamental pragmatics of life, lifespan contextualism, consisting of knowledge about the contexts of life and how these change over time, value relativism, which is knowledge that considers the relativism of values and life goals, and the recognition and management of uncertainty (Baltes & Smith, 2008; Baltes & Staudinger, 2000; Smith & Baltes, 1990). Recently, Staudinger and colleagues (Mickler & Staudinger, 2008; Staudinger, Dörner, & Mickler, 2005) developed a measure of personal wisdom, modeled after the Berlin Wisdom Paradigm, that inquires about participants' behavior, strengths, and weaknesses as a friend. The transcribed answers are again rated by independent judges, but the rating criteria concern the wisdom of the self rather than general wisdom. The five criteria are rich self-knowledge, the availability of heuristics for growth and self-regulation, which includes the expression and regulation of emotions and the development and maintenance of close social relationships, insight into the nature of interdependence and the causes of one's emotions and behavior, self-relativism, consisting of reflection, self-reflection, and the acceptance of self and others, and tolerance of ambiguity and uncertainty.

Brugman (2000) concentrates on the last aspect of the Berlin Wisdom Paradigm by defining wisdom as expertise in conquering the cognitive, emotional, and behavioral aspects of uncertainty and measuring it through the Epistemic Cognition Questionnaire (ECQ15), a 15-item self-report scale with three subscales that assess the acknowledgment of uncertainty, emotional stability despite uncertainty, and the ability to act in the face of uncertainty. By contrast, Kekes (1983) also understands wisdom as knowledge, but a special kind of knowledge that allows the wise person to comprehend the deeper interpretative meaning of generally known descriptive facts, such as "Humans are mortal." Similarly, McKee and Barber (1999) argued that wisdom requires the perception of things as they really are or seeing through the illusion of surface knowledge. Sternberg combines knowledge, values, interests, the environment, and the common good in his view of wisdom. According to Sternberg (1998, p. 347), wisdom is "the application of tacit knowledge as mediated by values toward the achievement of a common good through a balance among multiple (a) intrapersonal, (b) interpersonal, and (c) extrapersonal interests in order to achieve a balance among (a) adaptation to existing environments, (b) shaping of existing environments, and (c) selection of new environments."

Whereas many researchers emphasize the importance of knowledge in wisdom, others define wisdom as the balance between knowing and doubting (Meacham, 1990) or the recognition of the limits of personal knowledge (Kitchener & Brenner, 1990). Kitchener and Brenner's (1990) Reflective Judgment Interview presents ill-structured problems related to dilemmas of knowing in participants. Answers are rated with the wisest responses reflecting an awareness that personal knowledge is limited and, therefore, always includes an element of uncertainty, which leads to humility about one's own judgments.

Yet, other researchers view wisdom more comprehensively by including noncognitive and non-Western elements in their definition and assessment of wisdom. Takahashi and Overton (2002) conceptualize and measure wisdom as a combination of a cognitive analytic mode, consisting of knowledge and abstract reasoning skills assessed by subtests of the Wechsler Adult Intelligence Scale-Revised, and a noncognitive synthetic mode, which is measured by self-report scales of reflective understanding, emotional empathy, and emotional regulation. Moreover, several self-report measures of noncognitive wisdom have been developed, such as the 40-item Self-Assessed Wisdom Scale (SAWS), which combines critical life experiences, reflectiveness/reminiscence, openness to experience, emotional regulation, and humor (Webster, 2003, 2007), and the 18-item Adult Self-Transcendence Inventory (ASTI), which measures self-transcendent wisdom (Levenson et al., 2005). The ASTI is based on Curnow's (1999) review of the world's philosophical, religious, and psychological wisdom traditions, which concluded that wisdom comprises self-knowledge, detachment, self-integration, and self-transcendence. Personal self-transcendent wisdom was also assessed by ratings of participants' written examples of their own wisdom and its development in a study by Wink and Helson (1997). High wisdom ratings were characterized by insightful responses that transcended the personal and exhibited recognition of the complexity and limitations of knowledge, an integration of thought and emotion, and a concern with philosophical and spiritual issues. In the same study, Wink and Helson (1997) utilized 18 self-descriptive adjectives from the ACL to gauge the cognitive, reflective, and mature aspects of practical wisdom.

In an attempt to capture the cognitive and noncognitive elements of wisdom in a relatively parsimonious model, Ardelt (1997, 2003, 2004) developed the Three-Dimensional Wisdom Model (3D-WS), based on Clayton and Birren's (1980) research on implicit wisdom theories. The model corresponds to the integrative view of implicit wisdom theories (Glück & Bluck, 2011) and conceptualizes wisdom as an integration of cognitive, reflective, and compassionate personality qualities. Those three dimensions are considered necessary but also sufficient to characterize a wise person (Ardelt, 2004). The cognitive wisdom dimension represents a desire to know the truth and a deep and thorough understanding of life, particularly with regard to intrapersonal and interpersonal matters, including knowledge and acceptance of the positive and negative aspects of human nature, of the inherent limits of knowledge, and of life's unpredictability and uncertainty. The reflective wisdom dimension consists of the ability and willingness to see through illusion (McKee & Barber, 1999) by perceiving phenomena, events, and one's own self from multiple perspectives to transcend subjectivity and projections, which is the tendency to blame other people and circumstances for one's own faults and failures (Bradley, 1978; Green & Gross, 1979). Through mindful self-reflection, self-examination, and self-insight, subjectivity and projections can be transcended, which results in decreased self-centeredness, a deeper understanding of the human condition and life in general, and, consequently, greater sympathy and compassion for others, which describes the compassionate wisdom dimension. The 3D-WS has been assessed through personality rating scales, such as cognitive, reflective, and compassionate items from the California Q-Sort and Haan's Ego Rating Scale (Ardelt, 1997, 2000), and the self-reported 39-item Three-Dimensional Wisdom Scale (3D-WS), which measures cognitive, reflective, and compassionate personality qualities (Ardelt, 2003). Recently an abbreviated 12-item version of the 3D-WS, the 3D-WS-12, was developed (Thomas et al., in press).

Difference between Wisdom and Creativity

Sternberg (1985) conducted a study on implicit theories of wisdom, creativity, and intelligence by asking groups of college professors and laypersons to describe and rate the characteristics of the ideal wise, creative, and intelligent person. Results showed that participants perceived all three constructs as positively related to each other, but wisdom was deemed closer to intelligence than to creativity. The ideal wise person was characterized by sagacity, reasoning ability, the capacity to make expeditious use of information and to learn from ideas and the environment, good judgment skills, and perspicacity. The ideal creative person was described as possessing esthetic taste and imagination, being able and willing to think and act in unorthodox and unconventional ways, to make connections between ideas and things, to recognize similarities and differences, to combine ideas and information in a new way, to question societal norms and assumptions, to make decisions and take a stand but also be flexible if things do not work out, and to possess a certain drive for accomplishments and recognition. Whereas the ideal wise person was perceived as understanding life, willing to learn, and caring, the ideal creative person appeared more to challenge and question life to create something new.

Unfortunately, a uniform definition or *gold standard* to assess creativity and wisdom in products or persons does not exist. Hence, we need to take the different definitions and measurement approaches into account when studying the development, correlates, and effects of creativity and wisdom across the life course.

Development across the Life Course

Age and Creativity

Much of what is known about creativity across the life course is based on the study of eminent creators; that is, those rare individuals that history recalls as famous for their artistic or scientific works. In the 1970s and 1980s, Dean K. Simonton (1997) published several studies on the creative productivity across the lifespan of historically eminent individuals in a wide range of disciplines, ranging from math and science to literature, music, and painting. Unlike some previous studies, Simonton limited his research to eminent creators who lived at least to the age of 70, so that his estimates of peak productivity would not be biased toward youth by the short lifespan of some famous creators, such as John Keats, who died in his 20s. Simonton's basic finding was the *inverted backwards J*, that is, productivity appears to increase quickly in eminent creators from age 20 to an average peak of age 40 and decline slowly after that. Simonton also found that the peak varied dramatically from one creative domain to another. In abstract domains, such as math and physics, and in the production of short literary works, like lyric poems, creative productivity tends to peak early, at around age 30. In domains that require the integration of huge amounts of knowledge, such as philosophy and historical fiction, creative productivity tends to peak late, at around age 60.

Although Simonton found age differences in creative productivity, he did not discover age differences in the quality of creative products. When controlling for creative output, eminent creators were equally likely to produce high-quality products at any age. He also reported findings suggesting that motivated people can successfully begin participating in most creative domains at any age, although peak productivity will still occur relatively earlier for abstract domains than for knowledge-rich domains.

Simonton's research is positive in that it suggests that creativity is not limited to the early part of life. However, his eminent historical creators approach has a number of weaknesses. First, the vast majority of artists, writers, musicians, and scientists he examined were white males from Western Europe or North America, as most historically eminent creators recognized in Western culture have been white males. The creative domains examined were those usually considered fine arts or sciences by Western Europeans, and excluded Eastern art and traditional crafts. Thus, the research does not have much to say about the life course of creative women or non-Westerners, and it has virtually nothing to say about the value of everyday forms of creativity.

Studying craft participation, for example, is a way of studying little-c everyday creativity (Runco, 2007). Craft products tend to be produced by women, especially older women, in many cultures. This fact in itself might account for their devaluation by the fine arts community (Adams-Price & Steinman, 2007). Craft participation among middle-aged and older women might be motivated by economic need, in the case of third world women crafters (Dhamija, 1981), by the need for recreation, as in the case of middle-class Japanese wives who study painting (Creighton, 1995), or as an activity that can lead to increased social interactions, as in the case of women who attend quilting bees (Maidment & Macfarlane, 2011a, 2011b; Piercy & Cheek, 2004). Participation in craft activities cuts across social class and the sociocultural milieu.

If creativity is measured by divergent thinking, it is likely that it increases with age in tandem with intellectual development. Kleibeuker, De Dreu, and Crone (2013) reported that studies have not consistently found increases in divergent thinking in school children from middle to late childhood. However, they did find increases in fluency and flexibility on creative divergent thinking tasks from early to mid-adolescence, possibly due to the increasing cognitive control and attention associated with adolescence. Divergent thinking is generally found to be lower in late life than at earlier ages (Reese et al., 2001), although this was not necessarily true when older adults were allowed enough time to complete divergent thinking tasks (Foos & Boone, 2008).

Age and Wisdom

As with creativity, it is assumed that the development of wisdom takes time and grows with age (Kekes, 1983). However, it is not clear at what age wisdom might peak, whether it declines with age (Sternberg, 2005), and when the best products of wisdom come forth. Comparable to the study of eminent creators might be the study of eminent wise persons. Yet, most wisdom research to date concerns *little-w* rather than *Big-W* wisdom. When people are asked to nominate a wise person, they tend to nominate older men rather than women or younger individuals (Ardelt, 2008a; Baltes et al., 1995; Denney, Dew, & Kroupa, 1995). However, women are more likely to be nominated if researchers inquire about exemplars of interpersonal wisdom (Denney, Dew, & Kroupa, 1995). Nominees of the wisest person in history are overwhelmingly male religious and political figures, such as Jesus Christ, the Buddha, Muhammad, Jewish Rabbis, Mahatma Gandhi, Martin Luther King Jr., and Abraham Lincoln (Ferrari et al., 2011; Weststrate, Ferrari, & Ardelt, under review). Jesus was about 30 years old when he started to preach (Luke 3:23) and was martyred only a few years later, although the exact date is unknown. At the age of 29, Siddhārtha Gautama renounced the life of a householder to search for liberation from aging, illness, and death. After engaging in diverse and very extreme spiritual exercises that did not bring the desired results, he decided to practice the middle way and discovered the path to enlightenment and ultimate wisdom (Armstrong, 2001). At the age of 35, Siddhārtha Gautama became the Buddha, a fully enlightened being, and he continued to teach and impart wisdom to his followers for 45 years until his death at the age of 80 (Ñanamoli, 2001). Muhammad was 40 when he heard revelations from God. He started to share his prophecies at the age of 42 and taught for 20 years until his death at age 62 (Armstrong, 2006). Mahatma Gandhi conceived his ideas about noncooperation and nonviolence in a book on *Hind Swaraj* (Hindu home rule) that was published in 1909 when he was 40 years old (King, 2013). He became an important Indian leader at the age of 51 and remained a leader of the nonviolence movement until his assassination at the age of 78 (Gandhi, 2007). Martin Luther King Jr. was influenced by Gandhi and his nonviolence movement. He was 26 years old when he led the Montgomery Bus Boycott for racial equality (Walsh, 2003) and 34 years old when he delivered his famous "I have a dream" speech during the March on Washington (Hansen, 2003). Five years later, he was assassinated at the age of 39 (Lokos, 1968). Abraham Lincoln became president at the age of 52, led the nation during the American Civil War, and delivered the Gettysburg Address about the principles of equal rights, liberty, and democracy at the age of 54. He was assassinated at the age of 56 (Donald, 1995).

Overall, a review of these eminent wise persons reveals that the products of their wisdom became widely known during their early to middle adulthood. They also continued to impart wisdom until their death, with no indication that their wisdom declined with age. It is interesting to note, however, that many eminent wise persons were either condemned to death or assassinated, which hints at the potential revolutionary nature of wisdom.

In studies of little-w wisdom, evidence suggests that similar to the development of divergent thinking, wisdom is likely to increase during adolescence and young adulthood. Wisdom, assessed by the Reflective Judgment Interview, tended to grow from age 16 to age 32 in a longitudinal study, unless the highest score was already attained at age 28 (Kitchener & Brenner, 1990; Kitchener et al., 1989). In cross-sectional research, general wisdom-related knowledge was positively related to age until about 24 years, then remained relatively stable, and finally showed some decline after age 80 (Pasupathi, Staudinger, & Baltes, 2001; Staudinger, 1999). However, for study participants who scored high on moral reasoning, age was weakly positively related to wisdom-related knowledge across the age spectrum (Pasupathi & Staudinger, 2001). Similarly, in a longitudinal study by Wink and Helson (1997), practical wisdom tended to be greater at age 52 than age 27, particularly for individuals who became clinical psychologists, suggesting the potential for lifelong growth in wisdom for individuals who are intrinsically motivated to develop their personality (Staudinger & Kunzmann, 2005).

Wisdom, assessed by the 3D-WS and the SAWS, had a curvilinear relation with age in cross-sectional research, with lower mean level scores in young adulthood and old age and the highest average scores around midlife or later midlife (Bergsma & Ardelt, 2012; Thomas et al., in press; Webster, Westerhof, & Bohlmeijer, 2014). Another study showed that although older adults and young college students had similar average scores on the 3D-WS, older adults with a college degree tended to outperform current college students on the 3D-WS, whereas due to their lower average score on the cognitive wisdom dimension, the scores of older adults without a college degree tended to be lower than those of younger or older college-educated adults (Ardelt, 2010). As indicated by longitudinal research, early adulthood factors, such as socioeconomic status, the social environment, psychological mindedness, and openness to experience, have long-ranging positive effects on later life wisdom (Ardelt, 1998, 2000; Wink & Dillon, 2003; Wink & Helson, 1997).

Overall, research suggests that the seeds of both creativity and wisdom are planted early in life (Richardson & Pasupathi, 2005) and depend on an enriching and challenging educational and social experience, role models, social support, intrinsic motivation, and certain personality qualities (Edmondson, 2012; Helson & Srivastava, 2002; Hennessey & Amabile, 2010; Jordan, 2005; Richards et al., 1988; Simonton, 2000).

Wisdom, Creativity, and Personality

Both wise and creative people tend to be open to new experiences and interested in understanding their own internal life and that of others (Feist, 1998; Feist & Barron, 2003; Glück et al., 2013; Helson & Srivastava, 2002; Le, 2011; Levenson et al., 2005; Perrine & Brodersen, 2005; Silvia et al., 2014; Staudinger et al., 1998; Webster, Westerhof, & Bohlmeijer, 2014; Wink & Helson, 1997) and, therefore, are likely to transcend social boundaries, structures, and procedures (Simonton, 2000; Staudinger & Kessler, 2008). However, only wise people might have discovered the true *art of living*, that is, to live a life that is good for oneself, others, and society as a whole by transcending the ego-centered self (Ardelt, 2008b; Baltes & Staudinger, 2000; Csikszentmihalyi & Nakamura, 2005; Helson & Srivastava, 2002; Orwoll & Perlmutter, 1990; Sternberg, 1998). For example, wisdom-related knowledge was positively related to the importance of other-enhancing values, such as the well-being of friends, societal engagement, and the protection of the environment, and inversely to the importance of living a pleasurable, hedonistic life (Kunzmann & Baltes, 2003). Helson and Srivastava (2002) showed that relatively wise women were more likely than creative women to be rated as warm, compassionate, benevolent, caring, and accessible. Meaning-making was another salient personality characteristic of wise women compared to the originality and ambition of creative women. Moreover, empathy at age 21 had a positive effect on women's practical and transcendent wisdom at age 52 (Wink & Helson, 1997). The 3D-WS, SAWS, and ASTI have also been found to be positively associated with empathy and emotional competence (Glück et al., 2013).

In addition, wisdom, measured in a variety of ways, tends to be positively correlated with orientation toward personal growth, self-acceptance, autonomy, positive relations with others, generativity, self-transcendence, and ego development (Ardelt, 2008b, 2011; Glück et al., 2013; Helson & Srivastava, 2002; Le & Levenson, 2005; Staudinger, Lopez, & Baltes, 1997; Webster, 2003, 2007; Wink & Dillon, 2003; Wink & Helson, 1997). The 3D-WS and the SAWS were also positively correlated with forgiveness of self, others, and situations (Ardelt, 2011) and the 3D-WS also with emotional intelligence (Zacher, McKenna, & Rooney, 2013). Among the NEO personality scales, wisdom has been found to be positively associated with agreeableness, conscientiousness, extraversion, and low scores on neuroticism (Levenson et al., 2005; Webster, Westerhof, & Bohlmeijer, 2014).

By contrast, the creative personality appears to be less integrated and more complex than the wise personality, with signs of inner struggle and conflict. Feist's (1998) meta-analysis of 29 studies indicated that compared to nonartists, artists tended to be more open to new experiences, esthetic, creative, curious, imaginative, sensitive, original, self-confident, and self-accepting, but also more driven, ambitious, dominant, hostile, and impulsive and less cautious, conscientious, controlled, rigid, orderly, reliable, socialized, and conventional. In addition, the creative personality is characterized by independence, nonconformity, unconventionality, behavioral and cognitive flexibility, and risk-taking boldness (Simonton, 2000). Yet, a 44-year longitudinal study showed that male graduate students from 14 departments who were rated or scored high at age 27 on tolerance, psychological mindedness, personality integration, self-insight, good judgment, and likeability and low on mania and hostility tended to have greater lifetime creative achievements at age 72 (Feist & Barron, 2003). This latter finding suggests that wisdom and creativity might be more similar for some groups than others.

Wisdom, Creativity, and Demographic Characteristics

Whereas educational attainment and socioeconomic status tend to be positively correlated with wisdom measures that incorporate a cognitive domain (Ardelt, 2003; Ardelt & Edwards, in press; Bergsma & Ardelt, 2012), education is less likely associated with noncognitive assessments of wisdom (Glück et al., 2013; Webster, 2003), although there are exceptions (Webster, Westerhof, & Bohlmeijer, 2014). Even though individuals are more likely to nominate men than women as exemplars of wisdom, no gender differences in wisdom ratings or scores are generally found. For example, gender tends to be unrelated to general wisdom-related knowledge (Kunzmann & Baltes, 2003; Smith & Baltes, 1990), analytic and synthetic wisdom modes (Takahashi & Overton, 2002), and the 3D-WS, ASTI, and SAWS (Ardelt, 2003; Ardelt & Edwards, in press; Glück et al., 2013; Levenson et al., 2005; Webster, 2007; Webster, Westerhof, & Bohlmeijer, 2014). Findings related to race and ethnic differences in wisdom are more mixed. While there were no significant differences in 3D-WS scores between white and black older Americans (Ardelt, 2003; Ardelt & Edwards, in press) and in ASTI scores between Vietnamese American and European American students, European Americans tended to score significantly higher than Vietnamese Americans on the 3D-WS (Le, 2008) and also significantly higher than Japanese on the analytic and synthetic modes of wisdom (Takahashi & Overton, 2002). The reasons for these cultural differences have not been explored in depth yet.

Not a lot of research exists on the relationship between demographic characteristics and creativity. Most of the research on socioeconomic status and creativity comes from child and adolescent giftedness studies. Because it is well known that children from impoverished environments tend to perform more poorly than children raised in richer environments on standardized tests believed to measure intelligence (Bigelow, 2006; Brooks-Gunn, Klebanov, & Duncan, 1996), a few researchers have looked to see if children from impoverished environments also perform poorly on tests of creativity, such as the TTCT. Some studies indicate that children who attend schools in poor neighborhoods perform more poorly on creativity tests than children who attend schools in richer neighborhoods (Dai et al., 2012; Dudek, Strobel, & Runco, 1993). In fact, school quality was a better predictor of creativity test scores than parental education, but confidence and motivation were important predictors as well (Dai et al., 2012). Dudek, Strobel, & Runco (1993) suggested that lower scores for children from poor neighborhoods on creativity tests might be related to poorer verbal skills, which might also explain why girls tended to outperform boys on the verbal creativity tests. By contrast, race differences that are independent of socioeconomic status are generally not found on the TTCT (Glover, 1976; Torrance, 1971), although one study reported higher average creativity scores for lower socioeconomic status black children than middle-class white children (Kaltsounis, 1974).

Even less is known about the relationship between socioeconomic status and participation in creative activities in adulthood, although it would seem reasonable to expect that impoverished individuals would have less opportunity to engage in creative activities than persons who are not impoverished. However, it is relatively common for women from poor families in developing countries to earn or supplement the family income by creating and selling handicrafts, which in turn tends to increase their self-efficacy (e.g., Dhamija, 1981; Krishnaraj, 1992). It would be interesting to examine how earning money from crafts affects the well-being of poorer and older North American women.

Benefits in Later Life

Benefits of Creativity

Over the last several years, there has been considerable interest in examining the degree to which creative activities can benefit older adults, including both healthy older adults and older adults with dementia or other illnesses. Inspired by Gene Cohen's call for evidence-based research on the benefits of creative activities for older adults (Cohen, 2002; Cohen et al., 2006; Miller & Cohen, 2010), the National Center for Creative Aging (NCCA) was founded in 2001 under the auspices of the National Endowment for the Arts (NEA) to promote research and programs that encourage older adults to engage in creative activities and the arts. The NCCA tends to promote participation in fine arts activities as opposed to craft activities, which some people associate with simple activities suitable for nursing homes (Larson & Perlstein, 2003). For Cohen (2006), the best arts activities for older adults are those where older adults engage in challenging activities tutored by professional artists over a long period of time.

Cohen (2006) summarized the positive effects of long-term participation in creative activities as follows: creative activities give older adults a sense of control and mastery, opportunities for social engagement, and increased brain plasticity, all of which can lead to better health. Control and mastery come from the feeling of satisfaction gained from doing something new or better than before. Cohen suggested that this sense of control might improve immune system functioning and that social engagement, which comes from sharing the activity with others who are either an audience or cocreators, tends to reduce stress. Finally, participation in the arts tends to provide challenges, which can induce the formation of new synapses and dendrites, thus increasing brain plasticity.

For example, quilt-making had a number of psychological benefits for middle-aged and older women in Appalachian, Mormon, and Amish North American subcultures (Cheek & Piercy, 2004, 2008). Quilting helped older women maintain a sense of identity and self-efficacy, allowed them to feel that they were growing in skills, and connected them to other women with similar interests. Quilting groups might help older women achieve a sense of generativity, because they offer women the opportunity to share their quilt-related knowledge and skills with other women (Cheek & Piercy,

2008). Similarly, middle-aged and older women received several psychological benefits from making jewelry, either as a hobby or as a vocation (Adams-Price & Steinman, 2007). Women reported that jewelry-making increased their well-being and sense of meaning and added recognition from others, a sense of accomplishment/productivity, and a chance to relax and relieve stress. The psychological benefits were linked to the women's agentic generativity, the feeling of leaving one's mark on the world.

Interestingly, the movement toward involving older adults in arts activities seems to be more connected to the art therapy movement than to academic research on creativity (Stuckey & Nobel, 2010). Some proponents of creative aging view creative activities as a means to cope with health problems or other age-related deficits, but others are inspired by the concept of successful aging to look at the potential of older adults (Carr, Wellin, & Reece, 2009; Cohen, 2006; Fisher & Specht, 1999). This dichotomy mirrors the discussion in the aging literature about whether or not late-life gains are actual gains or merely compensation for losses (Flood & Phillips, 2007; Uttal & Perlmutter, 1989).

One benefit of late-life participation in creative activities appears to be the creation of meaning in older adults' lives (Carr, Wellin, & Reece, 2009). Although most creative endeavors contain a component of meaning, story-telling and the writing of poetry are probably the most obvious examples of meaning-making through creative activities. It could also be argued that participation in the traditional crafts of one's culture could be a way to create meaning within a cultural context.

Benefits of Wisdom

If wise individuals know the art of living, they should also know how to age and die well. Yet, some researchers have argued that the greater clarity and insight into the human condition and the aging process that wisdom provides, including the negative aspects of the human existence and growing older, might not necessarily be conducive to experiencing subjective well-being (Mickler & Staudinger, 2008; Staudinger et al., 2005; Staudinger & Glück, 2011). Indeed, the empirical evidence is mixed.

Studies of highly educated middle-aged and older white adults did not find significant correlations between wisdom, measured as practical wisdom, transcendent wisdom, personal wisdom, or expertise in uncertainty, and life satisfaction or the absence of depressive symptoms (Brugman, 2000; Mickler & Staudinger, 2008; Wink & Helson, 1997). Yet, studies of racially, educationally, and/or economically diverse samples of older adults show that wisdom, assessed by the combined ratings of cognitive, reflective, and compassionate personality qualities, the 3D-WS, or the combined analytic and synthetic wisdom modes, was positively related to life satisfaction, general well-being, or the absence of depressive symptoms (Ardelt, 2003; Le, 2011; Takahashi & Overton, 2002), even after controlling for current life circumstances, such as physical and subjective health, financial situation, socioeconomic status, physical environment, and social involvement (Ardelt, 1997; Ardelt & Edwards, in press). In addition, and similar to creative endeavors in old age, wisdom was associated with greater physical and subjective health, mastery, and purpose in life and less fear of death (Ardelt, 2000, 2003). In fact, feelings of mastery, control, and purpose in life tend to mediate the relation between wisdom and subjective well-being in old age either fully (Etezadi & Pushkar, 2013) or partially (Ardelt & Edwards, in press).

It appears that wise people are not only able to perceive reality as it is, but they can also learn from experiences and have the resources and confidence to master the vicissitudes of life (Glück & Bluck, 2013). For example, when faced by a problem or crisis, older wise exemplars first took a step back to relax and consider the situation. Then they engaged in active coping to rectify the situation to the best of their abilities, taking lessons learned in the past into account. By contrast, older nonwise exemplars avoided reflecting on the situation and were more likely to immediately use passive coping strategies, such as praying or accepting, when confronted by a problem, even if a more active approach would have been more appropriate (Ardelt, 2005).

Overall, the research suggests that creativity and wisdom are particularly beneficial in old age when objective circumstances might threaten subjective well-being, such as poor health or low socioeconomic status. For example, the positive relation between wisdom and subjective well-being was statistically stronger for older hospice patients and nursing home residents than relatively healthy older community residents after controlling for demographics, social involvement, and subjective health. Although well-being tended to be lower for hospice patients and nursing home residents than for community residents, the difference in average well-being scores became smaller with higher wisdom scores (Ardelt & Edwards, in press). Because aging comes with inevitable social, mental, and physical losses, it is conceivable that creative activities and wisdom become more valuable by providing a sense of mastery, control, and purpose in life, when other means to augment subjective well-being, such as traveling, going out, or entertaining, are no longer available.

Discussion

Although creativity and wisdom are held in high esteem, a generally agreed upon definition and assessment of these elusive constructs does not exist. This might explain some of the differences in the research findings. Yet, we are also able to draw some general conclusions: First, the associations between age and creativity and age and wisdom appear to be nonlinear, with initial increases in adolescence and early adulthood up to a certain point, followed by either a plateau or a later decline. The height of the summit and when it is reached depend on the individual, the domain of creative activity, and whether the quantity or quality of products or personality qualities of creativity and wisdom are studied. Second, both creativity and wisdom have been viewed as products, independent of the individuals who produced them. Yet, the more interesting question is how wise and creative individuals excel at living. Creative people are exceptional, because they create something that did not exist before, such as a painting, a sculpture, a poem, a novel, an invention, or a new way of solving a problem. Wise people do not necessarily create something new, but they are exceptional, because they understand the deeper meaning of old truths, such as "Love thy neighbor" or "Humans are mortal," and they act accordingly (Kekes, 1983) to create a life that is good for them, others, and the whole society. Wise individuals creatively apply their wisdom to deal with the challenges of life, provide advice, guidance, and help to others, and to the best of their ability, behave in ways that benefits rather than harms society. Their outstanding characteristic is their other-centeredness, which includes the ability to see phenomena and events from different points of view to gain a deeper understanding of the issues as well as deep compassion and concern for others. Creative individuals, by contrast, appear to be more complex and to have a less integrated and self-transcended personality than wise people. Yet, an intrinsic motivation to either create something new or to grow in wisdom seems to be essential for the manifestation of both creativity and wisdom. Finally, creativity and wisdom seem to be particularly beneficial during the later years of life by providing a sense of control, mastery, and life purpose that enhance subjective well-being in old age.

Although research on creativity and wisdom has proliferated during the past decades, we still do not know enough about the conditions that foster creativity and wisdom. More longitudinal studies are needed that trace the development of creativity and wisdom across the life course and explore childhood and adolescent predictors of later life creativity and wisdom. For example, it is possible that the emergence of creativity and wisdom depends on role models and a social support system. Other questions are whether creativity and wisdom can be learned in schools and universities (Hennessey & Amabile, 2010; Reams, 2015; Sternberg, 2001; Sternberg, Jarvin, & Grigorenko, 2009) and what might be the long-term benefits for students and society. Another interesting research area is the study of creativity and wisdom in organizations, particularly those that serve older adults, such as assisted living facilities and nursing homes (Geller, 2013; McBee, 2008). One promising approach is the TimeSlips creative storytelling program (Basting, 2003), which engages older adults with dementia and their caregivers in creative storytelling that does not rely on memory but brings meaning and enhanced well-being to the older adults' lives and more profound interactions with their caregivers (Fritsch et al., 2009; George & Houser, 2014; Phillips, Reid-Arndt, & Pak, 2010). A promising approach for wisdom development is the introduction of mindfulness training in assisted living facilities and nursing homes (Moss et al., 2015). Creativity and wisdom are clearly valuable throughout the life course but are especially beneficial in old age to enhance subjective well-being, particularly when circumstances are less than optimal.

Note

1. We would like to thank Jenna L. Schall for her help with the literature review.

References

Adams-Price, C. E., & Steinman, B. A. (2007). Crafts and generative expression: A qualitative study of the meaning of creativity in women who make jewelry in midlife. *The International Journal of Aging & Human Development, 65*(4), 315–333. doi: 10.2190/AG.65.4.c

Amabile, T. M. (1982). Social psychology of creativity: A consensual assessment technique. *Journal of Personality and Social Psychology, 43*(5), 997–1013. doi: 10.1037/0022-3514.43.5.997

Amabile, T. M. (1983). The social psychology of creativity: A componential conceptualization. *Journal of Personality and Social Psychology, 45*(2), 357–376. doi: 10.1037/0022-3514.45.2.357

Ardelt, M. (1997). Wisdom and life satisfaction in old age. *The Journals of Gerontology, Series B: Psychological Sciences, 52B*(1), P15–P27. doi: 10.1093/geronb/52B.1.P15

Ardelt, M. (1998). Social crisis and individual growth: The long-term effects of the Great Depression. *Journal of Aging Studies, 12*(3), 291–314. doi: 10.1016/S0890-4065(98)90005-6

Ardelt, M. (2000). Antecedents and effects of wisdom in old age: A longitudinal perspective on aging well. *Research on Aging, 22*(4), 360–394. doi: 10.1177/0164027500224003

Ardelt, M. (2003). Empirical assessment of a three-dimensional wisdom scale. *Research on Aging, 25*(3), 275–324. doi: 10.1177/0164027503025003004

Ardelt, M. (2004). Wisdom as expert knowledge system: A critical review of a contemporary operationalization of an ancient concept. *Human Development, 47*(5), 257–285. doi: 10.1159/000079154

Ardelt, M. (2005). How wise people cope with crises and obstacles in life. *ReVision: A Journal of Consciousness and Transformation, 28*(1), 7–19. doi: 10.3200/REVN.28.1.7-19

Ardelt, M. (2008a). Being wise at any age. In S.J. Lopez (Ed.), *Positive psychology: exploring the best in people* (Vol. 1: Discovering Human Strengths, pp. 81–108). Westport, CT: Praeger.

Ardelt, M. (2008b). Self-development through selflessness: The paradoxical process of growing wiser. In H.A. Wayment & J.J. Bauer (Eds.), *Transcending self-interest: Psychological explorations of the quiet ego* (pp. 221–233). Washington, DC: American Psychological Association.

Ardelt, M. (2010). Are older adults wiser than college students? A comparison of two age cohorts. *Journal of Adult Development, 17*(4), 193–207. doi: 10.1007/s10804-009-9088-5

Ardelt, M. (2011). The measurement of wisdom: A commentary on Taylor, Bates, and Webster's comparison of the SAWS and 3D-WS. *Experimental Aging Research, 37*(2), 241–255. doi: 10.1080/0361073X.2011.554509

Ardelt, M., & Edwards, C.A. (in press). Wisdom at the end of life: An analysis of mediating and moderating relations between wisdom and subjective well-being. *The Journals of Gerontology, Series B: Psychological Sciences and Social Sciences*. doi: 10.1093/geronb/gbv051

Armstrong, K. (2001). *Buddha*. New York: Penguin Group.

Armstrong, K. (2006). *Muhammad. A prophet for our time*. New York, NY: HarperCollins.

Baltes, P.B., & Smith, J. (2008). The fascination of wisdom: Its nature, ontogeny, and function. *Perspectives on Psychological Science, 3*(1), 56–64. doi: 10.1111/j.1745-6916.2008.00062.x

Baltes, P.B., & Staudinger, U.M. (2000). Wisdom: A metaheuristic (pragmatic) to orchestrate mind and virtue toward excellence. *American Psychologist, 55*(1), 122–136. doi: 10.1037/0003-066X.55.1.122

Baltes, P.B., Staudinger, U.M., Maercker, A., & Smith, J. (1995). People nominated as wise: A comparative study of wisdom-related knowledge. *Psychology and Aging, 10*(2), 155–166. doi: 10.1037/0882-7974.10.2.155

Basting, A.D. (2003). Exploring the creative potential of people with Alzheimer's disease and related dementia: Dare to imagine. In J.L. Ronch & J.A. Goldfield (Eds.), *Mental wellness in aging: Strengths-based approaches*. (pp. 353–367, xxvii, 386). Baltimore, MD: Health Professions Press.

Bergsma, A., & Ardelt, M. (2012). Self-reported wisdom and happiness: An empirical investigation. *Journal of Happiness Studies, 13*(3), 481–499. doi: 10.1007/s10902-011-9275-5

Bigelow, B.J. (2006). There's an elephant in the room: The impact of early poverty and neglect on intelligence and common learning disorders in children, adolescents, and their parents. *Developmental Disabilities Bulletin, 34*(1–2), 177–215.

Bluck, S., & Glück, J. (2005). From the inside out: People's implicit theories of wisdom. In R.J. Sternberg & J. Jordan (Eds.), *A handbook of wisdom. Psychological perspectives* (pp. 84–109). New York: Cambridge University Press.

Bradley, G.W. (1978). Self-serving biases in the attribution process: A reexamination of the fact or fiction question. *Journal of Personality and Social Psychology, 36*(1), 56–71. doi: 10.1037/0022-3514.36.1.56

Brooks-Gunn, J., Klebanov, P.K., & Duncan, G.J. (1996). Ethnic differences in children's intelligence test scores: Role of economic deprivation, home environment, and maternal characteristics. *Child Development, 67*(2), 396–408. doi: 10.2307/1131822

Brugman, G.M. (2000). *Wisdom: Source of narrative coherence and eudaimonia.* Delft, The Netherlands: Eburon.

Carr, D., Wellin, C., & Reece, H. (2009). A review of arts and aging research: Revealing an elusive but promising direction for the era of the Third Age. *Journal of Aging, Humanities, and the Arts, 3*(3), 199–221. doi: 10.1080/1932561090 3134496

Cheek, C., & Piercy, K.W. (2004). Quilting as age identity expression in traditional women. *The International Journal of Aging & Human Development, 59*(4), 321–337. doi: 10.2190/t1r0-d8tw-ml6y-vyyl

Cheek, C., & Piercy, K.W. (2008). Quilting as a tool in resolving Erikson's adult stage of human development. *Journal of Adult Development, 15*(1), 13–24. doi: 10.1007/s10804-007-9022-7

Clayton, V.P., & Birren, J.E. (1980). The development of wisdom across the life-span: A reexamination of an ancient topic. In P.B. Baltes & O.G. Brim Jr. (Eds.), *Life-span development and behavior* (Vol. 3, pp. 103–135). New York: Academic Press.

Cohen, G.D. (2002). *The creative age: Awakening human potential in the second half of life*. New York, NY: William Morrow.

Cohen, G.D. (2006). Research on creativity and aging: The positive impact of the arts on health and illness. *Generations, 30*(1), 7–15.

Cohen, G.D., Perlstein, S., Chapline, J., Kelly, J., Firth, K.M., & Simmens, S. (2006). The impact of professionally conducted cultural programs on the physical health, mental health, and social functioning of older adults. *The Gerontologist, 46*(6), 726–734. doi: 10.1093/geront/46.6.726

Creighton, M.R. (1995). Japanese craft tourism: Liberating the crane wife. *Annals of Tourism Research, 22*(2), 463–478. doi: 10.1016/0160-7383(94)00086-7

Csikszentmihalyi, M., & Nakamura, J. (2005). The role of emotions in the development of wisdom. In R.J. Sternberg & J. Jordan (Eds.), *A handbook of wisdom. Psychological perspectives* (pp. 220–242). New York: Cambridge University Press.

Curnow, T. (1999). *Wisdom, intuition, and ethics*. Brookfield, VT: Ashgate.

Dai, D.Y., Tan, X., Marathe, D., Valtcheva, A., Pruzek, R.M., & Shen, J. (2012). Influences of social and educational environments on creativity during adolescence: Does SES matter? *Creativity Research Journal, 24*(2–3), 191–199. doi: 10.1080/10400419.2012.677338

Denney, N.W., Dew, J.R., & Kroupa, S.L. (1995). Perceptions of wisdom: What is it and who has it? *Journal of Adult Development, 2*(1), 37–47. doi: 10.1007/BF02261740

Dhamija, J. (1981). Women and handicrafts: Myth and reality. *Seeds, 4*, 1–16.

Donald, D. H. (1995). *Lincoln*. New York, NY: Simon & Schuster.

Dudek, S. Z., Strobel, M. G., & Runco, M. A. (1993). Cumulative and proximal influences on the social environment and children's creative potential. *The Journal of Genetic Psychology: Research and Theory on Human Development, 154*(4), 487–499.

Edmondson, R. (2012). Intergenerational relations in the west of Ireland and sociocultural approaches to wisdom. *Journal of Family Issues, 33*(1), 76–98. doi: 10.1177/0192513x11420959

Erikson, E. H. (1963). *Childhood and society*. New York: Norton.

Etezadi, S., & Pushkar, D. (2013). Why are wise people happier? An explanatory model of wisdom and emotional well-being in older adults. *Journal of Happiness Studies, 14*(3), 929–950. doi: 10.1007/s10902-012-9362-2

Feist, G. J. (1998). A meta-analysis of personality in scientific and artistic creativity. *Personality and Social Psychology Review, 2*(4), 290–309. doi: 10.1207/s15327957pspr0204_5

Feist, G. J., & Barron, F. X. (2003). Predicting creativity from early to late adulthood: Intellect, potential, and personality. *Journal of Research in Personality, 37*(2), 62–88. doi: 10.1016/S0092-6566(02)00536-6

Ferrari, M., Kahn, A., Benayon, M., & Nero, J. (2011). Phronesis, sophia, and hochma: Developing wisdom in Islam and Judaism. *Research in Human Development, 8*(2), 128–148. doi: 10.1080/15427609.2011.568869

Fisher, B. J., & Specht, D. K. (1999). Successful aging and creativity in later life. *Journal of Aging Studies, 13*(4), 457–472. doi: 10.1016/S0890-4065(99)00021-3

Flood, M., & Phillips, K. D. (2007). Creativity in older adults: A plethora of possibilities. *Issues in Mental Health Nursing, 28*(4), 389–411. doi: 10.1080/01612840701252956

Foos, P. W., & Boone, D. (2008). Adult age differences in divergent thinking: It's just a matter of time. *Educational Gerontology, 34*(7), 587–594. doi: 10.1080/03601270801949393

Fritsch, T., Kwak, J., Grant, S., Lang, J., Montgomery, R. R., & Basting, A. D. (2009). Impact of TimeSlips, a creative expression intervention program, on nursing home residents with dementia and their caregivers. *The Gerontologist, 49*(1), 117–127. doi: 10.1093/geront/gnp008

Gandhi, T. A. (2007). *"Let's kill Gandhi!": A chronicle of his last days, the conspiracy, murder, investigation, and trial*. New Delhi, India: Rupa & Co.

Geller, S. (2013). Sparking the creative in older adults. *Psychological Perspectives, 56*(2), 200–211.

George, D. R., & Houser, W. S. (2014). "I'm a storyteller!": Exploring the benefits of TimeSlips creative expression program at a nursing home. *American Journal of Alzheimer's Disease and Other Dementias, 29*(8), 678–684. doi: 10.1177/1533317514539725

Glaveanu, V. P. (2013). Creativity and folk art: A study of creative action in traditional craft. *Psychology of Aesthetics, Creativity, and the Arts, 7*(2), 140–154. doi: 10.1037/a0029318

Glover, J.A. (1976). Comparative levels of creative ability among elementary school children. *The Journal of Genetic Psychology: Research and Theory on Human Development, 129*(1), 131–135.

Glück, J., & Bluck, S. (2011). Laypeople's conceptions of wisdom and its development: Cognitive and integrative views. *The Journals of Gerontology, Series B: Psychological Sciences and Social Sciences, 66B*(3), 321–324. doi: 10.1093/geronb/gbr011

Glück, J., & Bluck, S. (2013). The MORE life experience model: A theory of the development of wisdom. In M. Ferrari & N. Weststrate (Eds.), *The scientific study of personal wisdom: From contemplative traditions to neuroscience* (pp. 75–97). New York: Springer.

Glück, J., König, S., Naschenweng, K., Redzanowski, U., Dorner-Hörig, L., Strasser, I., et al. (2013). How to measure wisdom: Content, reliability, and validity of five measures. *Frontiers in Psychology, 4: 405*, 1–13. doi: 10.3389/fpsyg.2013.00405

Gough, H.G. (1979). A creative personality scale for the Adjective Check List. *Journal of Personality and Social Psychology, 37*(8), 1398–1405. doi: 10.1037/0022-3514.37.8.1398

Green, S.K., & Gross, A.E. (1979). Self-serving biases in implicit evaluations. *Personality and Social Psychology Bulletin, 5*(2), 214–217. doi: 10.1177/014616727900500219

Hansen, D.D. (2003). *The dream: Martin Luther King, Jr., and the speech that inspired a nation*. New York, NY: Ecco.

Helson, R., & Srivastava, S. (2002). Creative and wise people: Similarities, differences and how they develop. *Personality and Social Psychology Bulletin, 28*(10), 1430–1440. doi: 10.1177/014616702236874

Hennessey, B.A., & Amabile, T.M. (2010). Creativity. *Annual Review of Psychology, 61*, 569–598. doi: 10.1146/annurev.psych.093008.100416

Jordan, J. (2005). The quest for wisdom in adulthood: A psychological perspective. In R.J. Sternberg & J. Jordan (Eds.), *A handbook of wisdom. Psychological perspectives* (pp. 160–188). New York: Cambridge University Press.

Kaltsounis, B. (1974). Race, socioeconomic status and creativity. *Psychological Reports, 35*(1, Pt 1), 164–166. doi: 10.2466/pr0.1974.35.1.164

Kekes, J. (1983). Wisdom. *American Philosophical Quarterly, 20*(3), 277–286.

Kharkhurin, A.V. (2014). Creativity.4in1: Four-criterion construct of creativity. *Creativity Research Journal, 26*(3), 338–352. doi: 10.1080/10400419.2014.929424

King, M.E. (2013). Mohandas K. Gandhi and Martin Luther King, Jr.'s bequest: Nonviolent civil resistance in a globalized world. In L.V. Baldwin, P.R. Dekar, & V.L. Crawford (Eds.), *"In an inescapable network of mutuality": Martin Luther King, Jr. and the globalization of an ethical ideal* (pp. 152–216). Eugene, OR: Cascade Books.

Kitchener, K.S., & Brenner, H.G. (1990). Wisdom and reflective judgment: Knowing in the face of uncertainty. In R.J. Sternberg (Ed.), *Wisdom: Its nature, origins, and development* (pp. 212–229). New York: Cambridge University Press.

Kitchener, K.S., King, P.M., Wood, P.K., & Davison, M.L. (1989). Sequentiality and consistency in the development of reflective judgment: A six-year longitudinal study. *Journal of Applied Developmental Psychology, 10*(1), 73–95. doi: 10.1016/0193-3973(89)90015-4

Kleibeuker, S.W., De Dreu, C.K.W., & Crone, E.A. (2013). The development of creative cognition across adolescence: Distinct trajectories for insight and divergent thinking. *Developmental Science, 16*(1), 2–12. doi: 10.1111/j.1467-7687.2012.01176.x

Krishnaraj, M. (1992). Women craft workers as security for family subsistence. *Economic and Political Weekly, 27*(17), WS7–WS17.

Kunzmann, U., & Baltes, P.B. (2003). Wisdom-related knowledge: Affective, motivational, and interpersonal correlates. *Personality and Social Psychology Bulletin, 29*(9), 1104–1119. doi: 10.1177/0146167203254506

Larson, R.T.H., & Perlstein, S. (2003). Creative aging: A new field for the 21st century. *Teaching Artist Journal, 1*(3), 144–151. doi: 10.1207/S1541180XTAJ0103_04

Le, T.N. (2008). Age differences in spirituality, mystical experiences and wisdom. *Ageing & Society 28*, 383–411. doi: 10.1017/S0144686X0700685X

Le, T.N. (2011). Life satisfaction, openness value, self-transcendence, and wisdom. *Journal of Happiness Studies, 12*(2), 171–182. doi: 10.1007/s10902-010-9182-1

Le, T.N., & Levenson, M.R. (2005). Wisdom as self-transcendence: What's love (& individualism) got to do with it? *Journal of Research in Personality, 39*(4), 443–457. doi: 10.1016/j.jrp.2004.05.003

Levenson, M.R., Jennings, P.A., Aldwin, C.M., & Shiraishi, R.W. (2005). Self-transcendence: Conceptualization and measurement. *International Journal of Aging & Human Development, 60*(2), 127–143. doi: 10.2190/XRXM-FYRA-7U0X-GRC0

Lokos, L. (1968). *House divided: The life and legacy of Martin Luther King*. New Rochelle, NY: Arlington House.

Maidment, J., & Macfarlane, S. (2011a). Crafting communities: Promoting inclusion, empowerment, and learning between older women. *Australian Social Work, 64*(3), 283–298. doi: 10.1080/0312407x.2010.520087

Maidment, J., & Macfarlane, S. (2011b). Older women and craft: Extending educational horizons in considering wellbeing. *Social Work Education, 30*(6), 700–711. doi: 10.1080/02615479.2011.586568

McBee, L. (2008). *Mindfulness-based elder care: A CAM model for frail elders and their caregivers*. New York, NY: Springer.

McKee, P., & Barber, C. (1999). On defining wisdom. *International Journal of Aging and Human Development, 49*(2), 149–164. doi: 10.2190/8G32-BNV0-NVP9-7V6G

Meacham, J.A. (1990). The loss of wisdom. In R.J. Sternberg (Ed.), *Wisdom: Its nature, origins, and development* (pp. 181–211). New York: Cambridge University Press.

Mickler, C., & Staudinger, U.M. (2008). Personal wisdom: Validation and age-related differences of a performance measure. *Psychology and Aging, 23*(4), 787–799. doi: 10.1037/a0013928

Miller, W., & Cohen, G.D. (2010). On creativity, illness, and aging. *Journal of Aging, Humanities, and the Arts, 4*(4), 302–311. doi: 10.1080/19325614.2010.529397

Moss, A.S., Reibel, D.K., Greeson, J.M., Thapar, A., Bubb, R., Salmon, J., et al. (2015). An adapted mindfulness-based stress reduction program for elders in a continuing care retirement community: Quantitative and qualitative results from a pilot randomized controlled trial. *Journal of Applied Gerontology, 34*(4), 518–538. doi: 10.1177/0733464814559411

Mumford, M. D. (2003). Where have we been, where are we going? Taking stock in creativity research. *Creativity Research Journal, 15*(2–3), 107–120. doi: 10.1207/s15326934crj152&3_01

Ñanamoli, B. (2001). *The life of the Buddha. According to the Pali Canon*. Seattle, WA: BPS Pariyatti Editions.

Nassif, C., & Quevillon, R. (2008). The development of a preliminary creativity scale for the MMPI-2: The C scale. *Creativity Research Journal, 20*(1), 13–20. doi: 10.1080/10400410701839918

Orwoll, L., & Perlmutter, M. (1990). The study of wise persons: Integrating a personality perspective. In R. J. Sternberg (Ed.), *Wisdom: Its nature, origins, and development* (pp. 160–177). New York: Cambridge University Press.

Pasupathi, M., & Staudinger, U. M. (2001). Do advanced moral reasoners also show wisdom? Linking moral reasoning and wisdom-related knowledge and judgement. *International Journal of Behavioral Development, 25*(5), 401–415. doi: 10.1080/016502501316934833

Pasupathi, M., Staudinger, U. M., & Baltes, P. B. (2001). Seeds of wisdom: Adolescents' knowledge and judgment about difficult life problems. *Developmental Psychology, 37*(3), 351–361. doi: 10.1037//0012-1649.37.3.351

Perrine, N. E., & Brodersen, R. M. (2005). Artistic and scientific creative behavior: Openness and the mediating role of interests. *Journal of Creative Behavior, 39*(4), 217–236.

Phillips, L. J., Reid-Arndt, S. A., & Pak, Y. (2010). Effects of a creative expression intervention on emotions, communication, and quality of life in persons with dementia. *Nursing Research, 59*(6), 417–425. doi: 10.1097/NNR.0b013e3181faff52

Piercy, K. W., & Cheek, C. (2004). Tending and befriending: The intertwined relationships of quilters. *Journal of Women & Aging, 16*(1–2), 17–33. doi: 10.1300/J074v16n01_03

Reams, J. (2015). The cultivation of wisdom in the classroom. *Integral Review, 11*(2), 103–134.

Reese, H. W., Lee, L.-J., Cohen, S. H., & Puckett, J. M., Jr. (2001). Effects of intellectual variables, age, and gender on divergent thinking in adulthood. *International Journal of Behavioral Development, 25*(6), 491–500. doi: 10.1080/01650250042000483

Richards, R. (2007). Everyday creativity: Our hidden potential. In R. Richards (Ed.), *Everyday creativity and new views of human nature: Psychological, social, and spiritual perspectives*. (pp. 25–53). Washington, DC: American Psychological Association.

Richards, R., Kinney, D. K., Benet, M., & Merzel, A. P. (1988). Assessing everyday creativity: Characteristics of the Lifetime Creativity Scales and validation with three large samples. *Journal of Personality and Social Psychology, 54*(3), 476–485. doi: 10.1037/0022-3514.54.3.476

Richardson, M.J., & Pasupathi, M. (2005). Young and growing wiser: Wisdom during adolescence and young adulthood. In R.J. Sternberg & J. Jordan (Eds.), *A handbook of wisdom. Psychological perspectives* (pp. 139–159). New York: Cambridge University Press.

Runco, M.A. (2007). To understand is to create: An epistemological perspective on human nature and personal creativity. In R. Richards (Ed.), *Everyday creativity and new views of human nature: Psychological, social, and spiritual perspectives.* (pp. 91–107, xiii, 349). Washington, DC: American Psychological Association.

Silvia, P.J., Beaty, R.E., Nusbaum, E.C., Eddington, K.M., Levin-Aspenson, H., & Kwapil, T.R. (2014). Everyday creativity in daily life: An experience-sampling study of 'little c' creativity. *Psychology of Aesthetics, Creativity, and the Arts, 8*(2), 183–188. doi: 10.1037/a0035722

Simonton, D.K. (1994). *Greatness: Who makes history and why*. New York, NY: Guilford Press.

Simonton, D.K. (1997). Creative productivity: A predictive and explanatory model of career trajectories and landmarks. *Psychological Review, 104*(1), 66–89. doi: 10.1037/0033-295x.104.1.66

Simonton, D.K. (2000). Creativity: Cognitive, personal, developmental, and social aspects. *American Psychologist, 55*(1), 151–158. doi: 10.1037/0003-066x.55.1.151

Smith, J., & Baltes, P.B. (1990). Wisdom-related knowledge: Age/cohort differences in response to life-planning problems. *Developmental Psychology, 26*(3), 494–505. doi: 10.1037/0012-1649.26.3.494

Staudinger, U.M. (1999). Older and wiser? Integrating results on the relationship between age and wisdom-related performance. *International Journal of Behavioral Development, 23*(3), 641–664. doi: 10.1080/016502599383739

Staudinger, U.M., Dörner, J., & Mickler, C. (2005). Wisdom and personality. In R.J. Sternberg & J. Jordan (Eds.), *A handbook of wisdom. Psychological perspectives* (pp. 191–219). New York: Cambridge University Press.

Staudinger, U.M., & Glück, J. (2011). Psychological wisdom research: Commonalities and differences in a growing field. *Annual Review of Psychology, 62*(1), 215–241. doi: 10.1146/annurev.psych.121208.131659

Staudinger, U.M., & Kessler, E.-M. (2008). Adjustment and growth. Two trajectories of positive personality development across adulthood. In M.C. Smith (Ed.), *Handbook of research on adult learning and development* (pp. 239–268). New York: Routledge.

Staudinger, U.M., & Kunzmann, U. (2005). Positive adult personality development: Adjustment and/or growth? *European Psychologist, 10*(4), 320–329. doi: 10.1027/1016-9040.10.4.320

Staudinger, U.M., Lopez, D.F., & Baltes, P.B. (1997). The psychometric location of wisdom-related performance: Intelligence, personality, and more? *Personality and Social Psychology Bulletin, 23*(11), 1200–1214. doi: 10.1177/01461672972311007

Staudinger, U.M., Maciel, A.G., Smith, J., & Baltes, P.B. (1998). What predicts wisdom-related performance? A first look at personality, intelligence, and facilitative experiential contexts. *European Journal of Personality, 12*(1), 1–17. doi: 10.1002/(SICI)1099-0984(199801/02)12:1%3C1::AID-PER285%3E3.0.CO;2-9

Sternberg, R.J. (1985). Implicit theories of intelligence, creativity, and wisdom. *Journal of Personality and Social Psychology, 49*(3), 607–627. doi: 10.1037/0022-3514.49.3.607

Sternberg, R.J. (1998). A balance theory of wisdom. *Review of General Psychology, 2*(4), 347–365. doi: 10.1037/1089-2680.2.4.347

Sternberg, R.J. (2001). Why schools should teach for wisdom: The balance theory of wisdom in educational settings. *Educational Psychologist, 36*(4), 227–245.

Sternberg, R.J. (2005). Older but not wiser? The relationship between age and wisdom. *Ageing International, 30*(1), 5–26. doi: 10.1007/BF02681005

Sternberg, R.J., Jarvin, L., & Grigorenko, E.L. (2009). *Teaching for wisdom, intelligence, creativity, and success*. Thousand Oaks, CA: Corwin Press.

Stuckey, H.L., & Nobel, J. (2010). The connection between art, healing, and public health: A review of current literature. *American Journal of Public Health, 100*(2), 254–263. doi: 10.2105/ajph.2008.156497

Takahashi, M., & Overton, W.F. (2002). Wisdom: A culturally inclusive developmental perspective. *International Journal of Behavioral Development, 26*(3), 269–277. doi: 10.1080/01650250143000139

Takahashi, M., & Overton, W.F. (2005). Cultural foundations of wisdom: An integrated developmental approach. In R.J. Sternberg & J. Jordan (Eds.), *A handbook of wisdom. Psychological perspectives* (pp. 32–60). New York: Cambridge University Press.

Tanggaard, L. (2013). The sociomateriality of creativity in everyday life. *Culture & Psychology, 19*(1), 20–32. doi: 10.1177/1354067x12464987

Thomas, M. L., Bangen, K. J., Ardelt, M., & Jeste, D. V. (in press). Development of a 12-item abbreviated Three-Dimensional Wisdom Scale (3D-WS-12): Item selection and psychometric properties. *Assessment*. doi: 10.1177/1073191115595714

Torrance, E.P. (1962). *Guiding creative talent*. Englewood Cliffs, NJ: Prentice-Hall.

Torrance, E.P. (1971). Are the Torrance tests of creative thinking biased against or in favor of "disadvantaged" groups? *Gifted Child Quarterly, 15*(2), 75–80. doi: 10.1177/001698627101500201

Uttal, D.H., & Perlmutter, M. (1989). Toward a broader conceptualization of development: The role of gains and losses across the life span. *Developmental Review, 9*(2), 101–132. doi: 10.1016/0273-2297(89)90025-7

Walsh, F. (2003). *The Montgomery bus boycott*. Milwaukee, WI: World Almanac Library.

Webster, J.D. (2003). An exploratory analysis of a self-assessed wisdom scale. *Journal of Adult Development, 10*(1), 13–22. doi: 10.1023/A:1020782619051

Webster, J.D. (2007). Measuring the character strength of wisdom. *International Journal of Aging & Human Development, 65*(2), 163–183. doi: 10.2190/AG.65.2.d

Webster, J.D., Westerhof, G.J., & Bohlmeijer, E.T. (2014). Wisdom and mental health across the lifespan. *The Journals of Gerontology, Series B: Psychological Sciences and Social Sciences, 69*(2), 209–218. doi: 10.1093/geronb/gbs121

Weststrate, N. M., Ferrari, M., & Ardelt, M. (under review). Investigating implicit theories of wisdom through exemplars and prototypes.

Wink, P., & Dillon, M. (2003). Religiousness, spirituality, and psychosocial functioning in late adulthood: Findings from a longitudinal study. *Psychology and Aging, 18*(4), 916–924. doi: 10.1037/0882-7974.18.4.916

Wink, P., & Helson, R. (1997). Practical and transcendent wisdom: Their nature and some longitudinal findings. *Journal of Adult Development, 4*(1), 1–15. doi: 10.1007/BF02511845

Yang, S.-Y. (2001). Conceptions of wisdom among Taiwanese Chinese. *Journal of Cross-Cultural Psychology, 32*(6), 662–680. doi: 10.1177/0022022101032006002

Zacher, H., McKenna, B., & Rooney, D. (2013). Effects of self-reported wisdom on happiness: Not much more than emotional intelligence? *Journal of Happiness Studies, 14*(6), 1697–1716. doi: 10.1007/s10902-012-9404-9

Zeng, L., Proctor, R. W., & Salvendy, G. (2011). Can traditional divergent thinking tests be trusted in measuring and predicting real-world creativity? *Creativity Research Journal, 23*(1), 24–37. doi: 10.1080/10400419.2011.545713

CHAPTER THREE

Religion and Volunteering across the Life Course

Fengyan Tang

Volunteerism has traditionally been associated with religion in the United States. The high prevalence of volunteering in the United States is probably attributed to the importance of religion in life. With the strength of religious institutions, practices, and beliefs, the United States has resisted the trend toward secularity and is regarded as one of the most religious nations worldwide (Wald & Calhoun-Brown, 2014). A majority of Americans identify with some branch of the Christian faith, and about half of them have altered their religious affiliations at least once during their lifetime (Wald & Calhoun-Brown, 2014). The social context and power of religion has played a significant part in promoting volunteer engagement throughout the life course (Taniguchi & Leonard, 2011; Wilson, 2012), as the significance of prosocial behavior or helping others is a common tenet in many religious traditions (Wuthnow, 1991). Religious beliefs and values are a fertile source of volunteer motivations (Wilson, 2012). Early exposure to religion and youth religious involvement help to sustain and expand volunteer engagement in adulthood and later life (Caputo, 2009; Park & Smith, 2000). For older adults, religious social networks are particularly important for them to get involved in volunteering due to the role loss in other aspects of social life. This may explain why the main organization to which the volunteers devoted the most hours was a religious one; specifically, older adults were more likely than other aged Americans to volunteer for religious organizations (U.S. Bureau of Labor Statistics,

2014). Churches are probably the most important voluntary organizations for Americans (Wald & Calhoun-Brown, 2014).

With the growth of the aging population and the increase in life expectancy, an increasing number of older adults have engaged in various forms of volunteer work in order to continue a meaningful life into the extended years after retirement. Despite gender, race, and socioeconomic differences in volunteer engagement, a major issue is how to maximize positive outcomes of volunteering across population segments. As documented in an extensive body of literature, volunteer engagement has protective effects on health, especially in the older population (e.g., Li & Ferraro, 2006; Morrow-Howell et al., 2003). In particular, a public form of religiosity magnifies the salubrious effects of volunteering on middle- and older-aged adults' well-being (McDougle et al., 2014). Therefore, it is important to improve our understanding of the relationships between volunteering and various domains in religion across the life course.

The purpose of this chapter is to overview current knowledge about the relationship between formal volunteering and religion with its four dimensions, namely, religiosity, religious identity, religious socialization, and religious social networks. Following the definition of volunteering, the chapter presents recent statistics of volunteering prevalence and time commitment by age groups, and reviews the factors associated with volunteering across the life course. With the focus on the influences on volunteering, this chapter reviews typology in religion, operationalization of religion domains, and how the domains are related to volunteering. The chapter concludes that religious institutions are in a key position to facilitate individuals, especially older adults in volunteer engagement.

Formal Volunteering

The term volunteering or volunteerism is defined vaguely but used broadly, referring to a wide range of prosocial behaviors, that is, voluntary behaviors intended to benefit others, such as formal volunteer activities, informal helping behaviors, or voluntary association activities (Cnaan, Handy, & Wadsworth, 1996; Wilson, 2000). This chapter mainly addresses formal volunteering, as done in most of current literature. Formal volunteering has been finely defined by Snyder and Omoto (2008) as freely chosen, long-term, and deliberate helping activities that are engaged in without remuneration, often through formal organizations, and on behalf of causes or individuals who desire assistance. Nonetheless, the definition is still imprecise, because in the real world how to define an act as volunteering is really a matter of degree (see Cnaan, Handy, & Wadsworth, 1996; Wilson, 2012). Further, the linkage of volunteer work to formal originations is problematic, suggesting that communities and countries with poorly developed infrastructure in nonprofit organizations will have fewer volunteers, according to the definition provided above (Wilson, 2012).

In the United States, however, volunteering is indeed characterized by involvement with various types of organizations—religious and secular, governmental and nongovernmental, state and local, profit and nonprofit sectors (Tang, 2010). Particularly, religious organizations have long been the main organizations in which volunteers are actively involved (Boraas, 2003; U.S. Bureau of Labor Statistics, 2014). Besides, this definition contains four dimensions, namely, free choice, no or little remuneration, organizational structure, and intended beneficiaries, which are often used in defining volunteerism (e.g., Cnaan, Handy, & Wadsworth, 1996). Variations in these dimensions reflect the different ways of how to define a volunteer, from a broad to a narrow spectrum. For example, an individual decides to volunteer from his/her free will, receives no remuneration at all, and volunteers in a formal organization for the purpose of benefiting others, especially strangers. In this case, volunteer is defined in the purist way, that is, an individual whose volunteering activity incurs a high net-cost is more likely to be publicly perceived as a "purer" volunteer than a volunteer activity with a low net-cost (Cnaan, Handy, & Wadsworth, 1996).

Based on various definitions and operations of volunteering in the existing literature, an intermediate definition is suggested; that is, volunteers refer to those who choose to engage of their free will, receive no or little stipend, and work in a formal organization either for the benefit of others or for self-interest (Cnaan, Handy, & Wadsworth, 1996). Material rewards and intentions for volunteering are open for debates (Wilson, 2000). The intention for volunteering may not necessarily be fully delineated in the definition of volunteering; what is more important is that volunteering produces goods and services that definitely have market values (Wilson, 2000). Volunteering is a productive and worthwhile effort by citizens of all ages and backgrounds; the benefits of volunteering usually accrue to the individuals being helped and the community and society at large as well as to volunteers themselves.

Volunteering across the Life Course

Volunteering behavior varies over the life course, and the resources needed for and the factors linked to volunteering are different across the life stages. A variety of factors in terms of contextual, social background, personality, attitudinal, and situational variables are related to volunteering (Smith, 1994). Individual resources, including human, social, and cultural capital are essential for volunteer engagement (Tang, 2006; Wilson & Musick, 1997). Despite the plurality and diversity in these factors, Cnaan and Cascio (1999) conclude that three sets of key factors affect volunteer engagement and performance: demographic characteristics, personality traits and attitudes, and situational variables that include economics, culture, climates, urban and rural residence, and organizational characteristics (Herzog & Morgan, 1993; Smith, 1994). Although religion plays a vital role in volunteering, secular factors such as socioeconomic resources, personality traits, and attributes of the environment often have influential impacts on individual volunteer behavior, explaining why nonreligious people also volunteer and/or devote as much time to volunteering as religious people do. This section starts with the introduction of volunteering rates and amounts by age groups, followed by the description of age, cohort, and period effects on volunteering. Also introduced are race, gender, and socioeconomic differences in volunteering and the factors associated with volunteering across the early, middle, and late life stages.

Volunteering Rates and Hours by Age Groups

In every year since 2000, more than one quarter of the adult population aged 16 and over in the United States have been involved in various volunteer activities, reaching annual peaks of about 29 percent in 2003 to 2005, then falling slightly over years thereafter and to 25 percent in 2013 (Caputo, 2009; U.S. Bureau of Labor Statistics, 2014). These statistics indicate that volunteering is a significant social activity for millions of Americans. By age group, people aged 35 to 44 years were most likely to volunteer with a volunteer rate of 31 percent, followed by those aged 45 to 54 years (28%), 55 to 64 years (26%), 65 years and over (24%), and youth aged 16 to 24 years were least likely to volunteer (22%) based on the 2013 statistics (U.S. Bureau of Labor Statistics, 2014). The volunteer rates generally taper off as age increases for persons 35 years and older. The volunteer work patterns by age groups are considerably stable since 2000, as indicated from yearly statistics (Caputo, 2009; U.S. Bureau of Labor Statistics, 2014). Early years literature review for the period 1975–1992 also indicates that volunteering participation peaks in middle age, in the range of 35 to 55 years (Smith, 1994).

During the past 40 years, although the overall adult volunteer rates declined from 1974 to 1989, the volunteer rates for older adults aged 65 and older actually increased during the same period. In fact, older adults have been increasing their volunteer engagement through the last four decades, going from 14 percent in 1974 to 24 percent in 2013 (Corporation for National and Community Service, 2007; U.S. Bureau of Labor

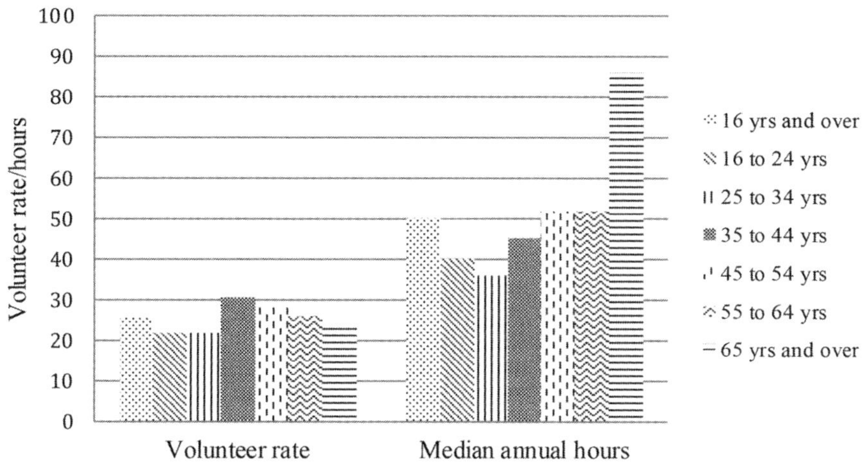

Figure 3.1 Volunteer rates and hours by age groups in 2013. (Note: For volunteer rate, *y*-axis represents percentage of volunteers across age groups; and for median annual hours, *y*-axis represents the number of hours volunteered during the past 12 months. *Source*: U.S. Bureau of Labor Statistics. (2014). Volunteering in the United States—2013. Retrieved from http://www.bls.gov/news.release/volun.nr0.htm)

Statistics, 2014). Although older adults are relatively fewer in number than younger people engaging in volunteer activities, older adult volunteers devote more hours to volunteer work than younger adults (Gallagher, 1994; Van Willigen, 2000). Some previous literature indicates that volunteer commitment by older adults was modest (Caro & Bass, 1995; Fisher & Schaffer, 1993). However, the Current Population Survey in September 2013 shows that volunteers aged 65 and over contributed the most hours to volunteer activities with a median of 86 hours, in contrast to younger people aged 35 to 44 years, who volunteered at a median of 45 hours (U.S. Bureau of Labor Statistics, 2014). Recent surveys also demonstrate that older adults are more likely than ever to contribute more time to volunteering once getting involved. The rapid and consistent increase in volunteering by older adults is probably attributed to the increasing size of the older population, the improved health status, and the prolonged life expectancy (Tang, 2010). Figure 3.1 shows volunteer rates and annual hours volunteered by age groups in 2013.

Age, Cohort, and Period Effects on Volunteering

Age differences in volunteering are confounded by cohort and period effects. A cohort effect refers to differences between generations that can be attributed to the unique experiences of each generation; a period effect refers to a change across a population that is essentially due to a historical event (Rosenberg & Letrero, 2006). Most scholars have agreed that the long civic generation born between 1910 and 1929 generally scored higher on most measures of social capital than later generations, including the silent generation born 1930–1945 and the baby boomer generation born 1946–1960 (Prisuta, 2003; Putnam, 2000). Social capital measures include participation in social clubs and voluntary associations, informal socializing, religious services attendance, and trust (Prisuta, 2003; Putnam, 2000). Despite the decreases in some social capital measures that correlate with volunteering, volunteer engagement among the older population has increased from cohort to cohort since the 1990s, and it is predicted that boomers would volunteer in larger numbers than members of previous cohorts during or after retirement (Einolf, 2009).

A period effect suggests that historical events, for example, the Great Depression of the 1930s, World Wars, the passage of Older American Act in 1965, shape current conditions and have an impact on volunteering (Rosenberg & Letrero, 2006). Although few studies are available to investigate the period effect of historical events, Penner (2005) documented that there was a dramatic increase in the number of volunteers following September 11, 2001 and that increases occurred for all kinds of charities and service organizations during a short period. Both natural and human-made disasters have effects on individual helping behavior, partly because of the influences of common external threats on people's sense of community and partly due to the exposure to the mass media that model altruistic public actions (Penner, 2005). Age, cohort, and period effects are interrelated to account for the changes in volunteering over time.

Race, Gender, and Socioeconomic Status (SES) Differences in Volunteering

Sociodemographics such as age, gender, race, marital status, health, education, income, and employment are related to volunteering. Particularly, gender, race, and social class are important indicators of human resources that enable people to volunteer or condition their interest in volunteer work (Wilson, 2012).

Gender. Gender differences in volunteering are confounded with the effects of employment and family characteristics (Taniguchi, 2006). Traditionally, a majority of women volunteers were not employed, whereas most men volunteers had full-time jobs and helped others in their spare time (Taniguchi, 2006). This gender pattern in volunteering has changed over the past several decades due to the rapid entry of women into the labor force and the major role played by women in family life and caregiving

(England, 2000; Taniguchi, 2006). Using a national sample of adults aged 25 to 74, Taniguchi (2006) found that whether men work full time or part time makes no difference in their volunteering efforts, whereas part-time employment promotes volunteering for women and that women but not men spend more time caring for the elderly and are likely to volunteer less. In late life, especially after retirement, volunteering might become a choice for both men and women, who are not different in volunteer engagement and amount (Cnaan & Cascio, 1999; Herzog & Morgan, 1993; Musick, Herzog, & House, 1999; Warburton, Le Broque, & Rosenmen, 1998). However, discrepancies exist in the literature; for example, a recent study found that older women are more likely than older men to volunteer and that gender rather than religiosity is a significant predictor of volunteering in later life (Manning, 2010). Also gender difference in types of volunteer work is observed. Women are more likely to engage in volunteer activity characterized as more caring, person-to-person tasks, while men tend to volunteer in political or public leadership positions (Rotolo & Wilson, 2007). In addition, women are more likely to volunteer in groups to support and complement their social and personal relationships, whereas men are more likely to individually engage in volunteer work that is complementary to their paid work (Wilson, 2000).

Race. Probably due to lower socioeconomic status (SES) and lack of resources, African Americans and Hispanics are not actively involved in formal volunteering (Smith, 1994). However, studies with different samples and analysis procedures yield mixed results. Some studies using bivariate analysis showed that non-Hispanic whites volunteered more, whereas multivariate results indicated that nonwhites, especially African Americans volunteered more after controlling for SES (Smith, 1994). Racial difference also exists in participation in types of formal voluntary organizations by birth cohorts (Miner & Tolnay, 1998). That is, in younger cohorts of African Americans and non-Hispanic whites have similar rates of voluntary organization participation, but older African Americans have lower rates of membership than their white counterparts in social service and job-related organizations (Miner & Tolnay, 1998). Racial differences in volunteering are more evident in the older generations than younger cohorts, probably because the discrimination and segregation experienced by older African Americans has resulted in restricted access to certain types of voluntary organizations among this elderly group (Miner & Tolnay, 1998). Further, evidence shows that African Americans are most likely to volunteer for neighborhood organizations and church groups that have historically been open to them (Miner & Tolnay, 1998). In addition, the African American church plays a more prominent role in its community, and church attendance has more influential impact on volunteering in African

Americans than in white Americans (Musick, Wilson, & Bynum, 2000). Church attendance has a negative effect on secular volunteering for whites only (Musick, Wilson, & Bynum, 2000). Thus we can see that religiosity, or church attendance in particular, affects volunteer engagement and types of voluntary organizations in which racial/ethnic groups are involved.

SES. SES is one of the most significant factors associated with volunteering. Education is associated with occupational status and income, and these variables constitute socioeconomic status (Warburton, Le Broque, & Rosenmen, 1998). The most salient factor is education which generates a higher standard of living and free time available for volunteering (Fisher, Mueller, & Cooper, 1991). Educated people usually have more resources, capabilities, and social networks than the less-educated to volunteer across lifespans. Household income is also positively related to volunteer engagement (Fisher, Mueller, & Cooper, 1991; Fisher & Schaffer, 1993; Gallagher, 1994). But the findings are mixed regarding the income effect on volunteer time. In addition, income makes little difference in voluntary organization involvement by older adults (Tang, 2008). Among various occupational categories, private sector blue-collar workers are least likely to volunteer, whereas professionals, managers, sales, and clerical employees participate in more volunteer work (Wilson & Musick, 1997b). Although little information is available regarding the interaction effects between religion and SES on volunteering, studies show that both factors are significantly predictive of volunteering efforts in terms of hours volunteered and the number of organizational types involved for volunteering (Tang, 2006). Religiosity may crosscut social class differences by providing compensating social resources and mobilizing beliefs (Musick, Wilson, & Bynum, 2000).

Factors Related to Volunteering across Life Stages

As we can observe, in general, volunteering rises from a lower participation rate at teenage years through early adulthood, peaks in middle age, and then declines in old age (Selbee & Reed, 2001). In addition to gender, race, SES, and other demographic characteristics, various factors are predictive of volunteer engagement and these factors vary in relation to volunteering across life stages. In early-life stages, family background and educational environment and activities play important roles in volunteering (Wilson, 2012). Children whose parents engage in volunteering and encourage them to do so are likely to volunteer, because parents likely pass civic engagement proclivities to their children (Caputo, 2009). On the other hand, disadvantages in childhood, including living in poverty, family instability, lack of parental supervision or warmth, weak parent-child attachment, and the absence of volunteer parental role models are associated with the reduced likelihood of volunteering in adulthood (Brown & Lichter, 2007). Years of schooling have a positive effect on volunteering; also students who attended private schools and catholic schools are more likely to volunteer after graduation than those from public schools (Wilson, 2012). The positive attitudes or feelings toward the school and the teachers as well as close relations with peers affect volunteering in young adulthood (Duke et al., 2009). In addition, participation in school-based extracurricular activities promotes volunteering in young adults (McFarland & Thomas, 2006). It can be seen that volunteering and other helping behaviors are rooted and cultivated in family and educational backgrounds.

Life events such as marriage, having a child, and employment have influences on the age-related pattern of volunteering (Li & Ferraro, 2006; Selbee & Reed, 2001). In early adulthood and middle age, married individuals, adults with school-aged children, and part-time workers are more likely to volunteer and to devote more hours than their counterparts, that is, those not married, those without children, and full-time workers or nonworkers (Selbee & Reed, 2001). As part of the socialization of school-aged children, parents are often involved in volunteering with schools, sports and religious organizations, because athletic, religious, and recreational organizations often rely on parents to run programs and fulfill organizational missions (Li & Ferraro, 2006). Other voluntary originations also provide a wide range of volunteer opportunities for social connection, civic participation, and other purposes. In middle age, people have settled into adult roles and built up the stakes in the community (Flanagan & Levine, 2010); therefore, they are likely to engage in volunteer activities that have connections with their family, community, and work roles. The need for volunteers in many aspects of social and civic life is cumulative in middle age, making it a peak time of volunteering (Li & Ferraro, 2006).

In later life, especially after retirement, it seems that older adults have more free time for volunteering than in earlier life stages. Two opposing theories have been proposed and applied in examining the relationships between volunteering and work/retirement behaviors: activity substitution theory and activity complement theory. Based on the activity substitution theory, older adults may take up formal volunteer work to compensate for age-related role loss, such as retirement, death of a spouse, and reduced family roles, as formal volunteering has compensatory effects on older adults' well-being (Mutchler, Burr, & Caro, 2003; Pavlova & Silbereisen, 2012). Previous research indicates that retirees and nonworkers, especially those who have volunteered before are likely to volunteer more extensively than those in the labor force (see Mutchler, Burr, & Caro,

2003). Contrastingly, the activity complement theory posits that volunteer activity and paid work are positively correlated and that retirement is associated with a decline in volunteering (Mutchler, Burr, & Caro, 2003). Older workers engage in volunteering through social networks embedded in the workforce and thus are able to make more time commitment to volunteering (Klumb & Baltes, 1999). Leaving the workforce leads to a decrease in social networks whereby retirees are less likely than those in the workforce to be asked or recruited for volunteering. Evidence from Denmark, Germany, Greece, and the Unites States shows that volunteer time decreased from age 50 to 74 when transition to retirement likely occurred (Komp, van Tilburg, & van Groenou, 2011). Both theories have been supported with empirical evidence to some extent, with indications that social networks and previous volunteer experience are significant predictors of volunteering in later life.

Obviously, the greatest threat to sustained volunteering in later life is health declines and functional impairment that make volunteering difficult (Li & Ferraro, 2006). It seems plausible that health is a significant predictor of volunteer engagement among older adults, whereas work and family responsibilities are more predictive of volunteering in middle age (Li & Ferraro, 2006). In addition, research indicates that reciprocal relationships exist between volunteering and health in older adults. Volunteering boosts personal well-being, including physical health, mental health, and life satisfaction; while older adults in good health are more likely to participate and spend more time in volunteering, which in turn enhances their well-being (Thoits & Hewitt, 2001).

To sum up, volunteering behavior in earlier life stages may affect the motivation for and incidence of volunteering in later life. It is very likely that adolescents with volunteer experience will volunteer in adulthood due to their access to pertinent resources and acquired skills for volunteering (Osterle, Johnson, & Mortimer, 2004). Those in early life who have internalized volunteering as a value, who have developed necessary skills, and who have made effective contributions as volunteers are more likely to volunteer in later life than those who have not had such experience (Bass & Caro, 2001), though the meaning of volunteering and resources needed for volunteer engagement differ across birth cohorts (Tang, 2006). Demographic changes, potential benefits from volunteering, personal values and attitudes, and changes in social structures give rise to volunteering by older Americans. Through volunteer work, older people can find a sense of fulfillment, maintain or improve their self-esteem and life satisfaction, and have more access to social support and resources than their nonvolunteering peers (Van Willigen, 2000). Therefore, volunteering is deemed as a way of health promotion in old age, as extensively evidenced with theoretical and empirical findings that older adults would benefit from volunteer engagement through maintaining or improving their social, physical, mental, and cognitive functioning.

Religion and Volunteering

In the 21st century, despite the secularization and modernization process in the industrial Western countries, the United States is viewed as one of the most religious nations (Ellison & MaFarland, 2013), having resisted the pressure toward secularity with its strength of religious institutions, practices, and beliefs (Wald & Calhoun-Brown, 2014). The overwhelming majority of Americans identify with some branch of the Christian faith, though some are not actually involved in the practice of that faith (Ellison & MaFarland, 2013). It is estimated that at least 80 percent of U.S. adults maintain a religious identity, preference, or affinity with some religious tradition and that between 50 and 60 percent are actual members of a religious congregation (see Ellison & MaFarland, 2013). Despite all the talk about decline in religiosity, the proportion of church members among persons aged 15 and over is almost the same today as it was in the 1950s; and churches are probably the most important voluntary organization that emphasizes joining-up and mobilization (Wald & Calhoun-Brown, 2014). In addition, recent decades have witnessed the heightened religious mobility, that is, an estimated 40 to 50 percent of Americans have altered their religious affiliations at least once during their lifetime, and many persons may change their religious allegiance multiple times (Wald & Calhoun-Brown, 2014). The social context and power of religion provide fertile sources for volunteer engagement in Americans, and the mobility in religion may affect religious and/or secular volunteering.

Resources, skills, and opportunities are not sufficient to involve people in volunteering; more importantly, altruistic values and moral/ethical orientations embedded in religion beliefs could provide strong motivations for volunteering and for engagement in other forms of civic service (Oesterle, Johnson, & Mortimer, 2004). Religion in all its forms has played a significant role in promoting volunteerism, most influentially in the United States (Taniguchi & Leonard, 2011; Wilson, 2012). Religious organizations are the main channel through which people are engaged in volunteering. Specifically, older adults, African Americans, people with less than a high school diploma, those not in the labor force, as well as married people with spouses present are more likely to volunteer for religious organizations than their counterparts (U.S. Bureau of Labor Statistics, 2014). It is commonly observed that Americans become more religious as they age

(Weeden & Kurzban, 2013), which may partly explain the steady increase in volunteering in older Americans. All major religions teach their members to care for others and help people in need (Wuthnow, 1991). As a form of cultural capital, religion is regarded as a valued resource embedded in social relations with productive and exchange capacities (Becker & Dhingra, 2001). Cultural capital refers to value or ethical resources, and membership in a religious organization has been used as a proxy for cultural capital (Wilson & Musick, 1997). Volunteers act out altruistic value or the desire to help others (Herzog & Morgan, 1993), which is in line with the central tenet of most religions.

Religious beliefs, attitudes, and sentiments are important sources of volunteer motivations (Wilson, 2012). Four types of cultural/religious capital are believed to promote volunteering: religiosity, namely, individual behaviors and attitudes toward religion; religious identity, namely, the sense or identification of belonging to a particular religious tradition or movement; religious socialization, namely, being exposed and influenced by religious values and behaviors during one's formative years; and religious social networks, namely, the access to and connection with churchgoers and/or other religious adherents of similar or like-minded religiosity (Caputo, 2009; Park & Smith, 2000). Religious beliefs and belonging, or conviction and community are highlighted as the mechanisms that link religion to volunteering (Lim & MacGregor, 2012). This section follows Park and Smith's (2000) typology of religious capital in discussion of its relation with volunteer engagement. Table 3.1 summarizes the definitions, measures, and the effects on volunteering.

Religiosity

Religiosity, as a form of cultural capital, refers to religious attitudes and behaviors obtained through religious practice or observation (Iannaccone, 1990; Park & Smith, 2000). It has been well known that religiosity promotes volunteering in the United States and other Western countries (Taniguchi & Thomas, 2011), due to the influences of Christianity (Johnson, 2013). In general, religious individuals are more active in volunteering and community participation than their secular counterparts, as documented in a large number of studies (see Lim & MacGregor, 2012). Indeed, Americans aged 40 and over who are actively involved in religious organizations and who attend religious services on a regular basis are most likely to volunteer (Wilson & Janoski, 1995). Volunteering for religious organizations can provide a great sense of meaning and purpose for middle- and older-aged adults (e.g., McDougle et al., 2014; Morrow-Howell et al., 2003; Piliavin & Siegl, 2007; Thoits & Hewitt, 2001).

Religious belief is strongly associated with individual motivation for volunteering, especially among Christians, as charity, service, and helping others are the central tenets of Christian denominations in the United States (Johnson, 2013). The strength and content of religious beliefs not only motivate volunteer behavior (Becker & Dhingra, 2001), but also influence the meaning of volunteering (Wuthnow, 1991; Wilson, 2000). Previous studies demonstrated mixed findings regarding the relationship between individual religious beliefs and motivations of volunteering for religious institutions (see Johnson, 2013). Some studies showed that motivation for religious institution volunteering increased along with the strength of individual religious beliefs (Hoge et al., 1998; Ladd, 1999), whereas other studies found no relationship between them (e.g., Park & Smith 2000; Wilson & Janoski, 1995).

Religious beliefs may also promote motivations for nonreligious institution volunteering as well (Wuthnow, 1991), probably because individuals with strong religious beliefs can find common grounds with nonreligious organizations that aim at voluntary activism and giving back (Johnson, 2013). Again, the results are mixed in the literature with some studies finding that religiosity increased secular helping and others finding no such relationship (e.g., Jackson et al., 1995). These studies suggest that personal religious beliefs may not be sufficient to serve as the mechanism through which religion promotes volunteering and that the measures of religiosity are neither valid nor reliable. Indeed, religiosity is most frequently studied in relation with volunteering in previous research; however, its operationalization has varied greatly, which contributes to the inconsistent findings across studies (Park & Smith, 2000). Among the various indicators, church attendance has been used as one of the major indicators of religiosity; others include church membership, prayer, the relative importance of faith, religious attitude toward giving one's time and money, and participation in church activities (see Park & Smith, 2000). Future research is needed to validate the operationalization of religiosity and test its association with volunteerism along with measures in other domains of religion.

Religious Identity or Affiliation

According to Park and Smith (2000), identification with personal religious labels is a sign of belonging to religious movements or traditions. Individuals with strong religious identity tend to align with values that are central to religious congregational volunteering (Ammerman, 2005; Johnson, 2013; Unruh & Sider, 2005). Although church members are more likely than nonmembers to engage in volunteer activities, not all members are equally engaged (Ruiter & De Graaf, 2006). There are denominational

Table 3.1 Four Dimensions in Religion and Effects on Volunteering

Dimension	Definition	Measures	Effects on Volunteering	References
Religiosity	Individual behaviors and attitudes toward religion	◦ Church attendance ◦ Church membership ◦ Prayer ◦ Importance of faith ◦ Attitude to giving one's time/money ◦ Participation in church activities	◦ Religious people are more active in volunteering than the nonreligious ◦ Mixed findings exist regarding the relationships between religious beliefs and motivations for or behaviors of volunteering	Becker & Dhingra, 2001 Jackson et al., 1995 Hoge et al., 1998 Ladd, 1999 Park & Smith, 2000 Wilson & Janoski, 1995 Wilson, 2000 Wuthnow, 1991
Religious Identity/ affiliation	Sense or identification of belonging to a particular religious tradition or movement	◦ Church affiliations ◦ Types within an affiliation ◦ Religion types (e.g., Protestants, Buddhists, Christians, etc.)	◦ Protestants volunteer more than Catholics ◦ Mainline Protestants are more likely to volunteer than Evangelicals and black Protestants ◦ Religion in forms other than Christianity also fosters volunteerism	Curtis, Baer, & Grabb, 2001 Driskell, Lyon, & Embry, 2008 Lam, 2002 Lim & MacGregor, 2012 Ruiter & De Graaf, 2006 Wilson & Janoski, 1995 Wuthnow, 1999

Religious socialization	Exposure to religious values and behaviors during one's formative years	◦ Family's importance of faith ◦ Influence of parents' religious identity ◦ Attendance at a religious high school/college	◦ Parents' affiliation is related to children's volunteer engagement ◦ Family's importance of faith is related to volunteering through a secular organization among churchgoing Protestants	Caputo, 2009 Park & Smith, 2000 Perks & Haan, 2011
Religious social networks	Access to and connection with churchgoers and/or other religious adherents of similar or like-minded religiosity	◦ Church attendance ◦ Christian family, friends ◦ Having a child in a Christian school ◦ Confide in congregation members ◦ Church member in network	◦ The number of Christian family and friends increases the odds of church-related volunteering ◦ Those having congregation members as close friends are more likely to volunteer ◦ Those who confide in fellow members are more likely to volunteer for congregational activities	Becker & Dhingra, 2001 Jackson et al., 1995 Lim & MacGregor, 2012 Musick, Wilson, & Bynum, 2000 Park & Smith, 2000 Ruiter & De Graaf, 2006

differences, in particular, the liberal and conservative divide, which shape the meaning of volunteer work and how church members devote their efforts to volunteering (Becker & Dhingra, 2001). Most congregations encourage informal help behaviors; however, they vary considerably in the degree to which they attach the importance to formal volunteering and other forms of civic engagement within and across denominations (Becker & Dehingra, 2001). In general, Protestants volunteer more than Catholics (e.g., Curtis, Baer, & Grabb, 2001; Lam, 2002; Ruiter & De Graaf, 2006; Wuthnow, 1991). This is probably because the Protestant church is less hierarchically structured than the Catholic Church and that smaller parishes are further divided in the Protestant Church (Suanet, van Groenou, & Braam, 2009). The less hierarchical structure and the smaller subdivisions would offer more possibilities for common church members to be involved in their congregations and volunteering activities (Ruiter & De Graaf, 2006; Suanet, van Groenou, & Braam, 2009). In addition, Protestants are not encouraged to pursue self-interests and thus likely have a sense of social responsibility (Lam, 2002). Social responsibility embedded in religious beliefs and values is important to foster volunteering for both religious and secular sectors.

Further, even within the same affiliation, there are differences in volunteer engagement; for example, some conservative Protestant denominations support only church volunteering but discourage secular volunteering, whereas liberal Protestant denominations encourage civic engagement and volunteering in the larger secular community (Wilson & Janoski, 1995; Wuthnow, 1999). It is noted that mainline Protestant churches are able to unite people from different regions, and demographics and their members usually have higher rates of secular volunteering and civic engagement (Driskell, Lyon, & Embry, 2008; Wuthnow, 1999). By contrast, Evangelical Protestants and black Protestants are less likely to be engaged in civic activities, including volunteering, than other denominations (Driskell, Lyon, & Embry, 2008).

Based on their analyses of data from 53 countries, Ruiter and De Graaf (2006) found that non-Christians were equally engaged in volunteer work as were Protestants, that is, people living in non-Christian countries volunteered to the same extent as did people in Christian countries (Ruiter & De Graaf, 2006). The study findings indicate that religion in forms other than Christianity or in countries other than the United States also fosters volunteerism. Using the Gallup World Poll data from 138 countries, Lim and MacGregor (2012) documented that compared with Catholics, respondents who identified themselves as Protestants, Buddhists, Christians, or other religion believers were more likely to volunteer, whereas Orthodox believers and atheists were less likely to engage in volunteering.

At the country level, when compared with Protestant religious culture, the Orthodox and Muslim religious cultures reduced the likelihood of individual volunteering (Lim & MacGregor, 2012). This study suggests that national religious contexts really matter in individual volunteering behaviors and that both individual religious identity and religious culture in a country account for the variance in individual volunteering behaviors.

Religious Socialization

Religious socialization refers to how one is raised in a religious background (Park & Smith, 2000). Exposure to religious values and behaviors in formative years could provide a powerful source of social capital that has an impact on one's proclivity to volunteer, because the practice of service to one's community usually starts from learning and adopting religious beliefs and behaviors from one's parents and family (Park & Smith, 2000). The measures of religious socialization include the influence of parents' religious identity, attendance at religious grade schools or high schools, and attendance at a Christian college (Caputo, 2009; Park & Smith, 2000). Religious socialization is linked to parents' religiosity and religious identity, indicating the "intergenerational transmission of religious proclivities and volunteer activities from parents to their adolescent children" (Caputo, 2009, p. 984). Further, exposure to religion and volunteering in formative years have an influence on religious involvement and civic engagement in adulthood. Through participation in religious organizations and educational institutions, children and youth can acquire an important form of cultural capital, that is, altruistic values and prosocial orientations that motivate volunteer work. Caputo (2009) found that parents' religious affiliation and fundamentalism (i.e., religious belief) were strongly predictive of youth's involvement in volunteering. Churches and religious organizations have traditionally served as an institutional and philosophical base for volunteering (Putnam, 2000), providing an important form of cultural capital that can be transferred across generations.

In an overview of volunteerism research, Wilson (2012) summarizes the relationship between religious socialization and volunteering across the life course: "early religious experiences socialize people into adult volunteer roles" (p. 182). Involvement in a religious organization as a youth positively predicts adult community participation, including volunteer engagement; in addition, the effect of youth religious involvement is not supplanted by adult religious involvement and other youth activities (Perks & Haan, 2011). In fact, youth religious involvement is a consistently stronger predictor of community participation than other factors such as gender, marital status, and nativity (Perks & Haan, 2011).

Religious Social Network

Religious social networks are "the relationships and connections between similar or like-minded religious individuals" (Park & Smith, 2000, p. 276). Religious networks usually occur within a religious organization. Churches and congregations are the main channels through which individual members can learn about volunteer opportunities and voluntary organizations recruit volunteers and plan helping activities. Congregations provide an organizational context that encourages and mobilizes volunteering behaviors (Wuthnow, 1991). Religious beliefs are primarily fostered in the context of religious community, and beliefs would hold no power if they are not ratified by a community of fellow believers (Stark & Bainbridge, 1996; Wuthnow, 1991). Therefore, most research has relied on religious attendance as a key indicator of social network. Other measures include the number of Christian family and friends, having a child in a Christian school (Park & Smith, 2000), trust in congregation members, being a church member in network (Becker & Dhingra, 2001), and having a churchgoing friend (Lim & MacGregor, 2012).

Church attendance is not only a main indicator of religiosity, but also a measure of the extent of involvement in church activities and one's connection with other members. Church members often meet in congregations, and religious attendance increases the likelihood of learning about volunteering opportunities or being asked to volunteer (Musick, Wilson, & Bynum, 2000; Ruiter & De Graaf, 2006). Although religion is a matter of individual faith, a person cannot become actively involved in volunteering and other forms of civic engagement without attending religious services or joining some kind of organized religious community. That is to say, a religious community is vital in encouraging volunteerism, building an environment that mobilizes its members to improve community services through volunteering and charitable behavior (Jackson et al., 1995). Church attendance has a significant influence on volunteering for both religious and nonreligious institutions through the formation of social networks and a sense of community (Park & Smith, 2000).

Social networks built in the congregations may serve as the mechanism through which religion fosters volunteerism and other prosocial behaviors. Congregations draw members into volunteering through their social networks and the fit between the congregation's identity and mission and individual members' beliefs and values (Becker & Dhingra, 2001). Social networks are related to both instrumental and emotional motives for volunteering (Becker & Dhingra, 2001). Instrumental motives are rational choices in weighing the costs and benefits of volunteering for a particular organization (Herzog, House, & Morgan, 1991); emotional motives pertain to one's sense of self and attachment to others (Hart, Atkins, & Ford 1996; Rochon, 1998; Schervish & Havens 1997; Teske, 1997). Through religious social networks, congregation members could increase their trust in and knowledge about a specific volunteer organization, and develop a sense of social responsibility to the organization for which their friends have volunteered; as a result, they are likely to be involved in the voluntary organization (McAdam & Paulsen, 1993; Wilson & Musick, 1997; Wilson, 2000). Becker and Dhingra (2001) found that church effect on volunteering actually operated through social networks rather than through religious beliefs and that the social networks formed within congregations made congregation members more likely to volunteer.

Religious social networks have spillover effects, that is, religious effect on volunteering may spread to nonreligious individuals through personal connections between the religious and the nonreligious (Lim & MacGregor, 2012). Social networks built within and out of the church can be relied on to motivate and recruit church members as well as their friends to volunteer for religious and/or secular organizations (Becker & Dhingra, 2001; Ruiter & De Graaf, 2006). A notable observation of networks in promoting volunteering is that "most formal volunteers are persuaded to volunteer by family members, coworkers, or fellow worshippers" (Wilson & Musick, 1997, p. 700).

In summary, the four dimensions in religion, namely, religiosity, religious identity, religious socialization, and religious social networks are closely intertwined to exert influences on volunteerism across the life course. Religiosity in terms of values, beliefs, attitudes, and behaviors is central to altruism and charity, providing a fertile source for volunteering motivation. Religious socialization, or the influence of parents' religiosity and identity, has an impact on youth religious involvement, which further predicts adult involvement in volunteering and the community. Social networks through a church provide opportunities for continuing volunteer engagement into late-life stages, which become more important for older adults to engage in volunteer work; churches and religious-related institutions are the main organizations for which older adults would like to volunteer.

Discussion

A variety of factors are associated with volunteering across the life course, including human, social, and cultural capitals. A human capital perspective posits that education, income, and health constitute one's stock of human capital that makes volunteering possible (Wilson, 2000). A social capital perspective argues that extensive social connections provide and increase volunteering opportunities (Oesterle, Johnson, & Mortimer, 2004; Wilson, 2000; Wilson & Musick, 1997). A cultural capital perspective posits that religiosity provides ethical resources and a philosophical base for volunteerism (Putnam, 2000). As members of one of the most religious countries in the world, Americans engage in a wide range of religious behaviors, including churchgoing, public and private devotional acts, and prosocial behaviors as well, including volunteerism and civic service. In the United States, religion has historically been linked to volunteerism, providing important resources of both cultural and social capitals. Volunteers live the altruistic or prosocial values in accordance with the main tenets of many religious affiliations. Social networks through religious involvement provide information, opportunity, pooled labor, and trust as important channels to volunteering (Wilson & Musick, 1997). Religious heritage and volunteering tradition can be passed down from generation to generation within the family. Altogether, religious values and behaviors, parental religious affiliation and fundamentalism, and social networks through churches promote volunteerism and other types of civic engagement. The social context and power of religion may have the most potent influence on volunteerism in Americans.

Volunteering is a lifelong behavior but with age-related patterns. People from teenagers to elders are eligible for volunteer work when they meet the qualification requirements with regard to capability, characteristics, and skills. However, variations exist in the antecedence, experience, and consequence stages among volunteers in different age groups. Life-course studies (e.g., Oesterle, Johnson, & Mortimer, 2004; Tang, 2006) indicate that the meaning and motivation of volunteering vary, and different resources are needed for volunteer engagement across life stages. Youth and younger adults draw upon more spiritual and social support to expand volunteering, whereas older adults increase the scope of voluntary organizations to which they are committed through church attendance or religious social networks (Tang, 2006).

The significance of religion in volunteering throughout the life course has been well established in the literature (Johnson, 2013). Yet knowledge is limited regarding how the four components in religion, that is, religiosity, religious identity, religious socialization, and religious social network are interrelated to each other and impact volunteer engagement throughout the life course. Also little is known about whether and how individuals change volunteer behavior tied to the influence of religion over the life course. All these investigations, of course, need to be based on better measurement of religion as a multidimensional concept, which may go beyond the four dimensions as documented here. Furthermore, research needs to focus more on contextual effects, especially the role of social networks in promoting volunteerism (Lim & MacGregor, 2012; Wilson, 2012). Religious social networks at individual, local, and national levels may serve as different mechanisms that link volunteerism, and may operate differently across age cohorts and over one's life course. Finally, researchers need pay attention to changing forms of volunteer work, such as online volunteering, informal volunteering, and some episodic and self-oriented behaviors (Wilson, 2012), which may have different associations with religion.

It is a recent trend that Americans, especially older adults, are likely to engage in and expand volunteer engagement. With the increasing size of the older population, the improved health status, and the prolonged life expectancy, how to make use of the time after retirement has become an important topic for older people themselves and gerontologists as well as society as a whole. Volunteering, as a form of productive activity, may lead older adults to successful aging and healthy aging. A variety of factors from individual attributes to social and historical contexts affect volunteering decision, experience, and consequence. Through volunteer work, older adults can create new meanings of old age and improve life satisfaction, thus enhancing their capability and status in social life. During the volunteer process, the importance of religion can never be overlooked. Religious institutions are in a key position to provide resources and support that encourage and sustain volunteer engagement by people of all ages, especially older adults.

References

Ammerman, N. T. (2005). Religious narratives, community service, and everyday public life. In M. Jo Bane, B. Coffin, & R. Higgins (Ed.), *Taking faith seriously* (pp. 146–174). Cambridge, MA: Harvard University.

Bass, S. A., & Caro, F. G. (2001). Productive aging: A conceptual framework. In N. Morrow-Howell, J. Hinterlong & M. Sherraden (Eds.), *Productive aging: Concepts and challenges* (pp. 37–78). Baltimore: The Johns Hopkins University.

Becker, P. E., & Dhingra, P. H. (2001). Religious involvement and volunteering: Implications for civil society. *Sociology of Religion, 62*, 315–335.

Boraas, S. (2003). Volunteerism in the United States. *Monthly Labor Review, 126*, 3–11.

Brown, J., & Lichter, D. (2007). Childhood disadvantage, adolescent development, and prosocial behavior in early adulthood. *Advances in Life Course Research, 11*, 149–170.

Caputo, R. (2009). Religious capital and intergenerational transmission of volunteering as correlates of civic engagement. *Nonprofit and Voluntary Sector Quarterly, 38*, 983–1002.

Caro, F. G., & Bass, S. A. (1995). Increasing volunteering among older people. In S. A. Bass (Ed.), *Older and active: How Americans over 55 are contributing to society* (pp. 71–96). New Haven, CT: Yale University.

Cnaan, R., & Cascio, T. (1999). Performance and commitment: Issues in management of volunteers in human service organizations. *Journal of Social Service Research, 24*(3/4), 1–37.

Cnaan, R. A., Handy, F., & Wadsworth, M. (1996). Defining who is a volunteer: Conceptual and empirical considerations. *Nonprofit and Voluntary Quarterly, 25*, 364–368.

Corporation for National and Community Service, Office of Research and Policy Development. (2007). *Volunteering in America: 2007 state trends and rankings in civic life*. Washington, DC: Author.

Curtis, J. E., Baer, D. E., & Grabb, E. G. (2001). Nations of joiners: Explaining voluntary association membership in democratic societies. *American Sociological Review, 66*, 783–805.

Driskell, R. L., Lyon, L., & Embry, E. (2008). Civic engagement and religious activities: Examining the influence of religious tradition and participation. *Sociological Spectrum, 28*, 578–601. doi: 10.1080/02732170802206229

Duke, N., Skay, C., Pettingell, S., & Borowsky, I. (2009). From adolescent connections to social capital: Predictors of civic engagement in young adulthood. *Journal of Adolescent Health, 44*, 161–168.

Einolf, C. (2009). Will the boomers volunteer during retirement? Comparing the baby boom, silent, and long civic cohorts. *Nonprofit and Voluntary Sector Quarterly, 38*, 181–199.

Ellison, C. G., & MaFarland, M. J. (2013). The social context of religion and spirituality in the United States. In K. I. Pargament (Ed.), *APA handbook of psychology, religion, and spirituality* (Vol. 1: Context, theory, and research, pp. 21–50). Washington, DC: American Psychology Association.

England, P. (2000). Marriage, the costs of children, and gender inequality. In L. J. Waite, C. Bachrach, M. Hindin, E. Thomson, & A. Thornton (Eds.), *The times that bind: Perspectives on marriage and cohabitation* (pp. 320–342). New York: Aldine de Gruyter.

Fisher, L. R., Mueller, D. P., & Cooper, P. W. (1991). Older volunteers: A discussion of the Minnesota Senior Study. *The Gerontologist, 31*, 183–194.

Fisher, L. R., & Schaffer, K. B. (1993). *Older volunteers: A guide to research and practice*. Newbury Park, NJ: Sage.

Flanagan, C., & Levine, P. (2010). Civic engagement and the transition to adulthood. *Future of Children, 20*, 159–179.

Gallagher, S. K. (1994). Doing their share: Comparing patterns of help given by older and younger adults. *Journal of Marriage and the Family, 56*, 567–578.

Hart, D., Atkins, R., & Ford, D. (1996). Urban America as a context for the development of moral identity in adolescence. *Journal of Social Issues, 54*, 513–530.

Herzog, A. R., & Morgan, J. N. (1993). Formal volunteer work among older Americans. In F. G. C. S. A. Bass & Y. Chen (Ed.), *Achieving a productive aging society* (pp. 119–142). Westport, CT: Auburn.

Herzog, A. R., House, J., & Morgan, J. (1991). Relation of work and retirement to health and wellbeing. *Psychology of Aging, 6*, 202–211.

Hoge, D. R., Zech, Z., McNamara, P., & Donahue, M. J. (1998). The value of volunteers as resources for congregations. *Journal for the Scientific Study of Religion, 37*, 470–480.

Iannaccone, L. R. (1990). Religious practice: A human capital approach. *Journal for the Scientific Study of Religion, 29*, 297–314.

Jackson, E. F., Bachmeier, M. D., Wood, J. R., & Craft, E. A. (1995). Volunteering and charitable giving: Do religious and associational ties promote helping behavior? *Nonprofit and Voluntary Sector Quarterly, 24*, 59–78. doi: 10.1177/089976409502400108

Johnson, J. B. (2013). Religion and volunteering over the adult life course. *Journal for the Scientific Study of Religion, 52*, 733–752.

Klumb, P. L., & Baltes, M. M. (1999). Time use of old and very old Berliners: Productive and consumptive activities as functions of resources. *The Journals of Gerontology, Series B: Social Sciences, 54B*, S271–S278.

Komp, K., van Tilburg, T., & van Groenou, M. (2011). Age, retirement and health as factors in volunteering in later life. *Nonprofit and Voluntary Sector Quarterly, 40*, 1–20. doi: 10.1177/0899764011402697

Ladd, G. W. (1999). Peer relationships and social competence during early and middle childhood. *Annual Review of Psychology, 50*, 333–359.

Lam, P. (2002). As the flocks gather: How religion affects voluntary association participation. *Journal for the Scientific Study of Religion, 41*, 405–422.

Li, Y., & Ferraro, K. F. (2006). Volunteering in middle and later life: Is health a benefit, barriers or both? *Social Forces, 85*, 497–519.

Lim, C., & MacGregor, C. A. (2012). Religion and volunteering in context: Disentangling the contextual effects of religion on voluntary behavior. *American Sociological Review, 77*, 747–780. doi: 10.1177/0003122412457875

Manning, L. K. (2010). Gender and religious differences associated with volunteering in later life. *Journal of Women & Aging, 22*, 125–135. doi: 10.1080/08952841003719224

McAdam, D., & Paulsen, R. (1993). Specifying the relationship between social ties and activism. *American Journal of Sociology, 99*, 640–667.

McDougle, L., Handy, F., Konrath, S., & Walk, M. (2014). Health outcomes and volunteering: The moderating role of religiosity. *Social Indicator Research, 117*, 337–351.

McFarland, D., & Thomas, R. (2006). Bowling young: How youth voluntary associations influence adult political participation. *American Sociological Review, 71*, 401–425.

Miner, S., & Tolnay, S. (1998). Barriers to voluntary organization membership: An examination of race and cohort differences. *The Journals of Gerontology, Series B: Social Sciences, 53B*, S241–S248.

Morrow-Howell, N., Hinterlong, J., Rozario, P., & Tang, F. (2003). Effects of volunteering on the well-being of older adults. *The Journals of Gerontology, Series B: Social Sciences, 58B*, S137–S145.

Musick, M.A., Herzog, A.R., & House, J.S. (1999). Volunteering and mortality among older adults: Findings from a national sample. *The Journals of Gerontology, Series B: Social Sciences, 54B*, S173–S180.

Musick, M., Wilson, J., & Bynum, W.B., Jr. (2000). Race and formal volunteering: The differential effects of class and religion. *Social Force, 78*, 1539–1571.

Mutchler, J.E., Burr, J.A., & Caro, F.G. (2003). From paid worker to volunteer: Leaving the paid workforce and volunteering in later life. *Social Forces, 8*, 1267–1293. doi: 10.1353/sof.2003.0067

Oesterle, S., Johnson, M.K., & Mortimer, J.T. (2004). Volunteerism during the transition to adulthood: A life course perspective. *Social Forces, 82*, 1123–1149.

Park, J.Z., & Smith, C. (2000). "To whom much has been given . . .": Religion capital and community voluntarism among churchgoing Protestants. *Journal for the Scientific Study of Religion, 39*, 272–286.

Pavlova, M.K., & Silbereisen, R.K. (2012). Participation in voluntary organizations and volunteer work as a compensation for the absence of work or partnership? Evidence from two German samples of younger and older adults. *The Journals of Gerontology, Series B: Psychological Sciences and Social Sciences, 167*, 514–524. doi: 10.1093/geronb/gbs051

Penner, L., Brannick, M.T., Webb, S., & Connell, P. (2005). Effects of volunteering of the September 11, 2001 attacks: An archival analysis. *Journal of Applied Social Psychology, 35*, 1333–1360.

Perks, T., & Haan, M. (2011). Youth religious involvement and adult community participation: Do levels of youth religious involvement matter? *Nonprofit and Voluntary Sector Quarterly, 40*, 107–129.

Piliavin, J.A., & Siegl, E. (2007). Health benefits of volunteering in the Wisconsin Longitudinal Study. *Journal of Health and Social Behavior, 48*, 450–464.

Prisuta, R. (2003). *Enhancing volunteerism among aging boomers*. Paper presented at the conference on Baby Boomers and Retirement: Impact on Civic Engagement. Available http://www.civicengagement.org/agingsociety/links/aarpboomers.pdf

Putnam, R.D. (2000). *Bowling alone: The collapse and revival of American community*. New York: Simon and Schuster.

Rochon, T.R. (1998). *Culture moves: Ideas, activism and changing values*. Princeton, NJ: Princeton University.

Rosenberg, E., & Letrero, I.L. (2006). Using age, cohort, and period to study elderly volunteerism. *Educational Gerontology, 32*, 313–334. doi: 10.1080/03601270600564088

Rotolo, T., & Wilson, J. (2007). Sex-segregation in volunteer work. *The Sociological Quarterly, 48*, 559–585.

Ruiter, S., & De Graaf, N. (2008). Socio-economic payoffs of voluntary association involvement: A Dutch life course study. *European Sociological Review, 25*, 425–442.

Schervish, P.G., & Havens, J.J. (1997). Social participation and charitable giving: A multivariate analysis. *Voluntas, 8*, 235–260.

Selbee, L.K., & Reed, P.B. (2001). Pattern of volunteering over the life circle. *Canadian Social Trends*, Statistics Canada—Catalogue No. 11-008, 1–5.

Smith, D.V. (1994). Determinants of voluntary association participation and volunteering: A literature review. *Nonprofit and Voluntary Sector, 23*, 243–263.

Snyder, M., & Omoto, A. (2008). Volunteerism: Social issues, perspectives and social policy implications. *Social Issues and Policy Review, 2*, 1–36.

Stark, R., & Bainbridge, W.S. (1996). *Religion, deviance, and social control*. New York: Routledge.

Suanet, B., van Groenou, M., & Braam, A. (2009). Changes in volunteering among young old in the Netherlands between 1992 and 2002: The impact of religion, age-norms, and intergenerational transmission. *European Journal of Ageing, 6*, 157–165.

Tang, F. (2006). What resources are needed for volunteerism? A life course perspective. *Journal of Applied Gerontology, 25*, 375–390.

Tang, F. (2008). Socioeconomic disparities in voluntary organization involvement among older adults. *Nonprofit & Voluntary Sector Quarterly, 37*, 57–75.

Tang, F. (2010). Volunteering by older adults in the Unites States. *The Journal of China Social Work, 3*, 289–300.

Taniguchi, H. (2006). Men and women's volunteering: Gender differences in the effects of employment and family characteristics. *Nonprofit and Voluntary Sector Quarterly, 35*, 83–101. doi: 10.1177/0899764005282481

Taniguchi, H. (2011). The determinants of formal and informal volunteering: Evidence from the American Time Use Survey. *Voluntas*. Advance online publication. doi: 10.1007/s11266-011-9236-y

Taniguchi, H., & Thomas, L.D. (2011). The influences of religious attitudes on volunteering. *Voluntas, 22*, 335–355. doi: 10.1007/s11266-010-9158-0

Teske, N. (1997). *Political activists in America: The identity construction model of political participation*. Cambridge: Cambridge University Press.

Thoits, P.A., & Hewitt, L.N. (2001). Volunteer work and well-being. *Journal of Health and Social Work, 42*, 115–131.

Unruh, H.R., & Sider, R.J. (2005). *Saving souls, serving society: Understanding the faith factor in church-based social ministry*. New York: Oxford University Press.

U.S. Bureau of Labor Statistics. (2014). *Volunteering in the United States—2013*. Retrieved from http://www.bls.gov/news.release/volun.nr0.htm

Van Willigen, M. (2000). Differential benefits of volunteering across the life course. *The Journals of Gerontology, Series B: Social Sciences, 55B*, S308–S318.

Wald, K.D., & Calhoun-Brown, A. (2014). *Religion and politics in the United States* (7th ed.). Lanham, MD: Rowman & Littlefield.

Warburton, J., Le Broque, R., & Rosenman, L. (1998). Older people—The reserve army of volunteers? An analysis of volunteerism among older Australians. *International Journal of Aging and Human Development, 46*, 229–245.

Weeden, J., & Kurzban, R. (2013). What predicts religiosity? A multinational analysis of reproductive and cooperative morals. *Evolution and Human Behavior, 34*, 440–445.

Wilson, J. (2000). Volunteering. *Annual Review of Sociology, 26*, 215–240.

Wilson, J. (2012). Volunteerism research: A review essay. *Nonprofit and Voluntary Sector Quarterly, 41*, 176–212. doi: 10.1177/0899764011434558

Wilson, J., & Janoski, T. (1995). The contribution of religion to volunteer work. *Sociology of Religion, 56*, 137–152.

Wilson, J., & Musick, M. A. (1997a). Who cares? Toward an integrated theory of volunteer work. *American Sociology Review, 62*, 694–713.

Wilson, J., & Musick, M. A. (1997b). Work and volunteering: The long arm of the job. *Social Force, 76*, 251–272.

Wuthnow, R. (1991). *Acts of compassion: Caring for others and helping ourselves.* Princeton, NJ: Princeton University Press.

Wuthnow, R. (1999). Mobilizing civic engagement: The changing impact of religious involvement. In T. Skocpol & M. P. Fiorina (Ed.), *Civic engagement in American democracy* (pp. 331–363). Washington, DC: Brookings Institution Press and Russell Sage Foundation.

CHAPTER FOUR

Biology and Aging: A Primer

Donna J. Holmes

The biology of aging—also referred to as *biogerontology* or *geroscience*—is a diverse field that includes an array of subdisciplines all focused very generally on basic biological aging processes (Holmes & Cohen, 2014; McDonald, 2014; Lithgow, 2013; Kennedy et al., 2014) (Table 4.1). Biologists generally define *aging* or *organismal senescence* as "a progressive, irreversible decline in physiological function, resilience and health associated with increasing chronological age" (Holmes & Cohen, 2014). The field as a whole seeks to understand aging in humans in broader biological perspective, and in comparison with aging in other groups of organisms, including wild animals in nature, as well as the laboratory species used most often as aging research models.

In humans and other homoeothermic (warm-blooded) vertebrate animals (mammals and birds), aging is generally associated with certain clinical syndromes, including: loss of fertility, declines in strength and mobility, frailty, sensory impairment (blindness, deafness, etc.), and changes in cognition and memory. Aging also is associated with an increased age-specific prevalence of particular diseases, including osteoarthritis, cardiovascular disease (CVD), cancers, diabetes, and dementias, including Alzheimer's disease—all of which contribute to increased probability of illness, functional disability, or death. These syndromes and diseases are sometimes referred to as *canonical aging syndromes* (Finch, 1990).

Table 4.1 demonstrates the enormous variation in methodologies and intellectual perspectives applied by biologists who specialize in aging. These include: evolutionary, comparative, and population-level approaches, some of which compare aging in different groups or populations of

Table 4.1 Disciplines Represented in the Biology of Aging

The biology of aging (*biogerontology* or *geroscience*) is a diverse field, characterized by scientists using a range of model organisms, approaches, and levels of analysis.

Population level

- Demography, population biology, and epidemiology
- Population genetics, for example:
  - exploring variability in specific molecular genetic markers of longevity and disease risk
- Evolutionary and comparative biology, for example:
  - comparing differences in lifespan and aging patterns in organisms in nature or the laboratory
  - including approaches like artificial selection experiments or laboratory breeding to isolate key aging phenotypes and genes

Organism level

- Physiological, for example:
  - nutritional interventions, drug administration, and the use of model laboratory organisms ranging from yeast, worms, and flies to mice, rats, and dogs
  - identifying mechanisms of organ- and system-level disease and dysfunction
  - identifying metabolic and cell-signaling pathways implicated in aging and disease

Cellular level

- employing cell lines in laboratory culture and establishing key metabolic or cellular processes that determine cell viability
- examining cells in vivo, in living organisms, to track aging-related changes in cell processes that are associated with disease and mortality risk

Molecular and genetic

- detecting molecules and pathways involved in aging-related changes and disease risk
- identifying key genes linked to disease, aging and lifespan

Sources: Finch, 1990, 2007; Rose, 1991; Carey, 1999; Austad & Holmes, 1999; Kirkwood & Austad, 2000; Conn, 2006; Masoro & Austad, 2005; Guarente, Partridge, & Wallace, 2008; Austad & Masoro, 2011.

organisms, or over evolutionary time frames; whole-organism or physiological approaches, as in experimental nutrition or drug intervention studies; and biochemical, molecular, or genetic studies examining the effects on aging of specific genes, molecules, or metabolic pathways (see, e.g.,

Finch, 1990, 2007; Conn, 2006; Pearson et al., 2008; Miller et al., 2011). While social and cultural variables often are not an explicitly stated or primary focus of biological aging studies, these factors nonetheless come into play in a variety of ways. For example, researchers who focus on the epidemiology and demography of aging consider historical, cultural, ethnic, and gender-related variables as major forces underlying patterns of human aging, mortality, longevity, and disease prevalence.

Aging, Lifespan, and the Global Population

A dramatic shift in the human lifespan has occurred across the globe over the past three centuries. Life expectancies (LEs) have increased dramatically since the industrial revolution (Olshansky & Ault, 1986; Olshansky et al., 1997; Vaupel, 2010). In the United States in 1850, the average LE at birth was only 35–40 years; by 1900 the average was still under 50 years. But by 2000, the LE at birth in the United States and many other countries had reached over 75 years. Average LE at birth now exceeds that in some countries, including Japan and Scandinavia. LE at older ages has risen considerably during this time period as well: a 65-year-old American man can now expect to live an additional 16 years; a woman, 20 years more, compared with only 13–15 years in 1940, as shown in Table 4.2 (reviewed in Olshansky et al., 1997; Crews, 2003; Vaupel, 2010).

This profound modern shift in human longevity is attributable almost entirely to cultural change, including advances in medicine, nutrition,

Table 4.2 Additional Years of Life Expectancy Remaining at Age 65 in the United States from 1950 to 2010 for Men and Women

	Additional Years of Life Remaining at Age 65 (Averages)	
Year	Males	Females
1950	12.8	15.0
1960	12.8	17.8
1970	13.1	17.0
1980	14.1	18.3
1990	15.1	18.9
2000	16.0	19.0
2010	17.7	20.3

Data represent averages for all races combined.

Source: National Center for Vital and Health Statistics.

sanitation, public safety, and other aspects of public health, rather than any alteration in the way humans age on a basic biological level. Recent changes in LE have depended a great deal on declines in infant and child mortality, as well as fewer deaths from infectious disease and improvements in public health and safety that affect people of all ages.

The increase in lifespan in most countries across the world is associated with an equally dramatic shift in the most prevalent causes of disease and death. In comparatively wealthy, industrialized cultures like the United States, we are much more likely than our recent ancestors to die of aging-related diseases like CVD, cancers, or dementias, or to be chronically disabled by conditions like respiratory disease, osteoarthritis, blindness, or hearing impairment. Obviously, these demographic and epidemiological shifts have a huge impact on the economic, medical, and social structures needed to support the health and well-being of older people and their caregivers. For these reasons, an integrative, interdisciplinary focus on the biology of aging has never been more critical for global public health.

Why Do We Age?

Evolutionary biology provides a robust theoretical framework to explain why aging occurs in humans and many other animal species, as well as why lifespans vary among species (Rose, 1991; Kirkwood & Austad, 2000; Cohen & Holmes, 2014). There is a persistent and commonly held idea among laypeople and nonspecialists that aging evolved to "make way for the young," or "for the good of the group"—in other words, the idea that older, less functional individuals sacrifice additional, more functional years to free up resources for the young. Although this idea has an unselfish appeal, it has long been discredited as an explanation for the existence of aging. In fact, evolutionary biologists generally do not view aging (organismal senescence) as the direct result of any adaptive physiological or developmental program.

In evolutionary terms, aging is most easily explained in sexually reproducing organisms like humans, which are incapable of reproducing via asexual means (such as budding or cloning). In these organisms, there is a clear genetic distinction between somatic (body or nonreproductive) and reproductive tissues and cells. *In genetic terms, reproduction is the only real measure of biological success, and only the reproductive segment of the lifespan is subject to the force of natural selection.* Physiological health and organismal integrity are actively promoted by selection only during reproductive lifespan of the individual, and not thereafter. As shown graphically in Figure 4.1, selection becomes weaker as reproduction becomes less likely.

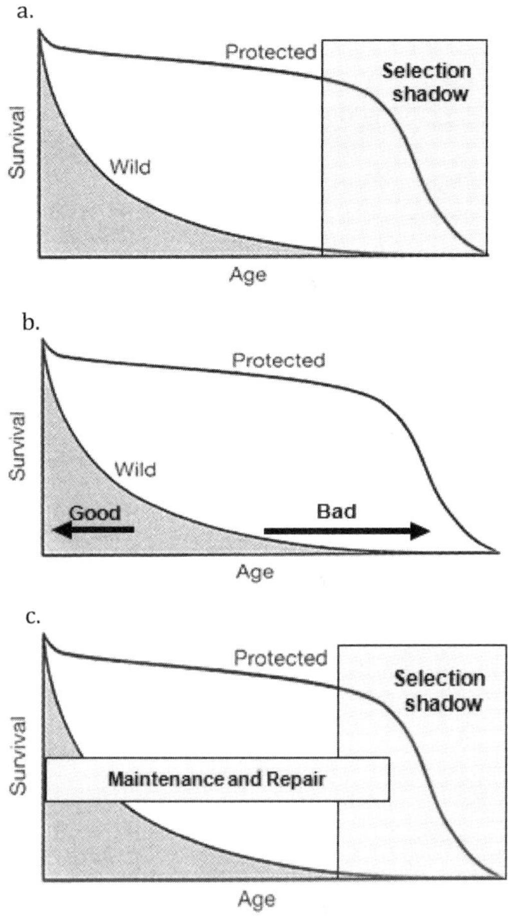

Figure 4.1 Evolutionary aging theory. Population- and species-level variation in the trajectory of aging and variation in longevity patterns result from natural selection for favorable *trade-offs between survival and reproduction*, driven by the force of mortality in a particular environment. (a) In the wild, most animals die of external causes before they show signs of aging, but captive animals protected against disease and death live more often into old age, beyond the force of natural selection in the wild (denoted by the "selection shadow"); (b) The *antagonistic pleiotropy theory* of aging predicts that pleiotropic genes (genes with multiple effects) beneficial early in life can cause or contribute to aging-related disease later on. In modern human and other populations protected against ancestral causes of mortality, harmful mutations that would otherwise be eliminated by natural selection can accumulate, contributing to aging (*mutation accumulation*). (c) According to *disposable soma* theory, organisms invest in effective maintenance and repair of somatic tissues only as long as they would be likely to survive and reproduce in the wild. (Adapted from Kirkwood, T. B.L., & Austad, S. N. [2000]. Why do we age? *Nature, 408*(6809), 233–238. doi: 10.1038/35041682 with permission from Nature; reprinted from Cohen and Holmes 2014 with permission from Elsevier Press.)

Seen in this way, aging is not programmed or adaptively optimized, but occurs as a by-product of selection to maximize the reproductive potential of organisms in a given population, given the average probability of dying in a given set of environmental conditions. Aging is expected to evolve when it is to an organism's genetic advantage to forgo longevity for its own successful reproduction in the short run.

This theoretical framework helps to explain why the risks of some diseases and disabilities associated with aging (e.g., cancers, CVD, osteoporosis, etc.) increase at older ages. The multisystem physiological failure that characterizes aging is the result of a *failure of natural selection* to promote continued investment in protection against disease, regulation of homeostasis, and repair of accumulated metabolic damage. Modern humans are well into the aging process by their 40th year, when fertility is waning in both men and women. By this time of life, most of our ancestors had fulfilled their reproductive potential. Relatively few humans in traditional, preindustrialized cultures have ever lived much over three decades (Crews, 2003; Finch, 2007). In short, the human body was not "designed" by natural selection to function optimally after the probability of successful reproduction has declined.

Human Lifespan in Comparative Perspective

Human aging can also be examined from the perspective of comparative biology, alongside the lifespans and aging patterns of other mammals, including other primate species. Modern humans are longer-lived and age considerably more slowly than either our closest primate cousins, the chimps and gorillas, or other mammals of similar body size (Ingram et al., 2006; Sonntag et al., 2012). The longest reliably documented human lifespan to date was attained by a French woman who lived to 122 years and died in 1997 (Allard et al., 1998).

In contrast, many other life forms, including fungi, plants, and some invertebrates, age much more slowly than we do, if they age at all. Galapagos tortoises and some deep-sea fishes, for example, have reliably documented lifespans of over 150 years. Some deep-sea clams, as well other wild invertebrates, plants, and fungi can live for up to several centuries. Some of these exceptionally slowly aging organisms are of great interest to biologists, since they may eventually yield some clues as to how intervene successfully in human aging.

Basic Approaches in the Biology of Aging

Many biologists approach their research using animal model systems developed specifically for laboratory studies. In most cases, these are species that have been domesticated and inbred for many generations, and are well suited for addressing particular biological questions in a laboratory setting. These include some organisms only distantly related to humans, like brewer's yeast, soil roundworms, and fruit flies, or laboratory rats and mice. Some aging biologists, on the other hand, utilize more closely related nonhuman primate species, like rhesus monkeys. Others study natural aging patterns in the field, focusing on wild animal populations.

A central aim of basic aging research is to identify key biological processes or laboratory interventions with the potential to be translational—that is, to lead to preventive or therapeutic innovations that promote human health and well-being. A sampling of basic aging processes currently under study is listed in Table 4.3. There is an intense focus on identifying and understanding basic mechanisms—genes or cell-signaling pathways, for example—that underlie variation in aging and longevity, as well as on why and how aging occurs in the first place.

Basic aging research tends to focus on aging of the whole organism, rather than on disparate diseases or physiological systems. While some of these studies (such as those using roundworms or flies, for example) may not seem relevant to humans, there is a clear emphasis on identifying common mechanisms for aging-related disease and mortality that are generalizable to a wide range of organisms, including humans. A basic tenet of the developing interdisciplinary *geroscience* approach to aging research is that identifying fundamental processes important in aging (e.g., inflammation, oxidative damage, protein instability, or physiological or cell-cycle dysregulation) will eventually reveal causative factors underlying multiple aging-related diseases and disabilities (e.g., cancers, diabetes, CVD, and Alzheimer's disease) (Lithgow, 2013; Kennedy et al., 2014).

Biologists focus on varying levels of causation in their approaches to aging research. Some processes and major questions currently under study are listed in Tables 4.1 and 4.3. Some researchers focus primarily on proximate causes and mechanisms of aging; that is, the physiological, cellular, and molecular processes underlying variation in lifespan and aging. Others concentrate on ultimate, evolutionary or population-level forces that give rise to aging patterns in the first place — for example, analyzing how natural selection acts to shape patterns of reproduction and survivorship and, as a result, variation in lifespan and aging trajectories, as discussed above (see, e.g., Kirkwood & Austad, 2000; Cohen & Holmes, 2014).

Aging in a given population of organisms can be quantified using *vital rate statistics*—preferably, in the form of continuously distributed age-specific rates of survival, death, or functional loss, as illustrated in Figure 4.2. Ideally, these statistics are generated using reliably documented ages at birth

Table 4.3 Seven Major Questions or Issues That Currently Represent a Major Research Focus of the Biology of Aging

1. Can safe, reliable interventions be developed for extending lifespan or healthspan in model animal systems and humans? Possible interventions:
   - Lifestyle-related
     - *Examples*: exercise and activity; stress reduction; improvements in safety
   - Nutritional
     - *Examples*: restricted calorie intake, specific supplements; neutraceuticals
   - Medical
     - Primary prevention, screenings
     - Medication, surgery, other pharmaceuticals, etc.
   - Genetic
     - Identification of key disease or aging genes
     - Direct genetic modification of lifespan or disease

     (genetic engineering can now significantly increase healthy lifespan in laboratory animals)
2. What "proximate" aging (or longevity) mechanisms and pathways can be identified that are shared across a broad range of organisms?
   - Genetic, biochemical, or physiological

     Examples: oxidative stress and damage; mitochondrial dysfunction; key cell-signaling and metabolic pathways; genetic damage; failure of cellular repair; disintegration of regulatory networks
3. What are the "ultimate" or evolutionary causes of aging and variation in lifespan?
   - How do lifespans and aging patterns compare between major groups of organisms and across the tree of life?
   - How is variation in lifespan within and between species shaped by natural selection and other evolutionary forces?
4. Which animal model systems are most useful for studies of basic aging mechanisms that could translate to humans?
   - Inbred, domesticated organisms are used for experimental manipulation of genes, cellular or physiological aging processes
   - Genetic manipulations can target key aging genes through creation of mutant or "knockout" laboratory animal strains

     Examples: Standard laboratory models: brewer's yeast (*Saccharomyces*), laboratory roundworms (*C. elegans*), fruit flies (*Drosophila*), and laboratory rats and mice

5. Which key molecules (genes or other aging "biomarkers") be used to predict lifespan, disease or mortality risk?
6. What are the major historical and demographic trends in longevity, aging, and disease risk in humans?
    - Demographic and epidemiological approaches used to examine historical changes using public health records
    - Comparison of populations, cultures, ethnic groups, and gender differences
7. What basic aging mechanisms can be identified that are specifically responsible for human disease ("translational" research)
    - *Examples*: medical issues, diseases or clinical syndromes associated with aging, and the underlying mechanisms for diseases, including CVD, cancers, frailty syndromes, dementia, etc.

Sources: Finch, 1990, 2007; Kirkwood & Austad, 2000; Masoro & Austad, 2005; Guarente, Partridge, & Wallace, 2008; Austad & Masoro, 2011; Holmes & Cohen, 2014; Kennedy et al., 2014.

and death. In basic demographic or statistical terms, aging can be detected in a population when there is a steady increase in age-specific death rates after sexual maturity. When age-specific survival or death rates are unavailable, other, cruder measures of aging or lifespan potential are often used. These include species-specific LEs or *maximum lifespan potentials*. These measures, however, can be biased by very large or small sample sizes, since the more the individuals surveyed, the greater the chance of finding very old individuals, even if they actually occur very rarely.

The most commonly used metric for longevity in human populations is *LE* at a particular age, equal to the average years of life remaining at that age in a given population or historical cohort. LE can be calculated from birth, at reproductive maturity, or at any stage later in life (for reviews, see Finch, 1990; Preston, Heuvelein, & Guillot, 2001). Table 4.2, for example, shows recent increases in LE at age 65 in the U.S. LE at birth is often used in the context of lifespan and aging. While this variable is certainly relevant for measuring historical changes in public health, it should be noted that LE at birth is very sensitive to mortality in infancy and childhood, and hence not the best measure of the probability of surviving to old age. The best metrics for aging rates and probability of death include slopes and other regression parameters derived from calculating mortality rates for many individuals, along with percentiles for age at death at various ages. In terms of best practice, appropriate statistical methods are chosen to fit the particular research question being addressed (see, e.g., Finch, 1990; Carey, 1999).

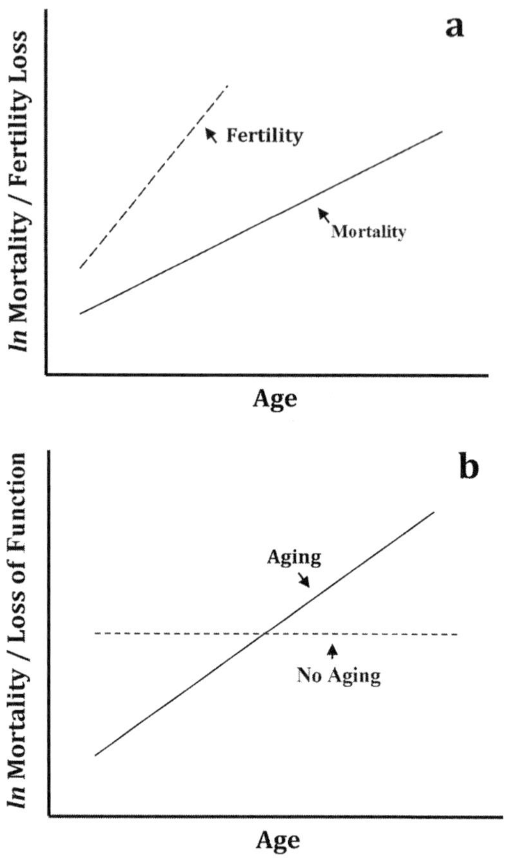

Figure 4.2 Aging can be quantified in a population by graphing linearized age-specific rates of mortality or loss of function. Death rates (a) or loss of reproductive function (b) are log-transformed and plotted against chronological age; the slopes of these functions represent aging rates. (No slope denotes no aging; steeper slopes denote faster aging rates.) Functional loss can occur at different rates for different physiological systems or capacities (e.g., reproduction, cardiovascular capacity, immune function). Evolutionary theory generally posits that aging results from the failure of natural selection to promote longer reproductive fitness, organismal maintenance, and survival. Natural selection acts via age-specific mortality pressure on a given population, which in turn shapes heritable patterns of aging in subsequent generations. As selection for successful reproduction wanes, aging-related defects accumulate, and rates of mortality increase. (Sources: Finch, 1990; Carey, 1999; Kirkwood & Austad, 2000. Reprinted from Cohen & Holmes, 2014 with permission from Elsevier Press.)

Aging is a complex process involving multiple, interactive physiological systems. *Chronological age* does not always reliably correlate with *biological age*, which ideally would predict the risk of dying of aging-related causes in the future. There are few physiological or molecular *biomarkers* of aging that can predict reliably how long an individual organism with particular phenotypic traits will live, or what will be the ultimate cause of death for a given individual. Individual humans vary a great deal in terms of their risk of death or disease at a particular chronological age. This holds true for individual laboratory animals, as well.

Biologists have nonetheless used a wide variety of parameters as aging biomarkers, including biochemical, cellular, and physiological variables, such as markers of oxidative or other metabolic damage to DNA and cell membranes, telomere shortening, disruption of homeostasis, insulin resistance, and inflammatory markers. Other, more function-based aging biomarkers are also used, including measures of physical agility, strength, and cognitive ability. For human aging studies, aging biomarkers have included measures from standard blood lab panels, like lipid profiles, markers of diabetes, and measures of infection and inflammation. Additional clinical tools often used currently in studies of human health and aging include assessment of cognitive performance, hand grip strength, gait, balance, and fall risk, and other measures of mobility and frailty, as well as the ability to independently perform activities of daily life such as bathing, preparing food, paying bills, and housework.

Attempts to derive one or a few reliable aging biomarkers have met with mixed or limited success (Ingram et al., 2001; Butler et al., 2004; Miller et al., 2001). Benchmarked aging biomarkers can be invasive, expensive, or difficult to obtain, and they can vary a great deal between species, making direct translation from animal models to humans difficult. Even within human populations, clinical markers are fairly crude predictors of the actual cause or probability of death. Nonetheless, basic geriatric assessments are generally useful for obtaining a picture of health, mobility, cognitive status, and independence in older adults (Ham et al., 2014).

Theories and Basic Mechanisms of Aging

While biologists can now successfully manipulate key genes or physiological processes in laboratory animals to alter the basic trajectory of aging, no one has yet successfully slowed the aging process in humans at a basic cellular level or molecular level. But there are robust working theories about how particular proximate physiological and cellular mechanisms are involved in determining lifespan and aging rates, as well as about the ultimate, or evolutionary, processes that are also at work, as described in Table 4.4. At least some, if not most, of these mechanisms are likely to be important in human aging, as well. A synopsis of current ideas about some promising key processes is provided below. Note that, in particular, aging researchers currently are focusing intensely on such phenomena as oxidative mitochondrial metabolism, cell-replication and signaling processes (such as those involved in cancer), and aspects of nutrient and metabolic signaling. There is also a great deal of interest in various forms of metabolic damage, including oxidative damage resulting from normal cellular processes.

Table 4.4 Basic Aging Mechanisms (Basic Biological Processes Currently under Study as Causative Mechanisms in the Biology of Aging)

Ultimate mechanisms:

- Evolution
  - *Natural selection; sexual selection; fitness trade-offs between reproduction and survival, etc., operating at the population level*

Proximate mechanisms:

- Developmental processes and physiological trade-offs
- Nutrition, energy metabolism, and growth, for example:
  - *Calorie restriction (CR) and CR mimics*
  - *Insulin and IGF-1 signaling (IIS)*
  - *Growth hormone (GH)*
  - *Sirtuins*
- Metabolic and oxidative damage
- Mitochondrial dysfunction and pathophysiology
- DNA damage and repair
- Cell replication and senescence
  - *Telomeres and telomerase*
- Inflammation
- Physiological dysregulation

Note that these include ultimate (evolutionary) as well as proximate (molecular, cellular, and physiological) mechanisms. These levels of explanations are not mutually exclusive, but complementary.

Sources: Rose, 1991; Finch, 2007; Kirkwood & Austad, 2000; Masoro & Austad, 2005; Guarente, Partridge, & Wallace, 2008; Austad & Masoro, 2011; Cohen & Holmes, 2014; Holmes & Cohen, 2014; Kennedy et al., 2014.

Evolution and Development

As discussed above, evolutionary or ultimate-level analysis focuses on changes in lifespan and aging in populations, and examines the force of natural selection in shaping age-specific mortality rates (and hence longevity and aging rates). In evolutionary terms, nonreproductive tissues are disposable, and are actively maintained only long enough to ensure successful reproduction. Aging is posited to result from *adaptive fitness trade-offs* between the probability of successful reproduction and the cost of long-term survival, maintenance, and repair. Natural selection has been shown in a large body of studies to shape trade-offs between reproduction, survival and lifespan in many sexually reproducing organisms (Rose, 1991; Kirkwood & Austad, 2000; Partridge, Gems, & Withers, 2005).

Developmental theories of aging also are closely tied to the concept of evolutionary fitness trade-offs. Traits that are beneficial early in life or contribute to successful maturation and reproduction in younger individuals can be harmful to older ones and increase susceptibility of aging-related disease (de Magalhaes & Church, 2005; Partridge, Gems, & Withers, 2005). For example, the growth and development of young organisms depends on the capacity of cells to replicate and proliferate rapidly. The same growth factors and hormones (e.g., estrogen and testosterone; growth hormone (GH); IGF-1) that integrate the growth and development of reproductive tissues can also trigger unregulated cell growth and cancers in older individuals.

Healthy, young, developing or reproducing animals exhibit *phenotypic plasticity*, the ability to respond flexibly to environmental demands, such as a scarcity or abundance of food, and to alter their physiology in an adaptive fashion accordingly (Gilbert & Epel, 2008; Stearns & Koella, 2008). Many animals, including humans, also exhibit *critical developmental periods* in which developing individuals are exquisitely sensitive to environmental cues. During these periods, environmental variation can not only alter early development, but also influence health and the trajectory of aging in adulthood (Ellison, 2005, Gluckman et al., 2009). For example, human infants born with abnormally low birth weights are at higher risk as adults for metabolic syndrome, which is associated with obesity, type 2 diabetes, and CVD risk, as well as a shortened lifespan from other causes (Hales & Barker, 1992). On the other hand, babies born to obese or diabetic mothers also are at higher risk of metabolic disease. In both humans and animal models, it is increasingly clear, moreover, that other nongenetic environmental factors, such as parental age and health, stress, endocrine disruptors, and environmental toxins, can alter early development and affect mortality rates and prevalences of aging-related disease over the adult life course (reviewed in Finch, 2007). For humans living well beyond our ancestral lifespans in a rapidly changing, industrialized modern setting, environmental variation can be so extreme as to make adaptive developmental responses physiologically impossible, as in the case of maternal and childhood obesity.

Nutrition, Energy Metabolism, and Growth

Nutrition, caloric intake, and the metabolic pathways employed in the body's use of fuel are known to play a key role in aging, disease susceptibility, and LE in laboratory animal models. Several of the most promising or influential research avenues and findings in this area are summarized below. While these lines of research have not yet resulted in the development of direct aging interventions, like medications, they are already helping to clarify why certain lifestyle interventions, like avoiding obesity and engaging in regular exercise, can help to extend healthy lifespan in humans.

Calorie restriction. Diets that are nutritionally complete but severely calorie-restricted (CR) have been shown in a great many studies to slow aging and extend lifespan in a wide range of species — from yeast and worms to laboratory mice and monkeys (reviewed in Weindruch & Walford, 1988; Anderson & Weindruch, 2012). The taxonomic breadth of the response to CR suggests that the underlying biological mechanisms are evolutionarily conserved. The metabolic pathways and genes implicated to date in the effects of CR include GH, insulin, and IGF-1, plus other proteins that regulate cell replication and stress resistance, like the sirtuins and mTOR (Haigis & Sinclair, 2011). Some of these like the mTOR signaling pathway, also play a role in aging-related diseases like Alzheimer's.

Some gene mutations, including those affecting levels of GH or IGF-1, can slow aging and extend lifespan in a way very similar to the effects of CR. Some exogenous compounds, including resveratrol from wine grapes and medications like rapamycin, a drug that suppresses the immune-rejection response to tissue transplants, have also been shown in some studies to mimic the effects of CR, or even to counteract the life-shortening effects of obesity in mice (Pearson et al., 2008; Haigis & Sinclair, 2011; Miller et al., 2011). CR mimics may act by triggering beneficial segments of the metabolic pathways involved in normal responses to CR.

Insulin, IGF-1 signaling, and growth hormone. Insulin and insulin-like growth factors, including IGF-1, are molecular regulators of energy metabolism, development, growth, and stress resistance. Insulin and insulin-like signaling pathways are seen in organisms as distantly related and dissimilar as yeast, worms, flies, mice and humans, and their functions include the modulation of lifespan and aging rate (Tatar, Bartke, & Antebi, 2003; Kopchick, Bartke, & Berryman, 2008). Mutations in genes controlling these processes have been found to cause major alterations in longevity and aging, including the receptor tyrosine kinase, DAF-2, which in turn regulates the forkhead transcription factor, DAF-16, in model organisms from diverse lineages. These cell regulatory pathways are likely to be important in human aging as well. Developmental disruptions of these pathways, as in obesity or fetal malnutrition, are likely to set the stage for aging-related diseases later in life.

GH regulates growth and metabolism in humans and other mammals and plays a major role in glucose metabolism and the determination of lifespan and aging rate (Brown-Borg, 2011, 2014). GH and IGF-1 pathways are highly interrelated, and both have prominent effects on growth rates, adult body size, metabolism, reproduction, and stress resistance. GH deficiencies and gene mutations have been strongly implicated in lifespan extension and slowed aging. Dwarf mouse mutants (Ames and Snell) genetically deficient in GH live much longer than normal lab mice. An artificially engineered transgenic GH-resistant mouse strain, GHR KO (Laron), is significantly smaller and lives up to 55 percent longer than wild-type mice. Interestingly, small body size in general is strongly associated with longer lifespan in a number of species, including mice, dogs, horses, and humans, supporting the idea that lower levels of GH, as well as IGF-1, may slow aging. By the same token, excess GH is associated with a variety of negative health outcomes, including CVD and cancer, as well as shortened life. Lifespan can be severely reduced in humans and mice with high levels of GH. GH therapy is currently being marketed as an antiaging therapy, as evidenced by ads in the popular media, but GH supplementation has never been shown in clinical trials to be beneficial, nor has it been approved by federal regulatory agencies.

TOR pathways. TOR, or target of rapamycin, is a metabolic enzyme that regulates many cell processes including growth, proliferation, motility, and protein synthesis. TOR activity is associated with aging in brewer's yeast, worms, and fruit flies in the laboratory (Kapahi & Kockel, 2011). In laboratory mice, rapamycin (an immunosuppressant drug that inhibits the mammalian counterpart of TOR, mTOR), has been shown reliably to extend lifespan. CR may exert its effects by decreasing TOR activity. Mammalian mTOR signaling has been implicated in the formation of amyloid and tau plaques associated with neuropathology in Alzheimer's disease. Naturally occurring compounds in foods, including resveratrol from wine grapes, curcumin, and caffeine, have been shown to inhibit mTOR in cells in vitro. But so far, no reliable antiaging effect has clearly been established for any nutritional supplement or compound affecting TOR pathways.

Sirtuins. Sirtuins, also known as Sir2 proteins, regulate multiple pathways in a wide taxonomic range of organisms, from bacteria to mammals. They regulate transcription, programmed cell death (apoptosis), and stress responses; they are also involved in mitochondrial energy production (Haigis & Sinclair, 2011). These proteins have been implicated in various aging processes and degenerative diseases, including Alzheimer's, cancer, and CVD. Transgenic lab mice that overexpress the sirtuin SIRT6 have been shown to live longer than controls (Kanfi et al., 2012). Resveratrol, a molecule with the potential to activate SIRT1, occurs naturally in red wine grapes. In some studies with laboratory mice, resveratrol drug mimics have extended lifespan; hence, resveratrol or similar compounds may eventually prove useful for intervening in aging in humans (Ingram et al., 2006; Pearson et al., 2008).

Metabolic Damage and Inflammation

The generation of metabolic energy for life occurs in the mitochondria of cells. During oxidative metabolism, the mitochondria generate unstable free radical molecules and reactive oxygen species (ROS). ROS production is influenced experimentally by calorie intake and other nutritional variables, as well as energetic and environmental demands (Wallace, 2008). ROS function normally in cells as signaling molecules, as well as playing an important role in regulating cell metabolism. They also have the potential to cause oxidative damage to the lipids, proteins, and DNA that make up the vital components of healthy cells, including the mitochondria. One long-standing idea about the origins of aging-related damage comes from research demonstrating that oxidative by-products of normal metabolism cause the types of cellular stress and damage that is associated with the degenerative diseases and functional losses that characterize aging (Harman, 1956; Van Remmen & Richardson, 2001; Muller et al., 2007).

CR has been shown to dampen ROS production and induce defenses against oxidative damage that may protect against cancers and other aging-related diseases. Additional support for the *free radical* and *oxidative damage hypotheses of aging* is provided by findings from mutant lab animal models showing associations between variation in levels of certain antioxidant enzymes, oxidative damage, and key genes that extend lifespan and slow aging (Van Remmen et al., 2004). These relationships, however, have not always been consistent with the prediction that cumulative oxidative damage is a primary cause of aging (see, e.g., Buffenstein et al., 2008).

Mutations in mitochondrial genes can accumulate in various tissues over the life course, causing aging-related declines in energy production, as well as damage and loss of cells, disease and pathophysiology (Allsopp et al., 1995; Kujoth et al., 2005). *The mitochondrial aging hypothesis* is conceptually linked with the free radical and oxidative theories of aging. It proposes that that mitochondrial function deteriorates over the lifespan because of oxidative damage to mitochondrial genes and membranes. Mitochondrial mutations are implicated in many diseases associated with aging, including cancers, Alzheimer's disease, diabetes, ocular cataracts and retinopathy.

Damage to DNA takes place spontaneously in cells of many animal tissues over time. According to the *DNA damage theory of aging*, aging is a consequence of the accumulation of unrepaired damage to nuclear or mitochrondrial DNA (Bohr et al., 2008). Such damage can affect normal cell replicative function, altering apoptosis (adaptive, programmed cell death), or resulting in cell loss, impaired cellular function, or transformation to cancerous cells. Oxidative damage is a proven cause of DNA damage. In humans and lab rodents, moreover, DNA oxidative damage products and breaks have been shown to accumulate with age and to correlate with aging-related memory loss and dementias, among other conditions.

Inflammation, a normal immune response to infection or injury, is another mechanism implicated in aging (Finch, 2007). Inflammatory processes, along with certain types of infections, are associated with many aging-related diseases. Inflammation is implicated in the formation of arterial plaque responsible for atherosclerosis ("hardening of the arteries"), a major component of CVD associated with heart attack and stroke. Obesity is also associated with enhanced levels of inflammation, ROS and reactive nitrogen species, and other primary aging processes (Chung et al., 2009).

Cell Replication and Senescence

Healthy, noncancerous cells maintained in culture, such as human fibroblasts (undifferentiated connective tissue cells), undergo a finite number of replications before reaching the *Hayflick limit*; after this, the cells "senesce" and stop replicating. (Note that this process is distinct from whole-organism aging or senescence.) In some aging-related diseases, like cancer, cells override the normal limits on replication and transform to undergo unregulated proliferation. Healthy cell replication is to a large extent controlled by telomeres and telomerase, as discussed below (Herbig et al., 2004). Certain other key cell-signaling genes, like tumor suppressors, also block the growth of precancerous cells.

Telomeres and telomerase. In vertebrate animals like humans, the ends of chromosomes are capped like the ends of shoelaces with repetitive DNA sequences called telomeres, which aid the cell in the copying of the terminal sequences of linear chromosomes. Small segments of telomeres are used up every time the cell replicates, until a point is reached where replication is no longer possible without serious errors. In healthy cell lines, the loss of telomere length triggers the Hayflick limit on replication and induces cell death. Telomere damage and shortening can be caused by oxidative stress, and some diseases of aging have been linked to changes in telomere length (Effros, 2003).

The enzyme telomerase maintains telomeres, prevents shortening, and sustains replicative potential. Longer, healthy telomeres have been suggested to protect against cancer and other aging-related diseases. Since the dysfunctional proliferation of cells can lead to cancer, and telomerase dysregulation likely plays a role in this, telomerase function has considerable potential as a target for chemotherapy. Some researchers have claimed that telomere length correlates with lifespan variation within populations of organisms or between species, or that it can predict the occurrence of aging-related disease and death. This idea remains controversial, however, and telomere shortening remains to be clearly shown to be a reliable biomarker of aging in any organism (von Zglinicki, Saretsky, & Passos, 2014).

Dysregulation of Physiology and Homeostasis

There is growing consensus that many of the mechanisms described here play some role in aging at least some of the time—others, on the other hand, may apply only in certain species under certain conditions. Oxidative damage, for example, may be important only when healthy regulatory control is lost. Inflammation may be a major cause of aging in modern humans, but is irrelevant in species lacking an inflammatory response. To accommodate the observed species differences in basic aging processes, some researchers have proposed theories of aging that fall under the heading of *complex systems theory*. According to this view, no individual molecule or mechanism plays an exclusive role in aging-related decline. Rather, aging is a higher-order phenomenon arising from failures of complex regulatory systems to maintain healthy organismal functioning, or homeostasis. This theory falls under a rubric that has been given different names, including allostatic load, homeostenosis, and physiological dysregulation (see, e.g., McEwen, 2002; Cohen et al., 2012).

Lifestyle, Health, and Aging

The probability of living a long and healthy life is determined to a significant extent by the genes we inherit from our parents. But the probability of enjoying a long *healthspan* or healthy, functional lifespan is influenced to an even greater extent by social and behavioral factors, including socioeconomic status, educational attainment, the complexity of positive social networks, and lifestyle and self-care patterns. Aging and death are inevitable for humans for the time being, but there is compelling clinical evidence that healthy activity levels, diet and other lifestyle choices, plus good preventive medical care, outweigh genetics in ensuring the likelihood of a long, active, and independent life (Huan et al., 2009).

Smoking and other tobacco use. Cigarette smoking and tobacco use are the number one risk factor for a shortened life. All over the world, smokers have much higher rates of lung cancer and chronic obstructive pulmonary disease (COPD) than nonsmokers. Public health agencies estimate that smoking shortens life by a decade or more, but that stopping smoking—even in middle age—adds healthy years.

Cardiovascular health. Heart attack, stroke, and other forms of CVD are the most common causes of death in older people. Men are at greater risk at all ages than women of dying of heart attack or stroke, but after menopause the risk of CVD in women increases to levels comparable to those in men of similar age. The risk of CVD can be significantly ameliorated by exercise, proper diet, and other healthy lifestyle choices. *Cigarette smoking is the number one risk factor for CVD worldwide, with obesity, poor nutrition, and lack of regular exercise coming in a close second.* Diabetes is also associated with CVD. Regular medical screenings, avoiding high blood pressure and unhealthy levels of blood lipids, as well as certain medications, like blood pressure–reducing drugs and statins, also can substantially reduce the risk of CVD.

Cancer screenings. Early cancer screenings are a proven tool for preventing cancer-related deaths, including screenings for breast, cervical, and colorectal cancers. Appropriately timed clinical screenings save hundreds of thousands of lives. No single, specific food or supplement has been identified that will prevent cancer altogether, but maintaining a healthy body weight and eating a healthy diet rich in fruits, vegetables, and whole grains, along with lean meats, nuts, and fish, undoubtedly helps to minimize cancer risk.

Diabetes prevention and management. Diabetes mellitus is a metabolic disease that involves dysregulated carbohydrate metabolism and abnormally high levels of glucose in blood and other tissues. Diabetes is associated with a number of other diseases of aging, including CVD, peripheral neuropathies, and blindness. Aging and obesity both increase the risk of type 2 (sometimes called "adult onset") diabetes. Early diagnosis and management through weight loss, diet, or medication can markedly decrease the risk of diabetes-related complications in older adults.

Nutrition, body weight, and physical activity. Healthy body weight, good nutrition, and regular physical activity all work together to extend both human lifespan and healthspan. Current dietary recommendations for sustaining health over the lifespan include avoiding excessive consumption of alcohol, good nutrition, regular exercise, and avoiding overnutrition. In half of the states in the United States, the majority of the population is now obese, based on measurement of body mass index. *Obesity is a major risk factor for a number of aging-related diseases, including CVD, cancer, and diabetes.* Regular physical exercise has been shown to be correlated with lower rates of dementias, cancer, and CVD; regular exercise may be even more important than avoiding becoming overweight.

Protection against infection. A hallmark of aging in humans and other mammals is a decline in the ability of the immune system to fight infections, and older adults are at a much greater risk of dying of such diseases as influenza, shingles, and pneumonia. Immunizations against these illnesses are widely available, and they protect older individuals effectively against infections. Hospital-borne, antibiotic-resistant strains of bacteria can be particularly risky to the health of older people.

Accident and frailty prevention. Loss of muscle mass, strength and agility, as well as loss of bone density, can contribute to generalized physiological *frailty syndromes* in older people. Falls and accidents can have especially serious emotional, social, and medical consequences for older adults. People generally fare better at older ages if they stay physically active and engage in activities designed to promote core body stability to prevent falls and other accidents.

Education, social networks, and mental health. There is growing evidence that older people who maintain a variety of family and other social connections are healthier and live longer than those who are isolated and have fewer social connections. The biological basis for this effect is not clear. Older people can be disproportionately prone to anxiety, depression, and negative stressors. Loss of a spouse or social support, isolation, relocation or other changes in living conditions, falls or other medical challenges all can adversely affect mental and physical health. Strategies for preventing, diagnosing, and treating mental illness are essential for sustaining health in older people.

For reasons not completely understood, formal education tends to promote health and longevity. Regular exercise, as well as social and cognitive enrichment, including regular engagement in activities involving memory and learning skills, could play a role in preventing or delaying normal cognitive aging and dementias, including Alzheimer's disease.

Social Variables and the Biology of Aging

The biology of aging may not at first appear to be concerned with social phenomena, nor linked directly to the social sciences. But a deeper look can reveal important, if underemphasized, interdisciplinary connections. Demographers, for example, focus on how human lifespan, mortality patterns, and rates of aging-related disease have changed over the course of history, as well as predicting future demographic change. They relate these changes, in turn, to changes in technology, safety, nutrition, and medicine, for example—that clearly impact human lifespan, disease rates, and other causes of death. Using similar approaches, epidemiologists calculate rates—either observed or projected—of aging-related disease, disability, and death, often contrasting groups within or between populations according to sex and gender influences, race/ethnicity, or socioeconomic and educational status. Gerontologists focusing on long-term demographic, clinical or genetic studies of aging, and or on health and lifespan in human populations identified to be unusually long-lived, often examine relationships among social factors and health—including education levels, familial and other social connections, and so on (Riley et al., 2000; Snowdon et al., 2003; Atzmon et al., 2006; Perls and Sebastiani, 2008; Avery et al., 2014). There is also a relatively recent, emerging focus on gender and sex differences in health, lifespan, and specific aging-related diseases, particularly sex differences in CVD that can lead to heart attack and stroke, as well as the chronic disease and disability that can be caused by disabling conditions like osteoarthritis and osteoporosis (for reviews, see Holmes, 2014; Goldman & Hatch, 1999; Goldman et al., 2013a).

Sex Differences in Aging

All over the world, women not only live longer, but die at lower rates than men of similar ages. This difference in LE is generally on the order of only a few years (reviewed in Austad, 2006; Austad, 2011; United Nations, 2011), but varies among geographical regions of the world. The longest average LEs on record are 86.4 and 79.6 years for Japanese women and men, respectively. The largest sex difference in median lifespans, eight years longer for women, is in the European region as a whole (World Health Organization, 2011). The widest gender gap in mean and median LEs at birth and older ages as a rule is seen in industrialized countries, where women have median LEs at birth up to 7–8 years longer and lifespans for both sexes are extended. In developing societies, where LEs for both sexes are shorter, the female longevity advantage tends to be narrower. The shortest lifespans and smallest female longevity advantages occur in developing, severely economically stressed or politically unstable regions. In Malawi, Africa in the 1990s, for example, mean LE at birth for women was 46.8 years, vs. 43.5 years for men; there were similar sex differences there for LEs at ages 50 and older.

Although death rates converge in men and women in their 60s and 70s, the female longevity advantage persists even at very old ages. The longest absolute lifespans have been recorded for women, as well as the longest averages, and more women than men are now living to reliably documented lifespans 100 years or more. (Note that, as mentioned previously, the world longevity record currently is 122 years. This extreme age was achieved by a Frenchwoman, Jeanne Calment.) This disparity is due in part to the fact that more women remain alive at older ages, increasing the probability of extremes in the data. Lifespans may continue to increase for both sexes, but there is debate currently regarding the upper biological limits to human lifespan (Vaupel, 2010; Olshansky, 2005).

Improvements in public health in industrialized countries have contributed immeasurably to increases in lifespan for both sexes since the mid-1800s. Much—but not all—of these increases can be attributed to lower rates of infant mortality and higher LEs at birth. But LEs at older ages have also increased a great deal. Over the past 100 years or so, as average longevity has increased and the risk of dying at all ages has dropped in industrialized countries, the differential in death rates between males and females has also shifted (Hoyert, 2012). From 1935 to 2010, the overall age-adjusted risk of dying for both sexes in the United States dropped by 60 percent (from 1,860.1 to 746.2 per 100,000 people). During this time, the female survival advantage, expressed as the female/male ratio of annual death rates, increased from 1.2 to 1.7 and then declined to 1.4 in 2010. This shift has been attributed in part to changes in rates of cigarette smoking by women and the associated risks of death and disease.

The persistent sex differential in LEs prompts the question of whether women actually age more slowly than men on a biological level. As noted earlier, aging in a particular population or subpopulation can be detected either as steady declines in survivorship with chronological age or increasing age-specific rates of mortality, as shown in Figure 4.2. To address this question, Austad (2011) compared sex differences in age-specific mortality data from Russian and Japan, two countries with considerably different female longevity advantages. This analysis, featured in Figure 4.3, reveals that the shapes of the mortality curves are quite similar for both sexes in both countries. Hence there is no indication that male and female aging rates differ in either case, suggesting that death rates for males simply start out higher early and remain higher throughout life.

Sex differences in longevity clearly are not unique to humans (see, e.g., Clutton-Brock & Isvaran, 2007). In some other primates, including the chimpanzee, the sex difference in lifespan is even more pronounced, with females also longer-lived (Austad, 2006). Sex differences in aging and LEs can be explained as a by-product of sex-specific evolutionary pressures

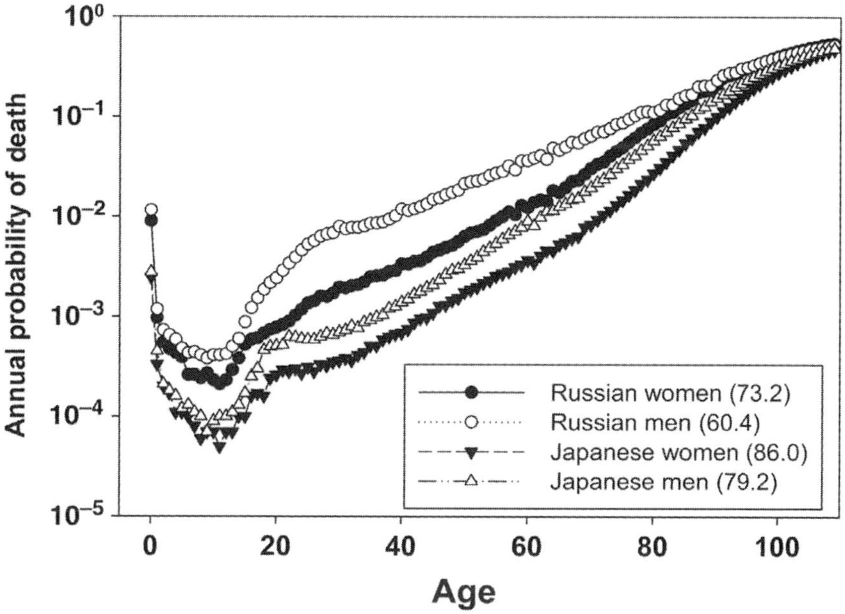

Figure 4.3 Comparison of age-specific mortality rates in men and women in Japan (a long-lived country) and Russia (a short-lived country). Mortality rates are expressed on a logarithmic scale as the annual probability of death. While mortality rates are lower for women than throughout the lifespan in both countries, the slopes of the mortality plots for men and women are similar, indicating that all four groups aged at similar rates. Note also the higher rates of mortality for younger males (especially Russian males). Numbers in parentheses in the legend represent life expectancies at birth. (Reprinted from Austad [2011] with permission. *Data source*: Human Mortality Database. www. mortality.org.)

(reviewed in Austad, 2006; Kruger & Nesse, 2006). Females and males are expected to evolve different strategies for investing in reproduction, and to make different genetic and physiological trade-offs between survival and reproduction to optimize reproductive success, and hence evolutionary fitness, over the entire lifespan (Promislow et al., 1992; Promislow, 2003; reviewed in Bonduriansky et al., 2008). Certain obvious physiological differences that can contribute to aging-related diseases like CVD and some cancers, including levels of hormones and growth factors, likely account at least in part for the lifespan differences seen.

Hormones as Factors in Sex Differences in Aging and Disease

Sex steroid hormones, including estrogen, progesterone, and testosterone, as well as stress hormones and growth factors like IGF-1 and GH, regulate healthy development and reproductive functions, and hence are essential for success in evolutionary terms. But these compounds also are clearly implicated as risk factors for some diseases in older animals and humans, particularly after the peak fertile years. Certain forms of breast cancer, for example, are fueled by estrogen, which promotes the proliferation of healthy cells and tissues, as well. Prostate cancer, a leading cause of death in older men, is promoted by the action of testosterone, a hormone essential for reproduction in the male.

The risks to health and longevity inherent in the hormonal regulation of development and reproduction are complicated, as is inherent in complex biological trade-offs. Under certain physiological circumstances, and at some points in the life cycle, estrogen, for example, has the capacity to protect the cardiovascular system (Moolman, 2006). After menopause, when estrogen production by the ovaries wanes, rates of increased risk for breast and other reproductive cancers for women drop overall, while the risk of death from heart attack and stroke continue to rise. Figures 4.4 and 4.5 show the differences between women and men in rates of aging-related diseases including the top killer, CVD. Men on average develop CVD about 10 years earlier, at around age 45, and are more likely to die of

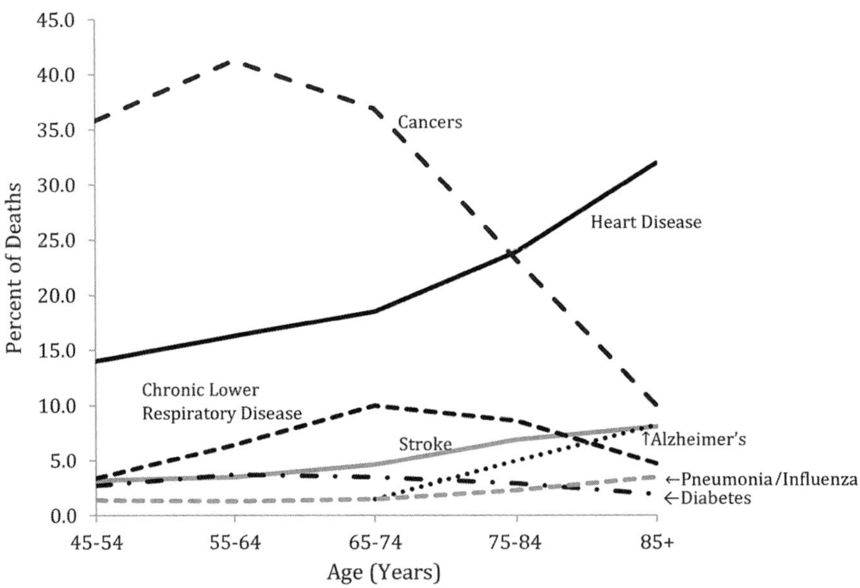

Figure 4.4 Percentage of deaths (prevalence) in women of seven leading causes of death in the United States (all races combined) in 2008. (Note increasing rates of CVD [heart disease and stroke] at older ages. Heron, M. [2012]. Deaths: Leading causes for 2008. *National Vital Statistics Reports, 60*(6): 1–94.)

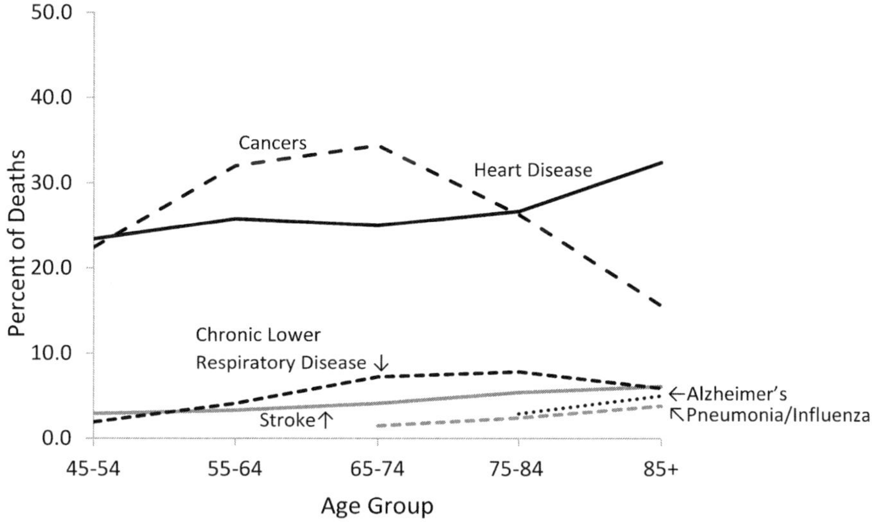

Figure 4.5 Percentage of deaths (prevalence) in men of seven leading causes of death in the United States (all races combined) in 2008. (Note increasing rates of CVD [heart disease and stroke] at older ages. Heron, M. [2012]. Deaths: Leading causes for 2008. *National Vital Statistics Reports, 60*(6): 1–94.)

a heart attack or stroke at all ages combined (Goldman & Hatch, 1999a; Heron, 2012). After menopause, however, women have a greater likelihood of dying from a heart attack, even after receiving similar medical treatment. Additional support for the cardioprotective effects of estrogen comes from the well-documented increased risk of death from CVD in women who undergo an early menopause following either surgical removal of the ovaries or spontaneous early menopause (Mendelsohn & Karas, 2005; Rocca et al., 2006; Stuenkel, 2012; Wellons et al., 2012). Conversely, the higher rates of CVD for adult men of all ages may be attributable, at least in part, to the lack of cardioprotection afforded by estrogen (but see Meilahn, 2000).

There is a large body of evidence suggesting that estrogen and progesterone can be neuroprotective, as well as cardioprotective (Brinton & Nilsen, 2003; Chen et al., 2006; L'Hermite et al., 2008). Estrogen and some progestins have been shown to protect against stroke and damage following traumatic brain injury. Lower levels of endogenous estrogen after menopause have been implicated in some studies in changes in memory and mood, as well as the risk of dementia (Mayeux & Gandy, 1999; Brinton & Nilsen, 2003; Maki & Henderson, 2012). Estrogens can modulate inflammation arising from the tissue damage associated with CVD or dementia, including the formation of atherosclerotic plaque and the brain proteins amyloid and tau that are associated with Alzheimer's disease and other dementias (Mikkola & Clarkson, 2002; Moolman, 2006; Nilsen et al., 2007).

Chromosomes and Sex Differences in Lifespan

An additional explanation suggested to be responsible for the higher vulnerability to mortality in human males is based on the human chromosomal system of sex determination and sex chromosome structure (Trivers, 1985; Bonduriansky et al., 2008). Humans have XY chromosomal sex determination, such that individuals with X and Y sex chromosomes become biological males. In humans, moreover, the X chromosome is much larger than the Y, and carries many more genes. From conception onward, human females (the XX sex) have an advantage over males, since any harmful gene variants on one X chromosome can be compensated for by a normal allele on the second X. Males, in contrast, have no such protection against deleterious gene alleles (Bull, 1983; Marshall Graves, 2008). This system has been invoked to explain, at least in part, males' greater vulnerability to death at all stages of the life cycle, as well as some sex-linked diseases. From a comparative standpoint, however, the relationships between sex determination mechanisms and sex differences in animal lifespans generally are not thoroughly understood, nor do they provide a complete explanation for sex differences in aging, LE, or health in humans.

While the exact biological and social reasons for the longevity advantage in women remain an open question, biologists continue to explore genetic, evolutionary, and physiological factors to explain sex differences in lifespan (reviewed in Austad, 2006, 2011; Holmes & Cohen, 2014). Public health scientists and some sociologists have focused on identifying environmental and cultural factors—including lifestyle and culturally imposed gender roles—that could be contributing to sex differences in health and longevity. No single approach — biological, behavioral, or social — has yet proven satisfactory for explaining these differences. A nuanced combination of some of these, as well as other standpoints, is used by public health scientists and epidemiologists to estimate sex- and gender-related risk factors for specific diseases.

Sex-Based Differences in Disease and Disability Rates

Older people in general show an increased prevalence of aging-related diseases, including CVD, the number one cause of death overall, as well as respiratory disease, cancers, diabetes, dementias, osteoarthritis and sensory deficits, including loss of vision and hearing. Human aging is also associated with loss of reproductive capacity, albeit more gradual in men than in women. The sexes diverge in interesting ways, however, in terms of the age-specific prevalence of, and mortality from, these conditions, as depicted in Figures 4.6 and 4.7 (Kochanek et al., 2011). Since women tend to live longer than and outnumber men in the aging population, the sheer number of older women with aging-related medical conditions is in and of itself an important public health issue (Yang & Leveille, 2013).

Although women tend to live longer and survive at higher rates at all ages than men, they also show higher rates of disabling conditions, including CVD, COPD, osteoarthritis and osteoporosis, blindness and hearing loss; see Figure 4.8: Results of the Cardiovascular Health Study in the United States (in which the effects of age, race, education, and marital status were controlled), which shows that women have higher rates of obesity, arthritis, and CVD, including coronary artery disease, congestive heart failure and stroke, as well as hearing problems, when compared with

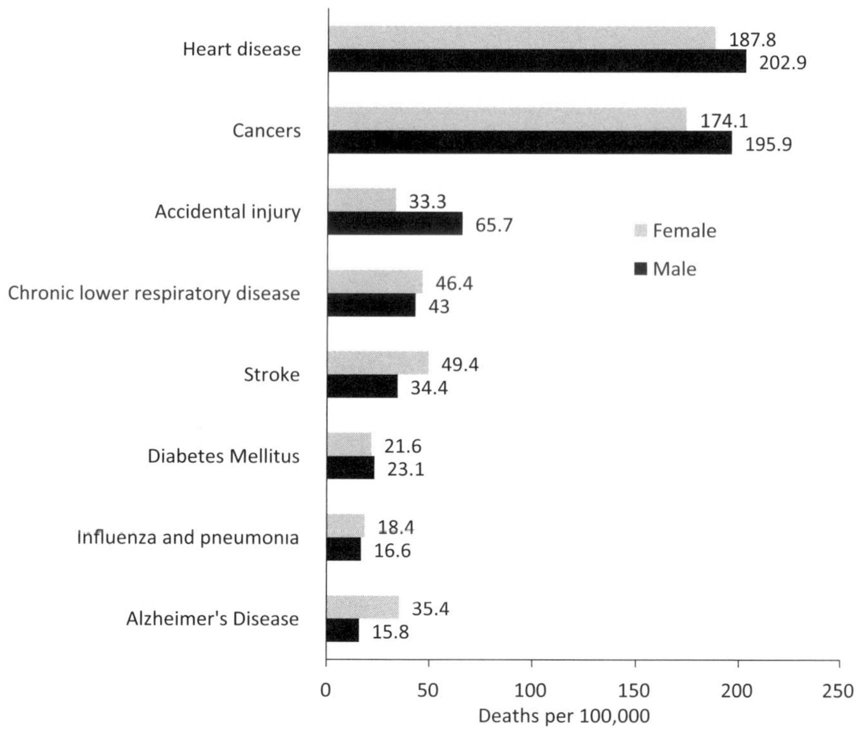

Figure 4.6 Death rates for men and women of different ages from eight of the most deadly diseases of aging in the United States in 2009. (Data are for all races combined, expressed as deaths/100,000 population. Kochanek et al. [2011]. Deaths: Final data for 2009. *National Vital Statistics Reports, 60*(3).)

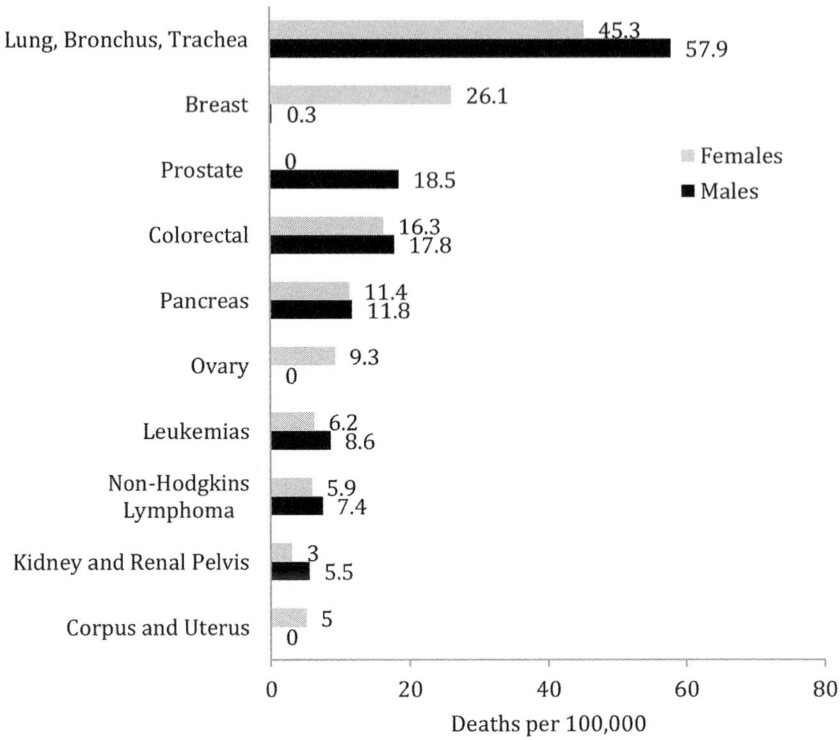

Figure 4.7 Death rates for men and women of different ages from 10 of the most deadly cancers in the United States in 2009. (Data are for all races combined, expressed as deaths/100,000 population. Kochanek et al. [2011]. Deaths: Final data for 2009. *National Vital Statistics Reports, 60*(3).)

men of the same age (Pan et al., 2009; Whitson et al., 2010). Women are also at higher risk of dementia. The drop in estrogen after menopause in midlife provides a plausible biological explanation for sex differences in prevalence of disabling osteoarthritis and osteoporosis. Where the other conditions are concerned, however, the explanation for the sex difference is less clear.

Other reasons for these sex differences in aging-related functional disabilities may include differences in physical training and strength, as well as women's self-perceived functional performance. Men and women have different psychological and social risk factors, as well as differences in their subjective experience of pain, dependency or stress, and these affect their risks of illness and disability. There are also gendered differences in styles of coping with medical issues and in attitudes toward and relationships with the medical system. All of these have the potential to affect sex

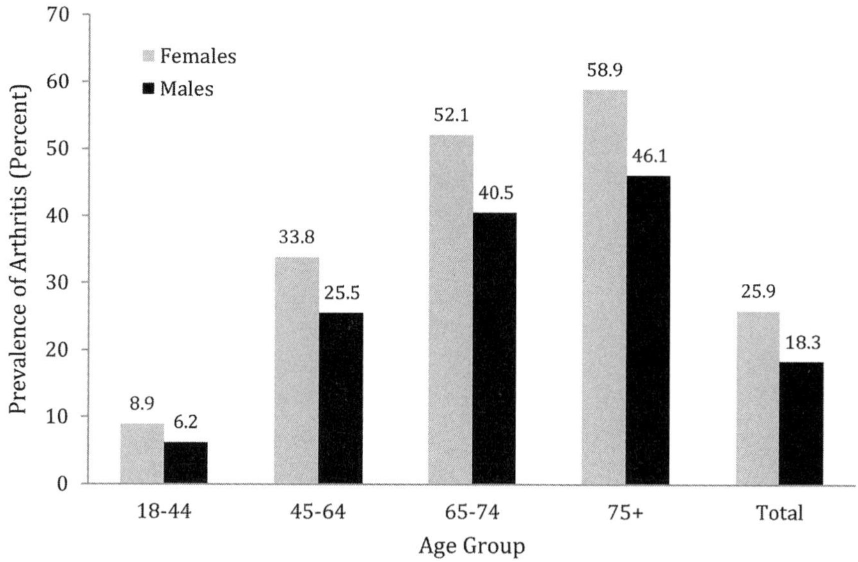

Figure 4.8 Prevalence of osteoarthritis in adult females and males of different age groups in the United States, 2007–2009. Note the higher prevalence of arthritis in older women. Prevalence is calculated as a percentage of each sex who reported they had received a diagnosis of arthritis from a medical provider. (Department of Health and Human Services, Women's Health U.S.A. 2011.)

differences in health, aging, and longevity in complex ways that are still poorly understood.

Obesity has been on the rise since the 1960s in the United States and other industrialized countries. Being significantly overweight is clearly a risk factor for aging-related diseases, including diabetes, CVD, dementias, and cancers. Women are far more likely to be overweight than men, with Hispanic and African American women at even greater risk. Dietary customs and cultural norms for body weight and appearance, as well as education and ideology about health and weight, also contribute significantly to the risk of obesity and associated conditions as women age.

Culture, Health, and Life Expectancy

Culturally influenced norms and behaviors undoubtedly contribute to sex differences in health, aging, and LE. These influences are difficult to separate from biological causes, particularly since they encompass an array of potential influences that includes economic status, education, access to medical support, lifestyle choices, and gender inequities. The causative influences on health of culturally influenced gender differences and roles are extremely complex: they are likely to include influences that are perceived or enacted by individuals, socially enforced, or all three.

Cultural innovations, including medical advances, have had a dramatic influence on human LE in sex- and gender-specific ways. Over the past two centuries, both sexes have exhibited dramatic declines in mortality in infancy (from birth to one year of age), and childhood diseases, as well as increases in LEs after age 50. Until very recent times, mortality from infections or other perinatal complications were major causes of mortality for women (Goldman & Hatch, 1999). Improvements in maternal health, prenatal and antenatal care account for much of the decrease in maternal and infant mortality rates since the mid-1800s. Since the mid-1900s in industrialized cultures, reliable contraceptives have also become widely available. Childbearing is generally delayed, and fertility overall has declined. In contrast, women living in traditional cultures with natural fertility cycles are either pregnant or lactating for most of the reproductive lifespan (Hrdy, 1999; Ellison, 2003). Women in traditional cultures with high rates of parity often have significantly shorter lives, as well (Jasienska, 2013), living beyond menopause only rarely. Since lifespans in industrialized countries now often extend to 80 years and beyond, modern women commonly spend up to a third of their lives in a postreproductive state. The full scope of this culturally produced reproductive shift on women's health is still being weighed, but it is clear that older women with aging-related medical issues comprise a growing segment of the population in industrialized countries. Strategies for sustaining women's health over a longer lifespan should be a major global priority (Goldman & Hatch, 1999a; Goldman, Troisi, & Rexrode, 2013b).

The Women's Health Movement

The women's movement in the United States and Europe brought to light long-standing effects of gender inequality on women's health (Goldman & Hatch, 1999b; Seaman & Wood, 1999; Goldman, Rexrode, & Troisi, 2013a) and stimulated a historical shift toward better access for women and their families to medical care and education, plus respect for our reproductive autonomy and rights to information about health and reproduction. The women's movement has also played a pivotal role in reducing rates of violence against women. Access to reproductive and health education, contraception, and legal abortions have all contributed to reductions in mortality rates of women of reproductive age, as well as infant deaths. Fertility rates have dropped to unprecedented low levels in industrialized countries over the past 50 years, as more women are delaying childbearing. All of these changes, along with longer LEs for women, have shifted dramatically the trajectory of the "normal" female life course, with most women expecting to live well beyond the age of menopause in their early 50s.

Since the 1980s, in the interest of correcting for historical gender bias in medical research and a lack of information on the health of older women, the U.S. National Institutes of Health has undertaken a series of very large, longitudinal studies focused on various aspects of the health of older women. These include the Heart and Estrogen/Progestin Replacement Study, referred to by the acronym HERS, which was designed to examine the effects of hormone replacement therapy on women's cardiovascular health, and the Women's Health Initiative, WHI, a 15-year trial exploring causes of death, disease, and disability in women after menopause. While some of the results of these large clinical studies have been controversial, their size and scope have made them invaluable for understanding health risks in older women.

Men and Mortality

Men are affected by their own sex-specific biological risk factors at older ages. All over the world, men engage in more risky behaviors, and are injured or die violent deaths at higher rates, as shown in Figure 4.9. Men on average are more likely to abuse substances, including tobacco, alcohol

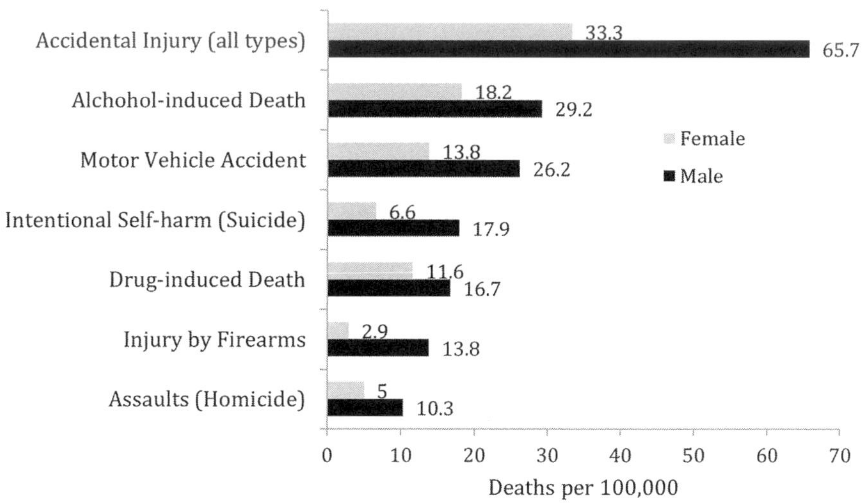

Figure 4.9 Rates of death by accident, substance abuse, or violence in women vs. men in the United States in 2009 (all races combined). (Note the higher rates of death in men by accidents of all types. Kochanek et al. [2011]. Deaths: Final data for 2009. *National Vital Statistics Reports, 60*(3).)

and other drugs, and they die more often from lung cancer, tuberculosis, and liver cirrhosis. Despite a historically male-centered medical paradigm, older men die at higher rates of CVD, including fatal heart attacks. This is, in part, likely to be due to the fact that men are less likely to seek regular medical support. Somewhat surprisingly, while women's rates of depression are higher than men's overall, men commit more suicides. Suicide is a significant risk to younger people, and young men between the ages of 15 and 24 are four to five times more likely to die than women of the same age (Kruger & Nesse, 2006; Austad, 2011).

Married men in the United States live longer, on average, than either single men or married women. Gender roles and other gender-specific social factors continue to change rapidly. More research into the complex interactions among cultural expectations, sex, gender, health, and longevity in both men and women should help to distinguish better among biological and cultural and lifestyle influences.

Gender Roles, Health, and Aging

Social factors with the potential to impact health and longevity include cultural norms and beliefs regarding gender differences and social roles (Goldman & Hatch, 1999b; Rowland Hogue, 2000; Denton et al., 2004; Goldman, Rexrode, & Troisi, 2013a). For example, social and psychosocial determinants of health, like life stressors, social and emotional resources, may play a greater role in women's health, while behavior and lifestyle factors like exercise and smoking, in contrast, seem to be more important for men (see, e.g., Denton & Walters, 1999; Denton et al., 2004). Culturally imposed gender roles can also negatively impact men's health (Verbrugge, 1986; Gryzwacz et al., 2012). The traditional masculine breadwinner role, along with cultural norms for masculinity, likely contributes to the higher risks of accidents, physical injury, participation in violent crime, substance abuse, and suicide affecting men worldwide. Gendered social norms could also help account for the fact that men less often seek medical or social support for health issues (National Center for Vital and Health Statistics, 2001). Men all over the world also smoke more than women and are at greater risk of mortality from lung cancer; note, however, that smoking rates for women are on the rise in many countries.

Discussion and Conclusions

The biology of aging is an integrative, interdisciplinary field unified by common objectives: to understand the basic mechanisms underlying aging and aging-related disease—and, ultimately, to intervene in the aging process to increase healthy human lifespan. While aging and the incidence and age-adjusted prevalences of associated diseases and disabilities clearly vary between men and women, and socially enforced gender roles are likely to underlie some portion of this variation, the actual nature of the interactions between the social and biological factors responsible are still rather poorly understood.

An evolutionary perspective on the biology of aging can be useful for understanding some sex differences in disease risk. Some physiological liabilities, such as the increased risk of cancer associated with reproductive hormones, are likely a result of sex-specific evolutionary trade-offs to maximize successful reproduction. The epidemiological sex steroid hormones are clearly responsible in part for sex differences in some diseases of aging, like reproductive cancers, and osteoporosis; less clear, however, is the part these hormones play in the risk of CVD.

Evolutionary analysis can also help to explain why aging occurs in humans in the first place, as well as why the risks of disease and death increase rapidly after the peak reproductive years have passed. Since the human lifespan in the United States has now increased well past that of our ancestors before the industrial revolution, aging-related health conditions are more likely to be the ultimate cause of death than ever before; the epidemiological shift in the common diseases of aging represents a major social and economic challenge for the new millennium all over the world. Paradoxically, while both LE and healthy lifespan have increased by several decades since 1900, a millennial epidemic of obesity, sedentary lifestyles, and diabetes now poses a new public health challenge. It is becoming increasingly clear that overnutrition and obesity can set the stage very early in life for "diseases of aging" associated with metabolic syndromes, like diabetes and CVD (Finch, 2007; Gluckman et al., 2009). In this sense, some aspects of aging may actually be triggered during prenatal development if the adaptive limits of healthy fetal developmental plasticity are exceeded. It remains to be seen if LEs continue to rise, if these diseases of modern abundance curtail this longevity increase, or if ultimately some intrinsic biological limit to human lifespan is reached.

References

Allard, M., Lebre, V., Robine, J., & Calment, J. (1998). *Jeanne Calment: From Van Gogh's time to ours: 122 extraordinary years*. New York: W. H. Freeman.

Allsopp, R. C., Chang, E., Kashefi-Aazam, M., Rogaev, E. I., Piatyszek, M. A., Shay, J. W., & Harley, C. B. (1995). Telomere shortening is associated with cell division in vitro and in vivo. *Experimental Cell Research, 220*(1), 194–200.

Anderson, R.M., & Weindruch, R. (2012). The caloric restriction paradigm: Implications for healthy human aging. *American Journal of Human Biology, 24*(2), 101–106. doi: 10.1002/ajhb.22243

Atzmon, G., Rincon, M., Schechter, C.B., Shuldiner, A.R., Lipton, R.B., Bergman, A., & Barzilai, N. (2006). Lipoprotein genotype and conserved pathway for exceptional longevity in humans. *PLoS Biology, 4*(4), e113. doi: 10.1371/journal.pbio.0040113

Austad, S.N. (2006). Why women live longer than men: Sex differences in longevity. *Gender Medicine, 3*(2), 79–92.

Austad, S.N. (2011). Sex differences in longevity and aging. In E.J. Masoro & S.N. Austad (Eds.), *Handbook of the biology of aging* (7th ed., pp. 479–495). New York: Academic Press.

Austad, S.N., & Masoro, E.J. (Eds.). (2006). *Handbook of the biology of aging* (6th ed.). New York: Academic Press.

Avery, P., Barzilai, N., Benetos, A., Bilianou, H., Capri, M., Caruso, C., . . . Kolovou, G. (2014). Ageing, longevity, exceptional longevity and related genetic and non-genetic markers: Panel statement. *Current Vascular Pharmacology, 12*(5), 659–661.

Bohr, V., Wilson, D., III, de Souza-Pinto, N., van der Pluijm, I., & Hoeijmakers, J. (2008). DNA repair and aging. In L.P. Guarente, L. Partridge, & D. Wallace (Eds.), *Molecular biology of aging* (pp. 309–346). New York: Academic Press.

Bonduriansky, R., Maklakov, A., Zajitschek, F., & Brooks, R. (2008). Sexual selection, sexual conflict and the evolution of ageing and life span. *Functional Ecology, 22*, 443–453.

Brinton, R.D., & Nilsen, J. (2003). Effects of estrogen plus progestin on risk of dementia. *JAMA-Journal of the American Medical Association, 290*(13), 1706.

Brown-Borg, H.M. (2011). Role of the somatotropic axis in mammalian aging. In E.J. Masoro & S.N. Austad (Eds.), *Handbook of the biology of aging* (7th ed., pp. 25–46). New York: Academic Press.

Brown-Borg, H.M. (2014). Endocrinology of aging and longevity. Reference modules in biomedical sciences. Retrieved from http://dx.doi.org/10.1016/B978-0-12-801238-3.00151-3

Buffenstein, R., Edrey, Y.H., Yang, T., & Mele, J. (2008). The oxidative stress theory of aging: Embattled or invincible? Insights from non-traditional model organisms. *Age (Dordrecht, Netherlands), 30*(2–3), 99–109. doi: 10.1007/s11357-008-9058-z

Bull, J.J. (1983). *Evolution of sex determining mechanisms*. Menlo Park, CA: Benjamin/Cummings.

Butler, R.N., Warner, H.R., Williams, T.F., Austad, S.N., Brody, J.A., Campisi, J., . . . Wright, W.E. (2004). The aging factor in health and disease: The promise of basic research on aging. *Aging Clinical and Experimental Research, 16*(2), 104–111.

Carey, J.R. (1999). Population study of mortality and longevity with Gompertzian analysis. In B.P. Yu (Ed.), *Methods in aging research* (pp. 3–24). New York: CRC.

Chen, S. H., Nilsen, J., & Brinton, R. D. (2006). Dose and temporal pattern of estrogen exposure determines neuroprotective outcome in hippocampal neurons: Therapeutic implications. *Endocrinology, 147*(11), 5303–5313.

Chung, H. Y., Cesari, M., Anton, S., Marzetti, E., Giovannini, S., Seo, A. Y., . . . Leeuwenburgh, C. (2009). Molecular inflammation: Underpinnings of aging and age-related diseases. *Ageing Research Reviews, 8*(1), 18–30. doi: 10.1016/j.arr.2008.07.002

Clutton-Brock, T. H., & Isvaran, K. (2007). Sex differences in ageing in natural populations of vertebrates. *Proceedings of the Royal Society B: Biological Sciences, 274*(1629), 3097–3104.

Cohen, A. A., & Holmes, D. J. (2014). Aging: Evolution. *Elsevier Reference Modules in Biomedical Sciences*. doi: 10.1016/B978-0-12-801238-3.00032-5

Cohen, A. A., Milot, E., Yong, J., Seplaki, C. L., Fülöp, T., Bandeen-Roche, K., & Fried, L. P. (2013). A novel statistical approach shows evidence for multi-system physiological dysregulation during aging. *Mechanisms of Ageing and Development, 134*, 110–117.

Conn, P. M. (Ed.). (2006). *Handbook of models for human aging*. New York: Academic Press.

Crews, D. C. (2003). *Human senescence: Evolutionary and biocultural perspectives*. Cambridge: Cambridge University Press.

de Magalhaes, J. P., & Church, G. M. (2005). Genomes optimize reproduction: Aging as a consequence of the developmental program. *Physiology (Bethesda), 20*, 252–259. doi: 20/4/252 [pii] 10.1152/physiol.00010.2005

Denton, M., Prus, S., & Walters, V. (2004). Gender differences in health: A Canadian study of the psychosocial, structural and behavioural determinants of health. *Social Science and Medicine, 58*, 2585–2600.

Denton, M., & Walters, V. (1999). Gender differences in structural and behavioral determinants of health: An analysis of the social production of health. *Social Science and Medicine, 48*, 1221–1235.

Ellison, P. T. (2003). *On fertile ground: A natural history of human reproduction*. Cambridge, MA: Harvard University Press.

Ellison, P. T. (2005). Evolutionary perspectives on the fetal origins hypothesis. *American Journal Human of Biology, 17*(1), 113–118. doi: 10.1002/ajhb.20097

Effros, R. B. (2003). Genetic alterations in the ageing immune system: Impact on infection and cancer. *Mechanisms of Ageing and Development, 124*, 71–77.

Finch, C. E. (1990). *Longevity, senescence, and the genome*. Chicago, IL: University of Chicago Press.

Finch, C. E. (2007). *The biology of human longevity: Inflammation, nutrition, and aging in the evolution of lifespans*. Amsterdam: Academic (Elsevier).

Gilbert, S., & Epel, D. (2008). *Ecological developmental biology*. Sunderland, MA: Sinauer Associates.

Goldman, M. B., & Hatch, M. C. (1999a). Chapter 1. Overview of women and health. In M. B. Goldman & M. C. Hatch (Eds.), *Women and health*. New York: Academic Press.

Goldman, M. B., & Hatch, M. C. (1999b). *Women and health*. New York: Academic Press.

Goldman, M.B., Troisi, R., & Rexrode, K. (2013a). *Women and health* (2nd ed.). New York: Academic Press.

Goldman, M.B., Troisi, R., & Rexrode, K. (2013b). Women's health in the 21st century. In M.B. Goldman, R. Troisi, & K. Rexrode (Eds.), *Women and health* (2nd ed., pp. 5–19). New York: Academic Press.

Gluckman, P.D., Hanson, M.A., Bateson, P., Beedle, A.S., Law, C.M., Bhutta, Z.A., . . . West-Eberhard, M.J. (2009). Towards a new developmental synthesis: Adaptive developmental plasticity and human disease. *The Lancet, 373*(9675), 1654–1657. doi: S0140-6736(09)60234-8 [pii] 333

Gryzwacz, J.G., Stoller, E.P., Brewer-Lowry, A.N., Bell, R.A., Quandt, S.A., & Arcury, T.A. (2012). Gender and health lifestyle: An in-depth exploration of self-care activities in later life. *Health Education and Behavior, 39*, 332–340.

Guarente, L., Partridge, L., & Wallace, D.C., (Eds.). (2008). *Molecular biology of aging*. New York: Cold Spring Harbor Laboratory Press.

Haigis, M.C., & Sinclair, D.A. (2011). Sirtuins in aging and age-related diseases. In E.J. Masoro & S.N. Austad (Eds.), *Handbook of the biology of aging* (7th ed., pp. 243–274). New York: Academic Press.

Hales, C., & Barker, D. (1992). Type 2 (non-insulin-dependent) diabetes mellitus: The thrifty phenotype hypothesis. *Diabetologia, 35*, 595–601.

Ham, R., Sloane, P., Warshaw, G., Potter, J., & Flaherty, E. (2014). *Ham's primary care geriatrics: A case-based approach* (6th ed.). New York: Elsevier Health Sciences.

Harman, D. (1956). Aging: A theory based on free radical and radiation chemistry. *Journal of Gerontology, 11*(3), 298–300.

Herbig, U., Jobling, W.A., Chen, B.P., Chen, D.J., & Sedivy, J.M. (2004). Telomere shortening triggers senescence of human cells through a pathway involving ATM, p53, and p21(CIP1), but not p16(INK4a). *Molecular Cell, 14*(4), 501–513. doi: S1097276504002564 [pii]

Heron, M. (2012). Deaths: Leading causes for 2008. *National Vital Statistics Reports, 60*(6): 1–94. Retrieved from http://www.ncbi.nlm.nih.gov/pubmed/22827019

Holmes, D. (2014). Sex and gender differences in life span, aging, and health. *Elsevier Reference Modules in Biomedical Sciences*. October 15, 2014. doi: 10.1016/B978-0-12-801238-3.00161-6

Holmes D.J., & Cohen A.A. (2014). Overview: Aging and gerontology. Reference Module in *Biomedical Sciences*. Elsevier. October 15, 2014. doi: 10.1016/B978-0-12-801238-3.00149-5

Hoyert, D.L. (2012). *75 years of mortality in the United States, 1935–2010*. (No. 88). Hyattsville, MD: National Center for Health Statistics.

Hrdy, S.B. (1999). *Mother nature: A history of mothers, infants, and natural selection*. New York: Pantheon.

Huan, J., Chang, M.D., Burke, A.E., & Glass, R.M. (2009). Preventive health care for older adults. *Journal of the American Medical Association, 302*(24), 2722. doi: doi:10.1001/jama.302.24.2722

Ingram, D.K., Nakamura, E., Smucny, D., Roth, G.S., & Lane, M.A. (2001). Strategy for identifying biomarkers of aging in long-lived species. *Experimental Gerontology, 36*(7), 1025–1034.

Jasienska, G. (2013). *The fragile wisdom: An evolutionary view on women's biology and health*. Cambridge, MA: Harvard University Press.

Kanfi, Y., Naiman, S., Amir, G., Peshti, V., Zinman, G., Nahum, L., . . . Cohen, H.Y. (2012). The sirtuin SIRT6 regulates lifespan in male mice. *Nature, 483*(7388), 218–221. doi: 10.1038/nature10815

Kapahi, P., & Kockel, L. (2011). TOR: A conserved nutrient-sensing pathway that determines life-span across species. In E.J. Masoro & S.N. Austad (Eds.), *Handbook of the biology of aging* (7th ed., pp. 203–214). New York: Academic Press.

Kennedy, B.K., Berger, S.L., Brunet, A., Campisi, J., Cuervo, A.M., Epel, E.S., . . . Sierra, F. (2014). Geroscience: Linking aging to chronic disease. *Cell, 159*(4), 709–713. doi: 10.1016/j.cell.2014.10.039

Kirkwood, T.B., & Austad, S.N. (2000). Why do we age? *Nature, 408*(6809), 233–238. doi: 10.1038/35041682

Kochanek, A.R., Xu, J., Murphy, S.L., Minino, A.M., & Kung, H. (2011). Deaths: Final data for 2009. *National Vital Statistics Reports, 60*(3).

Kopchick, J., Bartke, A., & Berryman, D. (2008). Extended life span in mice with reduction in the GH/IGF-1 axis. In L. Guarente, L. Partridge, & D. Wallace (Eds.), *Molecular biology of aging* (pp. 347–370). New York: Academic Press.

Kruger, D.J., & Nesse, R.M. (2006). An evolutionary life-history framework for understanding sex differences in human mortality rates. *Human Nature, 17*, 74–97.

Kujoth, G.C., Hiona, A., Pugh, T.D., Someya, S., Panzer, K., Wohlgemuth, S.E., . . . Prolla, T.A. (2005). Mitochondrial DNA mutations, oxidative stress, and apoptosis in mammalian aging. *Science, 309*(5733), 481–484.

L'Hermite, M., Simoncini, T., Fuller, S., & Genazzani, A.R. (2008). Could transdermal estradiol plus progesterone be a safer postmenopausal HRT? A review. *Maturitas, 60*(3–4), 185–201.

Lithgow, G.J. (2013). Origins of geroscience. *Public Policy & Aging Report, 23*(4), 10–11.

Mayeux, R., & Gandy, S. (1999). Alzheimer's disease. In M.B. Goldman & M.C. Hatch (Eds.), *Women and health* (pp. 1228–1238). New York: Academic Press.

Maki, P.M., & Henderson, V.W. (2012). Hormone therapy, dementia, and cognition: The Women's Health Initiative 10 years on. *Climacteric, 15*(3), 256–262.

Marshall Graves, J.A. (2008). Weird animal genomes and the evolution of vertebrate sex and sex chromosomes. *Annual Review of Genetics, 42*, 565–586.

Masoro, E.J., & Austad, S.N., Eds. (2005). *Handbook of the biology of aging* (6th ed.). New York: Academic Press.

McDonald, R.B. (2014). *Biology of aging*. New York: Garland Science, Taylor and Francis Group.

McEwen, B.S. (2002). Sex, stress and the hippocampus: Allostasis, allostatic load and the aging process. *Neurobiology of Aging, 23*(5), 921–939.

Meilahn, E. (2000). Hormonal milieu and heart disease. In M.B. Goldman & M.C. Hatch (Eds.), *Women and Health* (pp. 782–788). New York: Academic Press.

Mendelsohn, M.E., & Karas, R.H. (2005). Molecular and cellular basis of cardiovascular gender differences. *Science, 308*, 1583–1587.

Mikkola, T. S., & Clarkson, T. B. (2002). Estrogen replacement therapy, atherosclerosis and vascular function. *Cardiovascular Research, 53*(605–619).

Miller, R. A. (2001). Biomarkers of aging: Prediction of longevity by using age-sensitive T-cell subset determinations in a middle-aged, genetically heterogeneous mouse population. *The Journals of Gerontology, Series A: Biological Sciences and Medical Sciences, 56*(4), B180–186.

Miller, R., Harrison, D., Astle, C., Baur, J., Boyd, A., de Cabo, R., . . . Strong, R. (2011). Rapamycin, but not resveratrol or simvastatin, extends life span of genetically heterogeneous mice. *The Journals of Gerontology, Series A: Biological Sciences and Medical Sciences, 66A*(2), 191–201.

Moolman, J. (2006). Unravelling the cardioprotective mechanism of action of estrogens. *Cardiovascular Research, 69*(2006), 777–780.

Muller, F. L., Lustgarten, M. S., Jang, Y., Richardson, A., & Van Remmen, H. (2007). Trends in oxidative aging theories. *Free Radical Biology and Medicine, 43*(4), 477–503.

National Center for Vital and Health Statistics. (2001). Utilization of ambulatory care by women: United States, 1997–1998. *National Center for Vital and Health Statistics, Series 13*, 149.

Nilsen, J., Irwin, R. W., Gallaher, T. K., & Brinton, R. D. (2007). Estradiol in vivo regulation of brain mitochondrial proteome. *Journal of Neuroscience, 27*(51), 14069–14077.

Olshansky, S. J. (2005). Projecting the future of U.S. health and longevity. *Health Affairs (Millwood), 24*(Suppl. 2), W5R86–W5R89. doi: 10.1377/hlthaff.w5.r86

Olshansky, S. J., & Ault, A. B. (1986). The fourth stage of the epidemiologic transition: The age of delayed degenerative diseases. *Milbank Quarterly, 64*(3), 355–391.

Olshansky, S. J., Carnes, B., Rogers, R. G., & Smith, L. (1997). Infectious diseases—New and ancient threats to world health. *Population Bulletin, 52*(2), 1–52.

Pan, L., Galuska, D. A., Sherry, B., Hunter, A. S., Rutledge, G. E., Dietz, W. H., & Balluz, L. S. (2009). Differences in prevalence of obesity among black, white, and Hispanic Adults—United States, 2006–2008. *Morbidity and Mortality Weekly Report, 58*, 740–744.

Partridge, L., Gems, D., & Withers, D. J. (2005). Sex and death: What is the connection? *Cell, 120*(4), 461–472. doi: S0092-8674(05)00100-5 [pii] 10.1016/j.cell.2005.01.026

Pearson, K., Baur, J., Lewis, K., Peshkin, L., Price, N., Navas, P., . . . de Cabo, R. (2008). Resveratrol delays age-related deterioration and mimics aspects of dietary restriction in mice on a standard diet. *Cell Metabolism, 8*(2), 157–168.

Perls, T. T., & Sebastiani, P. (2008). Genetics of exceptional longevity. In L. Guarente, L. Partridge, & D. Wallace (Eds.). *Molecular biology of aging* (pp. 517–544). New York: Academic Press.

Preston, S. H., Heuvelein, P., & Guillot, M. (2001). *Demography: Measuring and modeling population processes*. Oxford: Wiley-Blackwell.

Promislow, D. E. L. (2003). Mate choice, sexual conflict, and evolution of senescence. *Behavior Genetics, 33*, 191–201.

Promislow, D. E. L., Montgomerie, R. D., & Martin, E. (1992). Mortality costs of sexual dimorphism in birds. *Proceedings of the Royal Society of London Series B. Biological Sciences, 250*, 143–150.

Tatar, M., Bartke, A., & Antebi, A. (2003). The endocrine regulation of aging by insulin-like signals. *Science, 299*, 1346–1351.

Riley, K.P., Snowdon, D.A., Saunders, A.M., Roses, A.D., Mortimer, J.A., & Nanayakkara, N. (2000). Cognitive function and apolipoprotein E in very old adults: Findings from the Nun Study. *The Journals of Gerontology, Series B: Psychological Sciences and Social Sciences, 55*(2), S69–S75.

Rocca, W.A., Grossardt, B.R., de Andrade, M., Malkasian, G.D., & Melton, J. (2006). Survival patterns after oophorectomy in premenopausal women: A population-based cohort study. *The Lancet, 7*, 821–828.

Rose, M.R. (1991). *Evolutionary biology of aging*. New York: Oxford University Press.

Rowland Hogue, C.J. (2000). Gender, race, and class: From epidemiological association to etiologic hypotheses. In M.B. Goldman & M.C. Hatch (Eds.), *Women and health* (pp. 15–23). New York: Academic Press.

Seaman, B., & Wood, S.F. (1999). Role of advocacy groups in research on women's health. In M.B. Goldman & M.C. Hatch (Eds.), *Women and health* (pp. 27–35). New York: Academic Press.

Snowdon, D. A. (1990). Early natural menopause and the duration of postmenopausal life. Findings from a mathematical model of life expectancy. *Journal of the American Geriatrics Society, 38*(4), 402–408. Retrieved from http://www.ncbi.nlm.nih.gov/pubmed/2329249

Sonntag, W.E., Csiszar, A., deCabo, R., Ferrucci, L., & Ungvari, Z. (2012). Diverse roles of growth hormone and insulin-like growth factor-1 in mammalian aging: Progress and controversies. *The Journals of Gerontology, Series A: Biological Sciences and Medical Sciences, 67*(6), 587–598. doi: 10.1093/gerona/gls115

Stearns, S. C., & Koella, J. C. (Eds.). (2008). *Evolution in health and disease* (2nd ed.). New York: Oxford University Press.

Stuenkel, C. (2012). Cardiovascular risk and menopause: Cause or consequence? *Menopause, 19*, 1067–1069.

Suh, Y., Atzmon, G., Cho, M.O., Hwang, D., Liu, B., Leahy, D.J., . . . Cohen, P. (2008). Functionally significant insulin-like growth factor I receptor mutations in centenarians. *Proceedings of the National Academy of Sciences of the United States of America, 105*(9), 3438–3442. doi: 0705467105 [pii] 10.1073/pnas.0705467105

Trivers, R.L. (1985). *Social evolution*. Menlo Park, CA: Benjamin/Cummings.

United Nations. (2011). *2009–2010 United Nations demographic yearbook*. New York: United Nations.

Van Remmen, H., Qi, W., Sabia, M., Freeman, G., Estlack, L., Yang, H., . . . Richardson, A. (2004). Multiple deficiencies in antioxidant enzymes in mice result in a compound increase in sensitivity to oxidative stress. *Free Radical Biology and Medicine, 36*(12), 1625–1634.

Van Remmen, H., & Richardson, A. (2001). Oxidative damage to mitochondria and aging. *Experimental Gerontology, 36*(7), 957–968.

Vaupel, J.W. (2010). Biodemography of human ageing. *Nature, 464*(7288), 536–542. doi: 10.1038/nature08984

Verbrugge, L. M. (1986). Role burdens and physical health of women and men. *Women and Health, 11*, 47–77.

Von Zglinicki, T., Saretsky, G., & Passos, J. (2014). Aging and telomeres. Reference Module in Biomedical Sciences. Retrieved from http://www.sciencedirect.com/science?_ob=ArticleListURL&_method=list&_ArticleListID=-816858873&_sort=r&_st=13&view=c&md5=153b6e46123ed908b38b5fbe397244d0&searchtype=a

Wallace, D. (2008). The human mitochondrion and pathophysiology of aging and aging-related diseases. In L. Guarente, L. Partridge, & D. Wallace (Eds.), *Molecular biology of aging* (pp. 1–38). Cold Spring Harbor, NY: Cold Spring Harbor Press.

Weindruch, R., & Walford, R.L. (1988). *The retardation of aging and disease by dietary restriction*. Springfield, IL: Charles C. Thomas.

Wellons, M., Ouyang, P., Schreiner, P., Herrington, D., & Vaidya, D. (2012). Early menopause predicts future coronary heart disease and stroke: The Multi-ethnic Study of Atherosclerosis. *Menopause, 19*(10), 1081–1087.

Whitson, H.E., Landerman, L.R., Newman, A.B., Fried, L.P., Pieper, C.F., & Cohen, H.J. (2010). Chronic medical conditions and the sex-based disparity in disability: The Cardiovascular Health Study. *The Journals of Gerontology, Series A: Biological Sciences and Medical Sciences, 65*(12), 1325–1331. doi: 10.1093/gerona/glq139

U.S. Department of Health and Human Services, Health Resources and Services Administration. (2011). *Women's health U.S.A., 2011*. U.S. Department of Health and Human Services.

World Health Organization. (2011). *World health statistics 2011*. Geneva: World Health Organization.

Yang, F.M., & Leveille, S.G. (2013). Morbidity, disability and mortality. In M.B. Goldman, R. Troisi, & K. Rexrode (Eds.), *Women and health* (2nd ed.). New York: Academic Press.

CHAPTER FIVE

Leading Causes of Morbidity and Mortality among Older Americans

Anna Zajacova and Vicki Johnson-Lawrence

The population of the United States is aging. By 2050, the number of adults aged 65 and older is projected to be 88.5 million, more than double compared to the 40.2 million in 2010 (Vincent and Velkoff 2010). This growth is driven by the large baby boomer cohorts born in 1946–1964, who started to turn 65 in 2011 (Ortman, Velkoff and Hogan 2014). As a proportion of the total population, adults 65 or older are projected to grow to 20 percent from the current 14 percent, and barely 5 percent in the early 20th century (Johnson et al. 2014). As medical and social interventions added *years to life*, drastically increasing life expectancy in the 20th century, the task now is to add *life to years* and improve the quality of life and health of the American older adults.

While today's older adults are healthier than ever before by most measures, health deteriorates at an accelerating pace with age. The prevalence of chronic disease, functional limitations, disability, and the risk of dying all increase with older age (NCHS 2013). The increasing rate of morbidity at old age, combined with the increasing size of older populations, significantly influence American lives: there is an increased burden on the health-care system, accompanied by the economic costs of medical care, as well as increased caregiving and economic burden on families and individuals called on to manage and control the long-term conditions and functional impairments of older Americans.

Chronic conditions such as heart disease, diabetes, cancer, and arthritis have profound systemic and person-level implications for the U.S.

health-care system as well as the well-being of older adults and their caregivers. The United States spends more on health care, both in dollars and as a proportion of GDP, than any other country in the world (WHO 2015a), but life expectancy and other key indicators of population health show worse outcomes than most other developed countries. About 75 percent of U.S. health-care spending is on patients with chronic conditions (CDC 2009a). This is in part because older adults are more likely to have chronic conditions, as well as experience other health problems that combine to make treatment more costly. For instance, the average medical expenditures are estimated to be 2.3 times higher for adults with diagnosed diabetes compared to adults without diabetes (CDC 2014). It is estimated that the direct medical expenditures exceed $313 billion annually for cardiovascular disease including stroke, $100 billion for cancer, $116 billion for diabetes, and $81 billion for arthritis (CDC 2009a). Total costs, including direct medical costs and indirect costs such as employment losses, disability, and premature deaths, are higher still. For example, the total cost of diabetes is estimated to be $245 billion annually (CDC 2014).

Definitions, Measurement, Data Sources

Health is a complex, multidimensional construct defined as a state of complete physical, mental, and social well-being and not merely the absence of disease or infirmity (World Health Organization 1948). Especially when we focus on older adults in developed countries, we often consider and measure two major dimensions of health status: (1) diseases, especially chronic conditions like heart disease and diabetes and (2) physical limitations and disability. *Morbidity* sometimes refers to both dimensions but usually refers specifically to diseases. In this chapter, we use morbidity to refer to diseases. We focus on six leading causes of morbidity: heart disease, cancer, diabetes, arthritis, chronic lower respiratory disease, and Alzheimer's, as well as their main health-behavioral antecedents.

Activity limitations and disability are critical aspects of health and important correlates of mortality (Üstün 2010). *Activity limitations* refer to difficulties a person may have in various activities due to physical or mental health problems. Limitations are often captured with activities of daily living (ADLs) and instrumental activities of daily living (IADLs). ADLs include basic self-care activities like bathing, dressing, or getting in and out of bed. IADLs comprise more complex activities critical for independent living, such as shopping, preparing meals, managing finances, and housework. *Disability* is a broad term that indicates the inability to carry out social roles due to underlying health limitations—it reflects a gap between the requirements of a social role and an individual's capacity within a particular environment. A discussion of limitations and disability is beyond the scope of this chapter. Interested readers can consult excellent studies of limitations and disability trends and disparities among older adults (Martin et al. 2010, Martin and Schoeni 2014, Schoeni et al. 2005, Schoeni, Freedman and Martin 2008, Seeman et al. 2010).

Mortality refers to death. Demographers have developed numerous ways to measure mortality, but the most intuitive measure is life expectancy. *Life expectancy* at birth represents the number of years an individual can expect to live assuming they experience the age-specific death rates present in the year of birth throughout their lives (Murphy, Xu and Kochanek 2013). Life expectancy is often used to indicate the overall health of a population (NCHS 2014).

Older adults, in this chapter, are defined as those 65 years or older unless indicated otherwise. As for *race/ethnicity*, the major groups in the United States are non-Hispanic white, non-Hispanic black, Hispanic, Asian or Pacific Islander (API), and American Indian or Alaska Native (AIAN). In this chapter, we largely focus on the first three groups. Many surveys do not include enough respondents from the last two groups to enable reliable estimates. For instance, for mortality estimates, it is estimated that the API and AIAN populations are underreported in death certificates by 7 percent for API and 30 percent for AIAN populations, making comparisons problematic (Murphy, Xu and Kochanek 2013).

Data Sources

The majority of statistics reported in this chapter are from large, national community-based population surveys such as the National Health Interview Surveys (NHIS), or from mortality statistics collected by the National Center for Health Statistics (NCHS). Morbidity information is self-reported in the surveys and has associated strengths and limitations. The strengths are that people know about their conditions and the surveys would be prohibitively expensive if morbidity data had to be measured or medical records collected. The limitations include systematic differences in reporting that may result in over reporting or underreporting of conditions, as well as differences in the definitions of chronic conditions across surveys. When studying older adults, national surveys present an additional barrier, in that they are often designed to represent the noninstitutionalized population. In other words, the surveys exclude adults in institutions such as nursing homes, which has the potential to underestimate the health problems among older adults, especially the oldest-old. About 4 percent of the older population—aged 65 and more—live in an institutional setting and thus are omitted from many national surveys. The proportion is strongly dependent on age so that the percentage of institutionalized individuals increases from about 1 percent among those aged 65–74 to 15 percent among those aged 85–94 and 33 percent among those aged 95 or older (Redfoot, Houser and AARP Public Policy Institute 2010). Some health problems are similar among community-dwelling older adults and their institutionalized counterparts—such as hypertension, heart disease, arthritis, and diabetes being among leading conditions—but there are also important differences. For instance, Alzheimer's disease and other dementias represent the second most prevalent set of conditions among residential-care persons, at 42 percent (Caffrey et al. 2012). Alzheimer's disease statistics are drawn from sources other than the self-reports in NHIS because too high a proportion of Alzheimer's patients live in institutional settings and thus are missed by the survey. This suggests that some statistics presented here may underestimate the *burden of disease*—the total impact of the health problems that encompasses morbidity, mortality, but also financial and other costs—among older Americans.

Conceptual Framework

Frameworks that tie together different parts of the morbidity and mortality process have been developed. Link and Phelan's (1996,1995) *Fundamental Causes* theory focuses on the key role of the underlying socioeconomic factors in shaping health—socioeconomic status (SES), operating through myriad mechanisms, shapes access to resources, including resources to maintain or improve health. Low SES means few resources to obtain desirable goods including health, putting people at *risk for risks* (Link and Phelan 1995): for instance, low SES puts individuals at risk for smoking via increased stress, fewer healthier alternatives to cope with the stressors, higher prevalence of smoking within one's social network that influences our own behavior, and increased advertising for cigarettes in low-income neighborhoods.

Other frameworks focus on the process from morbidity to disability (see Figure 5.1). In the 1960s, Nagi proposed a *Disablement Process* framework to describe the complex dynamic process of disablement, whereby an active pathology such as chronic illness leads to impairment—an abnormality at the organ or system level, which in turn may lead to activity limitations and disability (Nagi 1965, 1976). This framework does not imply direct causal effects from one factor to another. It also does not imply unidirectionality of effects or even time-dependency of the factors. The framework is a conceptual tool to consider the upstream factors from structural social influences to individual health behaviors and their links to health and longevity.

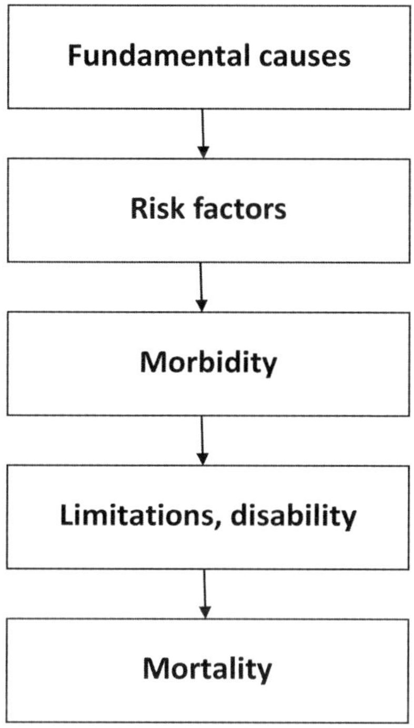

Figure 5.1 Conceptual framework (Authors' figure based on conceptualizations by Nagi [1965, 1976] and Verbrugge and Jette [1994] and Link and Phelan [1995])

For readers interested in a detailed treatment of the disablement process, we suggest the following sources for more information (Freedman, Martin and Schoeni 2002, Freedman et al. 2007, Manton, Gu and Lamb 2006, Martin, Schoeni and Andreski 2010, Martin and Schoeni 2014, Nagi 1965, 1976, Schoeni et al. 2005, Seeman et al. 2010, Verbrugge 1986, Verbrugge and Jette 1994).

Risk Factors for Morbidity and Mortality

Behavioral risk factors include smoking, alcohol use, physical activity, diet and nutrition, as well as a range of other behaviors such as avoiding impaired driving and use of seat belts. Four health behaviors—tobacco use, alcohol use, physical activity, as well as diet and nutrition—are linked to most burdens of chronic disease among American adults (CDC 2009a). Health behaviors are further tightly linked to biological risk factors such as obesity, blood pressure, and cholesterol levels. We will address the health behaviors and biological risk factors below; however, first a brief discussion of fundamental determinants of health is necessary.

Fundamental Determinants of Health

Underneath the individual level health-behavioral factors lie deeper, structural fundamental causes (Link and Phelan 1995). It is critical to consider these causes to recognize that the choices about health behaviors do not occur in a social vacuum but are structured and constrained by social factors (Cockerham 2005). These factors include SES of individuals and societal inequalities in access to resources, environmental factors such as presence of parks and safe sidewalks, health-care access and quality, community programs to enhance health, and a host of other influences that will enable making healthy choices—such as the availability of farmers' markets or supermarkets, public transportation, or reduced exposure to second-hand smoking or lead in household paint (Johnson et al. 2014, Link and Phelan 1995, Wilkinson 1996, Wilkinson and Marmot 2003).

At an even more fundamental level, health disparities are caused by social inequalities in access to resources (Link et al. 1998, Link and Phelan 1995). The factors noted above, such as safe and healthy environments, access to healthy diet, help with smoking cessation, are not distributed equally in the population. Social status, whether captured with education, income, or occupational prestige, is tightly linked with access to these types of resources and thus to health. It is therefore critical to always consider the underlying fundamental factors that shape access to resources for some and put others at *risk for risks*, which makes it easier for some compared to others to follow healthy lifestyles and minimize health risks.

Key mechanisms through which the fundamental effects of social status influence risk factors for morbidity and mortality include social stress and social support (Pearlin 1989). While there is a complex cognitive-emotional process through which stressors translate into perceived stress (Lazarus and Folkman 1984), in general stress impacts mental and physical health (Thoits 1995). The role of stress in health disparities has long been recognized (Antonovsky 1979). Numerous studies have documented a greater number of stressors among lower social classes; moreover, these stressors tend to be more enduring over time (Aneshensel 1992, Turner, Wheaton and Lloyd 1995). For nonwhite adults, the ongoing daily stress of racism contributes an additional salient burden on their health (Clark et al. 1999).

Health Behaviors

Health behaviors comprise a large set of mechanisms through which fundamental factors such as SES influence health. While health behaviors have been the focus of much public health intervention, it is necessary to contextualize these behaviors within the fundamental social factors in order to both understand them better and ultimately to design more effective prevention programs (Link and Phelan 1995, 1996, Link et al. 1998).

Tobacco Use

Tobacco use, primarily smoking, is the leading preventable cause of death among American adults. This behavior remains the leading cause of preventable morbidity and mortality, causing over 440,000 premature deaths (CDC 2008) and over $330 billion in direct and indirect costs annually (Mozaffarian et al. 2015).

The good news is that smoking has declined over time: at its prevalence peak in 1965, 42 percent of U.S. adults smoked as compared to just under 20 percent in 2011 (Garrett et al. 2011). The declining trends were particularly pronounced for men: among older men, for instance, 29 percent smoked in 1965, compared to 10 percent in 2011—the rates for older women have remained relatively constant, decreasing in that same time period slightly from 10 percent to 9 percent (FIFARS 2012). As the statistics above indicate, smoking is less prevalent at older ages—while 23 percent of adults 25–44 are smokers, so are 13 percent of those aged 65–74, and 6 percent of those aged 75 and older (Schoenborn, Adams and Peregoy 2013). Unfortunately, the progress on smoking has slowed or stalled in recent years. Smoking remains high in low-SES groups, as 6 percent of adults with postbaccalaureate education smoke, in contrast to 24 percent of those with less than a high school diploma, and a staggering 41 percent among general educational development (GED) recipients (Jamal et al. 2014).

Smoking has a strong SES gradient: low-educated and low-income adults are substantially more likely to smoke than their more-educated and higher-income counterparts. In terms of race/ethnicity, 22 percent of non-Hispanic white adults and 20 percent non-Hispanic black adults smoke, compared to 14 percent of Hispanic adults or 10 percent Asian Americans (Schoenborn, Adams and Peregoy 2013). Due to a complex set of social influences, women have always smoked less than men (Waldron 1991). The gender difference was particularly pronounced in the mid-1960s when about 33 percent of women and 52 percent of men smoked; since then, smoking declined to a prevalence rate of 15 percent among women and 20 percent among men (Garrett et al. 2011, Jamal et al. 2014).

Alcohol Use

Moderate alcohol use is likely not problematic and may even be beneficial to health (Rehm et al. 2003), but heavy regular use or binge-pattern use is detrimental to health. Excessive alcohol use is associated with nearly 90,000 deaths annually (CDC 2013a). The two main causes of death were alcoholic liver disease and motor vehicle accidents, but heavy alcohol use is a contributing factor to other causes of death as well. Economic costs of excessive alcohol use were estimated in 2006 to exceed $220 billion annually. This amount comprised loss of productivity, health-care costs, criminal justice costs, and losses in other economic areas (Bouchery et al. 2011).

Alcohol use declines with age. Among adults aged 65–74, 52 percent are current drinkers; at ages 75 and older, only 39 percent use alcohol (Schoenborn, Adams and Peregoy 2013). Yet, 8 percent of adults aged 65–74 report at least one episode of binge drinking—defined as having five or more drinks in a day—during the previous year. The race/ethnic and socioeconomic patterns in alcohol use are complex because the relationships pertaining to moderate use are not the same as relationships due to excessive use. One study noted that the rates of any current alcohol use in 2001–2002 were about 70 percent for whites, 53 percent for blacks, and 60 percent for Hispanics—among these drinkers, whites and blacks had higher rates of heavy drinking than Hispanics. To complicate matters further, the statistics differed substantially by gender and by whether the heavy drinking was daily or weekly (Chartier and Caetano 2010). The links between alcohol use and SES are similarly complex. Any current alcohol use is directly related to SES, meaning that adults with more education and higher income are more likely to be current drinkers—however, most of the current drinkers do not have the problematic heavy or binge-drinking patterns. For instance, alcohol use in general increased with education and with income, but binge drinking was highest among those with a GED certificate and was lowest among those with a high school diploma (Schoenborn, Adams, and Peregoy 2013).

Physical Activity

Physical activity has only relatively recently received deserved attention for its importance in many highly prevalent chronic conditions. Physical activity is associated with lower risk of most leading causes of morbidity and mortality including heart disease, diabetes, arthritis, some cancers, mental conditions like depression, cognitive functioning in old age, as well as levels of biological risk influenced by hypertension, cholesterol levels, and obesity (Elsawy and Higgins 2010, Nelson et al. 2007). Even among the oldest-old, physical functioning can be improved with physical activity (Butler et al. 1998). However, only 51 percent of older adults engaged in enough physical activity to meet federal guidelines released in 2008. The guidelines for older adults recommend at least 150 minutes of moderate-intensity aerobic activity, 75 minutes of vigorous-intensity aerobic activity, or an equivalent combination of each per week. Older adults should also engage in strengthening activities that involve all major muscle groups at least two days a week (Elsawy and Higgins 2010). Some reports find that only 33 percent of older adults met the guidelines for aerobic activity and fewer than 17 percent met the guidelines for muscle strengthening activity (Schoenborn, Adams and Peregoy 2013). On the positive side, the focus on exercise as an important health behavior seems to have increased physical activity in American adults since 1990 (Haskell et al. 2007).

Clear gender differences exist in physical activity among adults of all ages: men exercise more than women. Large race/ethnic disparities exist for physical activity: 51 percent of non-Hispanic white adults meet the physical activity guidelines compared to 42 percent of non-Hispanic black and 44 percent of Hispanic adults (Haskell et al. 2007). The SES patterns were similar for education and income: physical activity increased substantially at higher SES levels among adults of all ages, including older adults (Nelson et al. 2007, Schoenborn, Adams, and Peregoy 2013).

Diet and Nutrition

Healthy diets are important because of their close connection to chronic disease. Diet and nutrition are difficult to measure due to the complexities of the foods and meals we consume, as well as the day-to-day variation that complicates the recall and reporting among respondents. The overall picture, regardless of the specific measure, is that older Americans' nutrition fails to meet the recommendation for healthy diets (Krebs Smith et al. 2010). Often statistics use the consumption of fruits and vegetables as a marker of healthy nutrition. Using this marker, only a quarter of American adults meet the five-serving a day recommendation (BRFSS 2009). The USDA developed a more complex Healthy Eating Index (HEI), which takes into account the consumption of 10 categories such as whole grains, fatty acids, vegetables, seafood and plant proteins, and micronutrients like sodium (USDA 2010). Overall, older adults earned a score of 68 out of a maximum of 100 for the consumption of fruit, meat and beans, and total grains (Juan, Guenther and Kott 2009). The lowest scores were for the consumption of dark green vegetables and legumes, whole grains, and sodium intake. The diet of adults aged 75 and older was overall better than the diet of their younger—65–74 years—counterparts (FIFARS 2012). Not surprisingly, the HEI score of older adults who were not in poverty was higher than the score of older adults in poverty: 21 percent of the nonpoor had *good* diets while only 9 percent of poor older adults had HEI scores high enough to classify as having a *good* diet (Juan, Lino, and Basiotis 2004).

Biological Risk Factors

The three most widely known and perhaps most important biological chronic disease risk factors, also referred to as biomedical risk factors or biomarkers, include obesity, hypertension, and elevated blood cholesterol.

Obesity is calculated from an individual's height and weight using the formula for body mass index: BMI = weight in kg/height in m squared, and defined as BMI ≥ 30 (WHO 2015b). Among U.S. adults aged 60 and older, 35 percent are obese (Ogden et al. 2014). Obesity is a risk factor for all leading chronic conditions except chronic lower respiratory disease.

Hypertension, or high blood pressure, is defined as blood pressure 140/90 mmHg or above. Among older Americans, the prevalence of self-reported hypertension is high: 56 percent report having been diagnosed with hypertension (FIFARS 2012). Hypertension is a risk factor for heart disease and may also increase the risk for Alzheimer's disease.

Elevated cholesterol is defined as 240 mg/dL or above; levels between 200 and 240 mg/dL are considered borderline elevated. Among older Americans, only 24 percent have cholesterol levels under 200 mg/dL; 55 percent are in the borderline elevated range and 22 percent have high cholesterol (Shay et al. 2012). Elevated cholesterol is a strong risk factor for heart disease.

One way to conceptualize these factors within the framework used in this chapter is as biological consequences of unhealthy risk behaviors and antecedents of diagnosed chronic conditions. For instance, diet with excessive calories and a high proportion of simple carbohydrates may lead to impaired glucose tolerance, as well as obesity, and these two biological risk factors are strong predictors of diabetes. It is important to keep in mind that the associations among health behaviors, biological risk, and diseases are probabilistic rather than deterministic, and also that there are numerous other genetic, social, environmental, and biological predictors at all levels of the disablement process. It is also important to note that the causal directionalities across the three factors are complex and not simply unidimensional as our conceptual framework shows for parsimony. Finally, we note that various sources may put these biological risk markers among health behaviors—especially obesity (Hubert et al. 1983)—and they can be sometimes found among disease—especially hypertension, although the American Medical Association decided to officially categorize obesity as a disease in 2013 as well (American Medical Association 2013).

Morbidity

Morbidity refers to disease and illness. In this section, we review leading causes of morbidity among older American adults: heart disease, cancer, diabetes, arthritis, chronic lower respiratory disease, and Alzheimer's disease. These are conditions with highest burden in the population—a combination of having the highest prevalence among older adults, the salience of the disease to the patient, the direct and indirect costs associated with the disease, and being among the leading causes of death.

We note that all these leading causes of morbidity and mortality are chronic rather than acute conditions. Acute conditions are temporary illnesses such as colds, influenza, or pneumonia. The prevalence of acute conditions is actually lower among older adults than among younger adults—however, when they do occur among the elderly, they tend to be more severe, resulting in hospitalizations and deaths at higher rates than among younger adults (Thompson et al. 2004). Chronic conditions, also referred to as noncommunicable disease, are long-term, progressive, often incurable diseases that can be managed and lived with for a long time (Mendis 2014). Chronic diseases comprises most of the leading causes of disability and mortality among older Americans, as well as the bulk of health-care spending and cost increases (Thacker et al. 2006).

Throughout this chapter, we will discuss the often high levels of chronic conditions and large disparities in their prevalence. It is therefore useful to note up front that many older adults consider themselves to be relatively healthy. When asked how they judge their health in general, about 3 out of 4 people aged 65 and older rate their health as excellent, very good, or good (FIFARS 2012). At the same time, disparities are evident even for self-rated health: 78 percent of non-Hispanic white men and women report excellent to good health, compared to 62 percent of non-Hispanic black and 63 percent of Hispanic older adults (FIFARS 2012).

Trends in Morbidity

Understanding recent trends in the prevalence of morbidity and disability in the older population is important because it gives us a more dynamic picture of the health status of the population, including some indications of what we can expect in the near future with respect to older adults' morbidity and mortality.

Since the 1980s, the prevalence of disability and physical limitations among older adults has declined (Freedman et al. 2013, Freedman, Martin and Schoeni 2002, Martin, Schoeni and Andreski 2010). Surprisingly, there were no corresponding declines in chronic conditions (Crimmins and Beltrán-Sánchez 2011, Freedman et al. 2007, Martin et al. 2010). In fact, the prevalence of many conditions and multimorbidity has been increasing over time (Chatterji et al. 2015, Verbrugge and Liu 2014). The fact that the prevalence of chronic conditions has remained stable or even increased while disability declined over time suggests an improved ability to successfully manage chronic conditions, whether with medical interventions or with more effective environmental improvements like housing alternations. Advances in medical care, from pharmaceuticals to new diagnostic technologies and surgical procedures have improved the care of acute illnesses, which paradoxically increases the numbers of elderly with chronic conditions (Anderson 2010). At the aggregate level, population aging also contributes to the increases in morbidity among Americans. The prevalence of chronic disease is high in the U.S. population, but particularly so at older ages. About half of Americans have at least one chronic condition; the proportion rises to 91 percent among those aged 65 and older (Anderson 2010). Additionally, 73 percent of older Americans have two or more chronic conditions, a state referred to as multimorbidity (Barnett et al. 2012). The probability of having a chronic condition, as well as the number of conditions, increases with age—thus a greater proportion of Americans at older ages means a greater average prevalence of chronic disease (Anderson 2010).

Disparities in Morbidity

The average health levels in the older population mask profound inequalities across population groups. Health among older adults is not distributed equally. There are large systematic differences in health by gender, race/ethnicity, and SES whether measured by education, income, occupation, and other factors such as neighborhood where older adults reside. The term *systematic differences* refers to large and/or persistent differences in average levels of some characteristic or health outcome between population groups.

Race and ethnic inequalities are to a large extent but not completely due to systematic differences in SES: minority older adults, especially older blacks and Hispanics, have lower education and fewer economic resources on average than older whites (Williams and Collins 1995). Among Medicare beneficiaries, the proportion with two or more conditions was 69 percent among non-Hispanic white and non-Hispanic black respondents, 68 percent among Asian American respondents, and 66 percent among Hispanic respondents. However, black and Hispanic respondents were most likely to have at least six different chronic conditions (CMMS 2013).

Gender differences are somewhat complex. For some conditions, men have higher prevalence; for others, women do. For instance, among the top conditions in Medicare beneficiaries, women were more likely to have hypertension (61% vs. 54%), hypercholesterolemia (46% vs. 44%), and arthritis (35% vs. 22%). Men were more likely to have ischemic heart disease (36% vs. 27%) and diabetes (29% vs. 27%) (CMMS 2013). One way to see these gender differences in light of the longer life expectancy for women is that women have a higher prevalence of nonfatal though potentially debilitating conditions than men while men are more likely to be diagnosed with serious and potentially fatal conditions (Case and Paxson 2005, Macintyre, Hunt and Sweeting 1996). These differences arise from a combination of social and biological factors. One pronounced difference between older men and women is economic well-being: women aged 65 or older are about twice as likely as men to be poor (Meyer and Herd 2007). Other factors include chromosomal and hormonal differences, health behaviors, occupational risks, and social role differences (Gorman and Read 2006, Read and Gorman 2010).

SES differences are persistent, profound, and occur for most conditions in the same direction: socially and economically disadvantaged older adults are more likely to suffer from most conditions (CMMS 2013). For example, the age-adjusted prevalence of doctor-diagnosed diabetes among adults with family income over 400 percent of the poverty threshold was 8.5 percent as compared to 14.5 percent among adults with family incomes below the poverty threshold. Moreover, the socioeconomic inequalities appear to be increasing over time—for instance, educational disparities in various health outcomes have grown over the last several decades (Luo and Waite 2005, Montez et al. 2011, Schoeni et al. 2005).

Leading Chronic Conditions

Among adults aged 65 and older, leading chronic conditions include arthritis, which is reported by 51 percent of respondents; 30 percent report heart disease, 24 percent cancer, 22 percent chronic lower respiratory disease, and 20 percent report diabetes (see Figure 5.2). We review these leading causes of morbidity below. In addition, we also include Alzheimer's disease due to its high burden on the quality of life, mortality, economic costs, and rapid increases in the U.S. population. Because of the very nature of dementias, Alzheimer's disease patients are not interviewed in population health surveys at representative rates; therefore, the data tend to come from sources other than the self-reports we have for the other conditions.

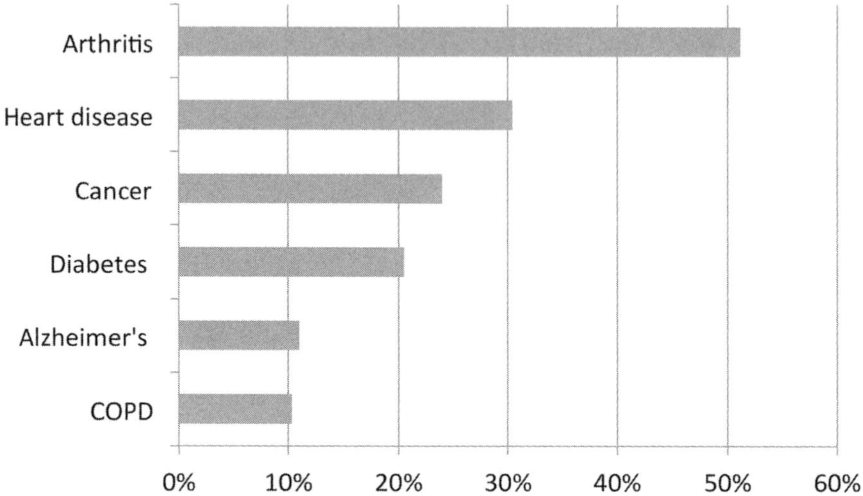

Figure 5.2 Prevalence of leading chronic conditions in U.S. adults aged 65 and older. (FIFARS [Federal Interagency Forum on Aging-Related Statistics], 2012; Alzheimer's Association 2014)

Heart Disease

Heart disease comprises a range of conditions of the heart and blood vessels, such as coronary heart/artery disease, heart attack, arrhythmia, and congestive heart failure. Many of these conditions are the result of atherosclerosis. Atherosclerosis is a condition that develops when a fatty substance referred to as plaque builds up in the walls of the arteries. This buildup hardens and narrows the arteries, making it harder for blood to flow through. Gradually or suddenly a plaque may partially or completely block the flow of blood in an artery. If this is an artery that supplies blood to the heart muscle, it is referred to as coronary heart disease or coronary artery disease.

Risk factors for heart disease include (1) high blood pressure, (2) high cholesterol, (3) diabetes, and (4) health behaviors including current smoking, physical inactivity, and unhealthy diet and obesity (CDC 2009a). A recent analysis determined that the population attributable fractions for heart disease mortality were 41 percent for high blood pressure, 14 percent for smoking, 13 percent for unhealthy diet and obesity, 12 percent for insufficient physical activity, and 9 percent for abnormal blood glucose levels (Go et al. 2014). Although death rates from heart disease have been declining steadily (FIFARS 2012), heart disease remains the leading cause of death in the United States (CDC 2009a). Moreover, there is some concern that the high levels of obesity and low levels of physical activity will cause a reversal of this trend and possible increases in heart disease deaths in the future (Mitka 2012).

Prevalence, Age Patterns, and Trends over Time

Among older Americans, about 30 percent report having heart disease (FIFARS 2012). This proportion has been relatively steady since the 1990s, with no systematic increases or decreases. Heart disease prevalence, as well as incidence, increase with age. For instance, coronary heart disease has been diagnosed in 20 percent of men and 10 percent of women aged 60–79 compared to 32 percent of men and 19 percent of women aged 80 or older (Mozaffarian et al. 2015).

Disparities in Heart Disease

The prevalence of heart disease is higher among men than among women except at the oldest ages when the gender pattern is reversed; the incidence of heart disease remains higher for men at all ages (Mozaffarian et al. 2015). With respect to race/ethnicity, the prevalence of heart disease is about 32 percent among older non-Hispanic white respondents, 25 percent among non-Hispanic black, and 22 percent among Hispanic respondents (FIFARS 2012). It is important to point out, however, that measured data or data on cardiovascular disease that includes hypertension is higher among non-Hispanic black respondents across the lifespan compared to non-Hispanic white adults (Mozaffarian et al. 2015). There is also a strong socioeconomic component whereby the prevalence of heart disease decreases with higher education or income in the population, in large part though different health behaviors such as smoking or healthy diet (Fiscella and Tancredi 2008, Winkleby et al. 1992).

Cancer

Cancer is a broad term for a range of over 100 diseases with different progression, symptoms, treatment options, and survival times. Biologically, cancer is caused by damage to the genes involved in cell replication. The three cancers with the highest incidence, as well as the highest number of deaths for each gender are lung, prostate, and colorectal for men; lung, breast, and colorectal for women (Siegel et al. 2014). Risk factors vary by cancer type but generally include (1) family history, (2) age, (3) smoking, (4) obesity, and (5) environmental exposure—such as sunburns or the use of tanning beds which are risk factors for melanoma (Tucker and Goldstein 2003). A recent study in *Science* showed that inherited predisposition and environmental factors account for only one-third of the variation in cancer risk; the majority is due to bad luck—random mutations that occur during DNA replication in normal stem cells (Tomasetti and Vogelstein 2015). Cancer remains one of the most prominent public health concerns in the United States and around the world. A recent study estimated the annual loss of productivity due to cancer between $9.6 and $16 billion among working-age adults in the United States (Guy et al. 2013). Cancer survivors report difficulties in multiple domains, from health-related quality of life (Brown, Lipscomb and Snyder 2001) to psychological problems such as depression and anxiety (Baker et al. 2005, Hewitt, Rowland and Yancik 2003). Despite improved diagnosis and treatment, cancer is the second leading cause of mortality in the United States and predicted to become the top leading cause of death in the next several years (Johnson et al. 2014).

Prevalence, Age Patterns, and Trends over Time

Thanks to earlier diagnosis and more effective treatment of many cancers, the number of cancer survivors in the U.S. population is estimated at 13 million and expected to reach 18 million within a decade (de Moor et al. 2013). Cancer is unique among the leading conditions in that we often focus on new cases—incidence—rather than prevalence. In 2014, 1,665,000 new cases of cancer were diagnosed and 586,000 deaths due to cancer occurred in the United States (Siegel et al. 2014). The incidence increases across the adult lifespan: among adults younger than 65, there are about 225 new cases per 100,000 annually while among older adults, there are about 2,040 cases (National Cancer Institute 2015). The age-adjusted incidence of cancer among older adults rose from the 1970s through the early 1990s and has been declining slightly since (National Cancer Institute 2015).

Disparities in Cancer

The lifetime probability of being diagnosed with cancer is slightly higher among non-Hispanic whites—41 percent—compared to 38 percent among non-Hispanic blacks and 37 percent among Hispanics (Howlader et al. 2014). There are large differences in the age at diagnosis, cancer sites, or survival, however. For example, non-Hispanic blacks are more likely to die of cancer than adults from any other race/ethnic group (CDC 2009a). With respect to gender, the lifetime probability of being diagnosed with cancer is higher in men (43 percent) than women (38 percent), and the lifetime probability of dying from cancer is also slightly higher in men: 23 percent compared to 19 percent among women (Howlader et al. 2014). Survival from cancer is higher for patients living in higher SES areas (Ward et al.

2004)—however, SES effects vary tremendously by cancer type. For instance, there is a strong SES inverse gradient for lung cancer because less-educated individuals smoke at higher rates, but breast cancer has a positive correlation with SES among women (Clegg et al. 2009).

Diabetes

A healthy body produces insulin, which is necessary for all cells in the body to accept the glucose as source of energy. *Diabetes* occurs when the body is unable to metabolize glucose, either because it does not produce insulin—Type I diabetes—or because the body produces sufficient insulin, but the cells are "resistant" to it or fail to respond to it—Type II. Nearly all cases of diabetes diagnosed among adults—90–95 percent—are Type II diabetes, previously referred to as adult-onset diabetes (CDC 2014).

The main risk factors for Type II diabetes are obesity and sedentary lifestyle. Diabetes increases the risk of heart disease, stroke, blindness and vision problems, kidney disease, and amputations (CDC 2014). Diabetes is also the seventh leading cause of mortality in the United States. Additionally it may be severely underreported on death certificates. For instance, among people with diabetes, only 10–15 percent had diabetes listed as the underlying cause (CDC 2014).

Prevalence, Age Patterns, and Trends over Time

Over 11 million older Americans, or 26 percent of the older U.S. population, have diabetes. About 28 percent of these individuals are undiagnosed and are thus not receiving any treatment. Moreover, 1.7 million new cases of diabetes are diagnosed annually in the United States; among older adults it's 400,000 new diagnoses annually. Even more worrisome, an additional 37 percent of U.S. adults have prediabetes, a condition when blood glucose levels are elevated but not high enough to be diagnosed a diabetes, as do 51 percent of adults aged 65 and older (CDC 2014).

As the statistics in the previous paragraphs indicate, the prevalence of Type II diabetes increases sharply with age. Over time, there has also been a dramatic rise in the prevalence of diabetes. In 1997–1998, the prevalence of diabetes for adults aged 65 and older was 13 percent; this proportion doubled in 15 years to 26 percent (FIFARS 2012).

Disparities in Diabetes

Among older adults, men have higher prevalence of diabetes than women: 23 percent versus 18 percent. There are large socioeconomic and race/ethnic differences in age-adjusted prevalence of diabetes as well. As with many other conditions, the prevalence of diabetes is higher among lower SES individuals (Mokdad et al. 2003). Among non-Hispanic whites and Asian Americans, the prevalence of diabetes is 8 percent and 9 percent, respectively; among Hispanic and non-Hispanic black populations, the prevalence is 13 percent, and among AIAN adults it is nearly 16 percent. Interestingly, the rates of prediabetes were comparable across major race/ethnic groups, suggesting there are systematic differences in how the disease develops over time (CDC 2014).

Arthritis

Arthritis is the most prevalent disease of the musculoskeletal system in older adults. Osteoarthritis, the most common form of arthritis, is a degenerative disease of the joints, typically knees, hips, hands, and lower back, that develops when the cartilage that protects the bones meeting at a joint wears away, resulting in inflammation, pain, and reduced movement. Risk factors for arthritis include overuse or injuries and obesity. Arthritis is not fatal but is the leading cause of disability among Americans (CDC 2009b): 19 percent of disabled individuals attributed their difficulties to arthritis or rheumatism, which exceeded back or spine problems—17 percent—and heart trouble—7 percent (CDC 2009b). Moreover it is estimated that the total cost of arthritis in terms of medical costs and lost earnings is about $130 billion annually (CDC 2013b).

Prevalence, Age Patterns, and Trends over Time

Arthritis is the second most common health complaint—after hypertension—among older adults: 51 percent of respondents aged 65 and older reported having been diagnosed with arthritis. The age-adjusted prevalence of arthritis has been relatively stable during the last decade (FIFARS 2012), but since arthritis prevalence increases with age (Lawrence et al. 2008), the aging of the U.S. population likely means increasing total burden of this disease in the future (CDC 2013b).

Disparities in Arthritis

Women report arthritis at higher rates than men: among older adults, about 56 percent of women and 45 percent of men have this condition (FIFARS 2012). The pattern of race/ethnic differences for arthritis differs from the pattern for other diseases, in that among older adults non-Hispanic whites are most likely to report arthritis (53%), followed by non-Hispanic black (51%) and Hispanic (44%) respondents (FIFARS 2012). However, non-Hispanic black adults were more likely to report severe pain or activity limitations due to arthritis compared to non-Hispanic white adults (CDC 2005). Finally, arthritis has a strong socioeconomic gradient. Among U.S. adults, the age-adjusted prevalence of arthritis is 26 percent among those with less than a high school diploma and 18 percent among those with at least a college degree (CDC 2013b).

Chronic Lower Respiratory Disease

This is a class of diseases that impact the lungs. The most fatal in this group is *chronic obstructive pulmonary disease* (COPD), which includes two underlying diseases: chronic bronchitis and emphysema. These diseases obstruct the flow of air within the respiratory system, causing difficulty breathing. Smoking is the primary risk factor for COPD; additional risks are from environmental exposures such as air pollution. COPD has a high morbidity and mortality burden: it is the third leading cause of death in the Unites States (Akinbami and Liu 2013).

Prevalence, Age Patterns, and Trends over Time

Among older adults, about 10 percent report having been diagnosed with COPD (FIFARS 2012). The prevalence of COPD has been declining slightly—although the declines were not statistically significant—in the U.S. population in recent years, partly because fewer adults are smoking (Akinbami and Liu 2013). With respect to age patterns, COPD prevalence increases for most of the lifespan and is highest among adults aged 65 and older—however, within this older adult group, the elderly aged 85+ have a lower prevalence than those aged 65–84 (Akinbami and Liu 2013). This may be a cohort effect—the oldest-old are cohorts that did not smoke at as high a rate as the cohorts that followed—or a selection effect whereby those with COPD die before reaching the oldest ages.

Disparities in COPD

The prevalence of COPD is significantly higher among women than men (Akinbami and Liu 2013). This is interesting given the lower smoking rates of women compared to men and suggests greater vulnerability of women with respect to the effects of smoking. Moreover, as the smoking differences between men and women decrease, the burden of COPD is shifting more to women. The race/ethnic differences for COPD are somewhat like those for arthritis: non-Hispanic white older adults have the highest prevalence (11%), compared to non-Hispanic black (8%), and Hispanic adults (7%). To some degree, this pattern reflects race/ethnic differences in smoking patterns as the primary risk factor for COPD (Schoenborn, Adams and Peregoy 2013). And finally, reflecting the strong socioeconomic patterning of greater smoking among low-SES individuals, the prevalence of COPD also has a close inverse relationship with SES (Viegi et al. 2000).

Alzheimer's Disease

Dementia is a general term for several conditions that cause a decline in memory and cognitive abilities. The most common type of dementia is *Alzheimer's disease*, a progressive and fatal condition (Alzheimer's Association 2014). The symptoms of Alzheimer's disease vary across patients but typically start with difficulties remembering new information. Later symptoms may include memory loss, difficulty planning complex actions or solving problems, trouble expressing oneself, confusion, poor judgment, and personality changes. The risk factors for Alzheimer's remain poorly understood but include (1) age, (2) genetic vulnerability—the gene apolipoprotein e4 (APOE e4) was found related to the probability of developing the disease, and (3) a range of behavioral and socioeconomic factors such as low education, past head trauma, smoking, and lack of physical activity (Lindsay et al. 2002). Alzheimer's is one of the leading causes of disability and the sixth leading cause of death in the United States (Alzheimer's Association 2014, Murphy, Xu and Kochanek 2013).

Prevalence, Age Patterns, and Trends over Time

The estimated prevalence of Alzheimer's in the older U.S. population is 11 percent, or about five million diagnosed individuals. As noted above, the incidence and prevalence of Alzheimer's rises sharply at the oldest ages. Among people aged 65 and older, the prevalence of Alzheimer's is estimated to double with every five years of age, so among adults aged 85 and older, 32 percent have Alzheimer's (Alzheimer's Association 2014). Because the disease occurs most frequently among the elderly, whose numbers and proportions in the U.S. population are rising rapidly, there will be a corresponding dramatic rise in Alzheimer's patients in the near future (Hebert et al. 2013).

Disparities in Alzheimer's Disease

The prevalence is higher in women than men although this is in part because women live longer than men on average, and age is the largest risk factor for Alzheimer's (Letenneur et al. 1999). Alzheimer's is more prevalent among African American and Hispanic older adults, compared to non-Hispanic whites and Asian Americans (Manly and Mayeux 2004). Finally, there is a strong SES component to Alzheimer's disease epidemiology: less-educated adults are at significantly higher risk of developing the disease than those with more education (Alzheimer's Association 2014).

Multimorbidity

The sections above described the leading chronic conditions in U.S. older adults. Most older adults, however, have more than one condition (CMMS 2013). *Multimorbidity*, which refers to the presence of two or more chronic conditions, adds additional complications to managing chronic disease and coordinating care across the different conditions, increases costs and risks of adverse outcomes, introduces medication interactions that result in complications of care, functional limitations, costly hospitalizations, lower health-related quality of life, and mortality (Anderson 2010, Fortin et al. 2007). The most prevalent multimorbidity combination is arthritis and hypertension among those with two conditions; the most common triad also includes diabetes.

Prevalence, Age Patterns, and Trends over Time

In 2010, about two thirds of U.S. adults aged 65 or older had multimorbidities; most of this age group had two or three conditions (CMMS 2013, Ward and Schiller 2013). The prevalence of multimorbidity increases steeply with age, so that among adults aged 85 years and older, 83 percent have two or more chronic conditions (CMMS 2013). The prevalence of multimorbidity has been increasing slightly, but significantly, throughout the first decade of the 21st century. The rise was observed in most demographic subgroups and across all ages, including in older Americans aged 65 and above (Ward and Schiller 2013).

Disparities in Multimorbidity

While women tend to report more conditions than men especially at earlier ages, there is a convergence among older adults such that some studies find men aged 65 and older to have a slightly higher probability of multimorbidity than women (Fortin et al. 2005, Ward and Schiller 2013). Black older adults have a higher prevalence than white older adults (Quiñones et al. 2011) while Hispanics are effectively comparable to non-Hispanic whites in the prevalence of multimorbidity (Ward and Schiller 2013). Not surprisingly, given that most individual chronic conditions are linked to SES, the prevalence of multimorbidity is also higher among adults of lower SES, whether measured by education or income. Among older Americans, for instance, adults without a high school diploma had a 46 percent higher probability of being multimorbid than their counterparts with a college diploma (Tucker-Seeley et al. 2011).

Mortality

One of the most widely used measures of population health is life expectancy at birth, which indicates the average—expected—number of years of life for individuals born in a given year. In 2010, life expectancy for U.S. adults was 78.7 years (Murphy, Xu and Kochanek 2013). For comparison, life expectancy 100 years prior in 1910 was about 50 years and in 1960 was about 70 years (Noymer 2005). Life expectancies at ages 65 and 85 have also been gradually increasing, meaning that older adults can expect to live longer than ever before. The life expectancy at age 65, for instance, is over 19 years (FIFARS 2012).

Mortality Risks across Age and Trends over Time

The risk of dying increases exponentially at older ages. The probability of dying within one year is 1.6 percent for an average 65-year-old person; it is 6 percent at age 80 and 27 percent at age 95 (Bell and Miller 2011). The life expectancy among Americans has been increasing steadily, by about 0.3 percent annually in recent years (Johnson et al. 2014). Mortality rates have been declining for most leading causes of death; the main drivers of the declining mortality are lower heart disease and cancer death rates. Between 1981 and 2009, the age-adjusted mortality among adults aged 65 and older declined for most leading causes: mortality due to cardiovascular and cerebrovascular disease dropped by over 50 percent—however, mortality due to chronic lower respiratory disease increased, as did deaths from Alzheimer's disease (Johnson et al. 2014, Murphy, Xu and Kochanek 2013).

Disparities in Mortality

The disparities in mortality across population groups in the United States are staggering. The disparities occur along socioeconomic, race/ethnic, gender, and geographic dimensions. If we look at major sex/race group combinations, for instance, then life expectancy in the early 21st century was nearly 87 years for Asian women, compared to 69 years for black men, a difference of 18 years (Murray et al. 2006). Or if we compared the most advantaged county-race combination versus the least advantaged combination, the life expectancy difference is 35 years (Murray et al. 2006).

With respect to sex, women's life expectancy of 81 years exceeds men's life expectancy of 76.2 years as is typical for most populations (Murphy, Xu and Kochanek 2013). Racial disparities persist for both genders although they have narrowed since 1990. Life expectancy at birth in 2010 was 4.7 years longer for white men than for black men; the difference was 8.2 years in 1990. White women's life expectancy was 3.3 years more than black women's; it was 5.8 years in 1990 (Kochanek, Arias and Anderson 2013). The disparities are caused by underlying differences in major chronic diseases and, among younger and middle-aged adults, in injuries (Murray et al. 2006). Hispanic males and females had longer life expectancy at birth than non-Hispanic white or non-Hispanic black males and females (Murphy, Xu and Kochanek 2013). The high life expectancy of Hispanic adults is referred to as the *Hispanic mortality paradox* because Hispanics have lower average education and income levels, which are typically associated with lower life expectancy (Crimmins, Kim and Vasunilashorn 2010, Markides and Eschbach 2011).

The mortality disparities are more pronounced among middle-aged adults and tend to decline at older ages (Murray et al. 2006). This may be in part because the overall higher mortality at older ages makes relative differences less obvious (Lynch et al. 2006), due to selection by prior mortality (Zajacova, Goldman and Rodriguez 2009), or due to cohort effects (Murray et al. 2006). In particular, the black-white gap decreases among older adults and even reverses among the oldest-old, so that among those who survive to age 85, black adults have slightly higher life expectancy compare to white adults: 6.8 vs. 6.6 years (FIFARS 2012).

An additional worrisome fact is that the disparities across most dimensions have increased over time (Murray et al. 2006, Pappas et al. 1993), and, moreover, the increased disparities reflect the *increase* in mortality for disadvantaged Americans (Ezzati et al. 2008). In the last two decades of the 20th century, 20 percent of women and 4 percent of men experienced a stagnation or decline in longevity, despite the continued increases in life expectancy for the population as a whole (Ezzati et al. 2008). This stagnation or rise in mortality was caused by the higher prevalence of cancer, COPD due to smoking, and diabetes (Ezzati et al. 2008).

Yoon et al. (2014) provided a different perspective on inequalities in leading causes of death. Focusing on deaths occurring prior to age 80, they compared the deaths in every U.S. state to the one that had the lowest mortality for this cause. This analysis enabled them to determine that if every state lowered mortality to the level of the lowest state, mortality would decline by between 21 percent for cancer and 38 percent for chronic lower respiratory disease and unintentional injuries.

Leading Causes of Mortality

Table 5.1 shows the top 10 leading causes of mortality in the United States, the proportion of all deaths due to each cause, as well as the sex and race death ratios due to each cause. Seven of these leading 10 are chronic diseases, and the top two—heart disease and cancer—comprise nearly half of all deaths in the United States (Johnson et al. 2014).

The list of leading causes of death has remained relatively stable for years. However, deaths due to heart disease, while still the leading group, have been declining to a point when, if current trends continue, cancers will become the leading cause of death in the next several years (Johnson et al. 2014). For nearly half a century, the third leading cause was cerebrovascular diseases—as of 2008: however, this cause was superseded by chronic lower respiratory disease (Johnson et al. 2014).

Table 5.1 Top 10 Leading Causes of Mortality, and Gender and Race Ratios for Each

Rank	Cause of Death	Percent of Total	Male:Female	Black:White
1	Diseases of heart (heart disease)	24.2	1.4	1.2
2	Malignant neoplasms (cancer)	23.3	1.6	1.3
3	Chronic lower respiratory diseases	5.6	1.4	1.2
4	Cerebrovascular diseases (stroke)	5.2	1.3	0.7
5	Accidents (unintentional injuries)	4.9	1.0	1.4
6	Alzheimer's disease	3.4	2.0	0.8
7	Diabetes mellitus (diabetes)	2.8	0.8	0.8
8	Nephritis, nephrotic syndrome and nephrosis (kidney disease)	2.8	1.4	2.0
9	Influenza and pneumonia	2.0	1.4	2.1
10	Intentional self-harm (suicide)	1.6	1.4	1.1

Source: Authors' summaries, based on data in Johnson et al. (2014).

The male:female ratio and the black:white ratio in Table 5.1 represent the risk of dying for one group relative to another group. For all leading causes except diabetes, the death rates were higher for men compared to women; and for 7 out of the 10 leading conditions the death rates were higher for black than white Americans. Death rates for the top two causes of death, heart disease and cancer, have declined since 2009. On a positive note, the black to white differences have narrowed slightly over time, to 4.1 years in 2010 although the age-adjusted death rate for the black population remains 1.2 times the rate for the non-Hispanic white population (Murphy, Xu and Kochanek 2013). The group with the highest life expectancy is Hispanic females, who can expect to live 83.8 years, followed by non-Hispanic white females with a life expectancy of 81.1 years, and Hispanic males at 78.5 years—however, caution is required because mortality for Hispanics is underreported by about 5 percent (Murphy, Xu and Kochanek 2013).

Conclusions

Throughout the 20th century, Americans added a tremendous number of years to life, in large part thanks to more effective medical and pharmaceutical interventions. Life expectancy is continuing to grow in the first part of the 21st century—at this point, however, the question of adding *life to years* is becoming increasingly urgent. What are the trends and inequalities in the health status, and perhaps quality of life, of older Americans?

The question of morbidity burden among older adults in the United States is critical not only because of the high burden of chronic diseases with respect to health-care cost, which is already higher in the United States than anywhere else in the world, but also due to other outcomes. Chronic diseases are expensive to treat, negatively impact quality of life, increase the probability of activity limitations and disability, are associated with increased use of health care, and predict higher mortality (Barnett et al. 2012, FIFARS 2012). With respect to health-care costs for older adults, 80 percent of all Medicare spending goes toward individuals with five or more conditions (Anderson 2010). Morbidity and poor health in general have profound consequences in different areas of life, including labor force participation. Older adults who experience health problems or health declines are more likely to exit the labor force (Mutchler et al. 1999). Those who remain in the labor force are more likely to change jobs, likely toward those where their limitations can be accommodated. About half of older workers in poor health who leave the labor force prematurely apply for disability benefits (Bound et al. 1999).

The challenges are enormous. American society is aging, with the proportion of older adults inching toward 20 percent. At the same time, as the trends in morbidity reviewed above showed, the prevalence of leading chronic conditions are not systematically declining and in some cases are increasing. Additionally, vast socioeconomic and race/ethnic disparities persist for many diseases and for mortality.

What are some directions toward solutions? One message is that prevention is key. Helping individuals lead healthier lives will decrease the incidence and prevalence of most chronic diseases and, in turn, disability. Successful prevention strategies however, must go beyond the individual and need to be oriented at the community, state, and national levels. This perspective is clear from the fundamental causes approach to health: upstream socioeconomic factors put individuals at *risk for risks* such as smoking or lack of physical activity (Link and Phelan 1995).

The American health-care system remains focused on diagnosis and curing acute diseases rather than the prevention and ongoing treatment of chronic disease (CDC 2009a). The U.S. health-care system therefore needs to be reoriented toward long-term care for patients with often multiple chronic diseases. Second, the system, which has achieved tremendous progress on curing acute illness and injury, must reorient itself from this focus toward preventing chronic illness onset and management. Third, health disparities must be reduced and eliminated. And finally, all health intervention needs to include the entire life course, as the risk factors for chronic illness develop years or decades prior to the diagnosis of a condition.

References

Akinbami, Lara J. and Xiang Liu. 2013. "Chronic Obstructive Pulmonary Disease among Adults Aged 18 and over in the United States, 1998–2009." *Women* 6:8.

Alzheimer's Association. 2014. "2014 Alzheimer's Disease: Facts and Figures." *Alzheimer's & Dementia* 10(2). Retrieved from https://www.alz.org/downloads/facts_figures_2014.pdf

American Medical Association. 2013, "Obesity as a Disease: AMA Adopts New Policies on Second Day of Voting at Annual Meeting." Retrieved March 18, 2015, 2015 (http://www.ama-assn.org/ama/pub/news/news/2013/2013-06-18-new-ama-policies-annual-meeting.page).

Anderson, Gerard. 2010. "Chronic Conditions: Making the Case for Ongoing Care." Princeton, NJ: Robert Wood Johnson Foundation.

Aneshensel, Carol S. 1992. "Social Stress: Theory and Research." *Annual Review of Sociology* 18:15–38.

Antonovsky, Aaron. 1979. "Health, Stress, and Coping." San Francisco, CA: Jossey-Bass.

Baker, Frank, Maxine Denniston, Tenbroeck Smith and Michele M. West. 2005. "Adult Cancer Survivors: How Are They Faring?" *Cancer* 104(S11):2565–76.

Barnett, Karen, Stewart W. Mercer, Michael Norbury, Graham Watt, Sally Wyke and Bruce Guthrie. 2012. "Epidemiology of Multimorbidity and Implications for Health Care, Research, and Medical Education: A Cross-Sectional Study." *The Lancet* 380(9836):37–43. doi: http://dx.doi.org/10.1016/S0140-6736(12)60240-2.

Bell, Felicitie C. and Michael L. Miller. 2011. "Life Tables for the United States Social Security Area 1900–2100: Actuarial Study No. 120." Washington, DC: US Social Security Administration.

Bouchery, Ellen E., Henrick J. Harwood, Jeffrey J. Sacks, Carol J. Simon and Robert D. Brewer. 2011. "Economic Costs of Excessive Alcohol Consumption in the U.S., 2006." *American Journal of Preventive Medicine* 41(5):516–24. doi: http://dx.doi.org/10.1016/j.amepre.2011.06.045.

Bound, John, Michael Schoenbaum, Todd R. Stinebrickner and Timothy Waidmann. 1999. "The Dynamic Effects of Health on the Labor Force Transitions of Older Workers." *Labour Economics* 6(2):179–202. doi: http://dx.doi.org/10.1016/S0927-5371(99)00015-9.

BRFSS. 2009, "Prevalence and Trends Data [Internet]." Atlanta, GA: Centers for Disease Control and Prevention. Retrieved March 31, 2015 (http://apps.nccd.cdc.gov/brfss/page.asp?cat=AC&yr=2007&state=US#AC).

Brown, Martin L., Joseph Lipscomb and Claire Snyder. 2001. "The Burden of Illness of Cancer: Economic Cost and Quality of Life." *Annual Review of Public Health* 22:91–113.

Butler, Robert N., Regina Davis, Carole B. Lewis, Miriam E. Nelson and Elton Strauss. 1998. "Physical Fitness: Benefits of Exercise for the Older Patient." *Geriatrics* 53(10):46–62.

Caffrey, Christine, Manisha Sengupta, Eunice Park-Lee and Lauren Harris-Kojetin. 2012. *Residents Living in Residential Care Facilities: United States, 2010*. Congress, NCHS data brief (http://www.cdc.gov/nchs/data/databriefs/db91.pdf).

Case, Anne and Christina Paxson. 2005. "Sex Differences in Morbidity and Mortality." *Demography* 42(2):189–214.

CDC. 2005. "Racial/Ethnic Differences in the Prevalence and Impact of Doctor-Diagnosed Arthritis—United States, 2002." *MMWR: Morbidity and Mortality Weekly Report* 54(5):119.

CDC. 2008. "Smoking-Attributable Mortality, Years of Potential Life Lost, and Productivity Losses—United States, 2000–2004." *MMWR: Morbidity and Mortality Weekly Report* 57(45):1226.

CDC. 2009a. *The Power of Prevention: Chronic Disease . . . The Public Health Challenge of the 21st Century Congress* (http://www.cdc.gov/chronicdisease/pdf/2009-Power-of-Prevention.pdf).

CDC. 2009b. "Prevalence and Most Common Causes of Disability among Adults—United States, 2005." *MMWR: Morbidity & Mortality Weekly Report* 58(16):421–26.

CDC. 2013a, "Alcohol and Public Health: Alcohol-Related Disease Impact (ARDI) Application." Retrieved February 12, 2015 (http://apps.nccd.cdc.gov/DACH_ARDI/Default/Default.aspx).

CDC. 2013b. "Prevalence of Doctor-Diagnosed Arthritis and Arthritis-Attributable Activity Limitation—United States, 2010–2012." *MMWR. Morbidity and Mortality Weekly Report* 62(44):869–71.

CDC. 2014. "National Diabetes Statistics Report: Estimates of Diabetes and Its Burden in the United States, 2014." Atlanta, GA: U.S. Department of Health and Human Services (http://www.cdc.gov/diabetes/pubs/statsreport14/national-diabetes-report-web.pdf).

Chartier, Karen and Raul Caetano. 2010. "Ethnicity and Health Disparities in Alcohol Research." *Alcohol Research & Health* 33(1–2):152.

Chatterji, Somnath, Julie Byles, David Cutler, Teresa Seeman and Emese Verdes. 2015. "Health, Functioning, and Disability in Older Adults—Present Status and Future Implications." *The Lancet*. doi: http://dx.doi.org/10.1016/S0140-6736(14)61462-8.

Clark, Rodney, Norman B. Anderson, Vernessa R. Clark and David R. Williams. 1999. "Racism as a Stressor for African Americans: A Biopsychosocial Model." *American Psychologist* 54(10):805–16. doi: 10.1037/0003-066X.54.10.805.

Clegg, Limin X., Marsha E. Reichman, Barry A. Miller, Benjamin F. Hankey, Gopal K. Singh, Yi Dan Lin, Marc T. Goodman, Charles F. Lynch, Stephen M. Schwartz, Vivien W. Chen, Leslie Bernstein, Scarlett L. Gomez, John J. Graff, Charles C. Lin, Norman J. Johnson and Brenda K. Edwards. 2009. "Impact of Socioeconomic Status on Cancer Incidence and Stage at Diagnosis: Selected Findings from the Surveillance, Epidemiology, and End Results: National Longitudinal Mortality Study." *Cancer Causes & Control* 20(4):417–35. doi: 10.1007/s10552-008-9256-0.

CMMS. 2013, "Chronic Conditions among Medicare Beneficiaries, Chartbook, 2012 Edition." Baltimore, MD: U.S. DHHS. (http://www.cms.gov/Research-Statistics-Data-and-Systems/Statistics-Trends-and-Reports/Chronic-Conditions/Downloads/2012Chartbook.pdf).

Cockerham, William C. 2005. "Health Lifestyle Theory and the Convergence of Agency and Structure." *Journal of Health and Social Behavior* 46(1):51–67. doi: 10.2307/4147653.

Crimmins, Eileen, JungKi Kim and Sarinnapha Vasunilashorn. 2010. "Biodemography: New Approaches to Understanding Trends and Differences in Population Health and Mortality." *Demography* 47(1):S41–64. doi: 10.1353/dem.2010.0005.

Crimmins, Eileen M. and Hiram Beltrán-Sánchez. 2011. "Mortality and Morbidity Trends: Is There Compression of Morbidity?" *The Journals of Gerontology, Series B: Psychological Sciences and Social Sciences* 66B(1):75–86. doi: 10.1093/geronb/gbq088.

de Moor, Janet S., Angela B. Mariotto, Carla Parry, Catherine M. Alfano, Lynne Padgett, Erin E. Kent, Laura Forsythe, Steve Scoppa, Mark Hachey and Julia H. Rowland. 2013. "Cancer Survivors in the United States: Prevalence across the Survivorship Trajectory and Implications for Care." *Cancer Epidemiology Biomarkers & Prevention*. doi: 10.1158/1055-9965.epi-12-1356.

Elsawy, Bassem and Kim E. Higgins. 2010. "Physical Activity Guidelines for Older Adults." *American Family Physician* 81(1):55–59.

Ezzati, Majid, Ari B. Friedman, Sandeep C. Kulkarni and Christopher J. L. Murray. 2008. "The Reversal of Fortunes: Trends in County Mortality and Cross-County Mortality Disparities in the United States." *PLoS Medicine* 5(4):e66.

FIFARS. 2012. "Older Americans 2012: Key Indicators of Well-Being." Washington, DC: U.S. Government Printing Office (http://www.agingstats.gov/main_site/data/2012_documents/docs/entirechartbook.pdf).

Fiscella, Kevin and Daniel Tancredi. 2008. "Socioeconomic Status and Coronary Heart Disease Risk Prediction." *Journal of the American Medical Association* 300(22):2666–68.

Fortin, Martin, Gina Bravo, Catherine Hudon, Alain Vanasse and Lise Lapointe. 2005. "Prevalence of Multimorbidity among Adults Seen in Family Practice." *Annals of Family Medicine* 3(3):223–28.

Fortin, Martin, Marie-France Dubois, Catherine Hudon, Hassan Soubhi and José Almirall. 2007. "Multimorbidity and Quality of Life: A Closer Look." *Health and Quality of Life Outcomes* 5:52–59. doi: 10.1186/1477-7525-5-52.

Freedman, Vicki, Brenda Spillman, Patti Andreski, Jennifer Cornman, Eileen Crimmins, Ellen Kramarow, James Lubitz, Linda Martin, Sharon Merkin, Robert Schoeni, Teresa Seeman and Timothy Waidmann. 2013. "Trends in Late-Life Activity Limitations in the United States: An Update from Five National Surveys." *Demography* 50(2):661–71. doi: 10.1007/s13524-012-0167-z.

Freedman, Vicki A., Linda G. Martin and Robert F. Schoeni. 2002. "Recent Trends in Disability and Functioning among Older Adults in the United States: A Systematic Review." *Journal of the American Medical Association* 288(24):3137–46.

Freedman, Vicki A., Robert F. Schoeni, Linda G. Martin and Jennifer C. Cornman. 2007. "Chronic Conditions and the Decline in Late-Life Disability." *Demography* 44(3):459–77. doi: 10.2307/30053097.

Garrett, Bridgette E., Shanta R. Dube, Angela Trosclair, Ralph S. Caraballo, Terry F. Pechacek, Centers for Disease Control and Prevention. 2011. "Cigarette Smoking—United States, 1965–2008." *MMWR: Morbidity and Mortality Weekly Report* 60(Suppl.):109–13.

Go, Alan S., Dariush Mozaffarian, Véronique L. Roger, Emelia J. Benjamin, Jarett D. Berry, et al. 2014. "Heart Disease and Stroke Statistics—2014 Update: A Report from the American Heart Association." *Circulation* 129(3):e28–e292. doi: 10.1161/01.cir.0000441139.02102.80.

Gorman, Bridget K. and Jen'nan Ghazal Read. 2006. "Gender Disparities in Adult Health: An Examination of Three Measures of Morbidity." *Journal of Health and Social Behavior* 47(2):95–110. doi: 10.2307/30040304.

Guy, Gery P., Donatus U. Ekwueme, K. Robin Yabroff, Emily C. Dowling, Chunyu Li, Juan L. Rodriguez, Janet S. de Moor and Katherine S. Virgo. 2013. "Economic Burden of Cancer Survivorship among Adults in the United States." *Journal of Clinical Oncology*. doi: 10.1200/jco.2013.49.1241.

Haskell, William L., I. Lee, Russell R. Pate, Kenneth E. Powell, Steven N. Blair, Barry A. Franklin, Caroline A. Macera, Gregory W. Heath, Paul D. Thompson and Adrian Bauman. 2007. "Physical Activity and Public Health: Updated Recommendation for Adults from the American College of Sports Medicine and the American Heart Association." *Medicine and Science in Sports and Exercise* 39(8):1423–34.

Hebert, Liesi E., Jennifer Weuve, Paul A. Scherr and Denis A. Evans. 2013. "Alzheimer Disease in the United States (2010–2050) Estimated Using the 2010 Census." *Neurology* 80(19):1778–83.

Hewitt, Maria, Julia H. Rowland and Rosemary Yancik. 2003. "Cancer Survivors in the United States: Age, Health, and Disability." *The Journals of Gerontology, Series A: Biological Sciences and Medical Sciences* 58(1):82–91.

Howlader, Nadia, Anne-Michele Noone, Martin Krapcho, Jessica Garshell and Daniel S. Miller. 2014, "Seer Cancer Statistics Review, 1975–2011," Bethesda, MD: National Cancer Institute. Retrieved March 20, 2015 (http://seer.cancer.gov/csr/1975_2011/).

Hubert, Helen B., Manning Feinleib, Patricia M. McNamara and William P. Castelli. 1983. "Obesity as an Independent Risk Factor for Cardiovascular Disease: A 26-Year Follow-up of Participants in the Framingham Heart Study." *Circulation* 67(5):968–77. doi: 10.1161/01.cir.67.5.968.

Jamal, Ahmed, Israel T. Agaku, Erin O'Connor, Brian A. King, John B. Kenemer and Linda Neff. 2014. "Current Cigarette Smoking among Adults—United States, 2005–2013." *MMWR: Morbidity and Mortality Weekly Report* 63(47):1108–12.

Johnson, Nicole Blair, Locola D. Hayes, Kathryn Brown, Elizabeth C. Hoo and Kathleen A. Ethier. 2014. "CDC National Health Report: Leading Causes of Morbidity and Mortality and Associated Behavioral Risk and Protective Factors—United States, 2005–2013." *MMWR: Surveillance Summaries* 63(4):3–27.

Juan, Wen Y., Mark Lino and P. Peter Basiotis. 2004. "Quality of Diets of Older Americans." *Nutrition Insights*.

Juan, Wen Y., Patricia M. Guenther and Phillip S. Kott. 2009. "Diet Quality of Older Americans in 1994–96 and 2001–02 as Measured by the Healthy Eating Index—2005." *Nutrition Insight 41*. Alexandria, VA: USDA, Center for Nutrition Policy and Promotion (http://www.cnpp.usda.gov/sites/default/files/nutrition_insights_uploads/Insight41.pdf).

Kochanek, Kenneth D., Elizabeth Arias and Robert N. Anderson. 2013. "How Did Cause of Death Contribute to Racial Differences in Life Expectancy in the United States in 2010." *NCHS Data Brief* 125.1–8.

Krebs Smith, Susan M., Patricia M. Guenther, Amy F. Subar, Sharon I. Kirkpatrick and Kevin W. Dodd. 2010. "Americans Do Not Meet Federal Dietary Recommendations." *The Journal of Nutrition*. doi: 10.3945/jn.110.124826.

Lawrence, Reva C., David T. Felson, Charles G. Helmick, Lesley M. Arnold, Hyon Choi, Richard A. Deyo, Sherine Gabriel, Rosemarie Hirsch, Marc C. Hochberg, Gene G. Hunder, Joanne M. Jordan, Jeffrey N. Katz, Hilal Maradit Kremers, Frederick Wolfe and Workgroup National Arthritis Data. 2008. "Estimates of the Prevalence of Arthritis and Other Rheumatic Conditions in the United States: Part II." *Arthritis & Rheumatism* 58(1):26–35. doi: 10.1002/art.23176.

Lazarus, Richard S. and Susan Folkman. 1984. *Stress, Appraisal, and Coping*. New York, NY: Springer Publishing Company.

Letenneur, Luc, Veronique Gilleron, Daniel Commenges, Catherine Helmer, Jean-Marc Orgogozo and Jean-Francois Dartigues. 1999. "Are Sex and Educational Level Independent Predictors of Dementia and Alzheimer's Disease? Incidence

Data from the Paquid Project." *Journal of Neurology, Neurosurgery & Psychiatry* 66(2):177–83. doi: 10.1136/jnnp.66.2.177.

Lindsay, Joan, Danielle Laurin, René Verreault, Réjean Hébert, Barbara Helliwell, Gerry B. Hill and Ian McDowell. 2002. "Risk Factors for Alzheimer's Disease: A Prospective Analysis from the Canadian Study of Health and Aging." *American Journal of Epidemiology* 156(5):445–53. doi: 10.1093/aje/kwf074.

Link, Bruce G. and Jo Phelan. 1995. "Social Conditions as Fundamental Causes of Disease." *Journal of Health and Social Behavior* Extra Issue: 80–94.

Link, Bruce G. and Jo Phelan. 1996. "Understanding Sociodemographic Differences in Health—the Role of Fundamental Social Causes." *American Journal of Public Health* 86(4):471–72.

Link, Bruce G., Mary E. Northridge, Jo C. Phelan and Michael L. Ganz. 1998. "Social Epidemiology and the Fundamental Cause Concept: On the Structuring of Effective Cancer Screens by Socioeconomic Status." *Milbank Quarterly* 76(3):375–402, 304–05.

Luo, Ye and Linda J. Waite. 2005. "The Impact of Childhood and Adult SES on Physical, Mental, and Cognitive Well-Being in Later Life." *The Journals of Gerontology, Series B: Psychological Sciences and Social Sciences* 60(2):S93–S101. doi: 10.1093/geronb/60.2.S93.

Lynch, John, George D. Smith, Sam Harper and Kathleen Bainbridge. 2006. "Explaining the Social Gradient in Coronary Heart Disease: Comparing Relative and Absolute Risk Approaches." *Journal of Epidemiology and Community Health (1979–)* 60(5):436–41. doi: 10.2307/40793976.

Macintyre, Sally, Kate Hunt and Helen Sweeting. 1996. "Gender Difference in Health: Are Things Really as Simple as They Seem?" *Social Science and Medicine* 42(4):617–24.

Manly, Jennifer J. and Richard Mayeux. 2004. "Ethnic Differences in Dementia and Alzheimer's Disease." Pp. 95–145 in *Critical Perspectives on Racial and Ethnic Differences in Health in Late Life*, edited by N. B. Anderson, R. A. Bulatao and B. Cohen. Washington, DC: National Academies Press.

Manton, Kenneth G., XiLiang Gu and Vicki L. Lamb. 2006. "Change in Chronic Disability from 1982 to 2004/2005 as Measured by Long-Term Changes in Function and Health in the U.S. Elderly Population." *Proceedings of the National Academy of Sciences* 103(48):18374–79. doi: 10.1073/pnas.0608483103.

Markides, Kyriakos S. and Karl Eschbach. 2011. "Hispanic Paradox in Adult Mortality in the United States." Pp. 227–40 in *International Handbook of Adult Mortality*. New York, NY: Springer.

Martin, Linda G., Vicki A. Freedman, Robert F. Schoeni and Patricia M. Andreski. 2010. "Trends in Disability and Related Chronic Conditions among People Aged Fifty to Sixty-Four." *Health Affairs* 29(4):725–31. doi: 10.1377/hlthaff.2008.0746.

Martin, Linda G., Robert F. Schoeni and Patricia M. Andreski. 2010. "Trends in Health of Older Adults in the United States: Past, Present, Future." *Demography* 47(1):S17–40. doi: 10.1353/dem.2010.0003.

Martin, Linda G. and Robert F. Schoeni. 2014. "Trends in Disability and Related Chronic Conditions among the Forty-and-over Population: 1997–2010." *Disability and Health Journal* 7(1, Suppl.):S4–S14. doi: http://dx.doi.org/10.1016/j.dhjo.2013.06.007.

Mendis, Shanthi. 2014. "Global Status Report on Noncommunicable Diseases 2014." Geneva, Switzerland: World Health Organization.

Meyer, Madonna Harrington and Pamela Herd. 2007. "Market Friendly or Family Friendly? The State and Gender Inequality in Old Age." New York, NY: Russell Sage Foundation.

Mitka, Mike. 2012. "Heart Disease and Stroke Deaths Fall, but Some Fear a Reverse in the Trend." *Journal of the American Medical Association* 307(6):550–52.

Mokdad, Ali H., Earl S. Ford, Barbara A. Bowman, William H. Dietz, Frank Vinicor, Virginia S. Bales and James S. Marks. 2003. "Prevalence of Obesity, Diabetes, and Obesity-Related Health Risk Factors, 2001." *Journal of the American Medical Association* 289(1):76–79.

Montez, Jennifer Karas, Robert A. Hummer, Mark D. Hayward, Hyeyoung Woo and Richard G. Rogers. 2011. "Trends in the Educational Gradient of U.S. Adult Mortality from 1986 through 2006 by Race, Gender, and Age Group." *Research on Aging* 33(2):145–71. doi: 10.1177/0164027510392388.

Mozaffarian, Dariush, Emelia J. Benjamin, Alan S. Go, Donna K. Arnett, Michael J. Blaha, Mary Cushman, Sarah de Ferranti, Jean-Pierre Després, Heather J. Fullerton and Virginia J. Howard. 2015. "Executive Summary: Heart Disease and Stroke Statistics—2015 Update. A Report from the American Heart Association." *Circulation* 131(4):434–41.

Murphy, Sherry L., Jiaquan Xu and Kenneth D. Kochanek. 2013. "Deaths: Final Data for 2010." *National Vital Statistics Reports* 61(4):1–118.

Murray, Christopher J. L., Sandeep C. Kulkarni, Catherine Michaud, Niels Tomijima, Maria T. Bulzacchelli, Terrell J. Iandiorio, Majid Ezzati and Thomas Novotny. 2006. "Eight Americas: Investigating Mortality Disparities across Races, Counties, and Race-Counties in the United States." *PLoS Medicine* 3(9). doi: http://dx.doi.org/10.1371/journal.pmed.0030260.

Mutchler, Jan E., Jeffrey A. Burr, Michael P. Massagli and Amy Pienta. 1999. "Work Transitions and Health in Later Life." *The Journals of Gerontology, Series, B: Psychological Sciences and Social Sciences* 54B(5):S252–61. doi: 10.1093/geronb/54B.5.S252.

Nagi, Saad Z. 1965. "Some Conceptual Issues in Disability and Rehabilitation." Pp. 100–13 in *Sociology and Rehabilitation*, edited by Marvin B. Sussman. Washington, DC: American Sociological Association.

Nagi, Saad Z. 1976. "An Epidemiology of Disability among Adults in the United States." *Milbank Quarterly* 54(4):439–67. doi: 10.2307/3349677.

National Cancer Institute. 2015. "Fast Stats: An Interactive Tool for Access to Seer Cancer Statistics." Surveillance Research Program.

NCHS. 2013. *Health, United States, 2012: With Special Feature on Emergency Care*. Congress.

NCHS. 2014. *Health, United States, 2013: Special Feature on Prescription Drugs*. Congress (http://www.cdc.gov/nchs/data/hus/hus13.pdf).

Nelson, Miriam E., W. Jack Rejeski, Steven N. Blair, Pamela W. Duncan, James O. Judge, Abby C. King, Carol A. Macera and Carmen Castaneda-Sceppa. 2007. "Physical Activity and Public Health in Older Adults: Recommendation from the American College of Sports Medicine and the American Heart Association." *Circulation* 116(9):1094–104.

Noymer, Andrew. 2005, "Life Expectancy in the USA, 1900–98." Retrieved March 25, 2015 (http://demog.berkeley.edu/~andrew/1918/figure2.html).

Ogden, Cynthia L., Margaret D. Carroll, Brian K. Kit and Katherine M. Flegal. 2014. "Prevalence of Childhood and Adult Obesity in the United States, 2011–2012." *Journal of the American Medical Association* 311(8):806–14.

Ortman, Jennifer M., Victoria A. Velkoff and Howard Hogan. 2014. *An Aging Nation: The Older Population in the United States.* P25-1140 Congress. Current Population Reports (http://www.census.gov/prod/2014pubs/p25–1140.pdf).

Pappas, Gregory, Susan Queen, Wilbur Hadden and Gail Fisher. 1993. "The Increasing Disparity in Mortality between Socioeconomic Groups in the United States, 1960 and 1986." *New England Journal of Medicine* 329(2):103–09.

Pearlin, Leonard I. 1989. "The Sociological Study of Stress." *Journal of Health and Social Behavior* 30(3):241–56. doi: 10.2307/2136956.

Quiñones, Ana R., Jersey Liang, Joan M. Bennett, Xiao Xu and Wen Ye. 2011. "How Does the Trajectory of Multimorbidity Vary across Black, White, and Mexican Americans in Middle and Old Age?" *The Journals of Gerontology, Series B: Psychological Sciences and Social Sciences* 66B(6):739–49. doi: 10.1093/geronb/gbr106.

Read, Jen'nan Ghazal and Bridget K. Gorman. 2010. "Gender and Health Inequality." *Annual Review of Sociology* 36(1):371–86. doi: 10.1146/annurev.soc.012809.102535.

Redfoot, Donald L., Ari Houser and AARP Public Policy Institute. 2010. "More Older People with Disabilities Living in the Community: Trends from the National Long-Term Care Survey, 1984–2004." Washington, DC: AARP Public Policy Institute (http://assets.aarp.org/rgcenter/ppi/ltc/2010-08-disability.pdf).

Rehm, Jürgen, Robin Room, Kathryn Graham, Maristela Monteiro, Gerhard Gmel and Christopher T. Sempos. 2003. "The Relationship of Average Volume of Alcohol Consumption and Patterns of Drinking to Burden of Disease: An Overview." *Addiction* 98(9):1209–28. doi: 10.1046/j.1360-0443.2003.00467.x.

Schoenborn, Charlotte A., Patricia F. Adams and Jennifer A. Peregoy. 2013. "Health Behaviors of Adults: United States, 2008–2010." *Vital and Health Statistics. Series 10, Data from the National Health Survey* 257:1–184.

Schoeni, Robert F., Linda G. Martin, Patricia M. Andreski and Vicki A. Freedman. 2005. "Persistent and Growing Socioeconomic Disparities in Disability among the Elderly: 1982–2002." *American Journal of Public Health* 95(11):2065–70.

Schoeni, Robert F., Vicki A. Freedman and Linda G. Martin. 2008. "Why Is Late-Life Disability Declining?" *Milbank Quarterly* 86(1):47–89. doi: 10.1111/j.1468-0009.2007.00513.x.

Seeman, Teresa E., Sharon S. Merkin, Eileen M. Crimmins and Arun S. Karlamangla. 2010. "Disability Trends among Older Americans: National Health and Nutrition Examination Surveys, 1988–1994 and 1999–2004." *American Journal of Public Health* 100(1):100–07. doi: 10.2105/AJPH.2008.157388.

Shay, Christina M., Hongyan Ning, Norrina B. Allen, Mercedes R. Carnethon, Stephanie E. Chiuve, Kurt J. Greenlund, Martha L. Daviglus and Donald M. Lloyd-Jones. 2012. "Status of Cardiovascular Health in US Adults: Prevalence Estimates from the National Health and Nutrition Examination Surveys (NHANES) 2003–2008." *Circulation* 125(1):45–56. doi: 10.1161/circulation aha.111.035733.

Siegel, Rebecca, Jiemin Ma, Zhaohui Zou and Ahmedin Jemal. 2014. "Cancer Statistics, 2014." *CA: A Cancer Journal for Clinicians* 64(1):9–29. doi: 10.3322/caac.21208.

Thacker, Stephen B., Donna F. Stroup, Vilma Carande-Kulis, James S. Marks, Kakoli Roy and Julie L. Gerberding. 2006. "Measuring the Public's Health." *Public Health Reports* 121(1):14–22.

Thoits, Peggy A. 1995. "Stress, Coping, and Social Support Processes: Where Are We? What Next?" *Journal of Health and Social Behavior* Extra Issue:53–79.

Thompson, William W., David K. Shay, Eric Weintraub, Lynnette Brammer, Carolyn B. Bridges, Nancy J. Cox and Keiji Fukuda. 2004. "Influenza-Associated Hospitalizations in the United States." *Journal of the American Medical Association* 292(11):1333–40.

Tomasetti, Cristian and Bert Vogelstein. 2015. "Variation in Cancer Risk among Tissues Can Be Explained by the Number of Stem Cell Divisions." *Science* 347(6217):78–81. doi: 10.1126/science.1260825.

Tucker, Margaret A. and Alisa M. Goldstein. 2003. "Melanoma Etiology: Where Are We?" *Oncogene* 22(20):3042–52.

Tucker-Seeley, Reginald D., Yi Li, Glorian Sorensen and S.V. Subramanian. 2011. "Lifecourse Socioeconomic Circumstances and Multimorbidity among Older Adults." *BMC Public Health* 11(1):313.

Turner, R. Jay, Blair Wheaton and Donald A. Lloyd. 1995. "The Epidemiology of Social Stress." *American Sociological Review* 60(1):104–26.

USDA. 2010. *Dietary Guidelines for Americans 2010 (7th Ed.).* Congress.

Üstün, T. Bedirhan. 2010. *Measuring Health and Disability: Manual for WHO Disability Assessment Schedule WHODAS 2.0.* Geneva, Switzerland: World Health Organization.

Verbrugge, Lois M. 1986. "From Sneezes to Adieux: Stages of Health for American Men and Women." *Social Science & Medicine* 22(11):1195–212.

Verbrugge, Lois M. and Alan M. Jette. 1994. "The Disablement Process." *Social Science and Medicine* 38(1):1–14.

Verbrugge, Lois M. and Xian Liu. 2014. "Midlife Trends in Activities and Disability." *Journal of Aging and Health* 26(2):178–206. doi: 10.1177/0898264313508189.

Viegi, Giovanni, Antonio Scognamiglio, Sandra Baldacci, Francesco Pistelli and Laura Carrozzi. 2000. "Epidemiology of Chronic Obstructive Pulmonary Disease (COPD)." *Respiration* 68(1):4–19.

Vincent, Grayson K. and Victoria A. Velkoff. 2010. *The Next Four Decades, the Older Population in the United States: 2010 to 2050.* P25-1138 Congress. Current Population Reports (http://www.census.gov/prod/2010pubs/p25-1138.pdf).

Waldron, Ingrid. 1991. "Patterns and Causes of Gender Differences in Smoking." *Social Science and Medicine* 32(9):989–1005.

Ward, Brian W. and Jeannine S. Schiller. 2013. "Prevalence of Multiple Chronic Conditions among US Adults: Estimates from the National Health Interview Survey, 2010." *Preventing Chronic Disease* 10:1–15.

Ward, Elizabeth, Ahmedin Jemal, Vilma Cokkinides, Gopal K. Singh, Cheryll Cardinez, Asma Ghafoor and Michael Thun. 2004. "Cancer Disparities by Race/Ethnicity and Socioeconomic Status." *CA: A Cancer Journal for Clinicians* 54(2):78–93.

WHO. 2015a. "National Health Account Database." Retrieved March 31, 2015 (http://apps.who.int/nha/database/ViewData/Indicators/en).

WHO. 2015b, "Overweight and Obesity: Fact Sheet No. 311: World Health Organization." Retrieved March 31, 2015 (http://www.who.int/mediacentre/factsheets/fs311/en/).

Wilkinson, Richard G. 1996. *Unhealthy Societies: The Afflictions of Inequality*. New York, NY: Routledge.

Wilkinson, Richard G. and Michael G. Marmot, eds. 2003. *Social Determinants of Health: The Solid Facts*. Copenhagen, Denmark: World Health Organization.

Williams, David R. and Chiquita Collins. 1995. "US Socioeconomic and Racial Differences in Health: Patterns and Explanations." *Annual Review of Sociology* 21:349–86.

Winkleby, Marilyn A., Darius E. Jatulis, Erica Frank and Stephen P. Fortmann. 1992. "Socioeconomic Status and Health: How Education, Income, and Occupation Contribute to Risk Factors for Cardiovascular Disease." *American Journal of Public Health* 82(6):816–20.

World Health Organization. 1948. "Preamble to the Constitution of the World Health Organization as Adopted by the International Health Conference." Paper presented at the New York, June, 19–22, 1946; signed on July, 22, 1946 by the representatives of 61 States (Official Records of the World Health Organization, no. 2, p. 100) and entered into force on April, 7, 1948.

Yoon, Paula W., Brigham Bastian, Robert N. Anderson, Janet L. Collins and Harold W. Jaffe. 2014. "Potentially Preventable Deaths from the Five Leading Causes of Death—United States, 2008–2010." *Morbidity and Mortality Weekly Report* 63(17):369–74.

Zajacova, Anna, Noreen Goldman and German Rodriguez. 2009. "Unobserved Heterogeneity Can Confound the Effect of Education on Mortality." *Mathematical Population Studies* 16(2):153–73.

CHAPTER SIX

Mental Health, Cognitive Ability, and Dementia across the Life Course

Donna D. McAlpine and Taeho Greg Rhee

Cognitive decline in abilities such as reasoning and memory begin quite early in adulthood and continue to decay throughout one's life course (Salthouse, 2010). Indeed, some decline in cognitive ability is expected as a function of normal biological aging. However, cognitive functioning that is impaired to the extent that it interferes with one's ability to carry out desired activities, be independent, sustain meaningful relationships, and to participate purposefully in life sharply increases in later life. The burden of severe cognitive impairment including the direct and indirect economic costs, diminished quality of life, increased morbidity and mortality, and deleterious impact on family and friends is tremendous (Alzheimer's Association [AA], 2014).

In contrast to observed trends in risk for cognitive impairments over the life course, the prevalence of other common mental health problems such as depression and anxiety appear to decline with age (Kessler et al., 2005). However, symptoms of other psychiatric disorders often cooccur with cognitive impairments (Gauthier et al., 2010; Lyketsos et al., 2002); for example, persons with cognitive disorders may also feel apathetic, agitated, or depressed. The comorbidity between types of mental health problems complicates diagnosis, diminishes quality of life, and adds to the burden of disorder.

While it is well documented that genetics plays a role in risk for cognitive impairments and other mental problems, we argue that variation in the trajectories of people who experience these problems is shaped by social context. Recognizing that the experience of cognitive impairment and other mental health problems for older adults varies with social circumstances allows us to understand differences in prevalence patterns, risks, and outcomes. Most importantly, a life-course framework identifies the important historical, developmental, and social factors that shape how we define mental disorders, who is at risk, and the consequences for individuals and their families (Elder, 1998; Halfon & Hochstein, 2002; Whalley, Dick, & McNeill, 2006).

The Epidemiology of Cognitive Impairments, Mental Health, and Illness

Mental health and mental illness are not simply antonyms and our definitions of what constitutes either vary by culture and time. Mental health is a holistic concept representing an individual's ability to cope or adapt to everyday changes and stress, perform important role functions, and feel that one's life is satisfying and fulfilling (U.S. Department of Health and Human Services, 1999; World Health Organization [WHO], 2014). Keyes (2007), for example, defines mental health in terms of characteristics such as feeling useful, having a sense of belonging and purpose, and feeling in control over the direction of life.

While it is now commonly acknowledged that there is a distinction between mental health and mental illness, much of the focus remains on mental illness or disorder. The *Diagnostic and Statistical Manual of Mental Disorders* (*DSM*), now in its fifth major iteration (*DSM-5*), is the major classification system used in the United States to define various types of mental disorders (American Psychiatric Association [APA], 2013). The classification of what constitutes a mental disorder and the symptoms that define each type of disorder are not merely the products of scientific discovery or consensus, but are instead partially the results of sharp political debates among interest groups (Mayes & Horwitz, 2005). The resulting delineations between categories of disorders and between symptoms that constitute each disorder in the DSM are, therefore, often somewhat arbitrary and amorphous. While recognizing that the difference between mental illness and mental health are often unclear and mental disorders are culturally and socially defined, *DSM-5* broadly defines mental disorder as "a syndrome characterized by clinically significant disturbance in an individual's cognition, emotion regulation, or behavior that reflects a dysfunction in the psychological, biological, or developmental processes underlying mental functioning" (APA, 2013, p. 20).

Earlier versions of the *DSM* were relatively agnostic to age of onset as a criterion to define disorder. The newest edition deliberately lays out the classification using a life-course perspective, beginning with disorders that typically first occur in early childhood such as developmental disorders progressing through the common disorders of adolescence and adulthood such as depression or anxiety to disorders that most often have first onset in later life including neurocognitive disorders (NCDs).

The major classification of NCD in the *DSM-5* replaced the classification of "delirium, dementia, amnestic and other cognitive disorders" in the previous version of the *DSM* (APA, 2000, p. 135). The authors decided to change the language, partially because the term dementia is stigmatized (Ganguli et al., 2011). Here we continue to use the term dementia, because, like the authors of the *DSM*, we recognize it continues to be widely used both by laypeople and health professionals. NCDs include delirium, a condition marked by sudden problems in awareness and attention. However, the focus of this review is on NCD that have a more gradual onset and are progressive and increase exponentially during later life.

According to the *DSM-5*, NCDs cover deficits in six areas: complex attention such as being easily distracted or having problems retaining new information; executive functions such as planning or decision-making skills; language including problems like forgetting words; learning and memory difficulties such as having problems keeping track of the day; perceptual motor skills such as difficulty following directions; and social cognition, which includes difficulty understanding or conforming to social norms. Most importantly, the most recent version of the *DSM* distinguishes between major neurocognitive disorder (major NCD), and mild or minor neurocognitive disorder (mild NCD). A diagnosis of major NCD, also referred to as dementia in previous versions of the *DSM*, requires evidence of a decline in at least one of the six areas of cognitive functioning that is also of concern to the individual or his or her social networks. The cognitive problems must substantially interfere with an individual's ability to independently perform everyday activities, not only occur during periods of delirium, and not be the result of another mental disorder, such as schizophrenia or depression. The diagnostic category of mild NCD was introduced in the *DSM-5* to cover declines in cognitive performance that do not meet the threshold of major NCD but are of concern to the individual, their social networks, or health professionals. To meet the diagnostic criteria for mild NCD, the decline in cognitive performance does not substantially interfere with being able to perform the tasks of daily life independently, but makes these activities more difficult. The *DSM-5* recognizes that "the distinction between major and mild NCD is inherently arbitrary, and the disorders exist along a continuum." (APA, 2013, p. 608).

The addition of mild NCD was greeted with some controversy. As Wakefield (2013) points out, one of the most publicly vocal critics of the *DSM-5* was Allen Frances, who was an editor of the previous version of the *DSM*. Frances objected to the expansion of *DSM-5* to include as disorders what might be considered normal emotions and behaviors. In specific reference to the inclusion of mild NCD, Frances (2012) explained:

> The everyday forgetting characteristic of old age will now be misdiagnosed as Minor Neurocognitive Disorder, creating a huge false positive population of people who are not at special risk for dementia. Since there is no effective treatment for this 'condition' (or for dementia), the label provides absolutely no benefit (while creating great anxiety) even for those at true risk for later developing dementia. It is a dead loss for the many who will be mislabeled.

Others support the inclusion of mild NCD, arguing that patients may be "comforted to know their healthcare providers recognize their problem" (Blazer, 2013, pp. 585–586) and may be able to offer some strategies to deal with minor changes in cognitive functioning. Further, there is some evidence that mild forms of cognitive impairment may be precursors to major NCD (AA, 2014), making the identification of mild NCD a promising strategy for early intervention.

It is clear that many people meet the criteria for mild cognitive impairments, although estimates vary widely based on the population surveyed and the measures used (Ward et al., 2012). In a recent national survey of 21 states, almost 13 percent of the population aged 45 and older reported they had experienced increased confusion or memory loss over the past year (Anderson et al., 2015), a crude, but conservative, estimate of what might be considered mild NCD under the *DSM-5*. Moreover, most persons with mild cognitive impairment do not progress to dementia (Petersen et al., 2014). There are reasons, therefore, to be concerned that the *DSM-5* may have overmedicalized cognitive disorders that are mild, transitory, or are a part of normal aging—although it is too soon to tell whether this will result in many more people getting unnecessary treatment and the diversion of resources from those who are more critically ill.

For both major and mild NCD, the *DSM-5* details a variety of subtypes that help specify etiology such as NCD due to Alzheimer's disease, Huntington's disease, Parkinson's disease, vascular disease, and traumatic brain injury (APA, 2013). Distinguishing between various types of NCD in the absence of specific diseases such as Huntington's is often difficult in practice because of a lack of clear biomarkers.

National and global estimates of the various subtypes of mild and major NCD have not caught up with *DSM-5* definitions, and estimates vary with the definitions of disorder that are employed and the populations that are studied (Wilson et al., 2011). One of the most rigorous studies in the United States is based on data collected in the Aging, Demographics, and Memory Study, a subsample of the National Health and Retirement Survey (Plassman et al., 2007, 2008). In this study, estimates of the prevalence of dementias and cognitive impairment are based on either in-home assessments or personal and proxy interviews. As shown in Table 6.1, about 14 percent of the population over the age of 70 meets the criteria for dementia, with Alzheimer's being the most common cause, affecting about 10 percent of the population. Cognitive impairments that do not meet the criteria for dementia are even more prevalent, impacting approximately 22 percent of the population. Extrapolating these prevalence estimates to the projected U.S. population in 2015 (U.S. Census Bureau Population Division, 2015), almost 4.1 million adults over the age of 70 are living with dementia, and a further 6.4 million are living with significant cognitive impairment that has not met the dementia threshold. It is also clear that the prevalence of both dementia and cognitive impairment significantly increase with age. After the age of 90, more than one in three older adults are living with dementia, and a further two in five are living with significant cognitive impairment. Globally, the prevalence of dementia is also very high, with an estimate of 35.6 million people in 2010 (World Health Organization [WHO] & Alzheimer's Disease International [ADI], 2012).

There is some controversy about whether the incidence of cognitive disorders has changed in recent years. Looking specifically at data from Medicare, the health insurance program that covers almost 100 percent of the population 65 years of age and older in the United States, some studies find an increasing incidence of Alzheimer's (Akushevich et al., 2013). In contrast, other studies conducted with community samples suggest that there has not been an increase in rates of Alzheimer's or other dementias and that instead incidence rates have been relatively stable or have even gone down (Rocca et al., 2011; Sheffield & Peek, 2011). For example, Sheffield and Peek (2011) examine changes in cognitive impairment from 1993 to 2004 using community-dwelling respondents to the Health and Retirement Survey, a large nationally representative study of older adults in the United States. Overall, they found that cognitive impairment declined from about 4 percent of the population over the age of 70 in 1993 to 2 percent in 2004. It is possible that the increase in incidence or prevalence of dementia that has been observed in studies using Medicare data may reflect increased case finding rather than a real increase in rates of disorder. Moreover, a decline in incidence of cognitive disorders may be due to the fact that more recent cohorts of older adults have higher educational achievement than did earlier cohorts (Dodge et al., 2013). However,

Table 6.1 Prevalence of Dementia and Cognitive Impairment without Dementia (CIND) in the United States by Age

	71–79 Years (95% CI)		80–89 Years (95% CI)		≥90 Years (95% CI)		Total (95% CI)	
Dementias								
All	5.0%	(2.6–7.3)	24.2%	(19.3–29.1)	37.4%	(25.5–49.3)	13.9%	(11.4–16.4)
Alzheimer's Disease	2.3%	(1.3–3.4)	18.1%	(13.5–22.7)	29.7%	(18.6–40.8)	9.7%	(7.6–11.9)
CIND								
	16.0%	(11.5–20.5)	29.2%	(24.3–34.1)	39.0%	(25.7–52.2)	22.2%	(18.7–25.7)

Note: Estimates of prevalence of dementia are based on data presented in Plassman et al. (2007); Estimates of prevalence of CIND are based on data presented in Plassman et al. (2008).

even if the incidence of cognitive impairments and dementia is steady or slightly decreasing, a matter still of some controversy, the numbers of persons with these problems will continue to increase with the aging of the population both in the United States and globally.

Most other major mental illnesses show a prevalence-pattern opposite of that observed for NCD in that most major mental illnesses have first onset early in life and the 12-month and life-time prevalence of common mental disorders such as depression, anxiety, and substance abuse appear to decline with age (Gum, King-Kallimanis, & Kohn, 2009; Kessler et al., 2005; Reynolds et al., 2015). Overall, about 23 percent of adults in the community meet the criteria for having an anxiety, mood, or substance use disorder in the past 12 months, compared to only 8.5 percent of persons aged 65 years and older (Gum, King-Kallimanis, & Kohn, 2009). The prevalence of schizophrenia in later life is between 0.3 percent and 1 percent, slightly lower than the prevalence among the total adult population (McAlpine, 2003). Rates of most common mental disorders also appear to decline across later life (Gum, King-Kallimanis, & Kohn, 2009; Reynolds et al., 2015). For example, Reynolds et al. (2015) estimate that persons aged 55 to 64 have about 4 times the odds of having a mood disorder than persons 85 years and older. Moreover, they find the same general pattern for anxiety, substance use, and personality disorders. However, these community studies underestimate the true prevalence of mental health problems because they do not include persons living in institutions. While estimates of the number of residents of nursing homes living with mental illness vary widely depending on the data set used, it is clear that the prevalence is higher than observed in community settings. For example, Bagchi, Verdier, and Simon (2009) estimate that between 16 percent and 45 percent of residents aged 65 or older living in nursing homes have a mental illness diagnosis. In another study, Grabowski et al. (2009) estimate that 27 percent of new admissions to nursing homes had a severe mental illness such as schizophrenia, bipolar disorder, or depression. Common mental illnesses such as depression or substance abuse are often accompanied by cognitive symptoms such as memory loss or difficulties with attention, making it sometimes difficult to distinguish between disorders.

It is also clear that other mental health problems often co-occur with dementia or cognitive impairment. The most commonly studied mental health problem among older adults is depression, because it is both prevalent and debilitating. Between about 2 percent and 6 percent of the population 65 years or older living in the community meet the criteria for having a recent episode of major depression (Gum, King-Kallimanis, & Kohn, 2009; Reynolds et al., 2015), and as many as 1 in 10 percent experience significant depressive symptomatology that does not meet the clinical threshold for disorder (Meeks et al., 2011). Rates of depression are even higher among persons with cognitive impairments. Using national data from the United States, for example, Steffens et al. (2009) estimate that while the rate of depression was about 8 percent for persons aged 71 years and older who did not have cognitive problems, it was 20 percent for persons with dementia and about 13 percent among persons with cognitive impairment that did not meet the threshold for dementia. While commanding less research attention, other studies suggest an association between mental health disorders such as alcohol abuse, anxiety and schizophrenia, and cognitive impairment in later life (Beaudreau & O'Hara, 2008; Hendrie et al., 2014; Mukamal et al., 2003).

The causal relationship between other mental health problems and cognitive impairments is complicated and difficult to establish with full certainty. Much of the research attention has focused on depression. It may be that a higher rate of depression among persons with cognitive impairments is a reaction caused by the stress of losing functioning and independence. It may also be that a third characteristic is associated with both risk of developing depression and cognitive impairment and thus confounds the relationship. Finally, it may be that depression is casually a risk factor for developing later cognitive disorders. Research has been robust in exploring this later possibility, which we explore further in the discussion of risk factors later in the chapter.

Many more individuals with NCD than meet the diagnostic criteria for a comorbid mental health problem experience significant psychiatric symptoms. Individuals with dementia face unique behavioral and psychological symptoms of dementia (BPSD), which is defined as "a heterogeneous range of psychological reactions, psychiatric symptoms, and behaviors occurring in people with dementia of any etiology" (Finkel & Burns, 2000). As shown on Table 6.2, BPSD is divided into two major clusters—behavioral and psychological symptoms clusters—and each cluster has two subgroups. In the behavioral symptoms cluster, two subgroups include aberrant motor behaviors and inappropriate behaviors. In the psychological symptoms cluster, two subgroups include mood-related symptoms and psychotic-related symptoms. The list of BPSD shown in Table 6.2 is not meant to be exhaustive, but is based on the current neuropsychiatric inventory (NPI), which is widely measured and collected in clinical practice and research (Gauthier et al., 2010). Co-occurring physical and mental conditions, as well as unmet needs, can cause BPSD in individuals with dementia.

Less attention has been paid to the association between cognitive impairment and mental health, if we conceptualize the former as much more than the absence of mental disorder. Given that the prognosis for

Table 6.2 Behavioral and Psychological Symptoms that Accompany Dementia

Behavioral Symptoms	Psychological Symptoms
Aberrant motor behaviors:	*Mood-related symptoms:*
– Pacing, kicking, hitting, pushing	– Depression/dysphoria
– Wandering	– Anxiety
– Fidgeting	– Apathy/indifference
– Hand-wringing	– Irritability/lability
– Other types of aberrant motor behaviors	
Inappropriate behaviors:	*Psychotic-related symptoms:*
– Agitation/aggression	– Delusions
– Disinhibition	– Hallucinations
– Euphoria/elation	
– Night-time behaviors (neuro-vegetative changes)	
– Appetite/eating changes (neuro-vegetative changes)	

Source: Adapted from International Psychogeriatric Association [IPA], 1996.

dementia is typically irreversible and the deficits associated with major NCD are many and profound, it is somewhat surprising that people with even severe dementia are mentally healthy on some measures. Much of the research on what might be considered mental health among persons with cognitive disorders has been done in the context of examining variation in quality of life. There are a variety of conceptualization and measures of quality of life, but broadly it "encompasses the individual's physical health, psychosocial well-being and functioning, independence, control over life, material circumstances and the external environment." (Bowling, 2005). One aspect of psychological well-being that contributes to quality of life, and can be considered a part of mental health, is life satisfaction. St. John and Montgomery (2010) in a study of community-dwelling older Canadians found that individuals with dementia or with cognitive impairment but no dementia reported slightly lower satisfaction with life in general and lower satisfaction with their material and social circumstances than did their counterparts with no cognitive impairments. While there were differences, they were modest—and overwhelmingly, the older adults in their study, irrespective of level of cognitive impairment, were satisfied with life. However, the study did not include people with severe dementia.

It is difficult to measure subjective dimensions of well-being for persons with severe dementia because cognitive impairments make awareness, insight, and communication difficult. However, there is a range of measures available to assess the subjective aspects of quality of life across the range of cognitive disorder, including severe disorder (Bowling et al., 2015). Some of the most important work is qualitative: research that involves asking patients with NCD what they value about life or what makes them satisfied and happy. In a synthesis of these studies, O'Rourke et al. (2015) identify six key themes that respondents with dementia identify as mattering for their quality of life: (1) connectedness to others and to one's environment; (2) positive relationships with others that provide a sense of being loved and cared about and which is reciprocal; (3) feeling a sense of purpose in life; (4) sense of wellness despite experience of significant symptoms; (5) feeling attached to the place or environment where one is living; and (6) having a sense of happiness or contentment. Importantly, it is these subjective assessments of life, rather than degree of impairment or disability itself that shape quality of life (Byrne-Davis, Bennett, & Wilcock, 2006; O'Rouke et al., 2015). Moreover, even persons with severe NCD express similar aspects of life such as relationships that they most care about and that shape their well-being (Cahill & Diaz-Ponce, 2011). Menne, Judge, and Whitlatch (2009) used 13 items to capture physical, emotional, interpersonal, and environmental domains of quality of life, and they found that being African American, having a nonspousal caregiver, more depressive symptoms, and less involvement in daily decision making were associated with poorer quality of life among individuals with dementia.

The Burden of Cognitive Impairment and Mental Health Problems

The overall burden of cognitive disability and mental illness includes their impact on individuals, their families and the overall community in terms of increased morbidity, mortality, diminished quality of life, lost productivity, and costs of health care and other services such as home and institutional care. There are a number of estimates of the economic impact of dementia (World Health Organization (WHO) & Alzheimer's Disease International (ADI), 2012; Wimo & Prince, 2010; Wimo et al., 2013; Yang et al., 2012); while they vary in assumptions about the prevalence of dementia, and in definitions of costs, they concur that the costs are enormous. A recent analysis by Wimo et al. (2013) estimates the global costs of dementia care, including both direct and indirect costs. Direct costs include expenditures associated with medical services such as medications, inpatient stays and visits to the doctor as well as expenditures associated with social care such as home care or nursing home care. Indirect costs of informal care include the estimated costs of unpaid care provided by family members. In 2010, they estimate that the total, worldwide economic costs for dementia care were 604 billion U.S. dollars, or about 1 percent of the world's gross national product. Approximately, 58 percent of these costs are attributable to direct medical and social costs and 42 percent to the cost of informal care. Not surprisingly, informal care represents a larger proportion of all costs in lower-income countries than in higher-income countries. The per capita costs of dementia-related care—$48,605 in U.S. dollars—are the highest in the world in North America (Wimo & Prince, 2010). In the United States, the total economic costs of dementia in 2010 was estimated to be between 159 billion and 215 billion dollars, with informal care comprising between 31 percent and 49 percent of the total costs (Hurd et al., 2013).

Another way to measure the burden of mental health problems is in terms of disability-adjusted life years (DALY), where DALY represents the years of healthy life lost to the disorder (World Health Organization (WHO), 2008). DALY takes into account both premature mortality and years spent in less than ideal health, and it is widely used to compare the impact of various types of health problems and interventions. In high-income countries, mental health disorders comprise 3 of the 10 leading causes of burden; depression ranks first, Alzheimer's disease and other dementias rank fourth, and alcohol abuse disorders rank as the fifth leading cause of disease burden (World Health Organization (WHO), 2008).

Having comorbid cognitive impairment and other mental health disorders such as depression is expected to increase the burden of either type of disorder. For example, mental health comorbidities increase the direct medical costs, especially inpatient care, for persons with cognitive conditions (Leibson et al., 2015).

Considerable research attention has focused on the caregiving burden, or the subjective and objective tasks associated with providing care for a person with a chronic health problem (Montgomery, Gonyea, & Hooyman, 1985). Objective burden includes the specific activities and resources involved in caregiving, such as time spent supervising someone, or helping with daily activities such as shopping and food preparation. Subjective burden refers to the emotions and feelings associated with the experience of caregiving (Montgomery, Gonyea, & Hooyman, 1985). Many of the responsibilities involved with caring for a person with mental health problems rest with family members. Perhaps not surprisingly, due to women's longer life expectancy and continued gendered expectations about who should fulfill caregiving roles (Walker, Pratt, & Eddy, 1995), the burden of caregiving disproportionately falls on women.

The objective burden is high for caregivers of persons with both severe and mild cognitive impairments. Using a nationally representative sample, Fisher et al. (2011) examined variation in the amount of time helping with specific activities or in supervision, physical and emotional strain, and perceived benefits of caregiving among individuals who reported that they had primary responsibility for caring for a family member with dementia, or CIND. Caregivers spent a considerable amount of time doing caregiving tasks; on average, approximately 9 hours per day for persons with dementia and 4 hours per day for CIND. Approximately 66 percent of caretakers reported significant physical strain and 71 percent significant emotional strain associated with their responsibilities; however, there were not significant differences between the two groups in perceived strain.

The objective and subjective tasks involved in caregiving have costs for the caregiver. Caregivers are at risk for depression and anxiety associated with the stress of being a caregiver (Covinsky et al., 2003; Seeher et al., 2013; Werner, 2012). In a study of caregivers of persons with moderate to severe dementia, for example, Covinsky et al. (2003) found that almost one-third of caregivers met the criteria for depression. Patient characteristics associated with increased risk for depression among caregivers include severity of dementia, behavioral problems (such as anger and aggression), and limitations in activities (Covinsky et al., 2003; Hooker et al., 2002). There are also important social group differences both in the types of caregiving and outcomes. Some studies find that depression is less common in caregivers of black compared to white patients with dementia (Covinsky et al., 2003; Janevic & Connell, 2001). Unfortunately, there has been insufficient research examining the burden associated with caring for persons with comorbid cognitive and other mental health disorders such as depression (Schulz & Martire, 2004).

Risk Factors

Research demonstrates that genetics play a role in the development of many mental illnesses, including cognitive disorders. There is a stronger link between genetic risk and early onset rather than later onset dementia (Loy et al., 2014). Overall, however, genetics alone explains very little of the variation in risk for dementia. For other mental disorders, that often co-occur with cognitive disorders, estimates of risk associated with heredity vary widely, although it is generally accepted that disorders such as schizophrenia have much higher heritability risk than disorders such as depression, although genetics in conjunction with environment probably play a part in the etiology of many types of mental disorders (Rutter, 2006).

While the genetic determinants of cognitive impairment and other mental illnesses continue to be vigorously examined in research, there is a growing body of literature about social determinants of risk and modifiable risk factors (Baumgart et al., 2015). Age, for example, while clearly a risk factor for NCD, is not modifiable. The focus of research and interventions has been on characteristics of individuals' circumstances in early life, their lifestyles and health behaviors, their physical and mental comorbidities, and their social environments that might be amenable to change and therefore reduce risk for later disorder. While this research literature is enormous, here we focus on general themes that have emerged and the most promising research directions.

Early Adversity and Disadvantage

A central tenet of life-course theory is that there are important developmental periods where experiences (both positive and negative) can shape outcome even years later (Elder, 1998). Simply put, what happens in early childhood matters for well-being across the life course. Overwhelming research on risks for common mental disorders such as depression or substance use shows that early-life adversities such as parental neglect and deprivation increase risk of having a mental disorder in childhood. In turn, having a mental disorder in childhood increases risk of having a mental disorder in adulthood (Mechanic, McAlpine, & Rochefort, 2014). The difficulty is, of course, that there is significant variation in the trajectories of children and predicting who will do well in adulthood and later life and who will not.

One of the most consistent findings in the literature is a strong inverse relationship between socioeconomic status (SES) and risk of mental health problems, where SES is usually operationalized as education, income, or occupation (Muntaner et al., 2004; Saraceno, Levav, & Kohn, 2005). For example, across studies persons from low-SES groups have a median of about 3.4 times higher prevalence of schizophrenia and 2.4 higher prevalence of depression compared to people of high SES (Saraceno et al., 2005). However, determining the causal direction between SES and mental disorders is difficult and both social selection and social causation explanations have some utility (Mechanic et al., 2014; Muntaner et al., 2004). Social selection implies that people with mental health problems are selected into lower SES attainment, based on having a mental health problem. For example, experiencing a mental disorder in childhood, adolescence or early adulthood makes it difficult to finish school, get a good job, or achieve a high income. Thus, early mental health problems may select a person into a lower SES than their more healthy peers. In contrast, social causation explanations for the inverse relationship between SES and the prevalence of mental disorders suggest that lack of material resources and the adversities and strains that come with low SES cause increased risk of disorder. Both social selection and causation probably operate for most major mental illnesses; but evidence suggests that social selection is more relevant for disorders such as schizophrenia, and social causation for disorders such as depression (Mechanic et al., 2014; Muntaner et al., 2004).

There is an emerging body of research examining the association between SES and cognitive impairments, but untangling causation is particularly tricky. While the evidence is not definitive, SES in early childhood—reflected in measures such as parental occupation or poverty in childhood—may be associated with measures of cognitive performance such as IQ in childhood (Borenstein, Copenhaver, & Mortimer, 2006). Others have examined the impact of childhood SES on cognitive performance in later life, but again the results are inconsistent and inconclusive (Borenstein et al., 2006).

The majority of research attention that links SES to cognitive impairments in later life has been focused on educational attainment. There is a growing body of research suggesting that persons with lower educational attainment are at greater risk for developing dementia or other cognitive impairments in later life than persons with higher levels of education (AA, 2014), although some researchers fail to find this association. There are a number of intriguing hypotheses to explain this association, but none are definitive (AA, 2014; Borenstein et al., 2006; Ngandu et al., 2007). First, it may be that educational attainment is a proxy for IQ and thus the observed relationship between educational level and cognitive performance in later life may be spurious. That is, IQ in childhood may select one into higher educational attainment and also be causally related to cognitive functioning across the life course. An alternative hypothesis is that education builds cognitive reserve so that more highly educated persons are able to compensate for declines in brain function in some areas. But it is also possible that pre-existing differences in cognitive reserve select people into various levels of educational achievement. The association between education and cognitive performance in later life may also be mediated by health behaviors and cardiovascular risk factors, although some research fails to support this hypothesis (Ngandu et al., 2007). Overall, we lack the scientific evidence to definitely draw conclusions about the causal connections between educational level and risk of cognitive disorders in later life. If causality is established, however, it would add compelling evidence for the importance of addressing inequality in early educational opportunities.

Race and Ethnicity

In general, epidemiological research suggests that across adulthood African Americans and Hispanics have similar or lower rates of common mental health disorders such as depression and substance use than whites (Breslau et al., 2005). However, the pattern is quite different for cognitive impairments later in life (AA, 2014; Sheffield & Peek, 2011). For example, compared to whites, the prevalence of Alzheimer's and other dementias is about twice as high among African Americans and about 1.5 times as high among Hispanics (AA, 2014). Research is less consistent about whether there are differences among racial groups in incidence of cognitive impairments (Barnes & Bennett, 2014).

Race and ethnicity are social, not biological, constructs and explanations for these trends likely lie in the social circumstances and experiences of persons from different racial and ethnic groups. One possible explanation for higher prevalence rates among African Americans is that the cognitive tests and measures used to diagnose cognitive impairments may be less valid measures of cognitive functioning in African Americans than in whites (Barnes & Bennett, 2014). However it is more likely that differences in rates of cognitive disorders across cultural groups are partially due to differences in cardiovascular risk factors, such as hypertension, that are associated with cognitive impairment (AA, 2014). Addressing the social factors such as poverty, stress, discrimination, and poor quality health care that put individuals from nonwhite ethnic/racial groups at risk for cardiovascular problems is necessary in order to address racial or ethnic disparities in prevalence of disorder.

Physical Health Comorbidities and Health Behaviors

Physical (also referred to as medical) and mental health conditions often co-occur. As Druss and Walker (2011, p. 4) conclude based on their review of the literature, "[c]omorbidity between medical and mental conditions is the rule rather than the exception." Individuals with mental health problems are also more likely to engage in health risk behaviors such as smoking than are their counterparts without mental health disorders (Druss & Walker, 2011).

Given the high rates of comorbidity between mental and medical problems, it is not surprising there is also a high prevalence of comorbid medical conditions among individuals with cognitive impairments (Bunn et al., 2014; Doraiswamy et al., 2002; Schubert et al., 2006). Common comorbid conditions include: hypertension, diabetes, visual impairment such as glaucoma and cataracts, stroke, heart disease and genitourinary, musculoskeletal and vascular disorders (Bunn et al., 2014; Doraiswamy et al., 2002; Schubert et al., 2006), and the number of comorbid conditions increases with age and severity of dementia. However, the prevalence of such chronic comorbid conditions in individuals with dementia varies by study setting or specific population of interest (Bunn et al., 2014).

The focus of research attention, however, has been on a cluster of cardiovascular risk factors that appear to be linked to risk for cognitive decline or dementia. While not conclusive, a large body of research suggests that factors such as hypertension, diabetes, smoking, physical activity, obesity, and diet contribute to higher risk of cognitive disorders or to differences in the progression of cognitive impairments (AA, 2014; Baumgart et al., 2015; Haan & Wallace, 2004). This has led to growing interest in the potential impact of targeting cardiovascular risk as a way to reduce either the prevalence or burden of dementia (Baumgart et al., 2015; Haan & Wallace, 2004; Lin et al., 2014). Cardiovascular risk, however, is shaped by social circumstances such as poverty and discrimination. Thus reducing cardiovascular risk factors that are associated with cognitive impairment requires addressing fundamental social determinants of health.

Depression

Finally, of the mental health conditions that co-occur with cognitive functioning, depression shows the strongest association with prevalence of cognitive impairment or dementia (AA, 2014; Byers & Yaffe, 2011; Ownby et al., 2006). However, findings are mixed depending on whether researchers examine early- or late-onset depression, the types of cognitive disorders assessed and the specific populations studied. At least two important lines of inquiry have emerged from this body of research. First, depression may be an earlier indicator or symptom of cognitive disorder, rather than a risk factor. If depression is a prodromal symptom interventions should focus on identification of depression as a means to intervene early before symptoms progress to severe cognitive impairment. Second, it is also possible that depression is an independent risk factor for cognitive impairment, a hypothesis supported by some research (Ownby et al., 2006). If depression is an independent risk factor, it is reasonable to expect that effectively treating depression may reduce the prevalence or progression of cognitive disorders, although this has yet to be demonstrated by research (Byers & Yaffe, 2011; Ownby et al., 2006).

Discussion: Promising Directions and Enduring Challenges

With the aging of the population, the challenges faced in identifying, treating, and improving outcomes for persons with mental health problems and cognitive impairments will only grow. Assuming the incidence of cognitive impairments and dementias remains relatively steady, by 2050 the number of people aged 65 years and older living with Alzheimer's will be almost 14 million (Hebert et al., 2013). Understanding and addressing the mental health needs of the aging population should be a public health priority.

Despite a burgeoning field of research, it is discouraging that there are no clearly effective, evidence-based prevention strategies for most mental disorders, including dementia. Even more discouraging is the observation that there is no compelling evidence that allows us to predict who will go from relatively minor cognitive impairments to irreversible, severe forms of dementia or who will have transitory compared to chronic mental health problems such as depression. There continues to be fundamental debates about the validity of diagnostic categories that are used to distinguish various mental illnesses and cognitive disorders from each other. The wide variety of definitions used and differences in the populations studied make it difficult to fully trust or make sense of the varied research findings. There is no cure for major mental illness, and the prognosis for major cognitive disorders is one of inevitable decline. Given these observations it is tempting to conclude that with the aging of the population the future is bleak for older individuals and their families living with these disorders. Fortunately, there are a number of promising directions that make such a conclusion premature.

First, the recovery movement in the field of mental health reminds us that the absence of disorder or complete remission of symptoms—or a cure—should not always be the priority for research or interventions (Slade, 2010). Recovery denotes "the development of new meaning and purpose in one's life as one grows beyond the catastrophic effects of mental illness" (Anthony, 1993, p. 527). A recovery lens forces us to focus on a central question: "working within the understood limits of biology and environment, what can be done to structure care and support so as to enhance patient functioning and promote the greatest quality of life possible?" (Mechanic et al., 2014, p. 245). Recovery, in the context of severe cognitive disorders, does not mean getting better because currently there are no effective treatments and the prognosis is one of inevitable decline. However, working within a recovery perspective focuses attention on interventions that can improve quality of life and is consistent with a patient-centered approach to health care (Hill et al., 2010).

The large amount of policy attention that is now being directed at addressing cognitive disorder in later life is also encouraging (Hoffman, 2014). One of the most important federal efforts is the National Alzheimer's Project Act, passed in 2011. The Act provided for the creation of a National Plan to address Alzheimer's and related diseases (U.S. Department of Health and Human Services, 2015). The Plan was released in 2012, and each year it is updated to monitor progress. The five central goals of the National Plan are ambitious (U.S. Department of Health and Human Services, 2015, p. 6): "Prevent and Effectively Treat Alzheimer's Disease by 2025; Enhance Care Quality and Efficiency; Expand Supports for People with Alzheimer's Disease and Their Families; Enhance Public Awareness and Engagement; and Track Progress and Drive Improvement."

While it is of course too soon to evaluate whether the Plan will meet these goals, it does provide leadership and directs needed attention and resources to cognitive disorders in later life. Moreover, it brings together individuals with these disorders, family members, researchers, providers, and other key stakeholders to help define the national research agenda and identify gaps in knowledge and practice.

Policy attention has also increasingly focused on alleviating the burden of caregiving (Feinberg & Reamy, 2011). The Affordable Care Act (ACA), the most recent national reform of health care, explicitly recognizes the importance of caregivers in a number of areas (Feinberg & Reamy, 2011). For example, the ACA emphasizes a model of care that includes family in assessments of quality. Family is also incorporated in shared-decision models and the coordination of care between providers and patients. The ACA includes provisions for providing support services to family caregivers to alleviate the burden (Feinberg & Reamy, 2011). While it will take to take to determine whether these reforms will have outcomes for individuals living with mental illness and their caregivers, they are promising (Mechanic et al., 2014).

Finally there are encouraging directions in our understanding of modifiable risk factors. Some suggest that addressing the burden of conditions such as diabetes, hypertension, and depression that are often comorbid with cognitive and other mental health disorders presents the most promising avenue for intervention (Lin et al., 2014; Haan & Wallace, 2004). Lin et al. (2014), for example, suggest that reducing the prevalence of obesity, diabetes, hypertension, and cardiovascular disease would substantially lower risk for dementia and delay onset, resulting in enormous health care saving. Of course, prevention of these types of disorders is difficult. Moreover, risk of developing conditions such as hypertension or diabetes is substantially higher among disadvantaged compared to advantaged groups (Lang et al., 2012). Successful prevention efforts, therefore, must address the fundamental social determinants of health that produce inequality, some of which have their roots in very early life—a difficult, but necessary challenge if we are to reduce the burden of cognitive disorders and other mental health problems in later life.

References

Akushevich, I., Kravchenko, J., Urkaintseva, S., Arbeev, K., & Yashin, A. I. (2013). Time trends of incidence of age-associated diseases in the US elderly population: Medicare-based analysis. *Age and Ageing, 42*, 494–500.

Alzheimer's Association (2014). Alzheimer's association report. 2014 Alzheimer's disease facts and figures. *Alzheimer's & Dementia, 10*, e47–e92.

American Psychiatric Association (2000). *Diagnostic and statistical manual of mental disorders (4th ed.) (DSM-IV-TR)*. Washington, DC: American Psychiatric Association.

American Psychiatric Association (2013). *Diagnostic and statistical manual of mental disorders (5th ed.) (DSM-5)*. Arlington, VA: American Psychiatric Association.

Anderson, L. A., Deokar, A., Edwards, V. J., Bouldin, E. D., & Greenlund, K. J. (2015). Demographic and health status differences among people aged 45 or older with and without functional difficulties related to increased confusion or memory loss, 2011 Behavioral Risk Factor Surveillance System. *Preventing Chronic Disease, 12*(E30), 140429. doi: http://dx.doi.org/10.5888/pcd12.140429

Anthony, W. A. (1993). Recovery from mental illness: The guiding vision of the mental health system in the 1990s. *Psychosocial Rehabilitation Journal, 16*(4), 11–23.

Bagchi, A. D., Verdier, J. M., & Simon, S. E. (2009). How many nursing home residents live with a mental illness? *Psychiatric Services, 60*, 958–964.

Barnes, L. L., & Bennett, D. A. (2014). Alzheimer's disease in African Americans: Risk factors and challenges for the future. *Health Affairs, 33*, 580–586.

Baumgart, M., Snyder, H. M., Carrillo, M. C., Fazio, S., Kim, H., & Johns, H. (2015). Summary of the evidence on modifiable risk factors for cognitive decline and dementia: A population-based perspective. *Alzheimer's & Dementia, 11*, 718–726.

Beaudreau, S. A., & O'Hara R. (2008). Late-life anxiety and cognitive impairment: A review. *American Journal of Geriatric Psychiatry, 16*, 790–803.

Blazer, D. (2013). Neurocognitive disorders in DSM-5. *American Journal of Psychiatry, 170*, 585–587.

Borenstein, A. R., Copenhaver, C. I., & Mortimer, J. (2006). Early-life risk factors for Alzheimer disease. *Alzheimer Disease and Associated Disorders, 20*(1), 63–72.

Bowling, A. (2005). *Aging Well: Quality of Life in Old Age*. New York, NY: Open University Press.

Bowling, A., Rowe, G., Adams, S., Sands, P., Samsi, K., Crane, M., . . . Manthorpe, J. (2015). Quality of life in dementia: A systematically conducted narrative review of dementia-specific measurement scales. *Aging & Mental Health, 19*, 13–31.

Breslau, J., Kendler K. S., Su, M., Gaxiola-Aguilar S., & Kessler, R. C. (2005). Lifetime risk and persistence of psychiatric disorders across ethnic groups in the United States. *Psychological Medicine, 35*, 317–327.

Bunn, F., Burn, A-M., Goodman, C., Rait, G., Norton, S., Robinson, L., Schoeman, J., & Brayne, C. (2014). Comorbidity and dementia: A scoping review of the literature. *BMC Medicine, 12*(1), 192.

Byers, A. L., & Yaffe, K. (2011). Depression and risk of developing dementia. *Nature Reviews Neurology*, 7, 323–331.

Byrne-Davis, L. M. T., Bennett, P. D., & Wilcock, G. K. (2006). How are quality of life ratings made? Toward a model of quality of life in people with dementia. *Quality of Life Research, 15*, 855–865.

Cahill, S., & Diaz-Ponce, A. M. (2011). "I have nobody here. I'd like to know where they all are": Can qualitative research detect difference in quality of life among nursing home residents with different levels of cognitive impairment. *Aging & Mental Health, 15*, 562–572.

Covinsky, K. E., Newcomer, R., Fox, P., Wood, J., Sands, L., Dane, K., & Jaffe, K. (2003). Patient and caregiver characteristics associated with depression in caregivers of patients with dementia. *Journal of General Internal Medicine, 18*, 1006–1014.

Dodge, H. H., Zhu, J., Lee, C., Chang, C. H., & Ganguli, M. (2014). Cohort effects in age-associated cognitive trajectories. *The Journals of Gerontology, Series A: Medical Sciences, 69*, 687–694.

Doraiswamy, P. M., Leon, J., Cummings, J. L., Marin, D., & Neumann, P. J. (2002). Prevalence and impact of medical comorbidity in Alzheimer's disease. *The Journals of Gerontology, Series A: Medical Sciences, 57A*, M173–M177.

Druss, B. G., & Walker, E. R. (2011). *Mental Disorders and Medical Comorbidity*. Princeton, NJ: Robert Wood Johnson Foundation, The Synthesis Project. Retrieved from: http://www.rwjf.org/content/dam/farm/reports/issue_briefs/2011/rwjf69438/subassets/rwjf69438

Elder, G. H., Jr. (1998). The life course as developmental theory. *Child Development 69*, 1–12.

Feinberg, L., & Reamy, A. M. (2011). *Health reform law creates new opportunities to better recognize and support family caregivers*. Washington, DC: AARP Public Policy Institute. Retrieved from: http://assets.aarp.org/rgcenter/ppi/ltc/fs239.pdf

Finkel, S. I., & Burns, A. (2010). Introduction. *International Psychogeriatrics*, 12 (suppl 1), 9–12.

Fisher, G. G., Franks, M. M., Plassman, B. L., Brown, S. L., Potter, G. G., Llewellyn, D., . . . Langa, K. M. (2011). Caring for individuals with dementia and CIND: Findings from the aging, demographics, and memory study. *Journal of the American Geriatrics Society, 59*, 488–494.

Frances, A. (2012). DSM-5 is a guide, not a bible: Simply ignore its 10 worst changes. *Huffington Post*. Retrieved from: http://www.huffingtonpost.com/allen-frances/dsm-5_b_2227626.html

Ganguli, M., Blacker, D., Blazer, D. G., Grant, I., Jeste, D. V., Paulsen, J. S., . . . The Neurocognitive Disorders Work Group of the American Psychiatric

Association's (APA) DSM-5 Task force (2011). Classification of neurocognitive disorders in DSM-5: A work in progress. *American Journal of Geriatric Psychiatry, 19*, 205–210.

Gauthier, S., Cummings, J., Ballard, C., Brodaty, H., Grossberg, G., Robert, P., & Lyketsos, C. (2010). Management of behavioral problems in Alzheimer's disease. *International Psychogeriatrics, 22*(3), 346–372.

Grabowski, D.C., Aschbrenner, K.A., Feng, Z., & Mor, V. (2009). Mental illness in nursing homes: Variations across states. *Health Affairs, 28*, 689–700.

Gum, A.M., King-Kallimanis, B., & Kohn, R. (2009). Prevalence of mood, anxiety, and substance-abuse disorders for older Americans in the National Comorbidity Survey-Replication. *American Journal of Geriatric Psychiatry, 17*, 769–781.

Halfon, N., & Hochstein, M. (2002). Life course health development: An integrated framework for developing health, policy, and research. *Milbank Quarterly, 80*, 433–479.

Haan, M.N., & Wallace, R. (2004), Can dementia be prevented? Brain aging in a population-based context. *Annual Review of Public Health, 25*, 1–24.

Hebert, L.E., Weuve, J., Scherr, P.A., & Evans, D.A. (2013). Alzheimer disease in the United States (2010–2050) estimated using the 2010 census. *Neurology, 80*(19), 1778–1783.

Hendrie, H.C., Wanzhu, T., Tabbey, R., Purnell, C.E., Ambuehl, R.J., & Callahan, C.M. (2014). Health outcomes and cost of care among older adults with schizophrenia: A 10-year study using medical records across the continuum of care. *American Journal of Geriatric Psychiatry,* 22, 427–436.

Hill, L., Roberts, G., Wildgoose, J., Perkins, R., & Hahn, S. (2010). Recovery and person-centered care in dementia: Common purpose, common practice? *Advances in Psychiatric Treatment, 16*, 288–298.

Hoffman, D. (2014). Alzheimer's disease legislation and policy: Now and in the future. *Health Affairs, 33*(4), 561–565.

Hooker K., Bowman, S.R., Coehlo, D.P., Lim, S.R., Kaye, J., Guariglia, R., & Li, F. (2002). Behavioral change in persons with dementia: Relationships with mental and physical health of caregivers. *The Journals of Gerontology, Series B: Psychological Sciences, 57B*, 453–460.

Hurd, M.D., Martorell, P., Delavande, A., Mullen, K.J., & Langa, K.M. (2013). Monetary costs of dementia in the United States. *The New England Journal of Medicine, 368*, 1326–1334.

International Psychogeriatric Association (IPA). (1996). Behavioral and psychological signs and symptoms of dementia: Implications for research and treatment. *International Psychogeriatrics, 8*(suppl. 3), 215–552.

Janevic, M.R., & Connell, C.M. (2001). Racial, ethnic, and cultural differences in the dementia caregiving experience: Recent findings. *Gerontologist, 41*, 334–347.

Kessler, R.C., Berglund, P., Demler, O., Jin, R., Merikangas, K.R., & Walters, E.E. (2005). Lifetime prevalence and age-of-onset distributions of DSM-IV disorders in the National Comorbidity Survey Replication. *Archives of General Psychiatry* 62, 593–602.

Keyes, C. L. M. (2007). Promoting and protecting mental health as flourishing: A complementary strategy for improving national mental health. *American Psychologist, 62*, 95–108.

Lang, T., LePage, B., Schieber, A, Lamy, S., & Kelly-Irving, M. (2012). Social determinants of cardiovascular diseases. *Public Health Reviews, 33*(2), 601–622.

Leibson, C. L., Long, K. H., Ransom, J. E., Roberts, R. O., Hass, S. L., Duhig, A. M., . . . Petersen, R. C. (Epub ahead of print). Direct medical costs and source of cost differences across the spectrum of cognitive decline: A population-based study. *Alzheimer's & Dementia*, doi: 10.1016/j.jalz.2015.01.007

Lin, P. J., Yang, Z., Fillit, H. M., Cohen, J. T., & Neumann, P. J. (2014). Unintended benefits: The potential economic impact of addressing risk factors to prevent Alzheimer's disease. *Health Affairs, 33*(4), 547–554.

Loy, C. T., Schofield, P. R., Turner, A. M., Kwok, J. B. J. (2014). Genetics of dementia. *Lancet, 383*, 828–840.

Lyketsos, C. G., Lopez, O., Jones, B., Fitzpatrick, A. L., Breitner, J., & DeKosky S. (2002). Prevalence of neuropsychiatric symptoms in dementia and mild cognitive impairment: Results from the Cardiovascular Health Study. *Journal of the American Medical Association, 288*, 1475–1483.

Mayes, R., & Horwitz, A. V. (2005). DSM-III and the revolution in the classification of mental illness. *Journal of the History of the Behavioral Sciences, 41*, 249–267.

McAlpine, D. D. (2003). Patterns of care for persons 65 years and older with schizophrenia. In C. I. Cohen (Ed.), *Schizophrenia into later life: Treatment, research, and policy* (pp. 3–18). Arlington, VA: American Psychiatric Publishing, Inc.

Mechanic, D., McAlpine, D. D., & Rochefort, D. A. (2014). *Mental health and social policy: Beyond managed care*. Boston, MA: Pearson Education, Inc.

Meeks, T., Vahia, I., Lavretsky, H., Kulkarni, G., & Jeste, D. (2011). A Tune in "a minor" can "b major": A review of epidemiology, illness course, and public health implications of subthreshold depression in older adults. *Journal of Affective Disorder, 129*, 126–142.

Menne, H. L., Judge, K. S., & Whitlatch, C. J. (2009). Predictors of quality of life for individuals with dementia: Implications for intervention. *Dementia, 8*, 543–560.

Moceri, V. M., Kukull, W. A., Emanuel, I., van Belle, G., & Larson, E. B. (2000). Early-life risk factors and the development of Alzheimer's disease. *Neurology, 54*(2), 415–420.

Montgomery, R. J. V., Gonyea, J. G., & Hooyman, N. R. (1985). Caregiving and the experience of subjective and objective burden. *Family Relations, 34*, 19–26.

Mukamal, K. J., Kuller, L. H., Fitzpatrick, A. J., Longstreth Jr., W. T., Mittleman M. A., & Siscovick, D. S. (2003) Prospective study of alcohol consumption and risk of dementia in older adults. *Journal of the American Medical Association, 289*, 1405–1413.

Muntaner, C., Eaton, W. W., Miech, R., & O'Campo, P. (2004). Socioeconomic position and major mental disorders. *Epidemiologic Reviews*, 26, 53–62.

Murray, L. M., & Boyd, S. (2009). Protecting personhood and achieving quality of life for older adults with dementia in the U.S. health care system. *Journal of Aging and Health, 21*(2), 350–373.

Ngandu, T., von Strauss, E., Helkala, E.-L., Winblad, B., Nissinen, A., Tuomilehto, J., . . . Kivipelto, M. (2007). Education and dementia: What lies behind the association? *Neurology, 69*, 1442–1450.

O'Rourke, H. M., Duggleby, W., Fraser, K. D., & Jerke, L. (2015). Factors that affect quality of life from the perspective of people with dementia: A metasynthesis. *Journal of the American Geriatrics Society, 63*, 24–38.

Ownby, R. L., Crocco, E., Acevedo, A., John, V., & Lowenstein, D. (2006). Depression and risk for Alzheimer Disease: Systematic review, meta-analysis and metaregression analysis. *Archives of General Psychiatry, 63*, 530–538.

Petersen, R. C., Caracciola, B., Brayne, C., Gauthier, S., Jelic, V., & Fratglioni, L. (2014). Mild cognitive impairment: A concept in evolution. *Journal of Internal Medicine, 275*, 214–228.

Plassman, B. L., Langa, K. M., Fisher, G. G., Heeringa, S. G., Weir, D. R., Ofstedal, M. B., . . . Wallace, R. B. (2007). Prevalence of dementia in the United States: The aging, demographics, and memory study. *Neuroepidemiology, 29*, 125–132.

Plassman, B. L., Langa, K. M., Fisher, G. G., Heeringa, S. G., Weir, D. R., Ofstedal, M. B., . . . Wallace, R. B. (2008). Prevalence of cognitive impairment without dementia in the United States. *Annals of Internal Medicine, 148*, 427–434.

Reynolds, K., Pietrzak, R. H., El-Gabalawy, R., Mackenzie, C. S., & Sareen, J. (2015). Prevalence of psychiatric disorders in U.S. older adults: Findings from a nationally representative survey. *World Psychiatry, 14*, 74–81.

Rocca, W. A., Petersen R. C., Knopman, D. S., Hebert, L. E., Evans, D. A., Hall, K. S., . . . White L. R. (2011). Trends in the incidence and prevalence of Alzheimer's disease, dementia, and cognitive impairment in the United States. *Alzheimer's Dementia, 7*(1), 80–93.

Rutter, M. (2006). *Genes and behaviors: Nature, nurture, and developmental influences: The challenge ahead for mental health*. Malden, MA: Blackwell Publishing.

Salthouse, T. A. (2010). *Major issues in cognitive aging*. Oxford, England: Oxford University Press.

Saraceno, B., Levav, I., & Kohn, R. (2005). The public mental health significance of research on socio-economic factors in schizophrenia and major depression. *World Psychiatry, 4*(3), 181–185.

Schubert, C. C., Boustani, M., Callahan, C. M., Perkins, A. J., Carney, C. P., Fox, C., Unverzagt, F., Hui, S., & Hendrie, H. C. (2006). Comorbidity profile of dementia patients in primary care: Are they sicker? *Journal of the American Geriatrics Society, 54*(1), 104–109.

Schulz, R., & Martire, L. M. (2004). Family caregiving of persons with dementia: Prevalence, health effects, and support strategies. *American Journal of Geriatric Psychiatry, 12*, 240–249.

Seeher, K., Low, L. F., Reppermund, S., & Broadaty, H. (2013). Predictors and outcomes for caregivers of people with mild cognitive impairment: A systematic literature review. *Alzheimer's & Dementia, 9*, 346–355.

Sheffield, K. M., & Peek, M. K. (2011). Changes in the prevalence of cognitive impairment among older Americans, 1993–2004: Overall trends and differences by race/ethnicity. *American Journal of Epidemiology*, 174, 274–283.

Slade, M. (2010). Mental illness and well-being: The central importance of positive psychology and recovery approaches. *BMC Health Services Research, 10*, 26.

St. John, P. D., & Montgomery, P. R. (2010). Cognitive impairment and life satisfaction in older adults. *International Journal of Geriatric Psychiatry, 25*, 814–821.

Steffens, D. C., Fisher, G. G., Langa, K. M., Potter, G. G., & Plassman, B. L. (2009). Prevalence of depression among older Americans: The Aging Demographics and Memory Study. *International Journal of Psychogeriatric, 21*, 879–888.

U.S. Census Bureau Population Division. (2015). *National population estimates for the 2010s. Monthly postcensal resident population, by singe year of age, sex, race and Hispanic origin*. Retrieved from: http://www.census.gov/popest/data/national/asrh/2014/2014-nat-res.html

U.S. Department of Health and Human Services. (1999). *Mental health: A report to the surgeon general*. Rockville, MD: U.S. Department of Health and Human Services. Retrieved from: http://profiles.nlm.nih.gov/ps/retrieve/ResourceMetadata/NNBBHS

U.S. Department of Health and Human Services. (2015). *National plan to address Alzheimer's disease: 2015 update*. Retrieved from: http://aspe.hhs.gov/daltcp/napa/NatlPlan2015.pdf

Wakefield, J. C. (2013). DSM-5: An overview of changes and controversies. *Journal of Clinical Social Work, 41*, 139–154.

Walker, A. J., Pratt, C. C., & Eddy, L. (1995). Informal caregiving to aging family members: A critical review. *Family Relations, 44*, 402–411.

Ward, A., Arrighi, H. M., Michels, S., & Cedarbaum, J. M. (2012). Mild cognitive impairment: Disparities of incidence and prevalence estimates. *Alzheimer's & Dementia, 8*, 14–21.

Werner, P. (2012). Mild cognitive impairment and caregiver burden: A critical review and research agenda. *Public Health Reviews, 34*(2), 1–15.

Whalley, L. J., Dick, F. D., & McNeill, G. (2006). A life-course approach to the aetiology of late-onset dementias. *The Lancet Neurology, 5*(1), 87–96.

Wilson, R. S., Weir, D. R., Leurgans, S. E., Evans, D. A., Hebert, L. E., Langa, K. M., . . . Bennett, D. A. (2011). Sources of variability in estimates of the prevalence of Alzheimer's disease in the United States. *Alzheimer's Dementia, 7*, 74–79.

Wimo, A., Jönsson, L., Bond, J., Prince, M., & Winblad, B. (2013). The worldwide economic impact of dementia 2010. *Alzheimer's & Dementia, 9*, 1–11.

Wimo, A., & Prince, M. (eds.) (2010). *World Alzheimer's report 2010. The global economic impact of dementia. Executive summary*. Retrieved from: http://www.alz.co.uk/research/files/WorldAlzheimerReport2010ExecutiveSummary.pdf

World Health Organization [WHO]. (2014). *Mental health: Strengthening our response*. World Health Organization: Fact Sheet No. 220. Retrieved from: http://www.who.int/mediacentre/factsheets/fs220/en/

World Health Organization (WHO). (2008). *The global burden of disease: 2004 update*. Retrieved from: http://www.who.int/healthinfo/global_burden_disease/2004_report_update/en/

World Health Organization (WHO) & Alzheimer's Disease International (ADI). (2012). *Dementia: A public health priority*. Retrieved from: http://www.who.int/mental_health/publications/dementia_report_2012/en/

Yang, Z., Zhang K., Lin, P., Clevenger, C., & Atherly, A. (2012). A longitudinal analysis of lifetime cost of dementia. *Health Services Research, 47*, 1660–1678.

CHAPTER SEVEN

Unpaid Care Work

Eliza K. Pavalko and Joseph D. Wolfe

Our focus in this chapter is on the unpaid care of ill or disabled adults, or what we refer to as unpaid care work. We use the term care work as opposed to the more commonly used term "caregiving." As pointed out by Harrington Meyer (2000), the term caregiving is misleading because it suggests that care is given by choice. It also obscures the reality of providing care, which is physically and emotionally demanding work, even if it is unpaid. Thus, we use the term care work and refer to those who do that work as care workers. The value and magnitude of unpaid care work is not fully appreciated, even though most adults provide care at some point in their lives and the value of that care is estimated at $450 billion. Estimates suggest that in 2015, about 43.5 million people are providing care to an ill or disabled adult, averaging 24 hours of unpaid care per week (National Alliance for Caregiving and AARP 2015). Although women are more likely to provide care, it is not just a woman's issue. Recent estimates are that 35–45 percent of those caring for ill or disabled adults are men (U.S. Bureau of Labor Statistics 2013, National Alliance for Caregiving and AARP 2015). Thus, a large portion of the U.S. population, both men and women, will provide unpaid care to an ill or disabled adult in their family.

Unpaid care work can be deeply rewarding, but it can also act as a disruptive and stressful event with the potential to cause both short- and long-term damage to families' financial, physical, and emotional well-being. The effects of unpaid care go well beyond individual lives to shape the U.S. health-care system and labor market. Our reliance on unpaid care to meet health needs has significantly increased in recent decades. The Congressional Budget office estimates that in 2011 care work from friends and family comprised 55 percent of the long-term care costs for the elderly (Congressional Budget Office 2013), and family care workers are increasingly responsible for a wide range of skilled nursing tasks that were once provided by trained medical professionals (Glazer 1990, Reinhard, Levine et al. 2012). The value of care work is also rising sharply, estimated at about $200 billion in 1996, $375 billion in 2007, and $450 billion in 2009 (Feinberg and Choula 2012). As a point of comparison, Medicaid spending in 2009, which includes both federal and state contributions for health and long-term care, was only $361 billion.

Care work is also relevant to the labor market. The most common ages for care work for the ill or disabled are between 45 and 55, which are the peak years for employment. A 2010–2011 Gallup poll estimates that 17 percent of employed Americans are providing unpaid care to an ill or disabled family member or friend, and that employed men are nearly as likely to be providing care as are employed women (Cynkar and Mendes 2011). The majority of those who are providing unpaid care while employed report that their responsibilities as care workers have an impact on their work performance and require some type of work accommodations (Witters 2011, Feinberg and Choula 2012). Unpaid care workers are also more likely to stop work or reduce hours, particularly if their workplace lacks the flexibility necessary to meet care needs. Employers thus bear the costs of unpaid care work through turnover and retraining costs that allow care workers to remain employed.

The prevalence of unpaid care work, along with its social and economic significance, makes it an important area of study. In this chapter, we review what we know about unpaid care of the ill or disabled. We begin by examining who provides care, paying special attention to how care work has changed over time and how it varies by gender, race/ethnicity, and socioeconomic status. We then review more fully the health and economic consequences of providing care. Finally, we turn our attention to the challenges of balancing unpaid care work with employment and the workplace policies that may help care workers balance competing demands on their time.

Age Variation and Social Change in Care Work

Care work is a critically important issue as demographic and social trends suggest a possible increase in the need for unpaid care work at the same time there is a decline in the supply of persons to provide that care. A major factor driving the future need for care is population aging. By 2050, one-fifth of the U.S. population will be 65 or older, compared to 12 percent in 2000 and 8 percent in 1950 (Congressional Budget Office

2013). Growth in the 85 and older population is expected to be especially dramatic because of population aging and increases in life expectancy. However, the number of disabled adults will heavily influence the future demand for care.

The number of Americans with a disability declined in the late 20th century, leading some to speculate that the need for care might decline. However, it is unclear whether this will be the case. Several positive changes, such as increased education, improved medical technology, and reduced tobacco use, suggest that disability rates could continue to decline, but increases in obesity and sedentary lifestyle are likely to negate any health benefits (Freedman, Crimmins et al. 2004, Chen and Guo 2008, Martin, Schoeni et al. 2010, Congressional Budget Office 2013). These countervailing forces suggest that reductions in disability, and thus the need for care, may stagnate or even reverse. At the same time, reductions in family size are shrinking the supply of people available to provide care. As noted by Uhlenberg and Cheuk (2008), "when mothers of the baby boom are in greatest need of care, i.e. when they are over age 80 around 2020, more than a fourth of them will have at least four children. However, 20 years later when baby boomers are over 80, only 10 percent of them will have four or more children." (p. 27). Taken together, these patterns suggest an upcoming deficit of care workers, but it remains difficult to predict precisely how these intersecting trends will impact the need for care workers.

The most dramatic increase in the elderly population will occur as the baby boom generation, currently in their 50s and 60s, ages into later life, but demographic and social changes of the last half century have already affected care work. We can thus consider how care work has been affected by large-scale social change in the past in order to gain insight into the likely future of care. Data from the 1984–1999 National Long-Term Care Surveys shows that from 1984 to 1994, the number of older persons with a disability, and the number with chronic disability living in the community, rose because of the aging of the population. However, the proportion of unpaid care workers declined during this period while the use of paid care rose (Spillman and Pezzin 2000). Analysis of similar data from 1994 to 1999 suggests a reversal in this trend, with paid care declining. Overall, while there were fluctuations, these data suggest that from 1984 to 1999 the rate at which spouses and children provided care remained fairly stable (Spillman and Black 2005). Since the late 1990s, the National Alliance for Caregiving (NAC) has also conducted comparable national surveys of care workers and found little change in the percentage of adults providing care between 1997 and 2009 (National Alliance for Caregiving and AARP 1997, 2009). Despite substantial changes in longevity, disability, family structure, health-care financing, and women's labor force participation, the proportion of those providing care at any point in time appears to have remained fairly stable between 1984 and 2009.

Comparisons of care work across birth cohorts provide further clarification of the effects of social change on care work. Cohorts also provide insight into how social trends, such as increases in women's employment, have impacted their unpaid care work. A series of studies of birth cohorts of women from New York State born between 1905 and the early 1930s found that women born in more recent cohorts were *more* likely to provide care, to have multiple spells of care work, and to provide care for parents or a disabled child than earlier cohorts, despite the increased employment among women in the later cohorts (Moen, Robison et al. 1994, Robison, Moen et al. 1995). Similarly, our analyses using a nationally representative sample of women born between 1922 and 1952 found little impact of employment on unpaid care work. We did find that the proportion of women providing care declined among more recent cohorts, but this decline only reflected changes at the lowest levels of care. The proportion of women providing moderate or intense levels of care, nine or more hours per week, was stable across cohorts (Pavalko and Wolfe 2015). Together, these studies suggest that families develop strategies for providing care when it is needed regardless of their employment demands, but they prioritize the most intense and necessary forms of care.

In sum, large-scale demographic changes are increasing the need for unpaid care while also decreasing the supply of care workers and the time they have available to provide care. These changes suggest a future deficit in care workers that, because of the reliance of the U.S. health-care system on unpaid care, could have disastrous consequences on families, health-care, and the labor force. However, several social changes in the last half of the 20th century suggested similarly dire situations, but families still appear to be providing care when it is most needed (Pavalko and Wolfe 2015). Although this may buffer the effects of a care deficit on the United States in general, it does not offer any protection to the financial, mental, and physical strains that occur when people try balancing unpaid care work of disabled adults with their other family and employment obligations. Thus, future research should focus on who provides care, the ways they provide it, and how it impacts their lives.

Who Cares? Social Inequalities in Care Work

Who provides care and how much care they provide is not evenly distributed across the population. One of the most documented and consistent findings is that women are more likely to provide care than men. National estimates indicate that about 60 percent of U.S. unpaid care workers are women (National Alliance for Caregiving and AARP 2015). In addition, women are more likely to help with personal care, devote more hours of care each week, spend more years providing care, and perform more care tasks (Pinquart and Sorensen 2006). Within families, daughters are about twice as likely as sons to provide care for a parent (Pillemer and Suitor 2014). There is also a gender gap in spousal care, with women receiving less care from their husbands than men receive from their wives (Noel-Miller 2011). While gender differences exist across different indicators of care, the magnitude of those differences is not large in many cases. For example, Pinquart and Sorensen (2006) conclude that, while gender differences in care work and its health effects are present, only gender differences in burden, depression, and amount of care are large enough to be of practical concern. Likewise, when considering a broad range of types of support, Kahn et al. (2011) find that the gender gap in most forms of care is modest and decreases with age.

With respect to the life course, unpaid care work is most prevalent during midlife. The NAC estimates that in 2015 the average age of care workers for people aged 18 and older was 49 (National Alliance for Caregiving and AARP 2015) compared to an average of 46 in 2004. Data from the 2011–2012 wave of the American Time Use Survey (ATUS), which focuses on care for those aged 65 and older, identify ages 45–54 as the most common ages of providing care (23%), followed closely by 55–64 (U.S. Bureau of Labor Statistics 2013). These age patterns are similar for men and women, although as we would expect, at any given age, women are slightly more likely to be providing care than are men. For example, between the ages of 45–54, the ATUS estimates that 26 percent of women and 20 percent of men are providing some type of elder care.

Both the forms and amount of care work vary across racial and ethnic groups. A meta-analysis of 116 empirical studies of racial/ethnic differences in care work reports that ethnic minority care workers provided more care than white care workers (Pinquart and Sorensen 2005). White-Means and Rubin (2008) found that blacks are more likely than whites to provide assistance with activities of daily living, but they did not find racial differences in assistance with instrumental activities of daily living or financial assistance. Racial variation in care work also intersects with gender and family structure, and family structure and socioeconomic resources account for most racial differences in care and kin support (Sarkisian and Gerstel 2004, White-Means and Rubin 2008). For example, black and white sons provide similar levels of care, whereas black daughters provide more care than white daughters. However, these differences can also differ by marital status (Laditka and Laditka 2001), suggesting a complex interaction between race and family structure.

Although there are fewer comparisons involving Hispanic populations, a 2008 study found that 36 percent of Hispanic households had at least one care worker compared to 25 percent of non-Hispanic households (Evercare 2008). They also found that the level of care work is more intense in Hispanic households, averaging more hours per week and help with more activities of daily living. There is also variation in care work among Latino subgroups. For example, Mexican Americans are thought to have particularly high rates of care workers because they have higher rates of disability and are less likely to rely on institutional care (Markides, Peek et al. 2013). The burden of care also varies by nativity as children of foreign-born elderly bare greater responsibility for care than children of U.S.-born elderly (Angel et al. 2014).

We know less about social class differences in care work, but the burden of care does appear greater for low-income families. The NAC/AARP study (2009) reports that low-income populations are more likely to rely on unpaid care, act as primary care workers, and live with care recipients. Income differences in caring also vary depending on the level of care. All income groups provide low levels of care, defined as between 1 and 4 hours of care, but this level of care is especially common among high-income families. In contrast, low-income families are twice as likely as moderate or high-income families to provide more than 30 hours of care per month. Low-income care workers face additional burdens when trying to combine unpaid care and employment. Lower-income jobs tend to have fewer options for flexible hours, are less likely to provide paid sick or vacation time, and low-income workers have fewer resources to support unpaid leave (Bianchi, Folbre et al. 2012).

A National Profile of Middle-Aged Care Workers

Several data sources provide broad estimates of care work across the U.S. population (see Folbre and Wolf 2012), but the experience and consequences of caring vary widely across the life course. To better understand the prevalence and distribution of care work among persons during their prime employment years, we turn to data from the 1979 cohort of the National Longitudinal Survey of Youth (NLSY79). The NLSY provides a nationally representative sample of 12,686 U.S. adults born between 1957 and 1964. Respondents were initially surveyed when they were aged 14–22 in 1979 and have continued to be followed through adulthood (U.S. Bureau of Labor Statistics 2015). In 2008, when they were 43–51, they were asked whether they regularly spent time caring for an ill or disabled household member or friend or relative outside the home.

Follow-up questions asked about the number of hours spent providing either type of care. The same set of questions was asked in 2010 and 2012, providing additional information on duration of care.

Descriptive information from the NLSY79 on care work and its distribution by gender, race/ethnicity, and income quartiles is shown in Table 7.1. Data are weighted to provide estimates of U.S. adults born between 1957 and 1964. As seen in Table 7.1, the profile of care work indicated by the NLSY79 is similar to that reported by the NAC/AARP. Between 2008 and 2012, 27 percent of men and women provide some type of care in at least one of the three surveys. Sixteen percent provide care in just one of the three surveys, while 4 percent are care workers in all three waves. Eleven percent of the sample cares for someone inside the household, whereas 19 percent provide care outside the home. Consistent with other care work surveys, the number of hours spent providing care is much greater among those providing care inside the home than it is for care outside the home. Care for persons living inside the home averages 33 hours per week, compared to an average of 11 hours per week for care of persons living outside one's home.

The second and third columns of Table 7.1 compare care work by gender. Midlife women are significantly more likely to provide care than midlife men, 34 percent versus 22 percent. While women are more likely to provide care inside and outside the home, the gender difference is much greater for care outside the home, with twice as many women than men reporting providing care outside the home. Among those caring inside the home, women average 37 hours of care per week, compared to 28 hours per week for men providing care. Among those caring outside the home, on the other hand, there is no difference between men and women in their hours spent caring. Furthermore, 15 percent of women provide care either inside or outside the home in two or more survey waves, but only 7 percent of men are providing care at multiple surveys.

We also find small racial/ethnic variation in unpaid care work. In the NLSY79, 33 percent of blacks report providing care, compared to 26 percent of whites and 29 percent of Hispanics. Blacks are significantly more likely than whites to provide care either inside or outside the home, and blacks are slightly more likely to provide care in multiple survey waves. In contrast to the Evercare (2008) survey discussed above, a slightly smaller percentage of Hispanics than blacks report providing any care, and a similar difference between the two groups is seen both for care inside and outside the home. The slight difference in care work between Hispanics and whites is not statistically significant. Among those providing care either inside or outside the home, there are no racial/ethnic differences in the hours of care reported.

Table 7.1 Descriptive Statistics of Caregiving by Gender, Race, and Income, NLSY79 (Weighted Data)

	Total	Women	Men	Hispanic	Black	White	Income Q1	Income Q2	Income Q3	Income Q4
Observed *N*	6,727	3,432	3,295	1,322	2,027	3,378	1,684	1,703	1,659	1,681
Average age (2008)	47	47	47	47	47	47	47	47	47	47
Any care										
Observed *N*	1,959	1,197	762	395	665	899	619	506	446	388
Percent	27	34[m]	22	29[b]	33[w]	26	36[i]	29[i]	26	23
Inside care										
Observed *N*	831	449	382	182	297	352	335	230	157	109
Percent	11	12[m]	10	13[w]	15[w]	10	20[i]	13[i]	9[i]	6
Hours per week	33	37[m]	28	31	34	33	43[i]	28	28	26
Outside care										
Observed *N*	1,339	901	438	247	455	637	377	331	331	300
Percent	19	26[m]	13	18[b]	23[w]	19	23[i]	19	19	17
Hours per week	11	11	10	13	11	10	13[i]	12[i]	11[i]	7
Years caring (%)										
0	73	66[m]	78	71[b]	67[w]	74	64[i]	71[i]	74	77
1	16	18[m]	14	17[b]	20[w]	15	19[i]	17	15	14
2	7	9	5	8	9[w]	7	11[i]	9[i]	6	5
3	4	6[m]	2	4	5	4	7[i]	3	4	3

– [m] denotes significantly different from men at the .05 level or smaller; [w] denotes significantly different from white at the .05 level or smaller, [b] denotes significantly different from black at the .05 level or smaller, and [i] significantly different from the fourth quartile of income at the .05 level or smaller.

– We pool data from the 2008, 2010, and 2012 waves for information on caregiving.

– The rows labeled "Hours per Week" only include information on individuals who reported providing care at any year, and if the respondent provided multiple years of care, we used their average hours of care.

Far more dramatic differences are found across income quartiles. Thirty-six percent of low-income respondents provide any type of care, while only 23 percent of high-income respondents provide care. Income differences are particularly large for care inside the home, with 20 percent in the lowest income quartile providing care inside the home compared to only 6 percent of those in the highest quartile. Low-income care workers also report spending far more hours of care both inside and outside the home. Among those providing care inside the home, low-income care workers report spending 43 hours on care per week, compared to an average of 26 hours among high-income care workers. Low-income care workers are also more likely than high-income care workers to provide care across multiple survey waves. These differences likely reflect both the poorer health and greater disability of adults in low-income households and the limited resources of low-income adults to pay for care.

Consequences of Care Work

Unpaid care, particularly if it is intense, has a range of effects on the care worker's physical health, well-being, and economic security. The consequences of caring for the care provider's health and well-being have been extensively studied. Following several decades of research on the health effects of care work that use a variety of measures of care work, health outcomes, and sample designs, a series of meta-analyses have evaluated the extent to which care work affects a range of physical and psychological outcomes (Pinquart and Sorensen 2003, Vitaliano, Zhang et al. 2003, Pinquart and Sorensen 2007). In terms of psychological health, the evidence shows that care workers experience more stress, depression, poorer subjective well-being, and lower self-efficacy than those not providing care (Pinquart and Sorensen 2003). Although physical health differences are not as large as they are for psychological outcomes, care providers also have worse physical health than those not providing care, particularly higher levels of stress hormones, antibodies, and worse self-assessed health (Pinquart and Sorensen 2003, Vitaliano, Zhang et al. 2003, Pinquart and Sorensen 2007). However, the magnitude of differences is modest between care workers and non-care workers for both physical and psychological health.

When comparing broad categories of care workers and non-care workers, the modest association between health outcomes and care work should not be a surprise. Care experiences, and thus the effects of those experiences, vary widely. Doing a few household chores or paying bills for an elderly or disabled parent is a different experience than providing medical and personal care for a spouse living in one's home, though both can be viewed as providing care. For example, health differences between care workers and noncare workers are much greater in studies that focus specifically on dementia care workers or among spousal care workers (Pinquart and Sorensen 2003), which reflects the much greater burden and stress associated with these forms of care. Living with the care recipient is also a factor. Care providers who do not live with the care recipient have better physical health than those who are caring for someone living inside their home. Interestingly, coresidence appears to have more of an impact on physical than mental health, suggesting that living with the care recipient may have a bigger impact on health behaviors such as sleeping, eating, and exercise and may also put the care worker at greater risk of injury from lifting and other physical tasks (Pinquart and Sorensen 2007).

The effects of care work on health and well-being also vary by gender, race, and social class. A meta-analysis of 229 studies finds that women care workers experience higher levels of depression and lower levels of subjective well-being and physical health than male care workers (Pinquart and Sorensen 2006). Again, however, the magnitude of these differences is small. Another meta-analysis found that Asian American, Hispanic, and black care workers all tend to have worse physical health than white care workers but that blacks reported less burden and depression than their white counterparts (Pinquart and Sorensen 2005). There is some evidence that race/ethnicity and income intersect with gender in their consequences for care worker health and well-being. One study, based on a national sample of midlife adults, found that nonwhite men care workers experience smaller increases in depression than non-Hispanic white men, but no racial/ethnic differences exist among women (Marks, Lambert et al. 2008). This study also found that low-income families put daughters providing care at greater risk for health problems than sons providing the same levels of care.

Much of researchers' attention has understandably been given to the negative health consequences of care work, but there are also positive effects of caring. A study of 1,229 care workers for persons with dementia found that study participants list a number of positive experiences, including feeling good about themselves, enabling them to appreciate life more, and strengthening their relationships with others (Tarlow, Wisniewski et al. 2004). Other studies have also found that care workers often feel a sense of personal gratification, appreciate being able to pay back support they may have received in the past, and enjoy a sense of personal growth (Henretta, Hill et al. 1997, Raschick and Ingersoll-Dayton 2004, Chesley and Moen 2006, Lin, Fee et al. 2012). However, as with health risks, the benefits of caring vary for men and women, with men often reporting greater benefits and growth from the experience (Chesley and Moen 2006, Lin, Fee et al. 2012).

While the consequences of care work for health and well-being have been extensively studied, there are still several important but largely unanswered questions about the health consequences of providing care. First, although we know a great deal about the contemporaneous and short-term effects of caring on health and well-being, there are surprisingly few studies examining health changes across the care work career and even fewer examining whether there are long-lasting health effects of providing care. Longitudinal studies do indicate changes in health across the care work career (Aneshensel, Pearlin et al. 1995, Pavalko and Woodbury 2000, Kim, Shaffer et al. 2014) as well as persistent health effects for some care workers even after care ends (Aneshensel, Botticello et al. 2004, Kim, Shaffer et al. 2014). However, we know little about which care experiences or statuses may promote resilience or whether any long-term effects of caring differ across health outcomes. Second, we are only beginning to understand how race, class, and gender may protect care workers or exacerbate the stresses they face. Much more work is needed to examine how experiences and consequences of care work vary across groups, and particularly how race, class, and gender intersect to shape the effects of care work. Finally, few studies examining the consequences of care work take into account the processes that influence who becomes a care worker in the first place, but several studies have found evidence that healthier adults are more likely to become care workers (McCann, Hebert et al. 2004, Roth, Haley et al. 2013). Closer attention to these selection processes is particularly important for clearly distinguishing both the positive and negative effects of providing care (Bianchi, Folbre et al. 2012).

Beyond its effects on health and well-being, a growing body of evidence identifies both short and long-term economic consequences of care work, particularly for women. Although employment does not affect whether or not women begin care work, doing that work increases the likelihood that women will reduce their employment (Pavalko and Artis 1997, Johnson and Lo Sasso 2006, Pavalko and Henderson 2006, Lilly, LaPorte et al. 2007, Berecki-Gisolf, Lucke et al. 2008). For example, Johnson and LoSasso (2006) estimate that women who help their parents over a two-year period reduce their work hours by 367 hours per year, a 41 percent drop. Pavalko and Artis (1997) also found that women who left the labor force to provide care did not immediately return after stopping care work. It is less clear whether similar effects of care work are found for men's employment, especially because much of the research on employment focuses on women. Studies comparing employment effects for men and women have been mixed. Data from the U.S. Health and Retirement Survey found care work did have an effect on employment for women but not men (Lee, Tang et al. 2014), while an Australian study found that being the primary care worker reduced the probability of employment by approximately 12 percentage points for both males and females (Nguyen and Connelly 2014). This study also found that secondary care workers, whether male or female, did not reduce their employment.

These short-term losses of income have significant long-term effects on lifetime income, as well as social security and pension benefits. Data from the Health and Retirement Survey suggests that a typical woman providing care loses a total of $324,044 due to reductions in work hours. This estimate includes $142,693 in lost wages, $131,351 in Social Security losses, and a conservative estimate of $50,000 in lost pension benefits (MetLife Mature Market Institute 2011). Income losses like these put care workers at an increased risk of poverty later in life. Wakabashi and Donato (2006), for example, found that women who were spending at least 20 hours per week assisting parents with personal care were 25 percent more likely to be living in poverty, 27 percent more likely to be receiving public assistance, and 46 percent more likely to be receiving Medicare eight years later. Although men are less likely than women to leave the labor force early to provide care, those who do also experience a substantial loss in wages and benefits—an average lifetime income loss of $283,716, including $89,107 in lost wages, $144,609 in Social Security, and $50,000 in pension (MetLife Mature Market Institute 2011).

The effects of care work on income are of particular concern for low-income women. Lee et al. (2014) demonstrate the reciprocal effects of income and unpaid care work over time, showing the vicious cycle it can create for low-income women. Unpaid care workers are more likely than noncare workers to experience income losses as a result of caring, and the limited financial resources of low-income families leave few options to hire outside help. Thus, women in low-income families are more likely to be called on to provide unpaid care and more likely to suffer economic loss from providing that care.

Challenges and Solutions for Addressing the Care Workers Dilemma

Given the growth in need for care and the increase in the time families spend at work (Jacobs and Gerson 2004), a major challenge will be to increase the compatibility of employment and unpaid care work. Compared to other industrialized countries, the United States offers relatively few protections that help spouses, sons, and daughters balance paid employment with unpaid care work. Most workplaces in the United States continue to assume that workers match the "ideal worker" norm and can provide full, uninterrupted commitment to paid work throughout their life (Williams 2000). This model assumes that the sometimes extensive unpaid work required to sustain a worker's own health and well-being as well as that of their family is provided by someone other than the worker, thus allowing them to devote their full energy to work. The problem with this model is that it does not match the reality of most workers' lives. In 2013, 69 percent of families in which at least one person was employed were either dual-earner married or single households (U.S. Bureau of Labor Statistics 2014). If a family member becomes ill or disabled in one of these households, there is no one available to provide unpaid care work without the competing demands of paid employment. That means that most unpaid care workers are employed and many employees are providing unpaid care.

What is the profile of employed care workers? To answer that question, we turn once again to the NLSY79 cohort, which provides nationally representative estimates of midlife men and women. Data are from the 2008–2012 surveys, when respondents were between 43–55 years of age. The first two columns of Table 7.2 compare employment between care workers and noncare workers in 2008. Those who were providing any type of care were slightly less likely to be employed, but 83 percent of middle-aged adults providing care were employed in 2008. Fifty-seven percent of employed care workers work in upper or lower white-collar occupations, and 81 percent are working full time. As we will discuss in more depth below, employee benefits that provide protection for time away from work and options for flexible hours can be particularly valuable for helping employees manage unpaid care demands. While most employed care workers have some paid sick or vacation time, 13 percent do not have any paid protection if they need to take a day away from work for unpaid care, and another 18 percent have fewer than 6 days of paid sick or vacation time per year available to them. Twenty-five percent of employed care workers lack job security if they take unpaid family leave, and only 55 percent have the option of flexible work hours to help manage the demands of care work.

The remaining columns in Table 7.2 compare work situations for men and women care workers and are separated by whether they are providing care to someone living inside or outside their home. One clear message from Table 7.2 is that combining unpaid care work with employment is not limited to any particular set of employees. Among those providing care to someone inside the home, men and women are equally likely to be employed. Employed care workers both inside and outside the home tend to work in a wide range of blue- and white-collar occupations. For both types of employed care workers, women are more likely than men to be working in lower white-collar or service occupations. Male care workers are slightly more likely to be employed full time, but 72 percent of women

Table 7.2 Employment Information by Location of Care and Gender, National Longitudinal Survey, 1979 Cohort (Weighted Data)

			Inside Care		Outside Care	
	No Care	Any Care	Women	Men	Women	Men
Observed *N*	4,767	1,959	449	382	901	438
Employed (%)	90[a]	83	76	81	80[m]	87
Occupation (%)						
Upper white	39[a]	30	26	21	32	34
Lower white	26	27	34[m]	12	39[m]	15
Skilled	11	10	2[m]	29	1[m]	17
Semi-skilled	10	12	8[m]	19	7[m]	21
Service	14[a]	20	31[m]	19	22	12
Employment type (%)						
Part time	13[a]	19	28[m]	12	28[m]	11
Full time	87[a]	81	72[m]	88	72[m]	89
Employee benefits (%)						
Any sick or vacation time	89[a]	87	97	98	95	97
6+ days sick or vacation Time	85[a]	82	96	96	93[m]	96
Family leave	74	75	69	69	77	73
Flexible hours	56	55	52	50	60[m]	61

- [a] significantly different from those who provide any care at the .05 level or smaller.
- [m] significantly different from men at the .05 level or smaller.
- Information on employment and occupation excludes those who are not working.
- Employment information for columns labeled "No Care" and "Any Care" is taken from the 2008 wave.
- Employment information for columns labeled "Inside Care" and "Outside Care" is taken from the first survey a respondent provides inside care.

who are employed care workers are also working full time. Employed men and women care workers tend to have similar levels of access to workplace policies and protections that are useful for juggling unpaid care and employment.

Information from other surveys suggests that the majority of employed care workers make some type of work accommodation to meet care demands, and many report that their unpaid care work affects their work performance (Witters 2011, Feinberg and Choula 2012, National Alliance for Caregiving and AARP 2015). The NAC survey found that 70 percent of employed care workers report making some work changes to accommodate their care demands. The most common changes are going in late, leaving early, or taking time off, which 66 percent reported, followed by 20 percent taking a leave of absence, 12 percent reducing their hours or taking a less demanding job, and 12 percent stopping work or retiring early (National Alliance for Caregiving and AARP 2009). The Gallup poll reports that 54 percent of employed care workers say that their unpaid care work has some impact on their work, and 19 percent report that it has a great impact, with 30 percent reporting missing six or more days of work in the past year in order to provide care (Witters 2011).

Reductions in work hours or labor force exits to provide care not only negatively impact the short and long-term income security of care workers, but they are also costly for employers. Twenty-four percent of employed care workers reduce hours, take a less demanding job, or stop work, which suggests that today's workplaces are not compatible with the realities of workers' lives. This incompatibility is expensive for employers because of the high cost of employee turnover. In the mid-2000s the Society for Human Resource Management estimated that it cost $3,500 to replace one $8.00 per hour employee and 30–50 percent of the annual salary of entry-level employees, 150 percent of middle-level employees, and up to 400 percent to replace specialized, high-level employees (Blake 2006).

Workplace Solutions

The incompatibility of employment and unpaid care work can be reduced significantly by workplace policies that improve workers' ability to care for family while also remaining employed. There are two categories of workplace policies designed to support care workers. The first includes workplace policies to provide flexibility and paid or unpaid time off from work to allow workers some time and flexibility to provide care. The second includes programs to provide workers with support and information, such as employee assistance programs and community referral services. Both types of programs are useful for helping employees who are caring for an ill or disabled adult, but policies that provide flexibility and time off work are particularly effective for helping workers meet family needs and remain employed. Below we review some of the most common workplace policies available to employed care workers and what we know about whether they are beneficial to employees.

Unpaid family leave. In the United States, unpaid family leave is mandated for eligible employees through the Family and Medical Leave Act (FMLA) of 1993. FMLA requires businesses with 50 or more employees to provide up to 12 weeks of unpaid leave for the birth or adoption of a child, to care for an ill family member, or for the worker's own health condition without loss of one's job. To be eligible, workers must have worked at that establishment for at least 12 months and have worked for at least 1,250 hours in the year prior to the leave.

While FMLA provides a basic level of protection nationally, some states and some companies provide more coverage than is mandated by law. Shortly after FMLA was enacted, 20–30 percent of private firms either offered more than 12 weeks of unpaid leave or offered leave to employees who had not met the exclusion criteria (Waldfogel 2001). Several states have also extended the family members who allow one to qualify for a leave. FMLA specifies that one can take an unpaid leave to care for one's child, spouse, or parent. Ten states have expanded this range of eligible family members. For example, as of 2012, nine states mandate FMLA protection to care for a partner, eight states include grandparents, in-laws and/or stepparents, and five states mandate FMLA coverage for care of nondependent adult children (Gornick, Howes et al. 2012). Only two states, California and New York, have expanded FMLA coverage to paid leave.

Evidence on the use and effectiveness of FMLA is mixed. Shortly after implementation, most firms reported that it is somewhat or very easy to comply with the law and that implementation did not adversely affect their productivity or profitability (Waldfogel 2001). Although many were covered by some type of family leave policy prior to the passage of the FMLA, its passage extended coverage to more workers. The National Compensation Survey reports that in 1990, 24 percent of private industry workers had access to unpaid family leave, compared to 85 percent with coverage in 2014 (Wiatrowski 2004, U.S. Bureau of Labor Statistics 2014). There is some evidence that unpaid leave may also help workers remain employed. A national study of midlife women found that employed care workers who had access to unpaid leave were more likely to still be employed two years later than those who did not have access (Pavalko and Henderson 2006).

While providing some protection, evidence also suggests that the overall impact of FMLA is modest. Most workers cannot afford to use unpaid leave, or if they do use it, do so for short periods of time. The median length of leave is 10 days, and 90 percent of leaves last 12 weeks or less (Waldfogel 2001). Even when a policy is formally available, informal workplace cultures may discourage its use (Blair-Loy and Wharton 2002). Finally, recent estimates suggest that firm compliance with the law may be lower than originally estimated, with between 23 and 46 percent of eligible firms not complying with the law (Armenia, Gerstel et al. 2014).

Paid leave. Paid leave is likely to be far more valuable to employees and effective for workplaces wishing to reduce turnover costs from employees who are providing unpaid care. Although there are currently national and local initiatives to expand paid leave, as of early 2015, only two states, California and New York, have extended family leave policies to provide paid leave. Nationally, 12 percent of private industry employees have access to paid family leave (U.S. Bureau of Labor Statistics 2014). Low-wage earners are the least likely to have access to family leave. Among workers earning wages in the lowest income quartile, only 5 percent had access to paid leave, while 22 percent of workers in the top quartile of earnings had access to paid leave (U.S. Bureau of Labor Statistics 2014). Low-income workers are most likely to have a family member needing care and are the least able to afford an unpaid leave, but they are also the least likely to have access to paid leave.

Given the scarcity of paid family leave for most workers, another valuable resource for workers balancing care work and employment is paid sick and vacation time. Several studies have found that women who were providing unpaid care and had access to sick or vacation time were less likely to leave the labor force than those whose jobs did not provide this benefit (Pavalko and Woodbury 2000, Pavalko and Henderson 2006). These benefits have historically been the most commonly available benefit for workers in private industry, with an average of eight days of sick leave a year (U.S. Bureau of Labor Statistics 2014). In 2014, 77 percent of private industry workers had access to paid vacations, 61 percent had paid sick leave, and 38 percent paid personal leave. Thus, while widely available, not all workers have even this minimal level of protection that can be essential for dealing with care emergencies.

Flexible hours. Giving workers more flexibility in when and where they do their work is another workplace strategy that may make it more feasible for care workers to remain employed. The Bureau of Labor Statistics estimates that 27.5 percent of U.S. workers have flexible work schedules, defined as flexibility in when one starts or stops work. Only 11 percent, however, have access to a formal flextime program at work (U.S. Bureau of Labor Statistics 2005). These varying definitions of what it means to have flexible hours makes it difficult to assess whether flextime is beneficial for care workers, but several studies have found modest effects on job turnover and emotional health (Chesley and Moen 2006, Pavalko and Henderson 2006).

However, several factors limit the effectiveness of flextime policies (Perlow and Kelly 2014). In many companies a formal policy may exist, but its implementation is left to the immediate supervisor, who may or may not support the policy. Workers also often face career repercussions and social stigma if they take advantage of flextime, particularly for personal or family needs (Leslie, Manchester et al. 2012, Williams, Blair-Loy et al.

2013). Although not specific to care workers, a growing body of evidence suggests that a more substantial cultural and structural shift in the organization of work time that gives workers control over when and how they get their work done may be more effective in reducing a variety of negative effects of work, including work-family conflict, job turnover, and poor health (Moen, Kelly et al. 2011, Kelly, Moen et al. 2014, Perlow and Kelly 2014).

Employee assistance programs. Employers are also increasingly offering employee assistance programs to provide employees access to referral or counseling services to deal with personal or family problems. Some explicitly include referral services for elder care. In 2008, 76 percent of public sector and 46 percent of private sector employees had an employee assistance program, and prevalence of these programs had roughly doubled since the late 1990s (Stoltzfus 2009). Unfortunately, there has been little to no evaluation of the effectiveness of these services for employees or the organizations that adopt them (Heathfield n.d.). While information and referral to other resources is likely to be useful to employees juggling unpaid care work, a limitation of assistance programs is that they do not address the time challenges faced by employed care workers, and thus may have limited effectiveness for reducing employee turnover.

Conclusions

Unpaid care work is not only essential for individuals and families; it is also a major component of our health-care system, providing more than half of the long-term care for the elderly. With an aging population, even small reductions in adults' ability to provide unpaid care could have major ramifications for the financing of health care. As the demand for care increases and the supply of family members to provide care declines, institutional support that allows adults to provide unpaid care while also maintaining paid work and family lives becomes even more critical. As this chapter has shown, providing unpaid care is most common in midlife, which corresponds to adults' peak years of employment. At any given time, it is estimated that 17 percent of adults are providing unpaid care while employed, and many will do so multiple times. Employees who are providing care to an ill or disabled family member are not isolated to any particular demographic group, as both men and women, and employees at all job levels are likely to provide care.

In this chapter, we have reviewed the implications of this care for the care worker's own health and economic well-being, and also a range of workplace policies that can make it more feasible for workers to remain employed while providing care. However, it is important to note that workplace policies, while valuable, are a limited solution. Even the most comprehensive workplace policies, such as sick and vacation days, are not uniformly available to all workers. Firms and supervisors adopt and implement these policies unevenly, and often the most vulnerable workers, which often include care workers, are the least likely to have protection. For this reason, truly effective support for care workers will also require reforms beyond the workplace. National policies and programs that provide more uniform and widespread coverage will be essential for assuring that unpaid care can be sustained without risking the care provider's long-term income security. Federal initiatives to make paid leave available to all care workers are one of the most important steps we could take to support them. Protection of paid sick and vacation time for all workers is also essential because they allow those providing care to manage emergencies.

Beyond initiatives to increase the availability of unpaid leave, it is also critical that we broaden forms of community support. The National Caregivers Support Program, a federally funded program to support family care workers, is one such example. This program provides information, assistance, and training for family care workers as well as respite care and other services. Programs and services vary across states, and the program remains underfunded (Wisensale 2008). A 2004 evaluation of the program found that in all states, funding levels were insufficient to meet caregiver needs, and services such as respite care are particularly underfunded (Feinberg et al. 2004). Expansion of this type of community support will become increasingly important as the demand for care increases. Providing multilevel support for care workers will be essential not only for individuals and families, but also for employers and the health-care system.

References

Aneshensel, C. S., et al. (1995). *Profiles in Caregiving: The Unexpected Career*. San Diego, CA, Academic Press.

Aneshensel, C. S., et al. (2004). "When Caregiving Ends: The Course of Depressive Symptoms After Bereavement." *Journal of Health and Social Behavior* 45(December): 422–440.

Angel, J. L., et al. (2014). "Nativity Status and Sources of Care Assistance Among Elderly Mexican-Origin Adults." *Journal of Cross-Cultural Gerontology* 29: 243–258.

Armenia, A., et al. (2014). "Workplace Compliance with the Law: The Case of the Family and Medical Leave Act." *Work and Occupations* 41: 277–304.

Berecki-Gisolf, J., et al. (2008). "Transitions into Informal Caregiving and Out of Paid Employment of Women in their 50s." *Social Science and Medicine* 67: 122–127.

Bianchi, S., et al. (2012). Unpaid Care Work. In *For Love and Money: Care Provision in the United States*. N. Folbre (Ed). New York, Russell Sage Foundation: 40–64.

Blair-Loy, M. and A.S. Wharton (2002). "Employees' Use of Work-Family Policies and the Workplace Social Context." *Social Forces* 80(3): 813–845.

Blake, R. (2006). Employee Retention: What Employer Turnover Really Costs Your Company. *WebProNews*.

Chen, H. and Z. Guo (2008). "Obesity and Functional Disability in Elderly Americans." *Journal of the American Geriatrics Society* 56(4): 689–694.

Chesley, N. and P. Moen (2006). "When Workers Care: Dual-Earner Couples' Caregiving Strategies, Benefit Use, and Psychological Well-Being." *American Behavioral Scientist* 49(9): 1248–1269.

Congressional Budget Office (2013). *Rising Demand for Long-Term Services and Supports for Elderly People*. Washington, DC.

Cynkar, P. and E. Mendes (2011). *More Than One in Six American Workers Also Act as Caregivers*. Washington, DC, Gallup.

Evercare (2008). *Hispanic Family Caregiving in the U.S.: Findings from a National Study*. Bethesda, MD.

Feinberg, L. F. et al. (2004). *The State of the States in Family Caregiver Support: A 50-State Study*. San Francisco: Family Caregiver Alliance and National Conference of State Legislators.

Feinberg, L.F. and R. Choula (2012). Understanding the Impact of Family Caregiving on Work. *Fact Sheet*. Washington, DC, AARP. 271.

Folbre, N. and D.A. Wolf (2012). Appendix: Measuring Care Work. In *For Love and Money: Care Provision in the United States*. N. Folbre (Ed.). New York, Russell Sage: 205–227.

Freedman, V.A., et al. (2004). "Resolving Inconsistencies in Trends in Old-Age Disability: Report from a Technical Working Group." *Demography* 41(3): 417–414.

Glazer, N.Y. (1990). "The Home as a Workshop: Women as Amateur Nurses and Medical Care Providers." *Gender & Society* 4: 479–499.

Gornick, J.C., et al. (2012). The Care Policy Landscape. In *For Love and Money: Care Provision in the United States*. N. Folbre (Ed.). New York, Russell Sage: 112–139.

Harrington Meyer, M., Ed. (2000). *Care Work: Gender, Class, and the Welfare States*. New York, Routledge.

Heathfield, S.M. (n.d.). Do EAP's Work or Just Make Employers Feel Good? About.com.

Henretta, J.C., et al. (1997). "Selection of Children to Provide Care: The Effect of Earlier Parental Transfers." *The Journals of Gerontology, Series B: Social Sciences* 52: 110–119.

Jacobs, J.A. and K. Gerson (2004). *The Time Divide: Work, Family, and Gender Inequality*. Cambridge, MA, Harvard University Press.

Johnson, R.W. and A.T. Lo Sasso (2006). "The Impact of Elder Care on Women's Labor Supply." *Inquiry* 43: 195–210.

Kahn, J.R., et al. (2011). "Help to Family and Friends: Are there Gender Differences at Older Ages?" *Journal of Marriage and the Family* 73(1): 77–92.

Kelly, E. L., et al. (2014). "Changing Work and Work-Family Conflict: Evidence from the Work, Family, and Health Network." *American Sociological Review* 79(3): 485–516.

Kim, Y., et al. (2014). "Prevalence and Predictors of Depressive Symptoms among Cancer Caregivers 5 Years after the Relative's Cancer Diagnosis." *Journal of Consulting and Clinical Psychology* 82: 1–8.

Laditka, J. N. and S. B. Laditka (2001). "Adult Children Helping Older Parents." *Research on Aging* 23(4): 429–456.

Lee, Y., et al. (2015). "The Vicious Cycle of Parental Caregiving and Financial Well-Being: A Longitudinal Study of Women." *The Journals of Gerontology, Series B: Psychological Sciences and Social Sciences*. 70(3): 425–431.

Leslie, L. M., et al. (2012). "Flexible Work Practices: A Source of Career Premiums or Penalties?" *Academy of Management Journal* 55: 1407–1428.

Lilly, M. B., et al. (2007). "Labor Market Work and Home Care's Unpaid Caregivers: A Systematic Review of Labor Force Participation Rates, Predictors of Labor Market Withdrawal, and Hours of Work." *Milbank Quarterly* 85(4): 641–690.

Lin, I.-F., et al. (2012). "Negative and Positive Caregiving Experiences: A Closer Look at the Intersection of Gender and Relationship." *Family Relations* 61: 343–358.

Markides, K. S., et al. (2013). Aging, Health, and Families in the Hispanic Population. *Kinship and Cohort in an Aging Society*. M. Silverstein and R. Giarusso. Baltimore, MD, Johns Hopkins University: 314–331.

Marks, N. F., et al. (2008). "Psychosocial Moderators of the Effects of Transitioning Into Filial Caregiving on Mental and Physical Health." *Research on Aging* 30(3): 358–389.

Martin, L. G., et al. (2010). "Trends in Health of Older Adults in the United States: Past, Present, Future." *Demography* 47(1): S17-S40.

McCann, J. J., et al. (2004). "Predictors of Beginning and Ending Caregiving During a 3-year Period in a Biracial Community Population of Older Adults." *American Journal of Public Health* 94(10): 1800–1806.

MetLife Mature Market Institute (2011). *The MetLife Study of Caregiving Costs to Working Caregivers: Double Jeopardy for Baby Boomers Caring for Their Parents*. Westport, CT.

Moen, P., et al. (2011). "Does Enhancing Work-Time Control and Flexibility Reduce Turnover? A Naturally Occurring Experiment." *Social Problems* 58(1): 69–98.

Moen, P., et al. (1994). "Women's Work and Caregiving Roles: A Life Course Approach." *The Journals of Gerontology, Series B: Social Sciences* 49(4): S176–S186.

National Alliance for Caregiving and AARP (1997). *Family Caregiving in the U.S.—Findings from a National Survey*. Bethesda, MD, National Alliance for Caregiving and AARP.

National Alliance for Caregiving and AARP (2009). *Caregiving in the U.S. 2009*. Bethesda, MD.

National Alliance for Caregiving and AARP (2015). *Caregiving in the U.S., 2015 Report*.

Nguyen, H. T. and L. B. Connelly (2014). "The Effect of Unpaid Caregiving Intensity on Labour Force Participation: Results from a Multinomial Endogenous Treatment Model." *Social Science and Medicine* 100: 115–122.

Noel-Miller, C. (2011). "Partner Caregiving in Older Cohabitating Couples." *The Journals of Gerontology, Series B: Psychological Sciences and Social Sciences* 66: 341–353.

Pavalko, E. K. and J. E. Artis (1997). "Women's Caregiving and Paid Work: Causal Relationships in Late Midlife." *The Journals of Gerontology, Series B: Psychological Sciences and Social Sciences* 52(4): S170–S179.

Pavalko, E. K. and K. A. Henderson (2006). "Combining Care Work and Paid Work: Do Workplace Policies Make a Difference?" *Research on Aging* 28: 359–374.

Pavalko, E. K. and J. D. Wolfe (2015). "Do Women Still Care? Cohort Changes in U.S. Women's Care for the Ill or Disabled." *Social Forces*. Epub.

Pavalko, E. K. and S. Woodbury (2000). "Social Roles as Process: Caregiving Careers and Women's Health." *Journal of Health and Social Behavior* 41(1): 91–105.

Perlow, L. A. and E. L. Kelly (2014). "Toward a Model of Work Redesign for Better Work and Better Life." *Work and Occupations* 41: 111–134.

Pillemer, K. and J. J. Suitor (2014). "Who Provides Care? A Prospective Study of Caregiving Among Adult Siblings." *The Gerontologist* 54(4): 589–598.

Pinquart, M. and S. Sorensen (2003). "Differences between Caregivers and Noncaregivers in Psychological Health and Physical Health: Meta-Analysis." *Psychology and Aging* 18(2): 250–267.

Pinquart, M. and S. Sorensen (2005). "Ethnic Differences in Stressors, Resources, and Psychological Outcomes of Family Caregiving: A Meta-Analysis." *The Gerontologist* 45(1): 90–106.

Pinquart, M. and S. Sorensen (2006). "Gender Differences in Caregiver Stressors, Social Resources, and Health: An Updated Meta-Analysis." *The Journals of Gerontology, Series B: Psychological Sciences* 61B(1): P33–P45.

Pinquart, M. and S. Sorensen (2007). "Correlates of Physical Health of Informal Caregivers: A Meta-Analysis." *The Journals of Gerontology, Series B: Psychological Sciences* 62B(2): P126–P137.

Raschick, M. and B. Ingersoll-Dayton (2004). "The Costs and Rewards of Caregiving among Aging Spouses and Adult Children." *Family Relations* 53: 317–325.

Reinhard, S. C., et al. (2012). Home Alone: Family Caregivers Providing Complex Chronic Care. *Research Report*. A.P.P. Institute. Washington, DC. 2012–10.

Robison, J., et al. (1995). "Women's Caregiving: Changing Profiles and Pathways." *The Journals of Gerontology, Series B: Social Sciences* 50B(6): S362–S373.

Roth, D. L., et al. (2013). "Family Caregiving and All-Cause Mortality: Findings from a Population-Based Propensity-Matched Analysis." *American Journal of Epidemiology* 178(10): 1571–1578.

Sarkisian, N. and N. Gerstel (2004). "Kin Support among Blacks and Whites: Race and Family Organization." *American Sociological Review* 69(4): 812–837.

Spillman, B.C. and K. J. Black (2005). *Staying the Course: Trends in Family Caregiving*. Washington, DC, AARP Public Policy Institute.

Spillman, B.C. and L.E. Pezzin (2000). "Potential and Active Family Caregivers: Changing Networks and the 'Sandwich Generation'." *The Milbank Quarterly* 78(3): 347–374.

Stoltzfus, E.R. (2009). *Access to Wellness and Employee Assistance Programs in the United States*.

Tarlow, B.J., et al. (2004). "Positive Aspects of Caregiving." *Research on Aging* 26(4): 429–453.

U.S. Bureau of Labor Statistics (2005). Workers on Flexible and Shift Schedules in May 2004. *News*.

U.S. Bureau of Labor Statistics (2013). Unpaid Eldercare in the United States—2011–2012. Data From the American Time Use Survey. *USDL-13-1886*.

U.S. Bureau of Labor Statistics (2014). Employment Characteristics of Families—2013. *USDL-14–0658*.

U.S. Bureau of Labor Statistics (2014). *National Compensation Survey: Employee Benefits in Private Industry in the United States, 2014, United States Department of Labor*.

U.S. Bureau of Labor Statistics (2015). "National Longitudinal Surveys." Retrieved February 26, 2015, from http://www.bls.gov/nls/nlsy79.htm.

Uhlenberg, P. and M. Cheuk (2008). Demographic Change and the Future of Informal Caregiving. *Caregiving Contexts: Cultural, Familial, and Societal Implications*. M.E. Szinovacz and A. Davey. New York, Springer: 9–34.

Vitaliano, P.P., et al. (2003). "Is Caregiving Hazardous to One's Physical Health? A Meta-Analysis." *Psychological Bulletin* 129(6): 946–972.

Wakabashi, C. and K.M. Donato (2006). "Does Caregiving Increase Poverty Among Women in Later Life? Evidence from the Health and Retirement Survey." *Journal of Health and Social Behavior* 47: 258–274.

Waldfogel, J. (2001). "Family and Medical Leave: Evidence from the 2000 Surveys." *Monthly Labor Review* 124(9): 17–23.

White-Means, S. and R.M. Rubin (2008). "Parent Caregiving Choices of Middle-Generation Blacks and Whites in the United States." *Journal of Aging and Health* 20: 560–582.

Wiatrowski, W.J. (2004). *Documenting Benefits Coverage for all Workers*. U.S.D. o. Labor, Bureau of Labor Statistics.

Williams, J. (2000). *Unbending Gender*. New York, Oxford University Press.

Williams, J.C., et al. (2013). "Cultural Schemas, Social Class, and the Flexibility Stigma." *Journal of Social Issues* 69: 209–234.

Wisensale, S.K. (2008). Caregiving Policies in the United States: Framing a National Agenda. *Caregiving Contexts: Cultural, Familial, and Societal Implications*. M.E. Szinovacz and A. Davey. New York, Springer: 215–233.

Witters, D. (2011). *Caregiving Costs U.S. Economy $25.2 Billion in Lost Productivity*. Washington, DC, Gallup.

CHAPTER EIGHT

Elder Abuse

Joah L. Williams, Melba Hernandez-Tejada, Emily S. Fanguy, and Ron Acierno

Changes in life expectancy over the last century are rapidly shifting the face of the global population. By 2050, for example, the number of people aged 65 or older is expected to triple to well over one billion, or 16 percent of the world's population (U.S. Department of Health and Human Services, 2011a). With the number of older adults expected to continue increasing over the coming decades, families and communities will be faced with the growing challenge of caring for the elderly. The majority of older adults will, of course, continue to reside independently in the community, often with the support of family and other community-based caregivers, while some will require more intensive care in the context of long-term care facilities such as nursing homes and assisted living facilities.

Each year 10 percent of independent, community-residing older adults in the United States will experience some form of elder abuse (Acierno et al., 2010). Older adults in both informal, domestic settings and formal settings involving community-based caregivers may be at risk of elder abuse, though each structure is associated with different forms of risk, and hence must employ different risk reduction strategies. In this chapter, we discuss the prevalence of elder abuse in its various forms, providing definitions of and describing risk factors for different types of abuse. We also discuss new strategies relevant to the prevention of elder abuse and highlight international efforts to raise awareness about elder abuse as a human rights issue.

Elder Abuse Research in a Historical Context

Early case reports of "granny battering" (Burston, 1975) first appeared in medical journals in the middle 1970s. In the years that followed, additional cases of "granny battering" were brought to national attention as older adult victims of abuse were invited to testify before a series of congressional subcommittees on aging (Gorbien & Eisenstein, 2005), increasing public awareness of the scope and impact of elder abuse. More than a decade would follow, though, before the first methodologically rigorous research emerged on the incidence of elder abuse in the United States. One of the first studies to report on the prevalence of elder abuse in the United States was conducted by Pillemer and Finkelhor (1988) using a random sample of community-dwelling older adults from the Boston area. Extrapolated results suggested that 32 older adults per 1,000, or 3 percent, experience some form of elder abuse, although the authors did not assess for financial exploitation and other commonly recognized forms of abuse that would likely yield higher estimates. Later, in the 1990s, the National Elder Abuse Incidence Study (NEAIS) was conducted by the American Public Health Services Association's National Center on Elder Abuse, which reported that an estimated 449,924 older adults in the United States aged 60 and over were victims of abuse or neglect in 1996 (Tatara, 1997). The NEAIS based its estimates, however, on Adult Protective Service records and sentinel reports of abuse and, thus, likely underestimated the actual incidence of elder abuse in that many incidents of abuse are never reported to authorities. It was not until the 2000s that the first large-scale efforts were made to explore the prevalence of elder abuse in nationally representative samples of older adults (Acierno et al., 2010; Laumann, Leitsch, & Waite, 2008), and we highlight these efforts in the next section, providing definitions and discussing the prevalence of elder abuse in its various forms.

Problem Definitions and Prevalence

Although elder abuse can take many forms, most widely accepted taxonomies include five categories of mistreatment: emotional/psychological abuse, financial exploitation, neglect, physical abuse, and sexual abuse. In some classification systems, the nature of the relationship between the older adult victim and the perpetrator is a key factor in determining whether these acts of mistreatment can be designated elder abuse in that, to be considered elder abuse, the mistreatment must occur within the context of a trust relationship (Bonnie & Wallace, 2003). Trust relationships are considered relationships where the older adult relies on or is in some way dependent on another person for care or basic needs and can include family members or professional caregivers. These events, however, can easily come from a nontrusted source, as in cases of assault when speaking of physical or sexual violence, or financial exploitation involving scamming and fraud. Therefore, in this section, we provide definitions of each category of elder abuse used in the National Elder Mistreatment Study (NEMS; Acierno et al., 2010), a large, epidemiological study of mistreatment against community-residing older adults aged 60 and over, perpetrated by individuals both known and unknown to the older adult. For the purposes of this chapter, we use the terms abuse and mistreatment interchangeably, and, of note, the Centers for Disease Control uses the term maltreatment.

The first category of mistreatment, emotional or psychological abuse, includes things like being yelled at, verbally attacked, or scolded in such a way that an older adult felt threatened or concerned about their safety. Emotional abuse can also include repeated acts involving verbal humiliation or embarrassment like calling an older adult stupid or even being ignored for days at a time. In the NEMS, almost 5 percent of older adults reported experiencing at least one severe episode of emotional abuse in the past year, with nearly 14 percent of older adults reporting some form of emotional abuse since reaching age 60. The National Social Life, Health, and Aging Project (NSHAP; Laumann, Leitsch, & Waite, 2008), an epidemiological survey of older adults aged 57 to 85 years, found even higher rates, with a 9 percent past year prevalence rate of emotional abuse in the form of being insulted or put down. These estimates suggest that emotional or psychological abuse may be the most common form of elder abuse, excluding lower-level financial abuse, such as not returning a few dollars change after shopping for groceries for an older relative for which the older relative paid. These figures indicate that older adults may be abused at much higher rates than previously thought.

Evidence suggests that the second most common form of elder abuse is financial exploitation. Older adults frequently have family members or other parties help them manage their finances and other assets, and it is in this context that financial exploitation typically occurs. In the NEMS, Acierno et al. (2010) distinguished between financial abuse by trusted others and financial exploitation by strangers and defined financial abuse as acts in which someone does not ask an older adult permission before spending their money or selling their property, withholds information about important financial decisions from an older adult, forges signatures in order to make important financial decisions without an older adult's consent, uses force or deception to make an older adult sign important financial documents, and/or steals money or property from an older adult.

Older adults can also be targeted by strangers in scams, which can include health insurance fraud, investment schemes, and false sweepstakes. These acts of financial exploitation are estimated to result in roughly $3 billion in annual financial loss (National Committee for the Prevention of Elder Abuse, 2011). Past year prevalence estimates of elder financial abuse range from greater than 3 percent in the NSHAP to 5 percent in the NEMS, excluding stranger fraud.

Elder neglect involves instances in which an older adult has one or more unmet needs of daily living and an identified individual responsible for meeting those needs repeatedly refuses to do so. Distinguish this from the identical situations of unmet needs for which there exists no designated legally or presumably responsible individual. The latter cases are not considered neglect, although one might argue that, in these instances, it is the State that bears the culpability for said abuse. Neglected older adults are those who lack transportation to medical appointments, have difficulty getting food or medicines, or even have difficulty preparing meals and taking medications as prescribed. Neglected older adults may also have difficulty keeping their residence clean and maintaining proper hygiene. Potential elder neglect in community-residing samples where a basic need is evident, and a person is formally or statutorily designated, legal or otherwise, as responsible, appears to be nearly as common as financial exploitation, with a past year prevalence rate of 5 percent in the NEMS.

While less common than other forms of mistreatment, community-residing elder physical and sexual abuse still occur at disturbing frequency when considering the size of the older adult population, with past year prevalence rates of just under 2 percent and 1 percent, respectively (Acierno et al., 2010). Elder physical abuse can include being struck by someone or threatened with a weapon, being physically restrained, or physically hurt in such a way that results in physical injuries. Elder sexual abuse includes acts such as forced, unwanted intercourse, being forced to undress or be photographed in states of undress, and molestation, which can be defined as being forced to touch someone else's breasts or genitals or having someone forcefully touch one's own breasts or genitals. Because of the highly stigmatizing nature of sexual abuse, it is likely that this event is underreported.

An Ecological Model of Elder Abuse

Although elder abuse is typically discussed as it relates to older adult victims of abuse and their abusers, we propose that elder abuse must be considered from a broader, ecological systems perspective (Bronfenbrenner, 1997) in order to maximize the impact of screening and prevention efforts.

That is, it may be artificial to separate out abuse by a trusted other from the same violent act perpetrated by a stranger. They are most certainly associated with different risk factors (Acierno et al., 2010), but the victim being hit on their body absorbing the blows very likely considers both problematic. The fact that risk factors overlap, and that experience of one form of violence increases the risk of the other, suggests that all forms of violence should be studied in an individual-in-the-environment context. The Ecological Model provides just such a framework for studying the individual-in-the-environment context. According to this model, human behavior and development is shaped by the interactions between the person, their immediate settings, and the social and cultural contexts in which these settings are embedded. The Ecological Model conceptualizes elder abuse as existing within these multiple interacting systems both within the community and the broader society (see Figure 8.1) and has been used in the conceptualization of elder abuse by Wolf (2000), the World Report on Violence and Health (Krug et al., 2002), and the 2013 Institute of Medicine (IOM) Workshop *Elder Abuse and its Prevention.* From the ecological

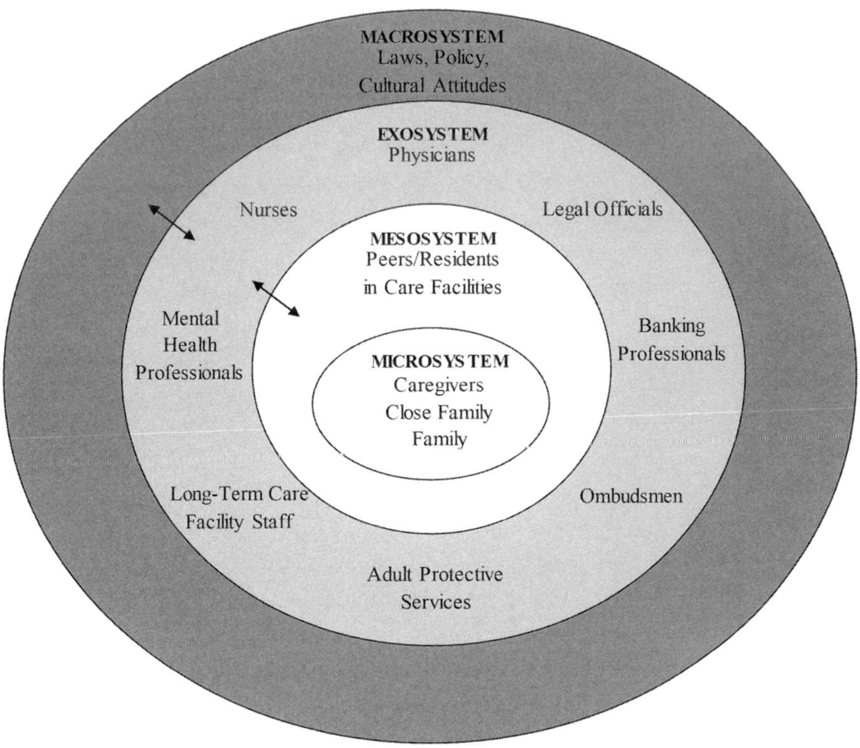

Figure 8.1 Ecological systems model of elder abuse

systems perspective, the microsystem and mesosystem, or contexts closest to the individual, can include such factors as caregivers, family members, or, in the case of long-term care facilities, fellow residents, and this level also includes personal characteristics such as age, gender, race, and health status that may confer risk for abuse. Acts of elder abuse may still be influenced by more distal contexts, or the exosystem, despite little or no direct interaction at this level. Associations between mistreatment and microsystem variables have been of particular interest, given that many of these potential risk factors are proximal and modifiable and, thus, viable targets for preventive intervention. Findings from previous research indicate that microsystem variables such as gender, race, socioeconomic status, psychiatric history, and substance use are associated with elder mistreatment as well as the outcomes of mistreatment, including criminal justice system participation (Bachman, 1994; Biggs et al., 2009; Hanson et al., 1995; Laumann, Leitsch, & Waite, 2008; Norris, 1992). Research on screening, prevention, and policy tend to focus on the exosystem and, to some extent, mesosystem variables. Very little funding and subsequent research has been directed toward these higher-level systems. In the following sections, we discuss these topics in relation to various levels of the older adult's ecological system.

Elder Abuse Risk Factors

In the last section, we noted that microsystem-level variables including age, gender, race, and psychiatric history are associated with elder mistreatment. In the NEMS community sample, for example, lower age was associated with increased risk for experiencing emotional and physical abuse. Lower age was also associated with increased risk for experiencing emotional or verbal abuse in the NSHAP (Laumann, Leitsch, & Waite, 2008)—a finding that the authors partially attribute to respondents possibly referencing routine family arguments in their reports. Although counter to the commonly accepted idea that abuse is more common among the oldest, most physically and psychologically impaired adults, it is important to note that both the NEMS and NSHAP lacked representative samples of institutionalized older adults who are generally older with more serious functional impairment.

Gender was also related to emotional abuse in the NSHAP in that women were found to be at greater risk for experiencing emotionally abusive behavior. The NSHAP also revealed important racial and ethnic differences with regard to financial mistreatment. For instance, in the NSHAP, African American elders reported higher rates of financial exploitation relative to Caucasian elders, while being Latino appears to be protective in that Latino elders endorsed lower rates of financial exploitation compared to Caucasian elders. One of the most important risk factors for elder abuse, though, appears to be social isolation, which is associated with increased risk for several forms of abuse including emotional abuse, neglect, physical abuse, and sexual abuse. The nature of the relationship between social isolation and elder abuse is certainly complex, but it stands to reason that, as in other forms of domestic violence, abusers may seek to isolate abused elders in order to conceal the abuse, thus creating further opportunities for future violence and limiting opportunities for intervention on behalf of the older adult. In terms of health and psychiatric factors, dementia and cognitive impairment are known risk factors for abuse. Indeed, in one recent study of community-residing older adults, 47 percent of those with dementia were found to have experienced some abusive event in the form of emotional abuse, physical abuse, or neglect (Wiglesworth et al., 2010). One reason for these elevated rates of abuse among adults with dementia is that, ironically, these adults may engage in more psychologically and physically aggressive behaviors toward their caregivers, who, in turn, may use restraints or other forceful methods when dealing with the older adult.

Perpetrator Characteristics

An important part of the process of understanding elder mistreatment is the study of perpetrator characteristics since the type of relationship between both can determine the length and extent of the abuse. For instance, strangers are not commonly the perpetrators, rather the abuser is a person well known by the victim, and in most cases is another family member.

Perpetrators, or those who commit emotional, physical, and sexual abuse, commonly share several characteristics. These include substance abuse around the time of mistreatment, a history of mental illness, unemployment, and social isolation, which is defined by less than three friends. Such aggressors are more often young men and are usually children or spouses of the victim.

According to Acierno et al. (2009) 56 percent of the perpetrators of emotional mistreatment are family members, just under 9 percent are strangers, 41 percent are unemployed, and 39 percent were socially isolated; while in the case of the perpetrators of physical mistreatment, a staggering 76 percent are family members and only 3 percent are strangers, over 51 percent of perpetrators were abusing some substance at the time of the mistreatment, and over 43 percent were socially isolated. With respect to sexual abuse, over 52 percent of the perpetrators were family members compared with only 3 percent strangers, and 53 percent were socially isolated. In the case of neglect and financial exploitation, a majority of the perpetrators were family members as well. As Pillemer and Finkelhor (1988) have indicated, the fact that high rates of spousal elder abuse occurs, contributes to the conceptualization that this is a crime that is more analogous to domestic violence than child abuse. Statistically, less than 8 percent of emotional abuse is perpetrated by strangers.

This epidemiological data lead us to conclude that treatment should focus not only on addressing the victim but also on considering how to address the perpetrators since the majority are family members, which makes it more difficult for the victim to follow legal pathways to stop the abuse. It is also remarkably noticeable that the perpetrators have issues that may be able to be addressed and produce a positive outcome and a secondary benefit by reducing elder mistreatment.

Health and Economic Impact of Elder Abuse

Elder abuse can have a serious impact on older adults' physical and psychosocial functioning. Abusive acts in and of themselves can result in minor injuries such as bruises and lacerations but are also associated with other, more serious medical problems including fractures, dementia, malnutrition, and death (Dong, 2005; Dong et al., 2009). While the full economic impact of these injuries is unknown, estimates suggest that direct medical costs associated with violent injuries to older adults may add up to as much as $5 billion annually (Mouton et al., 2004). In addition to physical injuries, recent evidence has shown that elder abuse is independently associated with emotional distress even after controlling for other known risk factors including physical health, social support, and prior trauma history (Cisler et al., 2012). This emotional distress is often reflected in higher rates of depression and anxiety among elder abuse victims relative to individuals with no history of abuse (e.g., Dong, Beck, & Simon, 2010; Dyer et al., 2000). The extreme emotional distress experienced in the context of elder abuse is likely to exacerbate other health problems and even increase risk for mortality (Amstadter et al., 2010; Dong et al., 2011), and healthcare providers working with older adults may be in a unique position to screen for and intervene in cases of elder abuse. In other words, they may do very well by their patients to ask questions that, historically, have been off limits because they were considered either disrespectful, or likely to upset patients. Such excuses for nonassessment have been jettisoned with respect to provider behaviors and domestic violence and should similarly be tossed with respect to elder abuse. Aforementioned studies point to the serious physical and emotional impact of elder abuse, but national epidemiological studies on the association between elder abuse and health/

mental health outcomes are needed to more fully understand the extent of this issue. At the time of this writing, there are no program announcements for such studies by any NIH institute, or by the CDC.

Elder Abuse Screening and Prevention—Challenges and Solutions

In 2011, the U.S. National Prevention Council published the National Prevention Strategy (U.S. Department of Health and Human Services, 2011b) with the aim of shifting health care in the United States from a focus on sickness and disease to one based on wellness and prevention. One of the priority areas highlighted in the National Prevention Strategy is the promotion of "Injury and Violence Free Living" across the lifespan, including the prevention of violence against older adults. One of the first steps in any successful prevention or intervention program is recognizing cues that raise suspicion about probable abuse or violence against individuals. In this section, we discuss screening strategies for detecting and identifying elder abuse and also describe intervention strategies relevant to health care and other community settings that serve older adults.

Screening and Assessment

Screening for elder abuse and neglect can be challenging, making routine screening difficult in some health-care settings. Despite these challenges, health-care providers are especially well positioned to identify possible cases of elder abuse in that older adults are frequent consumers of health-care services. Both the American Medical Association (1992) and the American Academy of Neurology (Schulman & Hohler, 2012) have issued position statements recommending that providers screen for elder abuse in clinical practice. In support of these recommendations, several brief assessment tools exist that are designed to be administered directly to an older adult him or herself. One such measure is the Hwalek–Sengstock Elder Abuse Screening Test (H–S/EAST; Neale et al., 1991), a 15-item measure that assesses aspects of abuse including physical abuse, exploitation, and neglect. Some of the questions on the H–S/EAST, however, are not specific to abusive behavior, such as often feeling sad and lonely, and clinicians using the H–S/EAST or any other screening measure, for that matter, must be sure to follow-up with more in-depth questioning if an older adult endorses a question that raises suspicion of probable abuse. Another screening measure designed to be administered directly to older adults is the Elder Abuse Suspicion Index (EASI; Yaffe et al., 2008). The EASI is a six-item measure that includes five items assessing for physical, emotional, and sexual abuse, financial exploitation, and neglect experienced during the 12 months prior to screening. The sixth item is intended to be completed directly by a clinician and prompts the clinician to document any visible signs of abuse, such as poor hygiene, bruises, or medication compliance issues.

Despite the clinical utility of brief screening measures like the H–S/EAST and the EASI, there are often significant barriers to directly screening older adults for elder abuse. Older adults with physical impairments, for example, may lack access to health-care providers or other individuals to whom they can potentially report the abuse, while older adults with cognitive impairments such as dementia may have memory impairments that limit their ability to recall abusive episodes. In response to such barriers, clinicians and health-care providers working with older adults may wish to obtain collateral information about possible abusive behaviors directly from an older adult's caregiver or other family members. While perhaps counterintuitive, several studies suggest that family and professional caregivers of older adults are often willing to report their own abusive behaviors when directly asked about such behaviors (Ben Natan, Matthews, & Lowenstein, 2010; Pillemer & Suitor, 1992). So, in addition to screening measures intended to be completed by older adults, researchers have also developed measures intended to be completed by caregivers that assess for potentially abusive caregiver behavior. The Caregiver Abuse Screen (CASE; Reis & Nahmiash, 1995), for example, is an eight-item measure for caregivers that assesses caregiver experiences such as "feeling that you are forced to be rough with" an older adult and "feeling you have to reject or ignore" an older adult. Although evidence suggests that abusers tend to score higher on the CASE than nonabusers, clearly not all abusive caregivers will be willing to disclose their own abusive behaviors, especially when such disclosure may have immediate, negative consequences, such as job loss or criminal prosecution (Acierno, 2003). Moreover, not all cognitively intact older adults may be willing to disclose their own victimization history. Thus, clinicians and health-care providers screening for elder abuse should consider several contextual factors beyond just older adult and caregiver self-reports of abuse.

One useful source of information to consider when assessing for possible elder abuse is the older adult's medical history. Elder abuse victims with dementia may have a history of multiple hospitalizations with irregular medical follow-up (Hansberry, Chen, & Gorbien, 2005) and may present to health-care settings with characteristic signs and injuries associated with specific types of abuse. For example, clinicians may notice malnutrition or dehydration in the case of neglected older adults (Dyer, Connolly, & McFeeley, 2003). Relatedly, physically abused older adults may present to emergency departments or acute care settings with injuries such as head injuries, bruises, and/or fractures (Clarke & Pierson, 1999; Jones et al., 1988) that can sometimes be distinguished from nonabusive injuries like fall-related injuries by location and injury type. That is, injuries sustained in the context of physical abuse that require medical treatment are more likely to be in the head and neck as a result of being choked or punched (Ziminski et al., 2013), while fall-related injuries are more likely to involve upper body injuries such as upper limb dislocation and breast contusions (Ziminski, Phillips, & Woods, 2012). So, considering an elder's medical history can be a useful adjunct to self and caregiver reports when screening for abuse.

Prevention and Intervention

Once a case of elder abuse is identified, there are several routes of intervention that can be considered. If the victim of elder abuse is determined to be vulnerable in the sense of having physical or cognitive impairments that limit their ability to protect themselves from further abuse, clinicians or other providers may need to report the abuse to Adult Protective Services in order to facilitate emergency intervention to keep the adult safe. However, state reporting laws should be consulted here, with respect to specific age and vulnerability parameters mandating report. For the most part, physicians, nurses, mental health professionals, professional caregivers, and others in the helping professions are typically subject to mandated reporting laws requiring them to report any suspected or confirmed case of elder abuse against a vulnerable adult. Laws on mandated reporting of abuse of demented, disabled, or obviously vulnerable older adults are akin to child abuse models where violence is perpetrated by an independent adult family member or caregiver against a dependent person, and, like Child Protective Services, Adult Protective Services may in serious cases of abuse remove an older adult victim of abuse from the custody of an abusive caregiver. By contrast, when both the victim and the perpetrator are independent, community-residing adults, a 69-year-old man and a 68-year-old woman, for example, intervention will in many ways depend on the wishes of the older adult victim, who may have legal rights to confidentiality. In other words, mandated reporting statutes for elder abuse are not consistent across all states, and one must be aware of state laws. An easy resolution to this issue is to place a call to Adult Protective Services, describe the situation without revealing any patient identifying information, and ask if you are a mandated reporter. In this sense, intervention with independent, community-residing adults is more akin to a domestic violence model, with the priorities of intervention often being to provide the older adult with information and referral about family violence and referrals for domestic violence shelters and counseling.

In line with the National Prevention Strategy, there is also an emerging interest in designing and evaluating programs geared toward the prevention of elder abuse—that is, preventing abusive acts against older adults before they happen or preventing further abuse in cases of repeat victimization. To this end, the IOM's Forum on Global Violence Prevention held a two-day public workshop on elder abuse and prevention (IOM and National Research Council (NRC), 2014) in April 2013. The goal of this workshop was to facilitate interdisciplinary dialogue on the causes of elder abuse and evidence-based prevention approaches, highlighting promising global prevention efforts. One approach to elder abuse prevention involves caregiver support interventions/respite care (see Pillemer et al., 2007) intended to reduce the stress of caregiving, a potentially important factor in elder abuse against dependent older adults. Caregiver stress appears, however, to be more related to the intensity of abuse once it occurs, rather than perpetration risk per se. In a preliminary evaluation of one such caregiver support intervention, Reay and Browne (2002) studied an education and anger management intervention program with 19 caregivers who either physically abused or neglected an elderly dependent. The education component of the program consisted of providing caregivers with information about local services, including adult day care services and caregiver support groups, as well as information about common caregiver stress reactions. Completing the program was associated with reductions in caregiver strain as well as caregiver depression and anxiety symptoms, with changes maintained at six-month follow-up.

Although caregiver interventions like the one just described show considerable promise in helping to address elder abuse, such interventions are limited in scope in that many caregivers will not receive these more structured types of programs. To increase the scope of prevention strategies, researchers and clinicians may be able to draw on prevention approaches used in related fields of interpersonal violence prevention, such as bystander-based interventions (see Banyard, 2011, for a discussion of bystander interventions applied in the context of sexual violence). Indeed, this makes sense when considering that social isolation and lack of social support is predictive of elder abuse, even after controlling for other risk factors (Acierno et al., 2010). The reason that bystander-based interventions may be especially appealing in the prevention of elder abuse is that such interventions move beyond a narrow focus on victim and perpetrator-specific behaviors previously conceptualized as microsystem-level variables and attempt to appeal to third party, mesosytem-level witnesses of potentially abusive events as allies in the effort to end elder abuse. In cases of elder abuse, potential third party witnesses might include individuals such as neighbors, local business people, health-care receptionists, public transportation personnel, and so on. In addition, education and motivation of noncaregiving family members, staff members at long-term care facilities, or even people like the older adult's banker who are distal parts of victims' microsystems may be able to detect situations, and once empowered, act where an older adult appears to be at risk of abuse.

In fact, the bystander intervention model has received recent attention from elder abuse researchers. Proposing a professional bystander intervention model for the detection of elder financial exploitation, Gilhooly et al. (2013) described five stages for bystander intervention that may be relevant for many types of elder abuse. These stages of intervention include: (a) noticing relevant cues suggestive of probable abuse, (b) construing the situation as abuse, (c) deciding the situation is a personal responsibility, (d) knowing how to deal with the situation, and (e) deciding to intervene. In practice, bystander-oriented programs can provide information and skills training relevant to each stage of intervention. For example, per stage a, bystander intervention programs for nursing home staff might teach staff members to recognize signs of physical abuse. Per stages d and e, the same program could help the staff members acquire skills necessary to intervene in high-risk situations where, say, an older adult resident appears to be at immanent risk of abuse or is actually being abused. As an illustration, such training could prepare staff members to safely intervene when a visibly upset patient with dementia is being yelled at by a fellow staff member. While no bystander intervention programs for elder abuse have been developed and evaluated to date, we encourage clinicians and researchers to consider this approach to prevention, as bystander intervention may play an important role in future efforts to prevent the mistreatment of elders.

Responding to Elder Abuse—Policy and Change

The issue of elder abuse has come to the attention of policy makers both nationally and internationally, with the result being increased public awareness and increased access to services for victims. In the United States, legislative efforts including the Older American Act and the Violence against Women Act (VAWA) have sought to expand funding for elder abuse services, education, and training (Dong & Simon, 2011). The Older American Act, for example, funds the National Center on Elder Abuse (http://www.ncea.aoa.gov/), a resource center that is part of the Department of Health and Human Services Administration on Aging that aims to provide information and resources on elder abuse to professionals and the general public and improve elder abuse research. In addition, the NCEA provides a listing of state reporting numbers for those needing to report a case of elder abuse or neglect. The Older American Act also establishes long-term care ombudsman programs intended to help provide advocates for residents in long-term care settings and help them resolve any reported issues related to elder mistreatment. Similarly, VAWA funds grants and services relevant to ending violence against women, including older women. In 2010, President Obama also signed into law the Elder Justice Act as part of the Affordable Care Act. Like the Older American Act and VAWA, the Elder Justice Act provides funds for state and local agencies to increase capacity to investigate and prosecute suspected cases of elder abuse as well as increase training for local ombudsmen programs to ensure timely and systematic response to cases of elder abuse (National Health Policy Forum, 2010).

Internationally, efforts to establish collaboration among leaders in the field of elder abuse and globally disseminate information regarding elder abuse prevention and practice have led to several major accomplishments. In 1997, representatives from several different countries established the International Network for the Prevention of Elder Abuse (INPEA), with the mission of promoting public awareness of elder abuse, promoting education and training of professionals working on behalf of elder abuse victims, and promoting advocacy and research on issues of elder abuse and neglect (Podnieks et al., 2010). To achieve this effort, INPEA has representatives from 32 countries worldwide and a representative to the United Nations (UN) and has launched several research activities with the World Health Organization and other organizations to better understand elder abuse in an international context. INPEA also worked to designate June 15 as World Elder Abuse Awareness Day, an event that is gaining popularity around the world as a means of increasing awareness about the prevalence and impact of elder abuse.

Discussion

The proportion of adults aged 60 and over is increasing rapidly across the world. With this increase in numbers comes increased relevance of the needs and issues confronting older adults, as well as associated needs and issues of their future caregivers. One area demanding immediate attention is elder abuse and mistreatment. Elder abuse can take the form of psychological, physical, sexual, neglectful, or financial mistreatment. Although older adults are the group least at risk of mistreatment by strangers, with probably the exception of financial mistreatment, the *past year* prevalence of elder abuse of community-residing older adults by known assailants is surprisingly high, at about 10 percent.

An Ecological Model to frame elder abuse helps to identify risk and protective factors and to direct screening and preventative measures toward those factors. For instance, the Ecological Model frames risk factors according to proximal spheres in a victim's life so that attention can be directed toward family and caretaker characteristics, community and provider characteristics, policies and legal frameworks, and ultimately the nation as a whole. To date, most focus has been on microsystem factors, or those factors in an individual's immediate environment, with one risk factor, social isolation and lack of social support, standing out among many others such as mental health needs of caretakers. Future work that also focuses on determining the health and mental health outcomes of elder mistreatment will help further prioritize intervention efforts; however, very little resources have been allocated to this area.

Given that research on elder abuse, particularly abuse of community-residing elders, is in its early stages, very little specific direction is available with respect to intervention. Nonetheless, screening and assessment, the first steps in any effort to intervene, are warranted. It is very likely that the most trusted professional group, health-care providers are in the best position to screen for elder abuse. Indeed, increased health services utilization associated with aging indicates that most victims will be in contact with providers at some point during their cycle of abuse. Several specific elder abuse measures were covered in this chapter. Not covered were techniques useful in persuading health-care providers to accept elder abuse screening as part of their clinical responsibility, as has been done for child abuse, and more recently domestic violence.

Hopefully, this chapter will bring increased awareness of the extent of the problem of elder abuse. Recent policy efforts at the national level certainly highlight increased public awareness of this problem and suggest that, in the coming years, there will be greater support for developing and disseminating evidence-based screening and intervention strategies for elder abuse. Even so, additional knowledge of the parameters of abuse, its effects on the elderly, and effective components necessary for intervention are badly needed in order to fully address this preventable problem of aging.

References

Acierno, R. (2003). Elder mistreatment: Epidemiological assessment methodology. In R.J. Bonnie & R.B. Wallace (Eds.), *Elder mistreatment: Abuse, neglect, and exploitation in an aging America* (pp. 261–302). Washington, DC: National Academies Press.

Acierno, R., Hernandez, M.A., Amstadter, A.B., Resnick, H.S., Steve, K., Muzzy, W., & Kilpatrick, D.G. (2010). Prevalence and correlates of emotional, physical, sexual, and financial abuse and potential neglect in the United States: The National Elder Mistreatment Study. *American Journal of Public Health, 100*, 292–297.

Acierno, R., Hernandez-Tejada, M.A., Muzzy, W., Steve, K. (2009). *National Elder Mistreatment Study* (final report to NIJ for grant 2007-WG-BX-0009). Retrieved from https://www.ncjrs.gov/pdffiles1/nij/grants/226456.pdf

American Medical Association. (1992). *AMA Council on scientific affairs: Diagnostic and treatment guidelines on elder abuse and neglect*. Chicago, IL: Author.

Amstadter, A.B., Begle, A.M., Cisler, J.M., Hernandez, M.A., Muzzy, W., & Acierno, R. (2010). Prevalence and correlates of poor self-rated health in the United States: The National Elder Mistreatment Study. *American Journal of Geriatric Psychiatry, 18*, 615–623.

Bachman, R. (1994). *Violence against women: A national crime victimization survey report*. (DOJ Publication No. NCJ 145325). Washington, DC: U.S. Government Printing Office.

Banyard, V.L. (2011). Who will help prevent sexual violence: Creating an ecological model of bystander intervention. *Psychology of Violence, 1*, 216–229.

Ben Natan, M., Matthews, P., & Lowenstein, A. (2010). Study of factors that affect abuse of older people in nursing homes. *Nursing Management, 17*(8), 20–24.

Biggs, S., Manthorpe, J., Tinker, A., Doyle, M., & Erens, B. (2009). Mistreatment of older people in the United Kingdom: Findings from the first national prevalence study. *Journal of Elder Abuse & Neglect, 21*, 1–14.

Bonnie, R.J., & Wallace, R.B. (Eds.). (2003). *Elder mistreatment: Abuse, neglect, and exploitation in an aging America*. Washington, DC: National Academies Press.

Bronfenbrenner, U. (1997). Ecology of the family as a context for human development: Research perspectives. *Developmental Psychology, 22*, 723–742.

Burston, G.R. (1975). Granny-battering. *British Medical Journal, 3*(5983), 592.

Clarke, M.E., & Pierson, W. (1999). Management of elder abuse in the emergency department. *Emergency Medicine Clinics of North America, 17*, 631–644.

Cisler, J.M., Begle, A.M., Amstadter, A.B., & Acierno, R. (2012). Mistreatment and self-reported emotional symptoms: Results from the National Elder Mistreatment Study. *Journal of Elder Abuse & Neglect, 24*, 216–230.

Dong, X. (2005). Medical implications of elder abuse and neglect. *Clinics in Geriatric Medicine, 21*, 293–313.

Dong, X.Q., Beck, T., & Simon, M. (2010). The associations of gender, depression, and elder mistreatment in a community-dwelling Chinese population: The modifying effect of social support. *Archives of Gerontology and Geriatrics, 50*, 202–208.

Dong, X., & Simon, M.A. (2011). Enhancing national policy and programs to address elder abuse. *JAMA, 305*, 2460–2461.

Dong, X.Q., Simon, M., Beck, T.T., Farran, C., McCann, J.J., Mendes de Leon, C., . . . Evans, D.A. (2011). Elder abuse and mortality: The role of psychological and social wellbeing. *Gerontology, 57*, 549–558.

Dong, X.Q., Simon, M., Mendes de Leon, C., Fulmer, T., Beck, T., Hebert, L., . . . Evans, D. (2009). Elder self-neglect and abuse and mortality risk in a community-dwelling population. *Journal of the American Medical Association, 302*(5), 517–526.

Dyer, C. B., Connolly, M. T., & McFeeley, P. (2003). The clinical and medical forensics of elder abuse and neglect. In R. J. Bonnie & R. B. Wallace (Eds.), *Elder mistreatment: Abuse, neglect, and exploitation in an aging America* (pp. 339–381). Washington, DC: National Academies Press.

Dyer, C. B., Pavlik, V. N., Murphy, K. P., & Hyman, D. J. (2000). The high prevalence of depression and dementia in elder abuse or neglect. *Journal of the American Geriatrics Society, 48*, 205–208.

Gilhooly, M. L. M., Cairns, D., Davies, M., Harries, P., Gilhooly, K. J., & Notley, E. (2013). Framing the detection of financial elder abuse as bystander intervention: Decision cues, pathways to detection and barriers to action. *Journal of Adult Protection, 15*, 54–68.

Gorbien, M. J., & Eisenstein, A. R. (2005). Elder abuse and neglect: An overview. *Clinics in Geriatric Medicine, 21*, 279–292.

Hansberry, M. R., Chen, E., & Gorbien, M. J. (2005). Dementia and elder abuse. *Clinics in Geriatric Medicine, 21*, 315–332.

Hanson, R. F., Kilpatrick, D. G., Falsetti, S. A., & Resnick, H. S. (1995). Violent crime and mental health. In J. R. Freedy & S. E. Hobfoll (Eds.), *Traumatic stress: From theory to practice* (pp. 129–161). New York: Plenum Press.

Institute of Medicine (IOM) and National Research Council (NRC). (2014). *Elder abuse and its prevention: Workshop summary*. Washington, DC: The National Academies Press.

Jones, J., Dougherty, J., Schelble, D., & Cunningham, W. (1988). Emergency department protocol for the diagnosis and evaluation of geriatric abuse. *Annals of Emergency Medicine, 17*, 1006–1015.

Krug, E., Mercy, J., Dahlberg, L., & Zwi, A. (2002). The world report on violence and health. *The Lancet, 360*, 1083–1088.

Laumann, E. O., Leitsch, S. A., & Waite, L. J. (2008). Elder mistreatment in the United States: Prevalence estimates from a nationally representative study. *The Journals of Gerontology, Series B: Psychological Sciences and Social Sciences, 63*, S248–S254.

Mouton, C. P., Rodabough, R. J., Rovi, S. L., Hunt, J. L, Talamantes, M. A., Brzyski, R. G., & Burge, S. K. (2004). Prevalence and 3-year incidence of abuse among postmenopausal women. *American Journal of Public Health, 94*(4), 605–612.

National Committee for the Prevention of Elder Abuse, Virginia Tech, MetLife Mature Market Institute. (2011). *The MetLife study of elder financial abuse: Crimes of occasion, desperation and predation against America's elders*. Westport, CT: Authors.

National Health Policy Forum. (2010). The Elder Justice Act: Addressing elder abuse, neglect, and exploitation. Retrieved from https://www.nhpf.org/uploads/announcements/Basics_ElderJustice_11-30-10.pdf

Neale, A. V., Hwalek, M. A., Scott, R. O., Sengstock, M. C., & Stahl, C. (1991). Validation of the Hwalek–Sengstock Elder Abuse Screening Test. *Journal of Applied Gerontology, 10*, 417–429.

Norris, F. H. (1992). Epidemiology of trauma: Frequency and impact of different potentially traumatic events on different demographic groups. *Journal of Clinical and Consulting Psychology, 60*, 409–418.

Pillemer, K., & Finkelhor, D. (1988). The prevalence of elder abuse: A random sample survey. *Gerontologist, 28*, 51–57.

Pillemer, K.A., Mueller-Johnson, K.U., Mock, S.E., Suitor, J.J., & Lachs, M.S. (2007). Interventions to prevent elder mistreatment. In L.S. Doll, S.E. Bonzo, D.A. Sleet, & J.A. Mercy (Eds.), *Handbook of injury and violence prevention* (pp. 241–254). New York: Springer.

Pillemer, K.A., & Suitor, J.J. (1992). Violence and violent feelings: What causes them among family caregivers? *Journal of Gerontology, 47*, S165–S172.

Podnieks, E., Penhale, B., Goergen, T., Biggs, S., & Han, D. (2010). Elder mistreatment: An international narrative. *Journal of Elder Abuse & Neglect, 22*, 131–163.

Reay, A.M., & Browne, K.D. (2002). The effectiveness of psychological interventions with individuals who physically abuse or neglect their elderly dependents. *Journal of Interpersonal Violence, 17*, 416–431.

Reis, M., & Nahmiash, D. (1995). Validation of the caregiver abuse screen (CASE). *Canadian Journal on Aging, 14*, 45–60.

Schulman, E.A., & Hohler, A.D. (2012). The American Academy of Neurology position statement on abuse and violence. *Neurology, 78*, 433–435.

Tatara, T. (1997). *The National Elder Abuse Incidence Study: Executive summary*. New York, NY: Human Services Press.

U.S. Department of Health and Human Services, National Institutes of Health, National Institute on Aging. (2011a). *Global health and aging* (NIH Publication No. 11-7737). Retrieved from http://www.who.int/ageing/publications/global_health.pdf

U.S. Department of Health and Human Services, Office of the Surgeon General, National Prevention Council. (2011b). *National Prevention Strategy*. Washington, DC: Author.

Wiglesworth, A., Mosqueda, L., Mulnard, R., Liao, S., Gibbs, L., & Fitzgerald, W. (2010). Screening for abuse and neglect of people with dementia. *Journal of the American Geriatrics Society, 58*, 493–500.

Wolf, R.S. (2000). The nature and scope of elder abuse: Changes in perspective and response over the past 25 years. *Generations, 24*, 6–12.

Yaffe, M.J., Wolfson, C., Lithwick, M., & Weiss, D. (2008). Development and validation of a tool to improve physician identification of elder abuse: The Elder Abuse Suspicion Index (EASI). *Journal of Elder Abuse & Neglect, 20*, 276–300.

Ziminski, C.E., Phillips, L.R., & Woods, D.L. (2012). Raising the index of suspicion for elder abuse: Cognitive impairment, falls, and injury patterns in the emergency department. *Geriatric Nursing, 33*, 105–112.

Ziminski, C.E., Wiglesworth, A., Austin, R., Phillips, L.R., & Mosqueda, L. (2013). Injury patterns and causal mechanisms of bruising in physical elder abuse. *Journal of Forensic Nursing, 9*, 84–91.

CHAPTER NINE

Nursing Homes and the Continuum of Care

Stephanie W. Burge

Like most of the industrialized world, the United States is undergoing an unprecedented demographic shift characterized by considerable population aging. Nearly 43.1 million Americans, approximately 14.1 percent of the population, exceed the age of 65, and American population aging will continue to accelerate in the 21st century, as baby boomers are now reaching ages that have historically been defined as elderly. In addition to general improvements in life expectancy—currently 81 for women and 76 for men (National Center for Health Statistics, 2014)—strides in medical diagnoses, treatment, and technology have significantly increased life expectancy for Americans already in their elder years. For example, women who reach the age of 65 can now expect to live an additional 20 years and men who reach commensurate ages have life expectancies of almost 18 more years (National Center for Health Statistics, 2014). While life expectancy has increased considerably, these years are also characterized by chronic conditions such as diabetes, chronic obstructive pulmonary disease (COPD), and arthritis, as well as increased risk of dementia and/or Alzheimer's disease and other functional impairments (Hung et al., 2011). As a result, the delivery and provision of long-term care—as well as its cost, quality, and fit with elders' needs—is centrally important to policy makers and scholars alike.

Discussions about delivery of long-term care tend to focus on residential long-term care, such as assisted living and nursing homes. Out of the nearly 6.3 million American elders needing long-term care, approximately 1.3 million reside in nursing homes (Harris-Kojetin et al., 2013). Long-term residential care offers a minority of long-term care services to the elderly population—nearly 80 percent of long-term care is unpaid, informal provision of care by family members (Congressional Budget Office, 2013; Levine et al., 2010). However, nursing homes have been a focal point for political discussion as well as scholarly interest for several reasons. First, costs associated with nursing home care are far higher than other types of long-term care service arrangements, especially when compared to home and community-based services (Kaye, Harrington, & LaPlante, 2010). For example, per-person costs associated with nursing home care expenditures are approximately five times as high when compared to elders residing in the community who receive home and community-based services, and differences in level of need for assistance account for only a small part of the difference in costs between institutional and noninstitutional care (Kaye, Harrington, & LaPlante, 2010). Collectively, nursing home-related expenditures totaled almost $156 billion in 2013, roughly 5 percent of all health-care spending in the United States for the year (Medicare Payment Advisory Commission, 2015). Second, in spite of the high costs of nursing home care, persistent questions about quality of care and culture continue to nag this venue of long-term care. Debates about nursing home quality and culture have ranged from how to best provide appropriate medical care in a less institutional, more home-like environment, to whether improvements in nursing home culture have measurable effects on resident outcomes (Shier et al., 2014; Zimmerman, Shier, & Saliba, 2014). Third, while nursing homes have historically housed elderly residents, contemporary portraits of nursing home residents represent a particularly vulnerable, frail, and impaired resident population (U.S. Department of Health and Human Services, Centers for Medicare and Medicaid Services, 2013), which makes quality of care an even more pertinent issue.

In this chapter, I review recent literature pertaining to the continuum of care offered in nursing homes and the resident populations they serve. First, I consider trends in nursing home utilization. Second, I briefly discuss literature that reviews predictors of nursing home placement. Next, I examine how nursing home residents fare with respect to functional health and cognitive status. To provide a frame of reference, I compare residents of nursing homes to elderly who live in residential care facilities, an often healthier and wealthier population. Then, I discuss the racial/ethnic composition of nursing home residents, with specific focus on barriers to nursing home access for minority elders. To better understand challenges in delivery of nursing home care, I conclude by reviewing literature on the history, purpose, and meaning of the culture change movement in nursing homes, as well as recent evidence on its efficacy with respect to improving resident outcomes.

Trends in Nursing Home Admission and Utilization

By nearly any measured outcome, both nursing home utilization rates and capacity have decreased considerably in the past two decades. First, in spite of increases in both the percentage of elderly and the absolute number of elderly in the United States, the actual number of nursing homes has declined considerably (Wiener, Anderson, & Brown, 2009). For example, in 1995, there were approximately 16,700 nursing homes operating in the United States (Strahan, 1997). By 2012, that number had shrunk by more than 1,000, with only 15,652 licensed and operating nursing homes (U.S. Department of Health and Human Services, Centers for Medicare and Medicaid Services, 2013). Between 1999 and 2008 approximately 16 percent of Medicaid and Medicare certified nursing homes closed (Feng et al., 2011), the majority of which were concentrated in communities with predominantly poor and minority populations. Another indicator of nursing home capacity, number of nursing home beds, tells a similar story (Strahan, 1997). In 1995, the nation's nursing homes housed approximately 1.8 million beds; however, by 2012, there were approximately 1.7 million nursing home beds (U.S. Department of Health and Human Services, Centers for Medicare and Medicaid Services, 2013). After standardizing the number of beds by population over the age of 65, which takes into account our increasing aging population, declines in nursing home capacity appear more stark. There were approximately 53 nursing home beds per 1,000 people over the age of 65 in 1995, but by 2012, that figure had declined to nearly 39 beds per 1,000. Even as capacity has declined, occupancy rates have also fallen in the same period, from approximately 87 percent in 1995 to 83 percent in 2012 (Strahan, 1997; U.S. Department of Health and Human Services, Centers for Medicare and Medicaid Services, 2013).

Another trend in nursing home utilization is the growing tendency for nursing homes to offer more medicalized nursing services. In particular, nursing homes are increasingly offering short-term stays to Medicare beneficiaries who need intense medical assistance for a brief period. The overwhelming majority of nursing homes are dually licensed as both nursing homes as well as skilled nursing facilities (Medicare Payment Advisory Commission, 2015). With a license to perform skilled nursing, nursing homes are eligible to admit short-term residents who have been recently discharged from a hospital, but who still need intensive medical services and care, as in the case of rehabilitation from an operation such as hip replacement. Under Medicare Part A, individuals who had a three day, medically required hospital stay and who are ready for discharge, but unable to return home, are eligible for up to 100 days of skilled nursing care. Approximately one in five of eligible Medicare beneficiaries seek short-term stays in skilled nursing facilities and nursing homes following discharge from the hospital (Carter, Garrett, & Wissoker, 2015).

Short-term skilled nursing residents represent a small, but growing portion of the nursing home population, accounting for 12 percent of all nursing home days in free-standing skilled nursing facilities in 2013 (Medicare Payment Advisory Commission, 2015). Undoubtedly, some of the growth in the short-term nursing home population reflects the higher reimbursement rate that Medicare pays for rehabilitative care, as compared to the reimbursement Medicaid offers for long-term nursing home residents, perhaps because short-term residents more frequently require additional services such as physical therapy (Medicare Payment Advisory Commission, 2015).

Although these short-term residents may not reside permanently in nursing homes, they still represent a more frail population than the larger pool of Medicare beneficiaries and thus are more comparable in health to the general long-term nursing home population than they are to community-dwelling elderly. For example, Medicare beneficiaries who are discharged from the hospital to skilled nursing facilities are over three times more likely to be over the age of 85, over twice as likely to report poor health, and over twice as likely to report at least some limitation in physical function with respect to activities of daily living (ADLs), as compared to the broader pool of Medicare beneficiaries (Medicare Payment Advisory Commission, 2015). Furthermore, as Mor et al. (2010) note, there is some cycling between short-term nursing home stays and hospitalization, which also suggests a fair amount of frailty in the population that temporarily resides in a nursing home following hospital discharge.

Undoubtedly, part of the decline in nursing home utilization has stemmed from increasing alternatives to nursing home care for elders who are less frail and exhibit greater physical function. In an endeavor to make long-term care both more affordable as well as to provide a better array of residential options to elders as they age, policy makers and scholars have emphasized the need to move away from institutionalized long-term care settings such as nursing homes and offer greater home and community-based services via Medicaid and Medicare (Wiener, Anderson, & Brown, 2009). Efforts to make other long-term care alternatives more feasible for elders capable of using such services are reflected in the changing patterns of allocated resources. For example, in 1995, only 19 percent of Medicaid long-term care spending focused on home and community-based services

(Feng et al., 2011). However, by 2008, approximately 42 percent of such spending was allocated to these services (Feng et al., 2011), and it is likely that with provisions outlined in the Affordable Care Act of 2010 this trend will continue (Shugarman, 2010).

Despite increased spending dedicated toward home and community-based services, historically, there has been a strong bias toward provision of long-term care in nursing homes rather than supplementing home care with other services, as reflected by the majority of nursing home residents who receive Medicaid benefits to cover at least part of costs associated with their care (Kaye, Harrington, & LaPlante, 2010; U.S. Department of Health and Human Services, Centers for Medicare and Medicaid Services, 2013). In large part, the bias toward institutional—rather than home-based—care has stemmed from state-to-state variation in Medicaid provision and benefits. Although Medicaid is a federal program, the administration of Medicaid to citizens is state governed. Consequently, there is significant difference in what Medicaid covers with respect to home and community-based services for long-term care from state to state. By contrast, provision of nursing home access to frail elders is a federally mandated function of Medicaid (Kaiser Commission on Medicaid and the Uninsured, 2013). Even though nursing home access is an entitlement under the Medicaid program, a large body of literature documents that nursing home quality varies according to the proportion of Medicaid residents, largely due to the fact that Medicaid reimbursement tends to be lower than fees paid by privately paying residents (Harrington, Swan, & Carrillo, 2007; Kelly, Liebig, & Edwards, 2008; Mor et al., 2011; Smith et al., 2007). In particular, the bias toward institutional care, as well as socioeconomic variation in nursing home access and quality, is likely to reinforce inequality in access to workable long-term care options. It seems likely that elders who have limited socioeconomic resources may be relegated to nursing home care rather than being able to bring in home and community-based support that might enable one to remain within the community, even as care needs increase. Moreover, needy elders may have fewer and poorer options when it comes to quality nursing home care, due to Medicaid's lower rate of reimbursement than other forms of payment such as private pay and long-term care insurance.

Growth of Residential Care Facilities

Concurrent with trends toward increasing availability of home and community-based services, there has been growth in the desirability, offerings, and capacity of residential care facilities, which are often called assisted living. These facilities offer what might be best viewed as an intermediary type of long-term care between home and community-based services and nursing homes. Residential care facilities generally offer a residential care setting as opposed to an institutionalized, medical environment, and provide minimal services including meals, supportive services, and 24-hour on-site supervision. Under the umbrella of assisted living, facilities may have state-granted specialty licenses that allow additional levels of care to populations with greater health and/or mental health needs, potentially allowing frail elders to age in place at a residential care facility for a longer period of time (Street, Burge, & Quadagno, 2009). However, these facilities generally have far fewer licensed nurses on staff than nursing homes, reflecting their less medical, more supervisory form of care. For example, in 2012, a full one-third of nursing home staff was licensed or registered nurses, as compared to fewer than 18 percent of staff in residential care facilities (Harris-Kojetin et al., 2013). Thus, it is possible that residential care facilities may have limited capacity to properly assist elders as their care needs intensify. In spite of the more limited medical offerings, for many elders, residing in assisted living is preferable to a nursing home (Ball et al., 2000; Street & Quadagno, 2004).

Although estimating growth in this type of long-term care facility has been difficult due to issues of varying definition and measurement (Mollica, Sims-Kastelein, & O'Keefe, 2008; Stevenson & Grabowski, 2010), evidence suggests that there was substantial growth in residential care facilities during the 1990s and early 2000s (Mollica, Johnson-Larmarche, & O'Keefe, 2005) although growth has flattened since the mid-2000s (Park-Lee et al., 2011). Using data from the 2012 National Survey of Long-Term Care Providers, a recent report from the National Center for Health Statistics estimates that there were nearly 22,200 residential care facilities in 2012, which represented approximately 1.4 times the number of licensed nursing homes at the time (Harris-Kojetin et al., 2013). Collectively, these facilities had capacity to serve nearly 851,400 residents, which is approximately half of the capacity that nursing homes offered in the same year (Harris-Kojetin et al., 2013). Consequently, capacity in a typical residential care facility is significantly smaller than the average nursing home; on average, a residential care facility can serve approximately 38 residents as compared to the 106 residents that may be served by the average nursing home (Harris-Kojetin et al., 2013).

Predictors of Nursing Home Admission

Given the diversity in long-term care arrangements, ranging from more institutional settings such as nursing homes to more intermediate arrangements such as residential care facilities and use of home and community-based services, there has been growing interest in factors that are associated with nursing home placement. Gerontologists have investigated myriad factors associated with nursing home institutionalization, some of which focus on physical and mental health status, medical intervention such as drugs designed to slow dementia progression, and family resources such as the availability of caregivers, economic resources, and sociodemographic characteristics.

Individuals who reside within nursing homes do so because their health requires care beyond what is available in a typical home environment within the community. Consequently, it is not surprising that physical limitations are associated with nursing home placement, and a variety of studies have linked increased physical impairment with nursing home admission among elders (Andel, Hyer, & Slack, 2007; Banaszak-Holl et al., 2004; Bharucha et al., 2004). Even limitation in instrumental ADL such as managing of finances, grocery shopping, and managing medications, which tends to precede inability to perform ADL, is also associated with enhanced odds of nursing home placement among elders who do not face cognitive impairment (Andel, Hyer, & Slack, 2007). However, it is worth noting that not all impairments are necessarily associated with nursing home admission. For example, recent meta-analyses investigating associations between physical health and nursing home placement have shown the relationship between incontinence and nursing home admission to be inconsistent (Luppa et al., 2010; Gaugler et al., 2009). Furthermore, low levels of physical impairment do not necessarily lead to nursing home placement, particularly since both residents and families tend to view nursing homes as the least preferred alternative in a spectrum of long-term care options (Ball et al., 2000). In a recent meta-analysis of predictors of nursing home placement, Gaugler et al. (2007) found that low levels of physical impairment—requiring assistance with one activity of daily living—were associated with only a slight increase in the odds of nursing home institutionalization among elders. However, elders who have more substantial physical impairment—requiring assistance with three or more ADLs—were over three times more likely to be placed in a nursing home than their less impaired counterparts.

While studies consistently demonstrate an association between decreased physical function and nursing home placement, cognitive impairment and/or onset of dementia are among the strongest predictors of nursing home placement. In fact, a recent meta-analysis of studies investigating nursing home institutionalization found that a dementia diagnosis, which tends to be linked to decreased ability to perform both instrumental and daily activities of living, was the most important predictor of nursing home placement (Luppa et al., 2010). In addition, greater levels of cognitive impairment—rather than the simple presence or absence of a dementia diagnosis—further increase the odds of nursing home placement among the elderly (Luppa et al., 2010). This relationship may intensify in part because of concomitant behaviors such as aggression and hallucinations, as well as accompanying physical function declines, which grow more prevalent in the later stages of dementia (Gaugler, Fang, Krichbaum & Wyman, 2009; Wattmo et al., 2011). Furthermore, increases in such behaviors and caregiving burden can leave family caregivers ill-equipped to manage such behaviors, which may in turn increase likelihood of nursing home placement (Gaugler et al., 2011). Other studies have linked mental health conditions such as depression (Harris, 2007) and mental illness such as schizophrenia with enhanced risk of nursing home placement, even after controlling for factors such as age, physical health and function, and socioeconomic status. Moreover, there is some evidence that nursing homes increasingly serve populations who are jointly diagnosed with dementia and mental health issues such as depression (Fullerton et al., 2009), which underscores these two conditions as risk factors that independently increase risk of nursing home admission.

While physical frailty, cognitive impairment, and mental health conditions are all significant predictors of nursing home placement among the elderly, each of these are associated with an individual's health status. However, what about social resources that may mitigate the need for nursing home care? Some studies have investigated living arrangements of frail elders and availability of familial care as factors that may delay onset of nursing admission. Past research has generally shown that living alone increases the risk that frail elders will be institutionalized (Gaugler et al., 2007; Wattmo et al., 2011), although part of this effect may be due to the fact that individuals living alone are not likely to be married and thus lack a spouse to be a caregiver. Family caregivers tend to promote longer times to nursing home entry among frail elders who have cognitive and physical limitations. For example, several studies have shown that being married delays entry into nursing home, although there has been some variation in the size of the effect depending on the data source considered (Freedman, 1996; Freedman et al., 1994; Gaugler et al., 2007; Miller & Weissert, 2000). In particular, some studies demonstrate that caregiving benefits conferred by spouses may be gendered, with men receiving greater benefit than women in terms of delayed transition to nursing home care (Noel-Miller, 2010; Stoller et al., 2008). Adult children, who may serve as caregivers, may also buffer the elderly from nursing home admission in the context of declining health (Bianchi et al., 2008; Choi et al., 2014; Wolff & Kasper, 2006). Furthermore, some evidence suggests that children may prove an even more valuable resource to women than men, who are more able to rely upon their wives for care as health may fail (Noel-Miller, 2010; Bianchi et al., 2008; Katz, Kabeto, & Langa, 2000). Of course, family caregiving is a resource that may be expended over time, as caregiver burnout may ensue, which may hasten the use of institutional care such as nursing homes for family members (Spilman & Long, 2009). Particularly in the case of adult children who are serving as caregivers, resources such as adult day care may lessen family caregiver burden and lower caregiver stress, which may delay nursing home placement for elderly parents (Cho, Zarit, & Chiriboga, 2009).

Nursing Home Resident Populations: Physical Function and Cognitive Impairment

In addition to declining utilization of nursing homes as a form of long-term care, nursing homes are increasingly a long-term care measure of last resort, as reflected by much higher rates of nursing home institutionalization among the oldest elder age groups as compared to younger elderly individuals. For example, in 2012, nearly 3 percent of the overall elderly population resided in nursing homes, but approximately 10 percent of those aged 85 and older lived in a nursing home (U.S. Department of Health and Human Services, Centers for Medicare and Medicaid Services, 2013). Interestingly, when comparing the age composition of long-term care facilities, residential care facilities such as assisted living serve significantly older populations than do nursing homes. Over half of residents in residential care facilities are over the age of 85 and almost one-third are between the ages of 75 and 84, as compared to 42 percent and 28 percent of nursing home residents, respectively (Harris-Kojetin et al., 2013). However, the age composition of residents tells only one side of the story, as nursing home resident populations experience significantly more frailty and functional limitations than residents in any other long-term care arrangement, including other residential care facilities such as assisted living (Harris-Kojetin et al., 2013).

Scholars and policy makers trying to understand resident profiles of physical function and frailty use a variety of measures including the extent to which residents need assistance performing ADLs such as eating, dressing, bathing, toileting, and transferring. Underscoring the relative frailty of nursing home residents relative to other long-term care populations, nearly two-thirds of nursing home residents required at least some assistance with three or more ADLs (U.S. Department of Health and Human Services, Centers for Medicare and Medicaid Services, 2013), as compared to just under 40 percent of residents who required similar levels of assistance in residential care facilities (Caffrey et al., 2012). There is also a positive relationship between ADL impairment and age in the nursing home population, with nursing home residents being successively more likely to suffer ADL impairment at each of the following age groups: young-old (65–74), middle-old (75–84), and oldest-old (85 or older) (U.S. Department of Health and Human Services, Centers for Medicare and Medicaid Services, 2013). For the more difficult physical tasks related to ADLs such as bathing or dressing, receiving some form of assistance is nearly ubiquitous among nursing home residents, as over 95 percent needed at least some assistance with bathing, while 9 out of 10 residents required at least some help with dressing in 2012 (CDC/NCHS, National Study of Long-Term Care Providers and Table 4 in Appendix B). By contrast, slightly less than three-quarters of residential care facility residents required assistance with bathing, and only about half required dressing assistance (Caffrey et al., 2012). Even for ADLs that are less physically intensive such as eating, nursing home residents are over three times more likely to need assistance compared to residential care facility residents, 56 percent vs. 18 percent, respectively (Harris-Kojetin et al., 2013). Measures related to other functional limitations such as incontinence also reveal that nursing homes currently serve a much more frail population than residential care facilities. Approximately 58 percent of nursing home residents experience either urinary or bowel incontinence, as compared to 39 percent of individuals who live in residential care facilities (Gorina et al., 2014).

Indicators related to cognitive impairment such as diagnoses of Alzheimer's disease and/or dementia, as well as diagnoses of depression also give insight into the extent to which nursing home residents differ from other types of long-term care residents in their need for care related to cognitive and mental health. Data from the National Study of Long-term Care Providers suggests that just less than 40 percent of individuals in residential care facilities have been diagnosed with Alzheimer's and/or related dementia, as compared to almost half of nursing home residents (Harris-Kojetin et al., 2013). When definitions of cognitive impairment are more inclusive and not restricted to formal diagnoses, some studies suggest that nearly two-thirds of nursing home residents experience at least some level of cognitive impairment (U.S. Department of Health and Human Services, Centers for Medicare and Medicaid Services, 2013). Although most data suggest that rates of elder cognitive impairment is greater in nursing homes than residential care facilities, one recent study suggests that assisted living may have a proportion of elders with cognitive impairment more similar to that of nursing homes (Zimmerman, Sloane, & Reed, 2014). In addition to high rates of cognitive impairment among nursing homes, a large proportion of nursing home residents have additional mental health diagnoses. For example, rates of diagnosed depression among nursing home residents are nearly twice that of residents in residential care facilities, 49 percent and 25 percent, respectively (Harris-Kojetin et al., 2013). Besides depression, other studies point to small, but significant proportions of nursing home residents who exhibit other mental illnesses including bipolar disorder and schizophrenia (Grabowski et al., 2009).

Nursing Home Populations: Racial/Ethnic Disparities in Access

Scholars investigating racial/ethnic inequality in access to nursing home care could use three different comparisons to investigate elder nursing home access by race/ethnic background. The first of these would be to compare relative proportions of racial/ethnic groups in nursing homes to the racial/ethnic composition of the broader population of elders. However, such a comparison assumes general equilibrium in physical and cognitive health impairments, an assumption which is questionable given other racial/ethnic disparities in access to health care (Nelson, Smedley, & Stith, 2009). A second comparison would be to compare racial/ethnic representation in nursing homes to the broader population of individuals needing long-term care, since evidence suggests that minority elders may have higher rates of illness, as well as physical and cognitive impairments that precipitate entry to long-term care (Ayse et al., 2012; Cooper et al., 2010; Haas, Krueger, & Rohlfsen, 2012; Warner & Brown, 2011). In fact, a recent study using data from the Health and Retirement Study showed that African American and Latino elderly have 1.5 times the level of ADL impairment and over 1.2 times the level of cognitive impairment compared to non-Hispanic white elders, which likely underscores their greater need for long-term care (Thomeer, Mudrazija, & Angel, 2015). A third comparison would be to compare racial/ethnic variation in nursing home access to other forms of long-term care, such as residential care facilities, which many elders view as preferable to nursing home care. In general, minority elders have fewer economic resources upon which to draw (DeNavas-Walt, Proctor, & Smith, 2009), a factor that may necessitate nursing home entry relative to other forms of long-term care that are less likely to be paid for via Medicaid.

Generally speaking, past literature on racial/ethnic variation in access to nursing homes has shown that minority elders experience lower levels of access (Akamigbo & Wolinsky, 2007; Angel et al., 2004; Smith et al., 2007) although some studies suggest this inequality may be eroding (Ness, Ahmed, & Aronow, 2004; Smith et al., 2008). In particular, the downward trend in nursing home utilization of the past few decades has been more characteristic of non-Hispanic white elders' use of nursing homes than it has been the case for minority elders. For example, a recent study by Feng et al. (2011), which used the National Minimum Data Set of nursing home admissions to investigate changes in the racial/ethnic composition of nursing home residents between 1999 and 2008, shows that nursing home admission decreased significantly for non-Hispanic white elders, but increased among Asian, Latino, and black elders, with rates of increase in admission ranging from approximately 54 percent for Asian and Latino elders to nearly 11 percent for black elders. Recent increases in the proportion of minority elderly residents in nursing homes do not necessarily suggest racial/ethnic equality in nursing home access, however. To further examine this issue, I draw upon data from the racial/ethnic composition of the overall elderly population, the resident population in nursing homes, and the resident population in residential care facilities.

In 2011, the racial/ethnic composition of the general elderly population was comprised of 79 percent of non-Hispanic white elders, 9 percent non-Hispanic black elders, 7 percent Hispanic elders, and 4 percent Asian elders (Administration on Aging, 2012). Initial comparisons to the nursing home population do not look that dissimilar from the general elderly population in terms of race/ethnic composition, with what appears to be slightly higher proportions of African American elders and slight underrepresentation of Hispanic elders in nursing homes than the general elder population. For example, in the same year, almost 79 percent of nursing home residents were non-Hispanic white, nearly 14 percent were black, approximately 5 percent were Hispanic, and nearly 2 percent were Asian (U.S. Department of Health and Human Services, Centers for Medicare and Medicaid Services, 2013). However, comparisons that account for disproportionate need for long-term care among elderly minority populations tell a different story. Using data from the Health and Retirement Study, a recent study finds that black elders and Hispanic elders have lower nursing home usage and these racial/ethnic disparities remain even after controlling for covariates such as ADL, IADL, and cognitive impairment, as well as disability, socioeconomic status, and family relationships (Thomeer, Mudrazija, & Angel, 2014). In fact, Thomeer et al. (2015) note that estimates of racial/ethnic variation in nursing home populations which fail to take into account levels of physical and cognitive impairment likely underestimate the level of racial/ethnic disparity in nursing home access.

Examining racial/ethnic diversity in residential care facilities is also suggestive of poorer access to workable, affordable, and quality long-term care arrangement for minority elders. Residential care facilities are generally viewed as preferable to nursing homes by elders, but tend to be paid for with private economic resources while nursing homes are far more likely to be paid for by Medicaid. Only one in five residential care facility residents use Medicaid for costs of services, as compared to nearly two-thirds of nursing home residents (Reeves & Musumeci, 2014; Kaye,

Harrington, & LaPlante, 2010). The resident population of residential care facilities is even more skewed toward overrepresentation of non-Hispanic white elders and underrepresentation of black elders and Latino elders. For example, over 87 percent of residential care facility residents are non-Hispanic white, as compared to 4 percent of non-Hispanic black residents and approximately 2 percent of Hispanic residents. The even greater underrepresentation of minority elders in residential care facilities relative to nursing home care is also suggestive that minority elders may face less access to good long-term care options than do non-Hispanic white elders.

Of course, as Thomeer et al. (2015) point out, it is difficult to ascertain the extent to which elderly minorities are underrepresented in nursing due to socioeconomic barriers as compared to racial/ethnic variation in cultural preferences for institutional and medical settings for long-term care in lieu of family provision of such care. On the one hand, past research demonstrates that Hispanic and black families are more likely to emphasize familial responsibility for eldercare than are non-Hispanic white families, which may underlie Hispanic and black elders' lower levels of nursing home utilization (Angel et al., 2004; Burton et al., 2010). However, on the other hand, a substantial body of research demonstrates racial/ethnic inequality with respect to health care over the life course (Conley, Strully, & Bennett, 2003; Haas, Krueger, & Rohlfsen, 2012), and there is also evidence that suggests the minority elders may face additional barriers in access to long-term care. For example, some studies suggest processes of institutional discrimination in access to nursing homes for minority elders (Falcone & Broyles, 1995; Fennell et al., 2012). For example, nursing homes continue to be both racially and socioeconomically segregated (Mor et al., 2004; Smith et al., 2007), and patterns of nursing home closures have been disproportionately located in communities with a higher proportion of poor and minority elders (Feng et al., 2011), suggesting that minority elders may have fewer options when it comes to long-term care.

Even among the nursing home options that are available to disadvantaged and minority elders, there is evidence that quality of care may be poorer in nursing homes that serve minority elders. Nursing homes located in communities characterized by high levels of poverty, residential race segregation, and other indicators of neighborhood disadvantage may offer inferior care relative to nursing homes in communities characterized by more socioeconomic advantage (Fennell et al., 2012; Mor et al., 2004). Some recent studies have linked the racial composition of nursing home residents to the quality of long-term care, finding that nursing homes with a higher proportion of minority residents having greater financial difficulty provide poorer quality of care than those with a smaller proportion of minority elders (Mor et al., 2004; Smith et al., 2007). In addition, other studies have found that Hispanic elders and black elders are disproportionately likely to reside within nursing homes that have poorer care quality relative to their non-Hispanic white peers (Fennell et al., 2010; Grabowski, 2004; Smith et al., 2007). There is also evidence which suggests that minority elders receive inferior preventative care in nursing homes as compared to their non-Hispanic white peers. For example, using data from the National Nursing Home Surveys, Luo et al. (2014) found that white residents had better outcomes with respect to pain management and key preventative vaccinations such as pneumococcal and influenza relative to their black peers. Studies that focus on other dimensions of preventative health care such as antidiabetic medications and anticoagulant medications, which are prescribed for those at risk for stroke, have found similar racial/ethnic disparities among nursing home residents (Allsworth et al., 2005; Christian, Lapane, & Toppa, 2003). Thus, continued attention is needed with respect to issues of both nursing home access, as well as quality of care for minority elders.

Nursing Homes: Culture Change, Implementation, and Prospects for Resident Outcomes

In the past two decades, there has been substantial scholarly and political emphasis on shifting culture within nursing homes from one that views nursing homes as an institutional and medical care setting to a culture that promotes a more home-like, residential setting that supports developmental growth at the later phases of the life course. Scholars studying the history of the culture change movement link the beginning of the movement to efforts by political and bureaucratic agencies, such as the Centers for Medicare and Medicaid Services and the Institute of Medicaid, and consumer advocacy groups, such as the National Citizen's Coalition for Nursing Home Reform, to bring greater public awareness to the issue of poor care quality in nursing homes (Koren, 2010). Passage of the Nursing Home Reform Act, via the Omnibus Budget Reconciliation Act of 1987, signified a considerable milestone in the movement, as this legislation instituted a shift in the legal definition of resident care from one that was primarily focused on medical intervention to a more holistic view of the residents' subjective well-being, including physical, mental, and psychosocial health (Koren, 2010). In the mid-1990s, a group of innovative providers, along with researchers, consumer advocacy groups, and regulators banded together to form the Pioneer Network. This network viewed its task as providing the groundwork for implementing person-centered care in nursing homes that focused holistically on the resident and reconceptualizing the nursing home as a residential space for long-term care to occur rather than a medicalized, institutional setting (Rahman & Schnelle, 2008).

Culture change advocates have argued that the provision of nursing home care should be resident-centered, and nursing homes that make greater efforts to focus on resident care holistically will not only promote physical health outcomes, but also improve resident quality of life and subjective well-being (Housen et al., 2009; Saliba & Schnelle, 2002). From the culture change movement, several different models of person-centered nursing home care developed during the latter part of the 1990s, each emphasizing different aspects of nursing home culture (Zimmerman, Shier, & Saliba, 2014), including the Eden Alternative, the Wellspring Model, and the Green House Model. The Eden Alternative focused on changing the institutional, nursing home environment in which elders reside into an age-integrated residential setting that more parallels community living via interaction with children, spaces that are green and lively with plant life, and interaction with animals. Proponents of the Eden Alterative view human growth and development in elders as best supported by an environment that is less like a medical setting and more like home (Zimmerman, Shier, & Saliba, 2014). By contrast, the Wellspring Model tackled a different component of nursing home culture, emphasizing the relationship between staff empowerment and resident care outcomes. In particular, the Wellspring Model emphasizes training and empowering direct care staff to aid in making decisions regarding resident care and the workplace environment, an approach viewed as critical to retaining quality staff (Rahman & Schnelle, 2008; Reinhard & Stone, 2001). Furthermore, the Wellspring approach highlighted the necessity to share best practices via a consortium of nursing homes with similar goals of culture change (Rahman & Schnelle, 2008). Finally, the Green House Model focused on scaling down nursing home care to a much more intimate environment, creating care communities of approximately 15 residents who coreside in small group homes, with a common care staff who provide assistance with both ADLs such as dressing and bathing, as well as instrumental ADLs such as cooking and cleaning. In an effort to promote person-centered care, the Green House Model also emphasizes resident direction in care and decision-making (Zimmerman, Shier, & Saliba, 2014).

In 2005, the Centers for Medicaid and Medicare instituted state-based government agencies called Quality Improvement Organizations to help address nursing home culture change, and in 2006, introduced a questionnaire, entitled Artifacts of Culture Change Tool, which was designed to help nursing homes perform self-assessments of their movement toward person-centered care (Rahman & Schnelle, 2008). To some extent, the 2010 Affordable Care Act has further reinforced the emphasis on nursing home culture change, as this piece of legislation took to task revision of long-term care delivered in nursing homes to be more person-centered and attached additional requirements of reporting of nursing home quality to better improve transparency related to quality of care so that consumers could be more informed about their long-term care choices (Grabowski et al., 2014b). Because such a large proportion of nursing homes depend on reimbursement from Medicare and Medicaid, it is possible that such efforts may help hasten the movement of nursing homes to institute culture change.

Besides trying to promote person-oriented care, advocates of nursing home culture change have focused on particular dimensions of nursing homes for which improvement is merited. In particular, nursing home culture activists and advocates have argued that person-oriented care needs to be multifaceted in order to be most effective and that a broad sweeping cultural shift in this form of long-term care will result in better resident outcomes (Grabowski et al., 2014; Koren, 2010; Shier et al., 2014). First, advocates argue that residents need greater input into their care, their living arrangements and environment, and schedule. For example, resident choice and self-direction in daily activities, food choices, and schedule are focal points for tailoring care to the resident. A second focal point emphasizes making the nursing home environment more home-like and less institutional. In this respect, nursing home culture movement leaders have argued that the nursing home setting needs to transform from a medical care setting to a more community-oriented residence. Third, advocates of culture change argue that relationships between residents, staff, family members, and the community need to be close and characterized by open exchange to best promote resident well-being. To some extent, the movement has also emphasized efforts to decentralize some aspects of decision making, especially as it relates to resident care by direct care staff, as a basis for empowering staff to better allocate their efforts with residents. As an extension of this, the culture change movement has argued that—to the extent possible—management and direct care staff need to engage in collaborative efforts to make decisions about both resident care and workplace culture. Lastly, advocates have argued that a necessary condition for culture change is measurement of progress to change, and as such have recommended data collection to assess nursing homes' relative progress on these initiatives.

While the culture change movement had its birth in the 1980s and 1990s, its implementation and studies endeavoring to collect evidence of its efficacy remain a 21st-century phenomenon. First, a relatively small proportion of nursing homes have undergone extensive restructuring to promote culture change by any definition or model (Grabowski et al., 2014a). For example, only about one-third of nursing homes are classified as implementing any version of culture change, and fewer than 15 percent have executed far-reaching measures to broadly shift nursing home culture to be more person-centered (Miller et al., 2014). Furthermore, the nursing homes which have engaged in greater efforts to improve nursing home culture and care are socially patterned: they are disproportionately nonprofit, have a higher proportion of private-pay residents, more and better trained staff, and better baseline quality before implementing these changes (Grabowski et al. 2014; Miller et al., 2014). So, to some extent, it is possible that while culture change in nursing homes may improve the lives of some residents, this movement may reinforce preexisting inequalities in nursing home experiences (Mor et al., 2004).

Several barriers have plagued nursing home efforts with respect to culture change, even for facilities that desire to engage in the process. For example, implementing culture change in facilities characterized by high levels of physical frailty and cognitive impairment may be quite difficult (Zimmerman, Shier, & Saliba, 2014), and nursing homes serve populations that are among the most frail (U.S. Department of Health and Human Services, Centers for Medicare and Medicaid Services, 2013). Consequently, the ability for resident care to be self-directed may be somewhat compromised by either physical or cognitive limitations. Indeed, many of implemented culture change efforts tend to refocus on either top-down changes or changes within staff, rather than incorporating the abilities and preferences of residents (Shura, Siders, & Dannefer, 2011). Second, many of the prescriptions for culture change indirectly imply increases in staffing levels, in an industry already characterized by high levels of staff turnover and job burnout (Collier & Harrington, 2008). Third, culture change requires significant monetary investment at the start of the process (Jenkens et al., 2011) and for many nursing homes the monetary investment needed to generate culture change seems too great for organizations that are both underresourced (Mor et al., 2004) and unsure about measures that have limited proven efficacy (Shier et al., 2014). Perhaps for this reason, relatively few nursing homes have gone through holistic processes of reorganization to implement culture change, instead favoring a more selective approach that picks and chooses between strategies that are tailored to the organization's specific concerns (Chapin, 2006; Elliot et al., 2014). Furthermore, because culture change may be thought of as a continual process rather than a dichotomous outcome, nursing homes that have been engaged in culture change longer tend to have made greater strides relative to those that have newly begun the process, underscoring the substantial investment of resources that culture change requires (Sterns, Miller, & Allen, 2010).

Theoretically, advocates of nursing home culture change argue that improved, person-centered care should have tangible payoffs in the form of improved and measurable resident outcomes. Such outcomes could be conceptualized as encompassing physical health, as well as subjective mental and cognitive well-being (Shier et al., 2014). However, identifying which resident outcomes to investigate, as well as figuring out how to appropriately measure such outcomes among frail and often impaired populations has been a difficult task for scholars, industry leaders, and political organizations (Castle & Ferguson, 2010; Shier et al., 2014). For example, some studies suggest that assessments of quality of life tend to diverge between residents, family, and staff (Crespo et al., 2012). Furthermore, given the high proportion of nursing home residents who experience cognitive impairment, adopting instruments for measuring resident outcomes related to culture change has also proven challenging. The Centers for Medicare and Medicaid Services, in an effort to better assess nursing home quality, provides a series of health-related measures that are designed to tap resident experiences in the aggregate. However, many of these focus on medical indicators—such as percent of residents experiencing a fall, percent reporting pain, percent given the flu vaccine, percent who had a catheter inserted, percent who were physically restrained—rather than assessing delivery of person-centered care and subjective satisfaction and well-being among residents (U.S. Department of Health and Human Services, Centers for Medicare and Medicaid Services, 2013). Furthermore, though culture change is not required by Medicare and Medicaid, assessments of quality using health-focused measures are regularly required. Consequently, some scholars have grown concerned that nursing homes may actively seek out healthier, low-care populations in an effort to improve quality ratings, perhaps at the expense of making legitimate efforts at culture change (Mukamel et al., 2009).

Figuring out how to measure practices that have been implemented to change nursing home culture has also proved problematic for scholars, since organizations have executed varied approaches to resident-centered care and culture change (Zimmerman, Shier, & Saliba, 2014). Conceptualization and measurement issues aside, studies often rely upon case studies, or small samples to demonstrate efficacy of a particular implementation strategy of culture change, which leaves the question of generalizability unanswered (Shier et al., 2014). In spite of these limitations, early studies suggest that at its best, culture change may positively affect residents' care and well-being (Grabowski et al., 2014b; Leedahl, Chapin, & Little, 2015; Sullivan et al., 2013; Kane et al., 2007; Ransom, 2000), and at its worst, culture change may have insignificant effects on resident outcomes (Coleman et al., 2002; Hill et al., 2011). Thus, while culture change may not always lead to improved resident outcomes, such changes are unlikely to result in poorer care. However, what is apparent is that these studies are far from underscoring the efficacy of nursing home culture change, which has the potential to undermine the strength of the movement, if industry leaders and government actors do not see evidence that the benefits of culture change outweigh the costs (Shier et al., 2014).

While it may be difficult to assess the efficacy of culture change on nursing home quality and resident quality of life and subjective well-being, some evidence suggests that various domains of organizational culture that tend to be focal points of the culture change movement may be associated with resident well-being. For example, residents' social integration within the nursing home environment is positively associated with both health and well-being. Residents who have close social ties with staff and other coresidents tend to report better physical and mental health outcomes (Leedahl, Chapin, & Little, 2015). Furthermore, while coresidents in nursing homes may not replace long-cherished and trusted friends from the community, these relationships are meaningful to residents' health and well-being to the extent that they promote a sense of belonging within the new residential environment of the nursing home (Leedahl, Chapin, & Little, 2015). The organizational culture and climate of nursing homes has also been shown to be associated with changes in residents' depressive symptoms. Cassie and Cassie (2012) found that residents who live in nursing homes that have implemented policies designed to promote more resident-centered care tend to have lower levels of depressive symptoms over time relative to their peers who are in less responsive and proficient nursing homes. However, it is important to note that approximately half of nursing home residents have cognitive impairment and cognitive impairment alone has important intersections with resident reports of quality of life (Abrahamson et al., 2012). Consequently, findings that generalize about the efficacy of various interventions may or may not apply to residents with high levels of cognitive impairment in the same way that they apply to residents with less cognitive impairment.

Discussion

In the past few decades, elders have shifted away from using nursing homes as a form of long-term care, even in the face of considerable population aging. Scholars and policy makers might make the argument that lower usage of nursing homes is a positive step in efforts to provide more balanced offerings of long-term care that better fit the constraints, needs, and desires of an aging American population. While there has been a significant increase in services rendered by home and community-based programs, as well as concurrent growth in elders served by residential care facilities, such services are unlikely to fill an important gap in the American long-term care solution, one that caters to the portion of the elderly population with substantial cognitive and physical impairment. Given trends in rates of cognitive impairment in the elderly and the expected increase in Alzheimer's disease and other dementias likely to accompany population aging, it is likely that nursing homes will remain significant to the long-term care system, even if relegated to the last phase of long-term care.

In this chapter, I have identified several critical issues that are likely to continue to characterize future discussions regarding the state of nursing homes in the future. First, issues regarding racial/ethnic inequality in access to nursing home care seem likely to be of continued interest for future study. With a growing percentage of minority elders, many of whom have experienced significant health inequality over the life course, inequality in access to affordable nursing home care will likely be a pressing issue for scholars and policy makers, as well as for families who seek workable solutions for long-term care of frail relatives. By nearly any account, minority elders have less access to nursing home care than levels of physical and cognitive impairment in this population suggest is needed. Bridging the racial/ethnic gap in access to nursing home care will require far more than merely moving admission rates, however. While increasing access to nursing home care may result in altered admission rates by race/ethnic groups, a more fundamental source of this inequality lies in the nursing home experience itself. Minority elders are disproportionately served by nursing homes with poorer quality, greater numbers of deficiencies, fewer mental health services, and poorer resident to staff ratios. Consequently, efforts to bring about greater equity of nursing home care will need to broadly redress these forms of inequality.

Second, given the vulnerable elder population that nursing homes serve, as well as the significant public expense associated with nursing home care, it seems inevitable that issues regarding nursing home quality will continue to be raised by policy makers, scholars, and American citizens. In recent years, advocates of the nursing home culture change movement have argued that moving to person-centered care in nursing homes will result in a more residential—rather than medical—experience for frail residents, improved care quality, and measurable change in resident health and well-being outcomes. However, progress toward nursing home culture change has been slow and only a small minority of nursing homes has undergone systematic culture change processes due to the considerable expense and effort required for such institutional upheaval. Furthermore, data showing nursing home culture change to significantly improve residents' health and well-being are scant, an issue that is further complicated by the fact that culture change has predominantly occurred in nursing homes already characterized by greater resources and better care quality. Inevitably, future research will continue to focus on the efficacy of culture change for resident outcomes, especially as it relates to extremely impaired and frail residents. Moreover, scholars and policy makers alike will likely seek effective ways to institutionalize culture change in a way that is sensitive to costs, given the already high expense of delivering long-term care within nursing homes. Consequently, it seems probable that the movement to resident-centered care will continue to be at the forefront of both scholarly and policy interest in the future.

References

Abrahamson, K., Clark, D., Perkins, A., & Arling, G. (2012). Does cognitive impairment influence quality of life among nursing home residents? *The Gerontologist, 52*, 632–640.

Administration on Aging. (2012). *A profile of older Americans, 2012*. U.S. Department of Health and Human Services. Washington, DC.

Akamigbo, A. B., & Wolinsky, F. D. (2007). New evidence of racial differences in access and their effects on the use of nursing homes among older adults. *Medical Care, 45*, 672–679.

Allsworth, J. E., Toppa, R., Palin, N. C., & Lapane, K. L. (2005). Racial and ethnic disparities in the pharmacologic management of diabetes mellitus among long-term care facility residents. *Ethnic Disparity, 15*, 205–212.

Andel, R., Hyer, K., & Slack, A. (2007). Risk factors for nursing home placement in older adults with and without dementia. *Journal of Aging and Health, 19*, 213–228.

Angel, J. L., Angel, R. J., Aranda, M. P., & Miles, T. P. (2004). Can the family still cope? Social support and health as determinants of nursing home use in the older Mexican-origin population. *Journal of Aging and Health, 16*, 338–354.

Ayse, A., Olfson, M., Siegel, M., Zurlo, K. A., Walkup, J. T., & Crystal, S. (2012). Racial and ethnic disparities in depression care in community-dwelling elderly in the United States. *American Journal of Public Health, 102*, 319–328.

Ball, M. M., Whittington, F. J., Perkins, M. M., Patterson, V. L., Hollingsworth, C., King, S. V., & Combs, B. L. (2000). Quality of life in assisted living facilities: Viewpoints of residents. *Journal of Applied Gerontology, 19*, 304–325.

Banaszak-Holl, J., Fendrick, A. M., Foster, N. L., Herzog, A. R., Kabeto, M. U., Kent, D. M., et al. (2004). Predicting nursing home admission: Estimates from a 7-year follow-up of a nationally representative sample of older Americans. *Alzheimer Disease and Associated Disorders, 18*(2), 83–89.

Bharucha, A. J., Pandav, R., Shen, C., Dodge, H. H., & Ganguli, M. (2004). Predictors of nursing facility admission: A 12-year epidemiological study in the United States. *Journal of the American Geriatrics Society, 52*, 434–439.

Bianchi, S. M., Hotz, J., McGarry, K., & Seltzer, J. A. (2008). *Intergenerational ties: Theories, trends, and challenges intergenerational caregiving*. Washington, DC: Urban Institute.

Burton, L. M., Bonilla-Silva, E., Ray, V., Buckelew, R., & Hordge Freeman, E. (2010). Critical race theories, colorism, and the decade's research on families of color. *Journal of Marriage and Family, 3*, 440–459.

Caffrey, C., Sengupta, M., Park-Lee E., et al. (2012). *Residents living in residential care facilities: United States, 2010*. NCHS data brief, no 91. Hyattsville, MD: National Center for Health.

Carter, C., Garret, B., & Wissoker, D. (2015). *Medicare's payments to skilled nursing facilities is as strong as ever*. Washington, DC: Medicare Payment Advisory Commission and Urban Institute.

Cassie, K. M., & Cassie, W. E. (2012). Organizational and individual conditions associated with depressive symptoms among nursing home residents over time. *The Gerontologist, 52*(6), 812–821.

Castle, N. G., & Ferguson, J. C. (2010). What is nursing home quality and how is it measured? *The Gerontologist, 50*, 426–442.

Chapin, M. (2006). *Creating innovative places: Organizational and architectural case studies of the culture change movement in long-term care* (Doctoral dissertation). Milwaukee, WI: University of Wisconsin-Milwaukee.

Cho, S., Zarit, S. H., & Chiriboga, D. A. (2009). Wives and daughters: The differential role of day care use in the nursing home placement of cognitively impaired family members. *The Gerontologist, 49*, 57–67.

Choi, H. J., Schoeni, R. F., Langa, K. M., & Heisler, M. M. (2014). Spouse and child availability for newly disabled older adults: Socioeconomic differences and potential role of residential proximity. *Journals of Gerontology, Series B: Psychological Sciences and Social Sciences*, doi:10.1093/geronb/gbu015

Christian, J. B., Lapane, K. L., & Toppa, R. S. (2003). Racial disparities in receipt of secondary stroke prevention agents among US nursing home residents. *Stroke, 34*, 2693–2697.

Coleman, M. T., Looney, S., O'Brien, J., Ziegler, C., Pastorino, C. A., & Turner, C. (2002). The Eden Alternative: Findings after 1 year of implementation. *The Journals of Gerontology, Series A: Medical Sciences, 57*, M422–M427.

Collier, E. (2008). Staffing characteristics, turnover rates, and quality of resident care in nursing facilities. *Research in Gerontological Nursing, 1*, 157–170.

Congressional Budget Office. (2013). *Rising demand for long-term services and supports for elderly people*. Washington, DC.

Conley, D., Strully, K. W., & Bennett, N. G. (2003). *The starting gate: Birth weight and life chances*. Berkeley, CA: University of California Press.

Cooper, C., Tandy, A. R., Balamurali, T. B., & Livingston, G. (2010). A systematic review and meta-analysis of ethnic differences in use of dementia treatment, care, and research. *The American Journal of Geriatric Psychiatry, 18*, 193–203.

Crespo, M., de Quirós, M. B., Gómez, M. M., & Hornillos, C. (2012). Quality of life of nursing home residents with dementia: A comparison of perspectives of residents, family, and staff. *The Gerontologist, 52*, 56–65.

DeNavas-Walt, C., Proctor, B. D., & Smith, J. (2009). Income, poverty, and health insurance coverage in the United States: 2003. Washington (DC): US Census Bureau; 2004. *Population Reports*, 60–226.

Elliot, A., Cohen, L. W., Reed, D., Nolet, K., & Zimmerman, S. (2014). A "recipe" for culture change? Findings from the THRIVE survey of culture change adopters. *The Gerontologist, 54*(Suppl. 1), S17–S24.

Falcone, D., & Broyles, R. (1994). Access to long-term care: Race as a barrier. *Journal of Health Politics, Policy and Law, 19*, 583–595.

Feng, Z., Fennell, M. L., Tyler, D. A., Clark, M., & Mor, V. (2011). Growth of racial and ethnic minorities in US nursing homes driven by demographics and possible disparities in options. *Health Affairs, 30*, 1358–1365.

Fennell, M., Clark, M., Feng, Z., Mor, V., Smith, D. B., & Tyler, D. A. (2012). Separate and unequal access and quality of care in nursing homes: Transformations of the research program for aging Hispanics. In J. L. Angel, F. Torres-Gil, & K. Markides (Eds.), *Aging, health and longevity in the Mexican-origin population* (pp. 207–225). New York: Springer.

Fennell, M. L., Feng, Z., Clark, M. A., & Mor, V. (2010). Elderly Hispanics more likely to reside in poor-quality nursing homes. *Health Affairs, 29*, 65–73.

Freedman, V. A. (1996). Family structure and the risk of nursing home admission. *The Journals of Gerontology, Series B: Social Sciences, 51*, S61–S69.

Freedman, V. A., Berkman, L. F., Rapp, S. R., & Ostfeld, A. M. (1994). Family networks: Predictors of nursing home entry. *American Journal of Public Health, 84*, 843–845.

Fullerton, C. A., McGuire, T. G., Feng, Z., Mor, V., & Grabowski, D. C. (2009). Trends in mental health admissions to nursing homes, 1999-2005. *Psychiatric Services, 60*, 965–971.

Gaugler, J. E., Duval, S., Anderson, K. A., & Kane, R. L. (2007). Predicting nursing home admission in the U.S.: A meta-analysis. *BMC Geriatrics, 7*, 13.

Gaugler, J. E., Fang, Y., Krichbaum, K., & Wyman, J. F. (2009). Predictors of nursing home admission for persons with dementia. *Medical Care, 47*, 191–198.

Gaugler, J. E., Wall, M. M., Kane, R. L., Menk, J. S., Sarsour, K., Johnston, J. A., . . . & Newcomer, R. (2011). Does caregiver burden mediate the effects of behavioral disturbances on nursing home admission? *The American Journal of Geriatric Psychiatry, 19*(6), 497–506.

Gorina Y., Schappert S., Bercovitz A., et al. (2014). Prevalence of incontinence among older Americans. National Center for Health Statistics. *Vital Health Statistics, 3*, 36.

Grabowski, D. C. (2004). The admission of blacks to high-deficiency nursing homes. *Medical Care, 42*, 156–161.

Grabowski, D. C., Aschbrenner, K. A., Feng, Z., & Mor, V. (2009). Mental illness in nursing homes: Variations across States. *Health Affairs, 28*, 689–700.

Grabowski, D. C., Elliot, A., Leitzell, B., Cohen, L. W., & Zimmerman, S. (2014a). Who are the innovators? Nursing homes implementing culture change. *The Gerontologist, 54*(Suppl. 1), S65–S75.

Grabowski, D. C., O'Malley, A. J., Afendulis, C. C., Caudry, D. J., Elliot, A., & Zimmerman, S. (2014b). Culture change and nursing home quality of care. *The Gerontologist*, 54(Suppl. 1), S35–S45.

Haas, S. A., Krueger, P. M., & Rohlfsen, L. (2012). Race/ethnic and nativity disparities in later life physical performance: The role of health and socioeconomic status over the life course. *The Journals of Gerontology, Series B: Psychological Sciences and Social Sciences, 67*(2), 238–248.

Harrington, C., Swan, J. H., & Carrillo, H. (2007). Nurse staffing levels and Medicaid reimbursement rates in nursing facilities. *Health Services Research,* 42(3p1), 1105–1129.

Harris, Y. (2007). Depression as a risk factor for nursing home admission among older individuals. *Journal of the American Medical Directors Association, 8*, 14-20.

Harris-Kojetin, L., Sengupta, M., Park-Lee, E., & Valverde, R. (2013). *Long-term care services in the United States: 2013 overview.* National health care statistics reports, no. 1. Hyattsville, MD: National Center for Health Statistics.

Hill, N. L., Kolanowski, A. M., Milone-Nuzzo, P., & Yevchak, A. (2011). Culture change models and resident health outcomes in long-term care. *Journal of Nursing Scholarship, 43*(1), 30–40.

Housen, P., Shannon, G. R., Simon, B., Edelen, M. O., Cadogan, M. P., Jones, M., Saliba, D. (2009). Why not just ask the resident? Refinement of a preference assessment tool (PAT) for nursing homes. *Journal of Gerontological Nursing, 35*, 40–49.

Hung., W. H., Ross, J. S., Boockvar, K. S., & Siu, A. L. (2011). Recent trends in chronic disease, impairment and disability among older adults in the United States. *BMC Geriatrics, 11*, 47.

Jenkens, R., Sult, T., Lessell, N., Hammer, D., & Ortigara, A. (2011). Financial implications of the Green House Model, *Senior Housing and Care Journal, 19*, 3–22.

Kaiser Commission on Medicaid and the Uninsured. (2013). Medicaid, a primer: Key information on the nation's health coverage program for low-income people (Report #7334-05). Washington, DC.

Kane, R. A., Lum, T. Y., Cutler, L. J., Degenholtz, H. B., & Yu, T. C. (2007). Resident outcomes in small-house nursing homes: A longitudinal evaluation of the initial green house program. *Journal of the American Geriatrics Society, 55*(6), 832–839.

Katz, S. J., Kabeto, M., & Langa, K. M. (2000). Gender disparities in the receipt of home care for elderly people with disability in the United States. *Journal of the American Medical Association, 284*, 3022–3027.

Kaye, H. S., Harrington, C., & LaPlante, M. P. (2010). Long-term care: Who gets it, who provides it, who pays, and how much? *Health Affairs, 29*(1), 11–21.

Kelly, C. M., Liebig, P. S., & Edwards, L. J. (2008). Nursing home deficiencies: An exploratory study of interstate variations in regulatory activity. *Journal of Aging & Social Policy, 20*(4), 398–413.

Koren, M. J. (2010). Person-centered care for nursing home residents: The culture-change movement. *Health Affairs, 29*(2), 312–317.

Leedahl, S. N., Chapin, R. K., & Little, T. D. (2015). Multilevel examination of facility characteristics, social integration, and health for older adults living in nursing homes. *The Journals of Gerontology, Series B: Psychological Sciences and Social Sciences, 70*(1), 111–122.

Levine, C., Halper, D., Peist, A., & Gould, D. A. (2010). Bridging troubled waters: Family caregivers, transitions, and long-term care. *Health Affairs, 29*, 116–124.

Luo, H., Zhang, X., Cook, B., Wu, B., & Wilson, M. R., (2014). Racial/ethnic disparities in preventative practice among US nursing home residents. *Journal of aging and health, 26*, 519–539.

Luppa, M., Luck, T., Weyerer, S., König, H., Brähler, E., Riedel-Heller, S.G. (2010). Prediction of institutionalization in the elderly. A systematic review. *Age and Ageing, 39*, 31–38.

Medicare Payment Advisory Commission. (2015). *Report to the Congress: Medicare payment policy*. March 2015, Washington, DC.

Miller, E.A., & Weissert, W.G. (2000). Predicting elderly people's risk for nursing home placement, hospitalization, functional impairment, and mortality: A synthesis. *Medical Care Research and Review, 57*, 259–297.

Miller, S.C., Cohen, N., Lima, J.C., & Mor, V. (2014). Medicaid capital reimbursement policy and environmental artifacts of nursing home culture change. *The Gerontologist, 54*(Suppl. 1), S76–S86.

Miller, S.C., Looze, J., Shield, R., Clark, M.A., Lepore, M., Tyler, D., . . . & Mor, V. (2014). Culture change practice in US nursing homes: Prevalence and variation by state Medicaid reimbursement policies. *The Gerontologist, 54*(3), 434–445.

Mollica, R., Johnson-Lamarche, H., & O'Keefe, J. (2005). *State residential care and assisted living policy*. Portland, ME: National Academy for State Health Policy.

Mollica, R. Sims-Kastelein K., & O'Keefe, J. (2008). *Assisted living and resident care policy compendium, 2007 update*. Portland, ME: National Academy for State Health Policy.

Mor, V., Gruneir, A., Feng, Z., Grabowski, D.C., Intrator, O., & Zinn, J. (2011). The effect of state policies on nursing home resident outcomes. *Journal of the American Geriatrics Society, 59*(1), 3–9.

Mor, V., Intrator, O., Feng, Z., & Grabowski, D.C. (2010). The revolving door of rehospitalization from skilled nursing facilities. *Health Affairs, 29*, 57–64.

Mor, V., Zinn, J., Angelelli, J., Teno, J.M., & Miller, S.C. (2004). Driven to tiers: Socioeconomic and racial disparities in the quality of nursing home care. *Millbank Quarterly, 82*, 227–256.

Mukamel, D.B., Ladd, H., Weimer, D.L., Spector, W.D., & Zinn, J.S. (2009). Is there evidence of cream skimming among nursing homes following the publication of the nursing home compare report card? *The Gerontologist, 49*, 793–802.

National Center for Health Statistics. (2014). *Health, United States, 2013: With special feature on prescription drugs*. Hyattsville, MD.

Nelson, A.R., Smedley, B.D., & Stith, A.Y. (Eds.). (2009). *Unequal treatment: Confronting racial and ethnic disparities in health care* (Vol. 1). Washington, DC: National Academies Press.

Ness, J., Ahmed, A., & Aronow, W.S. (2004). Demographics and payment characteristics of nursing home residents in the United States: A 23-year trend. *The Journals of Gerontology, Series A: Biological Sciences and Medical Sciences, 59*, 1213–1217.

Noel-Miller, C. (2010). Spousal loss, children, and the risk of nursing home admission. *The Journals of Gerontology, Series B: Psychological Sciences and Social Sciences, 65B*, 370–380.

Park-Lee, E., Caffrey, C., Sengupta, M., Moss, A.J., Rosenoff, E., & Harris-Kojetin, L.D. (2011). *Residential care facilities: A key sector in the spectrum of long-term care providers in the United States* (NCHS data brief, No. 78). Hyattsville, MD: National Center for Health Statistics.

Rahman, A.N., & Schnelle, J.F. (2008). The nursing home culture-change movement: Recent past, present, and future directions for research. *The Gerontologist, 48*, 142–148.

Ransom, S. Eden Alternative: The Texas Project. (2000). *Faculty publications—School of Health Administration*. Retrieved from https://digital.library.txstate.edu/handle/10877/4087

Reeves, E., & Musumeci, M.B. (2014). *Medicaid and long-term service supports: A primer*. The Kaiser Commission on Medicaid and the Uninsured, July 2014. Menlo Park: CA.

Reinhard, S., & Stone, R., (2001). Promoting quality in nursing homes. Washington, DC: American Association of Homes and Services for the Aging.

Saliba, D., & Schnelle, J.F. (2002). Indicators of the quality of nursing home residential care. *Journal of the American Geriatrics Society, 50*, 1421–1430.

Shier, V., Khodyakov, D., Cohen, L.W., Zimmerman, S., & Saliba, D. (2014). What does the evidence really say about culture change in nursing homes? *The Gerontologist 54, S1*, S6–S16.

Shugarman, L.R. (2010). Health care reform and long-term care: The whole is greater than the sum of its parts. *Public Policy & Aging Report, 20*, 3–7.

Shura, R., Siders, R.A., & Dannefer, D. (2011). Culture change in long-term care: Participatory action research and the role of the resident. *The Gerontologist, 51*, 212–225.

Smith, D. B., Feng, Z., Fennell, M. L., Zinn, J. S., & Mor, V. (2007). Separate and unequal: Racial segregation and disparities in quality across U.S. nursing homes. *Health Affairs, 26*, 1448–1458.

Smith, D. B., Feng, Z., Fennell, M. L., Zinn, J., & Mor, V. (2008). Racial disparities in access to long-term care: The illusive pursuit of equity. *Journal of Health Politics, Policy and Law, 33*, 861–881.

Spilman, B.C., & Long, S.K. (2009). Does high caregiver stress predict nursing home entry? *Inquiry, 46*, 140–161.

Sterns, S., Miller, S.C., & Allen, S. (2010). The complexity of implementing culture change practices in nursing homes. *Journal of the American Medical Directors Association, 11*, 511–518.

Stevenson, D.G., & Grabowski, D.C. (2010). Sizing up the market for assisted living. *Health Affairs, 29*, 35–43.

Stoller, E. P., & Miklowski, C. S. (2008). Spouses caring for spouses: Untangling the influences of relationship and gender. In M. E. Szinovacz, & A. Davey (Eds.), *Caregiving contexts: Cultural, familial, and societal implications* (pp. 115–131). New York: Springer.

Strahan, G.W. (1997). *An overview of the nursing homes and their residents: Data from the 1995 National Nursing Home Survey* (Advance Data from Vital and Health Statistics, No. 280). Hyattsville, MD: National Center for Health Statistics.

Street, D., Burge, S., & Quadagno, J. (2009). The effect of licensure type on the policies, practices, and resident composition of Florida assisted living facilities. *The Gerontologist, 49*, 211–223.

Street, D., & Quadagno, J. (2004). *Nursing home to assisted living transitions: An evaluation of the Medicaid NHTP pilot project and its implications for policy-makers.* Final report. Tallahassee: Pepper Institute on Aging, Florida State University.

Sullivan, J. L., Shwartz, M., Burgess, J. F., Jr., Peköz, E. A., Christiansen, C. L., Gerena-Melia, M., & Berlowitz, D. (2013). Person-centered care practices and quality in Department of Veterans Affairs nursing homes: Is there a relationship? *Medical Care, 51*, 165–171.

Thomeer, M. B., Mudrazija, S., & Angel, J. L. (2015). How do race and Hispanic ethnicity affect nursing home admission? Evidence from the Health and Retirement Study. *The Journals of Gerontology, Series B: Psychological Sciences and Social Sciences, 70*, 628–638.

U.S. Department of Health and Human Services, Centers for Medicare and Medicaid Services. (2013). *Nursing home data compendium, 2013 edition.*

Warner, D. F., & Brown, T. H. (2011). Understanding how race/ethnicity and gender define age-trajectories of disability: An intersectionality approach. *Social Science & Medicine, 72*, 1236–1248.

Wattmo, C. Wallin, A. K., Londos, E., & Minthon, L. (2011). Risk factors for nursing home placement in Alzheimer's disease: A longitudinal study of cognition, ADL, service utilization, and cholinesterase inhibitor treatment. *The Gerontologist, 51*, 17–27.

Wiener, J., Anderson, W. L., & Brown, D. (2009). *Why are nursing home utilization rates declining?* Centers for Medicare and Medicaid Services. Washington, DC.

Wolff, J. L., & Kasper, J. D. (2006). Caregivers of frail elders: Updating a national profile. *The Gerontologist, 46*, 344–356.

Zimmerman, S., Shier, V., & Saliba, D. (2014). Transforming nursing home culture: Evidence for practice and policy. *The Gerontologist, 54*(Suppl. 1), S1–S5.

Zimmerman, S., Sloane, P. D., & Reed, D. (2014). Dementia prevalence and care in assisted living. *Health Affairs, 33*, 658–666.

CHAPTER TEN

End-of-Life and End-of-Life Planning

Megumi Inoue, Sara Keary, and Sara M. Moorman

The circumstances surrounding death and dying have changed dramatically for Americans in the past century. In the past, death was a meaningful risk for persons of all ages, especially young children. In 1900, 12 percent of infants did not survive their first year, and half of the population had died by the age of 58 (Arias, 2014). Over the course of the century the risk of premature death declined; between 1935 and 2010, mortality risk dropped by over 50 percent for every age group except persons aged 85 and older (Hoyert, 2012). This statistic means that today, most decedents in the United States are among the oldest-old, and they die from the chronic diseases of old age—heart disease, cancer, and stroke—rather than infectious diseases or injuries.

These demographic changes have wrought changes in the medical treatment of dying persons, as well as in cultural understandings of the meaning of dying and death. Death is something to be staved off rather than something to be accepted as an inevitable fact of human existence (Zimmerman, 2007, 2012). Few people have spent time with a dying person, have witnessed a death, or have much personal or professional experience with loss of life (Christakis, 1999; Timmermans, 2005). In this respect, Americans are privileged compared to persons who live in parts of the world that experience armed conflict and socioeconomic underdevelopment. However, Americans' profound inexperience with death means that they often face difficulty making decisions about care for the dying.

Beyond the personal and familial difficulty of making end-of-life decisions, there are also societal concerns. Since the late 1970s, patients in their last year of life have consumed a quarter of annual Medicare costs, despite the fact that only 5 percent of Medicare beneficiaries die each year (Riley & Lubitz, 2010). In 2012, net federal spending on Medicare amounted to $466 billion (Congressional Budget Office, 2013). Medicare spending is projected to increase, given that members of the Baby Boom cohort, persons born between 1946 and 1964, will continue to age into eligibility for the program. Therefore, decisions about care for the dying lie in the public interest because they are decisions that taxpayers fund.

In this chapter, we frame these challenges and their potential solutions around three concepts: good death, bad death, and planned death. Good deaths are deaths that are as physically and psychologically comfortable as possible for patients and observers, while bad deaths are deaths that involve suffering and are disturbing to survivors. Increasingly, some form of planning occurs so as to reduce the likelihood of a bad death.

Natural Death, Good Death

Natural death, as defined by the National Association of Medical Examiners, is death that is "due solely or nearly totally to disease and/or the aging process" (Department of Health and Human Services, Centers for Disease Control and Prevention & National Center for Health Statistics, 2003, p. 21). What makes a death natural is that an illness has taken its course and individuals die of causes related directly to the disease process, rather than to, for example, medication used to treat the disease or its symptoms. Yet the layperson's definition of a natural death is quite different (Seymour, 1999). People imagine a natural death occurring at home, where the dying person can be surrounded by loved ones, with minimal medical intervention as needed to mitigate symptoms, and a balance between autonomous decisions among the patient and his or her family and the staff who are responsible for monitoring pain levels (Seymour, 1999). Scholars describe this type of death as *good*, or what is most desirable given that everyone must die (Steinhauser et al., 2000a, 2000b).

Good deaths can be had via (a) passive euthanasia, and/or (b) palliative care and hospice. Often these good deaths can also be correctly labeled natural deaths, so long as the progression of an illness is what ultimately caused the patient to die. However, although patients and families may invoke the term natural, they are typically referring to the quality rather than the cause of the death.

Passive Euthanasia

One of the fundamental ethical principles in medicine in the United States is respect for patient autonomy, which is a patient's right to direct his or her medical treatment. In the 1990 case *Cruzan v. Director, Missouri Department of Health* the Supreme Court of the United States upheld "a constitutional right to refuse life-sustaining medical treatment" (Larson & Eaton, 1997, p. 225). This right is known as *voluntary passive euthanasia*. The word *euthanasia* is from the Greek language and refers to a good and painless death, although it has come to be known as the intentional ending of life in order to relieve pain and suffering (Gordijn, 2004). Voluntary passive euthanasia implies allowing death by refusing or withdrawing life-sustaining treatment. Choosing to stop eating and drinking, disconnecting a respirator, or failing to perform cardiopulmonary resuscitation (CPR) all constitute different types of voluntary passive euthanasia (Gordijn, 2004).

Nonvoluntary passive euthanasia is also legal in the United States. The term refers to cases in which a patient is unable to communicate treatment preferences or lacks the capacity to express a choice for or against medical intervention (Ardelt, 2003). Among dying patients who require a medical decision, approximately 70 percent are incapacitated (Silveira, Kim, & Langa, 2010). In the case of nonvoluntary euthanasia, a physician decides to forego treatment after consulting a patient's family to determine that the

Table 10.1 Types of Euthanasia

	Passive	Active
Voluntary	Legal in the United States. Individuals have the constitutional right to refuse life-sustaining treatment (*Cruzan v. Director, Missouri Department of Health*, 1990).	Illegal in the United States. A physician is not permitted to administer a lethal dose of medication to a patient in an effort to end the patient's life, regardless of the patient's request (Rubin & Bernat, 2014).
Nonvoluntary	Legal in the United States. Treatment is forgone when a patient's wishes are unknown, and a terminal illness has progressed so that he or she cannot communicate a preference.	Illegal in the United States. An action is taken to cause death when a patient's wishes are unknown, and a terminal illness has progressed so that he or she cannot communicate a preference.

Note. Active forms of euthanasia are described in the section "Active Death" below.

patient would have chosen to forego treatment if he or she had the capacity. Choosing what the patient would have chosen if able is known as substituted judgment, and it is the legal standard because it has been deemed the best method to meet legal definitions of autonomy.

Palliative Care and Hospice

Passive euthanasia is commonly accompanied by palliative care. *Palliative care* is both a medical approach and a philosophical approach to care. Medically, its aims are to reduce distressing symptoms, to maximize quality of life and functional health, and to "neither hasten nor postpone death," although it may be used alongside medical interventions designed to prolong life (World Health Organization, 2014). The philosophy of palliative care is to "affirm life and regard dying as a normal process" (World Health Organization, 2014). Functionally, this philosophy means that care is provided by a team including professionals who can address the psychological and spiritual needs of both the patient and the family. Hospice care for the family may continue after the patient's death through bereavement counseling.

Therefore, there is a continuum of palliative care: It can occur concurrent with life-sustaining treatment for critically ill and/or dying patients. In cases of critical illness, palliative care includes management of symptoms such as insomnia, pain, and anxiety, as well as helping the patient and family to cope with the psychological, spiritual, and social consequences of critical illness. Starting palliative care early in the course of a serious illness may improve patients' quality of life, mood, and length of survival (Temel et al., 2010). However, this chapter primarily concerns *hospice*, one of the programs within the scope of palliative care. Hospices are organizations that provide palliative care at the end of life. In the United States, patients are eligible for Medicare reimbursement of hospice services when they have a prognosis of six months or less to live and have foregone treatment aimed at curing their illness or prolonging their life (National Hospice and Palliative Care Organization, 2014).

The primary benefits of hospice concern the clinical outcomes of patients and their families. Randomized, controlled trials—the gold standard in medical research—have demonstrated that patients receiving hospice care experience benefits including better mood, improved quality of life (Bakitas et al., 2009), greater satisfaction with their care experience, and fewer ICU admissions (Gade et al., 2008). Scores of additional studies demonstrate improvements in symptoms such as pain, in survival, in caregiver well-being, and other such outcomes (e.g., Meier, 2011). No studies have documented drawbacks to hospice care such as accelerated death.

In fact, for people dying of certain illnesses, hospice may *increase* survival time (Connor et al., 2007).

Of secondary benefit is that hospice may save money (Smith et al., 2014). One estimate is that a hospice stay of two weeks to one month saves Medicare $6,430 per patient (Kelley et al., 2013). Although savings may not be evident in all contexts (see Meng et al., 2013), hospice does not cost more than standard care.

Bad Death

Although good deaths can be had, most decedents do not have them. The prevalence of physical pain and other symptoms at the end of life has increased since the late 1990s (Singer et al., 2015). In a study of the family members of persons who died from dementia with a feeding tube inserted, 14 percent said that their consent to the tube was not sought, and 42 percent were consulted about this invasive treatment for fewer than 15 minutes (Teno et al., 2011). Although 61 percent of Americans aged 50 and older support legislation that would extend Medicare reimbursement to physicians who discuss end-of-life with their patients (Wilson & Crowley, 2014), and although patients who have such discussions report greater trust in their doctors (Keary & Moorman, 2015), this legislation has been stalled multiple times in Congress. Two major factors behind this alarming state of affairs are challenges in hospice care and the development and widespread use of life-sustaining technologies.

Challenges in Hospice Care

Hospice care has brought great relief and solace to many patients and families at the end of life. However, the U.S. health-care system does not use hospice to its fullest extent. In 2011, only 45 percent of U.S. decedents were under the care of hospice at the time of their death (NHPCO, 2014). In the same year, 70 percent of members of the public rated themselves as "not at all knowledgeable" about palliative care (Center to Advance Palliative Care, 2011a). Indeed, the extent of misunderstanding is such that over half of palliative care physicians have been accused of euthanasia or murder when providing palliative care, either by the family member of a patient or by another health-care provider (Goldstein et al., 2012). Three root problems include inequality of use, late initiation of services, and the dearth of palliative care education programs.

First, there are troubling disparities, most notably by race/ethnicity, in who benefits from hospice care. Patients of color are less likely to use hospice than white patients, and when they do use hospice, they receive services for a shorter time (Chung, Essex, & Samson, 2008; Connor et al., 2008). The disparity is not due to differences in cause of death by race or ethnicity (Connor et al., 2008), nor is it due to unavailability of hospice care in places where persons of color live (Silveira et al., 2011). Instead, persons of color are less likely than whites to be aware and recognize the benefits of hospice (Johnson, Kuchibhatla, & Tulsky, 2009). This cause suggests that the disparity may be preventable with improvements in education and outreach.

A second problem is also preventable: Patients often receive hospice only very late in the course of their illness. The median duration of hospice care is 19 days, and 35 percent of patients receive hospice care for less than a week (NHPCO, 2014). Even short durations of hospice save money (Kelley et al., 2013) and improve quality of life (Teno et al., 2007), but longer stays offer more benefits. Patients spend such short times in hospice because of overly optimistic prognoses on the part of physicians, patients, and families (Casarett et al., 2006; Christakis, 1999; Ford et al., 2008). Medicare will not reimburse for hospice services until a patient has agreed to forgo curative care, a decision that many are unwilling to make. However, Medicare is experimenting with reimbursement for palliative care alongside curative care, a move that could increase the amount of time patients receive palliative services (Centers for Medicare & Medicaid Services, 2014).

Well-trained health-care professionals can recognize terminal decline and the benefits of palliative care, leading to timely referral to and enrollment in a hospice (Welch et al., 2008). However, training and education are difficult to find. In 2011, there were only 2,887 physicians board-certified in palliative medicine in the United States (Center to Advance Palliative Care, 2011b). One estimate is that only 30 percent of U.S. medical schools require a course in palliative and hospice care, and that only 19 percent require students to complete a rotation (Van Aalst-Cohen, Riggs, & Byock, 2008). Notably, these figures concern only doctors, although nurses and other direct care workers also require training.

Life-Sustaining Technologies

In the 21st century, health-care systems in developed countries possess an unprecedented ability to sustain life among terminally ill patients using medical technologies. Many such technologies can maintain vital bodily functions, but they do not cure underlying illnesses, and they rarely restore the patient's quality of life. In fact, aggressive interventions often fail, and the patient dies or the interventions drastically lower the patient's quality of life. Nevertheless, life-sustaining treatments have become increasingly common since the mid-1980s: Among patients who died in the hospital in 1999, 30 percent had one or more life-sustaining treatments during their final hospitalization, compared to 18 percent in 1985 (Barnato et al., 2004).

As an example, consider one of the life-sustaining treatments with which the general public is most familiar: CPR. A mere 20 percent of patients who undergo CPR in a U.S. hospital survive to be discharged (Morrison et al., 2013). The figure is lower still for patients whose CPR occurs without the technology a hospital offers. Nor do survival-to-discharge figures account for the permanent cognitive and physical disabilities that often result from oxygen deprivation during cardiac arrest and physical trauma during chest compressions.

Yet nearly 4 in 10 members of the general public believe that 75 percent of patients who undergo CPR survive to be discharged from the hospital (Donohoe, Haefeli, & Moore, 2006). This mistaken belief is due in part to popular media. A U.K. study found that newspapers report disproportionately on cases in which patients survive to be discharged from the hospital (Field et al., 2011). A U.S. study found that in 90 percent of instances of CPR on television medical dramas, patients either explicitly survive to be discharged from the hospital or the show implies that they do (Diem, Lantos, & Tulsky, 1996). Once patients are accurately informed about their prognosis were they to undergo CPR, many who previously wanted CPR opt to complete a do-not-resuscitate (DNR) order, which requests that health-care professionals withhold CPR (Thorevska et al., 2005). Other life-sustaining treatments, including intubation and mechanical ventilation, artificial nutrition and hydration (i.e., a feeding tube), and dialysis, also have low success rates and are administered to patients who are unaware of the risks.

Thus, many life-sustaining treatments are futile. One working definition of *futile* reads:

> Any treatment that has no realistic chance of providing an effect that the patient would ever have the capacity to appreciate as a benefit, such as merely preserving the physiologic functions of a permanently unconscious patient, or has no realistic chance of achieving the medical goal of returning the patient to a level of health that permits survival outside the acute care setting of the medical center.
>
> (Schneiderman, 2011, p. 130)

Because identifying instances of futile care is both medically and ethically contentious, the amount and expense of futile care administered in the United States is difficult to determine. Nonetheless, health-care professionals provide life-sustaining treatments they believe to be futile. They do so for complex reasons, including inability to accept failure to save the patient; requests from the family to do all that is possible; institutional and legal delays to prevent malpractice lawsuits; miscommunication; and prognostic uncertainty (Jox et al., 2012; Palda et al., 2005).

Insufficiencies with hospice services and extensive use of life-sustaining technologies pose a number of problems to patients within the modern health-care system, as well as problems for society and the economy. Of course, solutions could be structural, population-level, public health approaches, such as expansion of funding for and education about hospice, and strict regulations on the use of aggressive treatments at the end of life. However, the solution actually pursued has been a much more individual-level fix: planning death, either via advance care planning (ACP) or via an active process such as physician-assisted suicide (PAS).

Planned Death

Advance Care Planning

ACP is the process of planning for future medical care in the event that (a) a person is no longer able to make or communicate his or her own medical decisions and (b) a medical doctor has declared the person's condition to be terminal or irreversible. ACP is an opportunity for individuals to identify and express which treatments they do or do not want for their end-of-life care so that health-care providers can give appropriate care. This process is especially critical in the practice of person-centered care, which ensures a person's needs, goals, values, family situation, and cultural preferences and traditions are respected and reflected in health service delivery (Feinberg, 2014; Greenlee, 2014).

ACP has three types: a living will, a durable power of attorney for health-care (DPAHC), and informal discussion. A living will specifies in writing the types of medical care a person does or does not want to receive under certain circumstances. For example, individuals can specify whether they would want to have life-sustaining treatment if they are in a coma and not expected to recover. A DPAHC is a designated individual permitted to make health-care decisions for an incapacitated person should decisions arise that are not covered in the living will. A living will and DPAHC are both legal documents, and together they are called an advance directive.

Health-care providers also encourage patients to hold informal discussions with their family members and health-care providers. Although informal discussions are not legally binding, they are still helpful for informing the family members or health-care providers who carry out a person's wishes (Mack et al., 2010). Talking about one's thoughts, values, and preferences for end-of-life care may help one's surrogate decision makers understand the values and preferences of a person so that they can make the right decisions when needed.

Because persons who have ACP are more likely than those without to express a desire to withhold or withdraw life-sustaining interventions and to receive palliative care, the completion of ACP can lower health-care costs in terminally ill patients' final days of life and offer patients opportunities to avoid unwanted treatment (Snyder, 2012; Emanuel, 1996). In fact, previous research has found that ACP specifying limited care is significantly associated with lower levels of Medicare spending, and persons who expressed a desire for limited treatment are less likely to die in a hospital and more likely to use hospice services (Nicholas et al., 2011). Receiving hospice care and dying at home can provide quality of life during individuals' final days that extensive life-sustaining care cannot provide.

Despite the value of ACP, there remain concerns and challenges. These include low rates of completion, accessibility of completed advance directives at the time of decision-making, effectiveness of advance directives in increasing surrogates' knowledge of a dying person's preferences, and levels of health literacy advance directives require.

In an attempt to encourage citizens to plan their end-of-life care to protect their autonomy, Congress passed the Patient Self-Determination Act (PSDA) in 1990. Under the PSDA, all Medicare and Medicaid funded facilities, such as hospitals, nursing homes, hospice agencies, home health agencies, and HMOs, are required to provide patients with written information on advance directives at the time of enrollment (Baker, 2002). Research findings indicate that the PSDA seems to have been successful at increasing public awareness and the use of advanced care planning, particularly among certain high-risk populations, such as older adults and persons in declining health (e.g., Resnick et al., 2009). However, while ACP has been conceptualized as a process that occurs over time that "seeks to discern an individual's evolving priorities, values, and goals of care, and to engage a proxy and others who may participate in future healthcare decisions" (Sabatino, 2014, p. 107), it typically occurs only after patients have been diagnosed with a terminal illness. Many patients die less than a month after having had their first conversation about ACP with a physician (Lopez-Acevedo et al., 2013; Mack et al., 2012).

Further, rates of ACP completion are alarmingly low in the general population. A recent estimate is that slightly over a quarter of U.S. adults aged 18 or older have an advance directive (Rao et al., 2014). Most people believe that they are too young and/or healthy to need plans for themselves (Pollack, Morhaim, & Williams, 2010) or that ACP would be upsetting to themselves or to family members (Schickedanz et al., 2009). White race, older age, higher educational attainment, and higher income have been repeatedly reported as robust predictors of having an informal discussion and advance directive (e.g., Alano et al., 2010; Carr & Khodyakov, 2007; Moorman & Inoue, 2013a). Findings on the effects of gender are inconclusive; some research has found that women are more likely than men to complete advance directives, but another study has found the opposite although women are more likely to engage in an informal discussion (e.g., Alano et al., 2010; Carr & Khodyakov, 2007).

Even when ACPs exist, they are not always available when they are needed. One study found that only 31 percent of patients who completed advance directives had them on their medical charts (Douglas & Brown, 2002). Patients often stow advance directives in safe deposit boxes along with wills and estate planning documents, or give them to geographically distant loved ones who cannot promptly alert doctors in an emergency.

ACP completers also fail to ensure that their appointed surrogate decision makers understand their care preferences. Surrogate decision makers' lack of knowledge of a dying person's treatment preferences is frequently found in research (e.g., Shalowitz, Garrett-Meyer, & Wendler, 2006). However, patients and surrogates *believe* that surrogates understand what patients want (Moorman, 2011). Ironically, the mismatch between what patients want and what surrogates believe that they want only increases with higher relationship quality (Moorman & Inoue, 2013b).

The last concern involves the level of health literacy that is required to execute advance directives (Fagerlin & Schneider, 2004). The average person does not know enough about illnesses, treatment options, and prognoses in order to specify care preferences. Many advance directives allow individuals to describe their personal values and to define quality of life, but someone must convert these general preferences into decisions about whether to administer specific treatments.

Active Death

Ironically, at the same time that technology has allowed for unprecedented ability to sustain life, it has also allowed for complex and contested ways of actively ending life. These include active euthanasia, PAS, and palliative sedation (PS). *Active euthanasia* refers to intentionally taking steps to end someone's life (Hooyman & Kiyak, 2010), primarily through the administration of a lethal dose of medication that is intended to cause death (Gordijn, 2004). Active euthanasia is different from passive euthanasia in that its goal is to directly result in death, whereas the goal in passive euthanasia is to stop preventing death (see Table 10.1).

Nonvoluntary active euthanasia is illegal in all countries and is viewed as murder. The only country that permits any form of nonvoluntary active euthanasia is the Netherlands, as outlined in the Groningen Protocol (Verhagen & Sauer, 2005). The Protocol permits physicians, with the agreement of a second physician and both parents, to euthanize newborns whose prognosis is certain and who are suffering unbearably. Some bioethicists support the Protocol (e.g., Lindemann & Verkerk, 2008; Manninen, 2006), while others oppose it (e.g., Jotkowitz, Glick, & Gesundheit, 2008; Kon, 2007). Little is available—at least in English—regarding public opinion. In the first five years of the Protocol, two babies, both of whom had epidermolysis bullosa, were euthanized (Verhagen, 2013). Additional cases may have gone unreported because the physician classified them as death during palliative care rather than euthanasia, as when pain medications or paralyzing medications were administered to ease symptoms (Verhagen, 2013).

Voluntary active euthanasia refers to when patients request euthanasia in order to end their life (Bergman Levy et al., 2013). Usually people who request euthanasia are experiencing unbearable pain and suffering. In the United States, no one is legally permitted to administer a lethal dose of medication to another person in an effort to relieve the suffering of the patient, regardless of the patient's request (Rubin & Bernat, 2014). Since the early 1990s, however, approximately 70 percent of Americans have said that in the case of terminal illness, physicians should be permitted to "end a patient's life by some painless means if the patient and his or her family request it" (McCarthy, 2014). Even when asked a more laden question, such as whether doctors should be permitted to "assist the patient to commit suicide if the patient requests it," approximately 60 percent approve (McCarthy, 2014).

Physician-assisted suicide is a form of voluntary active euthanasia that occurs when a "person helps another to actively end his or her life. It can include anything from providing a potentially lethal dose of medicine all the way to fully participating in a suicide" (Morhaim, 2012, p. 19). The term is usually used to mean instances in which a physician prescribes a patient a lethal dose of medication knowing that the patient intends to self-administer it (Hooyman & Kiyak, 2010). PAS is not a constitutionally protected right; the decision to legalize the practice is left to individual states (*Vacco v. Quill*, 1997; *Washington v. Glucksberg*, 1997). As of this writing, there are five states in the United States that allow a legal means through which people can choose PAS: Oregon, Washington, Montana, Vermont, and New Mexico (Ganzini, 2014; Eckholm, 2014). Oregon has had the law in place the longest, since 1997. Between 1997 and January 2015, 1,327 people received prescriptions to commit PAS, and

859 died by ingesting those medications (Oregon Public Health Division, 2015). Of those who died of PAS, roughly half were men and half were women, the median age was 71, 97 percent were white, and 46 percent had a college education or more (Oregon Public Health Division, 2015). There is no evidence that vulnerable persons, such as the uninsured or the mentally ill, were more likely to die than other persons (Battin et al., 2007). Interestingly, 90 percent of PAS decedents were enrolled in hospices, and nearly 80 percent were cancer patients (Oregon Public Health Division, 2015).

Palliative sedation, also known as "continuous deep sedation," is an intervention at the end of life that involves "the use of sedative medications to relieve intolerable and refractory distress by reduction in patient consciousness" (Morita et al., 2002, p. 452). The goal of PS is to achieve unconsciousness because "as far as is known, only such deep sedation is certain to prevent and treat the patient's physical and psychological suffering" (Billings, 2014, p. 213).

Perhaps the most controversial aspect of palliative sedation concerns the risk of sedating someone to the point of death. The *doctrine of double effect* suggests that intention is the most important aspect of the intervention. Even though there may be a known possibility of death, alleviating suffering and pain is the main intention of palliative sedation (Higgins & Altilio, 2008). An ethical consideration related to double effect is the concept of *proportionality*, which means that the benefits of an intervention should outweigh its burdens (Kirk & Mahon, 2010). This means that even though someone may suffer the burden of unconsciousness due to sedation, the benefit of pain alleviation is a more important result. When considering palliative sedation as a treatment for refractory distress, the idea of *imminence* is always considered. There is a general consensus that palliative sedation should be reserved as an intervention only when a physician has determined that a person has a very short period of time to left live, such as a few days (Billings, 2014).

PS was introduced in the mid- to late-1980s, and as a result of its novelty there remains a lack of conceptual understanding, clarity, protocol, and guidelines for its practice (Morita et al., 2002; Billings, 2014). In 1997, the Supreme Court indicated support for the use of PS. Justice Sandra Day O'Connor stated that "a patient who is suffering from a terminal illness and who is experiencing great pain has no legal barriers to obtaining medication, from qualified physicians, to alleviate that suffering, even to the point of causing unconsciousness and hastening death" (AMA, 2008, p. 3). Professional organizations waited another decade to weigh in. In 2008, the American Medical Association (2008, p. 2) along with the American Academy of Hospice and Palliative Medicine, came out in support of "the use of palliative sedation to the level of unconsciousness to relieve otherwise intractable suffering." In 2010, the National Hospice and Palliative Care Organization also indicated its support for palliative sedation as long as the terminal illness and imminence criteria were met (Kirk & Mahon, 2010). However, there is no single document outlining the implementation of PS practice guidelines on a national scale. Decisions regarding PS are ultimately left up to individual hospitals and hospices, although the practice does require informed consent from the patient or surrogate decision maker.

Physician and public attitudes about active euthanasia, PAS, and palliative sedation in the United States are, and will remain, contested. Physicians may face legal, personal, professional, and public conflict in agreeing to these options for their patients (Bergman Levy et al., 2013). Patients may also experience great turmoil, distress, and confusion about whether or not to pursue an active ending to the suffering caused by terminal illness. Further, terminally ill patients may not be cognizant of their conditions, and therefore may be unable to participate in medical decision making. Another layer of complexity is added to the challenges of ways of dying when surrogate decision makers are called upon to make choices about a loved one's end-of-life treatment approaches. Without clear clinical recommendations or consistent legal standards, these ways of dying remain complicated and controversial.

Discussion

In an era in which machines can sustain basic bodily functions such as circulation and respiration, dying persons—and we will all someday be dying persons—have important decisions to make. What quality of life do we desire? How much suffering are we willing to endure? Although individual patients have the autonomy to select treatment, these issues are societal as well as personal. Because taxpayers, via Medicare and Medicaid, bear part of the high financial cost of end-of-life care, they ought to have some say over what kinds of treatments are standard and to whom they are accessible. Further, societal debates about ethical and moral issues determine which types of death are legally permitted, and which constitute murder or manslaughter. Few Americans have experience with death and dying, yet they must become informed about the issues for their own well-being, often in the absence of accurate and thorough knowledge of the options. Educating Americans on these issues is necessary to ensure that we all have as much information as possible when the time comes for us to make decisions regarding our own ways of experiencing dying and death.

References

Alano, G.J., Pekmezaris, R., Tai, J.Y., Hussain, M.J., Jeune, J., Louis, B., . . . Wolf-Klein, G.P. (2010). Factors influencing older adults to complete advance directives. *Palliative and Supportive Care, 8*, 267–275. doi: 10.1017/S1478951510000064

American Medical Association (AMA). (2008). Sedation to unconsciousness in end-of-life care. *Report of the Council on Ethical and Judicial Affairs*. Report 5-A-08.

Ardelt, M. (2003). Physician-assisted death. In C.D. Bryant (Ed.) *Handbook of death and dying* (pp. 424–434). Thousand Oaks, CA: Sage Publications, Inc.

Arias, Elizabeth. (2014). *United States life tables, 2009*. Retrieved from http://www.cdc.gov/nchs/data/nvsr/nvsr62/nvsr62_07.pdf

Baker, M.E. (2002). Economic, political, and ethnic influences on end-of-life decision making: A decade in review. *Journal of Health and Social Policy, 14*, 27–39. doi: 10.1300/J045v14n03_02

Bakitas, M., Lyons, K.D., Hegel, M.T., Balan, S., Brokaw, F.C., Seville, J., . . . & Ahles, T.A. (2009). Effects of a palliative care intervention on clinical outcomes in patients with advanced cancer. *Journal of the American Medical Association, 302*, 741–749. doi:10.1001/jama.2009.1198

Barnato, A.E., McClellan, M.B., Kagay, C.R., & Garber, A.M. (2004). Trends in inpatient treatment intensity among Medicare beneficiaries at the end of life. *Health Services Research, 39*, 363–375. doi: 10.1111/j.1475-6773.2004.00232.x

Battin, M.P., van der Heide, A., Ganzini, L., van der Wal, G., & Onwuteaka-Philipsen, B.D. (2007). Legal physician-assisted dying in Oregon and the Netherlands: Evidence concerning the impact on patients in "vulnerable" groups. *Journal of Medical Ethics, 33*, 591–597. doi:10.1136/jme.2007.022335

Bergman Levy, T., Azar, S. Huberfeld, R., Siegel, A.M., & Strous, R.D. (2013). Attitudes toward euthanasia and assisted suicide: A comparison between psychiatrists and other physicians. *Bioethics, 27*(7), 402–408. doi:10.1111/j.1467-8519.2012.01968.x

Billings, J.A. (2014). Palliative sedation. In T.E. Quill & F.G. Miller (Eds.), *Palliative care and ethics* (pp. 209–230). New York, NY: Oxford University Press.

Carr, D., & Khodyakov, D. (2007). End-of-life health care planning among young-old adults: An assessment of psychosocial influences. *The Journals of Gerontology, Series B: Social Sciences, 62B*(2), 135–S141. doi: 10.1093/geronb/62.2.S135

Casarett, D., van Ness, P.H., O'Leary, J.R., & Fried, T.R. (2006). Are patient preferences for life sustaining treatment really a barrier to hospice enrollment for older adults with serious illness? *Journal of the American Geriatrics Society, 54*, 472–478. doi: 10.1111/j.1532-5415.2005.00628.x

Centers for Medicare & Medicaid Services. (2014). *Fact sheet: Medicare care choices model*. Retrieved from http://www.cms.gov/Newsroom/MediaReleaseDatabase/Fact-sheets/2014-Fact-sheets-items/2014–03–18.html

Center to Advance Palliative Care. (2011a). *2011 public opinion research on palliative care*. Retrieved from https://www.capc.org/media/filer_public/18/ab/18ab708c-f835–4380–921d-fbf729702e36/2011-public-opinion-research-on-palliative-care.pdf

Center to Advance Palliative Care. (2011b). *America's care of serious illness: A state-by-state report card on access to palliative care in our nation's hospitals*. Retrieved from www.capc.org/reportcard

Christakis, N. A. (1999). *Death foretold: Prophecy and prognosis in medical care*. Chicago: University of Chicago Press.

Chung, K., Essex, E., & Samson, L. F. (2008). Ethnic variation in timing of hospice referral: Does having no informal caregiver matter? *Journal of Palliative Medicine, 11*, 484–491. doi: 10.1089/jpm.2007.0149

Congressional Budget Office. (2013). *The 2013 long-term budget outlook*. Retrieved from http://www.cbo.gov/sites/default/files/cbofiles/attachments/44521-LTBO2013_0.pdf

Connor, S. R., Elwert, F., Spence, C., & Christakis, N. A. (2008). Racial disparity in hospice use in the United States in 2002. *Palliative Medicine, 22*, 205–213. doi: 10.1177/0269216308089305

Connor, S. R., Pyenson, B., Fitch, K., Spence, C., & Iwasaki, K. (2007). Comparing hospice and nonhospice patient survival among patients who die within a three-year window. *Journal of Pain and Symptom Management, 33*(3), 238–246. doi:10.1016/j.jpainsymman.2006.10.010

Cruzan v. Director, Missouri Department of Health, (88–1503), 497 U.S. 261 (1990)

Department of Health and Human Services, Centers for Disease Control and Prevention & National Center for Health Statistics. (2003). *Medical examiners' and coroners' handbook on death registration and fetal death reporting*. Retrieved from http://www.cdc.gov/nchs/data/misc/hb_me.pdf

Diem, S. J., Lantos, J. D., & Tulsky, J. A. (1996). Cardiopulmonary resuscitation on television: Miracles and misinformation. *New England Journal of Medicine, 334*, 1578–1582. doi: 10.1056/NEJM199606133342406

Douglas, R., & Brown, H. N. (2002). Patients' attitudes toward advance directives. *Journal of Nursing Scholarship, 34*(1), 61–65. doi: 10.1111/j.1547-5069.2002.00061.x

Donohoe, R. T., Haefeli, K., & Moore, F. (2006). Public perceptions and experiences of myocardial infarction, cardiac arrest, and CPR in London. *Resuscitation, 71*, 70–79. doi: 10.1016/j.resuscitation.2006.03.003

Eckholm, E. (2014, February 7). Aid in dying movement takes hold in some states. *The New York Times*. Retrieved from http://www.nytimes.com/2014/02/08/us/easing-terminal-patients-path-to-death-legally.html?_r=0

Emanuel, E. J. (1996). Cost savings at the end of life: What do the data show? *JAMA, 275*(24), 1907–1914. doi: 10.1001/jama.1996.03530480049040

Fagerlin, A., & Schneider, C. E. (2004). Enough: The failure of the living will. *Hastings Center Report, 34*(2), 30–42. doi: 10.2307/3527683

Feinberg, L. F. (2014). Moving toward person- and family-centered care. *Public Policy & Aging Report, 24*, 97–101. doi: 10.1093/ppar/pru027

Field, R. A., Soar, J., Nolan, J. P., & Perkins, G. D. (2011). Epidemiology and outcome of cardiac arrests reported in the lay press: An observational study. *Journal of the Royal Society of Medicine, 104*, 525–531. doi: 10.1258/jrsm.2011.110228

Ford, D. W., Nietert, P. J., Zapka, J., Zoller, J. S., & Silvestri, G. A., (2008). Barriers to hospice enrollment among lung cancer patients: A survey of family members and physicians. *Palliative and Supportive Care, 6*, 357–362. doi: 10.1017/S1478951508000564

Gade, G., Venohr, I., Conner, D., McGrady, K., Beane, J., Richardson, R. H., . . . & della Penna, R. (2008). Impact of an inpatient palliative care team: A randomized controlled trial. *Journal of Palliative Medicine, 11*, 180–190. doi:10.1089/jpm.2007.0055

Ganzini, L. (2014). Lessons learned from legalized physician-assisted death in Oregon and Washington. In T. E. Quill & F. G. Miller (Eds.), *Palliative care and ethics* (pp. 266–280). New York, NY: Oxford University Press.

Goldstein, N. E., Cohen, L. M., Arnold, R. M., Goy, E., Arons, S., & Ganzini, L. (2012). Prevalence of formal accusations of murder and euthanasia against physicians. *Journal of Palliative Medicine, 15*, 334–339. doi: 10.1089/jpm.2011.0234

Gordijn, B. (2004). Alzheimer disease and euthanasia. In R. B. Purtilo & H. A. M. J. ten Have (Eds.), *Ethical foundations of palliative care for Alzheimer disease* (pp. 218–225). Baltimore, MD: The Johns Hopkins University Press.

Greenlee, K. (2014). Making our own decisions about serious illness. *Public Policy & Aging Report, 24*, 81–85. doi: 10.1093/ppar/pru026

Higgins, P., & Altilio, T. (2008). Palliative sedation: An essential place for clinical excellence. *Journal of Social Work in End-Of-Life & Palliative Care, 3*(4), 3–30. doi:10.1080/15524250802003240

Hooyman, N. R., & Kiyak, H. A. (2010). *Social gerontology: A multidisciplinary perspective* (9th ed.). Boston, MA: Allyn and Bacon.

Hoyert, D. L. (2012). *75 years of mortality in the United States, 1935–2010*. Retrieved from http://www.cdc.gov/nchs/data/databriefs/db88.pdf

Johnson, K. S., Kuchibhatla, M., & Tulsky, J. A. (2009). Racial differences in self-reported exposure to information about hospice care. *Journal of Palliative Medicine, 12*, 921–927. doi: 10.1089/jpm.2009.0066

Jotkowitz, A., Glick, S., & Gesundheit, B. (2008). A case against justified non-voluntary active euthanasia (The Groningen Protocol). *The American Journal of Bioethics*, 8, 23–26. doi: 10.1080/15265160802513085

Jox, R. J., Schaider, A., Marckmann, G., & Borasio, G. D. (2012). Medical futility at the end of life: The perspectives of intensive care and palliative care clinicians. *Journal of Medical Ethics, 38*, 540–545. doi: 10.1136/medethics-2011-100479

Keary, S., & Moorman, S. M. (2015). Patient-physician end-of-life discussions in the routine care of Medicare beneficiaries. *Journal of Aging & Health*. Online before print. doi: 10.1177/0898264315569458

Kelley, A. S., Deb, P., Du, Q., Carlson, M. D. A., & Morrison, R. S. (2013). Hospice enrollment saves money for Medicare and improves care quality across a number of different lengths-of-stay. *Health Affairs, 32*, 552–561. doi: 10.1377/hlthaff.2012.0851

Kirk, T., & Mahon, M. (2010). NHPCO position statement and commentary on the use of palliative sedation in imminently dying terminally ill patients. *Journal of Pain and Symptom Management, 39*(5), 914–923. doi: 10.1016/j.jpainsymman.2010.01.009

Kon, A. A. (2007). Neonatal euthanasia is unsupportable: The Groningen Protocol should be abandoned. *Theoretical Medicine and Bioethics,* 5, 453–463. doi: 10.1007/s11017-007-9047-8

Larson, E. J., & Eaton, T. A. (1997). The limits of advance directives: A history and assessment of the patient self-determination act. *Scholarly Works.* Paper 260. Retrieved from http://digitalcommons.law.uga.edu/fac_artchop/260

Lindemann, H., & Verkerk, M. (2008). Ending the life of a newborn: The Groningen Protocol. *Hastings Center Report, 38*, 42–51.

Lopez-Acevedo, M., Havrilesky, L. J., Broadwater, G., Kamal, A. H., Aberneth, A. P., Berchuck, A., . . . Lee, P. S. (2013). Timing of end-of-life care discussion with performance of end-of-life quality indicators in ovarian cancer. *Gynecologic Oncology, 30*(1), 156–161. doi: 10.1016/j.ygyno.2013.04.010

Mack, J. W., Cronin, A., Taback, N., Huskamp, H. A., Keating, N. L., Malin, J. L., . . . Weeks, J. C. (2012). End-of-life care discussions among patients with advanced cancer: A cohort study. *Annals of Internal Medicine, 156*, 204–210. doi: 10.7326/0003-4819-156-3-201202070-00008

Mack, J. W., Weeks, J. C., Wright, A. A., Block, S. D., & Prigerson, H. G. (2010). End-of-life discussions, goal attainment, and distress at the end-of-life: Predictors and outcomes of receipt of care consistent with preferences. *Journal of Clinical Oncology, 28*(7), 1203–1208. doi: 10.1200/JCO.2009.25.4672

Manninen, B. A. (2006). A case for justified non-voluntary active euthanasia: Exploring the ethics of the Groningen Protocol. *Journal of Medical Ethics, 32*, 643–651. doi: 10.1136/jme.2005.014845

McCarthy, J. (2014). *Seven in 10 Americans back euthanasia.* Retrieved from http://www.gallup.com/poll/171704/seven-americans-back-euthanasia.aspx

Meier, D. E. (2011). Increased access to palliative care and hospice services: Opportunities to improve value in health care. *Milbank Quarterly, 89*, 343–380. doi: 10.1111/j.1468-0009.2011.00632.x

Meng, H., Dobbs, D., Weng, S., & Hyer, K. (2013). Hospice use and public expenditures at the end of life in assisted living residents in a Florida Medicaid waiver program. *Journal of the American Geriatrics Society, 61*(10), 1777–1781. doi: 10.1111/jgs.12459

Moorman, S. M. (2011). The importance of feeling understood in marital conversations about end-of-life health care. *Journal of Social and Personal Relationships, 28*(1), 100–116. doi: 10.1177/0265407510386137

Moorman, S. M., & Inoue, M. (2013a). Persistent problems in end-of-life planning among young and middle-aged American couples. *The Journals of Gerontology, Series B: Psychological Sciences and Social Sciences, 68*(1): 97–106. doi: 10.1093/geronb/gbs103

Moorman, S. M., & Inoue, M. (2013b). Predicting a partner's end-of-life preferences, or substituting one's own? *Journal of Marriage and Family, 75*(3), 734–745. doi: 10.1111/jomf.12030

Morhaim, D. (2012). *The better end: Surviving (and dying) on your own terms in today's modern medical world.* Baltimore, MD: The Johns Hopkins University Press.

Morita, T., Tsuneto, S., & Shima, Y. (2002). Definition of sedation for symptom relief: A systematic literature review and a proposal of operational criteria. *Journal of Pain and Symptom Management, 24*(4), 447–453. doi: 10.1016/S0885-3924(02)00499-2

Morrison, L. J., Neumar, R. W., Zimmerman, J. L., Link, M. S., Newby, K., McMullan, P. W., . . . & Edelson, D. P. (2013). Strategies for improving survival after in-hospital cardiac arrest in the United States: 2013 consensus recommendations. *Circulation, 127*, 1538–1563. doi: 10.1161/CIR.0b013e31828b2770

National Hospice and Palliative Care Organization. (2014). *The Medicare hospice benefit.* Retrieved from http://hospiceactionnetwork.org/linked_documents/get_informed/policy_resources/Medicare_Hospice_Benefit_print.pdf

Nicholas, L. H., Langa, K. M., Iwashyna, T. J., & Weir, D. R. (2011). Regional variation in the association between advance directives and end-of-life Medicare expenditures. *Journal of the American Medical Association, 306*(13), 1447–1453. doi: 10.1001/jama.2011.1410

Oregon Public Health Division. (2015). *Oregon's death with dignity act: 2014.* Retrieved from http://public.health.oregon.gov/ProviderPartnerResources/EvaluationResearch/DeathwithDignityAct/Documents/year17.pdf

Palda, V. A., Bowman, K. W., McLean, R. F., & Chapman, M. G. (2005). "Futile" care: Do we provide it? Why? *Journal of Critical Care, 20,* 207–213. doi: 10.1016/j.jcrc.2005.05.006

Pollack, K. M., Morhaim, D., & Williams, M. A. (2010). The public's perspectives on advance directives: Implications for state legislative and regulatory policy. *Health Policy, 96*, 57–63. doi: 10.1016/j.healthpol.2010.01.004

Rao, J. K., Anderson, L. A., Lin, F. C., & Laux, J. P. (2014). Completion of advance directives among U.S. consumers. *American Journal of Preventive Medicine, 46*(1), 46–70. doi: 10.1016/j.amepre.2013.09.008

Resnick, H. E., Schuur, J. D., Heineman, J., Stone, R., & Weissman, J. S. (2009). Advance directives in nursing home residents ≥65 years: United States 2004. *American Journal of Hospice and Palliative Medicine, 25*(6), 476–482. doi: 10.1177/1049909108322295

Riley, G. F., & Lubitz, J. D. (2010). Long-term trends in Medicare payments in the last year of life. *Health Services Research, 45*, 565–576. doi: 10.1111/j.1475-6773.2010.01082.x

Rubin, E. B., & Bernat, J. L. (2014). Voluntarily stopping eating and drinking. In T. E. Quill & F. G. Miller (Eds.), *Palliative care and ethics* (pp. 231–246). New York, NY: Oxford University Press.

Sabatino, C. P. (2014). Advance care planning tools that educate, engage, and empower. *Public Policy & Aging Report, 24*, 107–111. doi: 10.1093/ppar/pru018

Schickedanz, A. D., Schillinger, D., Landefeld, C. S., Knight, S. J., Williams, B. A., & Sudore, R. L. (2009). A clinical framework for improving the advance care planning process: Start with patients' self-identified barriers. *Journal of the American Geriatrics Society, 57*, 31–39. doi: 10.1111/j.1532-5415.2008.02093.x

Schneiderman, L. J. (2011). Defining medical futility and improving medical care. *Bioethical Inquiry, 8*, 123–131. doi: 10.1007/s11673-011–9293-3

Seymour, J. E. (1999). Revisiting medicalisation and "natural" death. *Social Science & Medicine, 49*, 691–704.

Shalowitz, D. I., Garrett-Mayer, E., & Wendler, D. (2006). The accuracy of surrogate decision makers. *Archives of Internal Medicine, 166*(5), 493–497. doi: 10.1001/archinte.166.5.493

Silveira, M. J., Connor, S. R., Goold, S. D., McMahon, L. F., & Feudtner, C. (2011). Community supply of hospice: Does wealth play a role? *Journal of Pain and Symptom Management, 42*, 76–82. doi: 10.1016/j.jpainsymman.2010.09.016

Silveira, M. J., Kim, S. Y. H., & Langa, K. M. (2010). Advance directives and outcomes of surrogate decision making before death. *New England Journal of Medicine, 362*, 1211–1218. doi: 10.1056/NEJMsa0907901

Singer, A. E., Meeker, D., Teno, J. M., Lynn, J., Lunney, J. R., & Lorenz, K. A. (2015). Symptom trends in the last year of life from 1998 to 2010: A cohort study. *Annals of Internal Medicine, 162*(3), 175–183. doi: 10.7326/M13-1609

Smith, S., Brick, A., O'Hara, S., & Normand, C. (2014). Evidence on the cost and cost-effectiveness of palliative care: A literature review. *Palliative Medicine, 28*, 130–150. doi: 10.1177/0269216313493466

Snyder, L. (2012). American College of Physicians ethics manual: Sixth edition. *Annals of Internal Medicine, 156*, 73–104.

Steinhauser, K. E., Christakis, N. A., Clipp, E. C., McNeilly, M., McIntyre, L. M., & Tulsky, J. A. (2000a). Factors considered important at the end of life by patients, families, physicians, and other care providers. *Journal of the American Medical Association, 284*(19), 2476–2482. doi:10.1001/jama.284.19.2476

Steinhauser, K. E., Clipp, E. C., McNeilly, M., Christakis, N. A., McIntyre, L. M., & Tulsky, J. A. (2000b). In search of a good death: Observations of patients, families, and providers. *Annals of Internal Medicine, 132*(10), 825–832. doi: 10.7326/0003-4819-132-10-200005160-00011

Temel, J. S., Greer, J. A., Muzikansky, A., Gallagher, E. R., Admane, S., Jackson, V. A., . . . & Lynch, T. J. (2010). Early palliative care for patients with metastatic non-small-cell lung cancer. *The New England Journal of Medicine, 363*, 733–742. doi: 10.1056/NEJMoa1000678

Teno, J. M., Mitchell, S. L., Kuo, S. K., Gozalo, P. L., Rhodes, R. L., Lima, J. C., & Mor, V. (2011). Decision-making and outcomes of feeding tube insertion: A five-state study. *Journal of the American Geriatrics Society, 59*(5), 881–886. doi: 10.1111/j.1532-5415.2011.03385.x

Teno, J. M., Shu, J. E., Casarett, D., Spence, C., Rhodes, R., & Connor, S. (2007). Timing of referral to hospice and quality of care: Length of stay and bereaved family members' perceptions of the timing of hospice referral. *Journal of Pain and Symptom Management, 34*, 120–125. doi: 10.1016/j.jpainsymman.2007.04.014

Thorevska, N., Tilluckdharry, L., Tickoo, S., Havasi, A., Amoateng-Adjepong, Y., & Manthous, C. A. (2005). Patients' understanding of advance directives and cardiopulmonary resuscitation. *Journal of Critical Care, 20*, 26–34. doi: 10.1016/j.jcrc.2004.11.002

Timmermans, S. (2005). Death brokering: Constructing culturally appropriate death. *Sociology of Health and Illness, 27*, 993–1013. doi: 10.1111/j.1467-9566.2005.00467.x

Vacco v. Quill, 117S.Ct. 2293; 138 L.Ed.2d 834 (U.S. 1997).

Van Aalst-Cohen, E. S., Riggs, R., & Byock, I. R. (2008). Palliative care in medical school curricula: A survey of United States medical schools. *Journal of Palliative Medicine, 11*, 1200–1202. doi:10.1089/jpm.2008.0118

Verhagen, E. (2013). The Groningen Protocol for newborn euthanasia: Which way did the slippery slope tilt? *Journal of Medical Ethics, 39*, 293–295. doi: 10.1136/medethics-2013-101402

Verhagen, E., & Sauer, P.J.J. (2005). The Groningen Protocol: Euthanasia in severely ill newborns. *The New England Journal of Medicine, 352*, 959–962. doi: 10.1056/NEJMp058026

Washington v. Glucksberg, 117S.Ct. 2258; 138 L.Ed.2d 772 (U.S. 1997).

Welch, L. C., Miller, S. C., Martin, E. W., & Nanda, A. (2008). Referral and timing of referral to hospice care in nursing homes: The significant role of staff members. *The Gerontologist, 48*, 477–484. doi: 10.1093/geront/48.4.477

Wilson, D. R., & Crowley, C. (2014). What patients and their families think about unwanted medical treatment. *Public Policy & Aging Report, 24*, 124–125. doi: 10.1093/ppar/pru033

World Health Organization. (2014). *WHO definition of palliative care*. Retrieved from http://www.who.int/cancer/palliative/definition/en/

Zimmerman, C. (2007). Death denial: Obstacle or instrument for palliative care? An analysis of clinical literature. *Sociology of Health and Illness, 29*, 297–314. doi: 10.1111/j.1467-9566.2007.00495.x

Zimmerman, C. (2012). Acceptance of dying: A discourse analysis of palliative care literature. *Social Science & Medicine, 75*, 217–224. doi: 10.1016/j.socscimed.2012.02.047

CHAPTER ELEVEN

Grief and Bereavement

Deborah Carr

Death is one of life's few certainties. All persons will die, and nearly all will survive the death of a loved one. Although death is universal, the timing, cause, and context of death vary widely over the life course (Carr, 2012). Consequently, the experience of bereavement, or losing a loved one through death, also varies widely over the life course and by gender. Grief is a typical reaction to the loss of a loved one, where survivors experience psychological and physical symptoms in the weeks and months that follow, and in some cases precede, the death (Rando, 1986; Weiss, 2008). The extent to which a bereaved person grieves, and the duration, nature and intensity of one's emotional distress is closely linked to the larger context of the death, one's relationship to the decedent, concurrent stressors, and one's coping resources (Bonanno et al., 2002; Carr, 2012). Survivors' reactions to loss vary widely, with some suffering from prolonged and even debilitating grief (Boelen & Prigerson, 2013), whereas others recover quickly, experiencing only short-lived symptoms of sadness (Bonanno et al., 2002).

In this chapter, I provide a brief overview of the nature of death and dying in the contemporary United States, which sets the stage for understanding the personal meaning and context of late-life bereavement. I then describe classic and contemporary work on grief and its subtypes. I then summarize research on distinctive types of family bereavement in late life, and show how and why the deaths of one's spouse, sibling(s), parent(s), and adult children affect the lives of older adults. Next, I focus in depth on the demographic, psychosocial, and contextual factors that shape grief in the face of one particular type of late-life bereavement: The loss of one's spouse/partner. This particular focus reflects the fact that the vast majority of research on late-life bereavement focuses on the specific case of widow(er)hood. Finally, I highlight unanswered questions regarding loss and bereavement among older adults and suggest avenues for future research.

Death and Dying in the United States: A Brief Historical Overview

In order to understand late-life bereavement, a brief overview of mortality patterns is necessary. When, how, and of which causes older adults die carry important implications for their survivors' emotional, physical, and financial well-being. An epidemiologic transition occurred over the past two centuries, in which infant and child deaths were replaced by late-life deaths, and infectious diseases were replaced by lifestyle-related chronic diseases as the leading causes of death (Olshansky & Ault, 1986; Omran, 1971). In the 19th and early 20th centuries, deaths occurred primarily due to infectious diseases, such as diphtheria and pneumonia; death occurred relatively quickly after the initial onset of symptoms. Throughout the 20th century, improved sanitation and nutrition, immunization for communicable diseases, effective treatments for infections, and other medical advances dramatically reduced mortality among younger persons, and increased life expectancy (IOM, 2014). While median life expectancy in 1900 was just 46 years old, it approached 80 years old in 2009 (Arias, 2014).

Today, death is largely a late-life phenomenon. Roughly three-quarters of the 2.4 million deaths in the United States in 2010 were to persons aged 65 and older (Federal Interagency Forum on Aging-Related Statistics, 2012). The leading causes of death among older adults are chronic and progressive illnesses including heart disease, cancer, chronic lower respiratory diseases, stroke, Alzheimer's disease, and diabetes (Federal Interagency Forum on Aging-Related Statistics, 2012). Late-life deaths today typically occur months or even years after the initial onset of chronic illness, thus the prolonged "living-dying interval" (Pattison, 1977) between diagnosis and death is typically marked by compromised quality of life, comorbid conditions, functional impairment, mobility limitations, impaired cognitive functioning, physical discomfort, and the need for assistance with activities of daily living (ADLs) and instrumental activities of daily living (IADLs). In 2009, more than 40 percent of persons aged 65 and older required assistance with ADLs or IADLs (Federal Interagency Forum on Aging-Related Statistics, 2012). The number of older Americans with serious cognitive impairment is also high and rising; the number of older adults suffering from Alzheimer's disease and related dementias is expected to grow from 5.5 million in 2010 to 8.7 million in 2030 (HHS/ASPE, 2013).

Because most late-life deaths occur following a period of chronic illness, the majority of older adults who experience the loss of a spouse, sibling, parent, or even an adult child typically have witnessed some suffering, have played a role as a caregiver, or have had the time to prepare practically and emotionally for the impending death. Caregivers to loved ones with dementia also must grapple with the loss of their loved one's ability to communicate and to be one's usual self prior to loss (Chan et al., 2013). In short, for most older bereaved persons, death is not an acute, sudden, and unexpected event, but is rather a slowly unfolding process. These dying trajectories carry implications for the nature and timing of grief.

Grief: Definitions and Subtypes

While bereavement refers to the objective situation of having lost a loved one through death, grief refers to the emotional or physical reactions of distress that one has in response to the loss. Grief has been described as "the cost we pay for being able to love in the way we do" (Archer, 1999, 5). Mourning, by contrast, refers to the public display or expression of grief, such as wearing black clothing or draping the coffins of deceased military personnel with American flags (Fontana & Keene, 2009). Rich anthropological research has documented cross-cultural differences in mourning practices, although the topic is beyond the scope of this chapter (see Robben, 2009).

As we shall see later in this chapter, the intensity and duration of one's grief symptoms vary widely based on who the decedent is, the cause of death, and a range of other personal and situational factors. Despite this heterogeneity, a core theme in grief research is distinguishing between normal grief and grief that is deemed complicated or prolonged (Prigerson et al., 2008; Shear et al., 2011). Although the boundaries demarcating these different types of grief are both fuzzy and controversial, a general assumption is that some sadness following the death of a loved one is normal and that grief symptoms are problematic only when they extend for prolonged periods of time, or inhibit one's daily functioning. For example, the types of grief viewed as most problematic and thus most in need of professional attention are chronic or prolonged grief (Shear et al., 2011), which is characterized by long-lasting symptoms associated with intense grief. Yet at the same time, individuals who show no symptoms of sadness historically were considered pathological. For example, delayed, inhibited, or absent grief were viewed as indications that an individual may not attach to significant others in a meaningful way, given that grief is a consequence of severed bonds to an important attachment object (e.g., Archer, 1999; Weiss, 2008).

One of the most hotly contested debates in grief research, theory, and practice over the past two decades has been the exclusion of bereavement in the *Diagnostic and Statistical Manual* (*DSM*; American Psychiatric Association, 2013). The *DSM* provides mental health practitioners with a definition and treatment guidelines for mental health disorders. In the *DSM-4*, American Psychiatric Association (1994), persons who experienced two months or more of sadness were excluded from receiving a major depression diagnosis if those symptoms were a result of a recent bereavement. This exclusion suggested that sadness for a delimited time period is normal in the face of a major loss and as such was not a pathological condition in need of treatment. However, in the *DSM-5*, American Psychiatric Association (2013), the bereavement exclusion was removed, and thus enables practitioners to diagnose (and medicate) some bereaved persons as suffering from major depressive disorder. Impassioned debates continue among researchers and practitioners, and hinge on competing notions about whether sadness is a normal reaction to loss, and whether untreated symptoms will fade with the passage of time or require more serious interventions (e.g., Shear, 2011, Wakefield & First, 2012). Some of the most compelling empirical evidence to date suggests that for older adults, in particular, most bereaved spouses experience brief spells of depressive symptoms but then quickly return to their preloss functioning (Bonanno et al., 2002), although a small minority experiences persistent and debilitating symptoms that require treatment (Shear et al., 2011).

Anticipatory Grief

Most writings on grief focus on a bereaved person's psychological and physiological responses after the death occurs. However, in the case of older adults, as noted earlier, the majority of deaths tend to occur after a prolonged illness. As such, one's feelings of loss, sadness, and loneliness may begin far earlier than the actual death, and may begin to unfold as one is caring for an ailing loved one, or watching the personhood of their loved one slip away as dementia symptoms take over (Chan et al., 2013; Rando, 1986). While these individuals may experience sadness during the dying process, they may ultimately be better prepared for the death when it arrives.

For example, researchers have administered grief surveys to caregivers when they were still providing care for their loved ones and found that predeath grief symptoms were highly correlated with feelings of distress (e.g., Meuser & Marwit, 2001). Several recent studies also show that those experiencing grief symptoms prior to the loss have reduced symptoms postloss, with some bereaved persons even reporting relief. For example, one study of older widows in Sweden found that 40 percent described the preloss period as more stressful than the postloss period. For these widows of men who died of cancer, preparatory grief involved emotional stress, intense preoccupation with the dying, longing for his/her former personality, loneliness, tearfulness, cognitive dysfunction, irritability, anger and social withdrawal, and a need to talk (Johansson & Grimby, 2012). However, they also reported resilience and effective coping after the loss, in part because the "living-dying interval" (Pattison, 1977) provided a time and space to prepare for the impending death.

Family Bereavement in Late Life

The primary types of family bereavement experienced by older adults are the deaths of spouses or romantic partners, siblings, parents, and adult children.

Spouse and Partner Loss

Spousal loss can occur at any age, yet in the United States and most wealthy nations today, it is a transition overwhelmingly experienced by persons aged 65 and older. Of the roughly 900,000 persons widowed annually in the United States, nearly three-quarters fall into this age category (Federal Interagency Forum on Aging-Related Statistics, 2012). Because life expectancy is roughly 79 for men and 84 for women, women are much more likely than men to become widowed (Miniño & Murphy, 2012). Among persons aged 65 to 74, 26 percent of women but just 7 percent of men are widowed; at ages 75 and more, these percentages jump to 58 percent of women and 21 percent of men. This stark gender gap also reflects the fact that widowers are far more likely than widows to remarry and thus may exit the widowed category. Widows are less likely than widowers to remarry because of a dearth of potential partners. Among persons aged 65 and older in the United States, the sex ratio is 1.5 women per every one man and by age 85, this ratio is more than 3 women per every man. As a result, few widows have the opportunity to remarry even if they would like to do so. Additionally, cultural norms encourage men to marry women younger than themselves, so widowed men may opt to remarry a younger woman, whereas older widows do not typically have that option (Federal Interagency Forum on Aging-Related Statistics, 2012). Qualitative interviews also show that older women who were caregivers to dying husbands, especially those dying from prolonged or treatment-intensive illness such as cancer are reluctant to remarry again and possibly resume the stressful role of caregiver (Bennett, Hughes, & Smith, 2003).

Far less is known about the number of bereaved persons following a long-term same-sex relationship. According to data from the 2010 U.S. Census, there are currently 605,000 same-sex households in the United States, 27 percent of whom identify as married. The average age of the partners in same-sex households is 48; roughly 13 percent are 65 or older, whereas 17 percent are between 55 and 64 (Lofquist, 2011). Thus a sizeable number of older gays and lesbians are at risk of losing a partner. As I discuss later in this chapter, gay and lesbian couples face both distinctive challenges yet possess protective resources as they cope with the loss of their partner.

Sibling Loss

Studies of sibling bereavement in late life are rare; most studies of the death of a brother or sister are focused on childhood and adolescence (e.g., Devita-Raeburn, 2004). This omission is troubling, given that most older adults have at least one living sibling, and most have emotionally close and mutually supportive relationships (White, 2001). Theoretical writings propose that the death of a sibling may have profound effects on older adults because "it marks an end to what is expected to be one of the longest and most intimate relationships of a lifetime" (Mahon, 1997).

One of the few empirical studies of adjustment to sibling loss in late life reveals that sibling death is linked with heightened depressive symptoms, and that this association is partly explained by the fear of death and sense of personal vulnerability that is triggered by a sibling's demise (Cicirelli, 2009). Because most siblings are close in age and spent their formative years together, the death of one sibling may render the other acutely aware of his or her own mortality. Relationships among surviving siblings typically grow closer following sibling death (Moss & Moss, 1989), and siblings with strained relationships may work to make amends, especially as they cope with the challenges of aging including illness, cognitive decline, and caregiving for parents (Hays, Gold, & Pieper, 1997).

Parental Loss

With rising life expectancy in recent decades, many older adults have at least one living parent, and the proportion of persons aged 65+ with a living parent is expected to increase further among future cohorts. Most older adults with a living parent will eventually face the death of that parent. However, very little is known about bereavement experiences of older adult children who survive the loss of very aged parents. Moss and Moss (1983–1984) attribute this research gap to the facts that late-life mortality is normative, and adult children have limited daily contact with their aging parent(s). As such, many presume that the daily lives of older adult children may not be disrupted by parental death, given a norm of residential independence in the United States and many other wealthy nations. However, adult children play an active role in end-of-life decision making (Carr & Khodyakov, 2007) and are the most common source of informal care to aging parents (Wolff & Kasper, 2006). Given adult children's high levels of engagement with their parents' health and health care, parental death remains "an unexpected crisis for most healthy, well-functioning adults" (p. 7) and also "represents a rite of passage into a new adult identity" (Umberson, 2003, p. 8).

A handful of studies have explored psychological reactions to late-life parental death and find wide variation based on the gender of parent and child, and nature of the late relationship. An estimated 45 percent of adult children experience somatic reactions to the death of a parent and roughly 10–15 percent report declines in overall health (Scharlach & Fredriksen, 1993). Symptoms of anxiety and depression often occur immediately after the death yet rarely persist in the longer term (Scharlach & Fredriksen, 1993). After six months, there is generally a significant decline in these emotional reactions to death (Pratt, Walker, & Wood, 1992). Umberson and Chen (1994) also found that adults who had recently lost a parent had significantly more frequent alcohol use and more depressive symptoms than their peers without a parental loss, and effects were largest for those who had positive relationships with their late parent. Grief symptoms also are linked to the nature of the death; some studies suggest that sudden deaths or deaths that the adult child feels partly responsible for are particularly likely to trigger symptoms of distress (Horowitz et al., 1984).

Other studies suggest that the toll of parental death is more severe when the second parent dies (Marshall, 2004). Some research also suggests that sibling relationships may grow closer upon the death of a second parent, as the surviving children must develop new rituals and practices to make up for those previously upheld by their parents, such as family holiday meals (Russo, 2010). In sum, while little is known about older adults' adjustment to elderly parents' deaths, the literature generally concludes that effects are short-lived, although the early weeks and months are marked by profound sadness and identity shifts, which are particularly acute when a second parent dies and the surviving child(ren) must assume the identity as the most senior member of their family line (Rosenblatt, 2000).

Child Loss

The death of a child is generally considered the most distressing event a parent can withstand, as it betrays that assumption of a natural order in which children outlive their parents (Hazzard et al., 1992). Extensive research explores the effects of parents' psychological and physical well-being, marital stability, and economic well-being following a child's death, with studies uniformly showing devastating effects that often linger for years (Klass, 1988). The bulk of this research is focused on the deaths of children under the age of 18 and shows that parental distress is particularly acute when the child's death was sudden due to causes such as SIDS, suicide, murder, or accidents (Institute of Medicine, 2003).

Far less research is focused on older adults' adjustment to the death of an adult child, although the general patterns that emerge are similar to those found earlier in the life course (Moss et al., 1986). However, the specific symptoms evidenced among surviving parents differ based on the expectedness and cause of their child's death, with sudden deaths such as murders and suicide eliciting symptoms of anger and shock, similar to PSTD. By contrast, deaths that occur following long chronic illnesses such as cancer are more often accompanied by anticipatory grief symptoms prior to the death (e.g., Shanfield, Benjamin, & Swain, 1984; Van Humbeeck et al., 2013). One way for older parents to adapt to the untimely death of an adult child is to maintain strong ties with their grandchild(ren) who were offspring of their now-deceased son or daughter and in doing so maintain their identity as a parent (Blank, 1998).

Surviving Spousal Bereavement: Risk and Protective Factors

Widowhood, or the loss of a spouse/romantic partner, is the most well-researched area of late-life family bereavement, reflecting the primacy of marriage in the lives of most older adults (Carr & Moorman, 2011). Older bereaved spouses vary widely in their social, emotional, and behavioral adjustment to loss. Some may have minor symptoms of depression and anxiety during the first six months following loss (Bonanno et al., 2002), whereas others may experience severe, debilitating, and persistent symptoms, including complicated and prolonged grief (Prigerson, Vanderwerker, & Maciejewski, 2008). Although myriad influences, including biological, psychological, social, and economic factors affect one's adjustment, I focus here on five sets of influences that recent studies have identified as particularly important: sociodemographic factors (age, cohort, gender, sexual orientation, and race) and four potentially modifiable factors: the nature of the late marital relationship, conditions surrounding the death, social support and integration, and other co-occurring losses and stressors.

Sociodemographic Influences on Partner Bereavement

The meaning, context, and personal consequences of spouse and partner bereavement vary based on one's social location, including one's age, birth cohort, gender, sexual orientation, and race/ethnicity. Although researchers have investigated extensively the ways that age and gender shape spousal bereavement, comparisons across other subgroups of older adults are rare. One reason for the limited research on race and sexual orientation differences in bereavement experiences reflect data availability. Most research on adjustment to late-life spousal loss focuses on mental and physical health symptoms during the first 12 to 18 months postloss, as symptoms typically fade after that time (e.g., Bonanno et al., 2002). However, given the relatively small number of recently bereaved persons in any cross-sectional study of bereavement, and the relatively low proportion of older adults identified as a sexual or racial minority, most data sets used to study spousal bereavement would not have adequate sample sizes to explore these particular points of intersectionality. For example, in 2010, only 9 and 7 percent of persons aged 65 or older identified as black or Latino, respectively (Federal Interagency Forum on Aging-Related Statistics, 2012), while only 2 percent identified as gay, lesbian, or bisexual (Gates & Newport, 2012).

Studying cohort differences also is challenging, as such studies would require not only multiple interviews with bereaved persons to track their adjustment over time but comparable interviews would need to be done at different points in historical time to capture the distinctive experiences of different birth cohorts. Taken together, research on subgroup differences in bereavement and grief underscore that spousal loss is not a monolithic experience and sheds light on the ways that social factors shape the quality of one's marriages and one's access to psychosocial, economic, and instrumental resources that may ease adjustment to loss.

Age. Spouse or partner bereavement has profoundly different meanings and consequences for older versus younger persons. Older adults have risk factors that render them particularly vulnerable to the emotional and physical health consequences of spousal loss, yet they also possess skills, experiences, social resources, and even cognitive capacities that enable them to adapt to loss. Older adults are more likely than younger persons to have experienced the deaths of significant other prior to spousal loss, and they may be better equipped to make sense of and cope with their most recent loss (Thompson et al., 1991). With older age, spousal loss may be at least somewhat expected. More than half of all women over age 65 in the United States are widowed (Federal Interagency Forum on Aging-Related Statistics, 2012); thus, older women may anticipate and prepare for the deaths of their husbands as they observe their peers experiencing spousal loss (Silverman, 2004). They also may turn to their widowed peers for emotional support and advice after their loss. By contrast, deaths to younger adults are more likely to occur suddenly and under very distressing circumstances, such as murders or accidents. Given that predictable, anticipated life transitions are less stressful than unexpected ones (George, 1993), older bereaved spouses may experience a less difficult readjustment than their younger counterparts.

Research also suggests developmental reasons why older adults tend to have less acute symptoms of depression in the face of loss, relative to their younger counterparts. Compared with younger adults, older adults have reduced emotional reactivity, or a greater capacity to manage or regulate their emotional states (Carstensen & Turk-Charles, 1994). As a result, their grief reactions also are shorter lived and less intense, compared with younger bereaved persons (Nolen-Hoeksema & Ahrens, 2002). Emotional reactivity declines in late life due to a variety of factors: biological decreases in autonomic arousal, the greater habituation of older adults to emotional life events, adherence to cultural expectations that the elderly should not be too emotional, and shifts in the relative salience of emotion versus cognition in late life (Carstensen & Turk-Charles, 1994). Older adults also are believed to possess wisdom, which may help minimize loss-related distress; they may respond to adverse life events with equanimity and acceptance (Baltes, Smith, & Staudinger, 1992).

In late life, bereaved heterosexual adults also may be better prepared to manage the practical tasks that were once managed by their late spouse. The boundaries demarcating traditional men's roles and women's roles in marriage become blurred as husbands and wives age. Although older married couples abide by a gender-typed division of household labor, just as younger couples do, this division may change as older adults face health declines and limitations to daily functioning (Szinovacz, 2000). The onset of physical health problems may render older adults less able to perform the specialized homemaking or home maintenance tasks they performed earlier in the life course. For instance, if a wife's physical limitations prevent her from preparing meals or cleaning, her husband may take over those duties. Likewise, cognitive decline in a husband may result in a wife's increased involvement in estate planning and other financial decisions that previously were managed by the husband. Older adults may gradually take on their spouses' tasks even prior to widowhood, and thus they may be better prepared on the death of a spouse (Carr, 2004).

Yet older adults also have important vulnerabilities. They are more likely than younger persons to experience co-occurring stressors that may overwhelm their ability to cope, including cognitive and physical declines;

financial strains; the deaths of friends and loved ones; and the loss of other important social roles, such as employment (Norris & Murrell, 1990). As noted earlier, because late-life deaths typically occur after a long illness, bereaved spouses often experienced a stressful period of caregiving and may see their loved one suffer for long periods prior to the death (Carr et al., 2001). As a result, older adults may be overwhelmed not only by their spouse's death but also by the acute and chronic stressors that accompany the death.

Cohort. Very little is known about generational or cohort differences in older widow(er)s' experiences. However, the nature of death and dying has changed dramatically over the past two centuries and these shifts, accompanied by other sweeping social changes in gender roles and family relations, have created a context in which loss is experienced very differently today than in the past.

No studies in the United States have directly compared cohorts of widow(er)s and their adjustment to loss. However, one recent study compared the psychological and social adjustment of two cohorts of widowed older women in Switzerland, one born in the early 1900s and widowed during the 1970s or earlier, the other born in the 1930s–1940s and widowed in the 2000s (Perrig-Chiello et al., 2015). These two cohorts of women faced very different opportunities for education and employment and also varied widely in the gender relations maintained in their households. The cohorts also differed with respect to the public benefits they received, reflecting the expansion of Switzerland's public pension system and expanded survivor and old-age benefits over the 20th century. The study showed that the two cohorts of women did not differ with respect to their emotional reactions to loss; the sadness and loneliness they experienced was comparable for the two cohorts. However, when other aspects of adaptation were considered including perceived financial strain and availability of social support, the more recent cohort fared considerably better, suggesting that while sadness may be a near universal consequence of spousal loss, other financial and social costs can be ameliorated through social programs or expansion in the social roles afforded to women.

Gender. The well-documented effects of spouse or partner loss on mental health (including depressive symptoms, loneliness, and anxiety) and on physical health outcomes (including mortality risk, disability, and functional limitations) are consistently larger for men than women (Lee & DeMaris, 2007), although one recent study suggests that with the passage of time, long-term widowed men and women do not differ significantly with respect to depressive symptoms (Sasson & Umberson, 2013). While romantic lore suggests that emotionally devastated widowers may die of a broken heart shortly after their wives die, research shows the loss of a helpmate and caretaker is a more plausible explanation for men's health declines following spousal loss. Wives monitor their husbands' diets, remind them to take daily medications, and urge them to give up vices like smoking and drinking (August & Sorkin, 2010). Widowers are more likely than married men to die of accidents, alcohol-related deaths, lung cancer, and chronic ischemic heart disease during the first six months after their loss, but not from causes less closely linked to health behaviors (Moon et al., 2011; Shor et al., 2012).

Widows, by contrast, often experience declines in their economic well-being, which may trigger anxiety and distress (Stroebe et al., 2006). Widows experience substantial declines in income from all sources, ranging from earned income to pensions to Social Security (Gillen & Kim, 2009). Within three years of the death of her husband, a widow's income drops by 44 percent on average (Holden & Kuo, 1996). More than half of older widows in poverty were not poor prior to the death of their husbands. Costs associated with burial, funeral, long-term and medical care, or estate-related legal proceedings can devastate the fixed income of older adults. Because current cohorts of older women typically tended to child-rearing and family responsibilities during their younger years, they have had fewer years of paid work experience and lower earnings than their male peers, on average. Older widows who try to reenter the labor force also may face age discrimination (Holden & Kuo, 1996), which in turn may compromise their emotional and financial well-being.

Sexual orientation. Relatively little is known about whether older gay men and lesbians adjust differently than heterosexual men and women to the loss of their long-term partners. However, mounting research suggests that older gay men and lesbians may face both distinctive challenges and advantages as they cope with loss. The stressors associated with loss may be particularly acute for gays and lesbians, who may also experience institutional and interpersonal discrimination due to their sexual orientation (Meyer, 2003). They may encounter conflict with their deceased partner's family, particularly with respect to the dispersion of personal possessions following death. Legal rights extended to heterosexual married couples have not typically been available for same-sex couples, including the opportunity to make health care and end-of-life decisions for ill partners. Bereaved same-sex partners may not receive sufficient emotional support upon loss because the end of their relationship is not recognized or acknowledged in the wider community (Green & Grant, 2008). The increasing legalization of marriage for same-sex individuals may gradually alleviate some of these stresses.

However, gay men and lesbians also have resources that may enable successful adjustment to partner loss. They have often created their own support networks of friends and selected family members. They also may be more likely than their heterosexual peers to enact flexible gender roles throughout the life course. Because they are not bound to traditional gender-typed family roles, they may be better prepared to manage the daily challenges and responsibilities faced by the newly bereaved (Almack, Seymour, & Bellamy, 2010).

Race. Research on racial differences in late-life spousal bereavement is sparse. This omission reflects the fact that few sample surveys include adequate numbers of older blacks, given their elevated risk of premature death (Federal Interagency Forum on Aging-Related Statistics, 2012). Studies of recently widowed older blacks are even more difficult, given that blacks are less likely than whites to marry, to remain married over the life course, or to remarry following an early-life marital dissolution (Federal Interagency Forum on Aging-Related Statistics, 2012). As such, we know very little about similarities and differences in how blacks and whites adjust to widow(er)hood. One prospective study of late-life spousal loss found that blacks and whites did not differ significantly with respect to depressive symptoms or yearning for their late spouse, although blacks had significantly fewer symptoms of anger and despair (Carr, 2004a). Blacks' lower levels of anger were largely explained by two important coping resources: their higher levels of religiosity and their greater reliance on their children for social and instrumental support relative to whites. By contrast, blacks' lower levels of despair were explained, in part, by the fact that they reported higher levels of preloss marital conflict than did whites. These findings are consistent with emerging evidence that bereavement experiences are most painful when the relationship lost was marked by closeness and warmth, rather than strain and conflict.

Nature of the Marriage or Romantic Relationship

Older adults' psychological adjustment to partner death varies based on the nature of the relationship lost. Early writings, based on the psychoanalytic tradition, proposed that bereaved persons with the most troubled marriages would suffer heightened and pathological grief (Parkes & Weiss, 1983). This perspective held that persons who had conflicted marriages would find it hard to let go of their spouses, yet also feel angry at the deceased for abandoning them. However, longitudinal studies that track married persons over time through the widowhood transition find that older persons whose marriages were marked by high levels of warmth and dependence and low levels of conflict experience elevated grief symptoms within the first six months postloss (Carr et al., 2000).

Although those with high-quality marriages may suffer a greater sense of sadness within the earlier months of loss, their strong emotional ties to the late spouse may prove protective in the longer term. Recent research suggests that those in high-quality marriages may be able to draw strength from continuing bonds with the decedent. Early work on grief suggested that bereaved persons needed to dissolve or relinquish their emotional ties to the deceased and get on with their lives (e.g., Freud 1917/1957), yet current research suggests that maintaining a psychological tie to the deceased is an integral part of adaptation (Field, 2008). Although some aspects of continuing bonds may be problematic for adjustment, researchers point to particular scenarios for which maintaining emotional ties to one's late spouse may be helpful. For instance, Rando (1993) observed that bereaved persons may think about what their late spouse might do, when faced with a difficult decision. Others may keep alive their spouse's legacy by recognizing the continuing positive influence the deceased has on one's current life. In this way, the warmth and closeness of the relationship may continue to be protective and affirming to the bereaved spouse.

Nature of the Death

Researchers have documented that adjustment to spouse or partner loss is affected by the timing and nature of the late spouse's death. As noted earlier, anticipated deaths tend to be less distressing than unanticipated ones. The knowledge that one's partner is going to die in the imminent future provides the couple with the time to address unresolved emotional, financial, and practical issues before the actual death. This preparation for death is believed to enable a smoother transition to widowhood. However, for older persons, anticipated deaths often are accompanied by long-term illness, painful images of a loved one's suffering, intensive caregiving, and neglect of one's own health concerns, thus taking a toll on one's health and emotional well-being (Carr et al., 2001).

Contrary to popular lore, there is no clear-cut evidence that caregivers show greater symptoms of distress than those who did not provide direct care to their late spouse. Emerging research shows that caregivers may even experience improved psychological health following the loss of their spouse, either because they are relieved of their stressful caregiving duties, they are no longer witnessing their loved one suffer, or they experience a sense of satisfaction, meaning, and accomplishment from caring for their loved one in his or her final days (Schulz, Boerner, & Herbert, 2008). However, family caregivers—who currently number more than 50 million in the United States alone—may require assistance prior to the death of their spouse (Caregiver Alliance, 2010). The threat of impending death, strain of caregiving work, and the loss of personal time and activities may be distressing in the days and weeks leading up to the death.

The quality of end-of-life care received by the decedent and place of death also affect the bereavement experience. Older adults who believe that their loved one was in pain or received problematic medical care at the end of life report greater anxiety and anger postloss than persons whose loved one had a good death (Carr, 2003). Use of hospice or palliative care services at the end of life is associated with better spousal bereavement outcomes (Christakis & Iwashyna, 1993), including fewer symptoms of depression (Ornstein et al., 2015). Site of care also matters. Teno and colleagues (2004) found that family members of recent decedents who received at-home hospice services were more likely than those who died at hospitals or nursing homes to say that their loved one received high-quality care, that they were treated with respect and dignity at the end of life, and that they and the patient received adequate emotional support. Ironically, however, more than three-quarters of Americans currently die in institutions (Federal Interagency Forum on Aging-Related Statistics, 2012); this carries implications for survivors' well-being.

Social Support and Integration

Emotionally intimate social relationships over the life course are an important resource as older adults adjust to spousal loss. One widely cited explanation for women's lower levels of distress following spousal loss relative to men's is that women maintain closer relationships over the life course than their male counterparts (Carr & Moorman, 2011). Older widows typically receive more practical and emotional support from their children than do widowers, given mothers' closer relationships with their children throughout the life course. Women also are more likely to have larger and more varied friendship networks than men, and these friendships are an important source of support as women cope with their loss (Ha, 2008). Men, by contrast, often seek social support in new romantic relationships, whether dating or remarriage (Carr, 2004b). Many researchers concur that one reason why women typically adjust better psychologically to loss than men is because they have closer social ties with their children, friends, and siblings.

For both widows and widowers, however, social isolation and limited contact can impede adjustment to loss. Social isolation often is due to structural factors. Older adults living independently may lack transportation, they may have physical limitations that impair their mobility, and they may be cut off physically from loved ones following a relocation to a new home or an assisted living facility. Even those who live close to their family may feel lonely because of family conflict, or because their family does not offer support of the type or amount that the widow(er) would like (Cacioppo & Cacioppo, 2014). The deaths of siblings and friends also may leave older bereaved spouses feeling isolated, as they have no one with whom to reminisce or share their private thoughts and feelings.

Other Stressors

Stress researchers agree that the psychological consequences of any one stressor may be amplified when experienced in conjunction with other losses or strains. For older bereaved persons, the death of a spouse is almost always accompanied by other strains and losses which may compromise their well-being, including financial strain, the loss of work and community roles including retirement and relocation, compromised mobility whether by walking or driving, health declines, decline or loss of sensory functions including vision and hearing, and even the loss of daily routines that gave one's life order and meaning. Widowhood often sets off a chain of secondary stressors, or stressors that result from the loss of a spouse; these secondary stressors in turn may compromise one's emotional and physical well-being. For widowers, the loss of a confidante, helpmate, and caregiver may be particularly harmful, whereas for widows, financial difficulties often are a source of distress (Stroebe et al., 2006).

Discussion and Future Research

This chapter has summarized the context of family bereavement in the contemporary United States, the general patterns of grief that emerge in the face of loss, and the distinctive challenges associated with spouse/partner, sibling, parent, and child loss in late life. However, our knowledge about family bereavement in late life is still in the nascent stages, especially with respect to sibling, parent, and child death, and with respect to race and sexual orientation differences in adjustment to spouse/partner loss. Moreover, much of what we know about bereaved spouses is based on current cohorts of older adults, who were born mainly in the early 20th century, married at midcentury, and experienced old age in the late 20th and early 21st centuries (e.g., Carr, Wortman, & Nesse, 2006). As such, extant research may not necessarily characterize the experiences of future cohorts of bereaved adults, especially the 75 million baby boomers born between 1946 and 1964 (Pruchno, 2012). The baby boomers are much more ethnically and racially diverse than prior cohorts, are more likely to have identified as gay or lesbian in early adulthood, and are more likely to have abided by egalitarian gender roles in the home than their predecessors. As such, in the future, researchers will be charged with exploring more fully the ways that race, ethnicity, and sexual orientation shape the experiences of older bereaved persons.

Demographic shifts over the past half-century have had profound effects on family structure, roles, and relationships, each of which may shape the experiences of spouse, child, sibling, or parent loss in late life (Manning & Brown, 2011). For example, declining fertility rates and increases in geographic mobility mean that future cohorts of older persons will have fewer children on whom they can rely for social support, and these children will be less likely than past generations to live close to their parents. For parents with only one child, the loss of that child may be particularly devastating emotionally, as it deprives one wholly of one's identity as parent (Klass, 1988) and may deprive parents of the one child who was a source of late-life emotional, instrumental, or financial support. Parental death may also be particularly difficult for adult children with no siblings, as they lack an important source of support and assistance.

Divorce and remarriage also may reshape the nature of family bereavement (Manning & Brown, 2011). Current and future cohorts of married couples are more likely than past generations to dissolve dissatisfying marriages through divorce; consequently, persons who remain married until late life may have higher levels of marital closeness and may suffer elevated grief following the loss of these close relationships (Carr et al., 2001). Likewise, older adults who have divorced and then remarry in late life may find spousal death to be particularly distressing, as they are being robbed of relatively new marriages and the promise of a future with their spouse. Emerging research shows, for example, that older women in second marriages report higher levels of marital happiness than their counterparts in long-term first marriages (Freedman, Cornman, & Carr, 2015). Remarriage also may be accompanied by the formation of reconfigured families which include step-children. Although stepchildren may be a source of support as older adults manage the loss of their spouses, emerging evidence suggests that stepchildren and parents often have conflicted interactions at the end of life, especially regarding caregiving responsibilities and the dispersion of the decedent's assets (Sherman, 2012; Sherman & Bauer, 2008).

Shifting gender roles also may reshape the bereavement experience of older heterosexual spouses. Current generations of young adult women have higher levels of education, more years of work experience, and more egalitarian divisions of labor in their families than do past cohorts. Thus, they may be less dependent on their husbands for income, home repair, and financial management tasks, whereas husbands may be less dependent on their wives for homemaking chores and emotional support (Spain & Bianchi, 1996). Under this scenario, future cohorts of widowed persons may experience much lower levels of anxiety than previous cohorts, as they have a greater comfort level in performing a range of household tasks.

Cultural contexts also may continue to powerfully shape experiences of loss and grief. The research described in this chapter has focused primarily on the United States or other Western, individualistic nations similar to the United States. Researchers should further explore how adjustment to familial loss may reflect a broader array of cultural contexts. Cultural factors, including patterns of household structure and filial piety, and attitudes toward life and death, may condition the experiences of older bereaved spouses, siblings, parents, and children. As practitioners develop policies and interventions for older bereaved persons, they must take into consideration the larger cultural, social, historical, and demographic backdrop against which family loss occurs.

Future research also should explore more fully the medical and technological contexts in which late-life death occurs. In particular, technological and medical advancements that extend the lifespan may create the need for more intensive family caregiving, a task that typically falls to wives, daughters, and mothers. Those who perform complex illness-related tasks at home in addition to personal care such as feeding, bathing, and toileting, may experience a crisis in caregiving that requires assistance or relocation of the patient outside the home (Waldrop & Meeker, 2011). Managing ventilators and feeding tubes, tending to pressure sores, and administrating medications are also linked to elevated symptoms of distress among family caregivers (Moorman & Macdonald, 2013). If women continue to bear the burden for personal care of ailing family members, then cohorts of women entering old age in the future may find their own emotional and physical well-being compromised. Further exploration of the way that social, cultural, and technological forces shape the bereavement experience will provide knowledge of theoretical and practical importance for future generations of bereaved older adults.

References

Almack, K., Seymour, J., & Bellamy, G. (2010). Exploring the impact of sexual orientation on experiences and concerns about end of life care and on bereavement for lesbian, gay, and bisexual older people. *Sociology*, *44*(5), 908–924.

American Psychiatric Association. (1994). *Diagnostic and statistical manual of mental disorders, (DSM-IV)*. Washington, DC: American Psychiatric Association.

American Psychiatric Association. (2013). *Diagnostic and statistical manual of mental disorders, (DSM-5)*. Washington, DC: American Psychiatric Association.

Archer, J. (1999). *The nature of grief: The evolution and psychology of reactions to loss.* London: Routledge.

Arias E. (2014). *United States life tables, 2009. National vital statistics reports, 62*(7). Hyattsville, MD: National Center for Health Statistics.

August, K.J., & Sorkin, D.H. (2010). Marital status and gender differences in managing a chronic illness: The function of health-related social control. *Social Science and Medicine, 71*(10), 1831–1838.

Baltes, P., Smith, J., & Staudinger, U. (1992). Wisdom and successful aging. In T. Sonderegger (Ed.), *Nebraska Symposium on Motivation* (Vol. 39, Psychology and aging, pp. 103–121). Lincoln: University of Nebraska Press.

Bennett, K.M., Hughes, G.M., & Smith, P.T. (2003). "I think a woman can take it": Widowed men's views and experiences of gender differences in bereavement. *Ageing International, 28*(4), 408–424.

Blank, J.W. (1998). *The death of an adult child: A book for and about bereaved parents*. New York: Baywood Publishing.

Boelen, P.A., & Prigerson, H.G. (2013). Prolonged grief disorder as a new diagnostic category in DSM-5. In M. Stroebe, H. Schut, and J. van den Bout (Eds.), *Complicated grief: Scientific foundations for health care professionals*. New York: Routledge.

Bonanno, G.A., Wortman, C.B., Lehman, D.R., Tweed, R.G., Haring, M., Sonnega, J., Carr, D., & Nesse, R.M. (2002). Resilience to loss and chronic grief: A prospective study from preloss to 18-months postloss. *Journal of Personality and Social Psychology, 83*, 1150–1164.

Cacioppo, J.T., & Cacioppo, S. (2014). Social relationships and health: The toxic effects of perceived social isolation. *Social and personality psychology compass, 8*(2), 58–72.

Caregiver Alliance. (2010). *Fact Sheet on Statistics*. Retrieved May 26, 2015 from http://www.caregiver.org/caregiver/jsp/content.

Carr, D. (2003). A good death for whom? Quality of spouse's death and psychological distress among older widowed persons. *Journal of Health & Social Behavior, 44*, 215–232.

Carr, D. (2004a). Black/White differences in psychological adjustment to spousal loss among older adults. *Research on Aging, 26*(6), 591–622.

Carr, D. (2004b). The desire to date and remarry among older widows and widowers. *Journal of Marriage and Family, 66*(4), 1051–1068.

Carr, D. (2004c). Gender, pre-loss marital dependence and older adults' adjustment to widowhood. *Journal of Marriage and Family, 66*, 220–235.

Carr, D. (2012). Death and dying in the contemporary United States: What are the psychological implications of anticipated death? *Social and Personality Psychology Compass, 6*(2), 184–195.

Carr, D., House, J.S., Kessler, R.C., Nesse, R., Sonnega, J., & Wortman, C.B. (2000). Marital quality and psychological adjustment to widowhood among older adults: A longitudinal analysis. *The Journals of Gerontology, Series B: Social Sciences, 55*, S197–S207.

Carr, D., House, J.S., Wortman, C.B., Nesse, R., & Kessler, R.C. (2001). Psychological adjustment to sudden and anticipated spousal death among the older widowed. *The Journals of Gerontology, Series B: Social Sciences, 56B*, S237–S248.

Carr, D., & Khodyakov, D. (2007). Health care proxies in late life: Whom do we choose and why? *Journal of Health and Social Behavior, 48*, 180–194.

Carr, D., & Moorman, S.M. (2011). Social relations and aging. In R.A. Settersten Jr., & J.L. Angel (Eds.), *Handbook of sociology of aging* (pp. 145–160). New York: Springer.

Carr, D., Nesse, R.M., & Wortman, C.B. (Eds.). (2006). *Spousal bereavement in late life*. New York: Springer Publishing Company.

Carstensen, L., & Turk-Charles, S. (1994). The salience of emotion across the adult life span. *Psychology and Aging, 9*, 259–264.

Chan, D., Livingston, G., Jones, L., & Sampson, E.L. (2013). Grief reactions in dementia carers: A systematic review. *International Journal of Geriatric Psychiatry, 28*(1), 1–17.

Christakis, N.A., & Iwashyna, T.J. (2003). The health impact on families of health care: A matched cohort study of hospice use by decedents and mortality outcomes in surviving, widowed spouses. *Social Science and Medicine, 57*, 465–475.

Cicirelli, V.G. (2009). Sibling death and death fear in relation to depressive symptomatology in older adults. *The Journals of Gerontology, Series B: Psychological Sciences and Social Sciences, 64*(1), 24–32.

DeVita-Raeburn, E. (2004). *The empty room: Surviving the loss of a brother or sister at any age*. New York: Simon and Schuster.

Federal Interagency Forum on Aging-Related Statistics. (2013). *Older Americans 2012: Key indicators of well-being*. Washington, DC: Department of Health and Human Services.

Field, N.P. (2008). Whether to relinquish or maintain a bond with the deceased. In M. Stroebe, R.O. Hansson, H. Schut, & W. Stroebe (Eds.), *Handbook of bereavement research and practice: 21st century perspectives* (pp. 133–162). Washington, DC: American Psychological Association (APA) Press.

Fontana, A., & Keene, J.R. (2009). *Death and dying in America*. Malden, MA: Polity.

Freedman, V., Cornman, J.C., & Carr, D. (2015). *Second time around: Second marriages, wellbeing and time use in late life*. Unpublished manuscript.

Freud, S. (1917/1957). Mourning and melancholia. In J. Strachey (Ed. and Trans.), *The standardized edition of the complete psychological works of Sigmund Freud* (pp. 152–170). London: Hogarth Press (Original work published 1917).

Gates, G.J., & Newport, F. (2012). *Special report: 3.4% of U.S. adults identify as LGBT*. Princeton, NJ: Gallup Poll. Retrieved May 30, 2015 from http://www.gallup.com/poll/158066/special-report-adults-identify-lgbt.aspx.

George, L.K. (1993). Sociological perspectives on life transitions. *Annual Review of Sociology, 19*, 353–373.

Gillen, M., & Kim, H. (2009). Older women and poverty transition: Consequences of income source changes from widowhood. *Journal of Applied Gerontology*, *28*(3), 320–341.

Green, L., & Grant, V. (2008). "Gagged grief and beleaguered bereavements?" An analysis of multidisciplinary theory and research relating to same sex partnership bereavement. *Sexualities, 11*(3), 275–300.

Ha, J. (2008). Changes in support from confidantes, children, and friends following widowhood. *Journal of Marriage and Family, 70*, 306–318.

Hays, J. C., Gold, D. T., & Pieper, C. F. (1997). Sibling bereavement in late life. *OMEGA: Journal of Death and Dying, 35*(1), 25–42.

Hazzard, A., Weston, J., & Gutterres, C. (1992). After a child's death: Factors related to parental bereavement. *Journal of Developmental & Behavioral Pediatrics, 13*(1), 24–30.

HHS/ASPE (Department of Health and Human Services, Assistant Secretary for Planning and Evaluation). (2013). *National plan to address Alzheimer's disease—2013 update*. Retrieved May 30, 2015 from http://aspe.hhs.gov/daltcp/napa/NatlPlan2013.shtml#intro.

Holden, K. C., & Kuo, H. H. D. (1996). Complex marital histories and economic well-being: The continuing legacy of divorce and widowhood as the HRS cohort approaches retirement. *Gerontologist, 36*(3), 383–390.

Horowitz, M. J., Weiss, D. S., Kaltreider, N., Krupnick, J., Marmar, C., Wilner, N., & DeWitt, K. (1984). Reactions to the death of a parent: Results from patients and field subjects. *Journal of Nervous and Mental Disease, 172*, 383–392.

Institute of Medicine (IOM). (2003). *When children die: Improving palliative and end-of-life care for children and their families*. Washington, DC: National Academies Press.

Institute of Medicine (IOM). (2014). *Dying in America: Improving quality and honoring individual preferences near the end of life*. Washington, DC: The National Academies.

Johansson, Å. K., & Grimby, A. (2012). Anticipatory grief among close relatives of patients at hospice and palliative wards. *American Journal of Hospice and Palliative Medicine, 29*, 134–138.

Klass, D. (1988). *Parental grief: Solace and resolution*. New York: Springer.

Lee, G. R., & DeMaris, A. (2007). Widowhood, gender, and depression: A longitudinal analysis. *Research on Aging, 29*, 56–72.

Lofquist, D. (2011). *Same sex couple households: American Community Survey briefs*. Washington, DC: U.S. Census Bureau. Retrieved June 10, 2013, from http://www.census.gov/prod/2011pubs/acsbr10–03.pdf

Mahon, M. M. (1997). Sibling bereavement: A concept analysis. *Death Studies, 21*(5), 477–499.

Manning, W. D., & Brown, S. L. (2011). The demography of unions among older Americans, 1980–present: A family change approach. In R. A. Settersten Jr. & J. L. Angel (Eds.), *Handbook of sociology of aging* (pp. 193–210). New York: Springer.

Marshall, H. (2004). Midlife loss of parents: The transition from adult child to orphan. *Ageing International, 29*(4), 351–367.

Meuser, T. M., & Marwit, S. J. (2001). A comprehensive, stage-sensitive model of grief in dementia caregiving. *The Gerontologist, 41*(5), 658–670.

Meyer, I. H. (2003). Prejudice, social stress, and mental health in lesbian, gay, and bisexual populations: Conceptual issues and research evidence. *Psychological Bulletin, 129*(5), 674–697.

Miniño, A. M., & Murphy, S. L. *Death in the United States, 2010*. NCHS data brief, no. 99. Hyattsville, MD: National Center for Health Statistics. 2012.

Moon, J. R., Kondo, N., Glymour, M. M., & Subramanian, S. V. (2011) Widowhood and mortality: A meta-analysis. *PLoS ONE* 6(8), e23465. doi:10.1371/journal.pone.0023465

Moorman, S. M., & Macdonald, C. (2013). Medically complex home care and caregiver strain. *The Gerontologist, 53*(3), 407–417.

Moss, M. S., Lesher, E. L., & Moss, S. Z. (1986). Impact of the death of an adult child on elderly parents: Some observations. *OMEGA: Journal of Death and Dying, 17*(3), 209–218.

Moss, M. S., & Moss, S. Z. (1983–1984). The impact of parental death on middle aged children. *OMEGA: Journal of Death and Dying, 14*(1), 65–75.

Moss, S. Z., & Moss, M. S. (1989). The impact of the death of an elderly sibling: Some considerations of a normative loss. *American Behavioral Scientist,* 33(1), 94–106.

Nolen-Hoeksema, S., & Ahrens, C. (2002). Age differences and similarities in the correlates of depressive symptoms. *Psychology and Aging, 17,* 116–124.

Norris, F. H., & Murrell, S. A. (1990). Social support, life events, and stress as modifiers to bereavement by older adults. *Psychology of Aging, 5*, 429–436.

Olshansky, S. J., & Ault, A. B. (1986). The fourth stage of the epidemiologic transition: The age of delayed degenerative diseases. *Milbank Quarterly, 64*, 355–391.

Omran, A. (1971). The epidemiologic transition: A theory of the epidemiology of population change. *Milbank Quarterly, 29*, 509–538.

Ornstein, K. A., Aldridge, M. D., Garrido, M. M., Gorges, R., Meier, D. E., & Kelley, A. S. (2015). Association between hospice use and depressive symptoms in surviving spouses. *JAMA Internal Medicine*. Online First.

Parkes, C. M., & Weiss, R. S. (1983). *Recovery from bereavement.* New York, NY: Basic.

Pattison, E. M. (1977). The living–dying process. In C. A. Garfield (Ed.), *Psychosocial care of the dying patient* (pp. 133–168). New York, NY: McGraw-Hill.

Perrig-Chiello, P., Spahni, S., Höpflinger, F., & Carr, D. (2015). Cohort and gender differences in psychosocial adjustment to late-life widowhood. *The Journals of Gerontology, Series B: Psychological Sciences and Social Sciences*, gbv004. Online First.

Pratt, C. C., Walker, A. J., & Wood, B. L. (1992). Bereavement among former caregivers to elderly mothers. *Family Relations, 41*, 278–283.

Prigerson, H. G., Vanderwerker, L. C., & Maciejewski, P. K. (2008). A case for inclusion of prolonged grief disorder in DSM-V. In M. Stroebe, R. O. Hansson, H. Schut, & W. Stroebe (Eds.), *Handbook of bereavement research and practice: 21st century perspectives* (pp. 165–186). Washington, DC: American Psychological Association (APA) Press.

Pruchno, R. (2012). Not your mother's old age: Baby Boomers at age 65. *The Gerontologist, 52*(2), 149–152.

Rando, T. A. (1986). *Loss and anticipatory grief*. New York: Lexington Books.

Rando, T. A. (1993). *Treatment of complicated mourning.* Champaign, IL: Research Press.

Robben, A. C. (Ed.). (2009). *Death, mourning, and burial: A cross-cultural reader.* New York: John Wiley & Sons.

Rosenblatt, P.C. (2000). *Parent grief: Narratives of loss and relationship*. Philadelphia, PA: Taylor & Francis.

Russo, F. (2010). *They're your parents, too!: How siblings can survive their parents' aging without driving each other crazy*. New York: Bantam.

Sasson, I., & Umberson, D.J. (2014). Widowhood and depression: New light on gender differences, selection, and psychological adjustment. *The Journals of Gerontology, Series B: Psychological Sciences and Social Sciences, 69*(1), 135–145.

Scharlach, A.E., & Fredriksen, K.I. (1993). Reactions to the death of a parent during midlife. *OMEGA, 27*, 307–319.

Schulz, R., Boerner, K., & Hebert, R.S. (2008). Caregiving and bereavement. In M. Stroebe, R.O. Hansson, H. Schut, & W. Stroebe (Eds.), *Handbook of bereavement research and practice: 21st century perspectives* (pp. 265–286). Washington, DC: American Psychological Association (APA) Press.

Shanfield, S.B., Benjamin, A.H., & Swain, B.J. (1984). Parents' reactions to the death of an adult child from cancer. *The American Journal of Psychiatry, 141*(9), 1092–1094.

Shear, M.K., Simon, N., Wall, M., Zisook, S., Neimeyer, R., Duan, N., . . . & Keshaviah, A. (2011). Complicated grief and related bereavement issues for DSM-5. *Depression and Anxiety, 28*(2), 103–117.

Sherman, C.W. (2012). Remarriage as context for dementia caregiving: Implications of positive support and negative interactions for caregiver well-being. *Research in Human Development, 9*(2), 165–182.

Sherman, C.W., & Bauer, J.W. (2008). Financial conflicts facing late-life remarried Alzheimer's disease caregivers. *Family Relations, 57*(4), 492–503.

Shor, E., Roelfs, D.J., Curreli, M., Clemow, L., Burg, M.M., & Schwartz, J. (2012). Widowhood and mortality: A meta-analysis and meta-regression. *Demography, 49*, 575–606.

Silverman, P.R. (2004). *Widow to widow: How the bereaved help one another*. New York: Routledge.

Spain, D., & Bianchi, S.M. (1996). *Balancing act: Motherhood, marriage and employment among American women*. New York: Russell Sage Foundation.

Stroebe, M.S., Folkman, S., Hansson, R.O., & Schut, H. (2006). The prediction of bereavement outcome: Development of an integrative risk factor framework. *Social Science and Medicine, 63*(9), 2440–2451.

Szinovacz, M.E. (2000). Changes in housework after retirement: A panel study. *Journal of Marriage and Family, 62*, 78–92.

Teno, J.M., Clarridge, B.R., Casey, V., Welch, L.C., Wetle, T., Shield, R., & Mor, V. (2004). Family perspectives on end-of-life care at the last place of care. *Journal of the American Medical Association, 291*, 88–93.

Thompson, L.W., Gallagher-Thompson, D., Futterman, A., Gilewski, M.J., & Peterson, J. (1991). The effects of late life spousal bereavement over a 30-month interval. *Psychology and Aging, 3*, 434–441.

Umberson, D. (2003). *Death of a parent: Transition to a new adult identity*. New York: Cambridge University Press.

Umberson, D., & Chen, M.D. (1994). Effects of a parent's death on adult children: Relationship salience and reaction to loss. *American Sociological Review, 59*, 152–168.

Van Humbeeck, L., Piers, R. D., Van Camp, S., Dillen, L., Verhaeghe, S. T., & Van Den Noortgate, N. J. (2013). Aged parents' experiences during a critical illness trajectory and after the death of an adult child: A review of the literature. *Palliative Medicine, 26*, 583–595.

Wakefield, J. C., & First, M. B. (2012). Validity of the bereavement exclusion to major depression: Does the empirical evidence support the proposal to eliminate the exclusion in DSM-5? *World Psychiatry, 11*(1), 3–10.

Waldrop, D., & Meeker, M. (2011). Crisis in caregiving: When home-based end-of-life care is no longer possible. *Journal of Palliative Care, 27*(2), 117–125.

Weiss, R. S. (2008). The nature and causes of grief. In M. S., Stroebe, R. O. Hansson, H. E. Schut, W. E. Stroebe, & E. I. Van den Blin (Eds.), *Handbook of bereavement research and practice: Advances in theory and intervention* (pp. 29–44). Washington, DC: American Psychological Association.

White, L. (2001). Sibling relationships over the life course: A panel analysis. *Journal of Marriage and Family, 63*(2), 555–568.

Wolff, J. L., & Kasper, J. D. (2006). Caregivers of frail elders: Updating a national profile. *The Gerontologist, 46*(3), 344–356.

APPENDIX A

Organizations for Older Persons

Elizabeth A. Daniele

Hundreds of organizations represent the rights, interests, and concerns of older Americans. They operate at the federal, state, and local levels. They are publically, privately, and user funded. This is a compilation of some of the organizations that address various aspects of aging. For every organization I included there are a dozen more I could have included. In selecting organizations to feature here, I highlight some with resources that are of particular note due to their relative rarity, such as Spanish language resources, visual aids, particularly accessible formats, toolkits, and data-rich sites. These descriptions are paraphrased from the organizations' own web pages. Each group is unique in terms of organizational history, trajectory, and online offerings.

AARP
http://www.aarp.org
With 37 million members, AARP works to improve the lives of individuals aged 50 and older. AARP is a nonpartisan organization with widely distributed publications and broadcasts; the website offers articles on a variety of topics. The associated AARP Foundation is a charitable organization dedicated to aiding older Americans in need.

Administration on Aging (AoA)
http://www.aoa.gov
Part of the U.S. Department of Health and Human Services, AoA publishes an annual *Profile of Older Americans*; keeps statistics in a database called AGing Integrated Database (AGID) that offers state profiles and data in accessible formats; compiles information on older minorities; and publishes aging-related census data. The AoA supports Eldercare Locator (www.eldercare.gov or +1-800-677-1116), a tool that enables individuals to search for services by geographic location or type of service sought.

Advancing Excellence in America's Nursing Homes
https://www.nhqualitycampaign.org/
In 2006, this campaign was founded by a coalition of 28 organizations interested in "making nursing homes better places to live, work, and visit." Their website provides resources on organizational and clinical aspects of nursing home services featuring steps to meet goals around staffing, person-centered care, pain management, and mobility in facilities.

Aging with Dignity
https://www.agingwithdignity.org
Inspired by Mother Teresa of Calcutta and her proclamation on the value of human interaction, this national nonprofit organization aims to protect the self-worth of aging adults especially toward the end of life. *Five Wishes* is a template for an advance directive living will available on their website in many languages.

AgingStats.gov: Federal Interagency Forum on Aging-Related Statistics
http://www.agingstats.gov/
This forum was begun in 1986 by federal agencies interested in sharing and refining data related to aging. Their website features reports on older Americans, brief descriptions of surveys relevant to gerontology, and links to additional statistical information.

Alliance for Aging Research
http://www.agingresearch.org
A nonprofit advocacy organization, the Alliance for Aging Research works to improve the lives of older adults through scientific advancement. Their website provides articles, publications, and blogs about topics such as caregiving, drug safety, various health conditions, and aging healthfully.

Alliance for Retired Americans
http://retiredamericans.org
Advocates for economic justice and civil rights for Americans since 2001, the Alliance for Retired Americans member population of 4.3 million includes many retired union members. Contact information for state chapters and selected weekly news and media clips are available on the website.

Alzheimer's Association
http://www.alz.org
With the aims of enhancing care, advancing research, and advocating, the Alzheimer's Association is a national organization with many local chapters, a helpline (+1-800-272-3900), support groups and message boards, and online resources for families and caregivers. Their website features tools that help individuals and their families make appropriate action plans

and find community resources. The Alzheimer's Association offers research grants, hosts an annual international conference to bring researchers of Alzheimer's together, and publishes the journal *Alzheimer's & Dementia*.

American Bar Association Commission on Law and Aging
http://www.americanbar.org/groups/law_aging.html
A small group of experts on aging and law nested within the national professional association for attorneys, this commission exists to support and obtain legal rights, human dignity, independence, and quality of life for older adults. They study legal issues related to housing, elder abuse, planning for incapacity, decisions around health care, dispute resolution, guardianship, and public benefit programs like Social Security.

American Federation for Aging Research (AFAR)
http://www.afar.org
This grant-giving organization supports healthful aging by funding biomedical research. The primary initiatives of AFAR include funding research related to healthy aging, drawing more primary care physicians toward working with older adults, increasing communication between scientific and clinical communities, and educating the public regarding medical findings.

American Geriatrics Society (AGS)
http://www.americangeriatrics.org
This nonprofit is comprised of professionals interested in improving "health, independence, and quality of life" for elders. AGS aims to provide excellent patient-centered care by expanding awareness of research about treatment for older adults, and increasing the populations of health-care professionals doing geriatric care, and using principles of geriatric medicine. They offer policy suggestions and founded the Health in Aging Foundation to increase public awareness about older adult health and care.

American Society on Aging (ASA)
http://www.asaging.org
This multidisciplinary organization exists to continually educate and disseminate information to professionals working with elders or those in aging-related fields. ASA publishes a scholarly journal entitled *Generations*, as well as a bimonthly newspaper, and a complementary online blog in addition to offering periodic webinars, continuing education trainings for those who work with older adults, and an annual conference.

ARCH National Respite Network and Resource Center
http://archrespite.org
This organization offers a tool for finding local respite services, a coalition that promotes maintaining these services in legislation and policy

initiatives, and a resource center replete with toolkit, webinars, and funding information related to respite over the lifespan.

Argentum (formerly Assisted Living Federation of America)
http://alfa.org
An association representing senior living communities, this organization advocates for excellence in senior care, choice, and independence. Argentum supports an online action center that enables individuals to contact their federal representatives and offers webinars and toolkits for those managing senior living communities.

Association for Gerontology in Higher Education (AGHE)
http://www.aghe.org
The dual missions of AGHE are to advance the study of gerontology and geriatrics education at institutions of higher education and to support faculty and students who study these topics. In existence since 1974, today the association publishes the journal *Gerontology & Geriatrics Education*. Their website also features suggestions of books that are appropriate for K–12 students.

The Bernard Osher Foundation
http://www.osherfoundation.org
Founded in 1977, today the Osher Foundation provides support for students returning to school and offers lifelong learning for older adults. Osher Lifelong Learning Institutes (OLLI) programs offer noncredit classes for adults aged 50 or older at 119 college and universities across the United States. The National Resource Center for Osher Lifelong Learning Institutes (http://nrc.northwestern.edu) offers a newsletter, a live feed of tweets, news stories, and an interactive map to find OLLI programs.

Brookdale Center for Healthy Aging
http://brookdale.org
An academic gerontology center since 1974 and affiliated with Hunter College, the Brookdale Center endeavors to better the lives of older adults through research on health problems common for older adults and professional development of individuals who work in human services, law, and other areas impacting elders. The Brookdale website offers toolkits dealing with fiscal issues at care facilities, emergency preparation, and how to address chronic disease.

Caregiver Action Network (CAN)
http://www.caregiveraction.org
Focusing on the more than 65 million persons who provide care to loved ones encumbered by disability, disease, chronic ailment, or old age, this

nonprofit organization prioritizes bettering the quality of life for the caregivers. Formerly known as the National Family Caregivers Association, goals of CAN include supporting resourcefulness of caregivers, reducing their stress and financial strains, and increasing respect for caregivers, as well as enhancing their senses of competence and confidence. The CAN website offers an online discussion forum, family caregiver toolbox, a list of other groups caregivers can use as resources, and volunteers who are trained to support and teach advocacy to caregivers.

The Center for Social Gerontology (TCSG)
http://www.tcsg.org
Founded in 1972 with a commitment to advancing individual autonomy of older adults and promoting incorporation of an increasingly larger population of older and very old Americans, TCSG continues as a nonprofit organization. TCSG aims to make changes through research, sharing information with policy makers and the public, and training future care providers.

Centers for Medicare & Medicaid Services (CMS)
http://www.cms.gov
Covering 100 million people with different types of insurance programs, CMS is an organization within the U.S. Department of Health and Human Services. Their website features sections on key regulations, news and publications, research reports and data, trainings, and creative solutions for health-care dilemmas. Additionally, the CMS website offers information about Medicare and Medicaid, how to coordinate these two services, and links to the Health Insurance Marketplace site which is replete with information about programs, forms, and application materials.

Death Cafés
http://deathcafe.com
Death Café is a social franchise with a website that guides individuals on how to use the name, join the online community, and represent the organization. Death Cafés are gatherings where individuals discuss death in group-directed fashion without an agenda or theme. These have been hosted in Europe, North America, and Australasia since 2011.

Eldercare Workforce Alliance
http://www.eldercareworkforce.org
Created to tackle the crisis of having a capable workforce to care for an aging U.S. population, this alliance of 31 organizations aims to improve quality of care to older Americans. They represent health-care providers, consumers, and family members who provide care.

Elderhostel Road Scholar Programs

http://www.roadscholar.org

Elderhostel is a nonprofit organization that started offering noncredit classes and overnight accommodations for adults in 1975. In 2009, they renamed their travel-based learning programs Road Scholar. Today these programs operate around the world and include a range of options such as outdoor excursions, traveling with a grandchild, exploring cities, and educational cruises.

Ethnic Elders Care Network

http://ethnicelderscare.net

Designed as a resource for those who provide care to ethnic elders with Alzheimer's disease, this site promotes cultural competence in care provision by increasing education for those who provide care and the wider population. The Ethnic Elders Care Network also promotes research, prevention, and treatment of Alzheimer's disease.

Family Caregiver Alliance (FCA)

https://caregiver.org

Representing those who provide long-term care for loved ones, FCA aims to support those individuals by providing education and support as well as advocating and producing research through their National Center on Caregiving. The FCA website features services listed by state, online discussion and support groups, and a number of research reports. They offer an informative training known as *Caregiving 101: Exploring the Complexities of Family Caregiving*.

Generations United

http://www.gu.org

With the goal of improving the lives of younger and older adults, Generations United advocates for intergenerational collaboration. Their website features information about relevant public policies, intergenerational issues, families that are headed by grandparents, a blog about successful intergenerational undertakings, and the Seniors4kids program that works to mobilize adults over 50 on behalf of children.

Gerontological Society of America (GSA)

https://www.geron.org

This organization exists to advance aging studies and share information between scientific and policy-making communities as well as educate the population at large. As the oldest and largest organization with an agenda of research, practice, and education, they publish the top scholarly journals and have a large meeting of professionals each year.

Gray Panthers

(Chapters in various cities maintain their own websites.)

Founded by Maggie Kuhn in 1970, today this intergenerational organization has a presence in various locations around the United States. The key values of this justice-oriented group, according to their Facebook page, are "honoring maturity, unifying the generations, active engagement, [and] participatory democracy" (https://www.facebook.com/GrayPanthers/info?tab=page_info).

Health Finder en español

http://www.healthfinder.gov/espanol/

A Spanish language resource for living well, this site offers a guide with advice on healthy living for different age groups, resources on a variety of health concerns or problems, and news about health. The Office of Disease Prevention and Health Promotion sponsor the site.

Healthy Aging

http://www.cdc.gov/aging/index.html

The target audience of this site is health professionals who want to learn more about the Healthy Aging program from the Centers for Disease Control and Prevention. The public health program is committed to finding ways to advance and safeguard the health of older adults as well preserve quality of life for the older adult population.

International Association of Homes and Services for the Ageing (IAHSA)

http://www.iahsa.net

Founded in 1994 as a means of facilitating communication between individuals with different professional expertise about aging, according to their website, the membership of IAHSA today includes specialists on housing, research, technology, and design. As an international network, their website features news headlines related to aging in many national contexts, designs from their biennial conference, and reports on topics such as technology and innovation.

Latino Center on Aging (LCA)

http://www.gerolatino.org

An advocacy organization in New York City since 1991, LCA recognizes linguistic, cultural, and fiscal barriers as restricting the health of Latino elders. LCA works to educate, advocate, and close gaps between service providers and older adult Latinos.

Leadership Council of Aging Organizations (LCAO)
http://www.lcao.org
Comprised of 72 national nonprofit organizations that provide services to elders, this coalition advocates for older Americans in policy arenas. Their website features items such as issues briefs and open letters to policy makers as well as news updates on relevant topics.

LeadingAge
http://www.leadingage.org
This large organization addresses a broad range of topics, and is comprised of 6,000 nonprofit member groups incorporating partners such as states, businesses, foundations, and researchers. LeadingAge is home to three centers, which focus on applied research, aging-related technology, and housing. The LeadingAge website provides a search engine to find services by geography and topic, learning and education materials, and information about their advocacy work and annual conferences.

Meals on Wheels America
http://www.mealsonwheels.org
Started in Philadelphia in 1954, today this organization helps 2.5 million seniors through over 5,000 independently operated programs across the country. More than 2 million Meals on Wheels volunteers facilitate the provision of services in efforts to ease isolation and hunger among older adults with reduced mobility. This program is supported in part by funding from the Older Americans Act.

Medicare Rights Center
http://www.medicarerights.org
Medicare Rights Center is a nonprofit dedicated to helping consumers obtain high-quality medical care, primarily through facilitating understanding of benefits provided by the Medicare system. They provide a telephone helpline (800–333–4114); an interactive online tool that answers questions about Medicare; fact sheets about enrollment, medication costs, dual enrollment, and cases of denial of services; and release audiovisual recordings on relevant topics presented by older adults.

National Adult Day Services Association (NADSA)
http://nadsa.org
In 1995, the National Institute on Adult Daycare was renamed National Adult Day Services Association to better include respite, day care centers,

and day health-care providers. Adult day centers provide social and/or health services for adults who need to be monitored outside the home. Such sites may provide social interactions, transportation, nutrition, personal care for daily living, and physical or mental stimulation. As a representative organization for these centers, NADSA offers advice on selecting a site and opening centers and also promotes an agenda encouraging increased access to this type of service.

National Alliance for Caregiving (NAC)
http://www.caregiving.org
A nonprofit coalition of national organizations dedicated to easing the strains on family members who are caregivers, this organization was founded in 1996. The aim of NAC is to advocate for policies to improve situations for caregivers, educate about caregivers' conditions, and promote research related to caregiving.

National Asian Pacific Center on Aging (NAPCA)
http://napca.org
With the aim of supporting Asian Americans and Pacific Islanders (AAPI) so they receive the same rights and benefits as other American seniors, this organization advocates at multiple levels, educates both their constituents and the broader population, and works to empower AAPI older adults. Their website features portals tailored for members of the community of AAPI older adults, their family members, service providers, and advocates or policy makers; offers relevant census data and research reports; and provides information on work and training opportunities as well as healthful aging. NAPCA has helplines in Chinese, Korean, Vietnamese, and English (http://napca.org/helpline/).

National Association for Hispanic Elderly (Asociación Nacional Pro Personas Mayores)
http://www.anppm.org
Established in 1975 to serve Hispanic and other low-income elders, this private nonprofit addresses services for older adults, employment and training programs, housing and neighborhood plans, and produces culturally relevant educational and outreach materials through its media center.

National Association of Area Agencies on Aging (n4a)
http://www.n4a.org
This umbrella organization of Area Agencies on Aging (AAAs) and Title VI Native American aging programs aims to enable older adults and individuals with disabilities stay in their homes and local communities. AAAs were

established under the Older Americans Act of 1973 to help elders live dignified, independent lives; today these variously named organizations facilitate planning, development, coordination, and provision of services across the nation. Serving eight million people nationwide, most AAAs support health of older adults through evidence-based programming, home and community-based services, insurance counseling, case management, and the five key areas required by the Older Americans Act: caregiving, elder rights, health and wellness, nutrition, and supportive services.

National Association of Nutrition and Aging Services Programs (NANASP)
http://www.nanasp.org
Since 1977, this membership organization has been advocating health and wellness among older Americans through support and promotion of nutrition programs funded by the Older Americans Act. The NANASP motto stresses local enactment of ideals that are national in scope. Their website contains links to advocacy letters, relevant news stories and government testimonies, conferences, the *NANASP Washington Bulletin*, and other publications.

National Academy of Social Insurance (NASI)
https://www.nasi.org
This nonprofit organization specializes in understanding and communicating the values of social insurance. The NASI website features information about Social Security, Medicare, Workers' Compensation, disability, Unemployment Insurance, long-term care, workforce issues and employee benefits, and income assistance.

National Association of States United for Aging and Disabilities (NASUAD)
http://www.nasuad.org
Founded in 1964 as the National Association of State Units on Aging, today this organization represents aging and disabilities services agencies from 56 state and territorial areas of the United States. The aim of the organization is to create, support, and advance state systems for delivery of services to homes and communities of individuals who are disabled or aged and their caregivers.

National Caregivers Library
http://www.caregiverslibrary.org/
Affiliated with Caregiving Ministries, which seeks to support the growing population of people who care for their loved ones, this library website is designed for caregivers. It offers resources such as checklists and articles on myriad topics from basics of caregiving and caring for oneself, to long distance care,

end-of-life, legal issues, transportation, and care facilities. The website features a section for employers that overviews the impact of caregiving on businesses.

National Caucus and Center on Black Aging (NCBA)
http://www.ncba-aged.org
Since 1970, this organization represents the concerns of minority and low-income seniors with aims of improving quality of life and drawing older minorities to the attention of other organizations that serve the public, such as legislators and policy makers.

National Center on Elder Abuse (NCEA)
http://www.ncea.aoa.gov
Funded by the U.S. government through the Administration on Aging, this center is designed to provide information related to elder mistreatment. Their website offers a listserv, and resources on best practices, news, research, and training for a target audience that includes advocates, health-care professionals, the general public, and those working in justice system and policy-making arenas.

National Consumer Voice for Quality Long-Term Care
http://theconsumervoice.org
Founded in 1975 as the National Citizens' Coalition for Nursing Home Reform and changing to the current name in 2010, today Consumer Voice represents seniors who use long-term care facilities. With information tailored for consumers, family members, and advocates, the Consumer Voice website provides an ombudsman location tool, resources about long-term care in an online clearinghouse, links to relevant news stories and current policy-related topics, a newsletter, and events like webinars and the annual conference.

National Clearinghouse on Abuse in Later Life (NCALL)
http://www.ncall.us
By educating and advocating, NCALL works to eradicate abuse of older adults. The mission statement of this organization reflects that elder abuse is a result of systemic conditions as well as philosophies, behaviors, and extant regulations. NCALL offers resources on the justice system and technology in formats such as webinars and information sheets.

National Committee to Preserve Social Security and Medicare Foundation (NCPSSM Foundation)
http://www.ncpssmfoundation.org
A nonprofit working to assure well-being and financial stability of older adults in the United States, NCPSSM advocates for broad support of

public welfare services for populations covered by Social Security and Medicare. The NCPSSM website notes that those with disabilities, the oldest-old, ethnic minorities, women, rural residents, and children are among the most vulnerable. This organization works to promote greater public understanding of both challenges to and benefits of Social Security and Medicare as well as increase awareness on these topics. The NCPSSM agenda to educate Americans includes an aim addressing media coverage of these public programs for older Americans.

National Council on Aging (NCOA)
https://www.ncoa.org
A nonprofit advocacy organization for adults over age 60, the National Council on Aging aims to improve the economic security of older adults that they may have secure and dignified later lives. This organization offers tools to learn about basic needs, economic security, and health benefits by sponsoring BenefitsCheckUp (https://www.benefitscheckup.org), EconomicCheckUp (https://www.benefitscheckup.org/esi-home/) and My Medicare Matters (https://www.mymedicarematters.org).

National Hispanic Council on Aging (NHCOA)
http://www.nhcoa.org
Founded in the late 1970s to improve quality of life among Latino elders, today NHCOA links affiliated community organizations across the continental United States and Puerto Rico through the Hispanic Aging Network, which enables dissemination of culturally appropriate programming. These organizations address issues of wellness, financial stability, and housing while emphasizing relevance of these topics for aging Latinos, for example, by focusing on diabetes prevention, promoting food security, advocating for paid family leave, and developing affordable housing options for low-income seniors.

National Indian Council on Aging (NICOA)
http://nicoa.org
This nonprofit organization was established in 1976 at the urging of members of the National Tribal Chairmen's Association to represent aging and elder American Indian and Alaska Natives at the national level. The aims of NICOA are to communicate and cooperate with community-based providers who serve and represent American Indian and Alaska Native elders; promote health and maximize effective health care by sharing information and offering technical assistance; and offer education resources salient for American Indian and Alaska Native elders, their caregivers, and advocates.

This organization also participates in the Senior Community Service Employment Program (SCSEP).

National Institute on Aging (NIA)
https://www.nia.nih.gov
This organization is under the National Institutes of Health (NIH) and focuses on research "dedicated to understanding the nature of aging, supporting the health and well-being of older adults, and extending healthy, active years of life for more people." The website features not only an alphabetized list of health topics, and also innovative publications to promote doctor-patient communication, resources explaining various aspects of exercise, posters promoting the value of physical activity, as well as resources in Spanish, and a subsection on dedicated to research and funding.

National Resource Center on LGBT Aging
https://www.lgbtagingcenter.org
Funded by a grant from the U.S. Department of Health and Human Services in 2010, this organization works to improve the services provided to lesbian, gay, bisexual, and transgender (LGBT) older adults. Their site features a number of webinar trainings on how to work with diverse populations as well as an interactive map to find resources by state and by topic. Their database features information on veterans, transgender themes, racial equity, intimate partner violence, and *en español* (Spanish language) resources.

National Resource Center on Native American Aging
https://www.nrcnaa.org
With the aim of bringing attention to concerns for aging Native populations, this organization works to improve services provided to Native elders and create better outcomes for the population served. This National Resource Center is funded by the Administration on Aging.

National Senior Citizens Law Center (NSCLC)
http://nsclcarchives.org
Created in 1972, this organization works to protect disadvantaged minorities so individuals of any background can live as contributing citizens without distraction from destitution or lack of health care. NSCLC educates and trains local advocates and litigates with the goal of defending the rights of low-income seniors. The NSCLC website offers information about relevant court cases, economic safety net programs like Supplemental Security Income (SSI) and Social Security, as well as information on

refugees and SSI benefits, cross-cultural health disparities and a subsection on language access.

NIH Senior Health

http://nihseniorhealth.gov

This website is a resource designed specifically for adults over age 60 with a compilation of health-related information subdivided into broad categories and offered in an accessible, alphabetized, easily navigable list format with summaries of each topic, options to gather additional information, and suggested complementary topics. In addition to providing access to some of the vast stores of information sustained by NIH, this website offers training materials for those who hope to teach older adults to use this particular resource.

National Shared Housing Resource Center (NSHRC)

(http://nationalsharedhousing.org)

Homesharing programs are based on geographic region, so local areas operate their own websites to coordinate interest in home sharing in a given state or county. The NSHRC website serves as a hub for such local programs and provides an accessible online directory that is a useful resource for finding regionally operated programs by state.

Office of Disability, Aging, and Long-Term Care Policy (DALTCP)

http://aspe.hhs.gov/office_specific/daltcp.cfm

This office evaluates programs and policies of the United States Department of Health and Human Services. DALTCP is also charged with investigating ways to advance the fiscal and general wellness of older Americans. The DALTCP subunits are Division of Behavioral Health and Intellectual Disabilities Policy, Division of Disability and Aging Policy, and Division of Long-Term Care Policy.

Older Women's League (OWL)

http://www.owl-national.org

Founded in 1980 to promote economic security for women over 40, today OWL represents over 75 million women of that demographic. The organization releases a report each May, entitled the annual *Mother's Day Report*, to highlight a key economic issue for that year. OWL identifies key concerns related to quality of life such as wellness, menopause, elder abuse, end-of-life, and some health-care initiatives.

Old Women's Project

http://www.oldwomensproject.org

A collective of three women from San Diego, California, that does not accept members but encourages participation from all females in various actions they have organized and other progressive protests and local rallies they have joined. The Old Women's Project website summarizes their aim: "to make visible how old women are directly affected by all issues of social justice, and to combat the ageist attitudes that ignore, trivialize or demean us."

Raging Grannies
(Various websites, e.g., http://raginggrannies.org/, http://raginggrannies.net, http://www.raginggrannies.com)
Founded in 1987 in Canadian British Columbia, this conglomeration of activist organizations uses performance-based tactics like costume and song to spread their vision for a just and peaceful society. Their protests have addressed gender equity, environmental concerns, affordability of health care, and economic justice.

Resource Centers for Minority Aging Research (RCMAR)
http://www.rcmar.ucla.edu
A National Institute on Aging grant funds seven centers across the United States with the aim of "bridging the gap between health disparity research and successful minority aging." The RCMAR website features publications by affiliates, conferences, funding opportunities, and links to the informative websites of each of the seven centers.

SeniorNet
http://www.seniornet.org
This nonprofit, member-supported organization has offered older adults education about computers and Internet usage since 1986. Their website features past newsletters, information about learning centers that offer classes on technology for adults aged 50 or older, and exercises on computer basics such as how to use a mouse.

Senior Community Service Employment Program (SCSEP)
http://www.doleta.gov/seniors/
Created under Title V of the Older American Act of 1965, today the U.S. Department of Labor Employment and Training Administration administers this federally funded program as a minimum-waged community service job-training program. It constitutes the largest program serving older adult workers in search of work or training. Individuals must be at least 55 years old, unemployed, and living in households with income at or below 125 percent of the federal poverty level in order to participate.

Services & Advocacy for Gay, Lesbian, Bisexual, & Transgender Elders (SAGE)
http://www.sageusa.org
This national group is the largest and longest running organization advocating and providing services to LGBT older adults. They have a presence

in 20 states as well as Washington, D.C., to support quality of life for LGBT adults, encourage positive representations of this population, increase understanding of aging in general, and advocate for aging LGBT adults.

Setting Priorities for Retirement Years (SPRY) Foundation
http://www.spry.org
With a focus on converting research related to aging into information that can be readily used and applied in a variety of settings, SPRY Foundation has a strong focus on education. Their site features publications as well as past initiatives.

Social Security Administration
http://www.ssa.gov
This federal agency coordinates Social Security services offered across the United States. The website offers information about benefits for disability, Supplemental Security Income, retirement, children, individuals after incarceration, children with disabilities, and government employees. Their online offerings also include information for racial and ethnic minorities, same-sex couples, women, wounded veterans, immigrants, deaf or hard of hearing, blind or visually impaired persons, as well as third-party representatives, planners, and professionals.

Stanford Geriatric Education Center (SGEC)
http://sgec.stanford.edu
Specializes in health care for older adults from diverse populations, this consortium provides information to health-care providers about the needs of ethnic minority elders and their loved ones. The SGEC website features webinars as well as a unique section with resources about "cultural and spiritual diversity in end of life care."

Well Spouse Association
http://www.wellspouse.org
Founded in 1988 by 10 individuals who were spouses to chronically ill individuals, this organization exists to support that demographic through local chapters, increase awareness among professionals and the public as to the role of healthy spouses, and to promote solutions that work for these families. The website features annual reports; articles on advocacy, navigating health-care systems, spousal caregiving, and humor; as well as a calendar of events that are organized by members.

APPENDIX B

Documentaries about Aging

Elizabeth A. Daniele

Of the hundreds of documentaries that focus on aging, this list features a handful created since 2000. Such films are particularly important given our aging nation. Many of the documentaries featured here highlight inequalities linked to race, class, gender, sexuality, and living arrangements. Topics include the experiences of ethnic minority elders, older adult sexuality for lesbian, gay, bisexual, and transgender (LGBT) and straight Americans, aging workers, elder care, and abuse of older adults. The films incorporate myriad perspectives on aging, politics, inequality, and social movements. Inclusion on this list does not reflect an endorsement. Films are generally paraphrased or summarized in my words, though in some cases the words of the film creator or production company are included.

"A Place to Live: The Story of Triangle Square"
88 minutes
This impressive documentary follows seven gay and lesbian seniors who want to live in Triangle Square in Los Angeles. Triangle Square was the first affordable housing designed specifically for LGBT elders in the United States. Fittingly opening with reflections on their individual life histories, the film draws attention to the experiences of low-income, older LGBT adults and captures elements of opening the unique facility.

Childs, C., Munro, S., Dromi, N. (Producers), & Coal, C. (Director). (2008). *A place to live: The story of Triangle Square* [Motion Picture]. United States: NoCo Media Group and Bittersweet Productions.

"The Age of Love"
79 minutes
This documentary follows seniors who participate in a unique speed dating event for adults over age 70. It raises questions about relationships, romance, aging bodies, and the human experience of loving.

Loring, S. (Producer & Director). (2014). *The age of love* [Motion Picture]. United States: Free Play Pictures.

"Ageless"
27 minutes
This documentary addresses the topic of media and mainstream depictions of beauty as embodied by youth.

Gwaltney, H. (Producer), Akhamie, A., Saylor, D. (Associate Producers), & Gwaltney, H. (Director). (2014). *Ageless* [Motion Picture]. United States.

"American Outrage"
33 minute- and 56- minute versions
This film features the story of Carrie and Mary Dann, two elder Western Shoshone sisters who have been fighting against the United States Government since the early 1970s for the right to stay on their land in Nevada.

Gage, B., & Gage, G. (Directors). (2008). *American outrage* [Motion Picture]. United States: Gage and Gage Films & Bullfrog Films.

"American Revolutionary: The Evolution of Grace Lee Boggs"
82 minutes
This documentary focuses on the life of Grace Lee Boggs, who has been an activist involved with many social movements throughout her 97 years of life, including civil rights, feminism, and environmental justice.

Libresco, C., Wilkin, A. (Producers), & Lee, G. (Producer & Director). (2013). *American revolutionary: The evolution of Grace Lee Boggs* [Motion Picture]. United States: Chicken and Egg Pictures.

"An Age for Justice: Elder Abuse in America"
16 minutes
In a short video produced by a coalition of groups for the Elder Justice Now campaign, the film highlights physical, fiscal, and emotional elder abuse—and uses vignettes about individuals to put a human face on these different types of mistreatment.

WITNESS. (2010, April 21). *An age for justice: Elder abuse in America* [Video file]. Retrieved from https://www.youtube.com/watch?v=-eaJXBj87to&feature=youtu.be

"Before You Know It"
110 minutes
This film offers a relatively intimate perspective of individual LGBT seniors' lives by following three older gay men: one who likes to cross dress but

does not do so publically until he moves to an LGBT retirement community, one who does community outreach for Services and Advocacy for GLBT Elders (SAGE) in Harlem when New York State approves gay marriage, and an owner of a long-standing gay bar in Texas. While the documentary addresses some universal aspects of aging, it also brings to the fore some unique challenges faced by older adults who identify as LGBT.

Bush, A., Giustini, S. (Producers), & Raval, P.J. (Producer & Director). (2013). *Before you know it* [Motion Picture]. United States: Untitled Films.

"Big Mama"
40 minutes
This award-winning film documents the trials of Viola Dees, an African American elder trying to raise her grandson, Walter, while navigating the foster care system. The film highlights the importance of love at different ages and some difficulties encountered by grandfamilies, such as health concerns and questions about when the state challenges a grandparent's competence.

Block, M., Nevins, S. (Executive Producers), & Seretean, T. (Producer & Director). (2000). *Big mama* [Motion Picture]. United States: California Newsreel.

"The Caretaker"
8 minutes
This short documentary is about an undocumented Fijian immigrant who is a caregiver for an ill, elderly Japanese American woman in California.

Rigby, T., & McLean, K. (Directors). (2012). *The caretaker* [Motion Picture]. United States: Public Broadcasting service (PBS).

"The Collector of Bedford Street"
34 minutes
This documentary focuses on Larry Selman, the filmmaker's neighbor who is an older community activist with an intellectual disability. When his uncle can no longer provide care, Larry's community comes together to ensure that he can stay in his apartment.

Elliott, A. (Producer & Director). (2002). *The collector of Bedford Street* [Motion Picture]. United States: Welcome Change Productions.

"Cut Back: Facing Ageism"
73 minutes
This documentary offers discussion of ageism in the workplace primarily through personal tales from individuals who have experienced such

discrimination. These individual testimonies are supplemented by commentary from experts and professionals who deal in this realm. The film has been divided into segments and is available in its entirety online at http://cutbackmovie.com.

Sahertian, P. (Producer & Director). (2009). *Cut back: Facing ageism* [Motion Picture]. United States: CHeZ MaTch.

"Do Not Go Gently"
57 minutes
This film explores the power and impact of creativity in later life by documenting experiences of three artists.

Littig, E. (Executive Producer), & Godoy, M. (Producer & Director). (2007). *Do not go gently* [Motion Picture]. United States: American Public Television.

"Fleeced: Speaking Out against Senior Financial Abuse"
30 minutes
Exposing the high rates of seniors who are scammed or taken advantage of in the financial realm, this film looks at the impacts of financial deception on elders.

Jacobs, K. (Producer). (2013). *Fleeced: Speaking out against senior financial abuse* [Motion Picture]. United States: National Community Reinvestment Coalition, & WFYI Productions.

"Gen Silent"
64 minutes
By following six LGBT older adults in Boston, Massachusetts, this film explores decisions around health care and aging. It explores the theme one professional calls "distrust of mainstream institutions" among a generation that lived through McCarthyism and the highly closeted gay culture in the 1950s. Because institutionalization was a common treatment for homosexuals in earlier eras, there may be hesitancy to go to such places as hospitals or long-term care facilities. Further, the topics of training health-care providers on awareness and sensitivity, as well as provider resistance and objection to caring for LGBT elders are discussed.

Atkin, B.J. (Executive Producer), & Maddux, S. (Director). (2011). *Gen silent* [Motion Picture]. United States: Interrobang! Productions

"Golden Years: Aging and the Elderly"
27 minutes
Looking at the impacts of an aging population in the United States, this film focuses on programming at a particular nursing home and highlights

the longevity revolution to discuss quality and quantity of life in later years.

Kasparian, Y. (2005). Golden years: Aging and the elderly [Television series episode]. In Kammen, G. (Producer) *The way we live*. United States: Intelecom.

"Kings Point"

40 minutes

This documentary tells the stories of men and women who moved to Florida many years ago and how they are managing in their retirement community as they age. As the film's website says, this film "explores the dynamic tension between living and aging—between our desire for independence and our need for community—and underscores our powerful ambivalence toward growing old" (http://www.kingspoint movie.com).

Wider, J., Wider, T. (Producers), & Gilman, S. (Producer & Director). (2012). *Kings point* [Motion Picture]. United States: Wider Film Projects, & HBO Documentary Films.

"Old People Driving: A Film about the End of the Road"

25 minutes

Alluding to the national love of driving automobiles and acknowledging what one interview subject refers to as the association of driving with independence, this film explores the topic of older adult drivers. The documentary features stories of two male drivers in their 90s and is interspersed with statistics about older drivers as compared to other age groups, relevant media clips, and commentary from experts as well as family and friends of these older drivers. The filmmakers highlight gendered aspects of decisions to give up driving and raise questions about the role of public policy in this sphere.

Haas, S. (Producer & Director). (2010). *Old people driving: A film about the end of the road* [Motion Picture]. United States: New Day Films.

"The 100+ Club"

30 minutes

This film challenges traditional ideas about what it means to be an older adult by introducing three individuals who have lived a century, but are still pursuing ambitions in the realms of athletics, writing, and theater production.

Brown, M. (Producer), & Lake, M. (Director). (2012). *The 100+ club* [Motion Picture]. Australia: Flickchicks.

"The Passage of Time"
69 minutes
Comprised of interviews with people of many ages, this documentary explores the meaning of aging through exploration of meanings of life and death. Available for free and in its entirety online (https://vimeo.com/119885830), this film may be a useful tool to open discussions about aging, life course, and mortality.

Habif, D.A. (Producer & Director). (2013). *The passage of time* [Motion Picture]. United States: Horizon Films.

"Raging Grannies"
33 minutes
This film is interspersed with educational performances and media spots, but comprised primarily of footage from activist actions and personal interviews with older women who are members of the San Francisco Bay Area Peninsula Raging Grannies group. This chapter of Raging Grannies is one among many worldwide, and they describe themselves as concerned with the welfare of children and families around the world. The film highlights their clever use of humor and their self-proclaimed nonthreatening image to draw attention to matters of injustice in their region.

Carranza, R. (Producer), & Walton, P. (Producer & Director). (2009). *Raging grannies* [Motion Picture]. United States: New Day Films.

"The Retirement Gamble"
55 minutes
This episode of Frontline investigates the American retirement system, focusing on how retirement savings are managed. The program suggests that Wall Street is winning profits at the expense of individuals.

Gaviria, M., Smith, M. (Writers), & Smith, M. (Director). (2013). The retirement gamble [Television series episode]. In Gaviria, M. (Producer) *Frontline*. United States: Public Broadcasting Service (PBS).

"The Sandwich Generation"
28 minutes
The terms sandwich generation refers to those who are caring for young children and aging parents. The filmmaker, Julie Winokur, and her husband document their personal journey in moving across the country with their two children to care for Winokur's elderly father, who has dementia.

Winokur, J. (Producer & Director). (2008). *The sandwich generation* [Motion Picture]. United States: Talking Eyes Media.

"The Self-Made Man"
53 minutes
This documentary raises questions about what the film's website calls rational suicide and the right-to-die, and what entrepreneur Bob Stern's suicide note calls quantity versus quality of life. It is comprised of photos and narratives about the Stern family, interviews with family and friends of Bob Stern, and footage of Bob speaking to a camera about not pursuing medical treatment for his illnesses.

Bernal Beach Films (Producer), & Stern, S. (Director). (2005). *The self-made man* [Motion Picture]. United States: New Day Films.

"Stages"
82 minutes
This film features older Puerto Rican women coming together with youth in a New York City community center to create a play about their lives. As the website mentions, the participants' work engages "themes of immigration, identity, aging and coming of age" (http://www.stagesmovie.com).

Meerkat Media Collective (Directors). (2009). *Stages* [Motion Picture]. United States: New Day Films.

"Still Doing It: The Intimate Lives of Women Over 65"
56 minutes
Opening with bold statements by women over age 65 about their excitement over sexual activity in their later lives, this film explores the topic of intimacy among a diverse group of older women in the United States. Tying in individual histories of marriage, religious practices, involvement with social movements, as well as contemporary interviews, these women speak very frankly about sexual urges and sexual activity in later life, female bodies in general, and aging bodies in particular.

Holtberg, D. (Producer), & Fishel, D. (Director). (2004). *Still doing it: The intimate lives of women over 65* [Motion Picture]. United States: Mind's Eye Productions.

"Ten More Good Years"
71 minutes
Through interviews with experts and LGBT elders, this film explores historical trends and pressing contemporary realities for an aging LGBT population.

Jacoby, M. (Producer & Director). (2007). *Ten more good years* [Motion Picture]. United States: LookOut Films.

"Two Raging Grannies"
78 minutes
Two elder women who have significant histories of involvement with social justice issues travel the United States asking questions that challenge the framework of infinite economic growth.

Falch, C. (Producer), & Bustnes, H. (Producer & Director). (2013). *Two raging grannies* [Motion Picture]. Denmark: Faction Film.

"We Got Us"
27 minutes
This film focuses on four older women who play mah-jongg together on a weekly basis. Filmed over 18 months, it reflects their views on themes of living and aging.

Brooker, J., (Producer & Director), & Harry, M. (Producer). (2001). *We got us* [Motion Picture]. United States: Docurama.

Index

About the Editors and Contributors

Editors

Madonna Harrington Meyer, PhD, is chair of sociology, Laura J. and L. Douglas Meredith Professor of Teaching Excellence, and faculty associate of the Aging Studies Institute, at Syracuse University. She is co-editor, with Ynesse Abdul-Malak, of the forthcoming *Grandparenting in the United States*. She is author of *Grandmothers at Work: Juggling Families and Jobs*, winner of the 2014 GSA Kalish Book Award. She is co-author with Pamela Herd of *Market Friendly or Family Friendly? The State and Gender Inequality in Old Age*, winner of the 2008 GSA Kalish Book Award. She is also editor of *Care Work: Gender, Labor, and the Welfare State*.

Elizabeth A. Daniele, MS, is a PhD student and fellow in sociology at Syracuse University. She is a co-editor of *Student Involvement and Academic Outcomes: Implications for Diverse Student Populations* (2015). She also co-authored a chapter about diversity in American graduate education in *International Perspectives in Higher Education Admission Policy: A Reader* (2015). She has a BA from Smith College and an MS in higher education administration from the University of Rochester.

Contributors

Ron Acierno, PhD, is professor and associate dean for research in the College of Nursing at the Medical University of South Carolina. He has two distinct research foci: Elder Mistreatment epidemiology and telemedicine for delivering evidence based mental health treatments. He led the National Institute of Justice/National Institute on Aging (NIA) funded *National Elder Mistreatment Study*, the largest risk factor and prevalence study of elder abuse to date, and authored the methodology chapter for the NIA core handbook *Elder Mistreatment: Abuse, Neglect, and Exploitation in an Aging America* (2003).

Carolyn E. Adams-Price, PhD, is an associate professor of psychology at Mississippi State University, and a research fellow at the National Strategic Planning and Analysis Research Center (NSPARC). She is the editor of *Creativity and Successful Aging: Theoretical and Empirical Approaches* (1998). She has a BA from the University of California at Santa Cruz, an MS from Brandeis University, and a PhD in life-span developmental psychology from West Virginia University. She is the author of 40+ journal articles and book chapters, mostly on aging.

Monika Ardelt, PhD, is associate professor of sociology and an advisory board member of the Center for Spirituality and Health at the University of Florida. She is a Brookdale National Fellow and a Fellow of the Gerontological Society of America. Dr. Ardelt developed the widely used *Three-Dimensional Wisdom Scale* (3D-WS; Ardelt, 2003) and is the coeditor of the book *Faith and Well-Being in Late Life: Linking Theories with Evidence in an Interdisciplinary Inquiry* (2009). Her research focuses on successful human development across the life course with particular emphasis on the relations between wisdom, religion, spirituality, aging well, and dying well.

Stephanie W. Burge, PhD, is associate professor of sociology at the University of Oklahoma. Her research on long-term care focuses on assisted living facilities and factors that promote elders' successful transition into long-term care, with emphasis on how residents' social relationships affect their perceptions of well-being and health. She has also studied admission and retention practices and policies of assisted living facilities. A second avenue of her research focuses on the transition to adulthood, highlighting gender differences in adolescents' educational and career plans, as well as the link between adolescent plans and eventual attainments in young adulthood.

Deborah Carr, PhD, is professor and former chair of sociology at Rutgers University. She has published widely on death, dying, and bereavement, with nearly 100 chapters and articles appearing in journals including *Journal of Health & Social Behavior* and *Journal of Marriage & Family*. She is the author or editor of several books including *Worried Sick: How Stress Hurts Us and How to Bounce Back* (2014), *Encyclopedia of the Life Course and Human Development* (2009), and *Spousal Bereavement in Late Life* (2006). Carr serves as editor-in-chief of *The Journals of Gerontology, Series B: Social Sciences* (2015–18).

Emily S. Fanguy is the program assistant for Project BEST at the National Crime Victims Research and Treatment Center at the Medical University of South Carolina. She received her Bachelor of Science in psychology from the College of Charleston in 2013.

Melba Hernandez-Tejada, DHA, is a research instructor at the Medical University of South Carolina and a research coordinator at the Ralph H. Johnson VA Medical Center. She has a master's degree in clinical psychology from Simon Bolivar University (Caracas, Venezuela) and Doctor of Health Administration from the Medical University of South Carolina. She has several publications on elder mistreatment, health disparities, and PTSD and telemedicine in veterans.

Donna J. Holmes, PhD, is an associate research professor and medical educator at the University of Idaho. She has authored 60 papers and book chapters, including commentaries on aging for *Science* and *Heredity*. She was the editor of the aging and gerontology section of Elsevier's 2014 *Reference Modules in Biomedical Sciences* and is coediting a forthcoming book, *Evolution and Human Health across the Life Span*. She is the 2016 chair of the Biological Sciences Section, Gerontological Society of America, and serves on the Executive Committee of the American Aging Association. She has an AB from Miami University and a PhD from Bowling Green State University.

Megumi Inoue, PhD, MSW, RN, is an assistant professor in the Department of Social Work at George Mason University. Her research focuses on health and aging, and she is particularly interested in end-of-life care and patients' autonomy in health-care settings. Dr. Inoue brings her extensive clinical experience as a social worker and a registered nurse to her understanding of research on end-of-life issues.

Vicki Johnson-Lawrence, PhD, is a social epidemiologist and assistant professor within the Department of Public Health and Health Sciences at the University of Michigan-Flint. Her work examines health inequities over the life course, and she specifically studies cooccurring chronic conditions within vulnerable populations.

Sara Keary, PhD, MSW, is a gerontological social worker with a clinical background in inpatient geriatric psychiatry, bereavement, and HIV/AIDS. Her research focuses on issues affecting LGBT older adults as well as advance care planning among older adult populations. She received her BASW and MSW from the University of Pittsburgh School of Social Work and her PhD in social work from Boston College.

Donna D. McAlpine, PhD, is an associate professor of public health at the University of Minnesota. She is coauthor, with David Mechanic and David A. Rochefort, of the sixth edition of *Mental Health and Social Policy. Beyond Managed Care* (2014). She received her PhD in sociology from Rutgers, The State University of New Jersey.

Sara M. Moorman, PhD, is an associate professor of sociology at Boston College. She is a fellow of the Gerontological Society of America and a member of the Institute on Aging at Boston College. Her research on marital quality and advance care planning has appeared in peer-reviewed publications including *The Gerontologist, The Journal of Aging and Health, The Journal of Marriage and Family, The Journal of Social and Personal Relationships, The Journals of Gerontology, Series B,* and *Research on Aging*. She earned her doctorate in sociology from the University of Wisconsin at Madison in 2009.

Eliza K. Pavalko, PhD, is the Allen D. and Polly S. Grimshaw Professor of sociology and Vice Provost for Faculty and Academic Affairs at Indiana University. Her research focuses on paid work, caregiving, and health across the life course. Recent articles include "Do Women Still Care? Cohort Changes in U.S. Women's Care for the Ill or Disabled" (with Joseph D. Wolfe) in *Social Forces*, "Double Time: Is Health Affected by a Spouse's Time at Work?" (with Sibyl Kleiner) in *Social Forces*, and "Social Inequality and Health Across the Life Course" (with Jennifer Caputo) in *American Behavioral Scientist*.

Taeho Greg Rhee, AM, is a PhD candidate at the Department of Pharmaceutical Care and Health Systems, College of Pharmacy, University of Minnesota, Twin Cities. His research interests include aging, determinants of and disparities in mental health, use of psychiatric medications, and patient safety. He holds an AB in economics and mathematics from Emory University and an AM in social service administration from the University of Chicago.

Fengyan Tang, PhD, is associate professor of social work at the University of Pittsburgh. She has published over 40 peer-reviewed journal articles and book chapters in the topics of productive engagement of older adults in volunteering, paid work, and caregiving. She also studies aging in place, service use, health disparities, minority aging, and subjective well-being in later life.

Joah L. Williams, PhD, is an assistant professor in the Department of Psychology at the University of Missouri, Kansas City. He received his PhD in clinical psychology from the University of Memphis in 2013 and recently completed a fellowship in child and adult trauma research at the Medical University of South Carolina's National Crime Victims Research and Treatment Center. He has broad research and clinical interests in the area of traumatic stress and has published several articles and book chapters on the consequences and treatment of interpersonal violence exposure.

Joseph D. Wolfe, PhD, is an assistant professor of sociology at the University of Alabama at Birmingham. In addition to care work, he studies the cumulative processes triggered by adversity that are capable of shaping health throughout the life course and across generations. His current research examines the relationship between multigenerational attainment and mortality, the importance of social ties for intergenerational stress proliferation, and the interactive effects of adversity and substance use on health.

Anna Zajacova, PhD, is an associate professor of sociology at University of Wyoming. Zajacova's background is in demography, sociology, and social epidemiology. She studies population health among adults in the United States, focusing especially on social determinants of health and mortality. Her recent research was published in the *Journal of Health and Social Behavior, American Journal of Epidemiology, The Gerontologist, Cancer,* and *the Journals of Gerontology.*

Multigrid Methods for Finite Elements

by

V. V. Şhaidurov
Computing Center,
Russian Academy of Sciences,
Siberian Branch,
Krasnoyarsk, Russia

KLUWER ACADEMIC PUBLISHERS
DORDRECHT / BOSTON / LONDON

A C.I.P. Catalogue record for this book is available from the Library of Congress.

ISBN 0-7923-3290-3

Published by Kluwer Academic Publishers,
P.O. Box 17, 3300 AA Dordrecht, The Netherlands.

Kluwer Academic Publishers incorporates
the publishing programmes of
D. Reidel, Martinus Nijhoff, Dr W. Junk and MTP Press.

Sold and distributed in the U.S.A. and Canada
by Kluwer Academic Publishers,
101 Philip Drive, Norwell, MA 02061, U.S.A.

In all other countries, sold and distributed
by Kluwer Academic Publishers Group,
P.O. Box 322, 3300 AH Dordrecht, The Netherlands.

This is an updated and revised translation of the original work
Multigrid Methods of Finite Elements,
Moscow, Nauka © 1989
Translated from Russian by N.B. Urusova

Printed on acid-free paper

Printed in the Netherlands

Contents

Preface

At present, the finite element method has become one of the most widespread and effective methods to solve a variety of problems in mathematical physics and engineering. Its popularity is connected with universality and simplicity of mathematical form for a wide range of problems, in combination with flexibility of numerical algorithms, enabling concrete properties of an individual problem to be considered. To no small degree, its success has been due to the development of high-speed computer techniques and by advances in the fields of projective methods and approximation theory.

The material for this book is based on a series of works of various mathematiciants, especially the monographs by P.G.Ciarlet, S.F.McCormick, L.A.Oganesyan and L.A.Rukhovets, G.I.Marchuk and V.I.Agoshkhov, G.Fix and G.Streng and W.Hackbusch, as well as on results of research carried out by the author at the Krasnoyarsk Computing Center of the Siberian Division of the Russian Academy of Sciences.

Traditional mathematical principles of the finite element method will be discussed briefly enough in view of the large number of monographs on the subject. A more detailed description is given of important technical problems which are not treated well in the literature, namely: triangulation techniques of two- and three-dimensional domains, efficient quadrature formulae, and using a mixed method as a systematic way to change burdensome main conditions in basis subspaces for natural ones. Such a substitution allows, for example, to simplify a treatment of the Dirichlet non-uniform boundary conditions, to reduce the biharmonic equation to a system of second-order equations and to remove the rather inconvenient requirement of solenoidality of basis functions in the Stokes and Navier-Stokes problems.

When considering specific problems, the simplest and most widespread finite elements were used, at the same time noting ways of using more complicated ones.

The greatest attention is paid to the numerical solution of algebraic problems with large sparse matrices following discretization by means of multigrid algorithms, first proposed by R.P.Fedorenko in 1961. These algorithms lead to a wide range of applications and, at the same time, such an unimproved property as a finite number of arithmetical operations per one unknown for achievment of the accuracy stipulated by the convergence order.

Hundreds of present publications reveal that the practical use of these methods are often ahead in efficiency of other direct and iterative methods.

This book presents a more detailed study of multigrid methods applied to concrete problems. It also includes some new results on the optimization of iterative parameters, solving generalized spectral problems, applying a mixed finite element method, and solving problems with peculiarities and curvilinear boundaries.

This book is intended for engineers and research workers using or developing the finite element method for solving practical problems. The material is discussed in such a way that the main parts may be applied, directly or by close analogy, to many more problems. The relatively self-contained and detailed discussion is intelligible to senior-year students of mathematics and engineering specialities.

The style and the material of the book underwent essential changes in comparison with Russian variant published in 1989. Discussions with collegues, new results of other scientists influenced the description. Besides, some proofs were specified and inaccuracies were corrected.

This work became possible due to a partial financial support of Mathematical Department of the Magdeburg Otto-von-Guericke University, Berlin Institute of Applied Analysis and Stochastics, Beijing Institute of Systems Science. The auther acknoleges them for the possibility to take part in several conferences, to work in excellent libraries, to discuss with collegues from many countries. The author is deeply grateful to G.I.Marchuk and other scientists including N.S.Bakhvalov, R.P.Fedorenko, L.Tobiska, V.G.Korneev, Q.Lin, E.G.D'jakonov, U.Langer, whose advice and remarks have led to improvement. The author also thanks S.N.Bogdanov, A.V.Smirnov for numerical experiments carried out and T.G.Belokopytova, N.B.Urusova, S.V.Belokopytov, J.Fuhrmann, S.Hengst for the help during the work at the manuscript.

V.Shaidurov

Introduction

The history of the finite element method goes back to the works of V.Ritz, I.G.Bubnov and B.G.Galerkin. The constructive foundation of the method is a variational form of the problem and the use of splines with small supports called finite elements. Applying this method to a differential problem gives a finite-dimensional system of linear (or non-linear) algebraic equations, the solution of which yields parameters of splines approximating a sought function.

Solving a concrete problem of mathematical physics by using this method usually involves 4 main stages:

1. a variational formulation of the problem;

2. a choice of finite elements and a triangulation of the geometrical domain, i.e., dividing the domain into small supports of finite elements of a given form;

3. an assembly of the system of algebraic equations, often by using quadrature formulae;

4. solving the algebraic equations obtained.

In spite of the fact that there exists a great number of books on the finite element method, when this method is constantly being developed, questions arise at each of these stages indicated above which are not discussed well in the literature. For the first stage, a mixed variational formulation becomes lately a means of greater importance. Its application permits to use simpler finite elements, to raise the accuracy and efficiency of the numerical realization of problems such as the biharmonic equation, and the Stokes and Navier-Stokes problems. As far as the second stage is concerned, there is no a systematic discussion of the automatic triangulation of geometrical domains, especially of three-dimensional ones. The requirement of the third stage for calculations to be efficient puts quadrature formulae at the forefront, which, as a rule, are little-used for calculations. Finally, the fourth stage is not in practice discussed in the literature on finite elements. This is due to the fact that systems solved by means of a great number of direct and iterative methods. The monograph by A.A.Samarski and E.S.Nikolaev [156] provides a good overview of these methods.

One of the most effective and rather universal iterative methods for solving the systems obtained has become lately the multigrid method. Two approaches form its algorithmic base. We can illustrate these by an example of a grid problem corresponding to a rather fine triangulation and having a large number of unknowns. The first approach consists in consecutively solving the grid problems similar to an initial problem but corresponding to coarser triangulations. Solving begins on the most coarse triangulation, where it can be made efficiently. Then the obtained solution is interpolated on a finer triangulation and used as an initial approximation having an accuracy close to a satisfactory one. Thus, much fewer iterations in the iterative process are needed to obtain the required accuracy. This approach was widely practised in the times of manual and mechanized calculations when one uses all the costly information obtained from the coarse grid if he was forced to pass on to a finer grid. The second approach was suggested by R.P.Fedorenko in his article [53]. It is based on a fast convergence of some iterative processes for higher harmonics, which permits to decrease their contribution into the error essentially within a few iterations. Lower harmonics converge far slower and so they make up the most part of the error. As a result, the error becomes some smoothly changing grid function for which a system of grid equations can be written with residual on the right-hand side. In principle, this system can be solved, and the error can be found, but such a way is rather expensive. Instead of this note that a differential problem with a sufficiently smooth solution can be brought in correspondence to this system. For this differential problem, we again construct a grid on a coarser triangulation (for example, two or three times coarser). Such a system can be solved more efficiently since the number of unknowns and equations, for example, in the two-dimensional case, is four or nine times less. By virtue of stated smoothness, its solution approximates the sought error on this triangulation well enough.

Now interpolate it (even if linearly) onto a finer triangulation. In view of smoothly changing the error will be found with a rather high accuracy. Further one can construct some more iterations to suppress the high-frequency component following an interpolation or repeat once again all the procedure of transition to a coarser triangulation. Solving a grid problem on a triangulation twice or three times coarser may be still expensive, so it also can be solved approximately by using the described technique of the transition to a coarser triangulation. This method for decreasing the dimension can be used until going on to the coarsest triangulation on which the solution can be obtained easily enough by using the direct method.

Though the multigrid method is relatively complicated in the algorithmic sense, in 1964 R.P.Fedorenko [54] managed to prove its convergence for the finite-difference analogue of Poisson equation on square.

In 1966 N.S.Bakhvalov [19] proved this method to be optimal in respect of the number of arithmetical operations needed to achieve the accuracy agreed with the convergence order.

According to asymptotical estimates of efficiency, the method was ahead of other known algorithms but for a time its quality was veiled in its complicated logic and hard mathematical substantiation.

At a certain stage of developing the finite element method, a new mathematical apparatus and program realizations sufficiently decreased expense of the algorithm and simplified its validating. That is why at the end of 70th an increase has begun and is still in progress in the amount of the literature on multigrid methods.

The monograph on the convergence theory of multigrid methods by W.Hackbush [68], owing to an abundance of the results accumulated and presented, should be defined as a reference book sooner. Therefore, when writing this book one of the purposes was to discuss systematically and to study in detail this promising method to be applied to the most frequently-used boundary problems of mathematical physics.

The structure and the substantiation of the multigrid method for finite elements are closely connected with the first three stages of discretization. This requires the material to be discussed in strict sequence.

Chapter 1 presents typical linear boundary problems of order 2 or 4, explanes how to pass from a classical operator formulation to a generalized variation formulation including the mixed one. For the discussion to be uniform, only one of the variation principles was considered, namely, the Bubnov-Galerkin method. Most of the results can be applied to Ritz method as well as to the method of least squares.

Chapter 2 treats general properties of finite elements and has a reference nature on the simplest and frequently-used finite elements as well as triangulation techniques of the two- and three-dimensional regions including a condensation of the triangulation near peculiar points and lines.

Chapter 3 deals with the convergence of the approximate solutions of the Bubnov-Galerkin method in the following sequence: approximation properties of finite elements, convergence conditions of approximate solutions, a choice of efficient quadrature formulae, approximation techniques for boundary and for main boundary conditions, and raising the accuracy of approximate solutions in terms of Richardson's extrapolation from different grids.

Chapter 4 gives a description and a substantiation of the convergence of several multigrid method modifications on a sequence of nested triangulations. The algorithms are given in the recurrent form with respect to different situations. At first, convergence conditions are discussed in terms of the abstract algebraic interpretation. It gives us a possibility to implement the theory to both the finite difference and the finite element methods. Then we specify this theory in terms of the finite element method. Therefore the multigrid methods have been classified with respect to the properties of the initial variational problems: for self-ajoint problem, non-self-ajoint one, spectral problem, mixed formulation, and so on.

The chapter also gives solutions of auxiliary problems for an optimization of iterative parameters. They permit a more speedly convergence of iterative algorithms in different norms. In the following sections this is confirmed by some numerical results.

Chapter 5 treats realizations of multigrid algorithms for elliptic equations of order 2. First, by an example of the two-dimensional Dirichlet problem a comparison is given between variant algorithms and among them have been chosen the optimal ones in respect of the number of arithmetical operations. Numerical experiments are given to illustrate these results.

A technique of constructing the nested grids for problems in a domain with curvilinear boundary has been considered as well as concrete realizations of iterative algorithms based on this technique.

Realizations of iterative algorithms have been discussed for the boundary problem with a peculiarity in the angle, when triangulation is locally condensed, as well as for the three-dimensional Dirichlet problem, the second and third boundary problem. Studying the three-dimensional problem does not show an essential distinction between it and the two-dimensional one in realization of multigrid algorithms as well as their substantiation and estimation of efficiency.

Also the spectral problem, it gives the generalized algebraic spectral problem $Au = \lambda Bu$ with symmetric non-diagonal matrices. The algorithm constructed on a sequence of triangulations permits to find an individual eigenvalue and corresponding eigenfunctions or groups of such functions in case of multiple eigenvalue, the previous eigenvalue and eigenfunctions being not calculated.

Chapter 6 explains, by concrete examples, how to generalize the results, so that they could be applied to non-linear equations and systems. In the first two sections, general results on the convergence of finite elements for non-linear problems with monotone-type operators have been discussed, as well as two typical non-linear problems applied in appendices have been solved by using multigrid algorithms. The solution of the planar elasticity problem shows possibility of generalizing the constructed algorithms and of their applying to elliptic systems. Among many well-known discretization methods of biharmonic equation has been considered a mixed formulation of the finite element method resulting in a system of two Poisson equations with coupled boundary conditions. The generalized formulation contains only first derivatives and so it is not necessary to use complex basis functions from the class $C^1(\Omega)$. The mixed formulation has also been used to discretize the stationary Stokes and Navier-Stokes problems. Here we used the simplest combination of the finite elements, linear elements for velocities and constant elements for pressure.

In the three last problems, the matrices of algebraic systems obtained have a spectrum with alternating signs, which is typical for the mixed formulation of the finite element method. However, the application of multigrid algorithms to them is as efficient as to positive-definite matrices.

A few words should be said about the discussing form. Formulae, theorems have two-digit numeration but lemmata, remarks have three-digit one own in each chapter. In the three last chapters, as it may seem, the material is discussed rather monotonously, especially when formulating stages of discretization and multigrid algorithms for algebraic equations obtained. It is due to brief repetitions of the most important points for the reader interested in solving a certain boundary problem to obtain the necessary information on studying a small amount of the preceding material.

Chapter 1

Elliptic boundary-value problems and Bubnov-Galerkin method

Section 1.1 of this short chapter presents formulation of the main problems studied in the book. Initially, each problem is stated in the differential operator form then a generalized formulation is given in the form of one or more integral identities. Solvability of the generalized problems follows from some abstract results also given in 1.1.

Section 1.2 concerns a general scheme of the Bubnov-Galerkin method for solving the generalized problems. Among several approaches to discretization used in the finite element method (the Ritz method, least-squares etc.), we have selected the most frequently used one. The theoretical results obtained may be applied to other discretization methods either directly or by close analogy between these methods.

1.1 Statements of differential problems and smoothness of solutions

In this section we first present notation and definitions of function classes and then one frequently used result of unique solvability of an abstract elliptic problem which is known as the Lax-Milgram lemma.

Afterwards, the main classes of boundary-value problems for elliptic equations and systems of order 2 and 4 are stated. Every problem is discussed according to the following plan. First a classical (operator) statement is given. Then a generalized formulation is deduced and is shown to be uniquely solvable. Finally, if the generalized solution is sufficiently smooth, it is proved to be the solution of the initial classical problem.

In a number of cases, it is shown that weakening of some requirements in the generalized problems results in a new formulation of the initial differential problem. For instance, discontinuities of first kind of coefficients of the principal part of the elliptic operator in the generalized form do not produce anything new; as for these in the operator form, they lead to the diffraction problem with conjunction conditions on discontinuity lines.

In the generalized third boundary-value problem, some modification of Green's formula permits one to obtain the boundary conditions with oblique derivative as natural one.

For the Neumann singular problem, introduction of an appropriate class of admissible (for the solution) functions results in the generalized problem with unique solution.

Finally, in the mixed method for the biharmonic equation, we succeeded in weakening the requirements of smoothness for the class of admissible functions from $W_2^4(\Omega)$ in the classical formulation to $W_2^1(\Omega)$ in the generalized mixed one. Later, we will show that this essentially simplifies the usage of the finite elements for solving the fourth-order elliptic equations.

Since this section includes results well-known to specialists in differential equations, they are given either without proof or with some short oversimplified foundation. But, in the both cases we give references to well-known sources where a detailed derivation is available.

1.1.1 Main notations of smoothness classes

We first recall some results from differential calculus.

Denote by $\mathbf{R}^n$ the *n-dimensional Euclidean space* of points $x = (x_1, \ldots, x_n)$ with the metric

$$|x - x'| = (\sum_{i=1}^{n}(x_i - x_i')^2)^{1/2}.$$

Take a set $\Omega \subset \mathbf{R}^n$ and a function $v : \Omega \to \mathbf{R}$. If at a point $a \in \Omega$ there exists a partial derivative with respect to x_i, we will denote it by

$$\partial_i v(a) \equiv \frac{\partial v}{\partial x_i}(a).$$

Our notation of *the gradient* of function v at this point, i. e., of the vector

$$(\partial_1 v(a), \ldots, \partial_n v(a))^T,$$

will be $\nabla v(a)$ or $\operatorname{grad} v(a)$. Symbol ^{T} stands for transposition. By $\partial_{ij} v(a) = \partial_i(\partial_j v(a))$ we denote the second derivatives, and for higher derivatives we will use multiindex notation. Given the *multiindex* $\alpha = (\alpha_1, \ldots, \alpha_n)$, $|\alpha| = \sum_{i=1}^{n} \alpha_i$. Then $\partial^\alpha v(a)$ denotes the derivative

$$\partial_1^{\alpha_1}(\partial_2^{\alpha_2} \ldots (\partial_n^{\alpha_n} v(a)) \ldots) \equiv \frac{\partial^{|\alpha|} v(a)}{\partial x_1^{\alpha_1} \ldots \partial x_n^{\alpha_n}}.$$

Let $\Omega \subset \mathbf{R}^n$ be a bounded domain, i. e., an open connected set with the boundary Γ and closure $\bar{\Omega} = \Omega \bigcup \Gamma$.

The space $D(\Omega)$ consists of all infinitely differentiable functions with supports in Ω.

$L_2(\Omega)$ is the Hilbert space of measurable functions $v : \Omega \to \mathbf{R}$, which are quadratically integrable on Ω with respect to the Lebesque measure. The norm is introduced into $L_2(\Omega)$ by the relation

$$\|u\|_{0,\Omega} \equiv (\int_\Omega u^2 dx)^{1/2}.$$

For an integer $m \geq 0$ *the Sobolev space* $W_2^m(\Omega)$ consists of functions $v \in L_2(\Omega)$ all partial derivatives of which (in the sense of generalized functions) $\partial^\alpha v$ belong to $L_2(\Omega)$ for $|\alpha| \leq m$. Introducing the norm in $W_2^m(\Omega)$

$$\|v\|_{m,\Omega} \equiv (\sum_{|\alpha| \leq m} \int_\Omega |\partial^\alpha v|^2 dx)^{1/2},$$

we obtain the Hilbert space.

Further, we will also use the semi-norm

$$|v|_{m,\Omega} \equiv \Big(\sum_{|\alpha|=m} \int_\Omega |\partial^\alpha v|^2 dx \Big)^{1/2}.$$

Closing the space $D(\Omega)$ with respect to norm $\|\cdot\|_{m,\Omega}$, we obtain the Hilbert space $\mathring{W}_2^m(\Omega)$. From the fact that Ω is bounded it follows that there exists a constant $c(\Omega)$ such that Friedrichs inequality is satisfied [132]:

$$|v|_{0,\Omega} \leq c(\Omega)|v|_{1,\Omega} \qquad \forall v \in \mathring{W}_2^1(\Omega). \tag{1.1}$$

Therefore, on the space $\mathring{W}_2^m(\Omega)$, the semi-norm $|\cdot|_{m,\Omega}$ is equivalent to the norm $\|\cdot\|_{m,\Omega}$.

Now we introduce definitions specifying smoothness of the boundary. Denote by $\bar{c}_x$ the cylinder

$$\{x \in \mathbf{R}^n : \sum_{i=1}^{n-1} x_i^2 \leq K^2, \quad -2LK \leq x_n \leq 2LK\}$$

with point 0 as the center and the radius K. The domain Ω will be called *strictly Lipschitz* [94] if $\forall x^0 \in \Gamma$ the coordinates $y_k = \sum_{l=1}^n c_{kl}(x_l - x_l^0)$ with the orthogonal matrix $(c_{kl})_{k,l=1}^n$ can be introduced so that the intersection of Γ and the cylinder $\bar{c}_y$ corresponding to the y-coordinates is given by the equation

$$y_n = \omega(y_n'), \qquad y_n' = (y_1, \ldots, y_{n-1}),$$

where $\omega(y_n')$ is the Lipschitz function for $|y_n'| \leq K$ with the Lipschitz constant which is not larger than L and

$$\bar{\Omega} \bigcap \bar{c}_y = \{y : |y_n'| \leq K, \quad \omega(y_n') \leq y_n \leq 2LK\}.$$

The numbers K and L are fixed for the domain Ω, therefore, the boundary Γ of the bounded domain can be represented by a finite number of local coordinate systems and mappings ω.

We call Γ the *X-class boundary* if the mappings $\omega : \{|y_n'| \leq K\} \to \mathbf{R}$ in the definition above are the X-class functions. For example, $X = C^m$ is a class of m times continuously differentiable functions.

Below, we will assume that Ω is a bounded strictly Lipschitz domain. Therefore, at almost each x on Γ there exists a unit external normal $\nu = (\nu_1, \ldots, \nu_n)^T$ to which the operator of (external) normal derivative corresponds

$$\partial_\nu \equiv \sum_{i=1}^n \nu_i \partial_i,$$

defined almost everywhere on Γ for smooth functions.

In the two-dimensional case, the vector $(\nu_2, -\nu_1)^T$ points to the direction tangent to Γ at point x (to the right of ν). Therefore, the operator of differentiating with respect to the tangent to Γ is expressed by the formula

$$\partial_\gamma \equiv \nu_2 \partial_1 - \nu_1 \partial_2.$$

Repeated derivatives will also be denoted by $\partial_{\nu\nu}u \equiv \partial_\nu(\partial_\nu u)$ and so on.

It is useful to remember another equivalent and more instructive definition of spaces $\overset{\circ}{W}{}_2^1$, $\overset{\circ}{W}{}_2^2$ [133]:

$$\begin{aligned}\overset{\circ}{W}{}_2^1(\Omega) &= \{v \in W_2^1(\Omega);\ v = 0 \quad \text{on} \quad \Gamma\},\\ \overset{\circ}{W}{}_2^2(\Omega) &= \{v \in W_2^2(\Omega);\ v = \partial_\nu v = 0 \quad \text{on} \quad \Gamma\}.\end{aligned}$$

We also introduce *the Urysohn (cutoff) function* $\omega_\delta \in C^2(\mathbf{R})$ with constant $\delta > 0$ satisfying next conditions $\omega_\delta'(x) \le 0$ on $(0, \infty)$, $\omega_\delta(x) = \omega_\delta(-x)$ and

$$\omega_\delta(x) = \begin{cases} 1 & \text{if} \quad |x| \le \delta, \\ 0 & \text{if} \quad |x| \ge 2\delta. \end{cases}$$

1.1.2 Solving two abstract problems

Let H be a Hilbert space with the inner product (u, v) and the norm $\|u\| = (u, u)^{1/2}$.

We introduce the following definitions.

A functional $\mathcal{L}(\cdot, \cdot) : H \times H \to \mathbf{R}$ will be called *the bilinear form* if it is linear in each of two arguments :

$$\mathcal{L}(\alpha_1 u_1 + \alpha_2 u_2, \beta_1 v_1 + \beta_2 v_2) = \sum_{i,j=1}^{2} \alpha_i \beta_j \mathcal{L}(u_i, v_j)$$
$$\forall u_i, v_j \in H, \quad \forall \alpha_i, \beta_j \in \mathbf{R}, \quad \text{where} \quad i, j = 1, 2.$$

Further we introduce a linear functional $f : H \to \mathbf{R}$ and require f and $\mathcal{L}$ to be continuous on their domains of definition. By virtue of linearity, continuity of functionals is equivalent to their boundedness [77]. Therefore, it is sufficient to assume that the following inequalities hold[1]:

$$|\mathcal{L}(u, v)| \le c\,\|u\|\,\|v\| \qquad \forall u, v \in H, \tag{1.2}$$
$$|f(v)| \le c\,\|v\| \qquad \forall v \in H. \tag{1.3}$$

Let us formulate the following abstract problem: *find an element $u \in H$ such that*

$$\mathcal{L}(u, v) = f(v) \qquad \forall v \in H. \tag{1.4}$$

An additional simple condition is sufficient to provide existence and uniqueness of a solution of this problem.

The bilinear form $\mathcal{L}(\cdot, \cdot) : H \times H \to \mathbf{R}$ is said to be *positive definite* in H (or H *-elliptic*) if for some $\mu > 0$

$$\mathcal{L}(v, v) \ge \mu \|v\|^2 \qquad \forall v \in H. \tag{1.5}$$

Now we formulate the following result on the solvability of the problem (1.4). It is known as *Lax-Milgram lemma.*

[1]We will use designation c_α with different symbols α or without them for constants which are independent of x, n, h and functions standing in the right-hand part of inequality.

Theorem 1.1 [40]. *Let the bilinear form* $\mathcal{L}(\cdot,\cdot) : H \times H \to \mathbf{R}$ *be continuous and positive definite in the Hilbert space* H *and let the functional* $f : H \to \mathbf{R}$ *be continuous in* H. *Then the problem* (1.4) *has a unique solution* $u \in H$.

Below, in this chapter we will show how a number of classical problems of mathematical physics can be reduced to the above formulation by choosing appropriate $\mathcal{L}$, f, H.

There can be more complex cases where bilinear form $\mathcal{L}$ can not be positive definite. Moreover, the spaces of admissible functions for the solution and test functions can not be the same, as, say, in the Petrov-Galerkin method. Namely: let H_1 and H_2 be two real Hilbert spaces with the inner products $(\cdot,\cdot)_{H_1}$, $(\cdot,\cdot)_{H_2}$ and the corresponding norms $\|\cdot\|_{H_1}$, $\|\cdot\|_{H_2}$. Let also $\mathcal{B}(u,v)$ be a continuous and, consiquently, bounded bilinear form on $H_1 \times H_2$:

$$|\mathcal{B}(u,v)| \le c_0 \|u\|_{H_1}\|v\|_{H_2} \qquad \forall u \in H_1, v \in H_2, \tag{1.6}$$

and $f(v)$ a linear continuous, i. e., bounded functional on H_2:

$$|f(v)| \le c_1 \|v\|_{H_2} \qquad \forall v \in H_2. \tag{1.7}$$

Let us consider the following abstract problem: *find an element* $u \in H_1$ *such that*

$$\mathcal{B}(u,v) = f(v) \qquad \forall v \in H_2. \tag{1.8}$$

The solvability of this problem often follows from the I.Babuška theorem which we formulate below for real spaces.

Theorem 1.2 [11]. *Assume that conditions* (1.6), (1.7) *are satisfied and*

$$\sup_{u\in H_1} \frac{|\mathcal{B}(u,v)|}{\|u\|_{H_1}} \ge c\,\|v\|_{H_2}, \qquad c > 0, \tag{1.9}$$

$$\sup_{v\in H_2} \frac{|\mathcal{B}(u,v)|}{\|v\|_{H_2}} \ge c_2\,\|u\|_{H_1}, \qquad c_2 > 0. \tag{1.10}$$

Then the problem (1.8) *has a unique solution* u^* *which obeys the estimate*

$$\|u^*\|_{H_1} \le c_1/c_2. \tag{1.11}$$

A mixed formulation is possible for several problems which consists in searching a saddle point of a sign-indefinite functional [47], [36].

Let V and W be real Hilbert spaces with the scalar products $(\cdot,\cdot)_V$, $(\cdot,\cdot)_W$ and with the norms $\|\cdot\|_V$, $\|\cdot\|_W$, respectively; $a(\cdot,\cdot)$ and $b(\cdot,\cdot)$ are continuous bilinear forms on $V \times V$ and $V \times W$; $f(\cdot)$, $g(\cdot)$ are the given continuous functionals on V and W. We state the following abstract mixed problem: *find a pair* $(u,\varphi) \in V \times W$ *such that*

$$a(u,v) \;+\; b(v,\varphi) = f(v) \qquad \forall v \in V, \tag{1.12}$$

$$b(u,\psi) \;=\; g(\psi) \qquad \forall \psi \in W. \tag{1.13}$$

Suppose that the following conditions are satisfied.

1. There exists a constant k such that

$$\sup_{v\in V\setminus\{0\}} b(u,\varphi)/\|v\|_V \geq k\,\|\varphi\|_W \qquad \forall\varphi\in W. \tag{1.14}$$

2. There exist constants γ and γ' such that

$$\sup_{u\in Z\setminus\{0\}} a(u,v)/\|u\|_V \;\geq\; \gamma\,\|v\|_V \qquad \forall v\in Z, \tag{1.15}$$

$$\sup_{v\in Z\setminus\{0\}} a(u,v)/\|v\|_V \;\geq\; \gamma'\,\|u\|_V \qquad \forall u\in Z, \tag{1.16}$$

where

$$Z=\{v\in V,\quad b(v,\varphi)=0\quad \forall\varphi\in W\}.$$

The last two conditions coincide for symmetric bilinear form a. Moreover, in the subsequent problems they will follow most often from V-ellipticity of the form a so that the most of effort would be to verify (1.14). In the literature, condition (1.14) is called *the Brezzi stability condition.*

Theorem 1.3 [36]. *With conditions* (1.14)-(1.16) *satisfied, problem* (1.12), (1.13) *is uniquely solvable.*

The problem (1.12), (1.13) can be reduced to (1.8). Namely, let

$$\tilde H = H_1 = H_2 = V\times W \quad\text{and}\quad (\cdot,\cdot)_{\tilde H}\equiv(\cdot,\cdot)_V+(\cdot,\cdot)_W.$$

The sum of (1.12) and (1.13) gives the following equivalent formulation: *find an element* $\tilde u=(u,\varphi)\in\tilde H$ *such that*

$$a(u,v)+b(v,\varphi)+b(u,\psi)=f(v)+g(\psi)\quad \forall\tilde v=(v,\psi)\in\tilde H. \tag{1.17}$$

Now let

$$\tilde{\mathcal B}(\tilde u,\tilde v)\equiv\tilde{\mathcal B}(u,\varphi;v,\psi)\equiv a(u,v)+b(v,\varphi)+b(u,\psi),$$

$$\tilde f(\tilde v)\equiv\tilde f(v,\psi)\equiv f(v)+g(\psi). \tag{1.18}$$

In these terms, the problem (1.17) is equivalent to the following one: *find an element* $\tilde u\in\tilde H$ *such that*

$$\tilde{\mathcal B}(\tilde u,\tilde v)=\tilde f(\tilde v)\qquad \forall\tilde v\in\tilde H. \tag{1.19}$$

As a result, conditions (1.9) and (1.10) for bilinear form $\tilde{\mathcal B}$ of problem (1.19) can be reformulated in the following form equivalent to (1.14)-(1.16) (see also [15]) and often called the Babuška conditions:

$$\sup_{(v,\psi)\in V\times W}\frac{|a(u,v)+b(v,\varphi)+b(u,\psi)|}{\|v\|_V+\|\psi\|_W}\geq c(\|u\|_V+\|\varphi\|_W),\quad \forall(u,\varphi)\in V\times W,\ c>0; \tag{1.20}$$

$$\sup_{(u,\varphi)\in V\times W}\frac{|a(u,v)+b(v,\varphi)+b(u,\psi)|}{\|u\|_V+\|\varphi\|_W}\geq c(\|v\|_V+\|\psi\|_W),\quad \forall(v,\psi)\in V\times W,\ c>0. \tag{1.21}$$

In these terms, we have such corollary of Theorem 1.2.

Theorem 1.4 *In problem* (1.12), (1.13) *let bilinear forms* a,b *be continuous on* $V\times V$ *and* $V\times W$ *and let linear functionals* f,g *be continuous on* V *and* W *respectively. With inequalities* (1.20) *and* (1.21) *satisfied, the problem* (1.12), (1.13) *has a unique solution.*

1.1.3 The Dirichlet problem for second-order elliptic equation

Consider a boundary value problem

$$Lu \equiv -\sum_{i,j=1}^{n} \partial_i(a_{ij}\partial_j u) + \sum_{i=1}^{n} \partial_i(a_i u) + au = f \quad \text{in} \quad \Omega, \tag{1.22}$$

$$u = 0 \quad \text{on} \quad \Gamma, \tag{1.23}$$

which is called *the homogeneous Dirichlet problem.* For coefficients of its principal part *the uniform ellipticity condition* is satisfied, i. e., there exist the constants μ_1, μ_2 such that

$$\mu_1|\xi|^2 \le \sum_{i,j=1}^{n} a_{ij}\xi_i\xi_j \le \mu_2|\xi|^2 \qquad \forall \xi \in \mathbf{R}^n, \forall x \in \bar{\Omega}. \tag{1.24}$$

Assume also that on Ω

$$a_{ij} = a_{ji}, \quad |a_i| \le c, \quad |a| \le c, \quad i,j = 1, \dots, n; \tag{1.25}$$

$$f \in L_2(\Omega). \tag{1.26}$$

Let us pass to generalized formulation of the problem. To this end, we multiply (1.22) by an arbitrary function $v \in \overset{\circ}{W}{}_2^1(\Omega)$ and use Green's first formula originating from the formula of integration by parts for generalized derivatives:

$$\int_\Omega \sum_{i,j=1}^{n} a_{ij}\partial_j u \partial_i v dx = -\int_\Omega \sum_{i,j=1}^{n} \partial_i(a_{ij}\partial_j u) v dx + \int_\Gamma \sum_{i,j=1}^{n} a_{ij} v \nu_i \partial_j u d\gamma. \tag{1.27}$$

Since the function v equals zero on Γ, we have

$$\mathcal{L}_1(u,v) = f_1(v), \tag{1.28}$$

where the linear functional $f_1 : \overset{\circ}{W}{}_2^1 \to \mathbf{R}$ and the bilinear form $\mathcal{L}_1(\cdot,\cdot) : \overset{\circ}{W}{}_2^1 \times \overset{\circ}{W}{}_2^1 \to \mathbf{R}$ are defined by the formulae

$$f_1(v) = \int_\Omega f v dx, \tag{1.29}$$

$$\mathcal{L}_1(u,v) = \int_\Omega \left(\sum_{i,j=1}^{n} a_{ij}\partial_j u \partial_i v + \sum_{i=1}^{n} a_i v \partial_i u + auv\right) dx. \tag{1.30}$$

The generalized formulation of the problem reads as follows [94].

Definition 1.1 *The function $u \in \overset{\circ}{W}{}_2^1(\Omega)$, satisfying the relation*

$$\mathcal{L}_1(u,v) = f_1(v) \qquad \forall v \in \overset{\circ}{W}{}_2^1(\Omega) \tag{1.31}$$

will be called a generalized solution of the Dirichlet problem (1.22), (1.23).

Let us check if the conditions of Theorem 1.1, which quarantee solvability of the problem, are satisfied. Apply the algebraic *Cauchy inequality* [94] to the main summands of the right-hand part:

$$|\sum_{i,j=1}^{n} a_{ij}\xi_i\eta_j| \leq |\sum_{i,j=1}^{n} a_{ij}\xi_i\xi_j|^{1/2} \cdot |\sum_{i,j=1}^{n} a_{ij}\eta_i\eta_j|^{1/2},$$

which is valid for any $\xi_i, \eta_j \in \mathbf{R}$. As for the rest of the summands, we apply (1.25) and the Cauchy-Bunyakovski inequality. As a result we obtain

$$|\mathcal{L}_1(u,v)| \leq \mu_2 |u|_{1,\Omega} |v|_{1,\Omega} + c\sqrt{n}\, |u|_{1,\Omega} |v|_{0,\Omega} + c|u|_{0,\Omega} |v|_{0,\Omega}.$$

Using the Friedrichs inequality (1.1), we obtain the relation

$$|\mathcal{L}_1(u,v)| \leq c|u|_{1,\Omega} \cdot |v|_{1,\Omega}. \tag{1.32}$$

This indicates the boundedness of the bilinear form $\mathcal{L}_1$ in the space $\overset{\circ}{W}{}_2^1(\Omega)$ with norm $|\cdot|_{1,\Omega}$.

It is even easier to show the boundedness of f_1 in $\overset{\circ}{W}{}_2^1(\Omega)$. Indeed, from the Cauchy-Bunyakovski and Friedrichs inequalities

$$|f_1(v)| \leq |f|_{0,\Omega} \leq c|f|_{0,\Omega}\, |v|_{1,\Omega}. \tag{1.33}$$

It remains only to check if $\mathcal{L}_1$ is positive definite. Substituting $v = u$ into (1.30) and using (1.24), we finally obtain

$$|\mathcal{L}_1(u,v)| \geq \mu_1 |u|_{1,\Omega}^2 + \int_\Omega (a - \frac{1}{2}\sum_{i=1}^{n} \partial_i a_i) u^2 dx. \tag{1.34}$$

Consider the frequently used case

$$a_i = 0, \quad i = 1, \dots, n; \qquad a \geq 0 \quad \text{on} \quad \bar{\Omega}. \tag{1.35}$$

Then

$$|\mathcal{L}_1(u,u)| \geq \mu_1 |u|_{1,\Omega}^2, \tag{1.36}$$

i. e., $\mathcal{L}_1$ is positive definite in $\overset{\circ}{W}{}_2^1(\Omega)$.

Thus, conditions (1.24)-(1.26), (1.35) are satisfied and the generalized problem is uniquely solvable.

Let us now see how the solutions of the initial and generalized problems are related. From (1.27)-(1.30) it follows that if u from $W_2^2(\Omega)$ is a solution of the initial differential problem, it will satisfy (1.31). This solution will coincide with the generalized solution because of the uniqueness of the latter. The inverse assertion is true only under definite smoothness conditions of initial data and the solution itself. Indeed, for all expressions in operator formulation (1.22) to make sense, differentiability of $a_{ij}\partial_j u$ is required. It is attained, for example, if a_{ij} is differentiable and u is sufficiently smooth. As far as the generalized formulation is conserned, it does not assume differentiability of the coefficients a_{ij} and expressions $a_{ij}\partial_j u$. This is rather important for diffraction problems, the coefficients of which may have discontinuities of first kind. They are due to the fact that the medium consists of two ore more materials with different physical properties.

Let us, for example, assume that domain Ω is divided by line S into subdomains Ω_1, Ω_2, the coefficients on each being differentiable. Obviously, the equation (1.22) does not hold along the line S, on which conjunction conditions connecting the solution pieces in subdomains Ω_1, Ω_2 must be imposed. The continuity of the solution as well as of the flow when crossing the line S is usually taken to be such conditions:

$$u(x)|_{\Omega_1} = u(x)|_{\Omega_2}, \quad x \in S, \tag{1.37}$$

$$\partial_c u(x)|_{\Omega_1} = -\partial_c u(x)|_{\Omega_2}, \quad x \in S. \tag{1.38}$$

The expression $u(x)|_{\Omega_i}$ here means the limit value $\lim u(x')$ when $x' \to x$ over domain Ω_i; $\partial_c u$ is the flow over S defined by the operator of co-normal derivative

$$u \to \partial_c u = \sum_{i,j=1}^{n} a_{ij}\nu_i \partial_j u \tag{1.39}$$

with an external normal to S.

Condition (1.37) can be derived from physical continuity of u; the second condition can also be formulated from physical reasons, but here it originates from another principles. Indeed, assume that the generalized solution u and the problem data satisfy along with (1.24)-(1.26) also the conditions $u \in W_2^2(\Omega_i)$ and $|\partial_j a| \le c$ on Ω_i ($i = 1, 2; j = 1, \dots, n$). Consider the following identity for arbitrary v from $\overset{\circ}{W}{}_2^1(\Omega)$:

$$\mathcal{L}_1(u,v) = \int_{\Omega_1 \bigcup \Omega_2} Lu \cdot v dx + \int_\Gamma \partial_c u \cdot v d\gamma + \int_S (\partial_c u|_{\Omega_1} + \partial_c u|_{\Omega_2}) v d\gamma. \tag{1.40}$$

This result follows from Green's formula for subdomains Ω_1, Ω_2. Since $v = 0$ on Γ, the integral over Γ vanishes. Choosing functions $v \in D(\Omega_1)$, we arrive at the equality

$$\int_{\Omega_1} Lu \cdot v dx = \int_{\Omega_1} f v dx. \tag{1.41}$$

Note that $Lu - f \in L_2(\Omega_1)$. Take sequence $v_n \in D(\Omega_1)$ converging to this function in the norm of $L_2(\Omega_1)$, put $v = v_n$ into (1.41) and let $n \to \infty$. Finally, $|Lu - f|_{0,\Omega_1} = 0$, i. e., $Lu = f$ almost everywhere in Ω_1 as an element of $L_2(\Omega_1)$. Similarly, $Lu = f$ in Ω_2. Applying the obtained equalities to (1.40), we arrive at the relation

$$\int_S (\partial_c u|_{\Omega_1} + \partial_c u|_{\Omega_2}) v d\gamma = 0. \tag{1.42}$$

Take a piece S_1 from S of the class C^2, which is away from Γ, and introduce in its small neighbourhood Ω' the natural coordinates $(y_1, \dots, y_n)^T$ with the normal Oy_n in the direction from Ω_1 to Ω_2. Rewrite the expression $\partial_c u|_{\Omega_i}$ for the whole Ω'. To this end, we define the values of v_i on Ω' by transfer along Oy_n. Inside Ω_i, the expression $\partial_c u|_{\Omega_i}$ is calculated as on S, while outside Ω_i it is prolongated evenly with respect to $y_n = 0$. As a result, we have a function $w \in W_2^1(\Omega')$ which on S_1 is equal to the expression between brackets in (1.42). Multiply this by the cutoff function $\xi \in C^2(\bar{\Omega})$, which is equal to one on S_1 and to zero on the neighbourhood boundary of Ω'. Substituting $v = \xi w$ into (1.42), we arrive at the equality

$$\int_{S_1} (\partial_c u|_{\Omega_1} + \partial_c u|_{\Omega_2})^2 d\gamma = 0, \tag{1.43}$$

which, as it follows from (1.38), holds almost everywhere on S_1. Since S_1 is arbitrary, (1.38) holds almost everywhere on S.

Thus, generalized formulations different from one other only by smoothness of coefficients, are essentially different when in the operator statement. Note that conditions (1.23) and (1.37) are important in the diffraction problem, i. e., they appear in the description of the class of admissible functions $\overset{\circ}{W}{}^1_2(\Omega)$ in which a solution is sought. The condition (1.38) is natural; we do not require that it holds for admissible functions, it may only hold approximately.

Now, a few words about possible smoothness of generalized solutions. Further we will see that the accuracy of approximate solutions obtained is related to it. It is inside the domain, where smoothness of the solution is established rather simply. Let us restrict ourselves to the case when $n = 2, 3$.

Theorem 1.5 [94]. *Let the problem* (1.31) *have unique generalized solution* $u \in \overset{\circ}{W}{}^1_2(\Omega)$, *conditions* (1.25), (1.26) *be satisfied, and on a strictly interior subdomain* Ω' *of the domain* Ω *the inequality*

$$|\partial_j a_{ij}| \leq c \qquad \forall i, j = 1, \dots, n \tag{1.44}$$

hold. Then the solution $u \in W_2^2(\Omega')$.

If the boundary Γ *or the dividing line of the media* S *have a smooth piece* S' *of the class* C^2, *then* $u \in W_2^2(\Omega')$ *for any subdomain* $\Omega' \subset \Omega$, *which is at positive distance from the rest of* S *and* Γ.

In the case $\Gamma \subset C^2$ *when* (1.44) *is satisfied on* Ω, *the solution* $u \in W_2^2(\Omega)$.

More accurate (limit) smoothness indices of the coefficients are given in [94].

It remains only to consider the smoothness of the solution near conic and corner points and corner lines, which often occurs in applications.

Let us begin with a two-dimensional case. Even here the expected smoothness $u \in W_2^2(\Omega)$ does not occur for all values of the angle. The disturbance of smoothness because of an unbounded increase of the second derivatives may be take place at points 1–4 as shown in Fig. 1.1. The value of the angles marked by 5 is less than π; they do not influence the fact that the solution u belongs to the class W_2^2 [146]. Below, in section 5.4, we return to the solution structure for special cases 1, 2, 4.

The three-dimensional case provides even more geometric singularities. Simple technologies for machine parts give, as a rule, different angles — two-sided, three-sided. Conic angles occur more seldomly. Also such natural objects as a river or sea coastal strip give acute edges. In addition, the angles appear at intersection of the boundary Γ and the interface of two media. Each of these kinds of angles may disturb the usually required smoothness $u \in W_2^2(\Omega)$, which will be illustrated below.

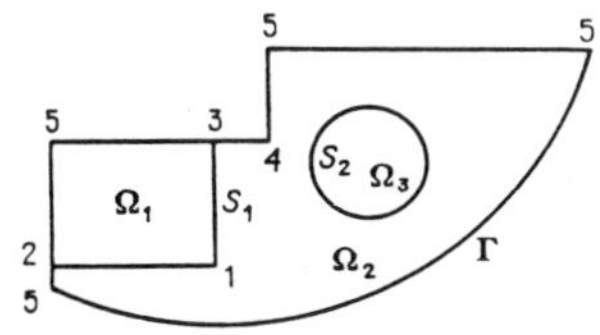

Figure 1.1: Three-component domain with dividing lines of media S_1, S_2

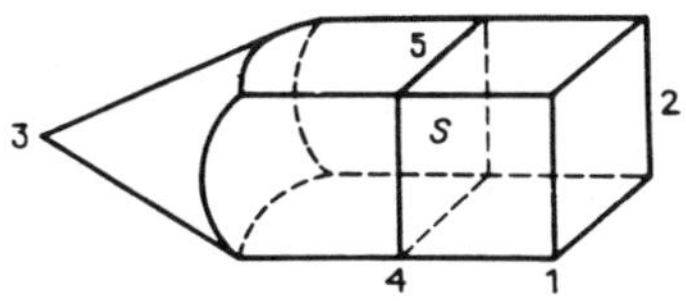

Figure 1.2: Three-dimensional domain with the surface S dividing two media

1.1.4 Boundary-value problems of third kind

Let us consider a case of natural boundary conditions. We will look for a solution of (1.22) satisfying the boundary condition of third kind

$$\partial_c u + \sigma u = g \quad \text{on} \quad \Gamma \tag{1.45}$$

with function $\sigma \geq 0$ on Γ.

Multiply (1.22) by an arbitrary function $v \in W_2^1(\Omega)$ and apply Green's formula (1.27). Using the notation introduced above, we rewrite

$$\mathcal{L}(u,v) = \int_\Omega Lu \cdot v dx + \int_\Gamma \partial_c u \cdot v d\gamma.$$

In equation above, replace Lu with f and the derivative with respect to the co-normal with $g - \sigma u$ according to (1.45). Then

$$\mathcal{L}_2(u,v) = f_2(v), \tag{1.46}$$

where

$$\begin{aligned} \mathcal{L}_2(u,v) &= \mathcal{L}_1(u,v) + \int_\Gamma \sigma u \cdot v d\gamma, \\ f_2(v) &= \int_\Omega f v dx + \int_\Gamma g v d\gamma. \end{aligned}$$

Thus we arrive at the following generalized formulation.

Definition 1.2 *The function $u \in W_2^1(\Omega)$ satisfying the relation* (1.46) $\forall v \in W_2^1(\Omega)$ *will called a generalized solution of the boundary-value problem of third kind* (1.22), (1.45).

Let us discuss solvability of this problem. Assume that conditions (1.25), (1.26) are satisfied and on Γ

$$0 < c_8 \le \sigma \le c_9, \qquad g \in L_2(\Gamma). \tag{1.47}$$

The space of traces of functions u from $W_2^1(\Omega)$ is compactly enclosed in $L_2(\Gamma)$ [94], and the estimate

$$|u|_{0,\Gamma} \le c_{10} \|u\|_{1,\Omega}. \tag{1.48}$$

holds. Hence,

$$\int_\Gamma \sigma u v d\gamma \le c_9 c_{10}^2 \|u\|_{1,\Omega} \|v\|_{1,\Omega}.$$

Adding the above and (1.32), we obtain

$$|\mathcal{L}_2(u,v)| \le c_{11} \|u\|_{1,\Omega} \|v\|_{1,\Omega}.$$

This estimate indicates continuity of the bilinear form $\mathcal{L}_2(\cdot,\cdot) : W_2^1 \times W_2^1 \to \mathbf{R}$. The continuity of $f_2 : W_2^1 \to \mathbf{R}$ is established similarly:

$$|f_2(v)| \le |f|_{0,\Omega} |v|_{0,\Omega} + |g|_{0,\Gamma} |v|_{0,\Gamma} \le c_{12} \|v\|_{1,\Omega}.$$

In order to prove that $\mathcal{L}_2$ is elliptic, we use another inequality established by Friedrichs [133] for any functions $u \in W_2^1(\Omega)$:

$$|u|_{0,\Omega}^2 \le c(|u|_{1,\Omega}^2 + |u|_{0,\Gamma}^2). \tag{1.49}$$

Assuming that conditions (1.35) hold, we rewrite the above using (1.36). Then

$$\begin{aligned} |\mathcal{L}_2(u,u)| &\ge \mu_1 |u|_{1,\Omega}^2 + c_8 |u|_{0,\Gamma}^2 \ge \\ &\ge \min(\mu_1/2c, c_8/c) |u|_{0,\Omega}^2 + (\mu_1/2) |u|_{1,\Omega}^2 \ge c_{13} \|u\|_{1,\Omega}^2. \end{aligned}$$

Thus, if conditions (1.24)-(1.26), (1.35) and (1.47) are satisfied, the generalized boundary-value problem of third kind has a unique solution.

Note that assuming that the generalized solution and the coefficients of the problem are sufficiently smooth, using (1.46) one can show that the initial operator statement holds. This can be proved as in subsection 1.1.3.

Let us consider one more point related to the oblique derivative. Let us restrict ourselves to two-dimensional case. Let the boundary condition

$$\partial_\nu u + \alpha \partial_\gamma u + \sigma u = g \quad \text{on} \quad \Gamma, \tag{1.50}$$

be set instead of (1.45) with known functions α, σ, g, $\sigma \ge 0$ on Γ. This boundary condition arises, for example, in problems of oceanology; the operator $\partial_\nu + \alpha\partial_\gamma$ does not coincide with the differentiation operator with respect to co-normal ∂_c. Nevertheless, applying another Green's formula for the same differential operator L one can turn the condition (1.50) into a natural one [106]. To this end, consider the identity

$$\partial_1(c\partial_2 u) - \partial_2(c\partial_1 u) = \partial_2 c \cdot \partial_1 u - \partial_1 c \cdot \partial_2 u. \tag{1.51}$$

which is valid for arbitrary functions $c \in C^1(\Omega)$ and $u \in W_2^2(\Omega)$. Multiply it by an arbitrary function $v \in W_2^1(\Omega)$ and integrate by parts:

$$\int_\Omega (\partial_1(c\partial_2 u) - \partial_2(c\partial_1 u))v dx = \int_\Omega (c\partial_1 u \cdot \partial_2 v - c\partial_2 u \cdot \partial_1 v)dx + \int_\Gamma c\partial_\gamma u \cdot v d\gamma.$$

Adding together these equality and (1.27), we arrive at the equation

$$\begin{aligned} \mathcal{L}(u,v) \quad + \quad & \int_\Omega (c\partial_1 u \cdot \partial_2 v - c\partial_2 u \cdot \partial_1 v + \partial_2 c \cdot \partial_1 u \cdot v - \partial_1 c \cdot \partial_2 u \cdot v)dx = \\ = \quad & \int_\Omega Lu \cdot v dx - \int_\Gamma (\partial_c u + c\partial_\gamma u)v d\gamma. \end{aligned} \tag{1.52}$$

Consider the expression between brackets in the boundary integral. Let us show that by choosing function c, this expression can be made proportional to $\partial_\nu u + \alpha\partial_\gamma u$ independently of the function u. Indeed, let

$$\partial_c u + c\partial_\gamma u = d(\partial_\nu u + \alpha\partial_\gamma u) \quad \text{on} \quad \Gamma. \tag{1.53}$$

Calculating the corfficients of $\partial_1 u$, $\partial_2 u$ at every point of Γ, we arrive at two linear equations in two unknowns:

$$\begin{aligned} \sum_{j=1}^{2} \nu_j a_{j1} + c\nu_2 &= d(\nu_1 + \alpha\nu_2), \\ \sum_{j=1}^{2} \nu_j a_{j2} - c\nu_1 &= d(\nu_2 - \alpha\nu_1). \end{aligned}$$

The determinant of the system matrix is equal to one, therefore, c and d are defined uniquely and, by virtue of the ellipticity condition (1.24), $0 \le \mu_1 \le d \le \mu_2$ on Γ and on Ω, because

$$\begin{aligned} d &= \sum_{i,j=1}^{2} \nu_i a_{ij} \nu_j, \\ c &= -\sum_{j=1}^{2} \nu_j a_{j1}(\nu_2 - \alpha\nu_1) + \sum_{j=1}^{2} \nu_j a_{j2}(\nu_1 + \alpha\nu_2). \end{aligned} \tag{1.54}$$

Taking (1.53), (1.50) into consideration, we rewrite the boundary integral in (1.52) as follows

$$\int_\Gamma (\partial_c u + c\partial_\gamma u)v d\gamma = \int_\Gamma d(g - \sigma u)v d\gamma.$$

Using the equality $Lu = f$ we rewrite (1.52) in the following form:

$$\mathcal{L}_3(u,v) = f_3(v), \tag{1.55}$$

where the bilinear form $\mathcal{L}_3(\cdot,\cdot) : W_2^1 \times W_2^1 \to \mathbf{R}$ and the functional $f_3 : W_2^1 \to \mathbf{R}$ are defined by the formulae

$$\begin{aligned} \mathcal{L}_3(u,v) \quad &= \quad \mathcal{L}_1(u,v) + \int_\Omega (c\partial_1 u \cdot \partial_2 v - c\partial_2 u \cdot \partial_1 v + \\ &+ \quad \partial_2 c \cdot \partial_1 u \cdot v - \partial_1 c \cdot \partial_2 u \cdot v)dx + \int_\Gamma d\sigma u v d\gamma, \\ f_3(v) \quad &= \quad f_1(v) + \int_\Gamma d g v d\gamma. \end{aligned}$$

Now, let us return to the initial formulation of the problem (1.22), (1.50). Define the function c from formula (1.54) and prolong it on Ω so that $c \in C^1(\bar{\Omega})$. For the sufficiently smooth functions α, v_i one can do it, for example, by transfer of the values of c along the normal and applying the cutoff function out of the boundary neighbourhood. The generalized formulation reads as follows: *find a function* $u \in W_2^1(\Omega)$ *satisfying relation* (1.55) $\forall v \in W_2^1(\Omega)$ *where function* d *is defined by equality* (1.54).

Thus, using the specially selected Green's formula, we have reduced the problem with oblique derivative to generalized formulation of the boundary-value problem of third kind with natural boundary conditions.

When the data and the solution u of the generalized problem are sufficiently smooth, one can show that u satisfies the initial problem in usual way.

1.1.5 The Neumann problem

Generally speaking, the Neumann problem is a special case of the boundary-value problem of third kind (1.22), (1.45) when $\sigma \equiv 0$ on Γ and thus the reasoning from the preceding part may be applied to it, as well. Here, we will consider a practically important case of the singular boundary-value problem, i. e., such combination of data for whose the operator of the differential problem is singular.

Let function u be a solution of equation

$$Lu \equiv -\sum_{i,j=1}^{n} \partial_i(a_{ij}\partial_j u) = f \quad \text{in} \quad \Omega \tag{1.56}$$

and satisfy the Neumann boundary condition

$$\partial_c u = g \quad \text{on} \quad \Gamma. \tag{1.57}$$

We see that constant functions $w = const$ appears in the kernel of the differential operator defined by the left-hand parts of (1.56), (1.57). This means that either the problem does not have any solution or it does have an infinitely large number of them, since along with the solution u, say, functions $u + \alpha w$ with an arbitrary constant α satisfy the equalities (1.56), (1.57).

Consider the problem of separation of a unique solution from many possible ones. We will choose the solution which is orthogonal to the constant function in $L_2(\Omega)$:

$$\int_\Omega u dx = 0. \tag{1.58}$$

Thus, it is not clear at this stage whether the requirement of uniqueness is reduced to the above condition or the kernel has larger dimension.

We show that condition (1.58) is sufficient for the generalized problem to be uniquely solvable. Define a space $\tilde{W}_2^1(\Omega)$ consisting of functions $u \in W_2^1(\Omega)$ which are orthogonal to one as in (1.58). Take a function $v \in \tilde{W}_2^1(\Omega)$ and identity (1.46):

$$\mathcal{L}_4(u, v) = f_4(v), \tag{1.59}$$

where

$$\mathcal{L}_4(u,v) = \int_\Omega \sum_{i,j=1}^n a_{ij}\partial_j u\, \partial_i v\, dx,$$
$$f_4(v) = \int_\Omega fv dx + \int_\Gamma gv d\gamma.$$

We obtain the following generalized formulation of Neumann singular problem: *find a function* $u \in \tilde{W}_2^1(\Omega)$ *satisfying* (1.59) $\forall v \in \tilde{W}_2^1(\Omega)$.

To apply Theorem 1.1, we assume that

$$|g|_{0,\Gamma} \le c_{14}, \qquad |f|_{0,\Omega} \le c_{15}. \tag{1.60}$$

Then the continuity of $f_4 : \tilde{W}_2^1 \to \mathbf{R}$ is established in the some way as it was established for f_2. The continuity of $\mathcal{L}_4 : \tilde{W}_2^1 \times \tilde{W}_2^1 \to \mathbf{R}$ follows from inequality (1.32) where $c = \mu_2$ because of the equality $a_i = a = 0$, i. e.,

$$|\mathcal{L}_4(u,v)| \le \mu_2 |u|_{1,\Omega} |v|_{1,\Omega} \le \mu_2 \|u\|_{1,\Omega} \|v\|_{1,\Omega}.$$

In order to determine the ellipticity of $\mathcal{L}_4$ we use *the Poincare inequality* [133]

$$|u|_{0,\Omega}^2 \le c_{16} |u|_{1,\Omega}^2 + c_{17}(\int_\Omega u dx)^2, \tag{1.61}$$

which is valid for arbitrary functions $u \in W_2^1(\Omega)$. If, in addition, $u \in \tilde{W}_2^1(\Omega)$, then by virtue of (1.58), it gives Friedrichs inequality (1.1). Applying this inequality together with (1.24) we obtain

$$|\mathcal{L}_4(u,u)| \ge \mu_1 |u|_{1,\Omega}^2 \ge \mu_1/2\,(|u|_{1,\Omega}^2 + c_{16}^{-1} |u|_{0,\Omega}^2) \ge c_{18} \|u\|_{1,\Omega}^2,$$

which means that bilinear form $\mathcal{L}_4$ is positive definite in $\tilde{W}_2^1(\Omega)$.

Thus, the conditions of uniform ellipticity (1.24) and boundedness (1.60) hold and the Neumann generalized problem (1.59) has a unique solution by Theorem 1.1.

The question whether this solution satisfies the initial differential problem (1.56), (1.57) is not so trivial and does not depend on the smoothness of f, g, u only. Indeed, let us show that the initial problem is not solvable for any conbination of functions f and g. Suppose that the problem (1.56), (1.57) has a solution $u \in W_2^2(\Omega)$. Using Green's formula (1.27) with function $v \equiv 1$ on Ω, we have the relation

$$\int_\Omega Lu dx = -\int_\Gamma \partial_c u d\gamma.$$

Applying formulae (1.56), (1.57), we find

$$\int_\Omega f dx = -\int_\Gamma g d\gamma. \tag{1.62}$$

Thus we obtained some necessary solvability condition of the initial problem which is not involved in the statement of the generalized problem.

We show that if (1.62) is satisfied and the data are sufficiently smooth, the generalized solution will also be a solution of the initial problem. Let $u \in C^2(\Omega), a_{ij} \in$

$C^1(\Omega), f \in C(\Omega)$. Take an arbitrary function $v \in W_2^1(\Omega)$ and apply Green's formula (1.27):

$$\mathcal{L}_4(u,v) = \int_\Omega Lu \cdot v dx + \int_\Gamma \partial_c u \cdot v d\gamma. \tag{1.63}$$

We now show that (1.59) holds for any function $v \in W_2^1(\Omega)$, not only for $\tilde{W}_2^1(\Omega)$. To this end, we write it in the form of the sum $v = v_1 + v_2$ where $v_1 \in \tilde{W}_2^1(\Omega)$ and $v_2 \equiv const$. For v_2, the equalities $\mathcal{L}_4(u,v_2) = f_4(v_2) = 0$ hold, the latter following from (1.62). For v_1, (1.59) holds, hence

$$\mathcal{L}_4(u,v) = \mathcal{L}_4(u,v_1) = f_4(v_1) = f_4(v).$$

Taking the above and (1.63) together, we get

$$\int_\Omega Lu \cdot v dx + \int_\Gamma \partial_c u \cdot v d\gamma = \int_\Omega f v dx + \int_\Gamma g v d\gamma \quad \forall v \in W_2^1(\Omega).$$

Further reasoning using the cutoff function ξ is analogous to the boundary-value Dirichlet problem. We finally come to the assertion that for the generalized solution $u \in W_2^2(\Omega)$, (1.56) holds almost everywhere inside Ω, while (1.57) holds almost everywhere on boundary Γ.

1.1.6 Elasticity problem

Let Ω be a bounded domain in $\mathbf{R}^3$ with the piecewise smooth boundary Γ. Consider a system of equations of linear elasticity theory

$$-\mu\Delta u - (\lambda + \mu)\,\text{grad div}\, u = f \quad \text{in} \quad \Omega, \tag{1.64}$$

where μ, λ are the positive constants called *Lame's coefficients* of the material, $u = (u_1, u_2, u_3)^T$ is *the displacement vector*, $f = (f_1, f_2, f_3)^T$ is the known *body force vector*, $\text{div}\, u = \sum_{i=1}^3 \partial_i u_i$. The boundary conditions

$$u = 0 \quad \text{on} \quad \Gamma \tag{1.65}$$

should be added to this equation. Here 0 is the zero vector in $\mathbf{R}^3$.

To simplify further computations, we introduce traditional notations. Symmetric matrices $(\epsilon_{ij}(u))_{ij=1}^3$ and $(\sigma_{ij}(u))_{ij=1}^3$ with the elements

$$\epsilon_{ij}(u) = (\partial_j u_i + \partial_i u_j)/2, \tag{1.66}$$

$$\sigma_{ij}(u) = \lambda(\sum_{k=1}^3 \epsilon_{kk}(u))\delta_{ij} + 2\mu\epsilon_{ij}(u), \tag{1.67}$$

where δ_{ij} is the Kronecker symbol, are called, respectively, *strain and stress tensors.*

Using the formula of integration by parts,

$$\int_\Omega \sigma_{ij}(u)\partial_j v_i dx = -\int_\Omega (\partial_j \sigma_{ij}(u)) v_i dx + \int_\Gamma \sigma_{ij}(u) v_i \nu_j d\gamma.$$

Summing over $i, j = 1, 2, 3$ and taking into account the symmetry of σ_{ij} and the definition of ϵ_{ij} on the left-hand part gives Green's formula

$$\int_\Omega \sum_{i,j=1}^{3} \sigma_{ij}(u)\epsilon_{ij}(v)dx = \int_\Omega \sum_{i=1}^{3}(-\sum_{j=1}^{3} \partial_j\sigma_{ij}(u))v_i dx + \int_\Gamma \sum_{i=1}^{3}(\sum_{j=1}^{3} \sigma_{ij}(u)\nu_j)v_i d\gamma, \tag{1.68}$$

which is valid for any u, v, where $u \in (W_2^2(\Omega))^3$, $v \in (W_2^1(\Omega))^3$.

In terms of the stress tensor, the system (1.64) takes the form:

$$-\sum_{j=1}^{3} \partial_j\sigma_{ij}(u) = f_i, \qquad i = 1, 2, 3. \tag{1.69}$$

We take an arbitrary vector-function $v = (v_1, v_2, v_3)^T \in (\overset{\circ}{W}{}_2^1(\Omega))^3$, multiply the equation by v_i, integrate it over Ω, and sum over $i = 1, 2, 3$. This yields

$$\int_\Omega \sum_{i=1}^{3}(-\sum_{j=1}^{3} \partial_j\sigma_{ij}(u))v_i dx = \int_\Omega f \cdot v dx. \tag{1.70}$$

Applying Green's formula (1.68) and using the fact that functions v_i are equal to zero on Γ, we finally obtain

$$\mathcal{L}_5(u, v) = f_5(v), \tag{1.71}$$

where

$$\begin{aligned} \mathcal{L}_5(u, v) &= \int_\Omega \sum_{i,j=1}^{3} \sigma_{ij}(u)\epsilon_{ij}(v)dx, \\ f_5(v) &= \int_\Omega f \cdot v dx. \end{aligned}$$

On the basis of (1.71) we formulate the generalized problem.

Definition 1.3 *The vector-function* $u = (u_1, u_2, u_3)^T \in (\overset{\circ}{W}{}_2^1(\Omega))^3$ *satisfying* (1.71) *for any vector-function* $v = (v_1, v_2, v_3)^T \in (\overset{\circ}{W}{}_2^1(\Omega))^3$ *is called the generalized solution of linear elasticity problem* (1.64), (1.65).

For vector-functions from $(W_2^m(\Omega))^3$, introduce the norm

$$\|v\|_{m,\Omega} = (\sum_{i=1}^{3} \|v_i\|_{m,\Omega}^2)^{1/2}.$$

Let us check whether the conditions of Theorem 1.1 of solvability of generalized problem hold. Assume that

$$\|f\|_{0,\Omega} \leq c_{19}. \tag{1.72}$$

Then the proof of boundedness of functional f_5 does not present any difficulties since the application of the Cauchy-Bunyakovski algebraic and then integral inequalities yields

$$|f_5(v)| = |\int_\Omega f \cdot v dx| \leq \int_\Omega (\sum_{i=1}^{3} f_i^2)^{1/2}(\sum_{i=1}^{3} v_i^2)^{1/2} dx \leq \|f\|_{0,\Omega} \cdot \|v\|_{0,\Omega} \leq c_{19}\|v\|_{1,\Omega}.$$

To prove that bilinear form $\mathcal{L}_5$ is bounded rewrite it in another form using the definitions of the tensors (ϵ_{ij}), (σ_{ij}) and the operation div:

$$\mathcal{L}_5(u,v) = \int_\Omega \{\lambda \operatorname{div} u \operatorname{div} v + 2\mu \sum_{i,j=1}^{3} \epsilon_{ij}(u)\epsilon_{ij}(v)\}dx. \quad (1.73)$$

Estimating each term on the right-hand part by means of the Cauchy-Bunyakovski inequality, we get

$$|\mathcal{L}_5(u,v)| \leq c_{20}\|u\|_{1,\Omega} \cdot \|v\|_{1,\Omega}.$$

To prove that $\mathcal{L}_5$ is elliptic, we use *the Korn inequality* [56]: there exists a constant $c(\Omega)$ such that if $v = (v_1, v_2, v_3)^T \in (\overset{\circ}{W}{}_2^1(\Omega))^3$ then

$$\|v\|_{1,\Omega} \leq c(\Omega)(\sum_{i,j=1}^{3} |\epsilon_{ij}(v)|_{0,\Omega}^2)^{1/2}. \quad (1.74)$$

Then from (1.73) it follows that

$$\begin{aligned}\mathcal{L}_5(u,u) &= \int_\Omega \{\lambda(\operatorname{div} u)^2 + 2\mu \sum_{i,j=1}^{3} \epsilon_{ij}^2(u)\}dx \geq \\ &\geq 2\mu \sum_{i,j=1}^{3} \int_\Omega \epsilon_{ij}^2(u)dx \geq 2\mu/c(\Omega)\|u\|_{1,\Omega}.\end{aligned}$$

Thus, when $\lambda, \mu > 0$ and (1.72) holds, all the conditions of Theorem 1.1 are satisfied and the generalized problem of linear elasticity has a unique solution in class $(\overset{\circ}{W}{}_2^1(\Omega))^3$.

Now consider the relation between solutions of the initial and generalized problems. Let first $u \in (W_2^2(\Omega))^3$ be a solution of the initial differential problem (1.64), (1.65). Then from (1.68)-(1.71) it follows immediately that u satisfies the generalized formulation. Thus the generalized solution, by virtue of its uniqueness, coincides with u.

The inverse is true only when the smoothness of the generalized solution is sufficient. Let, for example, $f \in (L_2(\Omega))^3$ and each component u_i of the generalized solution belong to $W_2^2(\Omega)$. Then, immediately from the definition of the class $\overset{\circ}{W}{}_2^1(\Omega)$, the boundary condition (1.65) follows. Using this boundary condition, the relation (1.70) follows from Green's formula. Take now some $i = 1,2,3$ and put into (1.70) $v_j = 0$ for $j \neq i$. Then

$$\int_\Omega -\sum_{j=1}^{3} \partial_j\sigma_{ij}(u)v_i dx = \int_\Omega f_i v_i dx.$$

Hence, as in subsection 1.1.3,

$$-\sum_{j=1}^{3} \partial_j\sigma_{ij}(u) = f_i \quad \text{almost everywhere in} \quad \Omega.$$

In view of the arbitrariness of $i = 1,2,3$ and the definition of tensors (ϵ_{ij}), (σ_{ij}) the above equality is equivalent to the initial notation of (1.64). Thus the generalized solution satisfies the initial differential problem.

Now consider some generalizations and modifications of this problem.

1. The body in region Ω may consist of two and more materials with different Lame's constants, which occurs in practice rather often. In this case, the generalized formulation (1.71) with piecewise constant λ, μ remains unchanged and also, as it is easy to see, admits a unique solution.

2. For this problem, the boundary condition (1.65) indicates a fixed boundary. How one should set a boundary condition corresponding to the boundary section that is not fixed? Let, as before, Γ_0 be a fixed boundary section and let $\Gamma_1 = \Gamma \setminus \Gamma_0$ be a not fixed one.

   Then

$$u = 0 \quad \text{on} \quad \Gamma_0. \tag{1.75}$$

On Γ_1, we assume that a force applied to the body with respect to the normal to Γ is the following

$$\sum_{j=1}^{3} \sigma_{ij}(u)\nu_j = g_i, \qquad i = 1, 2, 3, \quad \text{on} \quad \Gamma_1. \tag{1.76}$$

In the absense of such a force $g = (g_1, g_2, g_3)^T \equiv 0$. As the result, we obtain the elasticity problem with partially fixed boundary Γ_0: (1.64), (1.75), (1.76). Applying (1.68) - (1.71) to this problem gives the generalized problem of determining the vector-function u:

$$\mathcal{L}_5(u, v) = f_5(v) + \int_{\Gamma_1} g \cdot v d\gamma. \tag{1.77}$$

Every component u_i, v_i is supposed to belong to the class $\{w \in W_2^1(\Omega);\ w = 0$ on $\Gamma_0\}$. The Korn inequality [56] and unique solvability from Theorem 1.1 also hold for the problem provided that the measure of Γ_0 on Γ is positive.

Let us consider now whether the problem is uniquely solvable in case of $\Gamma_0 = \emptyset$. From physical point of view, the body is not fixed and in case of any interior load, its displacement as a rigid body is possible; this is described by

$$v = a \times x + b, \tag{1.78}$$

where a, b are constant vector in $\mathbf{R}^3$, and $a \times x$ is a vector product. There are 6 degrees of freedom in according to the number of components of the vectors a, b. From mathematical point of view the vectors v of the form of (1.78) appear in the kernel of the differential operator of the problem (1.64), (1.76) when $\Gamma_1 = \Gamma$. Introduce a six-dimensional space V of different vector-functions of the form (1.78) and construct an orthogonal complement to it in the space $(W_2^1(\Omega))^3$ (with the scalar product of the form $\int v \cdot u dx$). Denote this complement by $(\widetilde{W_2^1(\Omega)})^3$. Then the following generalized formulation holds: find $u \in (\widetilde{W_2^1(\Omega)})^3$ satisfying the relation

$$\mathcal{L}_5(u, v) = \int_\Omega f \cdot v dx + \int_\Gamma g \cdot v d\gamma \qquad \forall v \in (\widetilde{W_2^1(\Omega)})^3. \tag{1.79}$$

From the Korn inequality [56] and Theorem 1.1 this problem is solvable for any vector-functions f, g satisfying the condition

$$\|f\|_{0,\Omega} \leq c_{21}, \qquad \|g\|_{0,\Gamma} \leq c_{22}. \tag{1.80}$$

If, in addition

$$\int_\Omega f \cdot v dx + \int_\Gamma g \cdot v d\gamma = 0 \qquad \forall v \in (W_2^1(\Omega))^3, \tag{1.81}$$

then the sufficiently smooth generalized solution satisfies also the initial differential elasticity problem (1.64), (1.76) when $\Gamma_1 = \Gamma$.

3. For the homogeneous material, a decrease in the dimension of problems is possible in one of the directions. The simplest case is when displacement proceeds practically permanently in one of the directions, say, due to small thickness. In this case, we come to a planar elasticity problem in two independent space variables.

4. Studying plates and membranes with such properties as linear variation of stresses with respect to thickness, orthogonality of external forces to the surface etc. results (from integration (1.64) with respect to thickness) in boundary-value problems for equations of order 4 in two space variables. Some of them will be considered below.

1.1.7 The Dirichlet problem for biharmonic equation

Let Ω be two-dimensional bounded domain. Consider the boundary problem

$$\Delta^2 u = f \quad \text{in } \Omega, \tag{1.82}$$

$$u = 0 \quad \text{on } \Gamma, \tag{1.83}$$

$$\partial_\nu u = 0 \quad \text{on } \Gamma, \tag{1.84}$$

which describes the balance of a thin plate with fixed edge.

To pass to the generalized problem we assume that $u \in W_2^4(\Omega)$.

Take a function $v \in \overset{\circ}{W}{}_2^2(\Omega)$ and apply Green's formula

$$\int_\Omega \Delta u \Delta v dx = \int_\Omega \Delta^2 u v dx - \int_\Gamma \partial_\nu \Delta u v d\gamma + \int_\Gamma \Delta u \partial_\nu v d\gamma. \tag{1.85}$$

Multiply (1.82) by v, integrate over Ω and use in (1.85) the fact that functions v, $\partial_\nu v$ are equal to zero on Γ. We have

$$\mathcal{L}_6(u, v) = f_6(v), \tag{1.86}$$

where

$$\mathcal{L}_6(u, v) = \int_\Omega \Delta u \Delta v dx, \qquad f_6(v) = \int_\Omega f v dx.$$

Definition 1.4 *The function $u \in \overset{\circ}{W}{}_2^2(\Omega)$ satisfying equality* (1.86) *for any $v \in \overset{\circ}{W}{}_2^2(\Omega)$ is called the generalized solution of the Dirichlet problem* (1.82)-(1.84).

In order to study properties of the bilinear form $\mathcal{L}_6$ we take the equality

$$|\Delta v|_{0,\Omega} = |v|_{2,\Omega}, \qquad v \in \overset{\circ}{W}{}^2_2(\Omega),$$

which follows from formulae of integration by parts [40]. The norm $\|\cdot\|_{2,\Omega}$ in $\overset{\circ}{W}{}^2_2(\Omega)$ is equivalent to the semi-norm $|\cdot|_{2,\Omega}$, as it was mentioned already. Therefore,

$$c_{21}\|v\|_{2,\Omega} \leq |\Delta v|_{0,\Omega} \leq c_{22}\|v\|_{2,\Omega} \quad \forall v \in \overset{\circ}{W}{}^2_2(\Omega).$$

It follows that $\mathcal{L}_6$ is positive definite:

$$\mathcal{L}_6(u,v) = |\Delta u|^2_{0,\Omega} \geq c^2_{21}\|u\|^2_{2,\Omega}, \qquad u \in \overset{\circ}{W}{}^1_2(\Omega).$$

Using the Cauchy-Bunyakovski inequality gives, in turn, the boundedness

$$|\mathcal{L}_6(u,v)| \leq |\Delta u|_{0,\Omega} \cdot |\Delta v|_{0,\Omega} \leq c^2_{22}\|u\|_{2,\Omega}\|v\|_{2,\Omega}.$$

Assume that

$$f \in L_2(\Omega). \tag{1.87}$$

Then the bilinear functional f_6 is also bounded:

$$|f_6(v)| \leq |f|_{0,\Omega} \cdot |v|_{0,\Omega} \leq |f|_{0,\Omega} \cdot \|v\|_{2,\Omega}.$$

Thus, the assumptions of Theorem 1.1 are satisfied and, hence, when (1.87) holds, the Dirichlet generalized problem has a unique solution in $\overset{\circ}{W}{}^2_2(\Omega)$.

When f and generalized solution u are sufficiently smooth, one can show that u will also be a solution of the initial problem.

1.1.8 Boundary-value problems for plates

Besides the Dirichlet conditions

$$u = 0, \tag{1.88}$$

$$\partial_\nu u = 0, \tag{1.89}$$

the boundary conditions

$$\partial_{\nu\nu}u + \sigma(\partial_{\gamma\gamma}u - \frac{1}{\rho}\partial_\nu u) = 0, \tag{1.90}$$

$$\partial_\nu(\Delta u) + (1-\sigma)\partial_\gamma(\partial_{\nu\gamma}u) = 0, \tag{1.91}$$

are also possible. Here $1/\rho$ is the curvature of Γ at the given point, σ is the Poisson coefficient of plate material satisfying the inequality $0 < \sigma < 1/2$.

Conditions (1.90), (1.91) show that this boundary section is free. The combination (1.88), (1.90) standing for a given support is also possible on a part of boundary Γ.

Consider a case when the boundary Γ is a union of three parts $\Gamma = \Gamma_1 \bigcup \Gamma_2 \bigcup \Gamma_3$, on each different conditions are given:

on Γ_1 the plate is fixed, i. e., conditions (1.88), (1.89) hold;
on Γ_2 the plate has a support, i. e., conditions (1.88), (1.90) hold;
Γ_3 is free, i. e., conditions (1.90), (1.91) hold.

To take the conditions (1.90), (1.91) into account, we will do the same as in the problem with an oblique derivative: we will employ Green's formula. Namely, we take it in the following form:

$$\begin{aligned}\int_\Omega \Delta^2 u\cdot v dx &= \int_\Omega \{\partial_{11}u\partial_{11}v + (2-2\sigma)\partial_{12}u\partial_{12}v + \\ &+ \partial_{22}u\partial_{22}v + \sigma(\partial_{11}u\partial_{22}v + \partial_{22}u\partial_{11}v)\}dx - \\ &- \int_\Gamma \{\partial_\nu(\Delta u) + (1-\sigma)\partial_\gamma(\partial_{\nu\gamma}u)\}v d\gamma + \\ &+ \int_\Gamma \{\partial_{\nu\nu}u + \sigma(\partial_{\gamma\gamma}u - \frac{1}{\rho}\partial_\nu u)\}\partial_\nu v d\gamma. \end{aligned} \tag{1.92}$$

Introduce the following class of functions:

$$\tilde{W}_2^2(\Omega) = \{u \in W_2^2(\Omega), \quad u = 0 \quad \text{on} \quad \Gamma_1 \bigcup \Gamma_2, \quad \partial_\nu u = 0 \quad \text{on} \quad \Gamma_1\}.$$

To deduce the generalized formulation, we take an arbitrary function $v \in \tilde{W}_2^2(\Omega)$, multiply (1.82) by it and integrate over Ω. We get

$$\int_\Omega \Delta^2 uvdx = \int_\Omega fvdx.$$

Apply Green's formula (1.92) to the left-hand part and consider boundary integrals. On Γ_1 the integrals are equal to zero because of $\tilde{W}_2^2(\Omega) : v = \partial_\nu v = 0$ on Γ_1. On Γ_2 they also go to zero by virtue of $v = 0$ and (1.90). Finally, on Γ_3, the integrands are equal to zero because of (1.90), (1.91). As a result, the integrands vanish, which gives the formula

$$\mathcal{L}_7(u,v) = f_7(v), \tag{1.93}$$

where

$$\begin{aligned}\mathcal{L}_7(u,v) &= \int_\Omega \{\Delta u\Delta v + (1-\sigma)(2\partial_{12}u\partial_{12}v - -\partial_{11}u\partial_{22}v - \partial_{22}u\partial_{11}v)\}dx, \\ f_7 &= \int_\Omega fvdx.\end{aligned}$$

Such an addition to Green's formula is a result of physical analysis, and so there is nothing extraordinary in such a correspondence with boundary conditions (1.88)-(1.91).

Definition 1.5 *The function $u \in \tilde{W}_2^2(\Omega)$ satisfying relation* (1.93) *for any function $v \in \tilde{W}_2^2(\Omega)$ is called the generalized solution of the compound boundary-value problem for a plate.*

Estimating every term of bilinear form $\mathcal{L}_7$ by the Cauchy-Bunyakovski inequality, gives boundedness and continuity of bilinear form $\mathcal{L}_7(\cdot,\cdot) : \tilde{W}_2^2(\Omega) \times \tilde{W}_2^2(\Omega) \to \mathbf{R}$:

$$|\mathcal{L}_7(u,v)| \le c_{23}\|u\|_{2,\Omega}\|v\|_{2,\Omega}.$$

Moreover, assuming that

$$f \in L_2(\Omega), \tag{1.94}$$

we get the continuity of functional $f_7 : \tilde{W}_2^2(\Omega) \to \mathbf{R}$. To prove that $\mathcal{L}_7$ is positive definite, we modify the summands:

$$\begin{aligned}\mathcal{L}_7(u,u) &= \int_\Omega \{(\partial_{11}u)^2 + \sigma\partial_{11}u\partial_{22}u + (\partial_{22}u)^2 + 2(1-\sigma)(\partial_{12}u)^2\}dx \geq \\ &\geq (1-\sigma)\int_\Omega \{(\partial_{11}u)^2 + 2(\partial_{12}u)^2 + (\partial_{22}u)^2\}dx = (1-\sigma)|u|_{2,\Omega}^2. \end{aligned} \tag{1.95}$$

Now assume that the measure of Γ_1 in Γ is positive. Then, from [56] the inequality

$$\|u\|_{2,\Omega} \leq c_{24}|u|_{2,\Omega} \tag{1.96}$$

follows. In case $\Gamma_1 \neq \Gamma$, the proof is not so obvious as it was in the case $u \in \overset{\circ}{W}{}_2^2(\Omega)$. Applying this inequality to (1.95), we find

$$\mathcal{L}_7(u,u) \geq c_{24}^{-2}(1-\sigma)\|u\|_{2,\Omega}^2.$$

Thus, since $\sigma \in (0, 1/2)$, the form $\mathcal{L}_7$ is positive definite in $\tilde{W}_2^2(\Omega)$.

Therefore, all the conditions of Theorem 1.1 are satisfied and the generalized problem for a plate has a unique solution for any right-hand part $f \in L_2(\Omega)$.

1.1.9 The mixed method for biharmonic equation

Comparing last three problems, one can see that when passing from the three-dimensional elasticity problem to the plate problem, the integration with respect to thickness led to a simpler mathematical problem in two independent variables. The decrease of the dimension results in increase of the order of the equation, so second derivatives appear in the bilinear form. As a result, the application of the finite element method in practice, as we will see later, becomes complicated due to search for a solution in a more narrow class of functions, which imposes strict constraints on the applicability of different finite elements.

Now we ask whether it is possible to formulate the generalized problem for a plate so that the only first derivatives occur in the definition. A positive answer can be obtained by means of a mixed method whose essence consists in simultaneous search for solution and some expressions of it [40]. We will consider this method so as to solve the Dirichlet problem for the biharmonic equation, where it is evidently effective [6], [41], [61].

In addition to the solution u of problem (1.82)–(1.84), we introduce the function

$$v = -\Delta u \quad \text{on} \quad \bar{\Omega}. \tag{1.97}$$

Then (1.82) is equivalent to the equation

$$-\Delta v = f \quad \text{in} \quad \Omega. \tag{1.98}$$

To describe a required smoothness of the right-hand side, we introduce the Hilbert space $W_2^{-1}(\Omega)$ as the space dual of $\overset{\circ}{W}{}_2^1(\Omega)$. For this purpose, we use the relationship of duality $\langle\cdot,\cdot\rangle_\Omega$ between pairs of elements in $W_2^{-1}(\Omega)$ and $\overset{\circ}{W}{}_2^1(\Omega)$. We define the corresponding norm by

$$\|f\|_{-1,\Omega} = \sup_{v\in\overset{\circ}{W}{}_2^1(\Omega)\setminus\{0\}} \frac{\langle f,v\rangle_\Omega}{|v|_{1,\Omega}}.$$

The denotation of these spaces coincides with $H^{-1}(\Omega)$ from [106].

In this section, we assume that

$$f \in W_2^{-1}(\Omega). \tag{1.99}$$

Multiply (1.98) by an arbitrary function $\varphi \in \overset{\circ}{W}{}_2^1(\Omega)$ and (1.97) by $\psi \in W_2^1(\Omega)$. Integrate the obtained equalities by parts over Ω. Since functions u, φ are equal to zero on Γ, we obtain

$$\begin{aligned} &\int_\Omega (v\psi - \nabla u\cdot\nabla\psi)dx = 0,\\ &\int_\Omega \nabla v\cdot\nabla\varphi dx = \langle f,\varphi\rangle_\Omega. \end{aligned} \tag{1.100}$$

Introduce the space of pairs of function $V_2^1(\Omega) = W_2^1(\Omega)\times \overset{\circ}{W}{}_2^1(\Omega)$ with the norm

$$\|v,u\|_{V_2^1} = |v|_{0,\Omega} + |u|_{1,\Omega}$$

and define on it the bilinear forms

$$a_1(v,\psi) = \int_\Omega v\psi dx, \quad b_1(u,\psi) = -\int_\Omega \nabla u\cdot\nabla\psi dx$$

and the functional

$$f_8(\varphi) = -\langle f,\varphi\rangle_\Omega.$$

Definition 1.6 *The pair of functions $(v,u)\in V_2^1(\Omega)$ satisfying the relations*

$$\begin{aligned} a_1(v,\psi) + b_1(u,\psi) &= 0,\\ b_1(\varphi,v) &= f_8(\varphi), \qquad \forall(\psi,\varphi)\in V_2^1(\Omega), \end{aligned} \tag{1.101}$$

is called the generalized mixed solution of the Dirichlet problem for the biharmonic equation.

Thus, this formulation contains the first derivatives only.

Note that the bilinear form of problem (1.101) is not positive definite on $V_2^1(\Omega)$. Hence, Theorem 1.1 can not be applied. In order to prove a solvability of the problem, we first deduce an a priori estimate. Assume that (v,u) is a solution. Put $\varphi = u$, $\psi = v$ into (1.100). Then

$$\int_\Omega v^2 dx = \langle f,u\rangle_\Omega$$

and, hence

$$|v|_{0,\Omega}^2 \le \|f\|_{-1,\Omega}\, |u|_{1,\Omega}. \tag{1.102}$$

Now take $\varphi = 0$, $\psi = u$. We have

$$\int_\Omega (vu - \nabla u \cdot \nabla u)dx = 0.$$

Hence

$$|u|_{1,\Omega}^2 \le |u|_{0,\Omega} \cdot |v|_{0,\Omega}.$$

Combining the above with (1.102) we arrive at the inequality

$$|u|_{1,\Omega}^{3/2} \le \|f\|_{-1,\Omega}^{1/2}\, |u|_{0,\Omega}.$$

From the Friedrichs inequality (1.1), we get

$$|u|_{1,\Omega} \le c\|f\|_{-1,\Omega}. \tag{1.103}$$

Together with (1.102) this yields

$$|v|_{0,\Omega} \le c\|f\|_{-1,\Omega}. \tag{1.104}$$

Thus,

$$\|v, u\|_{V_2^1} \le c\|f\|_{-1,\Omega}. \tag{1.105}$$

We show that if the solution of the Dirichlet generalized problem (1.86) is smooth enough, the generalized mixed problem will have a unique solution.

Theorem 1.6 *Let $f \in W_2^{-1}(\Omega)$ and the solution of the Dirichlet generalized problem (1.86) belongs to $W_2^3(\Omega)$. Then the generalized mixed problem has the same unique solution $(v, u) \in V_2^1(\Omega)$.*

Proof. Let $u_1 \in W_2^3(\Omega) \bigcap \overset{\circ}{W}{}_2^2(\Omega)$ be a solution of the generalized Dirichlet problem (1.86). Assume that $v_1 = -\Delta u_1$ and take the inner product of this equality with an arbitrary function $\psi \in W_2^1(\Omega)$:

$$\int_\Omega v_1 \psi dx = -\int_\Omega \Delta u_1 \psi dx.$$

Applying Green's formula to the right-hand side and keeping in mind that $\partial_\nu u_1 = 0$ on Γ, we have

$$\int_\Omega (v_1 \psi - \nabla u_1 \cdot \nabla \psi)dx = 0.$$

Now take an arbitrary function $\varphi \in \overset{\circ}{W}{}_2^1(\Omega)$. Choose a sequence $\varphi_n \in D(\Omega)$ converging to it in norm $|\cdot|_{1,\Omega}$. Since $\varphi_n \in \overset{\circ}{W}{}_2^2(\Omega)$, from (1.86) we get the relation

$$\langle f, \varphi_n \rangle_\Omega = \int_\Omega \Delta u_1 \Delta \varphi_n dx = -\int_\Omega v_1 \Delta \varphi_n dx.$$

Applying Green's formula to the right-hand part and using the equality $\partial_\nu u_1 = 0$ on Γ, we obtain

$$\langle f, \varphi_n \rangle_\Omega = \int_\Omega \nabla v_1 \cdot \nabla \varphi_n dx.$$

Since $v_1 \in W_2^1(\Omega)$, $f \in W_2^{-1}(\Omega)$, we can pass to the limit at $n \to \infty$:

$$\int_\Omega \nabla v_1 \cdot \nabla \varphi dx = \langle f, \varphi \rangle_\Omega \qquad \forall \varphi \in \overset{\circ}{W}{}_2^1(\Omega).$$

Thus, (v_1, u_1) is a solution of the generalized mixed problem.

Now assume that there exists one more solution (v_2, u_2) of the mixed problem. Substitute both into (1.101) and subtract:

$$\begin{aligned} a_1(v_1 - v_2, \psi) + b_1(u_1 - u_2, \psi) &= 0, \\ b_1(\varphi, v_1 - v_2) &= 0, \qquad (\psi, \varphi) \in V_2^1(\Omega). \end{aligned}$$

Then any solution of this problem obeys a priori estimate (1.105):

$$|v_1 - v_2|_{0,\Omega} = |u_1 - u_2|_{1,\Omega} = 0.$$

Therefore $(v_1, u_1) = (v_2, u_2)$ in terms of equality of elements in $V_2^1(\Omega)$. □

Such attractive formulation (1.101) unfortunately has a drawback. Namely: the space $V_2^1(\Omega)$ is not closed with respect to norm $\|\cdot,\cdot\|_{V_2^1}$, since the first component belongs to $W_2^1(\Omega)$ but its norm is taken in $L_2(\Omega)$. The replenishing of space $V_2^1(\Omega)$ in this norm gives the pair $L_2(\Omega)\times \overset{\circ}{W}{}_2^1(\Omega)$ on which functional b_1 becomes unbounded.

We would have a stable variant of the formulation, for example, with the bilinear form

$$b_1(u, \psi) = \int_\Omega \Delta u \cdot \psi \, dx, \tag{1.106}$$

and the solution $(v, u) \in V_2^1(\Omega) = L_2(\Omega)\times \overset{\circ}{W}{}_2^2(\Omega)$. With these data, one can show that the problem (1.101) satisfies the I.Babuška conditions (1.20), (1.21) and the F. Brezzi ones (1.14)-(1.16). However, the bilinear form (1.106) loses main advantage: presence of the first derivatives only which permits to use simpler finite elements in discretization.

In section 6.4.1, we will return to formulation (1.101) and show that it can nevertheless be the basis for the application of the Bubnov-Galerkin method under some hypotheses about a triangulation and a degree of finite elements. Under these hypotheses, the formulation (1.101) becomes a corollary of another very specific but stable formulation from [15]. We will see this in subsection 6.4.1.

1.1.10 The Stokes problem

Let Ω be a two- or three-dimensional bounded domain. Consider a boundary-value problem which describes the motion of viscous incompressible fluid:

$$-\nu\Delta u + \operatorname{grad} p = f \quad \text{in} \quad \Omega, \tag{1.107}$$

$$\operatorname{div} u = g \quad \text{in} \quad \Omega, \tag{1.108}$$

$$u = 0 \quad \text{on} \quad \Gamma. \tag{1.109}$$

Here p is the unknown scalar function called *pressure*, the vector-function $u = (u_1, \dots, u_n)$ is *fluid motion velocity*; ν is a positive constant, called *viscocity kinematic coefficient* and the given vector-function $f = (f_1, \dots, f_n)$ describes external forces.

To pass to the generalized formulation, we assume that a solution u of this problem exists and

$$u \in (W_2^2(\Omega) \bigcap \overset{\circ}{W}{}_2^1(\Omega))^n, \qquad p \in W_2^1(\Omega). \tag{1.110}$$

Since the function p from (1.107) is defined up to additive constant, we will seek it not in $W_2^1(\Omega)$ but in space $\tilde{W}_2^1(\Omega)$ orthogonal to unit (see subsection 1.1.5).

Take an arbitrary function $q \in W_2^1(\Omega)$ and a vector-function $v \in (\overset{\circ}{W}{}_2^1(\Omega))^n$. Consider the scalar products (1.107) with v in $\mathbf{R}^n$ and (1.108) with q and integrate the both over Ω using Green's and Stokes formulae

$$-\int_\Omega v_i \Delta u_i dx = \int_\Omega \nabla u_i \cdot \nabla v_i dx \quad \forall v_i \in \overset{\circ}{W}{}_2^1(\Omega), \quad u_i \in W_2^2(\Omega), \tag{1.111}$$

$$\int_\Omega v \cdot \nabla p dx = -\int_\Omega \operatorname{div} v \cdot p dx \quad \forall v \in (\overset{\circ}{W}{}_2^1(\Omega))^n, \quad p \in W_2^1(\Omega). \tag{1.112}$$

As a result, we have

$$\begin{aligned} a_2(u,v) + b_2(p,v) &= f_9(v), \qquad v \in (\overset{\circ}{W}{}_2^1(\Omega))^n, \\ b_2(q,u) &= g_9(q), \qquad q \in \widetilde{L}_2(\Omega), \end{aligned} \tag{1.113}$$

where

$$\widetilde{L}_2(\Omega) = \{q \in L_2(\Omega); \int_\Omega q\, dx = 0\},$$

$$a_2(u,v) = \nu \int_\Omega \sum_{i=1}^n \nabla u_i \cdot \nabla v_i\, dx, \qquad b_2(p,v) = -\int_\Omega p \operatorname{div} v\, dx, \tag{1.114}$$

$$f_9(v) = \int_\Omega f \cdot v\, dx, \qquad g_9(q) = -\int_\Omega gq\, dx. \tag{1.115}$$

Let us implement formula (1.112) with $p = 1$, $v = u$. Then

$$\int_\Omega \operatorname{div} u\, dx = 0.$$

Because of (1.108) we need to assume that

$$\int_\Omega g\, dx = 0. \tag{1.116}$$

Definition 1.7 *The pair* $u \in (\overset{\circ}{W}{}_2^1(\Omega))^n$, $p \in \widetilde{L}_2(\Omega)$ *satisfying relations* (1.113) *is called the generalized mixed solution of the Stokes problem.*

In comparison with the preceeding section, the stability conditions of F.Brezzi and I.Babuška are satisfied. Consider, for example, the F.Brezzi conditions (1.14)–(1.16). Let us put $V = (\overset{\circ}{W}{}_2^1(\Omega))^n$, $W = \widetilde{L}_2(\Omega)$ and define

$$|u|_{k,\Omega} \equiv \left(\sum_{i=1}^n |u_i|_{k,\Omega}^2 \right)^{1/2}. \tag{1.117}$$

First, since bilinear form a_2 is symmetric, conditions (1.15) and (1.16) coincide. Second, any element $v \in (\overset{\circ}{W}{}_2^1(\Omega))^n$ obeys the equality

$$a_2(v,v) = \nu |v|_{1,\Omega}^2 = \nu \|u\|_V^2.$$

Inequalities (1.15), (1.16) follow it with constant $\gamma = \nu$, since $\forall v \in Z$

$$\sup_{u \in Z\setminus\{0\}} \frac{a_2(u,v)}{\|u\|_V} \geq \frac{a_2(v,v)}{\|v\|_V} = \nu\|v\|_V = \nu|v|_{1,\Omega}.$$

The verification of condition (1.14) is not so trivial, but is presented in many papers in various modifications (see, for example, [185], [78], [47], [58], [59]). We present only the final result.

Theorem 1.7 [58]. *Let Ω be a bounded domain with the Lipschitz-continuous boundary Γ. Then $\forall \varphi \in \tilde{L}_2(\Omega)$*

$$\sup_{v \in (\overset{\circ}{W}{}_2^1(\Omega))^n} \frac{(\varphi, \operatorname{div} v)}{|v|_{1,\Omega}} \geq k|\varphi|_{0,\Omega} \tag{1.118}$$

with constant $k > 0$ independent of φ.

Thus, all conditions of Theorem 1.3 are satisfied, which leads to the following deduction.

Theorem 1.8 [59]. *Let Ω be a bounded domain with the Lipschitz-continuous boundary Γ. Then problem* (1.113) *is uniquely solvable for any linear functionals f_9 continuous on $(\overset{\circ}{W}{}_2^1(\Omega))^n$ and g_9 continuous on $\tilde{L}_2(\Omega)$.*

Now we will show that smooth solution of the initial and generalized problems coincide.

Theorem 1.9 *Assume that $f \in (L_2(\Omega))^n$, $g \in \tilde{W}_2^1(\Omega)$ and let* (1.110) *hold for a solution of the Stokes problem* (1.107)–(1.109). *Then the generalized mixed problem* (1.113) *has the same solution with the function $p \in \tilde{L}_2(\Omega)$, the vector-function $u \in (\overset{\circ}{W}{}_2^1(\Omega))^n$ and this solution is unique.*

Proof. Repeating the above computations with Green's and Stokes formulae, we find that the same solution of the initial operator problem is also a solution of the generalized problem. Due to Theorem 1.8, this solution is unique. □

To describe the smoothness of data for the Stokes and other problems in further sections, we need the following spaces also.

$L_p(\Omega)$, $p \in [1,\infty]$, is the Hilbert space of measurable functions $v : \Omega \to \mathbf{R}$ with the finite norm

$$\begin{aligned} \|v\|_{0,p,\Omega} &\equiv \left(\int_\Omega |v|^p\,dx\right)^{1/p}, \qquad p \in [1,\infty), \\ \|v\|_{0,\infty,\Omega} &\equiv \sup_\Omega \text{ vrai } |v|, \qquad p = \infty. \end{aligned}$$

For an integer $m \geq 0$ the Sobolev space $W_p^m(\Omega)$, $p \in [1, \infty]$, consists of functions $v \in L_p(\Omega)$ all partial derivatives of which $\partial^\alpha v$ belong to $L_p(\Omega)$ for $|\alpha| \leq m$. The norm in $W_p^m(\Omega)$ is introduced by

$$\begin{aligned} \|v\|_{m,p,\Omega} &\equiv \left(\sum_{|\alpha| \leq m} \int_\Omega |\partial^\alpha v|^p \, dx \right)^{1/p}, \quad p \in [1, \infty), \\ \|v\|_{m,\infty,\Omega} &\equiv \max_{|\alpha| \leq m} \|\partial^\alpha v\|_{0,\infty,\Omega}, \quad p = \infty. \end{aligned} \tag{1.119}$$

When $p = 2$, we usually omit this subindex. Besides, we can omit subindex Ω too where it does not give a doubt, i. e.,

$$\|v\|_{m,2,\Omega} = \|v\|_{m,\Omega} = \|v\|_m.$$

For a vector-function $u = (u_1, \ldots, u_n)$, we put

$$\begin{aligned} \|u\|_{m,p,\Omega} &\equiv \left(\sum_{i=1}^n \|u_i\|_{m,p,\Omega}^p \right)^{1/p}, \quad p \in [1, \infty), \\ \|u\|_{m,\infty,\Omega} &\equiv \max_{1 \leq i \leq n} \|u_i\|_{m,\infty,\Omega}, \quad p = \infty. \end{aligned} \tag{1.120}$$

1.2 The general scheme of the Bubnov-Galerkin method

1.2.1 Solving the operator equations

Let H be a Hilbert space with an inner product $(\cdot, \cdot)$ and a norm $\|u\| = (u, u)^{1/2}$. Consider the equation

$$Lu = Au + Bu = f, \qquad f \in H, \tag{1.121}$$

where A, B are linear (possibly unbounded) operators in H with the domains of definition $D(A)$, $D(B)$. We assume that $D(A) \subseteq D(B)$ and $D(A)$ is dense in H.

Let us consider only the case when A is a symmetric positive definite operator, i. e., for all $u, v \in D(A)$ $(Au, v) = (u, Av)$, $(Au, u) \geq \gamma \|u\|^2$ with constant $\gamma > 0$. Introduce in $D(A)$ the inner product and the norm:

$$[u, v] = (Au, v), \qquad [\![u]\!] = [u, u]^{1/2}. \tag{1.122}$$

Completing $D(A)$ in H with respect to the given norm, we obtain the complete Hilbert space H_A which is called *the energetic space* generated by operator A. Accordingly, the norm in (1.122) is called *the energetic norm.*

Take the inner product of (1.121) with an arbitrary function $v \in D(A)$ in H. Then

$$(Au, v) \; + \; (Bu, v) = (f, v), \tag{1.123}$$
$$[u, v] \; + \; (Bu, v) = (f, v). \tag{1.124}$$

The last equality follows from (1.123) by virtue of (1.122). This equation is satisfied, for elements u, v belonging to the space H_A which is broader than $D(A)$. This enables one to obtain a generalized formulation of the initial problem.

Introduce a bilinear form and a linear functional:

$$\mathcal{L}(u,v) = [u,v] + (Bu,v), \qquad f(v) = (f,v). \tag{1.125}$$

Definition 1.8 *The function $u \in H_A$ satisfying the relation*

$$\mathcal{L}(u,v) = f(v) \qquad \forall v \in H_A. \tag{1.126}$$

is called the generalized solution of equation (1.121).

It is easy to see that solution of (1.121) will satisfy (1.126) as well. And vice versa, if there exists a generalized solution u, then if $u \in D(A)$ it would be also a solution of equation (1.121) because of completeness of $D(A)$ in H [115].

Now we formulate the Bubnov-Galerkin method corresponding to problem (1.126). To this end, the space H_A is approximated by a finite-dimensional subspace $H^h \subset H_A$ and the approximate problem is to find the element $u^h \in H^h$ such that

$$\mathcal{L}(u^h, v) = f(v) \qquad \forall v \in H^h. \tag{1.127}$$

Write (1.127) in the form of a system of linear algebraic equations. For this purpose, we introduce the basis ξ_i $(i = 1, \ldots, N)$ in H^h. Then u^h belongs to the subspace H^h if there exists a set of coefficients α_i such that

$$u^h = \sum_{i=1}^{N} \alpha_i \xi_i. \tag{1.128}$$

Using linearity of the functional f and the form $\mathcal{L}$ with respect to every argument, we can easily show that (1.127) is equivalent to the system

$$L^h U^h = F^h \tag{1.129}$$

with vector of unknowns $U^h = (\alpha_1, \ldots, \alpha_N)^T$, right-hand part $F^h = (f(\xi_1), \ldots, f(\xi_N))^T$ and quadratic matrix L^h of the dimension $N \times N$ with elements $L^h_{ij} = \mathcal{L}(\xi_j, \xi_i)$.

We first formulate solvability conditions of problems (1.127)-(1.129) in terms of the bilinear form $\mathcal{L}$ and the functional f.

Theorem 1.10 [40]. *Let the bilinear form $\mathcal{L}$ be bounded and positive definite in space H_A and let functional f be bounded in it. Then, the problems* (1.126), (1.127) *and the system* (1.129) *are uniquely solvable and the solution u^h_* of the Bubnov-Galerkin method obeys the estimate*

$$[\![u_* - u^h_*]\!] \le c \min_{v \in H^h} [\![u_* - v]\!]. \tag{1.130}$$

The positive definiteness of the form $\mathcal{L}$ quarantees, by virtue of Theorem 1.1, the unique solvability of the both problems — the initial (1.126) and the approximate (1.127). What will happen if we remove the condition of positive definiteness of $\mathcal{L}$ but demand that problem (1.126) is uniquely solvable? Then approximate problem (1.127) will be solvable only when the H_A space elements can be approximated sufficiently well. Namely, assume that the parameter h denotes an arbitrary element of some sequence tending to zero and every value of h corresponds to a subspace $H^h \subset H_A$. The sequence H^h is said to be *dense in the sense of limit* in H_A if for any element $v \in H_A$ there is a sequence of elements $v^h \in H^h$ such that

$$[\![v - v^h]\!] \to 0 \qquad \text{when} \quad h \to 0.$$

Theorem 1.11 [87], [115], [132]. *Let the problem* (1.126) *have a unique solution and let the operator* $A^{-1}B$ *be completely continuous in* H_A. *Also let the sequence of subspaces* H^h *be dense in the sense of limit in* H_A. *Then when* h *are small enough, the problem* (1.127) *and the system* (1.129) *are uniquely solvable,* $u_*^h \to u_*$ *in* H_A *when* $h \to 0$, *and the estimate* (1.130) *holds.*

Now we consider I.Babuška result used in cases where besides lack of positive definiteness of form $\mathcal{L}$, the different spaces of admissible functions for the solution u and test functions are possible. Let us return to the abstract problem (1.8): find the solution $u \in H_1$ such that

$$\mathcal{B}(u, v) = f(v) \qquad \forall v \in H_2. \tag{1.131}$$

We would remind that H_1, H_2 are two real Hilbert spaces with inner products and the norms corresponding to them; $\mathcal{B}$ is a continuous bilinear form on $H_1 \times H_2$ and f is a continuous linear functional on H_2 (see (1.6), (1.7)). Introduce two approximating finite-dimensional subspaces $H_1^h \subset H_1$, $H_2^h \subset H_2$ and consider the problem: *find* $u^h \in H_1^h$ *such that*

$$\mathcal{B}(u^h, v) = f(v) \qquad \forall v \in H_2^h. \tag{1.132}$$

Then analogue of Theorem 1.1 holds about a unique solution of problem (1.132) and an estimate is derived about possible closeness between the solutions of (1.132) and (1.131).

Theorem 1.12 [11]. *Let the conditions of Theorem 1.2 be satisfied and* u_* *be a solution of problem* (1.131). *Let besides*

$$\sup_{u \in H_1^h} \frac{|\mathcal{B}(u, v)|}{\|u\|_{H_1}} \geq c\|v\|_{H_2} \qquad \forall v \in H_2^h, \ c > 0; \tag{1.133}$$

$$\sup_{v \in H_2^h} \frac{|\mathcal{B}(u, v)|}{\|v\|_{H_2}} \geq c_3 \|u\|_{H_1} \qquad \forall u \in H_1^h, \ c_3 > 0. \tag{1.134}$$

Then there exists the unique solution u_*^h *of problem* (1.132) *satisfying the estimate*

$$\|u_* - u_*^h\|_{H_1} \leq (1 + c_0/c_3) \inf_{u \in H_1^h} \|u_* - u\|_{H_1}. \tag{1.135}$$

1.2.2 The spectral problem

Let us turn to the spectral problem

$$Au = \lambda Bu \tag{1.136}$$

of definition of eigenvalues λ and corresponding eigenfunction u. The condition introduced above that operator $A^{-1}B$ is completely continuous implies this time the discrete behaviour of the spectrum, i. e., the set of eigenvalues λ is at most countable (on complex plane) and does not have finite condensation points.

Consider only the case when both operators A, B are symmetric and positive definite. Take the inner product of the arbitrary function $v \in D(A)$ with (1.136) in H. Then

$$(Au, v) = \lambda(Bu, v). \tag{1.137}$$

As it was in the case of the space H_A, we introduce the energetic space H_B generated by the operator B with the inner product $[u, v]_B = (Bu, v)$ and the norm $[\![u]\!]_B = [u, u]^{1/2}$. Then (1.137) can be rewritten as

$$[u, v] = \lambda[u, v]_B. \tag{1.138}$$

Definition 1.9 *The pairs (λ, u) consisting of an eigenvalue λ and an eigenfunction $u \in H_A$ and satisfying* (1.138) *for any function $v \in H_A$ are called the generalized solutions of the spectral problem* (1.136).

Relation (1.138) along with every eigenfunction u is satisfied also for functions μu with arbitrary constant μ. To eliminate this degree of freedom, we will imply one representative satisfying the relation

$$[\![u]\!]_B = 1. \tag{1.139}$$

Theorem 1.13 [132]. *Let operators A, B be symmetric and positive definite and let $A^{-1}B$ be completely continuous in H_A. Then the generalized spectral problem has infinite number of eigenvalues $0 < \lambda_1 \leq \lambda_2 \leq \ldots \leq \lambda_i \leq \ldots$ and $\lambda_i \to \infty$ when $i \to \infty$. Each of the eigenvalues can be associated with one eigenfunction u_i so that all eigenfunctions form a system $\{u_i\}$ which is orthonormal in H_B, orthogonal in H_A, and complete in both spaces.*

We show how the correspondence between eigenvalues and eigenfunctions can be set up. In the case of the single eigenvalue λ_i, when the dimension of the subspace of the corresponding eigenfunctions equals one, we take one of the two functions normed in accordance with (1.139) and differed by sign as u_i. This eigenfunction is orthogonal to the eigenfunctions corresponding to other eigenvalues. Indeed, consider two solutions of the spectral problem μ_1, v_1 and μ_2, v_2 with $\mu_1 \neq \mu_2$. Then, according to (1.138)

$$\begin{aligned} [v_1, v_2] &= \mu_1[v_1, v_2]_B \qquad \text{when} \quad v = v_2, \\ [v_2, v_1] &= \mu_2[v_2, v_1]_B \qquad \text{when} \quad v = v_1. \end{aligned}$$

Since the inner products in H_A, H_B are symmetric, the relation defining orthogonality in H_B follows

$$(\mu_1 - \mu_2)[v_1, v_2]_B = 0.$$

Let now λ_i have multiplicity r, i. e., the dimension of the subspace of its eigenfunctions V_i equals to r. Choosing in V_i a basis orthonormal in H_B, we obtain the required set of functions which corresponds with the eigenvalues $\lambda_i = \lambda_{i+1} = \ldots = \lambda_{i+r-1}$.

Orthogonality of the basis constructed in H_A follows from equality (1.138) when $u = u_i$, $v = u_j$:

$$[u_i, u_j] = \lambda_i[u_i, u_j]_B = 0 \qquad \forall i \neq j.$$

We now formulate the Bubnov-Galerkin method for spectral problem (1.138). In the notation of subsection 1.2.1, we introduce a finite-dimensional subspace $H^h \subset H_A$. The approximate problem is then to find pairs $\lambda^h \in \mathbf{R}$, $u^h \in H^h$ satisfying the relation

$$[u^h, v] = \lambda^h [u^h, v]_B \qquad \forall v \in H^h. \tag{1.140}$$

For approximate eigenfunctions we will also use the normalization

$$[\![u^h]\!]_B = 1, \tag{1.141}$$

to eliminate unnecessary degree of freedom. Nevertheless, the factor ± 1 is arbitrarily choosen.

Let us reduce this statement to an algebraic generalized spectral problem. Introduce basis ξ_i $(i = 1, \dots, N)$ in H^h and find u^h in the form

$$u^h = \sum_{i=1}^{N} \alpha_i \xi_i. \tag{1.142}$$

Using linearity of inner products with respect to each argument gives the algebraic problem

$$L^h U^h = \lambda^h M^h U^h \tag{1.143}$$

on definition of eigenvalues λ^h and eigenvectors $U^h = (\alpha_1, \dots, \alpha_N)^T$ corresponding to them. The $N \times N$ matrices L^h and M^h with elements $L^h_{ij} = [\xi_j, \xi_i]$, $M^h_{ij} = [\xi_j, \xi_i]_B$ are symmetric and positive definite. Note that normalization (1.141) leads to the condition

$$(U^h)^T M^h U^h = 1. \tag{1.144}$$

Since spectral problem (1.140) has the same structure as initial problem (1.138), it obeys an assertion analogous to Theorem 1.13. Namely, the approximate spectral problem (1.140) has a finite set of eigenvalues $0 < \lambda^h_1 \leq \lambda^h_2 \leq \dots \leq \lambda^h_N$. Each of the eigenvalues λ^h_i can be associated with one eigenfunction u^h_i so that all eigenfunctions form a system $\{u^h_i\}$ orthonormal in H_B, orthogonal in H_A, and complete in H.

The correspondence between eigenvalues and eigenfunctions in (1.140) (or eigenvectors in (1.143)) is set up in the same way as in the initial problem (1.138).

Let us consider the convergence of eigenvalues and eigenfunctions of the Bubnov-Galerkin method when $h \to 0$ for sequence of subspaces H^h dense in the sense of limit in H_A. Let λ_i and λ^h_i be the i-th eigenvalues of problems (1.138) and (1.140), respectively. The convergence of λ^h_i to λ_i means that $\lambda^h_i \to \lambda_i$ when $h \to 0$. In order to show a convergence of eigenfunctions we first consider the single eigenvalue λ_i . Then, starting from certain h, i-th eigenvalue λ^h_i is also single due to convergence of neighbour eigenvalues $\lambda^h_{i\pm 1}$. Therefore λ^h_i is associated with one eigenfunction u^h_i for which the convergence means the condition

$$[\![u_i - u^h_i]\!] \to 0 \quad \text{when} \quad h \to 0. \tag{1.145}$$

But if λ_i is an eigenvalue of problem (1.138) of multiplicity r, then the convergence of u^h_i means that at every h in the r-dimensional eigensubspace V_i of the initial problem (1.138) there exists an eigenfunction w with a unit norm for which the relation

$$\inf_{w \in V_i, [\![w]\!]=1} [\![w - u^h_i]\!] \to 0 \quad \text{when} \quad h \to 0 \tag{1.146}$$

holds.

In these terms the main result on convergence of the spectral problem of the Bubnov-Galerkin method is given by

Theorem 1.14 [87], [132]. *Let operator A be symmetric and positive definite, operator $A^{-1}B$ be completely continuous in H_A, and let the sequence of subspaces H^h be dense in the sense of limit in H_A. Then eigenvalues of the Bubnov-Galerkin method converge to eigenvalues of spectral problem* (1.138). *If in addition operator B is symmetric and positive definite, then eigenfunctions converge as well.*

Assuming that B is symmetric, we try to avoid some problems not solved in many cases on the theoretical ground, rather than simplify computations. Recall them for non-symmetric B.

1. The known example of N.I.Polskii [132] shows that not all eigenfunctions of (1.136) can be approximated by the Bubnov-Galerkin method if B is non-self-adjoint.
2. In the initial problem, adjoined functions may be available. In this case the number of eigenvectors and adjoined vectors for some eigenvalues in the Bubnov-Galerkin method can change with every h and does not give any idea of real structure of eigensubspaces of the initial problem.
3. For differential problems with the real spectrum, the Bubnov-Galerkin method can yield complex eigenvalues so that it is to be realized over the complex value field.

1.2.3 The mixed method

Now, let us turn to the Bubnov-Galerkin method for the problem (1.12), (1.13) of definition of functions u, φ from the Hilbert spaces V, W

$$\begin{aligned} a(u,v)+b(v,\phi) &= f(v) \qquad \forall v\in V,\\ b(u,\psi) &= g(\psi) \qquad \forall \psi\in W. \end{aligned} \tag{1.147}$$

Recall that a, b are continuous bilinear forms on $V\times V$ and $V\times W$ satisfying conditions (1.14)-(1.16); f, q are the given continuous linear functionals on V and W.

Both spaces V and W are approximated by finite-dimensional subspaces $V^h\subset V$ and $W^h\subset W$.

As a result, the problem (1.147) reduces to the following: *find $u^h\in V^h$ and $\varphi^h\in W^h$ such that*

$$\begin{aligned} a(u^h,v)+b(v,\varphi^h) &= f(v) \qquad \forall v\in V^h,\\ b(u^h,\psi) &= g(\psi) \qquad \forall \psi\in W^h. \end{aligned} \tag{1.148}$$

Assume that conditions similar to (1.14)-(1.16) are satisfied:

1. there exists a constant $k>0$ such that

$$\sup_{v\in V^h\setminus\{0\}}\frac{b(v,\varphi)}{\|v\|_V}\ge k\|\varphi\|_W \qquad \forall\varphi\in W^h; \tag{1.149}$$

2. there exist constants $\gamma > 0$ and $\gamma' > 0$ such that

$$\sup_{u\in Z^h\setminus\{0\}} a(u,v)/\|u\|_V \geq \gamma\|v\|_V \qquad \forall v \in Z^h, \tag{1.150}$$

$$\sup_{v\in Z^h\setminus\{0\}} a(u,v)/\|v\|_V \geq \gamma'\|u\|_V \qquad \forall u \in Z^h, \tag{1.151}$$

where

$$Z^h = \{v \in V^h : b(v,\varphi) = 0 \qquad \forall \varphi \in W^h\}.$$

Then the following result holds.

Theorem 1.15 [47], [36]. *Let conditions of Theorem* (1.3) *be satisfied and let* (u_*, φ_*) *be the solution of problem* (1.147). *Moreover, let the discrete conditions* (1.149)-(1.151) *hold. Then problem* (1.148) *has a unique solution* (u_*^h, φ_*^h) *which obeys the estimate*

$$\|u_* - u_*^h\|_V + \|\varphi_* - \varphi_*^h\|_W \leq \sigma(\inf_{v\in V^h} \|u_* - v\|_V + \inf_{\psi\in W^h} \|\varphi_* - \psi\|_W) \tag{1.152}$$

with constant σ *independent of* f, q.

We remind that conditions (1.150) and (1.151) coincide for symmetric bilinear form a. Moreover, if the form a is positive definite, i. e.,

$$a(u,u) \geq \rho\|u\|_V^2, \quad \rho = \text{const} > 0, \quad \forall u \in V,$$

then conditions (1.150), (1.151) are satisfied with constants $\gamma = \gamma' = \rho$.

Now we formulate discrete stability conditions in the form of I.Babuška. Rewriting (1.17)-(1.18) as in subsection 1.1.2, we come first to abstract problem (1.19), then to its discretization in subspace $\tilde{H}^h = V^h \times W^h$: *find an element* $\tilde{u}^h \in \tilde{H}^h$ *such that*

$$\tilde{\mathcal{B}}(\tilde{u}^h, \tilde{v}) = \tilde{f}(\tilde{v}) \qquad \forall \tilde{v} \in \tilde{H}^h. \tag{1.153}$$

Application of Theorem 1.12 to this problem gives the following result.

Theorem 1.16 *Assume that conditions of Theorem 1.4 are satisfied and* (u_*, φ_*) *is a solution of problem* (1.147). *Assume also that*

$$\begin{aligned}\sup_{(v,\psi)\in V_h\times W_h} |a(u,v) \ &+\ b(v,\varphi) + b(u,\psi)|/(\|v\|_V + \|\psi\|_W) \geq \\ &\geq\ c(\|u\|_V + \|\varphi\|_W), \quad \forall (u,\varphi) \in V_h \times W_h, \end{aligned} \tag{1.154}$$

$$\begin{aligned}\sup_{(u,\varphi)\in V_h\times W_h} |a(u,v) \ &+\ b(v,\varphi) + b(u,\psi)|/(\|u\|_V + \|\varphi\|_W) \geq \\ &\geq\ c(\|v\|_V + \|\psi\|_W), \quad \forall (v,\psi) \in V_h \times W_h, \end{aligned} \tag{1.155}$$

where $c > 0$. *Then problem* (1.148) *has the unique solution* (u_*^h, φ_*^h) *satisfying the estimate* (1.152).

Introducing bases into subspaces V^h, W^h, we may recast (1.148) into a system of linear algebraic equations. To this end, we denote the elements of bases V^h and W^h by ξ_i $(i = 1, \dots, n_1)$ and η_i $(i = 1, \dots, n_2)$ where $n_1 = \dim V^h$, $n_2 = \dim W^h$ and

$N = n_1 + n_2$. Since u^h and φ^h belong to spaces V^h and W^h, there exist constants α_i and β_i such that

$$u^h = \sum_{i=1}^{n_1} \alpha_i \xi_i, \qquad \varphi^h = \sum_{i=1}^{n_2} \beta_i \eta_i.$$

Then the finding u^h, φ^h from (1.148) is equivalent to solving the system

$$L^h U^h = F^h \tag{1.156}$$

with the $N \times N$ square matrix L^h, vector of unknowns U^h and right-hand part F^h of dimension N:

$$L^h = \begin{bmatrix} A & B \\ B^T & 0 \end{bmatrix}, U^h = \begin{bmatrix} \alpha_1 \\ \vdots \\ \alpha_{n_1} \\ \beta_1 \\ \vdots \\ \beta_{n_2} \end{bmatrix}, F^h = \begin{bmatrix} f(\xi_1) \\ \cdots \\ f(\xi_{n_1}) \\ g(\eta_1) \\ \cdots \\ g(\eta_{n_2}) \end{bmatrix}. \tag{1.157}$$

Here 0 is the $n_2 \times n_2$ zero matrix, A and B are the $n_1 \times n_1$ and $n_1 \times n_2$ matrices with the elements

$$\begin{aligned} A_{ij} &= a(\xi_j, \xi_i), \qquad j = 1, \dots, n_1, \quad i = 1, \dots, n_1; \\ B_{ij} &= b(\xi_i, \eta_j), \qquad j = 1, \dots, n_2, \quad i = 1, \dots, n_1. \end{aligned}$$

Chapter 2

General properties of finite elements

Currently, a wide range of finite elements is known. An overview of them is provided, for example, in the monographs [134], [40], [9].

We will mainly dwell on properties of the simplest and most frequently used elements for solving the elliptic equations of order 2 and also touch two specific and more complex finite elements for solving the equations of order 4.

Besides usual finite-element properties necessary to define the order of approximation and the number of conditionality of the Bubnov-Galerkin method systems, we note the specific peculiarity which exhibits itself in sequences of nested grids. Namely, they admit a representation of basis functions on one grid in the form of linear combination of basis functions of another more fine grid. This property makes multigrid methods more simple and economic in use. Constructing the nested grids is therefore also treated, including that for domains with the curvilinear boundary.

In the two-dimensional case, we retain the traditional terms *simplex*, *square* and *rectangle* to label flat closed triangles and quadrangles with straight sides and corresponding properties. By the terms *curvilinear triangle*, *quadrangle* or, broadly, *polygon*, we will label the curvilinear configurations (on the plane and in the space) which are diffeomorphic[1] to a simplex, square or a flat polygon with straight sides, respectively. Note that diffeomorphism preserves angles (but not the values of them), so that a triangle cannot be diffeomorphic to a quadrangle. By *standard triangle*, we will mean the simplex in $\mathbf{R}^2$ with vertices $(0,0),(1,0),(0,1)$, and by *standard square*, the set $[0,1]^2$.

In the three-dimensional space, we leave unchanged the terms *simplex*, *cube* and *rectangle* to label polyhedra with flat faces — polygons with corresponding properties. We will sometimes use the terms *tetrahedron*, *hexahedron*, *octahedron* and *polyhedron* with the word *curvilinear* to denote the figures which are diffeomorphic in $\mathbf{R}^3$ to a simplex, cube or a usual octahedron, the polyhedron with flat faces — polygons with straight sides, respectively. By *standard tetrahedron* we will mean the simplex in $\mathbf{R}^3$ with vertices $(0,0,0),(1,0,0),(0,1,0),(0,0,1)$, and by *standard cube* the set $[0,1]^3$.

[1]Recall that diffeomorfism is a one-to-one and continuously differentiable mapping $f : M \to N$ of a differentiable manifold M into a differentiable manifold N, the inverse mapping f^{-1} being also continuously differentiable. If $f(M) = N$, M and N are said to be diffeomorphic.

2.1 Classification of finite elements

There exist various definitions of finite elements in the literature which are, generally speaking, equivalent from the point of view of practical use. We will consider the definition of the finite element as a triplet (ω, P, Φ) where

1. $\omega \subset \mathbf{R}^n$ is a bounded closed subset with the Lipschitz boundary and non-empty interjor;
2. P is the N-dimensional space of functions defined on ω;
3. Φ is the set of linearly-independent linear functionals $\varphi_i : P \to \mathbf{R}$ $(i = 1, \dots, N)$.

The subset ω is said to be a mesh or a cell. In the two-dimensional case, it is a triangle or quadrangle; in the three-dimensional case, it is a tetrahedron, a rectangular parallelepiped, etc. In some special cases, for the boundary to be approximated better, we suppose ω to have curvilinear sides.

In this study, P is, as a rule, a polynomial space. The linear functionals φ_i are said to be degrees of freedom. We will consider the most widely used version where $\varphi_i(p)$ are values of function p or its partial derivative at some points $a_j \in \omega$ $(j = 1, \dots, m)$ called nodes.

Definition 2.1 *The set Φ is said to be P-solvable if for any set of real numbers α_i $(i = 1, \dots, N)$ there exists a unique function $p \in P$ satisfying the conditions*

$$\varphi_i(p) = \alpha_i \qquad \forall i = 1, \dots, N. \tag{2.1}$$

Below, we will use only the finite elements which possess this property. In each, it is tantamount to the existence of such set of functions $p_i \in P$ $(i = 1, \dots, N)$, that

$$\varphi_i(p_i) = \delta_{ij} \qquad \forall i, j = 1, \dots, N. \tag{2.2}$$

By means of this basis, any function $p \in P$ can be written as

$$p = \sum_{i=1}^{N} \varphi_i(p) p_i. \tag{2.3}$$

The functions p_i are said to be the basis functions of the finite element; P is said to be its space of admissible functions.

When solving the concrete problem, one kind of finite elements is often chosen on whole set of cells ω_k. As a result, any finite element is defined by its cell ω_k — it gives automatically nodes for φ_i and a domain of definition for P. Then, it is convenient for the finite element to be identified with its cell ω_k. That is why in the literature on applications, the cells ω_k are often referred to as (finite) elements [115]. Sometimes, in applications, we will also follow this custom.

The most obvious classification of the finite elements can be accomplished with respect to the dimension of space $\mathbf{R}^n$. Further description applies mainly to the two-dimensional problems and only in some cases to the three-dimensional ones. The one-dimensional problems are not treated.

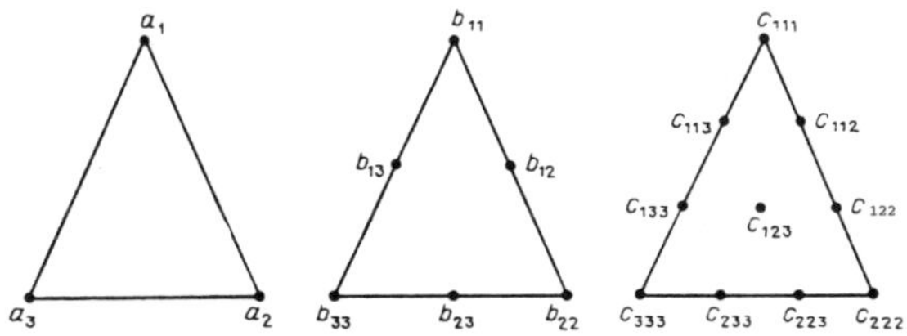

Figure 2.1: Nodes of triangular Lagrangian elements of the degree $k = 1, 2, 3$

In the two-dimensional case we consider elements with a triangular and rectangular cell; in the three-dimensional case we consider the cell as tetrahedron or rectangular parallelepiped. Finally, for every kind of cells, we will consider spaces P of polynomials of different degrees.

To describe these, we introduce the notation P_k (with integer $k \geq 0$) for the space of all the polynomials of degree not higher than k in $x = (x_1, \dots, x_n)$. In multiindex form, polynomials $p \subset P_k$ are $p(x) = \sum\limits_{|\alpha| \leq k} \gamma_\alpha x^\alpha$, where $\alpha = (\alpha_1, \dots, \alpha_n)$ is a multiindex. The dimension of space P_k is equal to the number of combinations of k elements from $n+k$, i. e., dim $P_k = C^k_{n+k}$.

If Ψ is a space of functions defined on $\mathbf{R}^n$, and set A lies in $\mathbf{R}^n$, then $\Psi(A)$ will denote the space obtained by restriction of $\mathbf{R}^n$ to A. For instance, $P_k(A) = \{p : A \to \mathbf{R}; p \in P_k\}$.

Note that due to the non-empty interior of ω, dim $P_k(\omega) =$ dim P_k.

We introduce also the notation Q_k (with integer $k \geq 0$) to denote a space of polynomials of degree not higher than k for each of the variables $x_1, \dots, x_n$. In multiindex form, the polynomials like $q \in Q_k$ are: $q(x) = \sum_{\alpha_i \leq k, i=1,\dots,n} \gamma_\alpha x^\alpha$, where $\alpha = (\alpha_1, \dots, \alpha_n)$ is a multiindex. It is obvious that dim $Q_k =$ dim $Q_k(\omega) = (k+1)^n$.

2.2 Two-dimensional finite elements

In the two-dimensional case, the most frequently used shape of the finite element mesh is a triangle. This is because of the fact that a two-dimensional region with piecewise differentiable boundary can be approximated by polygons which can be divided into a finite number of triangles. Some examples of the technique will be given at the end of this chapter. At the same time, there exist some boundary-value problems in the region composed of rectangles. In this case, it is more convenient to apply rectangular meshes.

2.2.1 Elements with a triangular mesh

Let a_1, a_2, a_3 be the vertices of a non-singular triangle $\omega \subset \mathbf{R}^2$ with coordinates $a_i = (a_{i1}, a_{i2})$ (Fig. 2.1, $k = 1$).

The first element, called *the Courant triangle*, is characterized by the triplet (ω, P, Φ), where $P = P_1(\omega)$ and $\Phi_1 = \{\varphi_i : \varphi_i(p) = p(a_i), i = 1, 2, 3\}$, or simpler: $\Phi_1 = \{p(a_i), i = 1, 2, 3\}$.

Since linear polynomial $p \subset P_1$ is completely defined by three values of $p(a_i)$, the set Φ_1 is P_1-solvable.

To define basis functions of this element, along with the Cartesian coordinates we introduce *barycentric coordinates* $\lambda_j = \lambda_j(x)$ $(j = 1, 2, 3)$. For every point $x = (x_1, x_2)$ they are introduced as a solution of the linear system

$$\sum_{j=1}^{3} a_{ij}\lambda_j = x_i, \qquad i = 1, 2,$$

$$\sum_{j=1}^{3} \lambda_j = 1. \tag{2.4}$$

Its matrix determinant equals twice the area of the triangle ω and therefore is not zero. As a result, this system has a unique solution for any $x \in \mathbf{R}^2$. By substituting into (2.4) we can show that the vertex $x = a_j$ corresponds to the solution $\lambda_i = \delta_{ij}$ $(i = 1, 2, 3)$. As a consequence, we have linear functions $\lambda \in P_1$ satisfying the condition

$$\varphi_j(\lambda_i) = \lambda_i(a_j) = \delta_{ij}, \qquad i, j = 1, 2, 3.$$

Thus, λ_i are the basis functions of the Courant element, i. e.,

$$p = \sum_{i=1}^{3} p(a_i)\lambda_i, \qquad p \in P_1. \tag{2.5}$$

The construction of polynomial p by its values at vertices a_i does not differ from the Lagrange interpolation, and so it is natural to call this element *the Lagrange element of degree* 1.

To define the Lagrange element of degree 2, we introduce besides vertices the midpoints of the sides of the triangle ω (see Fig. 2.1, $k = 2$):

$$b_{ij} = (a_i + a_j)/2, \qquad 1 \le i \le j \le 3. \tag{2.6}$$

Now *the element of degree* 2 is defined by the triplet $(\omega, P_2(\omega), \Phi_2)$, where $\Phi_2 = \{p(b_{ij}), 1 \le i \le j \le 3\}$. The number of degrees of freedom as well as the dimension of P_2 are equal to six. Hence, the set Φ_2 is P_2-solvable [40]. The basis functions of this element are expressed in terms of barycentric coordinates:

$$p = \sum_{i=1}^{3} \lambda_i(2\lambda_i - 1)p(b_{ii}) + \sum_{1 \le i < j \le 3} 4\lambda_i\lambda_j p(b_{ij}), \quad p \in P_2. \tag{2.7}$$

Finally, we introduce some additional points on the sides and the centre of gravity of the triangle (see Fig. 2.1, $k = 3$):

$$c_{ijk} = (a_i + a_j + a_k)/3, \qquad i, j, k = 1, 2, 3. \tag{2.8}$$

Now *the Lagrange element of degree* 3 is defined by the triplet $(\omega, P_3(\omega), \Phi_3)$, where $\Phi_3 = \{p(c_{ijk}), 1 \le i \le j \le k \le 3\}$. The total number of degrees of freedom is 10 and a complete polynomial from P_3 has the same number of coefficients. As a result, the set

Φ_3 is P_3-solvable [40]. Its basis functions are again expressed in terms of barycentric coordinates:

$$\begin{aligned} p &= \sum_{i=1}^{3} \frac{1}{2}\lambda_i(3\lambda_i - 1)(3\lambda_i - 2)p(c_{iii}) + \\ &+ \sum_{i\neq j;\, i,j=1}^{3} \frac{9}{2}\lambda_i\lambda_j(3\lambda_i - 1)p(c_{iij}) + 27\lambda_1\lambda_2\lambda_3 p(c_{123}), \quad p \in P_3. \end{aligned} \tag{2.9}$$

Such a construction can be carried out for polynomials P_k of an arbitrary degree k. For this purpose we introduce nodes

$$d_{i_1\ldots i_k} = (a_{i_1} + \ldots + a_{i_k})/k, \qquad i_1, \ldots, i_k = 1, 2, 3,$$

and the following set of functionals:

$$\Phi_3^{(k)} = \{p(d_{i_1\ldots i_k}), 1 \leq i_1 \leq i_2 \leq \ldots \leq i_k \leq 3\}.$$

Now *the Lagrange element of degree* k is defined by the triplet $(\omega, P_k(\omega), \Phi_3^{(k)})$. The number of degrees of freedom and the dimension of $P_k(\omega)$ are equal to $(k+1)(k+2)/2$ and one can easily show that $\Phi_3^{(k)}$ is P_k-solvable. This kind of elements is very useful in the connection with p- and hp-versions of finite element method [21]. In this book, k plays the same role as p in these versions.

Now let us consider two finite elements whose degrees of freedom besides values of $p(a)$ include values of partial derivatives at some nodes. We will therefore call them *the Hermitian elements.*

The first of these elements is of degree 3; it is defined by the triplet $(\omega, P_3(\omega), \Phi_4)$, where

$$\Phi_4 = \{p(a_i), \partial_1 p(a_i), \partial_2 p(a_i),\ i = 1, 2, 3;\ p(c_{123})\}.$$

The number of degrees of freedom is 10, which coincides with dimension of the space P_3. The set Φ_4 (like Φ_3) is P_3-solvable, i. e., three values p, $\partial_1 p$, $\partial_2 p$ at three vertices and p at the centre of gravity of the triangle are sufficient for defining polynomial p from P_3 unambiguously. The formula

$$\begin{aligned} p &= \sum_{i=1}^{3}(-2\lambda_i^3 + 3\lambda_i^2 - 7\lambda_1\lambda_2\lambda_3)p(c_{iii}) + 27\lambda_1\lambda_2\lambda_3 p(c_{123}) + \\ &+ \sum_{i\neq j,\, i,j=1}^{3} \lambda_i\lambda_j(2\lambda_i + \lambda_j - 1)\nabla p(c_{iii}) \cdot (c_{jjj} - c_{iii}), \quad p \in P_3, \end{aligned} \tag{2.10}$$

holds [40]. From the above, the form of the basis functions is clearly understood.

The last of the considered elements with triangular mesh is of degree 5. It is defined by the triplet $(\omega, P_5(\omega), \Phi_5)$, where

$$\begin{aligned} \Phi_5 = &\{p(a_i), \partial_1 p(a_i), \partial_2 p(a_i), \partial_{11} p(a_i), \partial_{12} p(a_i), \partial_{22} p(a_i) \quad (i = 1, 2, 3); \\ &\partial_\nu p(b_{12}), \partial_\nu p(b_{13}), \partial_\nu p(b_{23})\}. \end{aligned}$$

This element is often called *the Argyris triangle.* The number of its degrees of freedom is 21, which is in agreement with the number of coefficients of a polynomial of degree 5. This is a major precondition for the set Φ_5 to be P_5-solvable [40]. The form of the basis functions is rather involved and is usually given for a standard triangle.

Note that the last three degrees of freedom in Φ_5 corresponding to normal derivatives at the midpoints of the sides, can be eliminated. For preservation of solvability we decrease the dimension of the space of functions P_5 assuming a cubic behaviour of the normal derivative $\partial_\nu p$ along each of sides of ω. That is, we assume that $P_5'(\omega) = \{p \in P_5(\omega), \partial_\nu p \in P_3$ on each side of $\omega\}$ and $\Phi_5' = \{p(a_i), \partial_k p(a_i), \partial_{kl} p(a_i); k,l = 1,2; i = 1,2,3\}$. Then the triplet $(\omega, P_5'(\omega), \Phi_5')$ is usually called *the Bell triangle.* The set Φ_5' is P_5'-solvable. The basis functions are given for a standard triangle in [134]. The property $P_5' \supset P_4$ holds and plays an important role [40]. The approximation order of this element is less than that of the Argyris triangle. In practice, however, the smoothness properties of the solution which ensure maximal accuracy orders are, as a rule, unachievable for the both elements. Both yield nearly equal accuracy which is conditioned by the smoothness properties of the solution only. As a result, these rather complex elements are used to solve fourth-order equations when not only the basis functions but also their first derivatives are required to be continuous. Only these of all the elements enumerated in this section ensure the last property.

The following result is of interest [199]. In order that piecewise-polynomial function belongs to class C^q on an arbitrary triangulation, nodal parameters should consist of all the derivatives at the nodes up to order $2q$ inclusive. In the n-dimensional case, such polynomials are of degree $2^n q + 1$. In the two-dimensional case, this degree equals 5 for class C^1. Thus, the degree $k = 5$ cannot be reduced for admissible polynomials for these elements. So, even in principle, there are no more simple polynomials satisfying the condition for the first derivative to be continuous.

To find a way out, one can use two other kinds of the elements — the Clough-Tocher piecewise-polynomial elements or the Zienkiewicz rational-fractional singular elements [40]. But these both do not satisfy so-called nesting property (which will be introduced below) and would therefore greatly complicate multigrid algorithms. That is why we do not consider them.

2.2.2 Elements with a rectangular mesh

Let $a_{i,j}$ $(i,j = 0,1)$ be the vertices of a rectangle $\omega \subset \mathbf{R}^2$ with the sides parallel to the axis (Fig. 2.2, $k = 1$).

Let us introduce the Lagrange rectangular elements similar to the triangular ones. When $k = 1$, a bilinear finite element is characterized by the triplet $(\omega, Q_1(\omega), \Phi_6)$, where $\Phi_6 = \{p(a_{ij}), i,j = 0,1\}$. Four coefficients of the bilinear polynomial $p = d_{00} + d_{10}x_1 + d_{01}x_2 + d_{11}x_1x_2$ are uniquely defined by the values $p(a_{ij})$. Therefore the set Φ_6 is Q_1-solvable [40]. Let us describe the basis functions for the unit square $\omega = [0,1]^2$ only. Assume that

$$p_{ij}^1(x) = (-1)^{i+j}(1 - x_1 - i)(1 - x_2 - j).$$

Then

$$p = \sum_{i,j=0}^{1} p(a_{ij}) p_{ij}^1, \quad p \in Q_1(\omega). \tag{2.11}$$

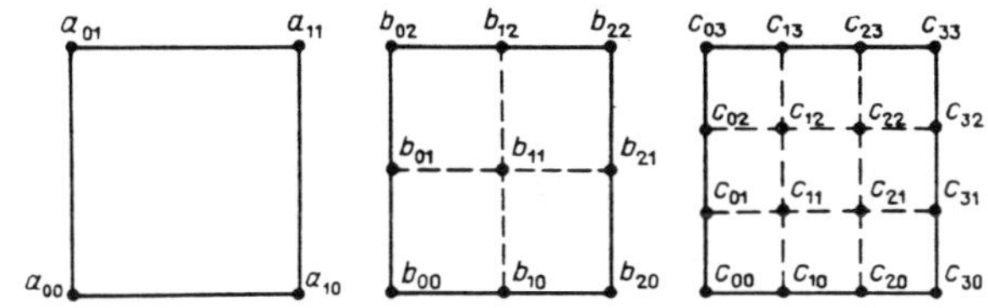

Figure 2.2: Nodes of rectangular Lagrangian elements of degree $k = 1, 2, 3$

To define an element of degree 2, we relabel the vertices of the rectangle $a_{ij} = b_{2i,2j}$ and introduce center and midpoints of the sides (see Fig. 2.2, $k = 2$):

$$b_{1j} = (b_{0j} + b_{2j})/2, \qquad b_{i1} = (b_{i0} + b_{i2})/2.$$

Now the Lagrange element of degree 2 on the rectangle ω is defined by the triplet $(\omega, Q_2(\omega), \Phi_7)$, where $\Phi_7 = \{p(b_{ij}), i, j = 0, 1, 2\}$. The number of degrees of freedom is 9; it agrees with the number of coefficients of a biquadratic polynomial. The set Φ_7 is, therefore, Q_2-solvable.

Finally, we introduce some additional points on the sides and inside the rectangle (see Fig. 2.2, $k = 3$):

$$\begin{aligned} c_{3i,3j} &= a_{ij}, \qquad i, j = 0, 1; \\ c_{sl} &= (1 - s/3)c_{0l} + (s/3)c_{3l}, \\ c_{sl} &= (1 - l/3)c_{s0} + (l/3)c_{s3}, \qquad s, l = 0, \dots, 3. \end{aligned}$$

Now the Lagrange rectangular element of degree $k = 3$ is defined by the triplet $(\omega, Q_3(\omega), \Phi_8)$, where $\Phi_8 = \{p(c_{ij}), i, j = 0, \dots, 3\}$. The number of degrees of freedom is 16, which coincides with the number of coefficients of a bicubic polynomial from $Q_3(\omega)$. The set Φ_8 is therefore Q_3-solvable.

We can carry out such a construction for arbitrary k. Let us introduce the nodes

$$\begin{aligned} d_{ki,kj} &= a_{ij}, \qquad i, j = 0, 1; \\ d_{sl} &= (1 - s/k)d_{0l} + (s/k)d_{kl}, \\ d_{sl} &= (1 - l/k)d_{s0} + (l/k)d_{sk}, \qquad s, l = 0, \dots, k, \end{aligned}$$

and the set of functionals

$$\Phi_8^{(k)} = \{p(d_{ij}), i, j = 0, \dots, k\}.$$

Then *the Lagrange rectangular element of* arbitrary *degree* k is defined by the triplet $(\omega, Q_k(\omega), \Phi_8^{(k)})$. The number of degrees of freedom and the dimension of $Q_k(\omega)$ are equal to $(k+1)^2$. One can easily show that $\Phi_8^{(k)}$ is Q_k-solvable.

Note that the values of function at the interior nodes of ω can be eliminated from degrees of freedom in the cases $k = 2, 3$. We have then a class of *the serendipity* or *incomplete Lagrange elements.*

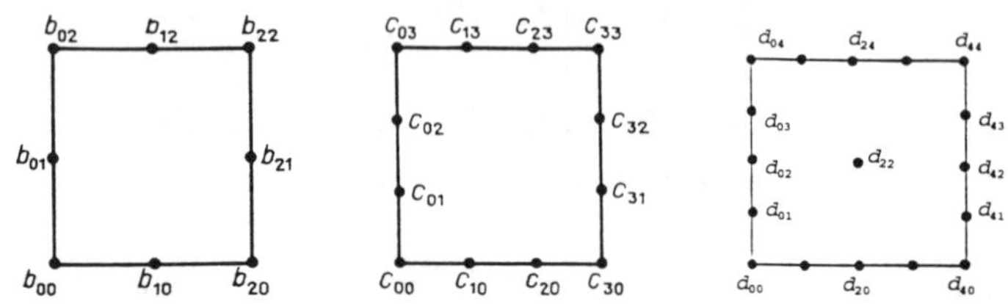

Figure 2.3: Nodes of serendipity elements of degree $k = 2, 3, 4$

For example, let us eliminate the point b_{11} (Fig. 2.3) from the nodes of the Lagrange element of degree 2 and introduce another class of polynomials Q_2' by discarding $x_1^2x_2^2$ in Q_2. The dimension of Q_2' equals 8 and agrees with the rest of the nodes. As a result, the set of functionals $\Phi_7' = \{p(b_{ij}), i, j = 0, 1, 2; (i, j) \neq (1, 1)\}$ is Q_2'-solvable. The basis of this element denoted below by (ω, Q_2', Φ_7') is given in [40]. Note that $Q_2' \supset P_2$ and so the possibility for approximation remains as before. This will be shown below.

We can exclude 4 interior nodes c_{ij} with $i, j = 1, 2$ from the Lagrange element of degree 3 (Fig. 2.3). As an admissible function set, let us take the space of polynomials Q_3' obtained by discarding the terms like $x_1^ix_2^j, (i, j) \in \{2, 3\}^2$ in Q_3. Introduce the functional set $\Phi_8' = \{p(c_{ij}), (i, j) \in \{0, 1, 2, 3\}^2 \setminus \{1, 2\}^2\}$. The number of degrees of freedom is 12 and equals the dimension of space Q_3'. The set Φ_8' is therefore Q_3'-solvable. The basis functions are also given in [40]. Note that $Q_3' \supset P_3$. Due to this fact, a decrease in the number of the nodes and degrees of freedom does not influence order of approximation.

So, both serendipity elements have the same order of approximation as the corresponding initial Lagrange elements, but the number of degrees of freedom is less. The dimension of a discrete algebraic problem for them is therefore also less, which is certainly their advantage in applications.

In the case $k \geq 4$, we cannot eliminate all interior nodes without a violation of the solvability. For $k \geq 4$ we take *the two-dimensional serendipity polinomial space*

$$Q_k' = P_k \oplus \{x_1^kx_2, x_1x_2^k\}.$$

The dimension of Q_k' equals $(k^2 + 3k + 6)/2$. The choice of the set of functionals is ambiguous. First of all, we have to retain $4k$ nodes on the boundary of mesh to control the continuity between elements as in $\Phi_8^{(k)}$. The rest of degrees of freedom is taken, for example, in one central node b_{11} (see Fig. 2.3, $k = 4$):

$$\Phi'^{(k)}_8 = \{p(d_{ij}),\ (i, j) \in (\{0, k\}\times\{0, \ldots, k\})\cup(\{0, \ldots, k\}\times\{0, k\}); \partial^\alpha p(b_{11}), |\alpha| \leq k-4\}.$$

This set has exactly $(k^2 + 3k + 6)/2$ degrees of freedom and is Q_k'-solvable. As a result, *the rectangular serendipity element of* arbitrary *degree* $k \geq 4$ is defined by the triplet $(\omega, Q'_k(\omega), \Phi'^{(k)}_8)$. Since $Q'_k \supset P_k$, this kind of elements has good approximation properties and is very useful in *hp*-version.

The rectangular Hermitian element, we will now consider, is one among many but often used. Sometimes it is called *the Bogner-Fox-Schmit rectangle* [40]. It is characterized by the triplet $(\omega, Q_3(\omega), \Phi_9)$, where

$$\Phi_9 = \{p(a_{ij}), \partial_1 p(a_{ij}), \partial_2 p(a_{ij}), \partial_{12} p(a_{ij}); i,j = 0,1\}.$$

The number of degrees of freedom is 16 again, which coincides with the dimension of Q_3. Hence, the set Φ_9 is Q_3-solvable. To define the basis functions on the unit square $\omega = [0,1]^2$, we introduce the following auxiliary functions

$$\begin{aligned} \varphi_0(t) &= 1 - 3t^2 + 2t^3, \qquad \varphi_1(t) = \varphi_0(1-t), \\ \psi_0(t) &= t^2 - t^3, \qquad \psi_1(t) = \psi_0(1-t). \end{aligned}$$

For $i, j = 0, 1$ we assume that

$$\begin{aligned} p_{ij}^{(0)}(x) &= \varphi_i(x_1)\varphi_j(x_2), \qquad p_{ij}^{(1)}(x) = \psi_i(x_1)\varphi_j(x_2), \\ p_{ij}^{(2)}(x) &= \varphi_i(x_1)\psi_j(x_2), \qquad p_{ij}^{(3)}(x) = \psi_i(x_1)\psi_j(x_2). \end{aligned}$$

Now

$$\begin{aligned} p = & \sum_{i,j=0}^{1} (p(a_{ij})p_{ij}^{(0)} + \partial_1 p(a_{ij})p_{ij}^{(1)} + \\ & + \partial_2 p(a_{ij})p_{ij}^{(2)} + \partial_{12} p(a_{ij})p_{ij}^{(3)}), \quad p \in Q_3(\omega). \end{aligned} \tag{2.12}$$

This is the only element among the above ones on rectangles which ensures not only the continuity of basis functions but also the continuity of their first derivatives. This makes it possible to apply it to solve fourth-order equations by conforming methods.

All the elements in this section are convenient to solve problems in the regions composed of rectangles or problems with natural boundary-value conditions. We will return to both of them later.

2.3 Three-dimensional finite elements

A tetrahedron or rectangular parallelepiped is the most widespread shape of the cell of the finite element in the three-dimensional case. The tetrahedron is used because a three-dimensional body with piecewise smooth surface is either a polyhedron itself or it can be approximated by polyhedra with a rather high order of accuracy. The polyhedron, in turn, can always be divided into a finite number of tetrahedra.

When solving the problems in the regions composed completely or partially of parallelepipeds, it is convenient to apply elements whose cells are shaped as a parallelepiped. The point is that one needs 5 or 6 times more tetrahedra than parallelepipeds of the same size for filling a volume, as we see in Fig. 2.4, 2.5. This leads to a larger number of finite elements applied to a discrete problem and correspondingly to increase in computation time and memory volume.

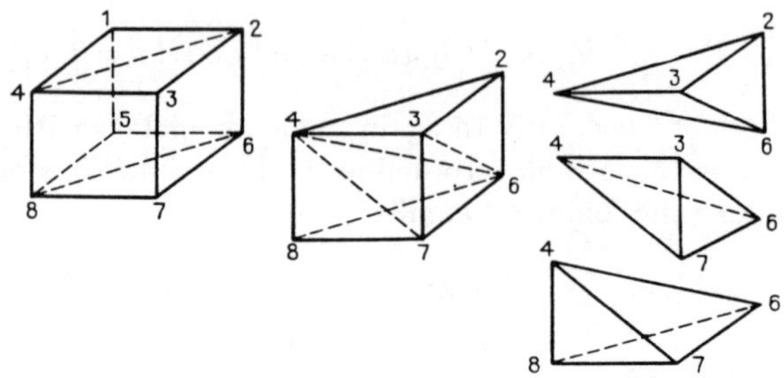

Figure 2.4: The division of rectangular parallelepiped into 6 tetrahedra

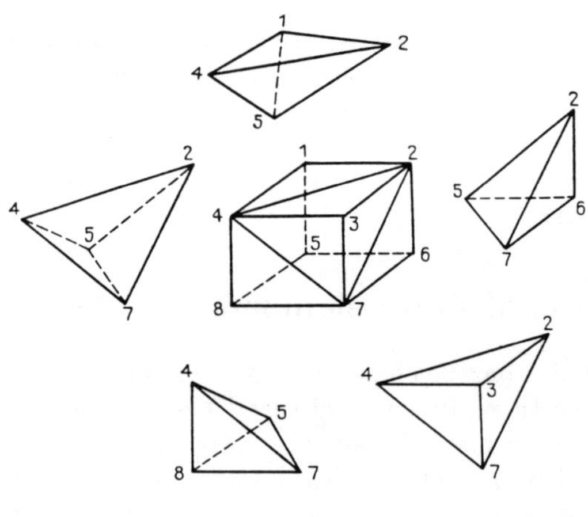

Figure 2.5: The division of rectangular parallelepiped into 5 tetrahedra

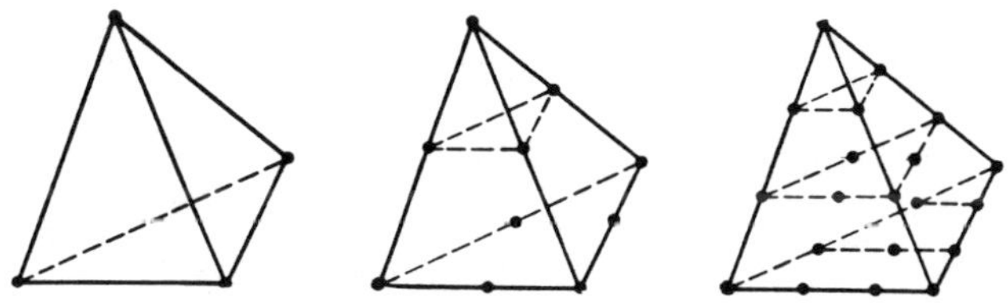

Figure 2.6: Nodes of the tetrahedral Lagrange elements of degrees $k = 1, 2, 3$

2.3.1 Elements with a tetrahedral cell

Let a_1, a_2, a_3, a_4 be the vertices of a non-singular tetrahedron $\omega \subset \mathbf{R}^3$ with coordinates $a = (a_{i1}, a_{i2}, a_{i3})$ (Fig. 2.6, $k = 1$).

Initially we will consider *the Lagrange element of degree* 1. It is characterized by the triplet $(\omega, P_1(\omega), \Phi_{10})$, where $P_1(\omega)$ is a set of linear polynomials in three arguments x_1, x_2, x_3 with a domain of definition ω; the set Φ_{10} consists of four functionals $\varphi_i : P_1(\omega) \to \mathbf{R}$ which associate polynomial p from $P_1(\omega)$ to its value at the point a_i, i. e., $\Phi_{10} = \{p(a_i), i = 1, 2, 3, 4\}$.

Since a linear polynomial in $\mathbf{R}^3$ is completely defined by four values of $p(a_i)$ at points a_i in general position, the set Φ_{10} is P_1-solvable.

Barycentric coordinates $\lambda_j = \lambda_j(x)$ $(j = 1, 2, 3, 4)$ are introduced into the tetrahedron as solution of the linear system of equations

$$\sum_{j=1}^{4} a_{ij}\lambda_j = x_i, \quad i = 1, 2, 3,$$

$$\sum_{j=1}^{4} \lambda_j = 1. \tag{2.13}$$

The matrix determinant of this system is proportional to the volume of the nonsingular tetrahedron ω and so is not zero. As a result, system (2.13) has a unique solution at any $x \in \mathbf{R}^3$. It is easy to verify that it obeys the condition

$$\lambda_i(a_j) = \delta_{ij}, \quad i, j = 1, 2, 3, 4.$$

λ_i are therefore the basis functions of this finite element:

$$p - \sum_{i=1}^{4} p(a_i)\lambda_i, \quad p \in P_1. \tag{2.14}$$

To define *the Lagrange element of degree* 2, we introduce midpoints of edges and relabel vertices of the tetrahedron ω (see Fig. 2.6, $k = 2$):

$$b_{ij} = (a_i + a_j), \quad 1 \leq i \leq j \leq 4. \tag{2.15}$$

Now the element of degree 2 is given by the triplet $(\omega, P_2(\omega), \Phi_{11})$, where $\Phi_{11} = \{p(b_{ij}),\ 1 \leq i \leq j \leq 4\}$. The number of degrees of freedom as well as the dimension of space $P_2(\omega)$ are equal to 10. The set Φ_{11} is therefore P_2-solvable [40]. The basis functions are expressed in terms of barycentric coordinates so that the following holds:

$$p = \sum_{i=1}^{4} \lambda_i(2\lambda_i - 1)p(b_{ii}) + \sum_{1\le i<j\le 4} 4\lambda_i\lambda_j p(b_{ij}), \quad p \in P_2. \tag{2.16}$$

Then we introduce some additional points on the edges and on centres of the sides of ω (see Fig. 2.6, $k = 3$):

$$c_{ijk} = (a_i + a_j + a_k)/3, \quad i,j,k = 1,2,3,4. \tag{2.17}$$

Now *the Lagrange element of degree* 3 on the tetrahedron ω is defined by the triplet $(\omega, P_3(\omega), \Phi_{12})$, where

$$\Phi_{12} = \{p(c_{ijk}), 1 \le i \le j \le k \le 4\}.$$

The total number of degrees of freedom is 20; the polynomial from P_3 has the same number of coefficients. As a result, the set Φ_{12} is P_3-solvable [40]. The basis functions of this element can be expressed in terms of barycentric coordinates:

$$\begin{aligned} p &= \sum_{i=1}^{4} \frac{1}{2}\lambda_i(3\lambda_i - 1)(3\lambda_i - 2)p(c_{iii}) + \sum_{i\ne j;\, i,j=1}^{4} \frac{9}{2}\lambda_i\lambda_j(3\lambda_i - 1)p(c_{iij}) + \\ &+ \sum_{1\le i<j<k\le 4} 27\lambda_i\lambda_j\lambda_k p(c_{ijk}), \qquad p \in P_3. \end{aligned} \tag{2.18}$$

We may construct such kind of element for an arbitrary degree k. For this purpose we introduce nodes

$$d_{i_1\dots i_k} = (a_{i_1} + \ldots + a_{i_k})/k, \qquad i_1, \ldots, i_k = 1,2,3,4,$$

and the set of functionals

$$\Phi_{12}^{(k)} = \{p(d_{i_1\dots i_k}), 1 \le i_1 \le i_2 \le \ldots \le i_k \le 4\}.$$

Now *the Lagrange element of degree* k is defined by the triplet $(\omega, P_k(\omega), \Phi_{12}^{(k)})$. The number of degrees of freedom and the dimension of $P_k(\omega)$ are equal to $(k+1)(k+2)(k+3)/6$ and one can easily show that $\Phi_{12}^{(k)}$ is P_k-solvable.

As for Hermitian finite elements on the tetrahedron, we will consider only one of degree 3. It has 8 nodes at the vertices and on centres of surfaces of the tetrahedron and is defined by the triplet $(\omega, P_3(\omega), \Phi_{13})$, where $\Phi_{13} = \{p(a_i), \partial_1 p(a_i), \partial_2 p(a_i), \partial_3 p(a_i), i = 1,2,3,4; p(c_{ijk}), 1 \le i < j < k \le 4\}$. It has 20 degrees of freedom as well as the Lagrange element of degree 3. The set Φ_{13} is therefore also P_3-solvable [40]. The basis functions of this element are defined by the following identity:

$$\begin{aligned} p &= \sum_{i=1}^{4}(-2\lambda_i^3 + 3\lambda_i^2 - 7\lambda_i \sum_{1\le j<k\le 4,\, j\ne i,\, k\ne i} \lambda_j\lambda_k)p(a_i) + \\ &+ 27 \sum_{1\le i<j<k\le 4} \lambda_i\lambda_j\lambda_k p(c_{ijk}) + \\ &+ \sum_{i\ne j;\, i,j=1}^{4} \lambda_i\lambda_j(2\lambda_i + \lambda_j - 1)\nabla p(a_i)\cdot(a_j - a_i), \quad p \in P_3. \end{aligned} \tag{2.19}$$

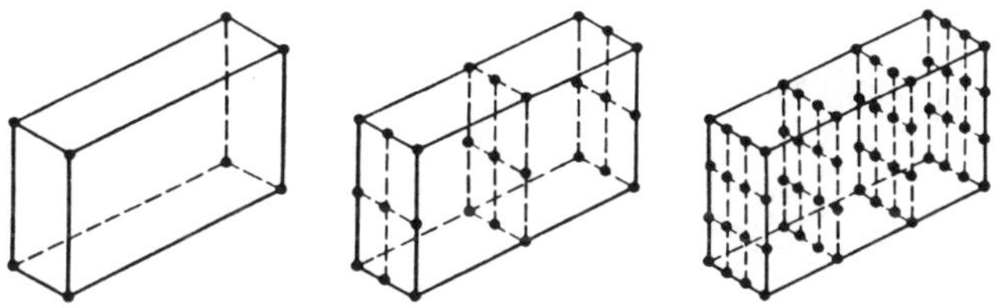

Figure 2.7: Nodes of the Lagrange elements of degrees $k = 1,2,3$ with a cell as a rectangular parallelepiped

2.3.2 Elements with a mesh shaped as a rectangular parallelepiped

For short, a rectangular parallelepiped will be called simply a rectangle where this does not lead to confusion.

Thus, let a_{ijl} $(i,j,l = 0,1)$ be the vertices of a rectangle $\omega \subset \mathbf{R}^3$ with faces parallel to the coordinate planes (Fig. 2.7, $k = 1$).

We first consider *the trilinear Lagrange finite element* characterized by the triplet $(\omega, Q_1(\omega), \Phi_{14})$, where $\Phi_{14} = \{p(a_{ijl}), i,j,l = 0,1\}$. The trilinear polynomial p from Q_1 has eight coefficients which are uniquely defined by values of $p(a_{ijl})$ at eight vertices of the rectangle. Therefore, the set Φ_{14} is Q_1-solvable [40]. For the unit cube $\omega = [0,1]^3$, the basis functions are defined by the equalities

$$p'_{ijl} = (-1)^{i+j+l}(1 - x_1 - i)(1 - x_2 - j)(1 - x_3 - l).$$

Hence

$$p = \sum_{i,j,l=0}^{1} p(a_{ijl})p'_{ijl}, \quad p \in Q_1(\omega). \tag{2.20}$$

To define *the Lagrange element of degree* 2, we relabel the vertices of the rectangle $a_{ijl} = b_{2i,2j,2l}$ and introduce the midpoints (Fig. 2.7, $k = 2$):

$$b_{1jl} = (b_{0jl} + b_{2jl})/2, \quad b_{i1l} = (b_{i0l} + b_{i2l})/2, \quad b_{ij1} = (b_{ij0} + b_{ij2})/2.$$

Now the Lagrange element of degree 2 on the rectangle ω is given by the triplet $(\omega, Q_2(\omega), \Phi_{15})$, where $\Phi_{15} = \{p(b_{ijl}), i,j,l = 0,1,2\}$. The number of degrees of freedom is 27; it coincides with the number of coefficients of a triquadratic polynomial from Q_2. As a result, the set Φ_{15} is Q_2-solvable [40].

To describe *the Lagrange element of degree* 3, we relabel the vertices and introduce some additional points on faces and inside the rectangle ω (Fig. 2.7, $k = 3$):

$$\begin{aligned}
&c_{3i,3j,3l} = a_{ijl}, \quad i,j,l = 0,1;\\
&c_{ijl} = (1 - i/3)c_{0jl} + (i/3)c_{3jl},\\
&c_{ijl} = (1 - j/3)c_{i0l} + (j/3)c_{i3l},\\
&c_{ijl} = (1 - l/3)c_{ij0} + (l/3)c_{ij3}, \quad i,j,l = 0,\dots,3.
\end{aligned}$$

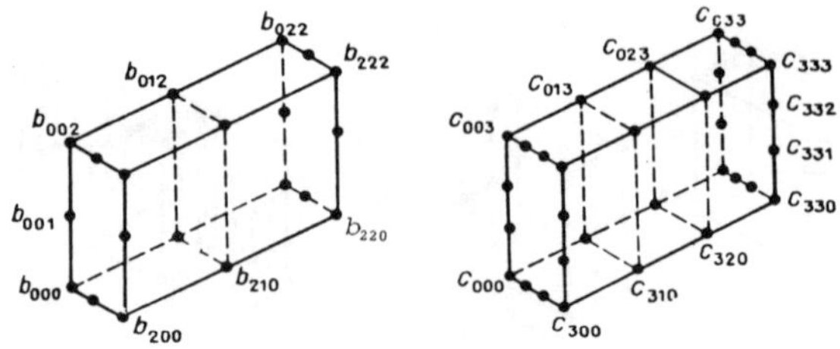

Figure 2.8: Nodes of serendipity elements of degrees $k = 2, 3$ with a cell as a rectangle parallelepiped

Then the Lagrange element for $k = 3$ on the rectangle $\omega \subset \mathbf{R}^3$ is defined by the triplet $(\omega, Q_3(\omega), \Phi_{16})$, where $\Phi_{16} = \{p(c_{ijl}), i, j, l = 0, \ldots, 3\}$. The number of degrees of freedom is 64, and a tricubic polynomial from Q_3 has 64 coefficients. Therefore, the set Φ_{16} is Q_3-solvable [40].

By analogy with the two-dimensional case, one may exclude superfluous degrees of freedom from two last elements and use the values of function at the vertices and on the edges of ω only.

Let us consider, for example, the nodes b_{ijl} of the Lagrange element of degree 2 in Fig. 2.7. Only 20 of these are placed on edges. In the functional set Φ_{15}, we only retain the values $p(b_{ijl})$ at these points (Fig. 2.8). Denote the functional set obtained by Φ'_{15} and restrict the class of polynomials Q_2. To this end, we introduce *the three-dimensional serendipity space of polinomials* Q'_2 which takes the form $P_1 Q_1$, i. e., $Q'_2 = \{pq; p \in P_1, q \in Q_1\}$. Then the dimension of Q'_2 is equal to 20, and the set Φ'_{15} is Q'_2-solvable. The basis of this serendipity element is given in [143]. Note that $Q'_2 \supset P_2$ and, hence, the approximating possibilities of this element is not worse than those of the initial Lagrange element with 27 degrees of freedom.

The Lagrange element of degree 3 has 32 nodes c_{ijl} (Fig. 2.8) at its vertices and on its edges. In Φ_{16}, we only leave the functionals in which the values of function p are taken at one of these nodes. Denote such functional set by Φ'_{16}. As an admissible function set, we take *the three-dimensional serendipity space of polynomials* Q'_3 of the form $q \sum_{i=1}^{3} p_i$, where $q \in Q_1$, and p_i is a quadratic polynomial in variable x_i. The dimension of Q'_3 equals 32 as well, which results in the Q'_3-solvability of the set Φ'_{16}. The basis of this serendipity element $(\omega, Q'_3(\omega), \Phi'_{16})$ is given in [142]. Note that $Q'_3 \supset P_3$ and so the approximating possibilities of this element compared with the original Lagrange element of degree 3 have not become poorer, while the number of degrees of freedom has been cut by half.

Thus the both serendipity elements have the same approximation order as the original Lagrange elements of the corresponding degree but their number of degrees of freedom is less. Therefore, serendipity incomplete elements are more preferable.

One can continue this sequence of serendipity elements for an arbitrary degree $k \geq 4$ by analogy with the two-dimensional case. But for the preservation of solvability, one has to introduce 6 multiple nodes in the centres of faces and, starting with $k = 6$, a multiple node in the centre of the cell besides simple nodes on edges.

2.4 Affine and isoparametric transformations

2.4.1 Curvilinear elements

An application of the above cited finite elements of degree $k > 1$ for the two-dimensional regions with a curvilinear boundary leads to a no considerable increase in the accuracy versus linear elements. The point is that an approximation of the boundary by broken straight lines gives the main contribution into the error of approximate solution in these cases, and this contribution remains unchanged at different k.

We come therefore to the problem of boundary approximation by more intricate broken curves or, what is the same, domain approximation by more intricate cells, in particular by curvilinear ones. But standard configurations are more suitable to discuss basis functions and quadrature formulae. These are usually the standard simplices and the rectangles $[0,1]^n$.

As a result, a need arises to transform an element cell. Let us describe these transformations. Let (ω, P, Φ) be some master finite element in variables $y \in \mathbf{R}^n$ with one of standard cells ω. Give the transformation of coordinates $F : y \in \omega \to \mathbf{R}^n$. Then ω is transformed to the cell $\tilde{\omega} = \{F(y), y \in \omega\}$. By selecting F, one can obtain a rather intricate shape of ω so that to approximate the requiered portion of the boundary well.

Note that evaluating an integral like $\int_{\tilde{\omega}} g(x)dx$, necessary to assemble a discrete system of the finite elements method, can be reduced to integration with respect to y-coordinates by means of the transformation F:

$$\int_{\tilde{\omega}} g(x)dx = \int_{\omega} g(F(y))Jdy, \tag{2.21}$$

where $J = \partial F/\partial y$ is the Jacobian of transformation F. Quadrature formulae like

$$\int_{\omega} g_1(y)dy \approx \sum_{i=1}^{L} g_1(y_i)\alpha_i, \tag{2.22}$$

with the nodes $y_i \in \omega$ and the weights α_i, are most often used for approximate evaluating the integrals on the right-hand side of (2.21). We have to know therefore certain values of F and its derivatives at y_i rather than the transformation F on the whole. Solving the discrete system of the finite elements method, we get an approximate solution $v^h(y)$ on ω. To restore the solution $u^h(x)$ on the initial subdomain $\tilde{\omega}$, we need (from theoretical point of view) to know the inverse operator $F^{-1} : \tilde{\omega} \to \omega$, since $u^h(x) = v^h(F^{-1}(x))$. In practice, however, there is a need for the function $u^h(x)$ at element nodes only. For quasi-linear problems, we need also the values of function v^n in the nodes of quadrature (2.22) during an iteration with respect to a non-linearity. That is to say, inverse transformation F^{-1} is not needed in most cases in practice.

Thus the curvilinear element will here be understood as a quadruple $F(\omega, P, \Phi)$. On the other hand, for theoretical and descriptive purposes, it is sometimes useful to represent it as the usual triplet $(\tilde{\omega}, \tilde{P}, \tilde{\Phi})$. Indeed, F converts $p(y) \in P$ into a function $\tilde{p}(x) = p(F^{-1}(x))$, and as a result we have the new space $\tilde{P} = \{\tilde{p}(x) = p(F^{-1}(x)), p \in P\}$. Similarly, functionals $\varphi_i(p) \in \Phi$ go over to $\tilde{\varphi}_i(\tilde{p}) = \varphi_i(\tilde{p} \circ F)$ giving the set $\tilde{\Phi} = \{\tilde{\varphi}_i(\tilde{p}), i = 1, \dots, N\}$. Thus, we in fact have the finite element $(\tilde{\omega}, \tilde{P}, \tilde{\Phi})$ with the space $\tilde{P}$ and the set of functionals $\tilde{\Phi}$ of rather complex structure.

Let us consider some practical aspect of constructing the transformation F. The most widely used kind of transformation is the affine one, when $F(y) = (F_1(y), \dots, F_n(y))$ and

$$F_i(y) = a_i \cdot y + b_i, \tag{2.23}$$

where $a_i = (a_{i1}, \dots, a_{in})$ and b_i are known constants.

A transformation like this is often used in theory and practice, since it allows to reduce different investigations and computer versions for various triangles, tetrahedra, parallelograms and parallelepipeds to one of the standard configurations. That is the reason why the basis functions for quadrangles and hexahedra were only given for a unit square and cube. However, it is impossible to convert by means of such a transformation, for example, a square to an arbitrary convex quadrangle. For this purpose, we must apply a more complex transformation F.

One of the successful techniques is to construct F by means of the same basis functions $p_i \in P$ which are used to describe an initial finite element. Such a transformation, *an isoparametric* one, has two virtues. From theoretical and algorithmic points of view, it remains within the scope of the material used and applies the constructed algorithms of interpolation for the initial element. From the standpoint of computation, polynomials p_i are analytically differentiable, simply to compute, and, as we can see from (2.21), produce no additional features in integrals and quadrature formulae.

Let us consider the case of the Lagrange finite elements where the main idea is stated most simply. Thus, let (ω, P, Φ) be an initial finite element in which functionals $\varphi_i \in \Phi$ can take the form

$$\varphi_i(p) = p(a_i), \quad i = 1, \dots, N, \tag{2.24}$$

where a_i are the nodes of the element. We look for a transformation F such that $F_i \in P$ and nodes $a_i \in \omega$ transform to the given nodes $b_i \in \tilde{\omega}$. Such transformation exists and is unique for P-solvable set Φ; by means of basis functions p_i, it is given by the relation

$$F(y) = \sum_{j=1}^{N} p_j(y) b_j. \tag{2.25}$$

Indeed, $F(a_i) = b_i$ by virtue of the property $p_j(a_i) = \delta_{ij}$ from (2.24) and (2.2).

If we impose no additional conditions on relative position of the nodes b_i, there is no guarantee that transformation F is reversible. We now consider some examples to study these conditions.

2.4.2 Isoparametric transformations of triangles

For the Courant triangle an isoparametric transformation coincides with an affine one. The initial simplex ω can therefore be converted into simplex $\tilde{\omega}$ only. Let us take simplex ω with vertices a_1, a_2, a_3 and barycentric coordinates λ_i in the notation of subsection 2.2.1. Then the transformation of ω into $\tilde{\omega}$ with vertices d_1, d_2, d_3 is given by

$$F(y) = \sum_{j=1}^{3} \lambda_j(y) d_j, \tag{2.26}$$

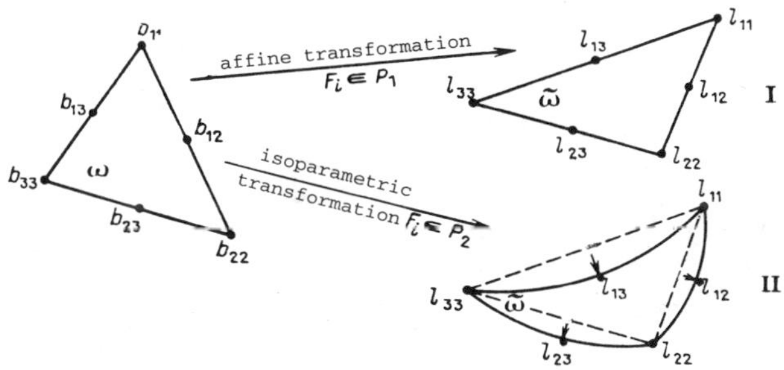

Figure 2.9: Transformations of the triangular Lagrange elements of degree 2

every vertex a_j transforms to d_j respectively. Here, the Jacobian is equal to the ratio of the areas of the triangles, i. e., $\partial F/\partial y = \mathrm{mes}(\tilde{\omega})/\mathrm{mes}(\omega)$. Therefore it does not vanish for any nonsingular simplices ω and $\tilde{\omega}$.

Consider now the Lagrange element of degree 2. Let b_{ij} be the nodes of the initial simplex ω, and l_{ij} the nodes of the mesh $\tilde{\omega}$ $(i,j = 1,2,3)$ corresponding to them (see Fig. 2.9). Then the transformation F is given by

$$F(y) = \sum_{i=1}^{3} \lambda_i(y)(2\lambda_i(y) - 1)l_{ii} + \sum_{1\leq i<j\leq 3} 4\lambda_i(y)\lambda_j(y)l_{ij}. \tag{2.27}$$

In the case of $l_{ij} = (l_{ii} + l_{jj})/2$ $(1 \leq i < j \leq 3)$ (Fig. 2.9, I), the mapping F becomes affine. The condition of non-singularity of the Jacobian is formulated as the non-singularity of simplices ω and $\tilde{\omega}$. In the general case (Fig. 2.9, II) for non-singularity of the Jacobian, the additional geometric condition is formulated in terms of the diameter of $\tilde{\omega}$ [134]:

$$| \, l_{ij} - (l_{ii} + l_{jj})/2 \, | \ll \mathrm{diam}(\tilde{\omega}), \tag{2.28}$$

or asymptotically so as to ensure the required approximation order [40]:

$$| \, l_{ij} - (l_{ii} + l_{jj})/2 \, | = O(\mathrm{diam}^2(\tilde{\omega})), \quad 1 \leq i \leq j \leq 3. \tag{2.29}$$

In the case of such a transformation, the straight side of simplex ω changes to a parabola passing through 3 given points [134]. Thus the most general shape of $\tilde{\omega}$ is a curvilinear triangle whose sides are parabola parts with 3 nodes on them satisfying the condition (2.28) or (2.29).

To ensure these conditions in practical problems, one can act, for example, as follows. Assume that we have to approximate the region of Fig. 2.9, II, where boundary arcs are curves parts from class C^2. Draw a chord joining the ends of arc l_{ii}, l_{jj} and erect a perpendicular at point $(l_{ii} + l_{jj})/2$. Denote the crossing point of the perpendicular and the arc by l_{ij}. As a result, when the diameter of ω is small, the condition (2.29) is satisfyed. If besides the arc is a curve part from class C^3, it will be approximated by the parabola through these three nodes with accuracy $O(\mathrm{diam}^3\tilde{\omega})$.

Finally, let c_{ijk} be the nodes of the Lagrange element of degree 3 on the initial simplex ω, and f_{ijk} the corresponding nodes of an isoparametric element with the cell

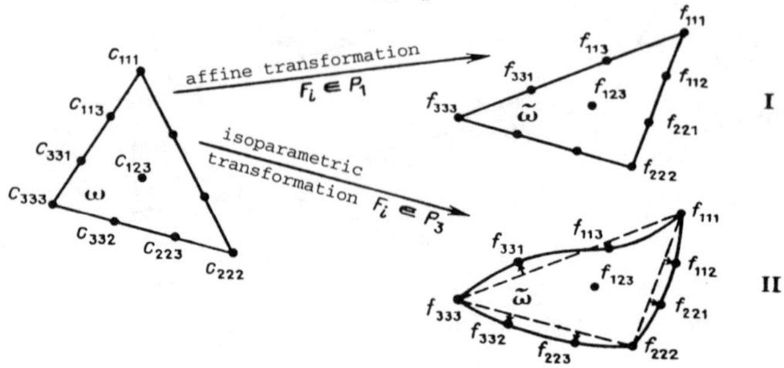

Figure 2.10: Transformation of the triangular Lagrange elements of degree 3

$\tilde{\omega}$ $(i, j, k = 1, 2, 3)$ (see Fig. 2.10). Then the transformation F is given by

$$F(y) = \sum_{i=1}^{3} \frac{1}{2}\lambda_i(y)(3\lambda_i(y) - 1)(3\lambda_i(y) - 2)f_{iii} +$$
$$+ \sum_{i\neq j;\, i,j=1}^{3} \frac{9}{2}\lambda_i(y)\lambda_j(y)(3\lambda_i(y) - 1)f_{iij} + 27\lambda_1(y)\lambda_2(y)\lambda_3(y)f_{123}. \qquad (2.30)$$

In the case $f_{ijk} = (f_{iii} + f_{jjj} + f_{kkk})/3$, $i, j, k = 1, 2, 3$ (Fig. 2.10, I), the mapping F becomes affine. The Jacobian $\partial F/\partial y = \mathrm{mes}(\omega)/\mathrm{mes}(\tilde{\omega})$ is non-singular together with the simplices ω and $\tilde{\omega}$. In the general case (Fig. 2.10, II) for non-singularity of the Jacobian, an additional geometric condition is formulated by analogy with (2.28):

$$\begin{aligned} &| f_{iij} - (2f_{iii} + f_{jjj})/3 | \ll \mathrm{diam}\, \tilde{\omega}, \quad i \neq j, \quad i, j = 1, 2, 3, \\ &| f_{123} - (f_{111} + f_{222} + f_{333})/3 | \ll \mathrm{diam}\, \tilde{\omega}. \end{aligned} \qquad (2.31)$$

In the case of such a transformation F, the straight side of ω changes to a cubic curve which passes through 4 given points [134]. Hence, the most general shape of the mesh $\tilde{\omega}$ is a curvilinear triangle whose sides are cubic curves.

To ensure the required approximation order, it is necessary that along with (2.31) some other asymptotic equalities (which are not obvious) are satisfyed [40]. Instead of discussing them, we show the construction that ensures their fulfilment. Let us assume that the region of Fig. 2.10, II is to be approximated and its boundary arcs are curves parts of class C^4. Draw a chord $f_{iii}, f_{jjj}, i \neq j$ and raise perpendiculars at points $(2f_{iii} + f_{jjj})$ and $(2f_{jjj} + f_{iii})$. Denote crossing points of the perpendiculars and the arc f_{iii}, f_{jjj} by f_{iij} and f_{jji} respectively. As a result, the cubic curve through 4 nodes $f_{iii}, f_{iij}, f_{jji}, f_{jjj}$ approximates the initial arc with accuracy $O(\mathrm{diam}^4\, \tilde{\omega})$. As soon as all the boundary nodes are constructed, the central node is determined by the rule

$$f_{123} = \frac{1}{6} \sum_{i,j=1;\, i\neq j}^{3} f_{iij}.$$

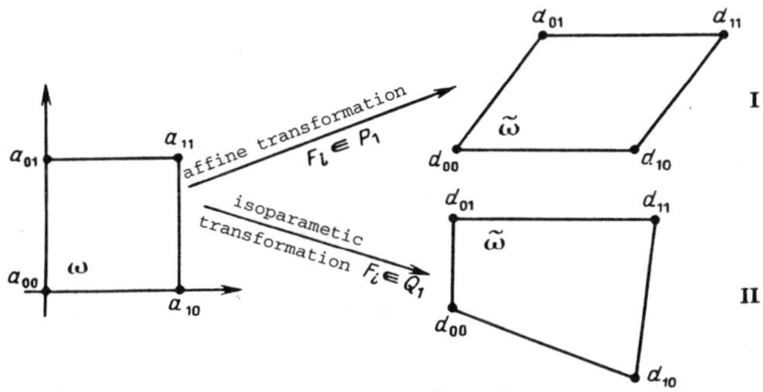

Figure 2.11: Transformation of a square cell of the Lagrange element of degree 1

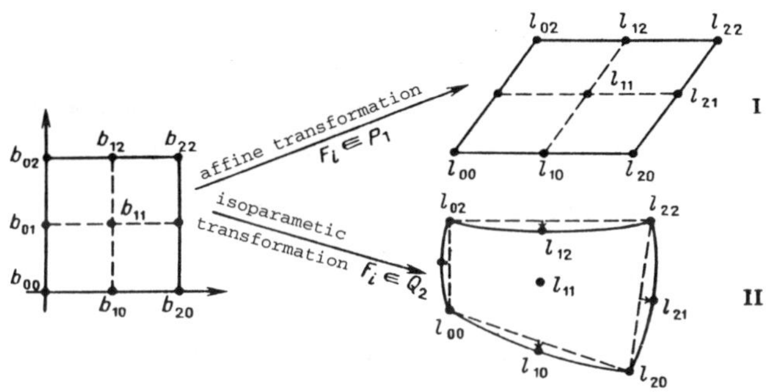

Figure 2.12: Transformation of a square cell of the Lagrange element of degree 2

2.4.3 Isoparametric transformation of a square

Consider a unit square ω with vertices a_{ij} $(i, j = 0, 1)$ (Fig. 2.11). The affine transformation yields a parallelogram $\tilde{\omega}$ in the most general case and can be determined by choosing the three vertices a_{ij}, their images, and using the formulae like (2.26). The Jacobian of such transformation equals $\text{mes}(\tilde{\omega})/\text{mes}(\omega)$ and is non-singular together with ω and $\tilde{\omega}$.

Take now a bilinear (which is isoparametric when $k = 1$) conversion of ω to $\tilde{\omega}$ with vertex images d_{ij} $(i, j = 0, 1)$ (Fig. 2.11, II). Then, in the notations of subsection 2.2.2, the transformation $F : \omega \to \tilde{\omega}$ is given by

$$F(y) = \sum_{i,j=0}^{1} p_{ij}^{1}(y) d_{ij}. \tag{2.32}$$

Broadly speaking, it is non-linear, but changes straight sides of ω to straight lines again. The most general shape of mesh $\tilde{\omega}$ is therefore an arbitrary quadrangle with straight sides. For non-singular ω, $\tilde{\omega}$, the Jacobian is a bilinear function and does not vanish if the quadrangle $\tilde{\omega}$ is convex [115]. Take now the Lagrange element of degree 2. Let b_{ij} be the nodes of an initial square $\tilde{\omega}$ and l_{ij} the corresponding mesh nodes of

$\tilde{\omega}$ $(i,j=0,1,2)$ (Fig. 2.12). Then the transformation $F:\omega\to\tilde{\omega}$ is given by

$$F(y)=\sum_{i,j=0}^{2} p_{ij}^{2}(y)l_{ij},\quad p_{ij}^{2}\in Q_2. \tag{2.33}$$

In the case of $l_{1j}=(l_{0j}+l_{2j})/2$ and $l_{i1}=(l_{i0}+l_{i2})/2$ when $i,j=0,1,2$, the mapping becomes subparametric i. e., $F_i\in Q_1$. As a result, we have the configuration dash-lined in Fig. 2.12, II. In this case, the condition of non-singularity of the Jacobian is formulated as the non-singularity and convexity of the quadrangle $\tilde{\omega}$.

In the general case for non-singularity of the Jacobian, an additional geometric condition is stated as follows. From given vertices l_{ij} $(i,j=0,2)$, we construct points $\tilde{l}_{1j}=(l_{0j}+l_{2j})/2, \tilde{l}_{i1}=(l_{i0}+l_{i2})/2$ $(i,j=0,1,2)$. The Jacobian $\partial F/\partial y$ is non-singular if the quadrangle with straight sides and vertices l_{ij} $(i,j=0,2)$ is convex and the following condition holds:

$$\mid \tilde{l}_{ij}-l_{ij}\mid \ll \operatorname{diam}\tilde{\omega},\quad (i,j)\in\{0,1,2\}^2\setminus\{0,2\}^2. \tag{2.34}$$

Asymptotically, in order to ensure the required approximation order, the above is replaced by [40]:

$$\mid \tilde{l}_{ij}-l_{ij}\mid = O(\operatorname{diam}^2\tilde{\omega}),\quad (i,j)\in\{0,1,2\}^2\setminus\{0,2\}^2. \tag{2.35}$$

In the case of such transformation, one of the variables x_1,x_2 is fixed on every side of the square ω. Therefore, straight sides transform to parts of parabola. Thus, the most general shape of the mesh $\tilde{\omega}$ is a curvilinear quadrangle with parts of parabolae passing through 3 given nodes.

To ensure validity of condition (2.35) for approximation of a curvilinear boundary, we propose the following. Assume that one needs to approximate the region II of Fig. 2.12 whose boundary arcs are curves of class C^3. Draw a chord to connect arc ends l_{0j} and l_{2j} and erect a perpendicular in the middle of the chord. Denote the crossing point of the perpendicular and the arc l_{0j},l_{2j} by l_{1j}. Points l_{i1} $(i=0,2)$ are constructed similarly. Determine a middle point by the rule $l_{11}=(l_{01}+l_{10}+l_{21}+l_{12})/4$. As a result, if the diameter of $\tilde{\omega}$ is small, the condition (2.35) holds and the parabolae through three given points approximate the initial curves with accuracy $O(\operatorname{diam}^3\tilde{\omega})$.

Similar construction and description holds for the serendipity element of degree 2, where the most general shape of $\tilde{\omega}$ is also a curvilinear quadrangle whose sides are parts of parabolae passing through 3 given nodes.

If we somewhat complicate the description, we obtain an isoparametric construction for complete and serendipity Lagrange element of degree 3. For these in the case of isoparametric transformation, the most general shape of $\tilde{\omega}$ is a curvilinear quadrangle with sides being parts of cubic curves passing through 4 given nodes.

When doing affine and isoparametric transformations of the three-dimensional Lagrange elements, no additional basic difficulties arise and all constructions can readily be extended from the two-dimensional case with a corresponding treatment. For example, an isoparametric transformation of a unit cube for the Lagrange element of degree 1 leads to a hexahedron whose edges remain straight line segments. But faces passing through them are not planar since they are described by bilinear functions.

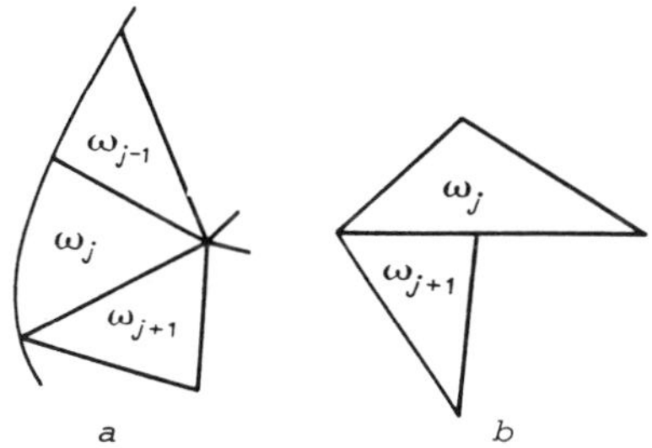

Figure 2.13: Joint of finite-element meshes: a — concordant, b — non-concordant

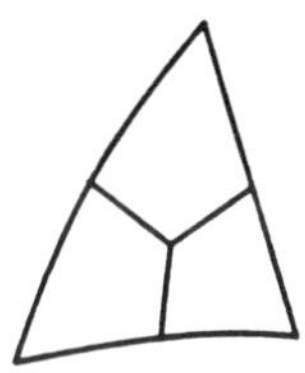

Figure 2.14: Division of a triangle into 3 quadrangles

2.5 Triangulation of two-dimensional domains

Let us consider a subdivision of the two-dimensional domain Ω:

$$\bar{\Omega} = \bigcup_{j=1}^{K^h} \omega_j. \tag{2.36}$$

The subdivision like this is called the *triangulation* of the domain and regarded as *concordant*, if any lateral side of mesh ω_j is a part of boundary or a lateral side of another mesh. Thus, the combination of Fig. 2.13, b is not concordant.

We will consider an elaborate subdivision of domains into triangles (with curvilinear sides possibly) for two reasons. First, for the canonical objects such as domains composed of rectangles and quadrangles (with curvilinear boundaries possibly), subdivision is not, by itself, an algorithmical problem. Actually, finite elements of a quadrangular shape are used just for these domains. Second, a non-singular triangle can easily be divided by segments of medians into 3 quadrangles, as in Fig. 2.14. Therefore, a subdivision into quadrangles can always be obtained from a subdivision into triangles. The opposite, i. e., dividing a quadrangle into two triangles is even more obvious. So subdivisions into triangles or quadrangles are considered to be somewhat equivalent.

There exist a number of ways which can be used for triangulation of domains. What is of special interest to us is automatization of the algorithm on the whole or

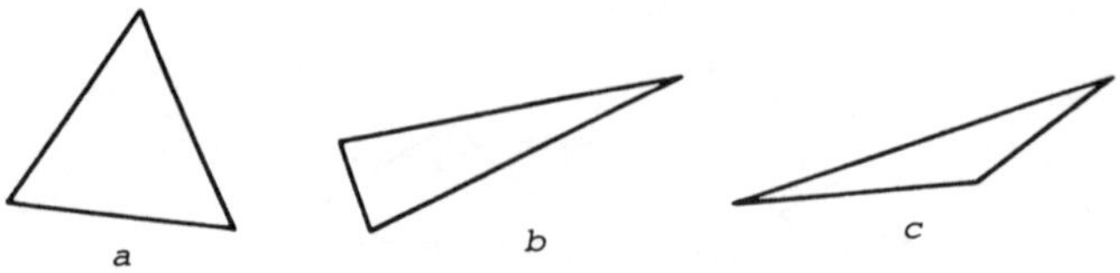

Figure 2.15: Possible forms of triangles: a — successful for both criteria (2.39), (2.40); b — successful for criterion (2.40) and unsuccessful for (2.39); c — unsuccessful for both criteria (2.39), (2.40)

its most labour-consuming parts. In some program packages of the finite-elements method, automatically constructed triangulation is then examined on the display and corrected manually. With the three-dimensional case, it is rather complicated both for package designer and for the user to organize such an examination. Therefore, to pass to three-dimensional problems smoothly, we will try to proceed without manual correction already in the two-dimensional case.

One can distinguish three, among many, independent algorithms often used in combination with one another.

In order to assess the triangulation quality, we recall the following. When approximating by triangular or quadrangular straight-sides finite elements, the estimate of the error includes, as a rule, the value [182], [40]

$$\rho(\omega)/\mathrm{diam}(\omega), \tag{2.37}$$

where $\rho(\omega)$ is the largest of the radii of circles inscribed in ω. Note that the smaller (2.37) is, the worse the approximation error under other conditions fixed. We must therefore construct such grids that (2.37) is as large as possible or, at least,

$$\rho(\omega)/\mathrm{diam}(\omega) \geq c_0 > 0 \tag{2.38}$$

uniformly over all the meshes ω_i ($i = 1, \dots, K^h$). For simplices, the above is equivalent to the following:

$$\min_{j=1,2,3} \sin \theta_{ji} \geq c_0 > 0, \tag{2.39}$$

where θ_{ji} is the j-th angle of simplex ω_i. In some cases [146], [167], the estimates of the approximation error can be proved with substitution of (2.37) for sine of an arbitrary angle in the simplex. If so, it is advisable to take the angle with maximal sine in every simplex ω_i. In this case, the triangulation is characterized by the relation

$$\max_{j=1,2,3} \sin \theta_{ji} \geq c_0 > 0, \quad i = 1, \dots, K^h. \tag{2.40}$$

A distinction between two criteria is that the second admits very acute angles but does not admit the angles which are too close to π (Fig. 2.15).

Note that in practice instead of quantities on the left-hand side of (2.39) and (2.40), the values proportional to them are calculated, namely:

$$2\,\mathrm{mes}\,\omega_i/a_i b_i \tag{2.41}$$

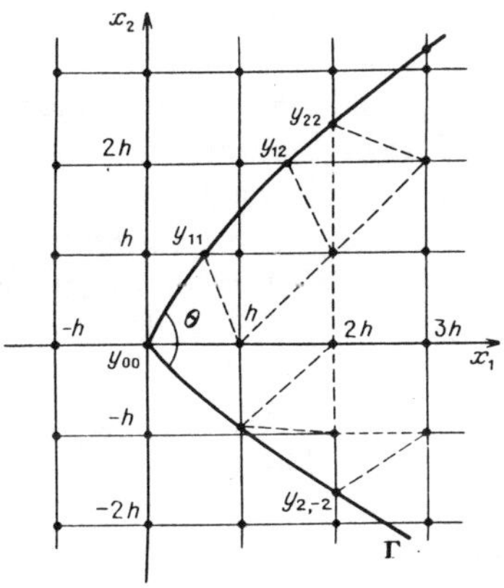

Figure 2.16: The boundary correction of nodes

or

$$2\,\mathrm{mes}\,\omega_i / b_i c_i, \tag{2.42}$$

where $a_i \le b_i \le c_i$ are the lengths of three sides of ω_i, $2\mathrm{mes}\,\omega_i$ is calculated by means of determinants [83].

To characterize a curvilinear triangle, we will use the corresponding quantities of the simplex constructed on the same three vertices (Fig. 2.9, II, 2.10, II).

2.5.1 The boundary-correction algorithm

Let Ω be a bounded domain in $\mathbf{R}^2$. We assume that its boundary Γ belongs to C^2 everywhere except at the origin of coordinates, where it forms the angle $\theta \in (0, 2\pi)$ (Fig. 2.16). The value of the angle included between crossing curves is supposed to equal the value of the angle between tangent lines drawn from the point of intersection.

Fix the parameter h and construct the coordinate grid $R_h^2 = \{x = (ih, jh); i, j = 0, \pm 1, \dots\}$. The point $x \in R_h^2$ is said to be *regular* if four closed straight segments joining it with four nearest points of the grid R_h^2 do not have common points with boundary Γ. Denote by R_h^r the set of all regular nodes of R_h^2 and by R_h^{ir} the set of all other, *irregular*, nodes. In Fig. 2.16, points $(2h, 0), (0, 2h)$ are regular, whereas $(h, 0), (0, 0), (0, h)$ are irregular.

Transform the grid R_h^2, using a certain operator T [125], [124]. If $x \in R_h^r$, then we put $T(x) = x$. Let now $x \in R_h^{ir}$. For it in the directions parallel to the axes, there exists a point $y \in \Gamma$, nearest to x, being at a distance $\le h$ from x. Denote this distance by $\delta(x)$. If $\delta(x) \le h/2$ and point y lies higher or to the right of x, we put $T(x) = y$. Put $T(x) = x$ in all other cases.

Thus, R_h^2 has been transformed into the set $\tilde{R}_h^2 = T(R_h^2)$. Natural enumeration of its points is as follows: $y_{ij} = T(x_{ij})$, where $x_{ij} = (ih, jh)$. For each couple $i, j = 0, \pm 1, \dots$, we will join sequentially points $y_{ij}, y_{i+1,j}, y_{i+1,j+1}, y_{i,j+1}$ and y_{ij}. Here, the arc of Γ connects two neighbouring points if they lie on Γ. But if at least one does not lie on Γ, they are connected by a straight line segment (Fig. 2.16).

As a result, we have a concordant subdivision of $\bar{\Omega}$ into triangles and quadrangles. The subsequent partition of quadrangles is obtained by drawing the diagonals. Note that for the sake of homogeneity, it should be done uniformly, e. g., at angle $\pi/4$ with the axis Ox_1. In irregular quadrangles, we draw the diagonal which leads to better, under the required criterion, values of the angles obtained.

In conclusion note that we intentially choose the vertex of the angle θ of the domain Ω so as to get to a node of the grid. With several angular points, we should observe that they all become nodes of the grid (possibly at the expense of non-uniform change of mesh-sizes).

Of the advantages of this algorithm, the uniformity of most of the set of the triangles obtained should be mentioned. The number of congruent triangles is equal to $O(h^{-2})$ and only $O(h^{-1})$ triangles are non-standard. In a number of cases, e. g., in the case of differential equations with constant coefficients, this facilitates calculations and storage of matrix elements of a discrete problem for regular nodes. When Γ is an interior boundary of triangulation (which holds in the diffraction problems), we will get a concordant subdivision on both sides of it. At last, natural enumeration and topological equivalence to regular grid permit effective application of two-stage methods with simple auxiliary operators [125]. What can be called disadvantage of this method is frequent reference to the boundary equation. If this is none too simple, it consumes much computer time.

2.5.2 The depletion algorithm

Let us consider the same domain Ω as in the preceding section. This time, we first introduce the set of boundary nodes $\Gamma_h = \{y_i \in \Gamma; j = 0, 1, \dots, m; y_m = y_0\}$ numbered consistently clockwise and forming an h-grid for it. *The h-grid of the set $S \subset R^h$* is here understood as a certain points of S being distant not smaller than $h/2$ from each other and such that the distance from any other point of S to these does not exceed h. All the angular points of boundary Γ must be included in Γ_h. Then, we introduce the set of interior nodes $\Omega_h \subset \Omega$ forming together with Γ_h the h-grid for $\bar{\Omega}$. For instance, one may take nodes of the grid $R_h^2 \bigcap \Omega$ which are at a distance not less than $h/2$ from the boundary (Fig. 2.17).

The main idea of this algorithm results from the concordant condition of triangulation: each arc $y_j y_{j+1}$ of boundary Γ is the edge of some triangular cell. In view of this fact, our algorithm is to use step-by-step one simple operation. Let us describe it. From the nodes Γ_h, we choose the y_j whose angle $\angle y_{j-1} y_j y_{j+1}$ is the smallest. In Fig. 2.17, it is the angle with the vertex y_0. Then we take the arc $y_j y_{j+1}$ and find the best of the triangles $\Delta y_j y_{j+1} x$ (from the angle criterion) by exhaustion of points $x \in \Gamma_h \bigcup \Omega_h$ being distant not larger than $3h/2$ from y_j. If $x = y_{j-1}$, we draw straight segment $y_{j-1} y_{j+1}$ cutting off triangle $\Delta y_{j-1} y_j y_{j+1}$ (e. g., $\Delta y_0 y_1 y_{m-1}$ of Fig. 2.17). If $x \neq y_{j-1}$, we draw straight segments $x y_j$, $x y_{j+1}$ and remove $\Delta y_j y_{j+1} x$ from $\bar{\Omega}$ (e. g., $\Delta y_1 y_2 x_{2,1}$ of Fig. 2.17). In both cases, we renumber then the boundary nodes and start this operation again on the reduced domain Ω and with revised set of boundary nodes $\tilde{\Gamma}_h$.

Note that these operations can lead to the multiply connectivity of domain $\bar{\Omega}$, especially at the last stages. So as to diminish computational expenditure, the process

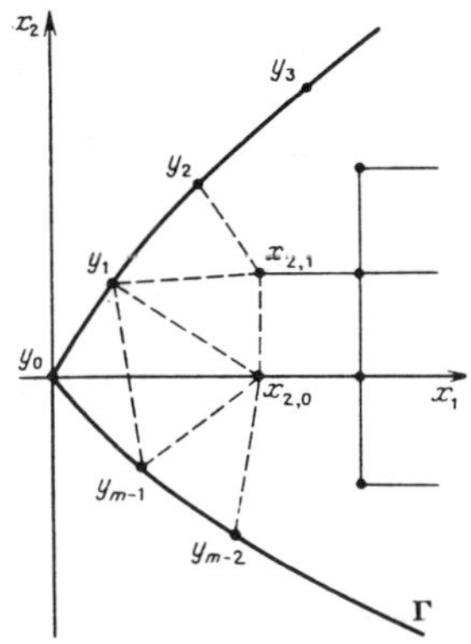

Figure 2.17: Depletion of triangles near the boundary

should be terminated as soon as regular points only remain in $\tilde{\Gamma}_h$. Triangulation ends by drawing the corresponding diagonals.

This method also ensures the uniformity of most of the set of the triangles obtained. Joining together two subdomains with common portion of the boundary (e. g., in the diffraction problems) does not present any difficulties as well. The logical intricacy of the algorithm is somewhat lower, the quality of triangulation is not worse than in the first case. Natural enumeration and topological equivalence to regular grid are missing. The work with the boundary equation is somewhat less laborious.

2.5.3 The breaking algorithm

Assume that some rough triangulation of domain Ω is already available and is required to be done refined. Consider breaking every triangular cell into 4 or 9 cells of smaller size.

When dividing into 4 parts, we connect by straight segments the midpoints of three sides of the triangle, including curvilinear ones (Fig. 2.18, *a*). It is clear that the initial triangle must not be too curved for performance of this operation. Moreover, the midpoints of curvilinear sides are determined approximately, so that, for example, the variant II of Fig. 2.9 with nodes l_{ij} is suitable.

When dividing into 9 parts, each side of the triangle is partitioned into 3 equal parts and each vertex is cut off by the straight segment passing through the nearest points obtained, as in Fig. 2.18, *b*. As a result, we have a hexagon. In it, we find a mean point of its vertices and join this point with these. Here again the above remarks are true about not great curvature of triangle ω and approximately determining the points on curvilinear sides (Fig. 2.10, II).

When dividing triangular cells of a concordant triangulation into equal number of parts, the triangulation obtained is also concordant, the maximal diameter of cells becoming two or three times less, respectively. One may repeat the breaking algorithm many times so as to effect the required fine triangulation. It is generally used after

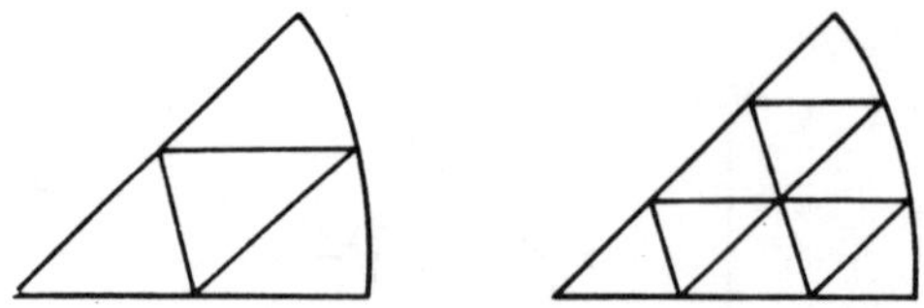

a b

Figure 2.18: The division of triangles into 4 and 9 parts

manually dividing the domain into a small number of triangular cells or after using one of the above algorithms with large mesh-size h.

When the sides of the initial triangle are straight lines, we obtain the triangles similar to the initial one. Therefore the property of uniformity is satisfied here in zones, i. e., in initial triangles with straight sides. It can also be used to reduce the computer time and volume of the memory when computing and storing the discrete system matrix.

This algorithm differs from the above cited ones in simple logical structure and does not need much time to be implemented on a computer. Moreover, breaking when repeated many times produces a sequence of naturally nested triangulations. The nesting property will be one of the main when discussing multigrid algorithms.

2.6 Triangulation of the three-dimensional domains

Let us consider subdividing a three-dimensional domain into the cell set (2.36). We will call it triangulation, as before. And, as before, it will be called concordant, if any lateral face of cell ω_i is a boundary portion or a lateral face of another cell ω_j.

Now consider subdividing the domain into tetrahedra (with curvilinear faces possibly). Subdividing into hexahedra will not be treated for the same reasons as in the two-dimensional case. Namely, in the present algorithms, hexahedra are either an intermediate stage or they can be obtained by cutting tetrahedra into 4 parts using pieces of planes passing through centers of adjacent faces and the middle point of the edge they form.

The most frequently used techniques for dividing the three-dimensional domains are the extentions of the three two-dimensional algorithms explaned in 2.5. In practice, they are used, as a rule, in combination with each other. We consider them separately.

In order to be able to characterize the quality of triangulation, we recall some facts. First we discuss finite elements in the form of tetrahedra and hexahedra with flat faces. The estimate of the approximation error on the cell ω includes, as a rule, the value [40]

$$\rho(\omega)/\operatorname{diam}\omega, \tag{2.43}$$

where $\rho(\omega)$ is the largest of the radii of spheres inscribed in ω. The smaller (2.43) is, the worse the approximation error, under other conditions fixed. Triangulation should therefore be performed such that (2.43) is isolated from zero:

$$\rho(\omega_i)/\operatorname{diam}\omega_i \geq c_0 > 0, \quad i = 1, \dots, K^h. \tag{2.44}$$

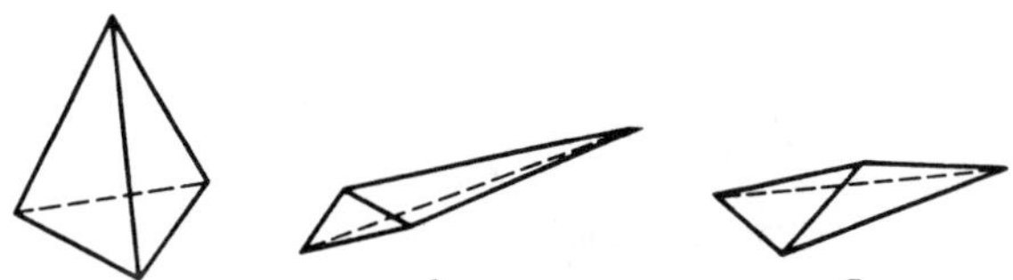

Figure 2.19: Possible forms of tetrahedra: form a is successful for both criteria (2.45), (2.46); b is acceptable under criterium (2.46) and poor under (2.45); c is poor for both criteria.

This inequality imposes several constraints on plane and dihedral angles in simplices, so that its formulation in terms of angles is inconvenient. Direct computation of (2.43) is possible but laborious. Therefore in practice instead of (2.43), we should take the value

$$6\,\mathrm{mes}\,\omega/abc, \tag{2.45}$$

where $6\,\mathrm{mes}\,\omega$ is calculated using determinants [83], and abc is the least product of lengths of the three edges which emerge from one vertex of simplex.

Sometimes by analogy with the two-dimensional case, the approximation error can be estimated in terms of

$$6\,\mathrm{mes}\,\omega/a'b'c' \tag{2.46}$$

instead of (2.43) or (2.45). Here $a'b'c'$ is the largest product of lengths of three edges emerging from one vertex of simplex.

Fig. 2.19 shows a difference of shapes of simplices in terms of two criteria. Roughly speaking, the second criterion needs only one good trihedral angle while the first one requires all the four trihedral angles to be good.

To characterize a curvilinear tetrahedron, we will use the values of (2.45), (2.46) pertaining to the simplex constructed on the same four vertices.

2.6.1 The boundary-correction algorithm

Let Ω be a bounded domain in $\mathbf{R}^3$ with boundary $\Gamma \subset C^2$. Fix the parameter h and plot the coordinate grid $R_h^3 = \{x = (ih, jh, kh);\ i, j, k = 0, \pm 1, \dots\}$. We will call point $x \in R_h^3$ *regular*, if six closed straight segments joining it to six nearest points of R_h^3 do not have common points with boundary Γ. Denote the set of regular nodes by R_h. The remainder will be called *irregular* and denoted by $R_h^{ir} = R_h^3 \setminus R_h^r$.

Transform R_h^3 with the help of operator T as follows. If $x \in R_h^r$, we put $T(x) = x$. Let now $x \in R_h^{ir}$. Then in the directions parallel to the axis, point $y \in \Gamma$ is found which is nearest to x and is at a distance $\leq h$ from x. Denote this distance by $\delta(x)$. In the case when $\delta(x) \leq h/2$ and one of the coordinates of y is larger than the corresponding coordinate of x, we put $T(x) = y$. $T(x) = x$ is put in all other cases.

Thus, we have constructed the operator $T : R_h^3 \to \tilde{R}_h^3$ with range $\tilde{R}_h^3 = T(R_h^3)$. Points $y_{ijk} = T(x_{ijk})$ have the same enumeration, as $x_{ijk} = (ih, jh, kh)$. For each fixed triplet of indices $i, j, k = 0, \pm 1, \dots$, we will consider eight points $y_{i+1/2\pm 1/2,\, j+1/2\pm 1/2,\, k+1/2\pm 1/2}$. They form a polyhedron (non-convex in general case), which is close to the initial cube.

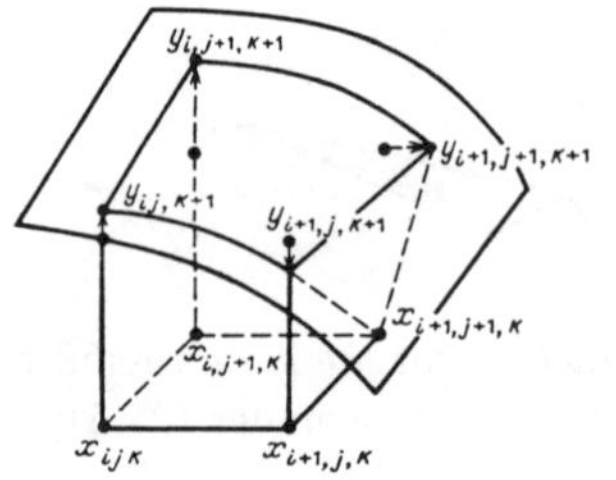

Figure 2.20: The boundary correction of nodes in three-dimensional case

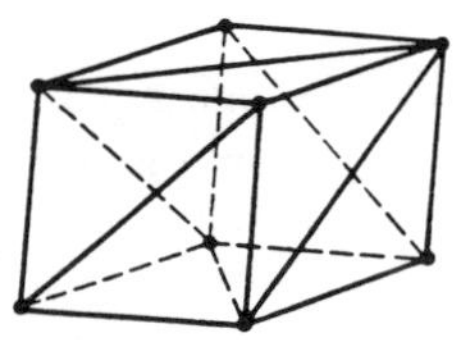

Figure 2.21: The variant of invalid diagonals

However, four points whose prototypes were on one cube face can now not lie in one plane. (For example, points $x_{i+1,j,k}$, $x_{i+1,j+1,k}$, $y_{i+1,j+1,k+1}$, $y_{i+1,j,k+1}$ of Fig. 2.20). Therefore it is more convenient that the polyhedron obtained (also the initial cube) should be recognized as dodecahedron with triangular (curvilinear possibly) faces.

Fig. 2.4 and 2.5 show two typical methods for dividing such a dodecahedron into tetrahedra. They depend on the way of drawing diagonals of lateral faces (or on the way of uniting the vertices in triplets defining lateral faces). The first method is more preferable for dividing cubes with regular vertices inside the domain. As for second one, crossing diagonals on parallel faces lead to different orientation of neighbouring cubes, which worses the homogeneity of triangulation. Show also the only way of drawing diagonals on faces (Fig. 2.21) when the cube cannot be divided into tetrahedra without introducing an additional node of triangulation.

In case when boundary Γ has angular points, it is necessary for them to be nodes of triangulation, possibly at the cost of non-uniform steps in each of the directions. In the case where boundary Γ has the edges which are join of smooth curvilinear faces, it is necessary in addition to move some neighbouring nodes x_{ijk} to these edges. In this case, the quality of triangulation usually becomes worse, and the algorithm gets more complicated because of plenty of possible situations.

Note among advantages of this algorithm the homogeneity, in the main, of triangulation, possible concordance of triangulation on two sides from the interior boundary, natural enumeration, and topological equivalence to the regular cubic grid.

2.6.2 The depletion algorithm

Let us consider the domain $\Omega \subset R^3$ with boundary Γ formed of crossing surfaces of class C^2. Below, when operating on three-dimensional domains, it will be convenient to consider these as topological polyhedra with possible curvilinear faces and edges and to use usual terminology with appropriate close meaning. It considerably facilitates understanding of the algorithms applied to polyhedra with flat faces, which are the most simple and frequently used methodological objects. For example, dihedral angle is the name we give to the configuration that results from crossing two (curvilinear) faces along some curve called an edge of this angle. Polyhedral angle is, respectively, the name given to the figure obtained by join of three and more faces with one common point called a vertex of this angle. To ensure measuring solid angles, let us show what is called its value. Let $x \in \Gamma$. Construct a cone using tangent lines to Γ from point x. On a unit sphere with x as a center, the cone cuts out some figure whose area is considered to be the value of (solid) angle of boundary Γ at point x. In the special case of an interior point of the smooth face, this value is equal to 2π. In the interior of Ω for the sake of homogeneity, it is supposed to equal 4π (the area of whole unit sphere).

To begin with, 4 disjoint sets have to be given in the following order:

1. Y_h are the angular points which are vertices of polyhedral angles and conic points;
2. R_h are the points lied on edges of dihedral angles;
3. G_h are the points lied on faces;
4. Ω_h are the points lied within Ω.

Here are properties they must possess:

1. Y_h involves all the angular points;
2. intersection between set $Y_h \bigcup R_h$ and each edge yields the h-grid for this edge;
3. intersection between set $Y_h \bigcup R_h \bigcup G_h$ and each face yields the h-grid for this face;
4. set $Y_h \bigcup R_h \bigcup G_h \bigcup \Omega_h$ is the h-grid for $\bar{\Omega}$.

After introducting these sets, we start to triangulate. The algorithm consists in step-by-step depletion of tetrahedra. It involves 5 stages.

1. We find point x_0 from $Y_h \bigcup R_h \bigcup G_h$ with the least solid angle. Note that search is made in every subsequent set only when the preceding one is empty. Hence, if Y_h has one point, it will just be taken as x_0.
2. At a distance $\leq \sqrt{3}h$ from x_0, we find point x_1 from $Y_h \bigcup R_h \bigcup G_h$ with the least solid angle. As before, search in R_h and G_h is made only when no appropriate points exist in the preceding set. In case there arises multivaluedness (within one of these sets), the point is taken which lies on the same edge as x_0 or (if not available) on the same face. If multivaluedness remains, one should take the point nearest to x_0.

3. In $Y_h \bigcup R_h \bigcup G_h \bigcup \Omega_h$ we take all the points which are distant less than $\sqrt{3h}$ from x_0, x_1 and choose from these a pair x_2, x_3 so that the following properties hold:
   (a) points x_0, x_1, x_2 lie on one smooth face of Γ;
   (b) point x_3 lies on the same side of this face as domain Ω;
   (c) the required value (2.44) or (2.45) of the quality criterion is maximum for simplex x_0, x_1, x_2, x_3.
4. We construct (curvilinear) tetrahedron with vertices x_0, x_1, x_2, x_3 and the following properties (Fig. 2.22, *a*, *c*, *e*):
   (a) if three vertices do not lie on one smooth face of boundary Γ, then the tetrahedron face corresponding to them is taken flat, otherwise it is taken as a boundary portion cut out of Γ by three other lateral faces of the tetrahedron.
   (b) if two vertices x_i, x_j lie on one edge R_k of boundary Γ, the tetrahedron edge $x_i x_j$ must be the part of R_k.
5. We remove the primary tetrahedron obtained from Ω. Remained body may have from one to three new faces (Fig. 2.22, *b*, *d*, *f*). In spite of the fact that they must be flat, their edges may be curvilinear also. When besides four vertices, one more point from $R_h \bigcup G_h \bigcup \Omega_h$ lies in the interior or on the surface of the tetrahedron constructed, this point is excluded from further consideration. After classifying the rest of the points, we obtain the new sets $\tilde{Y}_h, \tilde{R}_h, \tilde{G}_h, \tilde{\Omega}_h$ for the domain $\tilde{\Omega}$ with boundary $\tilde{\Gamma}$ and lesser volume. With these data, we again return to stage 1.

When h is small enough, e. g., when it is smaller than K and KL in the definition of the strict Lipschitz domain Ω, this procedure gives high-quality triangulation.

To complete our investigation of possible situations, we consider the conic points that do not have simple topological analogues in polyhedra. Assume, for instance, that the third stage of the present algorithm leads to the case of Fig, 2.23, *a*. Of course, the cone may be cut by the plane through x_1, x_2, x_3. This results in tetrahedron $x_0x_1x_2x_3$ with flat faces and of rather good quality (2.44) and (2.45). This may account for its choice for linear finite elements. As for isoparametric quadratic ones, it is not suitable for these because of the degeneration of plane angles at its foot. In this case, at the third stage, one should force to take point x_3 from Ω_h or Ω (see Fig. 2.23, *b* after withdrawing such a tetrahedron). Similar situations may arise when one or two edges leave a conic point. These situations are eliminated by adding two conditions at stage 3, namely:

(d) points x_0, x_1, x_2, x_3 do not lie on one face;

(e) no three of them lie on one edge.

These conditions also eliminate undesirable variants where h is large, related to the strong curvature of edges and faces.

Note that the domain Ω may become multiply connected, from consistently depletion, especially at the last stages, and the process remaines laborious up to the last tetrahedron. This is permissible when the cell-size is comparatively large. But for small h, this process should be terminated, as in the two-dimensional case. Namely:

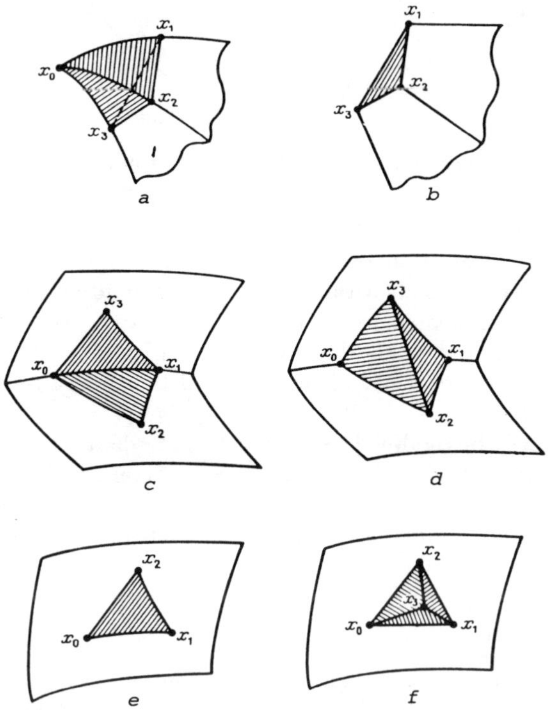

Figure 2.22: Construction of elementary tetrahedron and its withdrawing; typical cases.

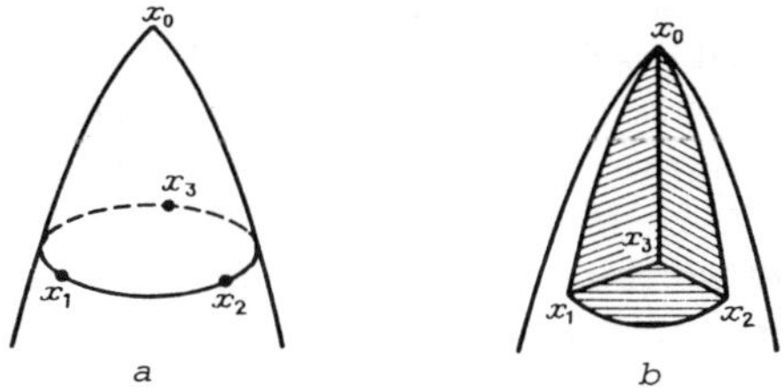

Figure 2.23: The elementary tetrahedron near the conic point

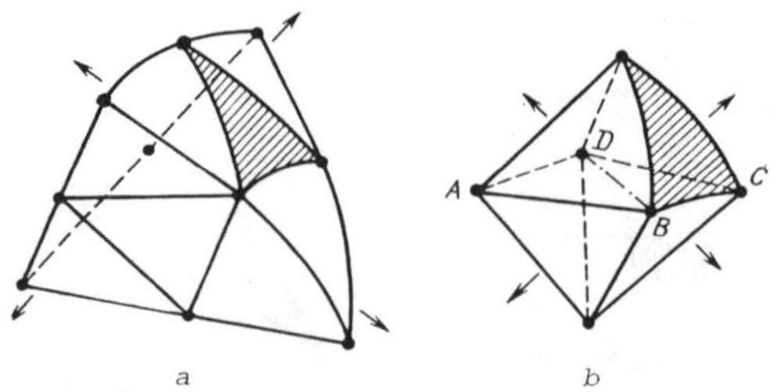

Figure 2.24: Stages of dividing of the tetrahedron into 8 parts

the h-grid in Ω should be taken regular, assuming $\Omega_h = \Omega \bigcap R_h^3$, where R_h^3 is the same set as in the preceding section with the exception that points being too close to Γ may be removed. As a result, the algorithm constructed should be terminated as soon as only these regular points remain in $\tilde{Y}_h \bigcup \tilde{R}_h \bigcup \tilde{G}_h$. Further triangulation is made using a certain subdivision of the cube into tetrahedra (Fig. 2.4, 2.5). This method ensures the overwhelming homogeneity of the obtained tetrahedra relative to parallel movement along the axes.

The algorithm can easily be modified to construct concordant triangulation with the interior boundary. Compared with the boundary-correction algorithm, this provides higher quality triangulation while its logical intricacy is somewhat less, especially in the case of edges and angles. But it does not provide natural enumeration as well as topological equivalence to a regular cubic grid.

2.6.3 The breaking algorithm

Assume that there exists some rough triangulation of domain Ω. It is required to make it finer. Consider the procedure of breaking every (curvilinear) tetrahedron into 8 or 27 tetrahedra of smaller size. The curvilinear faces are supposed to be given in parametric representation as smooth functions $x_i = x_i(\xi_1, \xi_2)$, $i = 1, 2, 3$.

Initially we consider the subdivision into 8 parts. Divide each of 4 tetrahedron faces into 4 parts by the rule of the two-dimensional breaking method (Fig. 2.18, a). To divide flat faces, we use straight segments in variables x_i. To curvilinear faces, we apply segments rectilinear in parametrical variables ξ_i. Then near each of the four tetrahedron vertices, we draw a surface through the midpoints of three edges emerging from this vertex, and along the lines obtained above (Fig. 2.24, a). These surfaces cut off 4 tetrahedra (with curvilinear faces possibly). In the octahedron that remains, we join together two vertices not lying on one face by a straight segment. There are three ways to join. We use the way giving the least length of straight segment thus obtained (segment BD of Fig. 2.24, b). This straight segment will be edge of four remaining tetrahedra of smaller size which result from drawing the faces through this edge and each of other four tetrahedron vertices along the edges already available.

To continue in this way, it is necessary that new curvilinear faces should be represented parametrically. For that purpose, we carry out the following construction. Let a_1, a_2, a_3 be the vertices of a two-dimensional simplex in variables ξ_1, ξ_2. Introduce barycentric coordinates $\lambda_1, \lambda_2, \lambda_3$. On the side a_2a_3, let us give the smooth function $g(\lambda_3)$ vanishing at the vertices a_2, a_3 (Fig. 2.25). Our aim is to define the smooth func-

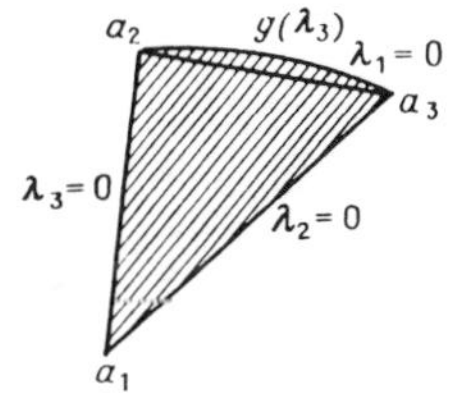

Figure 2.25: The construction of the surface through the given curve

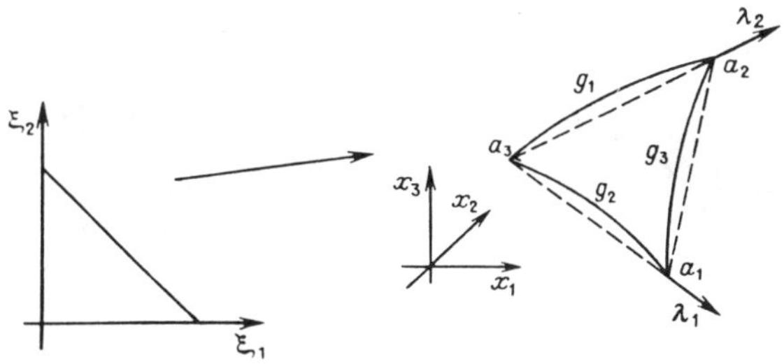

Figure 2.26: Construction of the parameterized surface passing through the curvilinear triangular contour

tion $z(\lambda_1, \lambda_2)$ which attains values $g(\lambda_3)$ on the side a_2a_3 and vanishes on the sides a_1a_2 and a_1a_3. There are many functions with such properties discussed in the literature. We consider the following one:

$$\begin{aligned} z(\lambda_1, \lambda_2) &= (1 - \lambda_1)g(1 - \lambda_2 - \lambda_1/2) + \\ &+ [g(\lambda_1/2) - g(1 - \lambda_1/2)](1 - \lambda_1 - \lambda_2) - g(\lambda_1/2)(1 - \lambda_1). \end{aligned} \tag{2.47}$$

Its choice is related to the fact that from the condition $g \in C^k[0,1]$ there follows $z \in C^k(\triangle a_1a_2a_3)$.

Let now three smooth curves be given in space in parametric representation which form the contour of a curvilinear triangle (Fig. 2.26). Take a standard simplex in the plane ξ_1, ξ_2 and introduce barycentric coordinates $\lambda_1, \lambda_2, \lambda_3$. Then, we construct the vector function $(x_i(\lambda_1, \lambda_2))_{i=1}^3$ each component of which is the sum of a linear function and three functions g_i of the form (2.47). Note that functions g_i are taken so that the surface defined parametrically by functions $x_i(\lambda_1, \lambda_2)$ passes through three given curves. This choice gives an unambiguous result, and a flat triangle for the flat initial contour.

In the specific case of the initial tetrahedron with flat faces only, such a subdivision gives 8 simplices. They all are equivolumed, but only 4 of them are similar to the initial tetrahedron. They can be divided into 3 different groups of congruent simplices.

For the tetrahedron to be divided into 27 parts, each of 4 faces should be divided into 9 parts by the rule explained in the two-dimensional breaking method (Fig. 2.18, *b*). Breaking is made by straight segments in variables x_i for flat faces and by straight segments in parametric variables ξ_j for curvilinear faces. Then near each of 4 tetrahedron vertices, a surface is passed through the points, being at a distance of one

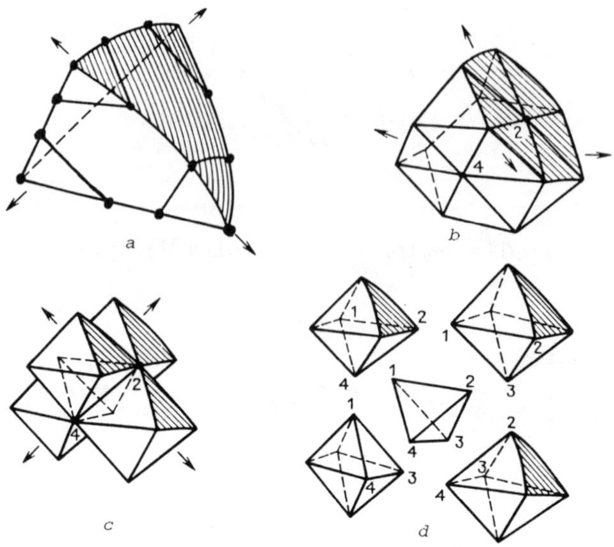

Figure 2.27: Breaking the tetrahedron into 27 parts

third the length of the edges emerging from this vertex, and along the lines constructed before (Fig. 2.27, *a*). These surfaces cut off 4 (curvilinear) tetrahedra (Fig. 2.27, *b*), which gives 4 hexagonal faces with mean points marked. Joining these points with one another gives a simplex. From each edge of this simplex, we pass two surfaces, so that they go through centres of hexagonal faces connected by this edge, and along the lines constructed earlier on these faces (Fig. 2.27, *c*). As a result, we have six more (curvilinear) tetrahedra. What remains is a combination of the simplex constructed and four octahedra contiguous to its faces (Fig. 2.27, *d*). Breaking the octahedra into 4 parts is made as before (Fig. 2.24, *b*).

In case the initial tetrahedron has only flat faces, such a subdivision gives 27 simplices. They are again divided into 3 different groups of congruent simplices.

Dividing all the tetrahedra of a concordant triangulation into an equal number of parts again yields concordant triangulation, the maximum diameter of cells being 2 or 3 times less, respectively. The breaking algorithm may be repeated over and over again so as to obtain the required refinement of triangulation. It is generally used either after manually dividing the domain into a small number of tetrahedra or after applying one of the above cited algorithms with large mesh-size h.

In the case of the initial tetrahedron with flat faces, breaking produces uniform triangulation in its interior. The breaking algorithm differs from those given above by simple logical structure and requirement of not so much computer time. In addition, when breaking is repeated many times, it yields a sequence of the triangulations naturally nested, which is used in multigrid algorithms.

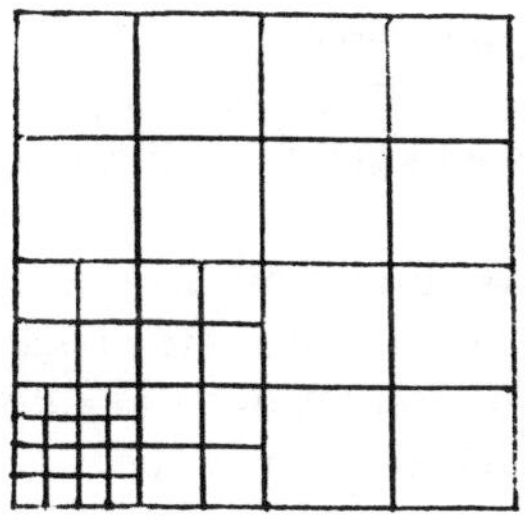

Figure 2.28: Voronoi subdivision and Delaunay triangulation: Full line — Voronoi polihedra, dotted lines — Delaunay triangules

2.7 Other algorithms and refinement of triangulation

The depletion algorithm essentially solves the problem of joining a given set of boundary nodes and irregular nodes near the boundary by straight segments so that a concordant triangulation with optimal angles of the triangles could be generated. Such general problem of joining an arbitrary given set of nodes proves conjugate to the subdivision of the domains into the Dirichlet cells or, what is the same, into the Voronoi polygons or polyhedra. This subdivision has use in crystallography, nuclear physics, and chemistry, and so an interest in algorithms for its construction has been maintained for many years. Let us first describe this subdivision and then construct according to it a triangulation with some optimal properties.

Let $p_1, \dots, p_l$ be fixed points in $\mathbf{R}^n$. Then a set of points in $\mathbf{R}^n$ being more close to p_i than to any other point p_j called *the Dirichlet cell* or *the Voronoi polygon (polyhedron)* with p_i as a center, i. e.,

$$V_i = \{x \in \mathbf{R}^n : \rho(x - p_i) \leq \rho(x - p_j), \quad j = 1, \dots, l\}, \tag{2.48}$$

where ρ is the distance in $\mathbf{R}^n$, not necessary Eucledian one. Let us analyse the two-dimensional case. Take an arbitrary point p_i. Another points p_j for which $V_i \bigcap V_j \neq \phi$ will be called its neighbours. Neighbourhood is called singular if this intersection involves only one point.

Assume that the Voronoi subdivision already exists. Let us construct *the Delaunay triangulation* dual to it. To accomplish this, we should join each point p_i and its non-singular neighbours by straight segments. That gives us a new subdivision. If it contains polygons with the number of vertices > 3, we should draw additional straight segments between singular neighbours such in number that no intersection occurs (Fig. 2.28).

As a result, we have a concordant triangulation with the following optimality property. Take two neighbouring triangles which form a strictly convex quadrangle. Then the least of six angles is not less than that we have when drawing the diagonal in the quadrangle in a different way or when choosing a different couple of the triangles contained this diagonal and with two other vertices [178].

At present, there exist a lot of papers which propose algorithms for constructing the Voronoi subdivision and the Delaunay triangulation (see, e.g., [29], [70] and the bibliography there). In the two-dimensional case, efficiency estimates of the constructed algorithms reach for the number of operations the threshold $O(l^2 \ln l)$ for l arbitrary given nodes and are not improved. In the case of the Delaunay triangulation in the $2h$-layer near the boundary, this threshold can be reduced to $O(l)$ both in the two- and three-dimensional cases.

It remains to settle the problem of preliminarily arranging the nodes of triangulation on the boundary of the domain and in its interior. This problem can be solved in different ways depending on final requirements on triangulation [184].

The original and fruitful direction is research in the field of application of mapping initial domains or their parts in such canonical regions as rectangles, triangles, circles, sectors, etc [46], [62]. For example, by mapping the domain on the rectangle, one can construct a triangulation which ensures the convergence of effective two-level iterative processes with direct solution on every iteration of auxiliary problems in the rectangle [126], [46].

Transformation of coordinates is often used to construct triangulations refining in the vicinity of special points or lines. Below, we discuss this problem.

Brief discussion of these approaches and their combinations is included in [184], [52] and references therein.

A number of specific questions arising in the three-dimensional case is discussed in [85], [89], [39], [70], [198], [149]. Note that using incomplete (serendipity) elements on polyhedra with the number of vertices < 8 for automatization has good prospects. In this case, a necessity of triangulation of the domain only into tetrahedra or cuboids no longer arises. Moreover, applying the three-dimensional algorithm of boundary correction does not, in fact, disturb homogeneity of numerical algorithms at subsequent stages.

Now, let us present somewhat more detailed discussion on the refinement of triangulation. In a number of cases, a solution of the differential problem has some singularities which result in an unbounded increase of derivatives. The discussion of this is presented in subsection 1.1.3 where angular points and boundary lines are concerned. A different class of singularities arises in the boundary layer for the equations with small parameter at higher derivatives. When solving such problems on a uniform triangulation, the order of convergence considerably decreases [182]. At the same time, one may give such a refinement of triangulation that the convergence order is restored without considerably increasing the number of nodes of triangulation (within a few percent) [167].

Let us consider refining the triangulation near a singular point in the two-dimensional case. For definitness, assume that it is placed at the origin of coordinates.

Note that refinement of triangulation can be obtained using any of the algorithms of 2.5, in which a different (not only Euclidean) distance should be taken. For example, let the mapping $f : \mathbf{R}^2 \to \mathbf{R}^2$ be given by

$$f_i(x) = x_i \mid x \mid^{-\alpha}, \quad i = 1, 2. \tag{2.49}$$

When $\alpha \in (0, 1)$, it leads to a tension of the plane in all directions from the origin of coordinates. Introduce the new distance ρ between points $x, y \in \mathbf{R}^2$ by

$$\rho(x, y) = \mid f(x) - f(y) \mid . \tag{2.50}$$

Using any of the algorithms of 2.5 with this distance gives a triangulation refining towards the origin of coordinates when $\alpha > 1$. The larger α is, the finer the grid becomes towards the singular point.

The uniformity of the rectangular grid in both coordinate directions becomes worse because of function (2.49) and so it is better to use this in a small vinicity of zero (whose diameter is, however, comparable with the dimensions of the domain). Gradual transition from the non-uniform grid to a uniform square grid can be made by use of the Urysohn function ω_δ from subsection 1.1.1. Put

$$\tilde{f}(x) = x + (f(x) - x)\omega_\delta(\mid x \mid).$$

The distance $\rho(x,y) = \mid \tilde{f}(x) - \tilde{f}(y) \mid$ is usual Euclidean beyond the sphere of radius 2δ and has the required extending properties inside the sphere with radius δ.

The grid should be made uniform along the axes. This is of importance for the use of rectangular finite elements. To this end, function f is defined by the formula

$$f_i(x) = x_i \mid x_i \mid^{-\alpha}, \quad i = 1,2. \tag{2.51}$$

Note that such constructions with the distance (2.50) are equivalent to another method. Using the transformation of coordinates $y = f(x)$, we change the domain Ω with boundary Γ into a domain $\tilde{\Omega}$ with boundary $\tilde{\Gamma}$. On the new domain $\tilde{\Omega}$, we construct a usual square grid. Then we use one of two given algorithms to match this grid to boundary Γ, or we break the already existent triangulation. Now using the transformation f^{-1}, inverse to f, we transform the constructed nodes and the topology of triangulation into the initial variables.

Let us act in this way to refine the grid near the curve. Assume, for example, that a smooth non-closed curve is given in parametric representation by two functions $\tilde{x}_i(t)$, $t \in [0,1]$; $i = 1,2$. Assume also that there exists a vector $a = (a_1, a_2)$ making an acute angle with the interior normal at any point of this curve.

Put $\tilde{x} = (\tilde{x}_1, \tilde{x}_2)$ and introduce new coordinates (s,t) in the belt which results from parallel transfer of the curve in the direction of vector a. For every x of this belt, parameters s, t are found by unique way:

$$x = \tilde{x}(t) + sa. \tag{2.52}$$

Actually, these are the new coordinates $(s,t) \in [0,\infty) \times [0,1]$. Introduce the transformation $g : (s,t) \to (s',t')$ by

$$t' = t, \quad s' = s^\alpha. \tag{2.53}$$

When $\alpha > 1$, it extends the belt in the direction s. In the (s',t') coordinates, we construct a uniform square grid, match it to the boundary by one of the algorithms and return consistently to the coordinates (s,t) and (x_1,x_2). We assumed that the boundary consists here, besides an image of Γ in the form $s' = 0$, of the broken line along which the triangulation is already constructed in the interior of the domain and near neighbouring portions of the boundary.

We have used here the second method related to the transformation of coordinates. Computation of the coordinates of grid nodes requires that formula (2.52) should be

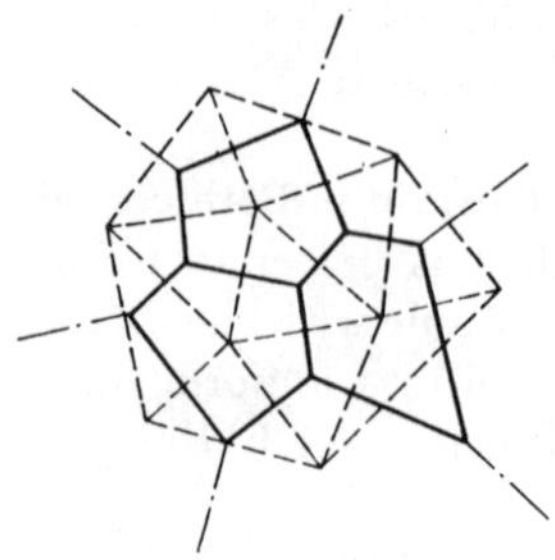

Figure 2.29: Local nonconcordant triangulation

applied many times and does not require the usage of inverse transformation. Of course, one can, according to the first approach, introduce distance (2.50) with the corresponding transformation f. But this would require the transformation, repeated many times, of coordinates (x_1, x_2) to (s, t), which is tantamount to the solution of a system like (2.52) for s, t with the right-hand side x. It can easily be done only for functions $\tilde{x}_i$ of rather simple structure. Thus the first approach is here ineffective.

The second method can easily be generalized to the three-dimensional case where refining the triangulation near the curvilinear surface is needed.

Sometimes, to intricate subdomains with disproportionate elements, one can apply a local breaking. It gives a compound triangulation non-concordant along some lines. This is of special importance for the homogenization problems. The usage of the Schwartz processes of subdomains alternation (without overlap) makes this method rather attractive [98]. To make this point clear, let us return to the problem with singular point. Let first a square grid with large cell-size be constructed and let then several cells near the singular point be broken into smaller square cells (s. f. Fig. 2.29). The concordant condition is then considered as being satisfied for elements of more intricate shape (ones composed of several squares or triangles) [95].

Chapter 3

On the convergence of approximate solutions

In this chapter we deal with estimates in various norms for the difference $u - u^h$ where u is a solution of the boundary value problem and $u^h \in H^h$ is a solution obtained by the Bubnov-Galerkin method. According to the theorems of section 1.2, the error satisfies the inequality

$$\|u - u^h\|_{m,\Omega} \leq c \inf_{w \in H^h} \|u - w\|_{m,\Omega}$$

with integer $m = 1, 2$. The search of the element w ensuring the infimum is a problem. Therefore we use the interpolant $I^h u \in H^h$ instead of the optimal function:

$$\|u - u^h\|_{m,\Omega} \leq c \, \|u - I^h u\|_{m,\Omega}.$$

First we will assume that the closed domain $\bar{\Omega}$ is a concordant union of the finite number of cells ω_k : $\bar{\Omega} = \bigcup_{k=1}^{K^h} \omega_k$. Then

$$\|u - I^h u\|_{m,\Omega} = (\sum_{k=1}^{K^h} \|u - I^h u\|^2_{m,\omega_k})^{1/2}.$$

Hence, the problem of estimating the error $\|u - u^h\|_{m,\Omega}$ amounts to the problem of estimating the values $\|u - I^h u\|_{m,\omega_k}$ on every finite element. We deal with it in section 3.1.

Section 3.2 gives the results on the convergence of the Bubnov-Galerkin method in different norms for the second- and fourth-order equations. Then, in section 3.3, we retrace the effect of the quadratures used for calculating the matrix elements and the right-hand side of the Bubnov-Galerkin system on order convergence. In section 3.4, the influence of another error is retraced, namely: approximation of the curvilinear boundary and of the values of functions given on it.

In section 3.5 we introduce the notion of nested basis functions which is rather important for multigrid algorithms and deal with the problem of increasing the accuracy of piecewise linear solutions of the Bubnov-Galerkin method due to solving the problem on two grids (Richardson extrapolation).

Finally, in section 3.6, we deal with the problem of conditionality of the discrete systems obtained.

3.1 Interpolation by finite elements

In this section we first treat the accuracy of interpolation by finite elements which can be achieved for a sufficiently smooth function on one cell. It is shown that the order of local approximation is connected with degree k of complete polynomials under the condition $P_k \subset P$. The second condition is of geometrical nature and connects accuracy with a cell form. It obstructs too narrow cells, too curved faces, and other cases of degeneration.

Then we transfer local concepts and interpolation properties from one finite element to their set interpolating the functions all over the domain Ω.

Finally, we deal with a procedure of the breaking of finite elements. It is an active part of multigrid algorithms as well as of their foundation. The most important property of this procedure, the nesting, consists in possible representation of basis functions on large cells in the form of linear combinations of basis functions on more fine subdivisions. The operators of restriction and interpolation from one triangulation to another are introduced.

3.1.1 Local interpolation

Let us introduce the concept 'interpolant' on the finite element (ω, P, Φ). Assume that derivatives up to order s are used in the definition of functionals $\varphi_i \in \Phi$ which are defined not only on $p \in P$ but on any function $v \in C^s(\omega)$. Put

$$I_\omega v = \sum_{i=1}^{N} \varphi_i(v) p_i, \tag{3.1}$$

where p_i are the basis functions of P. Since the set Φ is P-solvable, this representation is unique. We call it *the interpolant* of function v *in space* P.

The value $|v - I_\omega v|_{r,\omega}$ is of our interest. It can be most easily estimated for some standard cells, such as a standard triangle, a unit cube, etc. Therefore it is natural first to formulate an approximation criterion for the standard form, and then to trace effects of the transformation of this standard form into the required one.

Thus, let (ω, P, Φ) be a finite element with a standard cell ω. Assume that the element $(\tilde{\omega}, \tilde{P}, \tilde{\Phi}) = F(\omega, P, \Phi)$ is derived by the mapping $F : \omega \to \tilde{\omega}$ as in subsection 2.4.1. We call

$$I_{\tilde{\omega}} \tilde{v} = \sum_{i=1}^{N} \tilde{\varphi}_i(\tilde{v}) \tilde{p}_i \tag{3.2}$$

the interpolant of function $\tilde{v} \in C^s(\tilde{\omega})$ *in space* $\tilde{P}$.

Let us consider the following *completeness condition* with integer $k \geq 0$. For the element (ω, P, Φ), there exists an integer k such that $P_k(\omega) \subset P \subset W_2^{k+1}(\omega)$, i. e., the space P of admissible functions includes the set $P_k(\omega)$ of complete polynomials of degree k on ω.

From this, it is easy to see the following [40]. Let $W_2^{k+1}(\omega)$ be imbedded in $C^s(\omega)$, then $\forall r \leq k+1$, $\forall v \in W_2^{k+1}(\omega)$

$$|v - I_\omega v|_{r,\omega} \leq c(\omega, P) |v|_{k+1,\omega}. \tag{3.3}$$

Consider also the following *regularity condition* with integer $r \geq 0$. Let the mapping F be diffeomorphic and such that $v = \tilde{v} \circ F \in W_2^r(\omega)$ $\forall \tilde{v} \in W_2^r(\tilde{\omega})$. Let also there exist the constants $c_1, \ldots, c_4$ such that

$$h^r |\tilde{v}|_{r,\tilde{\omega}} \leq c_1 \|v\|_{r,\omega} \sup_\omega |J|^{1/2}, \qquad h = \operatorname{diam} \tilde{\omega},$$

$$|v|_{r,\omega} \leq c_2 h^r \|\tilde{v}\|_{r,\tilde{\omega}} \sup_\omega |J|^{-1/2}, \tag{3.4}$$

$$0 < c_3 \leq \sup_\omega |J| / \inf_\omega |J| \leq c_4. \tag{3.5}$$

These two conditions are sufficient to evaluate the order of approximation.

Theorem 3.1 *Assume that the completeness condition is satisfied for element (ω, P, Φ) with k such that $W_2^{k+1}(\omega)$ is imbedded in $C^s(\omega)$. Also assume that the regularity condition is satisfied for element $F(\omega, P, \Phi) = (\tilde{\omega}, \tilde{P}, \tilde{\Phi})$ for all $r \leq k+1$. Then*

$$|\tilde{v} - I_{\tilde{\omega}} \tilde{v}|_{r,\tilde{\omega}} \leq c(\omega, P) h^{k+1-r} \|\tilde{v}\|_{k+1,\tilde{\omega}} \qquad \forall \tilde{v} \in W_2^{k+1}(\tilde{\omega}). \tag{3.6}$$

Thus, we found justification for the persistence we showed in Chapter 2 while evaluating the maximum degree k of complete polynomials in the space P of admissible functions for every finite element.

In the case of the affine reversible mapping F, the regularity condition can be substantially simplified. Indeed, $\tilde{v} \circ F \in W_2^r(\omega)$ automatically for any $\tilde{v} \in W_2^r(\tilde{\omega})$, the Jacobian becomes constant and (3.5) holds with $c_3 = c_4 = 1$. Next, the Jacobi matrix $A = (a_{ij})$ (see (2.23)) satisfies the following estimates [40, Theorem 3.1.3]:

$$\|A\| \leq diam(\omega)/\rho(\tilde{\omega}), \qquad \|A^{-1}\| \leq diam(\tilde{\omega})/\rho(\omega), \tag{3.7}$$

where $\rho(\omega)$ is the diameter of the circle inscribed in ω. If one does not require to satisfy the regularity condition (3.4), then it follows from the general approximation theory [40, Theorem 3.1.4]

$$|v - I_{\tilde{\omega}} v|_{r,\tilde{\omega}} \leq c(\omega, P) h^{k+1} \rho^{-r}(\tilde{\omega}) |v|_{k+1,\tilde{\omega}}. \tag{3.8}$$

To eliminate $\rho^{-r}(\tilde{\omega})$, we suppose that

$$diam(\tilde{\omega})/\rho(\tilde{\omega}) \leq c. \tag{3.9}$$

It is just the inequality we call *the affine regularity condition.*

Theorem 3.2 *Assume that the completeness condition is satisfied for element (ω, P, Φ) with k such that $W_2^{k+1}(\omega)$ is imbedded in $C^s(\omega)$. Also assume that element $(\tilde{\omega}, \tilde{P}, \tilde{\Phi})$ obtained by affine transformation $F(\omega, P, \Phi)$ satisfies the affine regularity condition (3.9). Then for any $\tilde{v} \in W_2^{k+1}(\tilde{\omega})$*

$$|\tilde{v} - I_{\tilde{\omega}} \tilde{v}|_{r,\tilde{\omega}} \leq c(\omega, P) h^{k+1-r} |\tilde{v}|_{k+1,\tilde{\omega}}. \tag{3.10}$$

3.1.2 Global interpolation

The closure of domain Ω is here supposed to be a union of the finite number of cells ω_k, i. e.,

$$\bar{\Omega} = \bigcup_{k=1}^{K^h} \omega_k, \qquad \mathring{\omega}_k \cap \mathring{\omega}_l = \phi, \quad k \neq l, \tag{3.11}$$

where $\mathring{\omega}_k$ is the interior of the cell ω_k. Let us transfer the local concepts for one finite element to the set

$$\mathcal{F}^h = \{(\omega_k, P^k, \Phi^k)\}_{k=1}^{K^h}.$$

Thus the first step is taken, because Ω is just such a global analogue of the cell ω_h. We call the set A_h, a union of all nodes a_j^k of cells ω_k, the nodes of triangulation $\{\omega^k\}_{k=1}^{K^h}$:

$$A^h = \{a_j^k;\ j = 1, \dots, m_k,\ k = 1, \dots, K^h\},$$

common nodes of two and more cells are included only once. If such a node $a \in A^h$ belongs to two cells ω_k and ω_l, it is associated with two sets of functionals $\{\varphi_{aj}^k\}_{j=1}^{N_a^k}$ and $\{\varphi_{aj}^l\}_{j=1}^{N_a^l}$. We require these to coincide for functions $p \in C^s(\bar{\Omega})$:

$$\varphi_{aj}^h(p) = \varphi_{aj}^k(p) = \varphi_{aj}^l(p), \quad j = 1, \dots, N_a^h = N_a^k = N_a^l. \tag{3.12}$$

The condition that the above equalities are satisfied is called *the coherency condition* of the set $\mathcal{F}^h$. As a result, we have a global set of linearly independent functionals

$$\Phi^h = \{\varphi_j^h;\ j = 1, \dots, N^h\}. \tag{3.13}$$

Take function $v \in C^s(\bar{\Omega})$ and construct interpolant $I_{\omega_k} v$ on every ω_k. This results in the set of functions

$$\{I_{\omega_k} v\}_{k=1}^{K^h}. \tag{3.14}$$

If the point x lies inside some cell ω_k, it is associated with one value of $I_{\omega_k} v(x)$. If it lies on the boundary between ω_k and ω_l, it may be associated with two different values. This case cannot be omitted, because finite elements like these are also used in practice, for example, with piecewise constant basis functions [115]. We deal only with such sets (3.14) for which continuity is valid both inside and between the cells. Namely, the following *continuity conditions* must be satisfied:

$$1. \quad P^k \in C(\omega_k), \tag{3.15}$$

$$2. \quad I_{\omega_k} v = I_{\omega_l} v \quad \text{on} \quad \omega_k \cap \omega_l, \quad k, l = 1, \dots, K^h. \tag{3.16}$$

Now every point x is associated with only one value, and so the set (3.14) is equivalent to one function, hereafter denoted by $I_h v$. Note that thereby an operator $I_h : C^s(\bar{\Omega}) \to C(\bar{\Omega})$ is defined, hereafter called the (global) *interpolation operator*. We denote the linear space of all interpolants by P^h and call it *the trial functions space*. Obviously, this space is finite-dimensional. Its dimension is equal to N^h — the number of elements of the set Φ^h. It is natural to call these elements the degrees of freedom of the space P^h.

Introduce basis functions into the space P^h. To do this, one degree of freedom $\varphi_j^h \in \Phi^h$ is taken equal to unit and the rest of them, to zero. Then from the P^k-solvability of Φ^k, a function p_j^h can be constructed, obeing two conditions:

1) $p_j^h \in P^k$ as constriction on ω_k;

2) $\varphi_l^h(p_j^h) = \delta_{jl}$, where δ_{jl} is the Kronecker symbol.

$p_j^h \in C(\bar{\Omega})$ $(j = 1, \dots, N^h)$ from the continuity condition.

Consider now the node $\bar{a}$ to which the functional φ_j^h is associated. Denote by $J_{\bar{a}}$ the set of such integers r that $\bar{a}$ is a node of ω_r. Then from the linearity of the functionals, the basis function p_j^h is equal to zero on all the cells ω_k for which we have $k \notin J_{\bar{a}}$. The basis function support is therefore concentrated on a small number of cells:

$$\operatorname{supp} p_j^h = \bigcup_{r \in J_{\bar{a}}} \omega_r. \tag{3.17}$$

Note that interpolant $I_h v$ admits another, equivalent definition in terms of the basis functions:

$$I_h v = \sum_{j=1}^{N^h} \varphi_j^h(v) p_j^h. \tag{3.18}$$

Let us now check whether P^h belongs to classes $W_2^k(\Omega)$. Note that from the regularity condition (3.4), (3.5) it immediately follows that

$$P^h \subset L_2(\Omega) = W_2^0(\Omega). \tag{3.19}$$

Let now $P^k \subset W_2^1(\omega_k)$ $(k = 1, \dots, K^h)$. This, together with the continuity condition, leads to the following property [40]:

$$P^h \subset W_2^1(\Omega). \tag{3.20}$$

Now let the regularity condition and two more properties be satisfied, thus:

$$P^k \in C^1(\omega_k), \tag{3.21}$$

$$\partial_\nu(I_{\omega_k} v) = -\partial_\nu(I_{\omega_l} v) \quad \text{on } \omega_k \bigcap \omega_l,\ k, l = 1, \dots, K^h. \tag{3.22}$$

We call all the assertions (3.16), (3.21) and (3.22) the C^1-*continuity condition.* With this and using in addition the requirement

$$P^k \subset W_2^2(\omega_k) \quad \forall k = 1, \dots, K^h \tag{3.23}$$

we obtain the following [40]:

$$P^h \subset W_2^2(\Omega). \tag{3.24}$$

Let us now examine the accuracy of interpolation by operator I_h. Assume that $P^h \subset W_2^r(\Omega)$ with an integer $r \geq 0$. Also assume that $v \in W_2^{k+1}(\Omega)$, and $W_2^{k+1}(\Omega)$ is imbedded in $C^s(\bar{\Omega})$. Consider the value

$$\|v - I_h v\|_{r,\Omega} = (\sum_{k=1}^{K^h} \|v - I_h v\|^2_{r,\omega_k})^{1/2}. \tag{3.25}$$

As each term on the right-hand side is equal to $\|v - I_{\omega_k} v\|^2_{r,\omega_k}$, we can exploit the theorems of the preceding section. As a result we have the following [40].

Theorem 3.3 *Let $P^h \subset W_2^r(\Omega)$ and $W_2^{k+1}(\Omega)$ be imbedded in $C^s(\bar{\Omega})$, $k \geq r$. Let, besides, all finite elements (ω_l, P^l, Φ^l) $(l = 1, \dots, K^h)$ be regular with the integer $k+1$ for one and the same fixed finite element (ω, P, Φ) which satisfies the completeness condition with the integer k. Then*

$$\forall v \in W_2^{k+1}(\Omega) \qquad \|v - I_h v\|_{r,\Omega} \leq c(\omega, P)\, h^{k+1-r} \|v\|_{k+1,\Omega}. \tag{3.26}$$

Sometimes regularity cannot hold for only one "reference" finite element and so one has to take a whole set of them. In this case, there is some apprehension of the fact that constant $c(\omega, P)$ in (3.3) may tend to infinity when $h \to 0$. One should therefore here require not only completeness but also $c(\omega, P)$ to be uniformly bounded all over the "reference" family.

Theorem 3.4 *Let all finite elements (ω_l, P^l, Φ^l) $(l = 1, \dots, K^h)$ be regular with an integer $k+1$ for representatives of a set $\mathcal{F}^e = \{(\omega, P, \Phi)\}$ whose elements satisfy the completeness condition with the integer k and the constant $c(\omega, P)$ in (3.3) independing of $\omega \in \mathcal{F}^e$. Then, for any $v \in W_2^{k+1}(\Omega)$ provided that $W_2^{k+1}(\Omega)$ is imbedded in $C^s(\bar{\Omega})$ and $r \leq k+1$,*

$$\|v - I_h v\|_{r,\Omega} \leq c h^{k+1-r} \|v\|_{k+1,\Omega}. \tag{3.27}$$

To show a distinction between the theorems, we take the Courant triangular elements. As a pattern, we consider a Courant element on a standard triangle with vertices $(0,0)$, $(0,1)$, $(1,0)$. From the general approximation theory, the following inequality holds for $v \in W_2^2(\Omega)$:

$$\|v - I_\omega v\|_{r,\omega} \leq c\|v\|_{2,\omega} \quad \text{for} \quad r = 0, 1. \tag{3.28}$$

Let us consider images $\tilde{\omega}$ of various affine transformations of a standard triangle ω into $\tilde{\omega}$ assuming that $diam\, \tilde{\omega} = h$. It follows from the regularity condition (3.5) that

$$diam\, \tilde{\omega} / \rho(\tilde{\omega}) \leq c, \tag{3.29}$$

which is equivalent to condition (2.39) for all angles $\theta_{\tilde{\omega}i}$ of triangle $\tilde{\omega}$:

$$\sin \theta_{\tilde{\omega}i} \geq c > 0, \qquad i = 1, 2, 3. \tag{3.30}$$

At the same time, the estimate (3.28) can be proved by using direct calculations [146] for right triangles with vertices $(0,0)$, $(1,0)$, $(0,\delta)$ or $(0,0)$, $(\delta,0)$, $(0,1)$ where $\delta \in (0,1)$.

Note that constant c will be independent of δ. Let us then consider all possible affine transformations of this family into $\tilde{\omega}$ assuming that $diam\ \tilde{\omega} = h$. From the regularity condition (3.5) it follows that only one angle $\theta_{\tilde{\omega}i}$ with condition (3.30) is sufficient in the triangle $\tilde{\omega}$:

$$\exists i : \sin \theta_{\tilde{\omega}i} \geq c > 0. \tag{3.31}$$

Indeed, take the vertex of this angle in $\tilde{\omega}$ as an affine image of the right angle vertex in ω. Then, we can select ω from the "pattern" family so that the following inequality holds:

$$\frac{h^2}{4}c \leq |J| \leq h^2. \tag{3.32}$$

From this (3.4) immediately follows.

The same holds in the three-dimensional regions where two triangulation quality criteria are also needed. Therefore sections 2.5 and 2.6 treat two criteria — the one which is more strict, results from the general approximation theory, and the other which is not so strict, results from the uniform estimate (3.3) obtained for some "pattern" family by direct computations.

3.1.3 The breaking algorithm for finite elements and nesting of basis functions space

In this section, we consider nesting of trial functions spaces when the required triangulation is obtained by successively breaking some initial rough triangulation. This problem is of special importance for construction of the multigrid algorithms.

Let us continue studying the case where the closure of the domain Ω is the union of a finite number of cells (3.11).

Let us describe first the algorithm for breaking the finite elements set $\mathcal{F}^h$ which we will often use below. Fix $s = 2, 3$ and consider the general finite element $(\omega_k, P^k, \Phi^k) \in \mathcal{F}^h$. In the case of two- or three-dimensional simplex ω_k, we divide every edge into s parts and apply one of the algorithms for breaking simplices discussed in subsections 2.5.3, 2.6.3. The result is s^n simplices ω_{ki} $(i = 1, \ldots, s^n)$. On each we assume $P^{k,i} = P^k(\omega_{ki})$. Moreover, each simplex is affine-similar to ω_k, i. e., there exists an affine transformation $B_i : \omega_k \to \omega_{k,i}$. By using B_i, we get the new finite element $(\omega_{ki}, P^{k,i}, \Phi^{k,i}) = B_i(\omega_k, P^k, \Phi^k)$.

Remark 3.1.1 *In case $P^k = P_l(\omega_k)$, i. e., P^k is a constriction on ω_k of the space of complete polynomials of degree l, affine transformation again sends it to the complete polynomials space of degree l but with another domain of definition. $P^{k,i}$ will therefore be equal to $P_l(\omega_{ki})$.*

Breaking a two- or three-dimensional rectangular cell ω_k is performed in different ways. Divide the edges from one vertex into s parts and through the obtained points draw straight lines in the two-dimensional case, and planes parallel to lateral faces in the three-dimensional case. This gives s^n rectangles ω_{ki}. We know that rectangles ω_k and ω_{ki} are also affine-similar with transformation $B_i : \omega_k \to \omega_{ki}$. Using the latter, we obtain the new finite element $(\omega_{ki}, P^{k,i}, \Phi^{k,i}) = B_i(\omega_k, P^k, \Phi^k)$.

Remark 3.1.2 *The structure of this affine transformation involves a shift and a constriction along the rectangle sides. Let in the rectangle ω_k the local coordinates be introduced with the axes which are extensions of the rectangle edges leaving one vertex invarient. If P^k is a constriction $Q(\omega_k)$ of any linear space of polynomials Q, our affine transformation again transforms P^k in the same snace but with another domain of definition. $P^{k,i}$ will therefore coincide with $Q(\omega_{ki})$.*

In the case of the isoparametric element $(\omega_k, P^k, \Phi^k) = F_k(\tilde{\omega}_k, \tilde{P}^k, \tilde{\Phi}^k)$, whose pattern $(\tilde{\omega}_k, \tilde{P}^k, \tilde{\Phi}^k)$ has the cell $\tilde{\omega}_k$ shaped as simplex or rectangle, such subdivision is made for pattern itself.

Using the transformation F_k, we again obtain s^n finite elements $(\omega_{ki}, P^{k,i}, \Phi^{k,i}) = F_k(\tilde{\omega}_{ki}, \tilde{P}^{k,i}, \tilde{\Phi}^{k,i})$.

Thus in all three cases, one element generates s^n finite elements $(\omega_{ki}, P^{k,i}, \Phi^{k,i})$ $(i = 1, \dots, s^n)$. Note that such a subdivision of finite elements produces a new set of finite elements $\mathcal{F}^{h/s}$. This set has $K^{h/s}$ elements, s^n times more than K^h. Suppose that both sets satisfy the coherency and continuity conditions. Denote a space of trial functions and a set of functionals for $\mathcal{F}^h$ and $\mathcal{F}^{h/s}$ by P^h and Φ^h, $P^{h/s}$ and $\Phi^{h/s}$, respectively. Moreover, let $P^h \subset P^{h/s}$. Then, every basis function $p_k^h \in P^h$ is a linear combination of several basis functions $p_j^{h/s} \in P^{h/s}$. Indeed, $p_k^h \in P^{h/s}$ and, hence,

$$p_k^h = \sum_{j=1}^{N^{h/s}} \beta_{kj}^{h,h/s} p_j^{h/s}. \tag{3.33}$$

This basis function corresponds to some node $\bar{a} \in A^h$ and is therefore non-zero only on those cells ω_k where $r \in J_{\bar{a}}^h$ (see (3.17)). On all other cells as well as on their component parts $\omega_{k,i}$, it identically equals zero. Therefore, most of the weights $\beta_{kj}^{h,h/s}$ in (3.33) are equal to zero in view of the linearity of the functionals from $\Phi^{h/s}$ except those, whose nodes are found in the strict interior of the set $\bigcup_{k \in J_{\bar{a}}} \omega_k$. Obviously, their number does not depend on h/s and is related to the configuration of the subdivision (3.11). Let us introduce a special integer constant $q^{h/s}$ standing for the maximal (for all $k = 1, \dots, K^h$) number of the non-zero coefficients $\beta_{ij}^{h,h/s}$ in (3.33).

Note that thereby *the operation of interpolation* is defined as

$$I_{h/s}^h : \; P^h \to P^{h/s}. \tag{3.34}$$

On the functional level, it coincides with the identical transformation, since $\forall v \in P^h$ $v = I_{h/s}^h(v)$. On the algorithmical level, it leads to some arithmetical operations. The point is that one of the most common ways to store the function $v \in P^h$ is to memorize the vector of degrees of freedom α_k^h in the expansion of function v in terms of the basis:

$$v = \sum_{k=1}^{N^h} \alpha_k^h p_k^h. \tag{3.35}$$

The algorithmical image of function v in the space $P^{h/s}$ will then consist of $N^{h/s}$ degrees of freedom $\alpha_j^{h/s}$ calculated by the rule

$$\alpha_j^{h/s} = \sum_{k=1}^{N^h} \alpha_k^h \beta_{kj}^{h,h/s}. \tag{3.36}$$

This follows from (3.33), (3.35) and

$$v = \sum_{j=1}^{N^{h/s}} \alpha_j^{h/s} p_j^{h/s}. \tag{3.37}$$

Thus, the operation of interpolation is estimated, in the sense of its algorithmical complexity, by $(2q^{h/s} - 1)N^{h/s}$ arithmetical operations of multiplication and addition.

Relation (3.33) also permits to determine the transformation $R_h^{h/s} : P^{h/s} \to P^h$; we call it *operation of restriction.* Take the function $v \in P^{h/s}$ represented by formula (3.37) and compute the weights α_k^h by the rule

$$\alpha_k^h = \sum_{j=1}^{N^{h/s}} \beta_{kj}^{h,h/s} \alpha_j^{h/s}. \tag{3.38}$$

As a result, we have a function $w \in P^h$ represented in the form

$$w = \sum_{k=1}^{N^h} \alpha_k^h p_k^h. \tag{3.39}$$

Actually, this is the result of the operation of restriction $R_h^{h/s}(v)$. As to algorithmical complexity, this operation is estimated by $(2q^{h/s} - 1)N^h$ arithmetical operations.

There exists an obvious isomorphis between trial functions spaces P^h, $P^{h/s}$ and, respectively, arithmetical ones $\mathbf{R}^{N^h}$, $\mathbf{R}^{N^{h/s}}$ established by (3.35) and (3.37). We will therefore use the same notation $I_{h/s}^h$ and $R_h^{h/s}$ for vector mappings

$$I_{h/s}^h \quad : \quad \mathbf{R}^{N^h} \to \mathbf{R}^{N^{h/s}}, \tag{3.40}$$

$$R_h^{h/s} \quad : \quad \mathbf{R}^{N^{h/s}} \to \mathbf{R}^{N^h}, \tag{3.41}$$

defined by the rules (3.36) and (3.38).

Let us now obtain the conditions which ensure the nesting

$$P^h \subset P^{h/s}. \tag{3.42}$$

They can most easily be classified for the Lagrange finite elements.

Assume that the following requirements, which concerns spaces of admissible functions P^k and is hereafter called *the nesting condition*, are valid:

1. if ω_k is a simplex, then $P^k = P_l(\omega_k)$ with some integer $l \geq 1$;

2. if ω_k is a rectangle, then P^k is a constriction $Q(\omega_k)$ of some linear space of polynomials Q in local coordinates ω_k;

3. if the curvilinear element (ω_k, P^k, Φ^k) is obtained by (isoparametric) transformation F_k of the pattern $(\tilde{\omega}_k, \tilde{P}^k, \tilde{\Phi}^k)$, then condition 1 or 2, respectively, should hold for the pattern.

This, together with the global continuity and coherency conditions, is sufficient for the nesting (3.42) to hold.

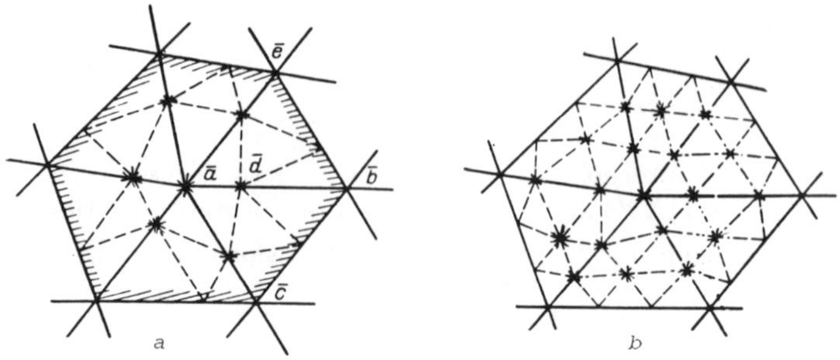

Figure 3.1: The fragment of triangulation after breaking into 4 and 9 parts

Theorem 3.5 *For the set $\mathcal{F}^h$ of the Lagrange finite elements and the set $\mathcal{F}^{h/s}$ obtained by breaking $\mathcal{F}^h$ into s^n parts, $s = 2, 3$, assume that the conditions of coherency, continuity, and for $\mathcal{F}^h$ also nesting condition, hold. Then, $P^h \subset P^{h/s}$.*

Proof. Let us take an arbitrary function $p^h \in P^h$. By virtue of the continuity condition, this function belongs to $C(\bar{\Omega})$.

Since all finite elements in $\mathcal{F}^{h/s}$ are also the Lagrange ones, the function p^h enters, due to continuity, the domain of definition of all functionals from $\Phi^{h/s}$. Let us check if it is contained in the set of admissible functions P of each element $(\omega, P, \Phi) \in \mathcal{F}^{h/s}$. If ω is a simplex, it is obtained by breaking some simplex ω_k of the set $\mathcal{F}^h$. From Remark 3.1.1, $P = P_l(\omega)$ and, hence, p^h belongs to it as a constriction on ω_k. If ω is a rectangle, a similar assertion follows from Remark 3.1.2. A curvilinear element is obtained by transformation $\mathcal{F}_k$, again one of the two Remarks 3.1.1, 3.1.2 is employed. Thus in all three cases, the function p^h is included, as a constriction on ω, in the space of admissible functions P of the element $(\omega, P, \Phi) \in \mathcal{F}^{h/s}$. As the set Φ is P-solvable, the function p^h is reconstructed on ω by values of functionals from $\Phi^{h/s}$ in a unique way. Therfore, since ω is arbitrary, p^h belongs to the linear space of functions such as (3.37) and, hence, to $P^{h/s}$. □

To illustrate this abstract reasoning, we consider simple examples in the two-dimensional case. Take first the Courant elements. Fig. 3.1,*a* shows a fragment of the triangulation of $\bar{\Omega}$ where the support of the basis function $p^h_{\bar{a}} \in P^h$ corresponding to node $\bar{a}$ is marked. It coincides with the set $\bigcup_{r \in J_{\bar{a}}} \omega_r$. Divide each triangulation edge into 2 parts (not necessary equal) and execute the breaking algorithm. The result is dotted in the same figure. Such breaking again generates a concordant triangulation. The continuity condition holds, since linear functions in each of neighbouring cells attain two equal values on the triangulation edge, are linear along it and, hence, coincide on it. The nesting condition is also valid and, hence, any function from P^h belongs to $P^{h/2}$. For example, basis function $p^h_{\bar{a}}$ corresponding to $\bar{a}$ is a linear combination of seven basis functions from $P^{h/2}$ whose nodes are indicated in Fig. 3.1, *a* by $*$. In the same way, the nodes of Fig. 3.1, *b* having non-zero weights in the expansion (3.33) for a basis function corresponding to the node $\bar{a}$, are marked when simplices are broken into 9 parts. Here there are 19 non-zero weights.

Consider now bilinear finite elements on rectangles and quadrangles. Fig. 3.2 shows a fragment of the triangulation of $\bar{\Omega}$ where the support of the basis function

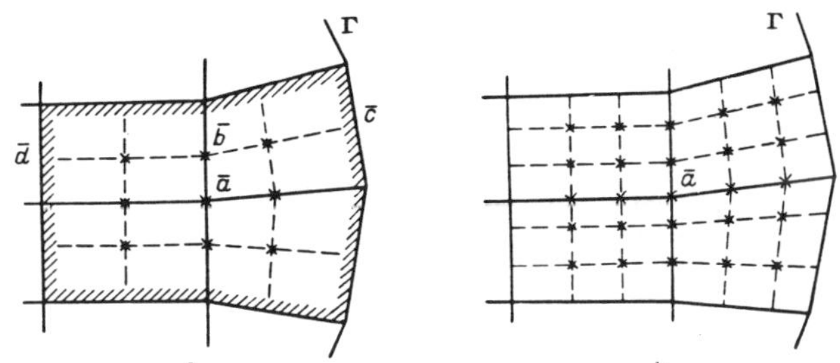

Figure 3.2: The fragment of quadrangular triangulation after breaking into 4 and 9 parts

$p^h_{\bar{a}} \in P^h$ corresponding to the node $\bar{a}$ is marked. It consists of four cells ω_r. Divide each triangulation edge leaving the node $\bar{a}$, into 2 parts (not necessary equal) and execute the algorithm for breaking into 4 parts. The result is dotted in the same figure. Rectangles are broken on two left-hand cells, their isoparametric images — on two right-hande ones. In the specific case of a bilinear element, the points $\bar{c}$, $\bar{d}$ divide its edges in the same ratio as point $\bar{b}$ does. Hence, points $\bar{c}$ and $\bar{d}$ cannot be taken arbitrary, unlike in the case of triangles. Such a subdivision will again produce a concordant quadrangular triangulation unless the quadrangles configuration comes into conflict with the choice of dividing points on the edges. One can avoid such a conflict if breaking all edges into equal parts.

On each triangulation edge between neighbouring cells ω_r and ω_k, the functions from P^r and P^k are linear and attain two equal values at the nodes of the triangulation. Therefore, both functions coincide on $\omega_r \bigcap \omega_k$, i. e., the continuity condition holds. The nesting condition is also valid and, hence, any function from P^h belongs to $P^{h/2}$. For instance, the basis function $p^h_{\bar{a}}$ is a linear combination of nine basis functions from $P^{h/2}$ whose nodes are marked in Fig. 3.2, *a*.

The same piece of a quadrangular triangulation is depicted at Fig. 3.2, *b*. But the breaking into 9 parts has been made. The nodes with non-zero weights in the expansion (3.33) for basis function $p^h_{\bar{a}}$ are marked again. This time, there are 25 of them.

The situation is somewhat different in the case of Hermitian elements. Consider, for example, the Hermitian element $(\omega, P_3(\omega), \Phi_4)$ with a triangular cell ω. Let us again refer to Fig. 3.1, *a*. Take any of the triangles, e. g., $\bar{a}\bar{b}\bar{c}$, and investigate after-effects of dividing into 4 parts. What is different from the case of the Lagrange elements for this subdivision is that trial functions from P^h do not, generally speaking, belong to the domain of definition of $\Phi^{h/2}$ and, hence, P^h is not nested in $P^{h/2}$. Indeed, let us take an arbitrary function $p^h \in P^h$ and consider the point $\bar{d}$. On triangles $\bar{a}\bar{b}\bar{c}$ and $\bar{a}\bar{b}\bar{e}$, it is associated with two different cubic polynomials. Note that at triangle $\bar{a}\bar{b}\bar{c}$, the value of derivative $\partial p^h/\partial x_2$ continuously depends, as it is readily seen from the expansion (2.10), on the values of function p^h and its derivatives at node $\bar{c}$, whereas at $\triangle\bar{a}\bar{b}\bar{e}$ on similar values at node $\bar{e}$. Therefore, they can always be choosen so that the derivatives $\partial p^h/\partial x_2$ at the point $\bar{d}$ are equal to optionally given numbers on both sides of the edge $\bar{a}\bar{b}$. Thus, the coherency condition (3.12) does not hold for function p^h at $\bar{d}$ and so it does not belong to the domain of definition $\Phi^{h/2}$.

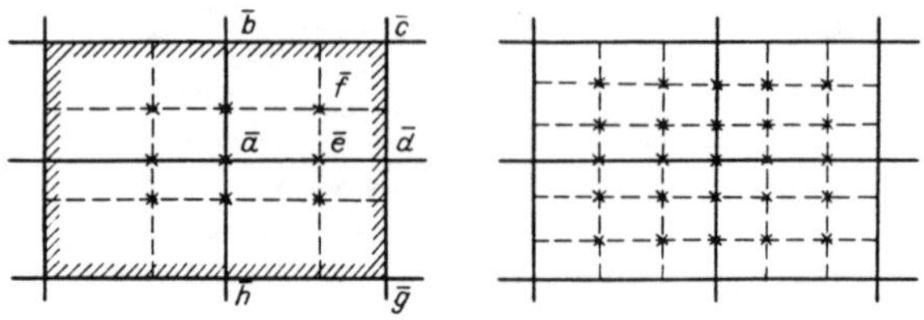

a b

Figure 3.3: The fragment of rectangular triangulation after breaking into 4 and 9 parts

The only exception to the foregoing Hermitian finite elements are bicubic elements on rectangles. In Fig. 3.3, a, we can see a fragment of a rectangular triangulation on which a support of four basis functions corresponding to $\bar{a}$ is marked. It is a union of four rectangles $\bigcup_{r \in J_a} \omega_r$. Divide each triangulation edge from the node $\bar{a}$ into two parts, not necessary equal, and draw stright lines parallel to the rectangles sides. The result is dotted in the same figure. Such a subdivision again generates concordant rectangular triangulation.

Let us prove that an arbitrary function from P^h, first, satisfies the C^1-continuity condition (3.21), (3.22), and second, belongs to the domain of definition $\Phi^{h/2}$. Indeed, take the arbitrary function $p^h \in P^h$. On rectangles $\bar{a}\bar{b}\bar{c}\bar{d}$ and $\bar{a}\bar{d}\bar{g}\bar{h}$ of Fig. 3.3, a, it is associated with two different functions from Q_3. Consider the edge $\bar{a}\bar{d}$. Along it, both functions are cubic polynomials in x_1. In view of the coherency condition (3.12), their values as well as their first derivatives (with respect to x_1) coincide at $\bar{a}$ and $\bar{d}$. This gives 4 conditions for 4 coefficients of cubic polynomials of one variable. Therefore they equal on $\bar{a}\bar{d}$. From this it follows that derivatives $\partial_1 p^h$ calculated as limits on different sides of $\bar{a}\bar{d}$, coincide along $\bar{a}\bar{d}$. The derivatives $\partial_2 p^h$ on $\bar{a}\bar{d}$ are also cubic polynomials in variable x_1 being the limits from both sides of $\bar{a}\bar{d}$. And again, in view of the coherency condition (3.12) at nodes $\bar{a}$, $\bar{d}$, the values of these polynomials and their first derivatives (with respect to x_1) coincide at $\bar{a}$ and $\bar{d}$. These 4 conditions are sufficient for cubic polynomials of one derivative to coincide along $\bar{a}\bar{d}$. From this, it follows that their derivatives with respect to x_1 also coincide along $\bar{a}\bar{d}$. Thus, the functions p^h, $\partial_1 p^h$, $\partial_2 p^h$, and $\partial_{12} p^h$ are continuous at $\bar{a}\bar{d}$. In view of the arbitrariness of the chosen triangulation edge, this results in (3.22) and the C^1-continuity condition.

The continuity of $\partial_{12} p^h$ at $\bar{a}\bar{d}$ is not needed here, but we need it to prove the nesting $P^h \subset P^{h/2}$. We first prove that p^h belongs to the domain of definition of $\Phi^{h/2}$. To this end, we take an arbitrary node from $A^{h/2}$. If it coincides with a node from A^h, e. g., with $\bar{a}$, then the functionals from $\Phi^{h/2}$ are all defined at it, as they coincide with functionals from Φ^h. If it is an interior point of some cell from $\mathcal{F}^h$ (e. g., f), the functionals from $\Phi^{h/2}$ are also defined in a unique way, since the function p^h is infinitely differentiable inside the cell. It remains only to consider the case where a node from $A^{h/2}$ is a point dividing the edge of the cells from $\mathcal{F}^h$ (e. g., $\bar{e}$). We know that as it lies on $\bar{a}\bar{d}$, the four required functionals from $\Phi^{h/2}$ are all defined at it unambiguously. Therefore, function $p^h \in P^h$ belongs to the domain of definition of functionals $\Phi^{h/2}$.

Moreover, for every element $(\omega, P, \Phi) \in \mathcal{F}^{h/2}$, the function p^h belongs to $P = Q_3(\omega)$ as a constriction on ω. Allowing the P-solvability of functionals Φ, we come to unique restoration of p^h on ω. Therefore $p^h \in P^{h/2}$.

This results in particular representation (3.33) of basis functions p_k^h in the form of a linear combination of basis functions $p_j^{h/2}$. Fig. 3.3, *a* shows the nodes $a \in A^{h/2}$ of basis functions p_k^h which are involved in (3.33) with non-zero weights $\beta_{kj}^{h,h/2}$ for four basis functions p_k^h of node $\bar{a}$. The number of these nodes is 9, and hence, the number of non-zero weights in (3.33) must be 36. In fact, their number is somewhat less. To illustrate this, we introduce the special notation for basis functions following from the representation of an arbitrary function $p \in P^h$:

$$p = \sum_{a \in A^h} (p(a)p_{\bar{a}1}^h + \partial_1 p(a)p_{\bar{a}2}^h + \partial_2 p(a)p_{\bar{a}3}^h + \partial_{12} p(a)p_{\bar{a}4}^h). \tag{3.43}$$

According to the conditions

$$\partial_1 p_{\bar{a}2}^h(\bar{a}) = \partial_2 p_{\bar{a}3}^h(\bar{a}) = \partial_{12} p_{\bar{a}4}^h(\bar{a}) = 0,$$

the weights for functions $p_{\bar{a}2}^{h/2}$, $p_{\bar{a}3}^{h/2}$, $p_{\bar{a}4}^{h/2}$ in (3.33) also vanish. Moreover, $\partial_2 p_{\bar{a}1}^h$ vanishes on the interval $\bar{a}\bar{d}$, and so the corresponding weight for function $p_{\bar{e}3}^{h/2}$ also become zero, etc. As a result, 29 non-zero weights are left for $p_{\bar{a}1}^h$ in (3.33). The same is true for three other basis functions of $\bar{a}$. The constant $q^{h/2}$ is therefore here equal to 29.

Fig. 3.3, *b* shows the same fragment of a rectangular triangulation where breaking was made into 9 parts. The nodes are again marked with non-zero weights in (3.33) for basis functions $p_{\bar{a}i}^h$ $(i = 1, 2, 3, 4)$. There are 25 such nodes. Hence, the number of non-zero weights must be 100. Their number is, in fact, less for each $i = 1, 2, 3, 4$ and the constant $q^{h/2}$ is equal to 89.

3.2 The convergence of the Bubnov-Galerkin method

With the above in mind, we now consider convergence of the Bubnov-Galerkin method, assuming that the domain Ω is exactly representated as a union of cells (3.11).

3.2.1 The solution of an operator equation

In order to state the main result on the accuracy of the Bubnov-Galerkin method solution, it remains only to combine the existing facts. Recall that we study the closeness of the solutions of two problems with $H^h \subset H_A$:

1. find $u \in H_A$:

$$\mathcal{L}(u, v) = f(v) \qquad \forall v \in H_A; \tag{3.44}$$

2. find $u^h \in H^h$:

$$\mathcal{L}(u^h, v) = f(v) \qquad \forall v \in H^h. \tag{3.45}$$

Theorem 3.6 [182]. *Assume that the bilinear form $\mathcal{L}$ is bounded and positive definite in the space H_A with the norm, equivalent to $W_2^m(\Omega)$ with some integer m, the functional f is bounded in H_A and the solution $u \in W_2^{k+1}(\Omega) \bigcap H_A$ for $k \geq m$. Also assume that the conditions of Theorem 3.3 or 3.4 with $r = m$ are satisfied for problem (3.45). Then, (3.45) has a unique solution $u^h \in H^h$ which obeys the condition*

$$\|u - u^h\|_{m,\Omega} \leq ch^{k+1-m}\|u\|_{k+1,\Omega}. \tag{3.46}$$

Thus the error is $O(h^{k+1-m})$ in a norm equivalent to an energetic one, where $2m$ is the order of the differential equation and k is the local order of accuracy of approximation by finite elements. Note that from the imbedding theorem, the error $|u - u^h|_{0,\Omega}$ will, at least, be of order $O(h^{k+1-m})$. But in the norm $|\cdot|_{0,\Omega}$, the accuracy order of interpolation is greater. We prove that the error $|u - u^h|_{0,\Omega}$ is also of a greater order. To this end, we use a method developed independently by J. A. Nitsche [139], J. P. Aubin [8], L. A. Oganesian, L. A. Rukhovetz [145].

Introduce the auxiliary (adjoint) problem: find a function $w \in H_A$ such that

$$\mathcal{L}(v, w) = (g, v) \qquad \forall v \in H_A, \tag{3.47}$$

where $g \in L_2(\Omega)$. Note that in the case of the symmetric bilinear form $\mathcal{L}$, the problems coincide when $f(v) = (f, v)$. Suppose that this problem is regular in the following sense: for any $g \in L_2(\Omega)$, the solution $w \in W_2^{2m}(\Omega) \bigcap H_A$ exists and is unique and the estimate

$$\|w\|_{2m,\Omega} \leq c|g|_{0,\Omega} \tag{3.48}$$

is valid.

Theorem 3.7 [40]. *Let for the problems (3.44) and (3.45) the conditions of Theorem 3.6 be satisfied and let the adjoint problem (3.47) be regular. Then for $k + 1 \geq 2m$*

$$|u - u^h|_{0,\Omega} \leq ch^{k+1}\|u\|_{k+1,\Omega}, \tag{3.49}$$

and for $m \leq k + 1 < 2m$

$$|u - u^h|_{0,\Omega} \leq ch^{2(k+1-m)}\|u\|_{k+1,\Omega}. \tag{3.50}$$

Proof. Assume $v = g = u - u^h$ in (3.47). Then $|u - u^h|_{0,\Omega}^2 = |(g, u - u^h)| = |\mathcal{L}(u - u^h, w)| = |\mathcal{L}(u - u^h, w - v^h)| \quad \forall v^h \in H^h$. By virtue of the boundedness of the bilinear form $\mathcal{L}$

$$|u - u^h|_{0,\Omega}^2 \leq c\|u - u^h\|_{m,\Omega}\|w - v^h\|_{m,\Omega}. \tag{3.51}$$

Let us take v^h as the interpolant of w in H^h, i. e., $v^h = I_h w$. Then from Theorem 3.3 or 3.4

$$\|w - v^h\|_{m,\Omega} \leq \begin{cases} ch^m\|w\|_{2m,\Omega}, & \text{if } k+1 \geq 2m, \\ ch^{k+1-m}\|w\|_{2m,\Omega}, & \text{otherwise.} \end{cases} \tag{3.52}$$

From Theorem 3.6 it follows that

$$\|u - u^h\|_{m,\Omega} \le ch^{k+1-m}\|u\|_{k+1,\Omega}. \tag{3.53}$$

Taking (3.48) and (3.51)-(3.53) together, we obtain the estimate

$$|u - u^h|^2_{0,\Omega} \le c\|u\|_{k+1,\Omega}|u - u^h|_{0,\Omega} \begin{cases} h^{k+1}, & \text{if } k+1 \ge 2m \\ h^{2(k+1-m)}, & \text{if } m \le k+1 < 2m \end{cases}$$

whence, actually, the statement of the theorem follows. □

Further, we will deal only with the case (3.49). Thus, on the natural additional assumption that the adjoint problem is regular, the error of the Bubnov-Galerkin method is, in L_2-norm, of the same order as the error of local interpolation.

Applying the results on n-diameters to the finite elements discussed, one can show that the obtained orders of accuracy cannot be improved [146], [40]. Namely, in the class $W_2^m(\Omega) \bigcap H_A$, there always exists a function u such that it obeys either

$$\inf_{v \in H^h} \|u - v\|_{m,\Omega} \ge ch^{k+1-m}\|u\|_{k+1,\Omega}, \qquad k+1 \ge m, \tag{3.54}$$

or

$$\inf_{v \in H^h} \|u - v\|_{0,\Omega} \ge ch^{k+1}\|u\|_{k+1,\Omega}. \tag{3.55}$$

In the case of the fourth-order equations, when $m = 2$, the requirement for the first derivatives to be estimated may arise. This estimate can be obtained either from multiplication inequalities for norms [94] or as in Theorem 3.7 and takes the form

$$\|u - u^h\|_{s,\Omega} \le ch^{k+1-s}\|u\|_{k+1,\Omega}, \tag{3.56}$$

where in our case $s = 1$.

Sometimes we need to estimate the norms of derivatives whose order is greater than in an energetic norm. In this case, the method of "inverse inequalities" is used [40]. It holds when realizing the ("inverse") assumption

$$h/diam\,\omega \le c \qquad \forall \omega \in \mathcal{F}^h. \tag{3.57}$$

The result is that the inverse inequalities take the form of the following constraint for the norms:

$$\|v\|_{1,\Omega} \le \frac{c}{h}|v|_{0,\Omega} \qquad \forall v \in H^h. \tag{3.58}$$

They lead to the estimate (3.56), where s can be larger than m [40].

The multiplication inequalities of [94] together with (3.58) give a simple method for obtaining the error estimates in the norms of $W_p^m(\Omega)$, where $p \in [1, \infty]$, in terms of error estimates in $W_2^m(\Omega)$ with various m.

3.2.2 The spectral problem

In this section, we discuss (without proof) the main results on the accuracy obtained when solving the spectral problem by the Bubnov-Galercin method. The discussion will concern the differential problem written in terms of bilinear forms $\mathcal{L}$ and b: *find a number λ and a function $u \in H_A$ such that*

$$\mathcal{L}(u,v) = \lambda b(u,v) \qquad \forall v \in H_A. \tag{3.59}$$

Here, $\mathcal{L}$ is a symmetric positive definite and bounded bilinear form in the space H_A with a norm equivalent to $W_2^m(\Omega)$, i. e., for any $u, v \in H_A$

$$\begin{aligned} c_1\|u\|_m &\le \|u\|_{H_A} \le c_2\|u\|_m, \\ \mathcal{L}(u,v) &\le c\|u\|_m\,\|v\|_m, \\ \|u\|_m^2 &\le c\mathcal{L}(u,u); \end{aligned} \tag{3.60}$$

b is the specific bilinear form in $L_2(\Omega)$ generated by the bounded positive function

$$b(u,v) = \int_\Omega buv\,dx, \quad 0 < c_3 \le b \le c_4. \tag{3.61}$$

Recall that the Bubnov-Galerkin method associates this problem with the discrete problem in space H^h dense in H_A in the sense of limit: *find a number λ^h and a function $u^h \in H^h$ such that*

$$\mathcal{L}(u^h,v) = \lambda^h b(u^h,v) \quad \forall v \in H^h. \tag{3.62}$$

We first formulate the statement for eigenvalues.

Theorem 3.8 [182]. *Assume that conditions* (3.60) *and* (3.61) *are satisfied for $\mathcal{L}$ and b, eigenfunctions of problem* (3.59) *belong to $W_2^m(\Omega)$, and conditions of Theorem* 3.3 *or* 3.4 *with $r = m$ are satisfied for problem* (3.62). *Then there is a constant δ such that for any integer l, we can find a small h_0 such that $\forall h \le h_0$*

$$\lambda_l \le \lambda_l^h \le \lambda_l + \delta h^{2(k+1-m)}\lambda_l^{(k+1)/m}, \tag{3.63}$$

where λ_l and λ_l^h are the l-th eigenvalues of problems (3.59) *and* (3.62), *respectively.*

First note that approximate eigenvalues are always larger than exact ones with the same number. Second, the error of approximation with respect to order is equal to the square of the error of the eigenfunction interpolant in an energetic or any other equivalent norm. Third, increasing the eigenvalue number results in increasing not only an absolute error but also a relative one, since for the converging case $(k+1)/m > 1$. This is why the eigenvalues of large orders are much more difficult to calculate. Finally, the requirement for h_0 to be sufficiently small is related to the fact that because of rather small dimension, the number of eigenvalues of the discrete problem (3.62) can be less than l. The eigenvalues with large numbers appear while sufficiently refining Ω and, hence, while increasing the dimension of problem (3.62).

For approximate eigenfunctions u_l^h, it is shown that their errors are of the same value as the errors of the operator equation from the preceding section, the only difference being that a dependence on l appears.

To avoid a superfluous degree of freedom, in both problems we again consider only normed eigenfunctions, i. e., such that

$$b(u,u) = 1. \tag{3.64}$$

Theorem 3.9 [182]. *When the assumptions of Theorem 3.8 are satisfied, for any eigenfunction u_l^h we can find a function u^h of problem (3.59) from the eigensubspace, corresponding to the eigenvalue λ_l, such that*

$$\|u_l - u_l^h\|_{m,\Omega} \leq ch^{k+1-m}\lambda_l^{(k+1)/2m}, \tag{3.65}$$

$$|u_l - u_l^h|_{0,\Omega} \leq c(h^{k+1} + h^{2(k+1-m)})\lambda_l^{(k+1)/2m}, \tag{3.66}$$

where the constants are independent of l and h.

In the most frequently used case where the local order of approximation $k+1$ obeys the inequality $k+1 \geq 2m$, the value between brackets on the right-hand side of (3.66) can be taken equal to h^{k+1}. Therefore in L_2-norm and in the norm equivalent to the energetic one, the order of error is the same as in the case of the operator equation.

Note a difficulty of calculating the higher fast oscilating eigenfunctions.

3.2.3 The mixed method

Let us now investigate the accuracy of a mixed method. Assume that there exist two problems, namely, the initial one:

$$\begin{aligned} a(u,v) + b(v,\varphi) &= f(v) \quad \forall v \in V, \\ b(u,\psi) &= g(\psi) \quad \forall \psi \in W, \end{aligned} \tag{3.67}$$

and the approximate one:

$$\begin{aligned} a(u^h,v) + b(v,\varphi^h) &= f(v) \quad \forall v \in V^h, \\ b(u^h,\psi) &= g(\psi) \quad \forall \psi \in W^h. \end{aligned} \tag{3.68}$$

The bilinear forms a, b and the functionals f, g satisfy the conditions of subsections 1.2.3 and 1.1.2.

Theorem 3.10 . *Let the norms $\|\cdot\|_V$, $\|\cdot\|_W$ in the spaces V, W be equivalent to the norms $\|\cdot\|_{m,\Omega_1}$ and $\|\cdot\|_{s,\Omega_2}$, respectively, and let for the finite-element approximations V^h, W^h the conditions of Theorem 3.3 or 3.4 with $r = m$ for V^h and $r = s$ for W^h be satisfied. Also assume that the conditions of Theorems 1.15 and 1.3 are satisfied for problems (3.67), (3.68) and that the solution of (3.67) exhibits the following smoothness: $u \in W_2^{m+k}(\Omega_1)$, $\varphi \in W_2^{s+k}(\Omega_2)$ for some $k > 0$. Then, (3.68) has the unique solution $u^h \in V^h$, $\varphi^h \in W^h$ which obeys the estimate*

$$\|u - u^h\|_{m,\Omega_1} + \|\varphi - \varphi^h\|_{s,\Omega_2} \leq ch^k(\|u\|_{m+k,\Omega_1} + \|\varphi\|_{s+k,\Omega_2}). \tag{3.69}$$

In the case $m \geq 1$, it is possible to use the dual argument principle as it was the case in 3.2.1 when justifying a higher accuracy of u^h in L_2-norm:

$$\|u - u^h\|_{0.\Omega_1} \leq ch^{k+m}(\|u\|_{m+k,\Omega_1} + \|\varphi\|_{s+k,\Omega_2}) \quad \text{when} \quad k \geq m. \tag{3.70}$$

Without discussing this method in the general case, we use it further in particular cases.

3.3 The use of quadrature formulae

Assembly of discrete algebraic systems (1.129), (1.143), (1.156) is connected with computation of integrals of coefficients and right-hand side. In overwelming majority of situations, one can not execute this integration exactly. Therefore, numerical integration is an important part of the finite elements method. In this section, the closure of domain Ω is supposed to be, as before, the union (3.11) of cells ω_k. Then, to compute the coefficients of algebraic system in the Bubnov-Galerkin method, we should use the quadrature scheme: every element of the matrix or the right-hand side takes the form

$$\sum_{k=1}^{K_h} \int_{\omega_k} \varphi(x)dx, \tag{3.71}$$

where the integral over a cell is approximated by the finite sum

$$\int_{\omega_k} \varphi(x)dx \approx \sum_{l=1}^{L} \alpha_{kl}\varphi(\beta_{kl}) \tag{3.72}$$

with weights $\alpha_{kl} \neq 0$ and nodes $\beta_{kl} \in \omega_k$.

3.3.1 Influence of isoparametric or affine transformations

As in subsection 2.4.1, when dealing with the isoparametric or affine-transformed element $(\tilde{\omega}, \tilde{P}, \tilde{\Phi}) = F(\omega, P, \Phi)$, one should return to its prototype — the master rectilinear element (ω, P, Φ). Then, for the arbitrary function $\psi : \omega \to \mathbf{R}$ and the superposition $\tilde{\psi}(x) = \psi(F^{-1}(x)) : \tilde{\omega} \to \mathbf{R}$ we have

$$\int_{\tilde{\omega}} \tilde{\psi}(x)dx = \int_{\omega} \psi(y)\frac{\partial F}{\partial y}(y)dy, \tag{3.73}$$

where the Jacobian $\partial F/\partial y$ is strictly positive on ω. Take a quadrature formula such as (3.72) on ω:

$$\int_{\omega} \varphi(y)dy \approx \sum_{l=1}^{L} \alpha_l\varphi(\beta_l). \tag{3.74}$$

Then, by virtue of (3.73), it induces a quadrature formula on $\tilde{\omega}$:

$$\int_{\tilde{\omega}} \tilde{\varphi}(x)dx \approx \sum_{l=1}^{L} \tilde{\alpha}_l\tilde{\varphi}(\tilde{\beta}_l), \tag{3.75}$$

where the weights and the nodes are defined by

$$\tilde{\alpha}_l = \alpha_l\frac{\partial F}{\partial y}(\beta_l) \quad \text{and} \quad \tilde{\beta}_l = F(\beta_l), \quad l = 1, \dots, L. \tag{3.76}$$

From this, it follows immediately that the regular transformation F converts the nonzero or positive weights α_l to the same weights $\tilde{\alpha}_l$, and the nodes β_l lying inside ω or on its boundary to the nodes of similar geometry on $\tilde{\omega}$.

So, we have two possibilities. Firstly, we may map a sell $\tilde{\omega}$ to the master sell ω as in subsection 2.4.1 and numerically integrate a transformed function over ω by (3.74). Secondly, we may use the quadrature formula (3.75) directly on $\tilde{\omega}$ which is induced by a formula on ω. In both cases, we deal with a quadrature formula on the master sell ω. Therefore, we dwell on quadrature formulae for master sells most commonly used: for the n-dimensional rectilinear simplex and the rectangle $[-1,1]^n$.

3.3.2 The ellipticity and the accuracy

This process of numerical integration generates the approximating bilinear form $\mathcal{L}_h(\cdot,\cdot)$ and the approximating functional $f_h(\cdot)$. As a result, we arrive at the problem of the definition of a solution $\tilde{u}^h \in H^h$ satisfying the identity

$$\mathcal{L}_h(\tilde{u}^h, v) = f_h(v) \quad \forall v \in H^h. \tag{3.77}$$

When approximating, two requirements are necessary: the ellipticity and the sufficient accuracy. The essence of the first is that the obtained bilinear form $\mathcal{L}_h$ must remain elliptic in $H^h \bigcap W_2^m(\Omega)$, i. e., there must be a constant c such that

$$\mathcal{L}_h(v, v) \geq c\|v\|^2_{m,\Omega} \quad \forall v \in H^h. \tag{3.78}$$

The second requirement is supported by the known result on the relationship of bilinear forms $\mathcal{L}$, $\mathcal{L}_h$ and functionals f, f_h of problems (1.127) and (3.77).

Theorem 3.11 [182]. *Let* (3.78) *be satisfied and for any* $v \in H^h \bigcap W_2^m(\Omega)$

$$|(\mathcal{L} - \mathcal{L}_h)(u^h, v)| + |(f - f_h)(v)| \leq ch^p \|v\|_{m,\Omega}. \tag{3.79}$$

Then the influence of an approximate integration in norm $\|\cdot\|_{m,\Omega}$ *takes the form:*

$$\|u^h - \tilde{u}^h\|_{m,\Omega} \leq ch^p. \tag{3.80}$$

Note that this inequality may give in addition an estimate of the change of the solution u^h (or u) obtained under a disturbance of the coefficients and the right-hand side of the differential equation.

A similar result is valid for the mixed method. Assume that an approximation of a boundary and integrals yields instead of (3.68) the following problem: find $\tilde{u}^h \in V^h$, $\tilde{\varphi}^h \in W^h$ satisfying the relations

$$\begin{aligned} a_h(\tilde{u}^h, v) + b_h(v, \tilde{\varphi}^h) &= f_h(v) \qquad \forall v \in V^h, \\ b_h(\tilde{u}^h, \psi) &= g_h(\psi) \qquad \forall \psi \in W^h. \end{aligned} \tag{3.81}$$

Here a_h, b_h are continuous bilinear forms on $V^h \times V^h$ and $V^h \times W^h$, and f_h, g_h are continuous functionals on V^h, W^h. Also assume that for a_h, b_h the properties are valid which are defined in (1.149)-(1.151) for bilinear forms a, b in spaces V^h, W^h.

These conditions guarantee, from Theorem 1.15, the unique solvability of (3.81). A closeness of the solutions $u^h, \tilde{u}^h$ and $\varphi^h, \tilde{\varphi}^h$ follows from approximating properties of

a_h, b_h, f_h, g_h:

$$\begin{aligned} &|(a-a_h)(v,w)| \le ch^p\|v\|_V\,\|w\|_V \qquad \forall v,w \in V^h,\\ &|(b-b_h)(v,\psi)| \le ch^p\|v\|_V\,\|\psi\|_W \qquad \forall v \in V^h, \psi \in W^h,\\ &|(f-f_h)(v)| \le ch^p\|v\|_V \qquad \forall v \in V^h,\\ &|(g-g_h)(\psi)| \le ch^p\|\psi\|_W \qquad \forall \psi \in W^h. \end{aligned} \tag{3.82}$$

Theorem 3.12 [36]. *Assume that both problems* (3.81) *and* (1.148) *satisfy the conditions* (1.149)-(1.151) *and obey the estimate* (3.82). *Then, the problem* (3.81) *has the unique solution* $\tilde{u}^h$, $\tilde{\varphi}^h$ *which obeys the estimate*

$$\begin{aligned} &\|u-\tilde{u}^h\|_V + \|\varphi-\tilde{\varphi}^h\|_W \le\\ &\le \|u-u^h\|_V + \|\varphi-\varphi^h\|_W + ch^p(\|u^h\|_V + \|\psi^h\|_W). \end{aligned} \tag{3.83}$$

From this theorem, or to be more accurate, from estimates (3.82), the constraints on accuracy of quadrature formulae follow.

The first requirement of ellipticity can be expressed in a different form on the level of the master element [21]. Here we dwell on two constraints which are tested most easily. As it is shown in Theorem 4.1.2 from [40], they are sufficient for the principal part of the equation (1.22). Moreover, one can argue their sufficiency for the principal part of equations (1.64), (1.82) by analogy with mentioned theorem.

Let a space P of admissible functions on the master element (ω, P, Φ) be included in the polinomial space $P_{k'}(\omega)$ and satisfy completeness condition with integer k, i. e.,

$$P_k(\omega) \subset P \subset P_{k'}(\omega). \tag{3.84}$$

Denote the set of functionals (degrees of freedom) like $p \to p(\alpha_l)$ by $\hat{\Phi} = \{p(\alpha_l), l = 1, \ldots, L\}$ where α_l are nodes of a quadrature formula. Then we assume that at least one of two constraints holds:

(i) *the quadrature formula is exact on the polinomial space* $P_{2k'-2m}(\omega)$;

(ii) *the set* $\hat{\Phi}$ *contains a* $P_{k'-m}(\omega)$*-solvable subset.*

Usually one more constraint is added:

(iii) *weights* α_l *are positive,* $l = 1, \ldots, L$.

Nevertheless, even if some quadrature formula has negative weights, we can use it under the first constraint for a continuous integrand function and a sufficiently small diameter of a sell $\tilde{\omega}$ (not ω!). Apropos of this, see Remark 3.1.1 below.

Now consider the constraint for accuracy of the quadrature formula:

(iv) *the quadrature formula is exact on the polinomial space* $P_{k'+k-2m}(\omega)$.

This constraint is sufficient to achieve the necessary accuracy when numerically integrating the principal part in (1.22), (1.64), (1.82). For integration of lower-order terms and the right-hand side, the requirements are usually weaker. These facts are argued in detail for $m = 1$ in [40].

Now we specially collect above information for simplices. For elements mentioned in Chapter 2 (exepting Bell's triangle), we have $P_k(\omega) = P = P_{k'}(\omega)$. In this case, constraints (i) and (iv) coincide and give the condition close to necessary one.

The situation is somewhat worse for rectangular elements on $[-1,1]^n$. For serendipity elements, we have the inclusion $Q'_k(\omega) \subset P_{k+n-1}(\omega)$. As a result, k' equals $k+n-1$

in constraint (iv) . This gives the requirements for the order of accuracy which are appropriate for $n = 2$ and slightly excessive for $n = 3$. For the complete element, the inclusion has a form $Q_k(\omega) \subset P_{nk}(\omega)$. Hence, k' equals nk, which is not constructive within the framework of (iv). Therefore, we employ results of Exercise 4.1.7 from [40] where the following inclusion is assumed as a basis:

$$P_k(\omega) \subset P \subset Q_k(\omega). \tag{3.85}$$

Then, the following constraint together with (iii) are sufficient for ellipticity:

(v) the set $\hat{\Phi}$ contains a $Q_k(\omega) \cap P_{nk-m}(\omega)$-solvable subset.

For the order of accuracy, the following constraint is sufficient:

(vi) the quadrature formula is exact on $Q_{2k-m}(\omega)$.

Finally, one more simple reason is useful. Let $\partial^m P$ denote the polinomial space of every possible partial derivatives of the order m for all elements of the space P and let $\dim \partial^m P$ be its dimension. Then one can prove ellipticity by analogy with Theorem 4.1.2 from [40] under (iii) and the following constraint:

(vii) the set $\hat{\Phi}$ contains a $\partial^m P$-solvable subset.

Hence,

(viii) the number L of nodes of the quadrature formula is not less than $\dim \partial^m P$.

3.3.3 The two-dimensional case

We first consider finite elements on simplices for the second-order equations ($m = 1$).

To preserve the order of accuracy which can be achieved by the Courant elements, the simplest quadrature formula No.1[1] with the central node from Table 3.1 or the threepoint formula No.2 are suitable. As to the number of references to φ, the first formula seems three times as effective. Indeed, denote by $op(\varphi)$ the number of arithmetical operations needed to calculate the function φ. Then, if $op(\varphi) \gg 1$, formulae No.1 and No.2 show $op(\varphi)$ and $3op(\varphi)$, respectively. But in fact, when calculating in a different way, the value $\varphi(x)$ at the triangulation node x is used, as a rule, in six cells. The virtual cost of three calculations of φ on a triangulation is therefore estimated as $0.5\,op(\varphi)$. Comparing this with the quantity evaluated earlier, we see that the second quadrature formula on a triangulation may be twice as effective than the first one in the case when $op(\varphi) \gg 1$.

It is sufficient for the Lagrange elements of degree 2 to use threepoint formula No.3 of Table 3.1 exact for polynomials from P_2. It has a minimum of the nodes which are, in addition, well arranged.

To preserve the accuracy of the Lagrange and Hermitian elements of degree 3, one should use the quadrature formula which is exact for polynomials from P_4. Such formula is provided in Table 3.1 under No.5. It has 10 nodes. Nine of them lie on sides, which diminishes its cost on a triangulation. In order that $f_h(\cdot)$ should integrate numerically, it is sufficient to use sevenpoint formula No.4, exact on P_3.

Remark 3.3.1 *This formula has negative weights α_i. We may attach no importance to this fact during numerical integration of the right-hand side $f_h(v)$. But this is important for integration in $\mathcal{L}_h$ because it is possible to violate the ellipticity of the approximate*

[1] Here and hereafter formula's number is the same as line's number in corresponding table.

Table 3.1: Quadrature formulae for the two-dimensional simplex

No	Number of nodes L	Space integrable exactly	Nodes β_l	Baricentric coordinates of nodes λ_1	λ_2	Weights α_l	Position of weights and cost	Reference
1	1	P_1	β_1	1/3	1/3	1/2	1 *op* 	[40] [160],
2	3	P_1	β_1	1	0	1/6	0.5 *op* 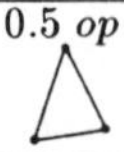	[160], [136]
			β_2	0	1	1/6		
			β_3	0	0	1/6		
3	3	P_2	β_1	1/2	0	1/6	1.5 *op* 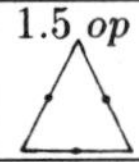	[40], [160], [183]
			β_2	1/2	1/2	1/6		
			β_3	0	1/2	1/6		
4	7	P_3	β_1	0	0	1/40	3 *op* 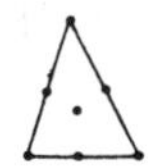	[40]
			β_2	1	0	1/40		
			β_3	0	1	1/40		
			β_4	1/2	1/2	1/15		
			β_5	1/2	0	1/15		
			β_6	0	1/2	1/15		
			β_7	1/3	1/3	9/40		
5	10	P_4	β_1	0	0	$-1/120$	4.5 *op* 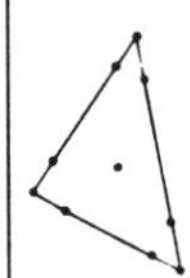	derived by author
			β_2	0	1	$-1/120$		
			β_3	1	0	$-1/120$		
			β_4	1/3	1/3	9/40		
			$\beta_5 - \beta_6$	$\frac{(3 \pm \sqrt{3})}{6}$	$\frac{(3 \mp \sqrt{3})}{6}$	1/20		
			$\beta_7 - \beta_8$	0	$\frac{(3 \pm \sqrt{3})}{6}$	1/20		
			$\beta_9 - \beta_{10}$	$\frac{(3 \pm \sqrt{3})}{6}$	0	1/20		

bilinear form $\mathcal{L}_h(\cdot,\cdot)$. When oscillations of coefficients a_{ij} are sufficiently small, this fact does not present difficulties [40]. *In practice, the level of littleness is established as follows. Let μ be the ellipticity constant of the bilinear form $\mathcal{L}$ and let ε be the maximal oscillation level of the coefficients a_{ij} in the principal part:*

$$\varepsilon \geq \max_{1 \leq i,j \leq n} \max_{x,x' \in \omega} |a_{ij}(x) - a_{ij}(x')|. \tag{3.86}$$

Then, for $\mathcal{L}_h(\cdot,\cdot)$ to be elliptic, it is necessary that

$$\varepsilon \sum_{l=1}^{L} |\alpha_l| \leq \mu/2n. \tag{3.87}$$

On a rough grid, this condition can be not satisfied. See also Exercise 4.1.2 *in* [40].

When further increasing the degree k of Lagrangian elements, it is necessary to use formulae exact on P_{2k-2} [40]. In principle, we can obtain such formulae with an arbitrary order by mapping the tensor Gaussian (or Lobatto) formulae from $[-1,1]^2$

Table 3.2: Quadrature formulae for the square $[-1,1]^2$

No	Number of nodes L	Space integrable exactly	Nodes β_l	Coordinates x_1	Coordinates x_2	Weights α_l	Position of weights and cost	Reference
1	1	P_1, Q_1	β_1	0	0	4	1 *op* 	[136]
2	4	P_1, Q_1	$\beta_1-\beta_4$	±1	±1	1	1 *op* 	[136]
3	5	P_3	$\beta_1-\beta_4$ β_5	±1 0	±1 0	1/3 8/3	2 *op* 	[136]
4	9	P_3, Q_3	$\beta_1-\beta_4$ β_5,β_6 β_7,β_8 β_9	±1 0 ±1 0	±1 ±1 0 0	1/9 4/9 4/9 16/9	4 *op* 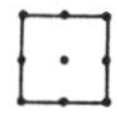	[136]
5	13	P_5	$\beta_1-\beta_4$ $\beta_5-\beta_8$ $\beta_9-\beta_{12}$ β_{13}	±1 ±1 $\pm\sqrt{\frac{3}{5}}$ 0	±1 $\pm\sqrt{\frac{3}{5}}$ ±1 0	$-5/9$ 5/9 5/9 16/9	6 *op* 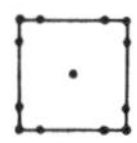	derived by author
6	12	P_5	$\beta_1-\beta_4$ β_5,β_6 β_7,β_8 $\beta_9-\beta_{12}$	±1 0 ±1 $\pm\sqrt{\frac{3}{13}}$	±1 ±1 0 $\pm\sqrt{\frac{3}{13}}$	16/225 8/45 8/45 169/225	7 *op* 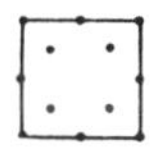	derived by author
7	16	P_5, Q_5	$\beta_1-\beta_4$ $\beta_5-\beta_8$ $\beta_9-\beta_{12}$ $\beta_{13}-\beta_{16}$	±1 ±1 $\pm\frac{1}{\sqrt{5}}$ $\pm\frac{1}{\sqrt{5}}$	±1 $\pm\frac{1}{\sqrt{5}}$ ±1 $\pm\frac{1}{\sqrt{5}}$	1/36 5/36 5/36 25/36	9 *op* 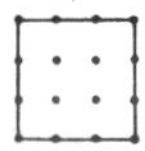	Cartesian product of Lobatto formula

into triangle [136]. But in [50], symmetrical formulae are derived for exact integration of P_k up to $k = 20$ which are significantly more economical than Gaussian or Lobatto products on the triangle.

Let us now consider finite elements with rectangular cells. We begin with the second-order equations ($m = 1$).

For the Lagrange element of degree 1, formula No.2 of Table 3.2 should be taken. It is exact for polynomials Q_1 and gives the same contribution as the error of approximation by bilinear finite elements. The quadrature formula (of a midpoint) No.1 gives the same accuracy. But its application does not yield the condition (3.78) for the approximate bilinear form $\mathcal{L}_h$ to be positive definite, because of the small number of the nodes. According to constraint (*iii*), no fewer than 3 nodes are needed. Thus, application of formula No.1 to $\mathcal{L}_h$ results in an unstable scheme. True, formula No.1 can be used to compute lower-order terms.

The Cartesian product of the twopoint quadrature Gauss formulae gives even greater accuracy [136]. It is exact on Q_3 and has as many nodes as formula No.2. But its application to equations with varying coefficients is 4 times as laborious. Indeed, every node of formula No.2 is, as a rule, a vertex of four triangulation quadrangles. Therefore, when $op(\varphi) \gg 1$ the virtual cost of formula No.2 on a quadrangular triangulation is $op(\varphi)$, whereas the cost of the Gauss quadrature formula is $4op(\varphi)$.

For the serendipity element of degree 2, the quadrature formula should be used which is exact for P_3 and has no fewer than 6 nodes for the positive definiteness of $\mathcal{L}_h(\cdot,\cdot)$ on the basis of constraints (iv), $(viii)$ [40]. Formula No.4 of Table 3.2 would be suitable. Its virtual cost on a quadrangular triangulation for varying coefficients can be brought to $4op(\varphi)$.

The Gauss fourpoint quadrature formula already mentioned is of the same accuracy, but it does not ensure the positive definiteness of $\mathcal{L}_h(\cdot,\cdot)$ because of the small number of the nodes.

For the serendipity element of degree 3, one should take a quadrature formula, exact on P_5, which has no fewer than 10 nodes for the positive definiteness of $\mathcal{L}_h$. Formula No.6 of Table 3.2 is suitable. For varying coefficients, its virtual cost may be carried to $7op(\varphi)$.

When solving second-order equations, the Hermitian element of degree 3 needs the quadrature formula exact on Q_5 and having no fewer than 15 nodes. Formula No.7 is acceptable.

For the serendipity elements of higher degree $k \geq 4$, it is sufficient to use formulae exact on P_{2k-1} according to constraint (iv). In principle, we can obtain appropriate formulae by the tensor product of the one-dimensional Gaussian or Lobatto formulae. For example, if we use the s-point one-dimensional formula, we receive the Gaussian formula exact on Q_{2s-1}, P_{2s-1} and the Lobatto formula exact on Q_{2s-3}, P_{2s-3}. In these cases, we can put $s = k$ for the Gaussian formula and $s = k+1$ for the Lobatto one. Their weights are positive, and the number of nodes is sufficient for validity of constraint (ii). Furthermore, in [51], symmetrical formulae are derived for exact integration of P_k up to $k = 21$ on the rectangle $[-1,1]^2$. They are more economical than Gaussian and Lobatto products.

When solving the fourth-order equations ($m = 2$) with the Hermitian element of degree 3, one should take the quadrature formula exact on Q_4 and having no fewer than 13 nodes on the basis of constraints (v), (vi). The result is that we again arrive at formula No.7.

3.3.4 The three-dimensional case

We first treat finite elements with cells ω shaped as simplices and dwell on the second order equations ($m = 1$) only.

The simplest quadrature formulae No.1 and 2 of Table 3.3 are suitable for the accuracy order of the Lagrange elements of degree 1. If $op(\varphi) \gg 1$, formula No.2 is preferable since each of its nodes is used, as a rule, in 24 cells (see Fig. 2.4). Its virtual cost on a triangulation is therefore 6 times as low than that of formula No.1.

Formula No.3 is adequate to the Lagrange elements of degree 2. Estimating its cost at $op(\varphi) \gg 1$, we take into account that the nodes lying at the edge midpoints enter

Table 3.3: Quadrature formulae for the three-dimensional simplex

No	Number of nodes L	Space integrable exactly	Nodes β_l	Baricentric coordinates of nodes λ_1	λ_2	λ_3	Weights α_l	Position of weights and cost	Reference
1	1	P_1	β_1	1/4	1/4	1/4	1/6	1 *op* 	[136]
2	4	P_1	β_1	0	0	0	1/24	1/6 *op* 	[136]
			β_2	1	0	0	1/24		
			β_3	0	1	0	1/24		
			β_4	0	0	1	1/24		
3	5	P_2	$\beta_1 - \beta_4$	the same as in No 2			1/120	7/6 *op* 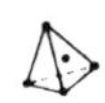	derived by author
			β_5	1/4	1/4	1/4	2/15		
4	11	P_3	$\beta_1 - \beta_4$	the same as in No 2			1/360	13/6 *op* 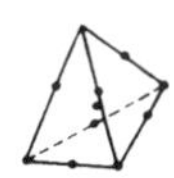	derived by author
			β_5	1/4	1/4	1/4	4/45		
			β_6	1/2	0	0	1/90		
			β_7	0	1/2	0	1/90		
			β_8	0	0	1/2	1/90		
			β_9	1/2	1/2	0	1/90		
			β_{10}	1/2	0	1/2	1/90		
			β_{11}	0	1/2	1/2	1/90		
5	21	P_4	$\beta_1 - \beta_4$	the same as in No 2			31/5040	31/6 *op*	derived by author
			β_5	1/4	1/4	1/4	16/315		
			β_6, β_7	$\delta_\pm$	0	0	2/315		
			β_8, β_9	0	$\delta_\pm$	0	2/315		
			β_{10}, β_{11}	0	0	$\delta_\pm$	2/315		
			β_{12}, β_{13}	$\delta_\pm$	$\delta_\mp$	0	2/315	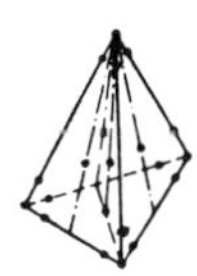	
			β_{14}, β_{15}	$\delta_\pm$	0	$\delta_\mp$	2/315		
			β_{16}, β_{17}	0	$\delta_\pm$	$\delta_\mp$	2/315		
			β_{18}	1/3	1/3	0	9/560		
			β_{19}	1/3	0	1/3	9/560		
			β_{20}	0	1/3	1/3	9/560		
			β_{21}	1/3	1/3	1/3	9/560	$\delta_\pm = \dfrac{\sqrt{2} \pm 1}{2\sqrt{2}}$	

in 6 cells on the average (see Fig. 2.4).

In order to preserve the accuracy of the Lagrange elements of degree 3, one should take quadrature formula No.5. Of all known quadrature formulae exact on P_4, it has the minimal number of nodes. Eleven nodes lie inside ω and, hence, its cost is relatively high for varying coefficients.

When further increasing the degree $k \geq 4$ of the Lagrangian elements, the formula exact on P_{2k-2} is sufficient for both ellipticity and accuracy on the basis of constraints (i), (iv). We can obtain such formulae with an arbitrary order by mapping the tensor Gaussian or Lobatto formulae from $[-1,1]^3$ into the simplex.

Let us now consider finite elements with the cubic cell $[-1,1]^3$.

For the Lagrange element of degree 1, formula No.2 of Table 3.4 should be taken. It retains the accuracy achieved in approximating by trilinear finite elements. The same accuracy is generated by quadrature formula of a midpoint No.1. But its application does not yield the condition (3.78) of the positive definiteness of the bilinear form $\mathcal{L}_h$ because of the small number of nodes. According to constraint (v), they are need to be no fewer than 7. Thus, application of formula No.1 allows to compute lower-order terms only.

We obtain even greater accuracy when using the Cartesian product of the twopoint quadrature Gauss formulae. It is exact on Q_3 and has the same number of the nodes — 8. But it is eight times as laborious than formula No.2 when applied to varying coefficients. Indeed, every node of formula No.2 is, as a rule, a vertex of eight triangulation hexahedra. Therefore at $op(\varphi) \gg 1$, the virtual cost of formula No.2 is estimated by $op(\varphi)$, whereas that of the quadrature Gauss formula is $8op(\varphi)$.

For the serendipity element of degree 2, one should take the quadrature formula which is exact on Q_3 and has no fewer than 17 nodes to ensure the positive definiteness of $\mathcal{L}_h$ on the basis of (vi) and (vii). Pay attention that the eightpoint Gaussian formula is not suitable for the reason of the little number of nodes. But the 27-point Lobatto formula (a tensor product) is acceptable.

For the serendipity element of degree 3, the quadrature formula should be taken which is exact on Q_5 and has no fewer than 29 nodes to ensure the positive definiteness of $\mathcal{L}_h$. Again, the 27-point Gaussian formula is not suitable, but the 64-point Lobatto formula is acceptable. Although both formulae have the same order of accuracy.

For the serendipity elements of degree $k \geq 4$, the quadrature formula should be exact on Q_{2k-1} on the basis of (vi). This time, the three-dimensional tensor product of the k-point Gaussian formula is acceptable because of a great number of nodes.

3.4 The approximation of boundary conditions

Currently there exist two approaches to the account of boundary conditions, distinguished from one another for different requirements for a triangulation. The first way is to approximate the boundary by triangulation cells as accurately as possible; which leads to isoparametric elements. The second way is to modify the Bubnov-Galerkin method so that basis functions could obey no boundary conditions, and a triangulation unconformable with boundary Γ could be used. The latter can be illustrated by the third boundary value problem where boundary conditions enter directly in a bilinear form, boundary functions are not required to satisfy boundary conditions, and so a

Table 3.4: Quadrature formulae for the cube $[-1,1]^3$

No	Number of nodes L	Space integ-rable exactly	Nodes β_l	Coordinates x_1	x_2	x_3	Weights α_l	Position of weights and cost	Reference
1	1	P_1, Q_1	β_1	0	0	0	8	1 *op* 	[136]
2	8	P_1, Q_1	$\beta_1-\beta_8$	±1	±1	±1	1	1 *op* 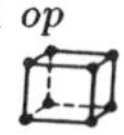	[136]
3	9	P_3	$\beta_1-\beta_8$	±1	±1	±1	1/3	2 *op* 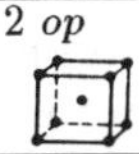	[136]
			β_9	0	0	0	16/3		
4	20	P_3	$\beta_1-\beta_8$	±1	±1	±1	-1	4 *op* 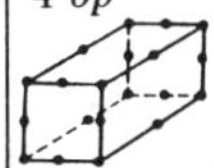	[136]
			$\beta_9-\beta_{12}$	±1	±1	0	4/3		
			$\beta_{13}-\beta_{16}$	±1	0	±1	4/3		
			$\beta_{17}-\beta_{20}$	0	±1	±1	4/3		
5	21	P_3	$\beta_1-\beta_8$	±1	±1	±1	1/6	5 *op* 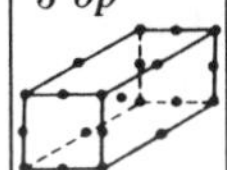	derived by author
			$\beta_9-\beta_{12}$	±1	±1	0	1/6		
			$\beta_{13}-\beta_{16}$	±1	0	±1	1/6		
			$\beta_{17}-\beta_{20}$	0	±1	±1	1/6		
			β_{21}	0	0	0	14/3		
6	33	P_5	$\beta_1-\beta_8$	±1	±1	±1	$-10/9$	8 *op* 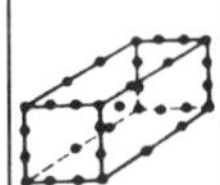	derived by author
			$\beta_9-\beta_{16}$	±1	±1	$\pm\sqrt{\frac{3}{5}}$	5/9		
			$\beta_{17}-\beta_{24}$	±1	$\pm\sqrt{\frac{3}{5}}$	±1	5/9		
			$\beta_{25}-\beta_{32}$	$\pm\sqrt{\frac{3}{5}}$	±1	±1	5/9		
			β_{33}	0	0	0	32/9		

uniform rectangular triangulation not necessary conformable with boundary Γ can be used.

3.4.1 A conformable triangulation and isoparametric elements

Let us first consider the approximation of the main boundary condition

$$u = g \quad \text{on} \quad \Gamma. \tag{3.88}$$

Subsections 2.4.2 and 2.4.3 explain how isoparametric elements are constructed near smooth portions of boundary Γ or near the dividing line between the media. In the two-dimensional case, an additional requirement should be added from section 2.5, namely: all angles of the boundary are vertices of (curvilinear) triangular and quadrangular cells. In the three-dimensional case, the angular and conic points are required to be vertices of tetrahedra or hexahedra, and, in addition, it is necessary to approximate the edges of dihedral (curvilinear) angles (see section 2.6). In all these cases, the equality

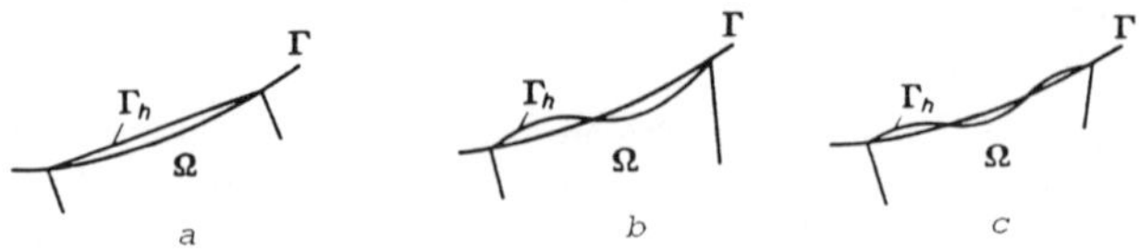

Figure 3.4: The isoparametric approximation of a boundary by portions of curvilines of the order $k = 1, 2, 3$

$u^h = g$ at those triangulation nodes which lie on Γ is sufficient for condition (3.88) to be satisfied (Fig. 3.4).

There are two theoretic problems to overcome. First, the triangulated domain Ω^h can not lie on $\bar{\Omega}$. Actually, this is the case in Fig. 3.4. Then, to investigate an approximate problem, one can pass to an extended domain $\tilde{\Omega} \supset \Omega \bigcup \Omega^h$, where he prolongates coefficients of the initial differential problem and applies Theorem 3.11 [40] to discrete problem with these coefficients. Recall that is only a theoretical approach. In practice, no extensions of a domain and coefficients are made, since their nodes lie on $\bar{\Omega}$ if quadrature formulae are chosen in the usual way.

Second, the Bubnov-Galerkin method cited above is formulated for uniform boundary conditions. To overcome this obstacle, we have to construct a function $v^h \in H^h$ which attains $v^h = g$ at the triangulation nodes, lying on Γ; and $v^h = 0$ at all interior nodes. The approximate solution u^h is then sought in the form $v^h + w^h$, where the function $w^h \in H^h$ satisfies the uniform boundary conditions. The system of the Bubnov-Galerkin method is stated immediately for it. A theoretical estimate of the closeness between functions w^h and $w = u - u^h$ is formed in the usual way. Here, an additional problem arises of the closeness between two solutions of a uniform differential equation which are distinguished by boundary values. Maximum principle settles this problem but not in the norms required. One should therefore take here the usual estimate for uniform elliptic equations [94], [106]:

$$\|u\|_{1,\Omega} \leq c|u|_{1/2,\Gamma}, \tag{3.89}$$

where the fractional norm on Γ is here introduced as a trace space on Γ of corresponding classes of functions defined on Ω [94] or as a norm of the interpolation space [106]. This estimate enables one to prove that the accuracy of a solution of the Bubnov-Galerkin problem with non-zero boundary values is the same as that for $g = 0$, provided that boundary Γ and function g are sufficiently regular.

Boundary conditions of the second and third kind are taken into account by means of additional terms immediately in the bilinear form and in the functional (see subsection 1.1.4), i. e., no additional conditions are here required to be imposed on basis functions. Therefore, isoparametric approximation of the domain results in applying the quadrature formulae for boundary integrals, and this is algorithmically different from the main boundary condition. Portions of boundary Γ are superseded with their approximations from Γ_h. A theoretical foundation of accuracy again includes a modification of the domain, an error of numerical integration; and uses Theorem 3.11 as a background. In the result, it is slightly different from that described for the first boundary value problem and gives a similar estimate of accuracy of an approximate solution. Namely, in the case of the isoparametric approximation of the domain, a choice on Γ_h of quadrature formulae of an appropriate degree leads to the same order of accuracy of the approximate solution u^h as that of the exact integration over Γ.

3.4.2 An unconformable triangulation and the penalty method

Further discussion of this section will be restricted (and this is not a matter of principle) to Poisson's equation

$$-\Delta u = f \tag{3.90}$$

and, respectively, to the bilinear form

$$\mathcal{L}(u,v) = \int_\Omega \nabla u \cdot \nabla v \, dx.$$

This time, let us assume that a regular simplex or rectangular triangulation has been constructed without regard to boundary Γ. For the second and third boundary value problems, there are again no principal difficulties to overcome — neither when constructing the Bubnov-Galerkin scheme nor when developing the theoretical foundation of approximation accuracy [182], [146].

Therefore, dwell upon the case of the first boundary condition (3.88). Taking the solution of the differential problem sufficiently smooth, we add to (3.88) the small term [12]:

$$U + d_h \, \partial_\nu U = g. \tag{3.91}$$

Here, the constant $d_h \to 0$ when $h \to 0$, and hence, the solution U converges to the initial u at $h \to 0$ [121]. As we have already seen in subsection 1.1.4, an application of boundary condition (3.91) to second-order equations changes the bilinear form and the functional by the terms, respectively,

$$S_1 = \int_\Gamma \frac{1}{d_h} uv d\gamma, \qquad S_2 = \int_\Gamma \frac{1}{d_h} gv d\gamma. \tag{3.92}$$

These terms are the penalty for unsatisfied boundary conditions. The name "penalty" given to the method is most obviously justified in the formula of the Ritz method.

The starting paper [12] investigates a balance between the penalty method error $u - U$ and the approximation error $U - U^h$ of the solution U^h of the Bubnov-Galerkin method for a disturbed problem. A recommendation is made for a choice of constant d_h:

$$d_h = ch^k, \tag{3.93}$$

where k is the order of approximation by finite elements in the norm $\|\cdot\|_{1,\Omega}$.

The last investigation of the method in [140] takes the boundary function somewhat smoother: $g \in W_2^k(\Gamma)$. Recall that from the fact that the solution belongs to class $W_2^k(\Omega)$, it only follows that $g \in W_2^{k-1/2}(\Gamma)$ [94]. The investigation of basis functions in $W_2^k(\Omega)$ and $W_2^k(\Gamma)$ from the standpoint of approximation makes other recommendations on a choice of g_h and gives improved estimates of convergence. We compare

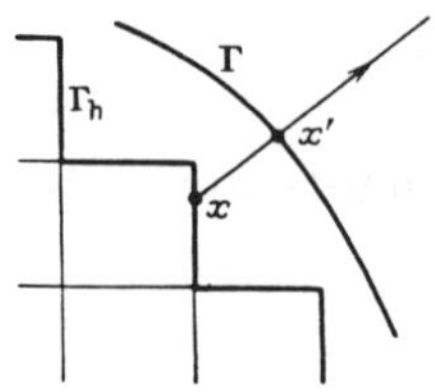

Figure 3.5: The drift of boundary values

them using a uniform rectangular grid for the two-dimensional Dirichlet problem and bilinear elements. The first approach yields

$$d_h = ch \tag{3.94}$$

and the estimates

$$|u - U^h|_{0,\Omega} \leq ch, \qquad |u - U^h|_{1,\Omega} \leq ch^{1/2}.$$

The second approach gives

$$d_h = ch^2 \tag{3.95}$$

and the corresponding estimates

$$|u - U^h|_{0,\Omega} \leq ch^2, \qquad |u - U^h|_{1,\Omega} \leq ch. \tag{3.96}$$

Note that the latter estimates are of the same order as on domains composed of rectangles.

At the same time, the fact that h in (3.95) is of higher degree leads to more complicated quadrature formulae for terms on the boundary since their order increases.

An approach provided in [146] gets round these difficulties — the complexity and somewhat higher requirements to the smoothness of g. It is supported by geometrical reasons which can be illustrated by a specific example of Poisson's equation and the above cited condition of bilinear elements on rectangles. To do this, we take a rectangular cell lying near the boundary Γ in Ω (Fig. 3.5). On its boundary Γ_h, the boundary condition is determined as follows. Take a point $x \in \Gamma_h$ and draw a ray from it in the direction of the external normal to Γ. It crosses the boundary Γ at a point x' (nearest to x) lying from x at the distance δ. Then, from the Taylor series expansion

$$u(x') = u(x) + \delta \partial_\nu u(x) + O(\delta^2).$$

Keeping in the mind that [155]

$$|\delta(x)| \leq ch \quad \forall x \in \Gamma_h,$$

we can discard $O(h^2)$ and substitute $g(x')$ for $u(x')$. As a result, we obtain the boundary condition

$$U(x) + \delta(x)\partial_\nu U(x) = g(x') \quad \text{on} \quad \Gamma_h. \tag{3.97}$$

Further it is transformed in the same way as described above for condition (3.91).

3.4.3 The mixed method

This method was first proposed in [13], where it is reffered to as the Lagrange multiplier method, because it is obtained as a problem which finds a minimum point of the corrected Ritz functional. The method has good prospects in magneto- and electrostatics (for reasons we will discuss later).

The first thing to be done to eliminate the main boundary conditions is to replace equality (3.88) with integral relation

$$\int_\Gamma (u-g)\psi d\gamma = 0 \qquad \forall\psi \in L_2(\Gamma). \tag{3.98}$$

Second, it follows from Green's formula for the arbitrary function $v \in W_2^1(\Omega)$ that

$$\mathcal{L}(u,v) - (f,v) = \int_\Gamma \partial_\nu u v d\gamma, \tag{3.99}$$

and the boundary integral is non-zero. Take two functions $u \in W_2^1(\Omega)$, $\varphi \in L_2(\Gamma)$ and consider the following system

$$\mathcal{L}(u,v) \; + \; \int_\Gamma \varphi v d\gamma = (f,v) \qquad \forall v \in W_2^1(\Omega), \tag{3.100}$$

$$\int_\Gamma u\psi d\gamma \; = \; \int_\Gamma g\psi d\gamma \qquad \forall\psi \in L_2(\Gamma). \tag{3.101}$$

According to (3.98), (3.99), this generalized problem has the solution (u,φ), where u is a solution of the Dirichlet problem (3.88) for the Poisson equation (3.90) and $\varphi = -\partial_\nu u$ on Γ. As shown in [13], it is unique.

For this problem to be solved approximately, we introduce two finite-dimensional spaces of peacewise polynomials (studied earlier) on the regular triangulation of $\bar{\Omega}$ and Γ. Denote these by H^h and G^h, respectively. As a result, the functions from H^h can satisfy no additional boundary conditions. On the whole, the dimension of the Bubnov-Galerkin system obtained increases, since two functions $u^h \in H^h$, $\varphi^h \in G^h$ satisfy the problem

$$\mathcal{L}(u^h,v) \; + \; \int_\Gamma \varphi^h v d\gamma = (f,v) \qquad \forall v \in H^h, \tag{3.102}$$

$$\int_\Gamma u^h\psi d\gamma \; = \; \int_\Gamma g\psi d\gamma \qquad \forall\psi \in G^h. \tag{3.103}$$

The number of additional unknowns is less by an order than that of unknowns in a traditional statement. In the two-dimensional case, for example, the dimension of H^h is equal to $O(h^{-2})$ on a regular triangulation, whereas the dimension of G^h is $O(h^{-1})$. In the three-dimensional case, these dimensions are equal to $O(h^{-3})$ and $O(h^{-2})$ respectively. In the case when Γ is represented parametrically, the construction of space G^h does not presents any difficulties.

When choosing a degree of approximating polynomials in H^h and G^h, one should be guided by the requirement that the order of approximation of all terms on the left-hand side of (3.102) and (3.103) be the same; and he should be guided by the reasons of section 3.3, when choosing quadrature formulae. This results in the unique solvability of the problem (3.102), (3.103).

Let us now show why this method is attractive in certain problems in magneto– and electrostatics. A number of these seeks to determine the surface gradient of the solution of the Dirichlet problem. It is of special importance for problems of breakdown. In this case, the use of simple basis functions within the scope of the methods provided in this section, would not be acceptable. For instance, in case the Courant elements are applied on a conformable (isoparametric) triangulation, convergence of surface gradient can not occur at all. The mechanics of this condition is discussed at length in [25]. It is shown that the error owing to the rough approximation of the boundary has a behaviour of a boundary layer of the width $\approx h$ and is concentrated just in component $\partial_\nu(u - u^h)$.

The mixed method is therefore preferable here because it gives possibility for simple finite elements on a regular triangulation to get an acceptable accuracy of computation of $\partial_\nu u$. For example, the accuracy obtained for the Courant elements in H^h and piecewise constant elements in G^h is as follows:

$$|\partial_\nu u - \varphi^h|_{0,\Gamma} \leq ch^{1/2}, \qquad |u - u^h|_{0,\Omega} \leq ch^2. \tag{3.104}$$

Increasing of the smoothness and the order of polynomials used in H^h and G^h, results in correspondingly increasing the order of convergence. In case the solution exhibits lesser accuracy, $W_2^{-1/2}(\Gamma)$ should be substituted for $L_2(\Gamma)$ [106].

3.5 The Richardson extrapolation

When solving the boundary value problems on polygonal domains, the Richardson extrapolation plays an important role as a method for increasing the accuracy of approximate solutions [121]. In short, the essence of this method is, first, to use simple finite elements of rather low order of approximation on two or more grids and, second, to form a linear combination of the obtained approximate solutions; which gives the high accuracy of the corrected solution. Instead of discussing the general theory, we consider a specific example of the method and discuss then its merits and dismerits.

Let it be required to solve the problem (1.22)-(1.23) in a two-dimensional polygonal domain Ω: find a function $u \in \overset{\circ}{W}{}_2^1(\Omega)$ such that

$$\mathcal{L}_1(u, u) = f_1(v) \qquad \forall v \in \overset{\circ}{W}{}_2^1(\Omega). \tag{3.105}$$

In order to discretize this problem, we use the Courant finite elements.

With this in mind, we triangulate the domain Ω using the breaking algorithm. We first perform rough subdivision of closed domain $\bar{\Omega}$ into a small number of closed triangles, hereafter called *zones*. Denote the maximal length of side by l_0. Recall that a triangulation like that is called concordant if any side of the triangle is a boundary part or a side of another triangle.

Breaking the initial triangles is further carried out for each taken separately. To accomplish this, take $n \geq 2$ and divide every side of the triangle into n parts. Draw three sets of straight lines parallel to the sides of the triangle through the obtained points. As a result, we obtain n^2 equal elementary triangles similar to the initial one with the coefficient $1/n$ (Fig. 3.6).

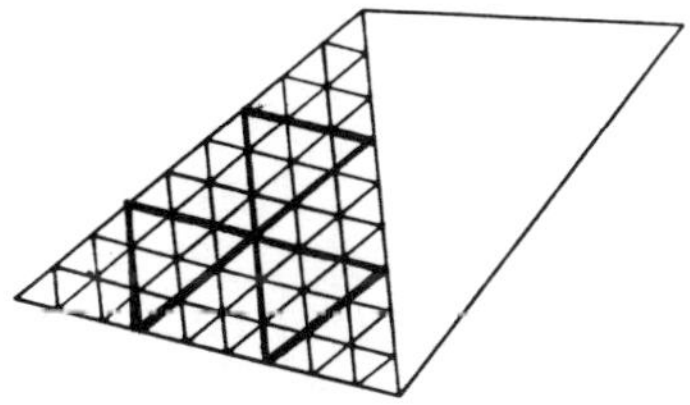

Figure 3.6: Stages of the polygon triangulation

Suppose that the initial subdivision is concordant. Then, dividing every initial triangle also yields a concordant subdivision where the maximal length of the edge does not exceed $h = l_0/n$. Denote by $\mathcal{T}_h$ the set of all elementary triangles we constructed.

Denote then by $\bar{\Omega}_h$ the union of all vertices of triangles $T \in \mathcal{T}_h$. Assume $\Omega_h = \bar{\Omega}_h \bigcap \Omega$. For every point $y \in \Omega_h$, introduce a basis function $\varphi_y \in \overset{\circ}{W}{}_2^1(\Omega)$ equal to unit at node y and to zero at all other nodes of $\bar{\Omega}$ and linear on every elementary triangle. Denote the linear span of this system of functions by H^h.

In accordance with the Bubnov-Galerkin method, we will seek an approximate solution $u^h \in H^h$ in the form of the sum

$$u^h(x) = \sum_{y \in \Omega_h} \alpha_y \varphi_y(x) \qquad \text{on} \quad \bar{\Omega}, \tag{3.106}$$

where $\{\alpha_y\}$ are certain constants defined by the identity

$$\mathcal{L}_1(u^h, v) = f_1(v) \qquad \forall v \in H^h. \tag{3.107}$$

As $\mathcal{L}_1$ and f_1 are linear in all arguments, the above identity is equivalent to the system of algebraic equations

$$\sum_{y \in \Omega_h} \alpha_y \mathcal{L}_1(\varphi_y, \varphi_z) = f_1(\varphi_z) \qquad \forall z \in \Omega_h. \tag{3.108}$$

The approximate solution u^h obtained is unique and piecewise linear, i. e., linear on every elementary triangle $T \in \mathcal{T}_h$. Recall that, from the material provided above and approximating properties of the Courant elements, the obtained solution has the first order of accuracy in the norm of $\overset{\circ}{W}{}_2^1(\Omega)$ and the second order in L_2-norm:

$$|u - u^h|_{1,\Omega} \leq c_1 h \|u\|_{2,\Omega}, \tag{3.109}$$

$$|u - u^h|_{0,\Omega} \leq c_2 h^2 \|u\|_{2,\Omega}. \tag{3.110}$$

As it was shown in [146], these estimates cannot be improved in the sense of power of h on class of functions u from $W_2^2(\Omega)$.

Let us now describe the Richardson extrapolation. To this end, we construct the additional subdivision $\mathcal{T}_{h/2}$ and the corresponding space $H^{h/2}$, and find the solution $u^{h/2} \in H^{h/2}$ of the Bubnov-Galerkin method

$$\mathcal{L}_1(u^{h/2}, v) = f_1(v), \qquad v \in H^{h/2}. \tag{3.111}$$

The obtained solution $u^{h/2}$ satisfies also estimates such as (3.109) and (3.110). The nodal parameters of functions u^h, $u^{h/2}$ are defined on grid $\bar{\Omega}_h$. Form a linear combination [121]:

$$\tilde{u}^h(x) = \frac{4}{3}u^{h/2}(x) - \frac{1}{3}u^h(x), \qquad x \in \bar{\Omega}_h. \tag{3.112}$$

The obtained values $\tilde{u}^h$ will approximate the function u at the nodes of $\bar{\Omega}_h$ much better than either of the functions u^h and $u^{h/2}$. Generally speaking, quantitative performance of improved accuracy can be given in the grid norm, but one of the advantages of the finite elements method — simple representation over the entire domain — seems then to be lost. Therefore, let us add the construction by the following. Assume for simplicity that n is divisible by 3. Consider the subdivision $\mathcal{T}_{3h}$ of the domain Ω (see Fig. 3.6). Each triangle T of $\mathcal{T}_{3h}$ involves 10 nodes of $\bar{\Omega}_h$; the grid function $\tilde{u}^h$ is defined in these nodes. Construct the cubic Lagrange interpolation function by these nodes. Denote the function obtained on $\bar{\Omega}$ by $\tilde{u}^h(x)$ again, the class of functions like that, which are zero on Γ, by $\tilde{H}^h$. Note that, because of the properties of the Lagrange elements described in subsection 3.1.2, function $\tilde{u}^h$ belongs to $C(\bar{\Omega})$ and $\overset{\circ}{W}{}^1_2(\Omega)$. But its main advantage is that [173]

$$|u - \tilde{u}^h|_{1,\Omega} \leq c_3 h^3 \|u\|_{4,\Omega}, \tag{3.113}$$
$$|u - \tilde{u}^h|_{0,\Omega} \leq c_4 h^4 \|u\|_{4,\Omega}. \tag{3.114}$$

The same estimates can be obtained, when using the Lagrange elements of degree 3 immediately in the Bubnov-Galerkin method on one grid. As here, we have solved two systems but with simple piecewise linear basis functions.

The second way is preferred in a number of cases. Indeed, for a particular problem, it is much easier, especially with regard to the programmer work, to construct a system of the Bubnov-Galerkin method with the Courant elements rather than with the Lagrange cubic elements. As far as automatized packages of programes are concerned, only a few contain the Lagrange elements of degree 3; but they all contain the Courant or bilinear elements. So in this case also, the Richardson extrapolation can remove a search for a package with high degree elements and its adaptation for a necessary class of problems.

Let us introduce some operators of prolongation and restriction, which will be useful below. Let $u^h \in H^h$ be a piecewise linear function with vector $U^h \in \mathbf{R}^{N^h}$ of values $u^h(x)$ in nodes $x \in \Omega_h$. Recall that u^h equals 0 at boundary nodes. Using the division $\mathcal{T}_{3h}$, construct the cubic Lagrangian interpolation function with 10 nodes in each of triangle $T \in \mathcal{T}_{3h}$. Denote the received function by $\bar{u}^h$. Then compute the vector $U^{h/2} \in \mathbf{R}^{N^{h/2}}$ of values $\bar{u}^h(x)$ at nodes $x \in \Omega_{h/2}$. Thereby, we introduce some operator of interpolation $\tilde{I}^h_{h/2} : U^h \to U^{h/2}$ or, more generally,

$$\tilde{I}^h_{h/2} \; : \; \mathbf{R}^{N^h} \to \mathbf{R}^{N^{h/2}}. \tag{3.115}$$

This operator is more intricate than $I^h_{h/2}$ from (3.40). Consider also the operator $\tilde{R}^h_{h/2}$ which is conjugate to $\tilde{I}^h_{h/2}$ in the Euclidean scalar product:

$$\tilde{R}^{h/2}_h = (\tilde{I}^h_{h/2})^*. \tag{3.116}$$

We call $\widetilde{R}_h^{h/2}$ the operator of restriction from $\mathbf{R}^{N^{h/2}}$ to $\mathbf{R}^{N^h}$. Of course, these operators may be constructed by the same way for another breaking of h to h/s with any integer $s \geq 2$.

The use of the Richardson extrapolation is based on the following series:

$$u^h = u^I + h^2 v^I + h^4 \xi^h \qquad \text{on} \quad \bar{\Omega}. \tag{3.117}$$

Here u^h is the solution (3.106) of the problem (3.107); $u^I = I_h u$ is the interpolant in H^h of the solution u of the problem (3.105); and $v^I = I_h v$ is the interpolant in H^h of some smooth function v remaining unchanged at all h. The remainder term satisfies the following estimates when $u \in W_2^4(\Omega)$:

$$|\xi^h|_{0,\Omega} \leq c_5, \qquad |\xi^h|_{1,\Omega} \leq c_6 h^{-1}. \tag{3.118}$$

The expansion (3.117) is difficult to prove, and this is the most laborious part in justifying the suitability of the Richardson extrapolation [173].

Note that this expansion can also be used to justify the a posteriori Runge criterion for analyzing the convergence or to prove the superconvergence of derivatives of u^h.

The estimates of the remainder term are most widely used in the uniform metric [100], where they take the following form at $u \in W_\infty^4(\Omega)$:

$$\max_{\Omega} |\xi^h| \leq c_7 \ln^2 h. \tag{3.119}$$

This permits estimates like (3.113) and (3.114) to be proved in the uniform norm with an additional logarithmic factor. For instance, we obtain the inequality

$$\max_{\bar{\Omega}_h} |u - \tilde{u}^h| \leq c_8 h^4 \ln^2 h \max_{|\alpha| \leq 4; x \in \bar{\Omega}} |\partial^\alpha u(x)| \tag{3.120}$$

instead of (3.114).

Similar estimates have also been proved for bilinear finite elements, curvilinear domains, and some nonlinear problems [100]–[104].

This method is of interest for solving the spectral problem: find $\lambda \in \mathbf{R}$ and function $u \in \overset{\circ}{W}{}_2^1(\Omega)$ satisfying the equality (see subsection 1.1.5)

$$\mathcal{L}_4(u, v) = \lambda (u, v)_b \qquad \forall v \in \overset{\circ}{W}{}_2^1(\Omega), \tag{3.121}$$

where

$$(u, v)_b = \int_\Omega buv dx, \qquad 0 < c_9 \leq b \leq c_{10}.$$

To solve this problem numerically, we will proceed as before. That is, we construct the triangulation $\mathcal{T}_h$, introduce the space H^h, and try to find the approximate solution $\lambda^h \in \mathbf{R}$, $u^h \in H^h$ using the Bubnov-Galerkin method:

$$\mathcal{L}_4(u^h, v) = \lambda (u^h, v)_b \qquad \forall v \in H^h. \tag{3.122}$$

Let us consider the k-th eigenvalue of the differential problem. Take the case where this is simple. In this case, it is associated with one eigenfunction u_k. It will be regarded as normalized so that $(u_k, u_k)_b = 1$.

Find the k-th eigenvalue λ_k^h of algebraic spectral problem (3.122). Since the eigenvalues of the Bubnov-Galerkin method converge to those of the differential problem, we can assert that λ_k^h is also simple when h is small enough. Then λ_k^h is associated with only one "eigenfunction" u_k^h normalized so that $(u_k^h, u_k^h)_b = 1$. The term "eigenfunction" here focuses our attention on the fact that, in essence, u_k^h is the interpolant in H^h of the eigenvector of the generalized algebraic problem but not the eigenfunction of the differential operator. The sign $\pm$ can be chosen for the approximate solution u_k^h in such a way that the following estimates hold [192]:

$$\begin{aligned} |u_k - u_k^h|_{1,\Omega} &\le c_{11} h \|u_k\|_{2,\Omega}, \\ |u_k - u_k^h|_{0,\Omega} &\le c_{12} h^2 \|u_k\|_{2,\Omega}, \\ |\lambda_k - \lambda_k^h| &\le c_{13} h^2 \|u_k\|_{2,\Omega}. \end{aligned} \tag{3.123}$$

Next we construct the triangulation $\mathcal{T}_{h/2}$, introduce the space $H^{h/2}$, and state the algebraic spectral problem: find $\lambda^{h/2} \in \mathbf{R}$ and $u^{h/2} \in H^{h/2}$ such that

$$\mathcal{L}_4(u^{h/2}, v) = \lambda(u^{h/2}, v)_b \qquad \forall v \in H^{h/2}. \tag{3.124}$$

The result is that the k-th eigenvalue is here also simple (at sufficiently small h), i. e., it is assigned to one eigenfunction $u_k^{h/2}$ which also obeys estimates like (3.123) and is normalized so that $(u_k^{h/2}, u_k^{h/2})_b = 1$. Of the two possible signs, such one is chosen that $(u_k^{h/2}, u_k^h)_b \approx 1$ holds.

The eigenfunctions are extrapolated in the same way described earlier. Namely, if there is a need only for grid values, the result of extrapolation holds on $\bar{\Omega}_h$ in the form

$$\tilde{u}_k^h(x) = \frac{4}{3} u_k^{h/2}(x) - \frac{1}{3} u_k^h(x). \tag{3.125}$$

But if we require the approximation over the entire domain $\bar{\Omega}$, we use, in addition, the cubic Lagrange interpolation extending the definition of function $\tilde{u}_k^h$ to the whole domain $\bar{\Omega}$. As a result, the obtained k-th approximate eigenvalue $\tilde{u}_k^h$ satisfies the estimates [173]

$$\begin{aligned} |u_k - \tilde{u}_k^h|_{1,\Omega} &\le c_{14} h^3 \|u_k\|_{4,\Omega}, \\ |u_k - \tilde{u}_k^h|_{0,\Omega} &\le c_{15} h^4 \|u_k\|_{4,\Omega}. \end{aligned} \tag{3.126}$$

In the uniform metric, an estimate with the logarithmic factor [101] occurs as in (3.120).

This approach can also be applied to eigenvalues by calculating

$$\tilde{\lambda}_k^h = \frac{4}{3} \lambda_k^{h/2} - \frac{1}{3} \lambda_k^h. \tag{3.127}$$

Then the following estimate is valid [173]:

$$|\tilde{\lambda}_k^h - \lambda_k| \le c_{16} h^4 \|u_k\|_{4,\Omega}. \tag{3.128}$$

With given eigenfunction $\tilde{u}_k^h$, we can also compute an approximate eigenvalue from the Rayleigh ratio:

$$\lambda_k^R = \mathcal{L}_4(\tilde{u}_k^h, \tilde{u}_k^h) / (\tilde{u}_k^h, \tilde{u}_k^h)_b. \tag{3.129}$$

Then, from the general Theorem 7.2 from [192] and the estimate (3.126), we have

$$|\lambda_k - \lambda_k^R| \le c_{17} h^6 \|u_k\|_{4,\Omega}. \tag{3.130}$$

Hence, an additional expenditure on computing the Rayleigh relation pays off here in full. It should be noted that the calculation of (3.129) is equivalent to the multiplication of two sparse matrices by vectors.

Let us now discuss the extrapolation effect in case the differential problem has a multiple eigenvalue λ_r. Assume that it obeys the relation

$$\lambda_{l-1} < \lambda_l = \lambda_{l+1} = \ldots = \lambda_k < \lambda_{k+1}, \qquad l \le r \le k. \tag{3.131}$$

The signs of strict inequality indicate that λ_k, λ_l are separated from λ_{l-1}, λ_{k+1}. Let us consider eigenvalues of algebraic spectral problem (3.122) with these numbers. This time, the following relations hold (when h is small enough):

$$\lambda_{l-1}^h < \lambda_l^h \le \lambda_{l+1}^h \le \ldots \le \lambda_k^h < \lambda_{k+1}^h. \tag{3.132}$$

Sometimes neighbouring quantities coincide at all or certain h; sometimes they do not, whatever h; in spite of the fact that they tend to one limit. Therefore, instead of individual eigenfunctions (even if they are all different) corresponding to eigenvalues $\lambda_l^h, \ldots, \lambda_k^h$ of (3.122), it is necessary to take the whole subspace of dimension $k - l + 1$ being the linear span of the "eigenfunctions"

$$u_l^h, \ldots, u_k^h. \tag{3.133}$$

Take these in the orthonormal form:

$$(u_i^h, u_j^h)_b = \delta_{ij}, \qquad i, j = l, \ldots, k. \tag{3.134}$$

Similarly, find "eigenfunctions" of spectral problem (3.124) and construct the orthonormal basis

$$u_l^{h/2}, \ldots, u_k^{h/2}. \tag{3.135}$$

Since the forming both these bases is random in nature, we have rather unlike functions u_r^h and $u_r^{h/2}$ for $r = l, \ldots, k$. Therefore extrapolation does not give here the correction effect.

Let us act as follows. Instead of (3.135), we take a basis most close to (3.133). To this end, we fix a certain number $l \le r \le k$ and consider the function

$$z_r^{h/2} = \sum_{i=l}^{k} \gamma_i u_i^{h/2}.$$

Now we choose the weights γ_i so that

$$(z_r^{h/2}, u_i^h)_l = \delta_{ri}.$$

Normalizing this vector, we obtain the required function

$$\bar{u}_r^{h/2} = z_r^{h/2} / (z_r^{h/2}, z_r^{h/2})_b. \tag{3.136}$$

Finally, the procedure of extrapolation is formulated as follows:

$$\tilde{u}_r^h(x) = \frac{4}{3}\bar{u}_r^{h/2}(x) - \frac{1}{3}u_r^h(x). \tag{3.137}$$

It is performed either at the nodes of grid $\bar{\Omega}_h$ or on the entire domain $\bar{\Omega}$ after using interpolation by the Lagrange cubic elements. For the obtained approximate eigenfunctions, the following assertion holds. At h sufficiently small in the eigensubspace of spectral problem (3.121) corresponding to the multiple eigenvalue $\lambda_k = \ldots = \lambda_l$, we can find a function u_r such that

$$\begin{aligned} |\tilde{u}_r^h - u_r|_{1,\Omega} &\leq ch^3\|u_r\|_{4,\Omega}, \\ |\tilde{u}_r^h - u_r|_{0,\Omega} &\leq ch^4\|u_r\|_{4,\Omega}. \end{aligned} \tag{3.138}$$

Regarding the extrapolation of eigenvalues, the reasoning which applies to simple eigenvalues is valid here as well. Namely, the extrapolation of the eigenvalues (3.127) yields the estimate (3.128); using the Rayleigh ratio (3.129) yields the improved estimate (3.130). In conclusion, turn our attention to advantages and disadvantages of the Richardson extrapolation. The former are the result of using the simplest finite elements to achieve the high order of accuracy. The disadvantage is that the extrapolation can be used quite successfully only on piecewise regular grids. For example, to justify the accuracy of the Lagrange cubic elements, the angle criterion should hold only for each individual triangle. For the extrapolation to be applied successfully, it is necessary that neighbouring triangles should be equal or very like [173], at least, in large zones. Therefore this fact should be taken into account when constructing the triangulation before the Richardson extrapolation.

3.6 The conditionality of linear equations systems and diagonal normalization

Let us consider some properties of the linear algebraic equations system to be solved in the Bubnov-Galerkin method:

$$L^h U^h = F^h. \tag{3.139}$$

Here $L^h = \{L_{ij}^h\}_{ij=1}^{N^h}$ is the square symmetric matrix with elements $L_{ij}^h = \mathcal{L}(\varphi_i^h, \varphi_j^h)$, $U^h = (\alpha_1^h, \ldots, \alpha_{N^h}^h)^T$ is a vector of unknowns, and $F^h = (F_1^h, \ldots, F_{N^h}^h)^T$ is the vector of the right-hand side. The ratio (*the number of conditionality*)

$$\kappa = |\lambda_{\max}(L^h)/\lambda_{\min}(L^h)| \tag{3.140}$$

of a maximum to a minimum in magnitudes of the matrix eigenvalues is of importance for us. The number κ is of special consequence as index of the rate of convergence of iterative methods and of the round-off errors effect in direct methods [193].

Let us first treat (3.140) in the case of the regular triangulation where the values of all angles and the ratio $h_{\min}/h_{\max}$ of lengths of the triangulation edges are different from zero by a constant independent of h. Then, for a correct-posed variational problem in the form (3.44) or (3.67), and upon a correct choice of finite elements, the following estimate holds, as a general rule:

$$\kappa \leq c_1 h_{\min}^{-2m} / |\lambda_1(\mathcal{L})|. \tag{3.141}$$

Here $\lambda_1(\mathcal{L})$ is the smallest (in absolute value) eigenvalue of the initial continuous problem, and c_1 increases when the geometry of elements becomes singular. For example, this is proved in [182] for some particular cases with a symmetric and positive-definite bilinear form $\mathcal{L}$.

This estimate permits two conclusions to be made.

First, the conditionality number is much larger for fourth-order equations where $2m = 4$, rather than for second-order ones where $2m = 2$. Therefore, if possible, instead of solving fourth-order equations one should solve systems of second-order equations. This can be done by using the mixed method.

Second, estimate (3.141) becomes unsatisfactory in case of any degeneration. For example, triangles satisfying the weakened criterion (3.109) of chapter 2 can give $h_{\min} \ll h$ and, hence, the ill conditionality. Similarly, this is the case when applying any grid refinement algorithm locally.

In some cases, it is sufficient to normalize matrix L^h. We show how to do this. It should be noted here that the Gerschgorin disks give a rather good estimate of the maximal eigenvalue of matrix L^h [182].

Lemma 3.6.1 [193]. *Any eigenvalue of the matrix L^h is situated at least at one of the circles of the radius*

$$\sum_{j \neq i, j=1}^{N^h} |L_{ij}^h| \tag{3.142}$$

with the centre L_{ii}^h and the number $i = 1, \ldots, n$.

Hence, in particular

$$|\lambda_{\max}(L^h)| \leq \max_{1 \leq i \leq N^h} \sum_{j=1}^{N^h} |L_{ij}^h|. \tag{3.143}$$

In many occasions, we may improve the conditionality number by diagonal normalization. Introduce the diagonal matrix $\mathcal{D}^h = diag(d_1, \ldots, d_{N^h})$ with the elements

$$d_l = \max_{1 \leq i \leq N^h} \sum_{j=1}^{N^h} |L_{ij}^h| / \sum_{j=1}^{N^h} |L_{lj}^h| \tag{3.144}$$

and multiply (3.139):

$$\mathcal{D}^h L^h U^h = \mathcal{D}^h F^h. \tag{3.145}$$

As a result, we have a problem in which (3.143) holds again for the maximal eigenvalue; the minimal one increases greately in many occasions, and the conditionality number of the obtained matrix $\mathcal{D}^h L^h$ is $O(h^{-2})$, as in the case of the regular triangulation. This result is not here proved at length, but we will return to it in some particular cases.

As we will see later, the diagonal normalization permits improving the conditionality number for second-order equations with strongly varying coefficients a_{ij}; for the mixed method, and for fourth-order equations when altering the elements, corresponding to values of the function and its derivatives, to make their powers the same.

In conclusion, two results are provided which will be frequently used in the further description.

For each vector W^h with components $W_j^h (j = 1, \dots, N^h)$, we put in correspondence a prolongation w^h from H^h, i. e., the function

$$w^h(x) = \sum_{j=1}^{N^h} W_j^h \varphi_j^h(x) \quad \text{on} \quad \Omega. \tag{3.146}$$

This prolongation generates the vector norm

$$\|W^h\|_h = |w|_{0,\Omega}. \tag{3.147}$$

It is useful, for our further reasoning, to compare this and the weighted Euclidean norm

$$\|W^h\| = (\sum_{j=1}^{N^h} (W_j^h)^2 h^n)^{1/2}. \tag{3.148}$$

They turned out to be equivalent.

Theorem 3.13 *The estimate*

$$c_7\|W^h\| \le \|W^h\|_h \le c_8\|W^h\| \tag{3.149}$$

holds for any choice of affine regular finite elements with one generating element.

Proof. Let us examine an arbitrary cell ω and the expression

$$(w^h, w^h)_\omega = \sum_{j,l \in J_\omega} W_j^h W_l^h (\varphi_j^h, \varphi_l^h)_\omega, \tag{3.150}$$

where J_ω are the indices of degrees of freedom at the nodes of ω. For affine regular finite elements, the basis functions φ_j^h, φ_l^h are obtained from affine transformation F of initial basis functions $\tilde{\varphi}_i$ on master cell $\tilde{\omega}$ of standard shape. The matrix $\tilde{M}$ with the elements $\tilde{M}_{ij} = (\tilde{\varphi}_i, \tilde{\varphi}_j)_{\tilde{\omega}}$ is Gram's matrix. Since $\{\tilde{\varphi}_i\}$ are linear independent, the matrix $\tilde{M}$ is non-generate, symmetric, and positive definite. Hence, its eigenvalues are positive including a minimum and a maximum:

$$0 < c_2 \le \lambda_{\min}(\tilde{M}) \le \lambda_{\max}(\tilde{M}) \le c_3. \tag{3.151}$$

Obviously, the constants c_2, c_3 are independent of h. From the affine regularity condition (3.9) it follows that the matrix M with the elements $M_{ij} = (\varphi_i^h, \varphi_j^h)$ is different from $\tilde{M}$ by the factor $c_4 h^n$. Therefore, from (3.150) and (3.151) it follows that

$$c_2 c_4 h^n \sum_{j \in J_\omega} (W_j^h)^2 \le \sum_{j,l \in J_\omega} W_j^h W_l^h (\varphi_j^h, \varphi_l^h)_\omega \le c_3 c_4 h^n \sum_{j \in J_\omega} (W_j^h)^2.$$

Now take a sum over all $\omega \in \mathcal{F}$:

$$(w^h, w^h) = \sum_{\omega\in\mathcal{F}} (w^h, w^h)_\omega.$$

Let c_5 and c_6 be, respectively, the minimal and the maximal number of elements ω which meet at one node. Then

$$(w^h, w^h) \leq \sum_{\omega\in\mathcal{F}} c_3c_4 \sum_{j\in J_\omega} (W_j^h)^2 \leq c_6c_3c_4h^n \sum_{i=1}^{N^h} (W_i^h)^2,$$

$$(w^h, w^h) \geq c_2c_4c_5h^n \sum_{i=1}^{N^h} (W_i^h)^2.$$

From this we just arrive at (3.149). □

Let us now state an estimate for the maximal eigenvalue of matrix L^h.

Theorem 3.14 *The estimate*

$$|\lambda_{\max}(L^h)| \leq c_9h^{n-2m} \tag{3.152}$$

holds for any choice of affine regular finite elements of class $W_2^m(\Omega)$ with one generating element and bilinear form $\mathcal{L}$ bounded in $W_2^m(\Omega)$.

Proof. For the bounded bilinear form (in the notation of Theorem 3.13)

$$|\mathcal{L}(w^h, w^h)| \leq c_{10}\|w^h\|_{m,\Omega}^2. \tag{3.153}$$

Let us consider an arbitrary cell $\omega \in \mathcal{F}$ and the expression

$$\|w^h\|_{m,\omega}^2 = \sum_{i,j\in J_\omega} W_i^h W_j^h \sum_{|\alpha|\leq m} (\partial^\alpha\varphi_i^h, \partial^\alpha\varphi_j^h)_\omega. \tag{3.154}$$

Take the generating element on the master cell $\tilde{\omega}$ with basis functions $\tilde{\varphi}_i$. The expressions

$$(\partial^\alpha\tilde{\varphi}_i, \partial^\alpha\tilde{\varphi}_j)_{\tilde{\omega}}$$

are finite, as $\tilde{\varphi}_i$ belongs to class $W_2^m(\tilde{\omega})$. Considering the regularity condition (3.4), (3.5), we arrive at the estimate

$$|\sum_{|\alpha|\leq m} (\partial^\alpha\varphi_i^h, \partial^\alpha\varphi_j^h)_\omega| \leq c_{11}h^{-2m}|\sum_{|\alpha|\leq m} (\partial^\alpha\tilde{\varphi}_i^h, \partial^\alpha\tilde{\varphi}_j^h)_{\tilde{\omega}}|.$$

Summing over all α yields

$$\max_{i,j\in J_\omega} |\sum_{|\alpha|\leq m} (\partial^\alpha\varphi_i^h, \partial^\alpha\varphi_j^h)| \leq c_{12}h^{-2m}. \tag{3.155}$$

Let c_{13} be the maximal number of basis functions corresponding to one cell. Then, from (3.154), (3.155), and (3.143)

$$\|w^h\|_{m,\omega}^2 \leq c_{12}h^{-2m} \sum_{i,j\in J_\omega} W_i^h W_j^h \leq c_{12}c_{13}h^{-2m} \sum_{i\in J_\omega} (W_i^h)^2.$$

Take a sum over all $\omega \in \mathcal{F}$ and combine this and (3.153):

$$|\mathcal{L}(w^h, w^h)| \leq c_6 c_{12} c_{13} h^{-2m} \sum_{i=1}^{N^h} (W_i^h)^2. \tag{3.156}$$

Hence it follows that the maximal eigenvalue satisfies (3.152) with constant $c_9 = c_6 c_{12} c_{13}$. Indeed, assume that the orthonormed eigenvector V^h corresponds to $\lambda_{\mathbf{max}}$ with a prolongation $v^h \in H^h$. Then

$$(V^h)^T L^h V^h = \lambda_{\mathbf{max}} (V^h)^T V^h = \lambda_{\mathbf{max}}.$$

From (3.156),

$$|\mathcal{L}(v^h, v^h)| = |(V^h)^T L^h V^h| \leq c_9 h^{n-2m}$$

follows. Comparing these inequalities, we obtain (3.152). □

Chapter 4

General description of multigrid algorithms

In section 4.1, we deal with the auxiliary results of solving the problems of iterative parameters optimization. In four following sections, the description of multigrid algorithms is performed at an abstract algebraic level. It gives the possibility to utilize the main results both to finite-element schemes and finite-difference ones. Here we use designations and approaches closed to works [31], [68]. For example, in these works, the abstract algebraic results are transformed into terms of finite-difference schemes for the second-order elliptic equations. In section 4.2, the basic multigrid algorithm for suppression of error of approximate solution is formulated and the full nested algorithm is described on the sequence of ascending levels. In section 4.3, we study the convergence of multigrid algorithms (to be more precise, multilevel) for problems with a self-ajoint positive definite operator. First, the convergence is stated for an arbitrary smoother and then the description is elaborated for generalized Jacoby-type smoothing processes. The point is that we succeed in finding the optimal iterative parameters so that the multiplier of error suppression in various norms is better (with respect to number m of iterations) than in the large majority of iterative smoothers. One can see this advance comparing various smoothers in monograph [68]. Even if the convergence rate is the same with some other iterative procedure, this smoother is usually simpler in computations. For example, one may use only elementary matrices of stiffness and mass without their storage and assembling.

This type of iterations does not rule out the appearance of more effective smoothers for concrete problems where particular properties may be used.

As an example, this section demonstrate that the error suppression in multigrid methods is thoroughly connected with the discretisation accuracy: the higher accuracy, the higher rate of suppression. Therefore, this rate is studied in conditions of insufficient, standard, and improved accuracy. The last situation is usual in hp-version of finite-element method with not great powers p of polinomials.

In section 4.4, the convergence rate of multigrid algorithm is studied for self-ajoint operators with the sign-indefinite spectrum. And, finally, in section 4.5 this rate is discussed in a more general case for problems with non-self-ajoint operators without positive definitness. As we refuse positive definitness and then self ajointness, we just lose in the convergence rate.

The remaining sections of this chapter deal with the natural criteria for finite-element methods. For example, in section 4.6, the abstract algebraic criteria of sections 4.3–4.5 are transformed into usual conditions of the finite-element method with Lagrangian elements for a bilinear form corresponding to second-order differential equations. The multigrid algorithm in combination with the Richardson extrapolation is constructed in section 4.7, which obtains high accuracy solutions in terms of simple finite elements of a rather low order of approximation. Section 4.8 offers algorithms for solving the problems with self-ajoint singular operators. From these, an algorithms are stated and justified, in section 4.9, for solving the spectral problem of determining the certain eigenvalues and eigenfunctions including multiple ones, for a self-ajoint operators. Section 4.10 presents the most general modification of multigrid algorithm for Lagrangian and Hermitian elements and equations of order $2s$, which uses a diagonal pre-conditioner of a discrete system. Finally, section 4.11 provides a particular multigrid algorithm, with a diagonal pre-conditioner as well, for the mixed method.

As compared with the works [30], [68], [109], the convergence has been proved directly for optimal iterative parameters. This results in improved theoretical estimates of the convergence rate. The problem of iterative parameters optimization can be solved so as to improve the suppression of the error in various norms.

4.1 Solving the problems of parameters optimization

Let us consider the following problem: *find real parameters* τ_i $(i = 0,\dots,m-1)$ *minimizing the quantity*

$$\max_{x\in[0,d]} |x \prod_{i=0}^{m-1} (1-\tau_i x)|. \tag{4.1}$$

The expression within the modulus sign has the form $x - x^2 p_{m-1}(x)$, where $p_{m-1}(x)$ is some polynomial in x of degree $m-1$. Therefore, a more general problem than (4.1) can be formulated: *find a polynomial* $p_{m-1}(x)$ *minimizing the quantity*

$$\max_{x\in[0,d]} |x - x^2 p_{m-1}(x)|. \tag{4.2}$$

This is really a more general problem because the expression in (4.2) can, in principle, have complex roots, whereas that in (4.1) cannot.

As a result, we have the general Chebyshev problem of minimizing the deviation of polynomial $x^2 p_{m-1}(x)$ from the given continuous function x.

Theorem 4.1 *The set of values*

$$\tau_k = \frac{1+\cos\alpha}{d(\cos\alpha - \cos(2k+3)\alpha)}, \quad k = 0,\dots,m-1, \quad \alpha = \pi/(2m+2), \tag{4.3}$$

is a solution of problem (4.1). *This solution is unique and yields a minimum of* (4.1) *equal to*

$$q_0 \equiv \frac{d}{m+1}\mathrm{tg}\frac{\alpha}{2}. \tag{4.4}$$

Proof. Let us consider a system of polynomials $x^2, x^3, \dots, x^{m+1}$. It does not satisfy Haar's condition [1] on the number of roots on $[0,d]$, and so general results of the Chebyshev theory of alternance are not applicable to it. Take therefore a sufficiently

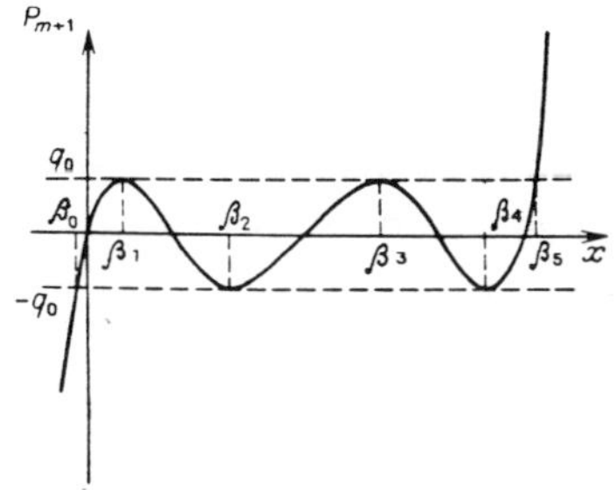

Figure 4.1: The polinomial $P_{m+1}(x)$ with $m = 4$

small positive ε, for example, let $\varepsilon \leq d \sin \alpha/2 \sin 3\alpha/2$, and consider the set $M = [\varepsilon, d]$. Then, by virtue of Haar's theorem [1], the minimization problem

$$\min_{\alpha_i \in \mathbf{R}} \max_{x \in M} |x - \sum_{i=2}^{m+1} \alpha_i x^i| \tag{4.5}$$

has a unique solution. We will not carry out the standard but rather tedious calculations to find it. We only write down certain solution and show that it satisfies the sufficient conditions. Take the Chebyshev polynomial of the first kind and degree $m+1$ normalized as follows:

$$P_{m+1}(x) = -q_0 \cos\{(m+1)\arccos(\cos\alpha - x(1+\cos\alpha)/d)\}. \tag{4.6}$$

It has the roots

$$\omega_k = d(\cos\alpha - \cos(2k+1)\alpha)/(1+\cos\alpha), \qquad k = 0, 1, \dots, m.$$

It is easy to see that $P_{m+1}(0) = 0$, $P'_{m+1}(0) = 1$. This enables (4.6) to be expressed in terms of quantities being minimized in (4.5) and (4.2). Besides, with chosen ε, on M there is a set of $m+1$ points

$$\beta_1 < \dots < \beta_i = d(\cos\alpha - \cos 2i\alpha)/(1+\cos\alpha) < \dots < \beta_{m+1} = d,$$

at which

$$P_{m+1}(\beta_i) = (-1)^{i+1} q_0 = (-1)^{i+1} \max_M |P_{m+1}|,$$

i. e., the polynomial attains maximal values alternating in sign (see Fig. 4.1). Therefore, according to [43] (theorems 7.1, 7.2), the sufficient conditions of the best approximation hold. And hence, P_{m+1} is the unique solution of the optimization problem (4.5). Since its roots are all real and one of them is equal to zero, P_{m+1} can be written in the form of the expression within the modulus sign in (4.1).

Thus, the solution to (4.1) on the interval $[\varepsilon, d]$ has been found. It has the form of (4.3) at any sufficiently small $\varepsilon > 0$. Is there any other solution which conforms to $\varepsilon = 0$? Assume the contrary. Let there exists a set of τ_i with which (4.1) on the interval $[0, d]$ is less or equal to q_0. Take $\varepsilon \leq d \sin\alpha/2 \sin 3\alpha/2$. Then on the interval $[\varepsilon, d]$ there exists another polynomial $\widetilde{P}_{m+1}$ such as (4.1) which obeys the inequality $\widetilde{P}_{m+1} \leq P_{m+1}$ on $[\varepsilon, d]$. However, by virtue of what is already proved, $\widetilde{P}_{m+1} = P_{m+1}$ on $[\varepsilon, d]$ and, hence, on $\mathbf{R}$. □

Remark 4.1.1 . *It should be noted that the obtained polynomial is a solution of the optimization problem* (4.1) *for a whole series of intervals like* $[a, d]$ *where* $\beta_0 = -d\mathrm{tg}^2\alpha/2 \leq a \leq \beta_1$ *(see Fig.* 4.1 *). Subsequently, this fact will be of importance for negative* a*. Its proof is constructed by literally repeating the justification of Theorem* 4.1 *when using the set* $M = [a, -\varepsilon] \bigcup [\varepsilon, d]$ *where* $\varepsilon < \min\{-\beta_0, \beta_1\}$*. Therefore*

$$|P_{m+1}(x)| \leq q_0 \qquad \forall x \in [-d\,\mathrm{tg}^2\alpha/2, d]. \tag{4.7}$$

Let us consider the polynomial

$$Q_m(x) = \frac{1}{x} P_{m+1}(x) = \prod_{i=1}^{m} (1 - \frac{x}{\omega_i}). \tag{4.8}$$

On the interval $(-\infty, \omega_1]$, it is a monotone decreasing function and $Q_m(0) = 1$. Therefore, $Q_m(x) \geq 1/2$ for all x less than some positive ε. This ε is dependent only on m. Using the inequality

$$Q_m(x) \geq 1 - \sum_{i=1}^{m} \frac{x}{\omega_i} \qquad \forall x \geq 0 \tag{4.9}$$

we obtain the estimate

$$\varepsilon \geq \frac{\omega_1}{2m} \geq \frac{d \sin\alpha \sin 2\alpha}{2m} = \gamma_m.$$

Hence,

$$Q_m(x) \geq 1/2 \qquad \forall x \leq \gamma_m.$$

On the interval $[-d\mathrm{tg}^2\alpha/2, d]$

$$|Q_m(x)| \leq \frac{\mathrm{ctg}\alpha/2}{m+1} \leq 1.28 \equiv q_1 \qquad \forall m \geq 1, \tag{4.10}$$

and on the interval $[0, d]$

$$|Q_m(x)| \leq 1 \qquad \forall m \geq 1. \tag{4.11}$$

Indeed, this inequality holds on the interval $[-d\mathrm{tg}^2\alpha/2, \omega_1]$ as Q_m are monotone, while on the rest interval $[\omega_1, d]$ this follows from the inequality

$$|Q_m(x)| = \frac{1}{x}|P_{m+1}(x)| \leq \frac{q_0}{\omega_1} \leq \frac{1}{2(m+1)\sin 2\alpha} \leq \frac{1}{4}. \tag{4.12}$$

Consider now the polynomial

$$S_{m-1}(x) = \frac{1}{x}(1 - Q_m(x)). \tag{4.13}$$

On the interval $(-\infty, 0]$, it is positive and monotone decreasing. The maximum of $|S_{m-1}|$ on the interval $[-d\mathrm{tg}^2\alpha/2, 0]$ is therefore achieved at the left end. From this, in view of (4.11), we have

$$\begin{aligned}|S_{m-1}(x)| &\leq S_{m-1}(-d\cdot \mathrm{tg}^2\frac{\alpha}{2}) \leq \\ \leq \frac{0.28}{d\mathrm{tg}^2\alpha/2} &\leq 0.46\frac{(m+1)^2}{d} \qquad \forall x \in [-d\mathrm{tg}^2\frac{\alpha}{2}, 0].\end{aligned} \tag{4.14}$$

On the interval $[0, d]$ from (4.9) the inequality

$$1 - Q_m(x) \leq \sum_{i=1}^{m} \frac{x}{\omega_i}$$

follows. Moreover, by virtue of (4.8), (4.12),

$$1 - Q_m(x) \geq 0 \qquad \forall x \in [0, d].$$

Taking two inequalities above, we have

$$0 \leq S_{m-1}(x) \leq \sum_{i=1}^{m} \frac{1}{\omega_i} = S_{m-1}(0) \leq S_{m-1}(-d\cdot \mathrm{tg}^2\frac{\alpha}{2}) \qquad \forall x \in [0, d].$$

Therefore, taking (4.14) into account, we arrive at the estimate

$$|S_{m-1}(x)| \leq q_2 \equiv \frac{0.28}{d}\mathrm{ctg}^2\frac{d}{2} \leq 0.46\frac{(m+1)^2}{d} \qquad \forall x \in [-d\mathrm{tg}^2\frac{\alpha}{2}, d]. \tag{4.15}$$

The function P_{m+1} is a result of linear transformation of the argument and of the normalizing the Chebyshev polynomial

$$T_{m+1}(x) = \cos\{(m+1)\arccos x\}. \tag{4.16}$$

To this end, one should shift the argument in T_{m+1} so that one of the roots became zero and carry out then normalizing. As T_{m+1} has $m+1$ real roots, together with P_{m+1} a whole set of functions can be obtained for $k = 1, \ldots, m+1$:

$$P_{m+1}^k(x) = -q_0^k \cos\left\{(m+1)\arccos\left(\cos\alpha_k - \frac{x}{d}(1+\cos\alpha_k)\right)\right\} \tag{4.17}$$

with the parameters

$$\alpha_k = \frac{(2k-1)\pi}{2(m+1)}, \qquad q_0^k = (-1)^{k+1}\frac{d}{m+1}\mathrm{tg}\frac{\alpha_k}{2}, \tag{4.18}$$

each of whose is defined on the interval $[-d\cdot \mathrm{tg}^2\alpha_k/2, d]$, where it is a polynomial of the form

$$P_{m+1}^k(x) = x\prod_{i=1}^{m}(1 - \frac{x}{\omega_i^k}) \tag{4.19}$$

with the roots

$$\omega_i^k = \frac{d(\cos\alpha_k - \cos\alpha_i)}{1+\cos\alpha_k}. \tag{4.20}$$

They can therefore be extended over the whole real axis and

$$|P_{m+1}^k(x)| \le |q_0^k| \qquad \text{on} \qquad [-d\mathrm{tg}^2\alpha_k/2, d]. \tag{4.21}$$

It should be noted that P_{m+1}^k coincides with P_{m+1} (discussed above) when $k = 1$, with $|q_0^k|$ being here the smallest.

Each of the polynomials P_{m+1}^k solves the optimization problem

$$\max_{x\in[a,d]} |x \prod_{i=0}^{m-1}(1-\tau_i x)| \tag{4.22}$$

for a corresponding set of intervals.

Theorem 4.2 *At any $k = 1, \dots, m+1$, inverse values of non-zero roots of polynomial P_{m+1}^k solve the optimization problem* (4.22) *for intervals* $[a, d]$ *with the left-hand boundary a satisfying the inequality*

$$-d\mathrm{tg}^2\alpha_k/2 \le a < -d\,\mathrm{tg}^2\,\alpha_{k-1}/2. \tag{4.23}$$

We do not construct the proof of this theorem as well as of the following one since these proofs differ from that of Theorem 4.1 only in the set M.

One of the important points of (4.22) occurs when solving the systems with a spectrum of alternating signs when $a = -d$.

Theorem 4.3 *The set of inverse values of non-zero roots of polynomial P_{m+1}^{k+1} is the solution of* (4.22) *on the interval* $[-d, d]$ *when $m = 2k$ is even:*

$$\begin{aligned} \tau_i &= d^{-1}\cos^{-1}(2i+1)\pi/2(m+1), \quad i = 0, 1, \dots, k-1; \\ \tau_i &= d^{-1}\cos^{-1}(2i+3)\pi/2(m+1), \quad i = k, \dots, 2k-1. \end{aligned} \tag{4.24}$$

When $m = 2k+1$ is odd, $\tau_m = 0$ is added to the set (4.24).

Take now one more problem which differs from (4.1) in the weight factor: *find numerical parameters τ_i $(i = 0, 1, \dots, m-1)$ minimizing the quantity*

$$\max_{x\in[0,d]} |\sqrt{x} \prod_{i=0}^{m-1}(1-\tau_i x)|. \tag{4.25}$$

Considering the expression within the modulus sign, we again arrive at the problem which consists in the search of a polynomial $P_{m-1}(x)$ minimizing the deviation

$$\max_{x\in[0,d]} |\sqrt{x} - x\sqrt{x}P_{m-1}(x)| \tag{4.26}$$

from continuous function $\sqrt{x}$.

Theorem 4.4 *The set of inverse values of non-zero roots σ_i of the function*

$$K_m(x) = (-1)^m p_0 \cos((2m+1)\arccos\sqrt{x/d}) \tag{4.27}$$

with

$$p_0 = \sqrt{d}/(2m+1) \tag{4.28}$$

is a solution of (4.25), *i. e.,*

$$\tau_i = \sigma_i^{-1} = d^{-1}\cos^{-2}\pi(2i+1)/2(2m+1), \qquad i = 0,1,\dots,m-1. \tag{4.29}$$

Proof. Let us consider the system of generalized polynomials $x^{1.5}, x^{2.5}, \dots, x^{m+0.5}$. Take $0 < \varepsilon < \gamma_m = d\cos^2\pi m/(2m+1)$ and the set $N = [\varepsilon, d]$. The minimization problem

$$\min_{\alpha_i \in \mathbf{R}} \max_{x \in N} |x - \sqrt{x}\sum_{i=1}^{m} \alpha_i x^i| \tag{4.30}$$

has a unique solution in terms of Haar's theorem [1]. We prove that function (4.27) is the solution. Indeed, it is defined on the interval $[0,d]$, where it is the product of $\sqrt{x}$ by a polynomial of degree m. All $m+1$ roots of this function

$$\sigma_k = d\cos^2\frac{\pi(2k+1)}{2(2m+1)}, \qquad k = 0,1,\dots,m, \tag{4.31}$$

are found on the interval $[0,d]$ and $\sigma_m = 0$. From the condition

$$\lim_{x\to 0}\frac{1}{\sqrt{x}}K_m(x) = 1$$

the equality

$$K_m(x) = \sqrt{x}\prod_{i=0}^{m-1}(1 - \frac{x}{\sigma_i}) \tag{4.32}$$

follows. Thus, the right-hand side of (4.32) has the form of the expression to be minimized in (4.25). Moreover, with chosen ε, there is on N the set of $m+1$ points

$$\gamma_m < \dots < \gamma_k = d\cos^2 k\pi/(2m+1) < \dots < \gamma_0 = d,$$

at which

$$K_m(\gamma_i) = (-1)^{m-i}p_0 = (-1)^{m-i}\max_N |K_m|,$$

i. e., K_m attains its extrema alternating in sign. Therefore, on the basis of [43], the sufficient conditions of the best approximation are satisfied. Thus, K_m is the unique solution of the optimization problem (4.30). Since all roots of K_m are real and one of them equals zero, K_m, as stated, has the form of the expression within the modulus sign in (4.25). We have thus found the solution of (4.25) on the interval $[\varepsilon, d]$ when ε is sufficiently small. A transition to $\varepsilon = 0$ is made in the same way as in Theorem 4.1. □

Remark 4.1.2 *Due to properties of elementary functions on a complex plane*

$$K_m(x) = -p_0 \operatorname{sh}((2m+1)\operatorname{arsh}\sqrt{-x/d}), \qquad x \le 0. \tag{4.33}$$

By virtue of (4.27) *and* (4.33) *on the interval* $[\gamma_{m+1}, d]$ *where* $\gamma_{m+1} = -d \cdot \operatorname{sh}(\ln(1+\sqrt{2}))^{1/(2m+1)}$, *there are* $m+2$ *points* γ_k *at which the maximum of the modulus of function* K_m *equals* p_0. *This permits to prove, in analogy with Theorem* 4.4, *that* K_m *gives the least deviation from zero, among functions of the form* (4.32), *on the intervals* $[a, d]$ *where*

$$\gamma_{m+1} \le a \le 0.$$

Here

$$|K_m(x)| \le p_0 \quad on \quad [\gamma_{m+1}, d]. \tag{4.34}$$

The following polynomial will be also of value for us:

$$N_m(x) = K_m(x)\,/\,\sqrt{x} = \prod_{i=0}^{m-1}(1 - \frac{x}{\sigma_i}). \tag{4.35}$$

It is proved by analogy with Q_m that

$$|N_m(x)| \;\le\; \ln^{-1}(1+\sqrt{2}) \le p_1 \equiv 1.14 \qquad \forall x \in [\gamma_{m+1}, d], \tag{4.36}$$

$$|N_m(x)| \;\le\; 1 \qquad \forall x \in [0, d]. \tag{4.37}$$

Consider one more optimization problem useful for solving the systems with a spectrum of alternating signs: *find numerical parameters* τ_l $(l = 0, 1, \ldots, m-1)$ *minimizing the quantity*

$$\max_{-d \le x \le d} |\,|x|^{1/2} \prod_{l=0}^{m-1}(1 - \tau_l x^2)|. \tag{4.38}$$

An analytical solution of this problem is expressed in terms of elliptic functions and is not applicable for practical use. An iterative process was therefore constructed in cooperation with E.I.Ogorodnikov to find parameters $\bar{\tau}_l$ of the standard interval $[0, 1]$. The results are presented in Table 4.1 for $m = 1, \ldots, 10$ with 9 digits after point. For other values of d, $\tau_l = \bar{\tau}_l/d^2$.

This problem is obviously equivalent to another one with $\mu = 1/4$: *find numerical parameters* τ_l $(l = 0, 1, \ldots, m-1)$ *minimizing the quantity*

$$\max_{0 \le x \le d^2} |x^\mu \prod_{l=0}^{m-1}(1 - \tau_l x)|, \qquad 0 < \mu \le 1/2. \tag{4.39}$$

As in Theorem 4.9, we find that this problem has a unique solution for set $M = [\varepsilon, d]$ and optimal parameters τ_l are real. What is happen if we use the nonoptimal parameters from (4.25) for the interval $[0, d^2]$:

$$\tau_l = d^{-2}\cos^{-2}(\pi(2l+1)/2(2m+1)), \qquad l = 0, 1, \ldots, m-1. \tag{4.40}$$

Table 4.1:

m	Values of parameters $\bar{\tau}_l$ for $d = 1$				
1	1.4846636724				
2	3.7965985807	1.1296333572			
3	7.5012710302	1.7720161807	1.0601507064		
4	12.563920885	2.7275830504	1.3804716245	1.0347446886	
5	18.979798663	3.9576687803	1.8551723980	1.2308809733	1.0226340660
6	26.747658892 1.0159175530	5.4540395394	2.4520487448	1.5258038895	1.1562946414
7	35.867057469 1.1132869846	7.2140131283 1.0118051543	3.1622612039	1.8940495403	1.3610798011
8	46.337803634 1.2652815136	9.2364918645 1.0860784358	3.9825019344 1.0091044690	2.3273007400	1.6169658911
9	58.159804051 1.4560362713	11.520955682 1.2040410274	4.9112859049 1.0677126347	2.8221090046 1.0072355773	1.9165101357
10	71.333009092 1.6790287897	14.067131556 1.3529793282	5.9478601520 1.1622576184	3.3768132979 1.0547049724	2.2563664381 1.0058886556

Let us leave the denotations K_m, N_m for polinomial (4.32), (4.35) with the roots $\sigma_i = 1/\tau_i$ on the interval $[0, d^2]$. Then

$$\max_{[0,d^2]} |x^\mu \prod_{l=0}^{m-1} (1 - \tau_l x)| = \max_{[0,d^2]} |K_m(x)|^{2\mu} |N_m(x)|^{1-2\mu} \le s_0 \equiv (\frac{d}{2m+1})^{2\mu}, \quad (4.41)$$

$$\max_{[0,d^2]} | \prod_{l=0}^{m-1} (1 - \tau_l x)| = \max_{[0,d^2]} |N_m(x)| = 1. \quad (4.42)$$

Thus, parameters (4.40) are quasi-optimal because they give the same optimal power in the value $s_0 = O(m^{-2\mu})$.

4.2 An abstract setting the multigrid algorithms

We describe the general multigrid algorithms in an abstract algebraic form. It makes it possible take into consideration both the finite element method and in principle difference schemes. Moreover, below we will utilize algebraic criteria of convergence. It is engendered by the use of h-, p- and hp-versions of the finite element method. In contrast to other criteria dealing with approximation properties, the algebraic criteria have general form for these versions.

4.2.1 The algebraic formulation of the multigrid algorithms

Assume that we have a sequence of finite-dimensional spaces

$$M_0, M_1, \dots, M_k \tag{4.43}$$

with inner products denoted by $(\cdot,\cdot)_i$ correspondingly in M_i. Assume also that we have the "interpolation" operators

$$I_i : M_i \to M_{i+1}, \qquad i = 0, \dots, k-1; \tag{4.44}$$

the "restriction" operators

$$R_i : M_i \to M_{i-1}, \qquad i = 1, \dots, k; \tag{4.45}$$

and the inversible operators

$$L_i : M_i \to M_i, \qquad i = 0, \dots, k. \tag{4.46}$$

The main purpose of our algorithms is to solve the problem on M_k: *given* $f_k \in M_k$, *find* $v_k \in M_k$ *such that*

$$L_k v_k = f_k. \tag{4.47}$$

But the proper feature of the multigrid algorithms consists in the necessity of solving auxiliary problems at lower levels. Therefore, we formulate an MG_i-algorithm for approximating the solution of the problem

$$L_i v_i = f_i, \quad \text{given} \quad f_i \in M_i \tag{4.48}$$

at any level $i \in [0, k]$. We begin with an initial guess w_0 and produce as a result another approximation (expected to be rather close to v_i) denoted by $w_1 = MG_i(w_0, f_i)$.

MG_i**-algorithm.** If $i = 0$ then

$$w_1 = MG_0(w_0, f_0) = L_0^{-1} f_0, \tag{4.49}$$

initial guess w_0 does no matter and MG_0 is finished. For $i > 0$ the algorithm is defined as follows:

A_1 (pre-smoothing). Let $u_0 = w_0$ and define u_{m_1} by

$$u_{l+1} = u_l - \mathcal{D}_{i,l+1}(L_i u_l - f_i), \qquad l = 0, 1, \dots, m_1 - 1; \tag{4.50}$$

A_2 (restricting). Let

$$g_{i-1} = R_i(L_i u_{m_1} - f_i); \tag{4.51}$$

A_3 (coarse-grid solving). Let $\tilde{w}_0 = 0 \in M_{i-1}$ and repeat MG_{i-1}-algorithm γ times:

$$\tilde{w}_s = MG_{i-1}(\tilde{w}_{s-1}, g_{i-1}), \qquad s = 1, \dots, \gamma; \tag{4.52}$$

A_4 (correcting). Let

$$y_0 = u_{m_1} - I_{i-1}\tilde{w}_\gamma; \tag{4.53}$$

A_5 (post-smoothing). Define y_{m_2} by

$$y_{l+1} = y_l - \mathcal{D}_{i,l+m_1+1}(L_i y_l - f_i), \qquad l = 0, 1, \ldots, m_2 - 1. \tag{4.54}$$

Finally, we set

$$w_1 = MG_i(w_0, f_i) = y_{m_2} \tag{4.55}$$

as a result of the MG_i-algorithm.

Here $\mathcal{D}_{i,l}$ $(l = 1, \ldots, m_1 + m_2)$ are some linear operators; we consider their form later. Later we also illustrate possible choices of the remaining integers m_1, m_2, γ.

Three steps $A_2 - A_4$ taken together are usually named *the coarse-grid correction.*

Now we formulate the full (nested) multigrid FMG-algorithm for solution of the sequence of problems (4.48) including the highest level (4.47) as the final stage.

FMG-**algorithm.**

1. Set $\tilde{u}_0 = L_0^{-1} f_0$.

2. For $i = 1, 2, \ldots, k$ do as follows:

   2.1 set $\tilde{u}_i = I_{i-1}\tilde{u}_{i-1}$;

   2.2 repeat the MG_i-algorithm t times:

$$\tilde{u}_i := MG_i(\tilde{u}_i, f_i). \tag{4.56}$$

After k-th step we come to the final result $\tilde{u}_k$ which is some approximation of the solution v_k of (4.47) at the level k.

4.2.2 The multigrid operator of error suppression

Fix integer $i \in [1, k]$ and let $e_0 = w_0 - v_i$ be the error of the initial guess w_0 for the exact solution v_i of problem (4.48) and $e_1 = w_1 - v_i$ be the error of the final approximation w_1. In principle, we can fulfil the MG_i-algorithm for any e_0 and receive the unique result w_1 and the corresponding error e_1. By such a way we have some operator $B_i : \ e_0 \to e_1$. We will name it the operator of error suppression. Let us show that B_i is linear and find its explicit form. For this purpose, we introduce the operators

$$J_i^{(m_1)} = (I - \mathcal{D}_{i,m_1} L_i) \ldots (I - \mathcal{D}_{i,1} L_i) \tag{4.57}$$

$$J_i^{(m_2)} = (I - \mathcal{D}_{i,m_1+m_2} L_i) \ldots (I - \mathcal{D}_{i,m_1+1} L_i). \tag{4.58}$$

Here and further the operator I stands for identity operator with appropriate dimension.

Lemma 4.2.1 *The operator B_i of error suppression in the MG_i-algorithm is definite, linear for any e_0, independent of f_i, w_0 and has the form*

$$B_i = J_i^{(m_2)}(I - I_{i-1}(I - B_{i-1}^{\gamma}) L_{i-1}^{-1} R_i L_i) J_i^{(m_1)}. \tag{4.59}$$

Proof. We prove this result by induction with respect to i. For $i = 0$, we solve the problem (4.48) directly (s. f. (4.49)) and the error is equal to zero. So, the operator B_0 of error suppression is a null operator. Now suppose that B_{i-1} is definite, linear for any error at the level $i-1$ and independent of f_{i-1} and the initial guess.

At the stage A_1, we denote the error of the iterative approximation u_l by $\sigma_l = u_l - v_i$. Then we subtract v_i from both sides of (4.50) and use (4.48):

$$\sigma_{l+1} = \sigma_l - \mathcal{D}_{i,l+1} L_i \sigma_l, \qquad l = 0, \dots, m_1 - 1. \tag{4.60}$$

By induction, we find the equality

$$\sigma_{m_1} = J_i^{(m_1)} e_0 \tag{4.61}$$

with notation (4.58). At the stage A_2, we again use (4.48).

$$g_{i-1} = R_i L_i \sigma_{m_1}. \tag{4.62}$$

Denote the solution of the problem

$$L_{i-1} \tilde{w}_* = g_{i-1} \tag{4.63}$$

by $\tilde{w}_*$, i. e.,

$$\tilde{w}_* = L_{i-1}^{-1} R_i L_i \sigma_{m_1}. \tag{4.64}$$

At the stage A_3 in the MG_{i-1}-algorithm, we use the zero initial guess. So the initial error δ_0 is equal to $\tilde{w}_*$. On applying MG_{i-1} once, we come to the result $\tilde{w}_1$ with the error $\delta_1 = B_{i-1}\delta_0 = B_{i-1}\tilde{w}_*$. After γ applications the error of approximation $\tilde{w}_\gamma$ is equal to $\delta_\gamma = B_{i-1}^\gamma \tilde{w}_*$, i. e.,

$$\tilde{w}_\gamma = \tilde{w}_* - \delta_\gamma = (I - B_{i-1}^\gamma)\tilde{w}_*. \tag{4.65}$$

At the stages A_4, A_5, we denote the error of y_l by $\rho_l = y_l - v_i$. Subtracting v_i from both sides of (4.53), we arrive at the equality

$$\rho_0 = \sigma_{m_1} - I_{i-1}\tilde{w}_\gamma.$$

Use here (4.65) and (4.64):

$$\begin{aligned} \rho_0 &= \sigma_{m_1} - I_{i-1}(I - B_{i-1}^\gamma)\tilde{w}_* = \\ &= (I - I_{i-1}(I - B_{i-1}^\gamma)L_{i-1}^{-1} R_i L_i)\sigma_{m_1}. \end{aligned} \tag{4.66}$$

By analogy with the stage A_1,

$$\rho_{m_2} = J_i^{(m_2)} \rho_0. \tag{4.67}$$

Combine (4.67), (4.66) and (4.61):

$$\rho_{m_2} = J_i^{(m_2)} \{I - I_{i-1}(I - B_{i-1}^\gamma)L_{i-1}^{-1} R_i L_i\} J_i^{(m_1)} e_0. \tag{4.68}$$

Since $e_1 = \rho_{m_2}$, the statement (4.59) is proved. □

4.3 The convergence in the symmetric variant

In this section and below, we suppose that the symmetric variant has the following five features:

$$\text{the operators } L_i \text{ are self-adjoint and positive-definite;} \tag{4.69}$$

$$I_{i-1} = R_i^* \tag{4.70}$$

and

$$J_i^{(m_1)} = J_i^{(m_2)*} \tag{4.71}$$

in the sense of inner products $(\cdot,\cdot)_i$;

$$L_{i-1} = R_i L_i I_{i-1}. \tag{4.72}$$

Finally, put $J_i \equiv J_i^{(m_1)}$ and suppose

$$J_i L_i = L_i J_i \qquad (\text{hence,} \quad J_i^* L_i = L_i J_i^*). \tag{4.73}$$

With this supposition, the convergence is proved rather simply and the convergence estimations are more accurate (see, for example, [31], [30], [108]).

4.3.1 The regular case

We first reduce the convergence criterion to one inequality not used in the literature before. Then we illustrate the proof of this criterion from the other known convergence conditions. Finally, we demonstrate the possibility for the choice of iterative parameters in Jacobi-type iterations. As a result we obtain better convergence estimates than without the optimal choice.

Along with the inner product $(\cdot,\cdot)_i$ in M_i, let us introduce the L_i-inner product

$$[u,v]_i = (L_i u, v)_i \qquad \forall u,v \in M_i \tag{4.74}$$

and the corresponding norms

$$\|u\|_i = (u,u)_i^{1/2}, \qquad [\![u]\!]_i = [u,u]_i^{1/2}. \tag{4.75}$$

Now, we construct some operator which is useful in the further description. For this purpose, take any $u \in M_i$, solve the equation

$$L_{i-1} v = R_i L_i u \tag{4.76}$$

and set

$$w = u - I_{i-1} v. \tag{4.77}$$

This algorithm gives us an operator $Q_i : \ u \to w$. It acts as follows:

$$Q_i = I - I_{i-1} L_{i-1}^{-1} R_i L_i \tag{4.78}$$

with the identical operator I and simulates an appearance of the main part of the error in the multigrid method. Namely, instead of solving the problem

$$L_i u = f_i \tag{4.79}$$

we solve the auxiliary one

$$L_{i-1} v = R_i f_i \tag{4.80}$$

on a more coarse grid or a lower level. The obtained solution v is then interpolated onto the fine grid or the high level again: $\tilde{u} = I_{i-1} v$. And finally, we compute the difference between the exact solution u and an approximate one $\tilde{u}$.

Lemma 4.3.1 *Under conditions* (4.69), (4.70), (4.72) *the operator Q_i is a self-adjoint projector from M_i into orthogonal complementary of $I_{i-1}M_{i-1}$ up to M_i in the inner product $[\cdot,\cdot]_i$.*

Proof. First, we show that w from (4.77) is orthogonal to any $z \in I_{i-1}M_{i-1}$. Let $y \in M_{i-1}$ such that $z = I_{i-1}y$. Use (4.77), (4.69)–(4.72) and finally (4.76):

$$\begin{aligned}(L_i w, z)_i &= (u - I_{i-1}v, L_i I_{i-1} y)_i = (R_i L_i u, y)_{i-1} - \\ &- (v, L_{i-1} y)_{i-1} = (R_i L_i u - L_{i-1} v, y)_{i-1} = 0.\end{aligned}$$

Thus w is orthogonal to z and due to the arbitrariness of z, we proved that w is orthogonal to $I_{i-1}M_{i-1}$.

Second, we show that Q_i is a projective operator. For this purpose, we compute from (4.78):

$$Q_i^2 = I - 2I_{i-1}L_{i-1}^{-1}R_i L_i + I_{i-1}L_{i-1}^{-1}R_i L_i I_{i-1} L_{i-1}^{-1} R_i L_i.$$

The last summand is simplified due to (4.72) and gives the previous one with another multiplier what leads to the required equality:

$$Q_i^2 = I - I_{i-1}L_{i-1}^{-1}R_i L_i = Q_i. \tag{4.81}$$

Third, we show that Q_i is self-adjoint. Use (4.78), (4.69), (4.70):

$$\begin{aligned}[Q_i u, v]_i &= ((L_i - L_i I_{i-1} L_{i-1}^{-1} R_i L_i)u, v)_i = \\ &= (L_i u, v)_i - (L_i u, I_{i-1} L_{i-1}^{-1} R_i L_i v)_i = (L_i u, Q_i v)_i = \\ &= [u, Q_i v]_i. \square\end{aligned}$$

Applying these operators, we may formulate the convergence criterion: *there is constant $c^* > 0$ such that $\forall i = 1, \dots, k$ $\forall v \in M_i$*

$$[\![v]\!]_i^2 - [\![J_i v]\!]_i^2 \geq c^* [\![Q_i J_i v]\!]_i^2. \tag{4.82}$$

Now we prove the convergence of *the symmetric V-cycle.*

Theorem 4.5 *Let the conditions* (4.69)–(4.73), (4.82) *be valid for the MG_i-algorithm with $\gamma = 1$. Then*

$$[\![B_i]\!]_i = \sup_{v \in M_i \setminus \{0\}} [\![B_i v]\!]_i / [\![v]\!]_i \leq \frac{1}{1 + c^*}. \tag{4.83}$$

Proof. First prove that the operators B_i are self-adjoint in the inner products $[\cdot,\cdot]_i$ under conditions (4.69)–(4.73). Use the induction in i. For $i = 0$ $B_0 \equiv 0$ and the result is valid. Then suppose that B_{i-1} is self-adjoint in the inner product $[\cdot,\cdot]_{i-1}$. Then $L_{i-1}B_{i-1}$ and $B_{i-1}L_{i-1}^{-1} = L_{i-1}^{-1}(L_{i-1}B_{i-1})L_{i-1}^{-1}$ are self-adjoint in $(\cdot,\cdot)_{i-1}$. Now use the explicit formulation (4.59). Then $\forall v, w \in M_i$

$$[B_i v, w]_i = (L_i J_i^*(I - I_{i-1}(I - B_{i-1})L_{i-1}^{-1}R_i L_i)J_i v, w)_i.$$

Use (4.73), (4.69), (4.70) and the self-adjointness of $B_{i-1}L_{i-1}^{-1}$ in connective order:

$$\begin{aligned}[B_i v, w]_i &= (L_i J_i v, J_i w) - (L_{i-1}^{-1}R_i L_i J_i v, R_i L_i J_i w) + \\ &+ (B_{i-1}L_{i-1}^{-1}R_i L_i J_i v, R_i L_i J_i w) = \\ &= (L_i v, J_i^*(I - I_{i-1}(I - B_{i-1})L_{i-1}^{-1}R_i L_i)J_i w)_i = \\ &= (L_i v, B_i w)_i = [v, B_i w]_i.\end{aligned} \tag{4.84}$$

It proves the self-adjointness of B_i in $[\cdot,\cdot]_i$.

Since M_i is finite-dimensional

$$[\![B_i]\!]_i = \sup_{v \in M_i \setminus \{0\}} |[B_i v, v]_i| / [\![v]\!]_i. \tag{4.85}$$

Now let us prove the inequality

$$0 \le \frac{[B_i v, v]_i}{[v, v]_i} \le \varepsilon \equiv \frac{1}{1 + c^*} \qquad \forall v \in M_i \setminus \{0\} \tag{4.86}$$

by induction. For $i = 0$ $B_0 \equiv 0$ and (4.86) is valid for any $c^* \in (0, \infty)$. Suppose that B_{i-1} satisfies (4.86) . Then put $w = v$ in (4.84) and use (4.78):

$$[B_i v, v]_i = [J_i^* Q_i J_i v, v]_i + (B_{i-1}L_{i-1}^{-1}R_i L_i J_i v, R_i L_i J_i v)_{i-1} =$$

$$= [Q_i J_i v, J_i v]_i + [B_{i-1}L_{i-1}^{-1}R_i L_i J_i v, L_{i-1}^{-1}R_i L_i J_i v]_{i-1}.$$

Due to (4.86), (4.69), (4.70), (4.78), (4.80)

$$\begin{aligned}0 \le [B_i v, v]_i &\le [Q_i J_i v, J_i v]_i + \varepsilon(R_i L_i J_i v, L_{i-1}^{-1}R_i L_i J_i v)_{i-1} = \\ &= (1 - \varepsilon)[Q_i J_i v, J_i v]_i + \varepsilon[J_i v, J_i v]_i = \\ &= (1 - \varepsilon)[\![Q_i J_i v]\!]_i^2 + \varepsilon[\![J_i v]\!]_i^2.\end{aligned} \tag{4.87}$$

Now use (4.82) and the equality $(1 - \varepsilon)/c^* = \varepsilon$:

$$[B_i v, v]_i \le \varepsilon[\![v]\!]_i^2. \tag{4.88}$$

That proves (4.86) and (4.85). □

Remark 4.3.1 *We may use, in principle, another version of the V-cycle and the W-cycle. But estimates would be the same or worse than (4.83). Further, parallel realization of the V-cycle is more convenient than that of the W-cycle. Therefore we will not investigate another version of the MG-algorithm and will try to use the symmetric V-cycle in all the cases where it is justified.*

4.3.2 The verification of the convergence criterion

In this section we show that criterion (4.82) follows from some known inequalities which may be more convenient for verification. We start with algebraic properties and, firstly, consider the following "approximation" assumption [6]: *there exists a constant* $c_1 > 0$ *such that*

$$[Q_i v, v]_i \leq c_1 \|L_i v\|_i^2/\lambda_i^* \qquad \forall v \in M_i. \tag{4.89}$$

In this section λ_i^* will denote the largest eigenvalue of L_i or some appropriate upper bound identical throughout the description. Secondly, we consider the "smoothing" assumption: *there exists a constant* $c_2 > 0$ *such that*

$$\|L_i J_i v\|_i^2/\lambda_i^* \leq c_2(\llbracket v \rrbracket_i^2 - \llbracket J_i v \rrbracket_i^2) \qquad \forall v \in M_i. \tag{4.90}$$

Lemma 4.3.2 *Assumptions* (4.89), (4.90) *imply* (4.82) *under conditions* (4.69), (4.70), (4.72) *with the constant* $c^* = (c_1 c_2)^{-1}$.

Proof. It follows from Lemma 4.3.1 that the operator Q_i is projective and self-adjoint in the inner product $[\ ,\ ]_i$. Therefore

$$[Q_i v, v]_i = \llbracket Q_i v \rrbracket_i^2. \tag{4.91}$$

Stand $J_i v$ for v in (4.89) and use (4.90)(4.91):

$$\llbracket Q_i J_i v \rrbracket_i^2 \leq c_1 \|L_i J_i v\|_i^2/\lambda_i^* \leq c_1 c_2(\llbracket v \rrbracket_i^2 - \llbracket J_i \rrbracket_i^2). \tag{4.92}$$

Dividing by $c_1 c_2$ the both parts of (4.92) we receive (4.82) □

In most of articles the smoothing procedure J_i consists of m identical iterations (4.50) with the matrix $\mathcal{D}_i = \mathcal{D}_{i,j}$, $j = 1, \ldots, 2m$; $m = m_1 = m_2$. In this case the "smoothing" assumption may be formulated in a step-wise manner: *there exists a constant* $c_3 > 0$ *such that*

$$\|v\|_i^2/\lambda_i^* \leq c_3(\mathcal{D}_i v, v)_i \qquad \forall v \in M_i. \tag{4.93}$$

Let us introduce *the iterative operator* $K_i = I - \mathcal{D}_i L_i$ *of one step.* Note that $J_i = K_i^m$. Use its notation and stand $L_i v$ for v in (4.93). Then we come to another form of (4.93): *there exists a constant* $c_3 > 0$ *such that*

$$\|L_i v\|_i^2/\lambda_i^* \leq c_3[(I - K_i)v, v]_i \qquad \forall v \in M_i. \tag{4.94}$$

Lemma 4.3.3 *Let* (4.69), (4.94) *hold and the operator* K_i *be symmetric, nonnegative in the inner product* $[\cdot,\cdot]_i$ *and let* $\llbracket K_i \rrbracket_i \leq 1$. *Then* (4.90) *is valid with the constant* $c_2 = c_3/2m$.

Proof. We use some inequalities from [31]. Namely, "since the spectrum of K_i is contained in the interval $[0, 1]$" in the sense of the inner product $[\cdot,\cdot]_i$,

$$[(I - K_i)K_i^{2m} v, v]_i \leq \frac{1}{2m} \sum_{j=0}^{2m-1} [(I - K_i)K_i^j v, v]_i = \frac{1}{2m}[(I - K_i^{2m})v, v]_i. \tag{4.95}$$

Transform both sides of (4.95):

$$[(I - K_i)J_i v, J_i v]_i \le \frac{1}{2m}([\![v]\!]_i^2 - [\![J_i v]\!]_i^2). \tag{4.96}$$

Then stand $J_i v$ for v in (4.94) and use (4.96):

$$\|L_i J_i v\|_i^2/\lambda_i^* \le c_3[(I - K_i)J_i v, J_i v]_i \le \frac{c_3}{2m}([\![v]\!]_i^2 - [\![J_i v]\!]_i^2). \quad \square$$

Now we show that the lucky choice of parameters in Jacobi-type iterative process gives a better result in the sense of dependence of c_3 on the number m of iterations.

Recall that λ_i^* is the upper bound of the largest eigenvalue of L_i. In practice we may compute λ_i^* by using Gershgorin's circles. Usually this way gives the value of λ_i^* which exceeds λ_i by several percents only. This results in a slight increase in the number of iterations m, as we will see later. Therefore we may use λ_i^* not only in the theory but also in algorithms.

So let us use the pre-smoothing and post-smoothing iterations:

$$A_1'. \qquad u_{l+1} = u_l - \tau_l(L_i u_l - f_i), \tag{4.97}$$

$$A_5'. \qquad y_{l+1} = y_l - \tau_l(L_i y_l - f_i), \qquad l = 0, 1, \dots, m-1, \tag{4.98}$$

instead of (4.50), (4.55). We choose special scalar parameters

$$\tau_l = \frac{(\lambda_i^*)^{-1}\cos^2\beta}{\cos^2(2l+1)\beta - \sin^2\beta}, \qquad \beta = \frac{\pi}{2(2m+1)}, \qquad l = 0, 1, \dots, m-1 \tag{4.99}$$

as a solution of some optimization problem.

Theorem 4.6 *Let* (4.69) *be valid and let the Jacobi-type iterative operator* J_i *be defined by formulae* (4.97), (4.98) *with parameters* (4.99). *Then* (4.90) *holds with the constant*

$$c_2 = \operatorname{tg}^2\frac{\pi}{2(2m+1)}. \tag{4.100}$$

Proof. Let us introduce the polynomials

$$N(\lambda) = \prod_{l=0}^{m-1}(1 - \tau_l\lambda) \tag{4.101}$$

and

$$M(\lambda) = (1 + \frac{\lambda}{c_2\lambda_i^*})N^2(\lambda) \tag{4.102}$$

with parameters (4.99), (4.100). Then use the transformation of coordinates

$$x = \lambda_i^* \sin^2\beta + \lambda\cos^2\beta \tag{4.103}$$

and show that

$$M(\lambda) = K^2(x) \equiv \cos^2((2m+1)\arccos\sqrt{x/\lambda_i^*}), \qquad x \in [0, \lambda_i^*]. \tag{4.104}$$

Indeed, the roots of $K(x)$ are equal to $\lambda_i^* \cos^2(2l+1)\beta$, $l = 0, \ldots, m$. Transformation (4.103) associates them with exact roots of the polynomial $M(\lambda)$ which are equal to the inverse values of τ_l and $-c_2\lambda_i^*$. Moreover, the simple root $x = 0$ is associated with the simple root $-c_2\lambda_i^*$ and multiplicity of the other roots is equal to 2 for both polynomials. Then we can compute that $M(0) = K^2(\lambda_i^* \sin\beta) = 1$. Therefore (4.104) is valid.

Since $\lambda \in [0, \lambda_i^*]$, we get $x \in [\lambda_i^* \sin^2\beta, \lambda_i^*]$. In this interval, function (4.104) is computable and

$$0 \le M(\lambda) \le 1. \tag{4.105}$$

From the explicit form of $M(\lambda)$, it follows that

$$\frac{\lambda}{\lambda_i^*} N^2(\lambda) \le c_2(1 - N^2(\lambda)) \qquad \forall \lambda \in [0, \lambda_i^*]. \tag{4.106}$$

Let $v \in M_i$ be an arbitrary vector. Since L_i is self-adjoint, there exists a system of eigenvectors $g_1, \ldots, g_{n_i}$ where n_i is the dimension of M_i. Each g_i corresponds to some eigenvalue λ_i and the system is orthogonal in the inner product $(\cdot,\cdot)_i$. Let

$$v = \sum_{j=1}^{n_i} \alpha_j g_j \tag{4.107}$$

be the decomposition of v in this system. Then

$$\|L_i J_i v\|_i^2 = \sum_{j=1}^{n_i} (\alpha_j \lambda_j N(\lambda_j))^2,$$

$$[\![v]\!]_i^2 = \sum_{j=1}^{n_i} \alpha_j^2 \lambda_j,$$

$$[\![J_i v]\!]_i^2 = \sum_{j=1}^{n_i} (\alpha_j N(\lambda_j))^2 \lambda_j.$$

Use these equations and (4.106) for $\lambda = \lambda_j$:

$$\begin{aligned} \frac{1}{\lambda_i^*}\|L_i J_i v\|_i^2 &= \sum_{j=1}^{n_i} \alpha_j^2 \lambda_j \cdot \frac{\lambda_j}{\lambda_i^*} N^2(\lambda_j) \le \\ &\le \sum_{j=1}^{n_i} \alpha_j^2 \lambda_j \cdot c_2(1 - N^2(\lambda_j)) = c_2([\![v]\!]_i^2 - [\![J_i v]\!]_i^2). \ \square \end{aligned}$$

Remark 4.3.2 *The constant* (4.100) *is least which may be proved in* (4.90). *There are no other iterative parameters* τ_l *(even complex) which give us the constant* c_2 *less or equal to* $\mathrm{tg}^2\beta$ *in estimate* (4.106). *This statement follows from the uniqueness of the polynomial with the least deviation from zero.*

Remark 4.3.3 *Combining the results of Theorem* 4.5, 4.6 *and Lemma* 4.3.2, *we come to the following estimate in energetic norm of error suppression for operators* B_i*:*

$$[\![B_i]\!]_i \leq 1/(1 + c_1^{-1}\mathrm{ctg}^2\pi/2(2m+1)) \tag{4.108}$$

for smoothing procedures (4.97)–(4.99). *For large* m*, the right-hand side asymptotically tends to the value*

$$c_1\pi^2/4(2m+1)^2 = O(m^{-2}). \tag{4.109}$$

For the trivial choice of iterative parameters

$$\tau_l = 1/\lambda_i^*, \qquad l = 0, 1, \dots, m-1,$$

instead of (4.99) *in the procedures* (4.97), (4.98), *we should have only* $[\![B_i]\!]_i = O(m^{-1})$.

Remark 4.3.4 *The choice* (4.99) *in our symmetric case gives a very good rate of convergence in comparison with other smoothing procedures* [68]. *On the other hand, the Jacobi-type iterations are convenient from many points of view. For example, we may fulfil multiplication by the matrix* L_i *without storage of its elements. We may use only stiffness matrices for each element. This is very convenient for parallel computations.*

Therefore we dwell on this type of iterations and will not investigate other types.

4.3.3 The non-regular case

The criterion (4.89) is not valid for problems with the insufficient approximation properties and we need utilize another weaker one.

Before, we introduce fractional powers of self-adjoint operators. Let L be some self-adjoint positive-definite operator in an n-dimensional space M. There exists a system of eigenvectors $g_1, \dots, g_n$ and a corresponding set of eigenvalues $\lambda_1, \dots, \lambda_n$. Let $v \in M$ be an arbitrary vector. Since the system $\{g_j\}$ is linearly independent, we may construct a decomposition

$$v = \sum_{j=1}^{n} \alpha_j g_j. \tag{4.110}$$

The operator L acts on v as follows:

$$Lv = \sum_{j=1}^{n} \alpha_j L g_j = \sum_{j=1}^{n} \alpha_j \lambda_j g_j. \tag{4.111}$$

For any positive value λ and real β we will consider λ^β in the sense of main value which is real and positive too. Accordingly, we introduce the linear operator $L^\beta : M \to M$ by the formula

$$L^\beta v = \sum_{j=1}^{n} \alpha_j \lambda_j^\beta g_j. \tag{4.112}$$

Due to (4.111) this definition coincides with the usual properties when β is integer, positive or negative.

Now we may formulate the weaker criterion: *there exist constants* $\alpha \in (0,1]$ *and* $c_4 > 0$ *such that* $\forall v \in M_i$

$$[\![Q_i v]\!]_i^2 = [Q_i v, v]_i \leq \frac{c_4}{(\lambda_i^*)^\alpha} \|L_i^{(1+\alpha)/2} v\|_i^2, \quad i = 1, \ldots, k. \tag{4.113}$$

When $\alpha = 1$, (4.110) coincides with (4.89).

In the paper [31] the similar criterion is presented which looks as follows in our notation: *there exist constants* $c_4 > 0$ *and* $\alpha \in (0,1]$ *such that* $\forall v \in M_i$

$$[Q_i v, v]_i \leq \frac{c_4}{(\lambda_i^*)^\alpha} \|L_i v\|_i^{2\alpha} [\![v]\!]_i^{2(1-\alpha)}. \tag{4.114}$$

Let us show that (4.114) follows from (4.113) with the same constants α, c_4. Let $v \in M_i$ be an arbitrary vector. Transform $L_i^{(1+\alpha)/2}$ with the help of (4.107), use the orthogonality of system $\{g_i\}$ and the Hölder inequality:

$$\begin{aligned} \|L_i^{(1+\alpha)/2} v\|_i^2 &= \sum_{j=1}^{n_i} \lambda_j^{1+\alpha} \alpha_j^2 = \\ &= \sum_{j=1}^{n_i} (\lambda_j \alpha_j)^{2\alpha} (\lambda_j^{1/2} \alpha_j)^{2(1-\alpha)} \leq \\ &\leq \left(\sum_{j=1}^{n_i} (\lambda_j \alpha_j)^2 \right)^\alpha \left(\sum_{j=1}^{n_i} (\lambda_j^{1/2} \alpha_j)^2 \right)^{(1-\alpha)} = \\ &= \|L_i v\|_i^{2\alpha} [\![v]\!]_i^{2(1-\alpha)}. \end{aligned}$$

Thus, left-hand side of (4.113) is smaller than left-hand side of (4.114). □

The criterion (4.114) is simpler to be verified because it does not use any fractional powers of L_i. But the criterion (4.113) contains the weaker norm in the right-hand side than (4.114).

In the non-regular case, the convergence of the usual V-cycle becomes worse in practice and theoretical estimates of the convergence rate become dependent on the number k of the levels [31]. The simplest recommendation consists in utilization of the W-cycle [68] which converges in this case. From the point of view of the computational complexity, the standard configuration of the W-cycle is similar to the V-cycle with the number of smoothing iterations which increases twice from one level to another. The V-cycle is simpler than the W-cycle from many points of view. Therefore we again try to use the symmetric V-cycle but with nonstationary number of iterations as in [31], [174], i. e., m will depend on the number of level i and will increase with decreasing i.

We proceed by close analogy with the article of J.H.Bramble, J.E.Pasciak [31]. But we use another (better) type of the smoothing procedure and need to alter the proof.

Theorem 4.7 *Let the conditions* (4.69)–(4.73) *and one of* (4.113) *or* (4.114) *be valid for the* MG_i*-algorithm with* $\gamma = 1$ *and the Jacobi-type smoothing iterative procedures be defined by the formulae* (4.97), (4.98) *with parameters* (4.99). *Assume also that the* *amount m of smoothing iterations depends on the number i (i. e., $m = m(i)$) and satisfies*

$$1 < \beta_0 \le \frac{2m(i-1)+1}{2m(i)+1} \le \beta_1 \qquad \forall i = 2, \dots, k. \tag{4.115}$$

Then

$$[\![B_i]\!]_i \le \frac{\sigma}{\sigma + \omega(i)} \tag{4.116}$$

with the constants

$$\sigma = \left(\frac{\tilde{\sigma} + 3^\alpha}{\tilde{\sigma}}\right)^{\frac{1-\alpha}{\alpha}} \tilde{\sigma}; \tag{4.117}$$

$$\tilde{\sigma} = 1.23\, \alpha \beta_1^2 c_4^{1/\alpha} \left(\frac{1-\alpha}{\beta_0^{2\alpha} - 1}\right)^{\frac{1-\alpha}{\alpha}} 3^{\alpha-1}; \tag{4.118}$$

$$\omega(i) = \mathrm{ctg}^{2\alpha}(\pi/2(2m(i)+1)). \tag{4.119}$$

Proof. We use induction in number of the level i. For $i = 0$, we have $[\![B_0]\!]_0 = 0$ due to the direct method; and (4.116) holds for any positive σ, $\omega(0)$. Assume that

$$[\![B_{i-1}]\!]_{i-1} \le \frac{\sigma}{\sigma + \omega(i-1)} = \varepsilon_{i-1} \tag{4.120}$$

is valid for some $i \in [1, k-1]$ with constants (4.117)–(4.119).

Let $v \in M_i$ be an arbitrary vector. Repeating the calculations (4.86)–(4.87), we obtain the inequality

$$[B_i v, v]_i \le (1 - \varepsilon_{i-1})[\![Q_i J_i v]\!]_i^2 + \varepsilon_{i-1}[\![J_i v]\!]_i^2. \tag{4.121}$$

Since (4.113) implies (4.114), we can implement (4.114) in any case. Substitute $J_i v$ for v in (4.114):

$$[\![Q_i J_i v]\!]_i^2 \le \frac{c_4}{(\lambda_i^*)^\alpha} \|L_i J_i v\|_i^{2\alpha} [\![J_i v]\!]_i^{2(1-\alpha)}. \tag{4.122}$$

Now use J.H.Young's inequality in the following form:

$$c^\alpha d^{1-\alpha} \le \alpha \gamma c + (1-\alpha) d \gamma^{-\frac{\alpha}{1-\alpha}} \tag{4.123}$$

which is valid for $c \ge 0$, $d \ge 0$ and arbitrary $0 < \gamma < \infty$. Taking

$$c = \|L_i J_i v\|_i^2 / \lambda_i^*,$$

$$d = [\![J_i v]\!]_i^2,$$

we have

$$[\![Q_i J_i v]\!]_i^2 \le c_4 \alpha \gamma \|L_i J_i v\|_i^2 / \lambda_i^* + c_4(1-\alpha)\gamma^{-\frac{\alpha}{1-\alpha}} [\![J_i v]\!]_i^2. \tag{4.124}$$

We recall that inequality (4.90) is valid with the constant

$$c_2 = c_2(i) = \mathrm{tg}^2(\pi/2(2m(i)+1)). \tag{4.125}$$

Using it in (4.124), we obtain:

$$[\![Q_iJ_iv]\!]_i^2 \le c_2c_4\alpha\gamma([\![v]\!]_i^2 - [\![J_iv]\!]_i^2) + c_4(1-\alpha)\gamma^{-\frac{\alpha}{1-\alpha}}[\![J_iv]\!]_i^2. \tag{4.126}$$

Now combine (4.126) and (4.121):

$$\begin{aligned} [B_iv,v]_i &\le (1-\varepsilon_{i-1})c_2c_4\alpha\gamma([\![v]\!]_i^2 - [\![J_iv]\!]_i^2) + \\ &+ ((1-\varepsilon_{i-1})c_4(1-\alpha)\gamma^{-\frac{\alpha}{1-\alpha}} + \varepsilon_{i-1})[\![J_iv]\!]_i^2. \end{aligned} \tag{4.127}$$

To simplify terms in (4.127), we take a positive number γ such that

$$\varepsilon_{i-1} = \alpha\gamma(1-\varepsilon_{i-1})c_4c_2(i). \tag{4.128}$$

With this γ let us show that

$$(1-\varepsilon_{i-1})c_4(1-\alpha)\gamma^{-\frac{\alpha}{1-\alpha}} \le \varepsilon_i - \varepsilon_{i-1}. \tag{4.129}$$

From the fact that the function $\mathrm{tg}x/x$ changes in the limits $[1, 1.103]$ for $x \in [0, \pi/6]$, it follows that

$$\beta_0^{2\alpha} \le \frac{\omega(i-1)}{\omega(i)} \le (1.11\beta_1)^{2\alpha}. \tag{4.130}$$

Now we proceed as in the paper [31]. First we calculate the left-hand side of (4.129), using explicit form of its ingredients and the estimate (4.130):

$$\begin{aligned} &\frac{\omega(i-1)}{\sigma+\omega(i-1)}\, c_4\,(1-\alpha)\left\{\frac{\alpha\omega(i-1)c_4}{\sigma\omega^{1/\alpha}(i)}\right\}^{\frac{\alpha}{1-\alpha}} \le \\ &\le \frac{1-\alpha}{\sigma+\omega(i-1)}\left\{1.11^2\beta_1^2c_4^{1/\alpha}\alpha/\sigma\right\}^{\frac{\alpha}{1-\alpha}}. \end{aligned} \tag{4.131}$$

The direct computation of the right-hand side of (4.129) gives

$$\varepsilon_i - \varepsilon_{i-1} \ge \frac{\sigma\omega(i)(\beta_0^{2\alpha}-1)}{(\sigma+\omega(i))(\sigma+\omega(i-1))}. \tag{4.132}$$

From (4.131), (4.132) we see that (4.129) holds if

$$(1-\alpha)(1.11^2\beta_1^2c_4^{1/\alpha}\alpha)^{\frac{\alpha}{1-\alpha}} \le (\beta_0^{2\alpha}-1)\sigma^{\frac{\alpha}{1-\alpha}}\frac{\sigma\omega(i)}{\sigma+\omega(i)}. \tag{4.133}$$

Transform right-hand side of (4.133). Due to the monotonicity of $\omega(i)$,

$$\sigma\frac{\omega(i)}{\sigma+\omega(i)} \ge 3^\alpha\frac{\sigma}{\sigma+3^\alpha}. \tag{4.134}$$

It follows from (4.117) that

$$\sigma^{\frac{\alpha}{1-\alpha}}\frac{\sigma}{\sigma+3^\alpha} \geq \tilde{\sigma}^{\frac{\alpha}{1-\alpha}}. \tag{4.135}$$

The last two inequalities give

$$(\beta_0^{2\alpha}-1)\sigma^{\frac{\alpha}{1-\alpha}}\frac{\sigma\omega(i)}{\sigma+\omega(i)} \geq (\beta_0^{2\alpha}-1)3^\alpha\tilde{\sigma}^{\frac{\alpha}{1-\alpha}}. \tag{4.136}$$

But the definition of $\tilde{\sigma}$ implies

$$(1-\alpha)(1.23\beta_1^2 c_4^{1/\alpha}\alpha)^{\frac{\alpha}{1-\alpha}} = (\beta_0^{2\alpha}-1)3^\alpha\tilde{\sigma}^{\frac{\alpha}{1-\alpha}}. \tag{4.137}$$

The last two expressions imply (4.133), (4.132), (4.129). Let us combine (4.127)–(4.129) and use the inequality $\varepsilon_{i-1} \leq \varepsilon_i$:

$$[B_i v, v]_i \leq \varepsilon_{i-1}([\![v]\!]_i^2 - [\![J_i v]\!]_i^2) + \varepsilon_i [\![J_i v]\!]_i^2 \leq \varepsilon_i [\![v]\!]_i^2. \tag{4.138}$$

Since the operator B_i is self-adjoint and positive-definite in the inner product $[\cdot,\cdot]_i$,

$$[\![B_i]\!]_i \leq \varepsilon_i. \quad \square$$

4.3.4 The more regular case

We saw that *the more* regular problem we consider, *the better* rate of convergence with respect to the number m of iterations in smoothing processes. Namely, the norm of suppression operator for large m looks like $O(m^{-2\alpha})$ for $\alpha \in (0,1]$. Do we have such a situation also for $\alpha > 1$? For example, criterium (4.113) for $\alpha > 1$ is fulfiled for finite elements of higher degrees in h-version and especially in p- and hp-versions. It gives us the first part of criterium (4.82).

In principle, we may formulate the optimization problem: find such iteration parameters τ_l in (4.101) which give the least constant c_2. The theoretical reasonings allow us to solve this problem in explicit form for $\alpha = (l+1)/2$, $l = 1,2,\ldots$. For another α we may solve this problem numerically. In principle, we have to put $c_2 = O(m^{-2\alpha})$. But this problem is very hard in both theoretical and numerical sence. Therefore, we show another simpler way. It gives us the value c_2 which is not optimal but has the optimal order $O(m^{-2\alpha})$.

Put

$$\alpha^* = \begin{cases} \alpha, & \text{if } \alpha \text{ is integer,} \\ [\alpha]+1 & \text{else.} \end{cases}$$

Suppose that (4.69) is valid. We will use the Jacobi-type iterations (4.97), (4.98) with $m = \alpha^* p$, integer $p > 1$ and multiple parameter α^*: $\forall j = 0,1,\ldots,m-1$ put $j' = [j/\alpha^*]+1$ and

$$\tau_j = \tau'_{j'} = \frac{(\lambda_i^*)^{-1}\cos^2\beta}{\cos^2(2j'+1)\beta - \sin^2\beta}, \qquad \beta = \frac{\pi}{2(2p+1)}. \tag{4.139}$$

In other words, we repeat the procedures (4.97), (4.98) α^* times with parameters (4.99) and $m = p$. Thus in the new procedure, the iterative polinomial $N_m^*(\lambda)$ has a form

$$N_m^*(\lambda) = N_p^{\alpha^*}(\lambda) \tag{4.140}$$

where

$$N_p(\lambda) = \prod_{j'=0}^{p-1}(1 - \tau'_{j'}\lambda). \tag{4.141}$$

Theorem 4.8 *Let* (4.69) *be valid,* $\alpha \geq 1$, *and Jacobi-type operator* J_i *be defined by formula* $J_i = N_m^*(L_i)$ *with parameters* (4.139), $m = \alpha^* p$, *integer* $p \geq 1$. *Then*

$$\|L_i^{(1+\alpha)/2} J_i v\|_i^2/(\lambda_i^*)^\alpha \leq c_3([\![v]\!]_i^2 - [\![J_i v]\!]_i^2) \qquad \forall v \in M_i \tag{4.142}$$

holds with the constant

$$c_3 = \mathrm{tg}^{2\alpha}\frac{\pi}{2(2m/p+1)} \leq (\frac{\sqrt{3}p}{2m})^{2\alpha}. \tag{4.143}$$

Proof. For polinomial $N_p(\lambda)$ we proved the estimate (4.106):

$$\frac{\lambda}{\lambda_i^*}N_p^2(\lambda) \leq c_2(1 - N_p^2(\lambda)) \qquad \forall\lambda \in [0, \lambda_i^*]. \tag{4.144}$$

Divide both sides by $N_p^2(\lambda)$, raise it to the power α and use the inequality $(1-x)^\alpha \leq 1 - x^\alpha$ at $x \in [0,1]$. As a result, we have

$$(\frac{\lambda}{\lambda_i^*})^\alpha \leq c_2^\alpha \frac{1 - N_p^{2\alpha}(\lambda)}{N_p^{2\alpha}} \leq c_2^\alpha \frac{1 - N_p^{2\alpha^*}(\lambda)}{N_p^{2\alpha^*}(\lambda)}. \tag{4.145}$$

Here we actively applied the estimate $N_p^2(\lambda) \leq 1 \quad \forall\lambda \in [0, \lambda_i^*]$ proved in 4.1. Due to (4.140) we proved by (4.145) the inequality

$$(\frac{\lambda}{\lambda_i^*})^\alpha N_m^{*\,2}(\lambda) \leq c_2^\alpha(1 - N_m^{*\,2}(\lambda)) \qquad \forall\lambda \in [0, \lambda_i^*]. \tag{4.146}$$

Now we use the decomposition (4.107) with respect to eigenvectors $g_1, \ldots, g_{n_i}$ and the equality

$$\|L_i^{(1+\alpha)/2} J_i v\|_i^2 = \sum_{j=1}^{n_i}(\alpha_j \lambda_j^{(1+\alpha)/2} N_m^*(\lambda_j))^2. \tag{4.147}$$

It gives us together with (4.146):

$$\|L_i^{(1+\alpha)/2} J_i v\|_i^2/\lambda_i^{*\alpha} = \sum_{j=1}^{n_i}\alpha_j^2\lambda_j \cdot (\frac{\lambda_j}{\lambda_i^*})^\alpha N_m^{*\,2}(\lambda_j) \leq \tag{4.148}$$

$$\leq \sum_{j=1}^{n}\alpha_j^2\lambda_j c_2^\alpha(1 - N_m^{*\,2}(\lambda_j)) = c_2^\alpha([\![v]\!]_i^2 - [\![J_i v]\!]_i^2). \tag{4.149}$$

It proves (4.142) with the constant $c_3 = c_2^\alpha$. □

Another part of the criterium has the same form as (4.113): *there exist constants* $\alpha \geq 1$ *and* $c_6 > 0$ *such that* $\forall v \in M_i$

$$[\![Q_i v]\!]_i^2 \leq \frac{c_6}{(\lambda_i^*)^\alpha} \|L_i^{(1+\alpha)/2} v\|_i^2, \qquad i = 1, \dots, k. \tag{4.150}$$

Combine together (4.142) and (4.150) we go to the convergence criterium (4.82) and estimate (4.84) of Theorem 4.5 with constant

$$c^* = (c_3 c_6)^{-1} = c_6 \mathrm{ctg}^{2\alpha} \frac{\pi}{2(2m/p+1)} = O(m^{2\alpha}). \tag{4.151}$$

So

$$[\![B_i]\!]_i \leq \frac{1}{1+c^*} = O(m^{-2\alpha}). \tag{4.152}$$

Note again, that the choice (4.139) of iterative parameters τ_j is not optimal. One can try to improve the constant c^* in (4.151) but not the order 2α which is unimproved.

4.4 A convergence for symmetric sign-indefinite operators

In this section, we continue the study of the case which is specified by features (4.70), (4.71), (4.72), (4.73). Instead of (4.69) we suppose that

$$L_i \quad \textit{is self-adjoint and inversible operators}, \quad i = 0, 1, \dots, k. \tag{4.153}$$

4.4.1 The convergence theorem

Along with each self-adjoint operator L_i in M_i, let us introduce a positive-definite operator Λ_i as follows. Let $g_1, \dots, g_n$ be the orthogonal system of eigenvectors and $\lambda_1, \dots, \lambda_n$ be the corresponding set of eigenvalues of the operator L_i. Here λ_i may be negative or positive. Let $v \in M_i$ be an arbitrary vector and let (4.110) be its decomposition into system $\{g_i\}$. The operator L_i acts on v as in (4.111) and we introduce operator Λ_i by formula

$$\Lambda_i v = \sum_{j=1}^{n} \alpha_j |\lambda_j| g_j. \tag{4.154}$$

Note that any power Λ_i^β is commutative with initial operator L_i. Denote also

$$S_i = L_i \Lambda_i^{-1} \tag{4.155}$$

which is a unitary operator.

Now we introduce the Λ_i-inner product

$$[u, v]_i = (\Lambda_i u, v)_i \qquad \forall u, v \in M_i \tag{4.156}$$

and the corresponding norm

$$\|u\|_{U_i} = [u, u]_i^{1/2}, \tag{4.157}$$

Moreover, we introduce an additional vector norm $\|\cdot\|_{\mathcal{F}_i}$ in M_i. Taking the various norms $\|\cdot\|_{\mathcal{F}_i}$, we later produce the whole scale of estimates corresponding to regularity.

We will examine the convergence of W-cycle in the norm (4.156), i. e., γ is equal to 2 in MG-algorithm and we study the norm

$$\|B_i\|_{U_i} \equiv \sup_{u \in M_i \setminus \{0\}} \frac{\|B_i u\|_{U_i}}{\|u\|_{U_i}}. \tag{4.158}$$

Naturally, for a sign-indefinite operator, the number of the convergence criteria is more than for a positive-definite one.

First we suppose that

$$\|J_i\|_{U_i} \leq c_J \qquad \forall i = 1, \ldots, k. \tag{4.159}$$

In most numbers of our iterative processes we get $c_J = 1$ as we will see later. Further, we require the fulfilment of inequality

$$\|u\|_{U_{i-1}} \leq c_I \|I_{i-1} u\|_{U_i} \qquad \forall u \in M_{i-1},\ i = 1, \ldots, k. \tag{4.160}$$

We will state it below for different choices of $\|\cdot\|_{U_i}$ in concrete problems. Then we require the main assumption in the form

$$\|L_i^{-1} - I_{i-1}\, L_{i-1}^{-1}\, R_i\|_{U_i \leftarrow \mathcal{F}_i}\, \|L_i J_i\|_{\mathcal{F}_i \leftarrow U_i} \leq \eta(m) \qquad \forall i = 1, \ldots, k \tag{4.161}$$

with the function $\eta(m)$ which is independent of i and tends to 0 when $m \to \infty$. Recall that m is a number of iterations in pre- and post-smoothing and the norms of operators are defined as follows:

$$\|L\|_{U_i \leftarrow \mathcal{F}_i} \equiv \sup_{u \in M_i \setminus \{0\}} \frac{\|Lu\|_{U_i}}{\|u\|_{\mathcal{F}_i}}; \tag{4.162}$$

$$\|L\|_{\mathcal{F}_i \leftarrow U_i} \equiv \sup_{u \in M_i \setminus \{0\}} \frac{\|Lu\|_{\mathcal{F}_i}}{\|u\|_{U_i}}. \tag{4.163}$$

Theorem 4.9 *Let the conditions* (4.153), (4.70)–(4.73), (4.159)–(4.161) *be valid for the MG_k-algorithm with $\gamma = 2$ (symmetric W-cycle). Then for any $\xi \in (0,1)$ there exists m_0 such that $\forall m \geq m_0$*

$$\|B_i\|_{U_i} \leq \xi \qquad \forall i = 0, 1, \ldots, k. \tag{4.164}$$

Proof. Put

$$c_B \equiv c_I^2 (c_J + 1)^2, \tag{4.165}$$

$$\xi_* \equiv \min\{\xi, 1/2\, c_B\} \tag{4.166}$$

and choose m_0 such that $\forall m \geq m_0$

$$\eta(m) \leq \sqrt{\xi_*/2}. \tag{4.167}$$

Then due to (4.167), (4.166)

$$\eta^2(m) + \xi_*^2 c_B \le \xi_*. \tag{4.168}$$

Instead of (4.164) we will show that

$$[B_i v, w]_i \le \xi_* \, \|v\|_{U_i} \, \|w\|_{U_i} \qquad \forall v, w \in M_i, \tag{4.169}$$

from which (4.164) follows. We use induction. For $i = 0$ the identity $B_0 \equiv 0$ holds and (4.169) is valid for any $\xi_* \in (0,1)$. Suppose that for any $m \ge m_0$ (4.169) is valid for $i-1$. Let use (4.59) and fulfil some computations:

$$\begin{aligned}
[B_i v, w]_i &= [J_i^*(I - I_{i-1}(I - B_{i-1}^2)L_{i-1}^{-1}R_i L_i)J_i v, w]_i = \\
&= (I - I_{i-1}(I - B_{i-1}^2)L_{i-1}^{-1}R_i L_i)J_i v, J_i \Lambda_i w)_i = \\
&= (Q_i J_i v, J_i \Lambda_i w)_i + (B_{i-1}^2 L_{i-1}^{-1} R_i L_i J_i v, R_i J_i \Lambda_i w)_i = \\
&= (Q_i^2 J_i v, J_i \Lambda_i w)_i + [B_{i-1}^2 L_{i-1}^{-1} R_i L_i J_i v, \Lambda_{i-1}^{-1} R_i J_i \Lambda_i w]_{i-1}
\end{aligned}$$

Now use induction assumption related to B_{i-1} and the explicit form of Q_i:

$$\begin{aligned}
[B_i v, w]_i &\le ((L_i^{-1} - I_{i-1}L_{i-1}^{-1}R_i)L_i J_i v, (I - L_i I_{i-1} L_{i-1}^{-1} R_i)J_i \Lambda_i w)_i + \\
&+ \xi_*^2 \|L_{i-1}^{-1} R_i L_i J_i v\|_{U_{i-1}} \|\Lambda_{i-1}^{-1} R_i J_i \Lambda_i w\|_{U_{i-1}} \le \\
&\le [(L_i^{-1} - I_{i-1}L_{i-1}^{-1}R_i)L_i J_i v, S_i(L_i^{-1} - I_{i-1}L_{i-1}^{-1}R_i)J_i \Lambda_i w]_i + \\
&+ \xi_*^2 \|L_{i-1}^{-1} R_i L_i J_i v\|_{U_{i-1}} \cdot \|\Lambda_{i-1}^{-1} R_i J_i \Lambda_i w\|_{U_{i-1}}.
\end{aligned} \tag{4.170}$$

Now we use (4.160):

$$\begin{aligned}
&\|L_{i-1}^{-1} R_i L_i J_i v\|_{U_{i-1}} \le c_I \| I_{i-1} L_{i-1}^{-1} R_i L_i J_i v\|_{U_i} \le \\
&\le c_I \|(L_i^{-1} - I_{i-1}L_{i-1}^{-1}R_i)L_i J_i v\|_{U_i} + c_I \|J_i v\|_{U_i}.
\end{aligned}$$

On the basis of (4.161) and (4.159), we have

$$\|L_{i-1}^{-1} R_i L_i J_i v\|_{U_{i-1}} \le c_I(\eta(m) + c_J)\|v\|_{U_i}. \tag{4.171}$$

Analogously, we get the following inequality with the help of a unitary operator S_i:

$$\|\Lambda_{i-1}^{-1} R_i J_i \Lambda_i w\|_{U_{i-1}} \le c_I(\eta(m) + c_J)\|w\|_{U_i}; \tag{4.172}$$

$$\|(L_i^{-1} - I_{i-1}L_{i-1}^{-1}R_i)L_i J_i v\|_{U_i} \le \eta(m)\|v\|_{U_i}; \tag{4.173}$$

$$\|S_i(L_i^{-1} - I_{i-1}L_{i-1}^{-1}R_i)J_i \Lambda_i w\|_{U_i} \le \eta(m)\|w\|_{U_i}. \tag{4.174}$$

Combining (4.170)–(4.174), we put the inequality

$$[B_i v, w]_i \le \{\eta^2(m) + \xi_*^2 c_I^2 (\eta(m) + c_J)^2\}\|v\|_{U_i}\|w\|_{U_i}. \tag{4.175}$$

From (4.167) it follows that $\eta(m) \le 1$. Therefore the multiplier on the right-hand side of (4.175) is evaluated with the help of (4.165), (4.168):

$$\eta^2(m) + \xi_*^2 c_I^2(\eta(m) + c_J)^2 \le \eta^2(m) + \xi_*^2 c_B \le \xi_*.$$

Combining it with (4.175), we go to (4.169). Take $w = B_i v$ and use (4.166). Then we come to inequalities

$$\|B_i v\|_{U_i} \leq \xi_* \|v\|_{U_i} \leq \xi \|v\|_{U_i},$$

which proves (4.164). □

Examine situation when $m \to \infty$. Then we have $\xi_* = \xi$ for large m, and on the ground of (4.167), we may take

$$\xi = O(\eta^2(m)). \tag{4.176}$$

That is better than estimate $\xi = O(\eta(m))$ which may be put for asymmetric W-cycle without post-smoothing iterations.

4.4.2 Convergence in an ordinary situation

As we will see later, the ordinary situation may be characterized by the choice

$$\|v\|_{\mathcal{F}_i} = \|v\|_i \tag{4.177}$$

and the estimate

$$\|L_i^{-1} - I_{i-1} L_{i-1}^{-1} R_i\|_{U_i \leftarrow \mathcal{F}_i} \leq \frac{c_L}{(\lambda_i^*)^{1/2}}. \tag{4.178}$$

Here, c_L is independent of i and λ_i^* is either spectral radius of L_i or its appropriate upper estimate

$$\lambda_i^* \geq \max_{\lambda \in Sp(L_i)} |\lambda|. \tag{4.179}$$

In this case we recommend the following type of smoothing iterations:

$$A_1''. \quad u_{l+1} = u_l - \tau_l L_i (L_i u_l - f_i), \tag{4.180}$$

$$A_5''. \quad y_{l+1} = y_l - \tau_l L_i (L_i y_l - f_i), \qquad l = 0, 1, \ldots, m-1. \tag{4.181}$$

In principle, the parameters τ_l are to be chosen by means of the solution of optimization problem (4.38) with $d = \lambda_i^*$. But we take the simpler "quasioptimal" iterative parameters (4.40) giving the same order of smallness for the error reduction:

$$\tau_l = (\lambda_i^*)^{-2} \cos^{-2}(\pi(2l+1)/2(2m+1)), \qquad l = 0, 1, \ldots, m-1. \tag{4.182}$$

We show that for this type of iterations, we have the estimate

$$\frac{1}{(\lambda_i^*)^{1/2}} \|L_i J_i\|_{\mathcal{F}_i \leftarrow U_i} \leq \frac{1}{\sqrt{2m+1}}. \tag{4.183}$$

Theorem 4.10 *Let* (4.153) *be valid and iterative parameters* τ_l *in the processes* (4.180), (4.181) *be chosen by means of* (4.182). *Then* (4.183) *holds.*

Proof. Let $v \in M_i$ be an arbitrary vector. Since L_i is self-adjoint, we may take the decomposition (4.110) with respect to eigenfunctions. Introduce the polinomial

$$N(\lambda) = \prod_{l=0}^{m-1} (1 - \tau_l \lambda^2). \tag{4.184}$$

With this designation, we may describe the iterative operator as

$$J_i = N(L_i). \tag{4.185}$$

Then

$$\begin{aligned} \|v\|_{U_i}^2 &= \sum_{j=1}^{n_i} (\alpha_j |\lambda_j|^{1/2})^2, \\ \|L_i J_i v\|_{\mathcal{F}_i}^2 &= \sum_{j=1}^{n_i} (\alpha_j \lambda_j N(\lambda_j))^2. \end{aligned} \tag{4.186}$$

From (4.41), the inequality holds

$$\frac{|\lambda|}{\lambda_i^*} N^2(\lambda) \leq \frac{1}{2m+1} \qquad \forall \lambda \in [-\lambda_i^*, \lambda_i^*]. \tag{4.187}$$

Now perform some computations:

$$\begin{aligned} \frac{1}{(\lambda_i^*)^{1/2}} \|L_i J_i v\|_{\mathcal{F}_i} &= \left(\sum_{j=1}^{n_i} \alpha_j^2 |\lambda_j| \frac{|\lambda_j|}{\lambda_i^*} N^2(\lambda_j) \right)^{1/2} \leq \\ &\leq \frac{1}{\sqrt{2m+1}} \left(\sum_{j=1}^{n_i} \alpha_j^2 |\lambda_j| \right)^{1/2} = \frac{1}{\sqrt{2m+1}} \|v\|_{U_i}. \end{aligned}$$

Devide both side by $\|v\|_{U_i}$ and take supremum. That gives (4.183). □

Combining (4.178), (4.183), we come to inequality (4.161) with

$$\eta(m) = \frac{c_L}{\sqrt{2m+1}}. \tag{4.188}$$

If we would use the usual choice

$$\tau_l = 1/(\lambda_i^*)^2$$

then we have

$$\eta(m) = \frac{c_L}{(4m+1)^{1/4}} \left(\frac{4m}{4m+1} \right)^m \approx \frac{c_L e^{-1/4}}{(4m+1)^{1/4}}.$$

Of course, for $m \geq 2$, the value (4.188) is better.

Note that the optimal parameters are expressed from Table 4.1 by formula $\tau_l = \bar{\tau}_l/(\lambda_i^*)^2$ and give the better error reduction. But for $m \geq 10$ the gain is slight in comparison with the computational cost of them and the estimate (4.42) becomes hypotetical.

4.5 General case. Convergence in initial norm

In this section we will examine the most general case when the operators L_i are neither self-adjoint nor positive-definite. We suppose only (4.70) and

$$L_i \quad \textit{are inversible operators}, \quad i = 0, 1, \dots, k. \tag{4.189}$$

4.5.1 Convergence criteria

In this case we will use non-symmetric W-cycle without post-smoothing iterations. The obtained results are some reformulation of the known results by W. T. Hackbusch [68]. The difference consists in a main convergence criterium and other outline of the proof. This criterium makes it possible to eliminate the dependence of parameters h, p which is convenient for p- and hp-versions. Other plan of proof allows to pass to the more effective symmetric W-cycle with post-smoothing iterations wherever it is possible under sypposition (4.72).

We keep only convergence in the norm

$$\|u\|_i = (u, u)_i^{1/2} \tag{4.190}$$

which follows from the initial inner product $(\cdot, \cdot)_i$. For any operator $L : M_i \to M_i$, introduce its norm

$$\|L\|_i = \sup_{u \in M_i \setminus \{0\}} \frac{\|Lu\|_i}{\|u\|_i}. \tag{4.191}$$

We use assumptions which are similar to (4.159)–(4.161). Namely, (4.159) transforms into

$$\|J_i\|_i \leq c_J \qquad \forall i = 1, \dots, k. \tag{4.192}$$

Inequality (4.160) becomes two-sided:

$$\underline{c}_I \|I_{i-1} u\|_i \leq \|u\|_{i-1} \leq \bar{c}_I \|I_{i-1} u\|_i \qquad \forall u \in M_{i-1}, \quad i = 1, \dots, k. \tag{4.193}$$

And (4.161) is rewriten in different norm:

$$\|L_i^{-1} - I_{i-1} L_{i-1}^{-1} R_i\|_i \cdot \|L_i J_i\|_i \leq \eta(m) \qquad \forall i = 1, \dots, k \tag{4.194}$$

with function $\eta(m)$ which is independent of i and tends to 0 at $m \to \infty$. Here $m = m_1$ is number of pre-smoothing iteration. The number of post-smoothig iteration m_2 is equal to 0.

Theorem 4.11 *Let the conditions* (4.70), (4.189), (4.192)–(4.194) *be valid for the* MG_k*-algorithm with* $\gamma = 2$, $m_1 = m$, $m_2 = 0$ (*asymmetric* W*-cycle*). *Then for any* $\xi \in (0, 1)$ *there exists* m_0 *such that* $\forall m \geq m_0$

$$\|B_i\|_i \leq \xi \qquad \forall i = 0, 1, \dots, k. \tag{4.195}$$

Proof. Put

$$\begin{aligned} c_B &\equiv \underline{c}_I^{-1}(\bar{c}_I + c_J), \\ \xi_* &\equiv \min\{\xi, 1/2\ c_B\} \end{aligned} \tag{4.196}$$

and choose m_0 such that $\forall m \geq m_0$

$$\eta(m) \leq \xi_*/2. \tag{4.197}$$

Then due to (4.197), (4.196)

$$\eta(m) + \xi_*^2 c_B \leq \xi_*. \tag{4.198}$$

Use induction. For $i = 0$ the identity $B_0 \equiv 0$ holds and (4.195) is valid for any $\xi \in (0, 1)$. Suppose that $\forall m \geq m_0$ inequality (4.195) is valid for $i - 1$. First we show instead of (4.195) that $\forall m \geq m_0$

$$(B_i v, w)_i \leq \xi_* \|v\|_i \|w\|_i \qquad v, w \in M_i. \tag{4.199}$$

Let us use (4.59) for this case; after some computations

$$\begin{aligned} (B_i v, w)_i &= ((I - I_{i-1}(I - B_{i-1}^2)L_{i-1}^{-1} R_i L_i) J_i v, w)_i = \\ &= ((I - I_{i-1} L_{i-1}^{-1} R_i L_i) J_i v, w)_i + (I_{i-1} B_{i-1}^2 L_{i-1}^{-1} R_i L_i J_i v, w)_i \leq \\ &\leq \|L_i^{-1} - I_{i-1} L_{i-1}^{-1} R_i\|_i \cdot \|L_i J_i\|_i \cdot \|v\|_i \cdot \|w\|_i + \\ &+ \|I_{i-1} B_{i-1}^2 L_{i-1}^{-1} R_i L_i J_i v\|_i \cdot \|w\|_i \leq \\ &\leq \eta(m)\|v\|_i\|w\|_i + \underline{c}_I^{-1}\xi_*^2 \|L_{i-1}^{-1} R_i L_i J_i v\|_{i-1}\|w\|_i. \end{aligned} \tag{4.200}$$

Now

$$\|L_{i-1}^{-1} R_i L_i J_i v\|_{i-1} \leq \bar{c}_I \|(I - I_{i-1} L_{i-1}^{-1} R_i L_i) J_i v\|_i + \|J_i v\|_i \leq (\bar{c}_I \eta(m) + c_J)\|v\|_i.$$

Combine this inequality with (4.200):

$$(B_i v, w)_i \leq \{\eta(m) + \xi_*^2 \underline{c}_I^{-1}(\bar{c}_I \eta(m) + c_J)\}\|v\|_i\|w\|_i. \tag{4.201}$$

From (4.197) it follows that $\eta(m) \leq 1$. Therefore the multiplier in the right-hand side of (4.201) is evaluated with the help of (4.198), (4.196):

$$\eta(m) + \xi_*^2 \underline{c}_I^{-1}(\bar{c}_I \eta(m) + c_J) \leq \eta(m) + \xi_*^2 c_B \leq \xi_*.$$

Combining it with (4.201), we obtain (4.199).

Take $w = B_i v$ and use (4.196):

$$\|B_i v\|_i \leq \xi_* \|v\|_i \leq \xi \|v\|_i.$$

It proves (4.195). □

Remark 4.5.1 *In cases of a deficient regularity or finite elements of higher order, one can modify criterion* (4.194) *into the more useful form:*

$$\|(L_i^{-1} - I_{i-1} L_{i-1}^{-1} R_i) L_i J_i\|_i \leq \eta(m) \qquad \forall i = 1, \ldots, k. \tag{4.202}$$

The proof of Theorem 4.11 *somewhat changes in* (4.200) *only. The result* (4.195) *stays the same.*

Let us examine a situation when $m \to \infty$. Then for a large m we have $\xi_* = \xi$ and because of (4.197) we can take

$$\xi = O(\eta(m)). \tag{4.203}$$

4.5.2 A case of ordinary accuracy

In this section we investigate the situation for operators which are neither self-adjoint nor positive-definite. There are many iterative smoothing procedures which are very efficient in special cases. We will not examine many possibilities and present a procedure with wide range of utilizations. Namely, we investigate the following type of pre-smoothing procedure:

$$A_1'''. \qquad u_{l+1} = u_l - \tau_l L_i^*(L_i u_l - f_i), \qquad l = 0, \dots, m-1, \tag{4.204}$$

where L_i^* adjoint of L_i in the inner product $(\cdot, \cdot)_i$. We choose parameters τ_l in such a way as to reach the least multiplier of suppression in dependence of number m.

To this end, introduce the designation μ_i^* for either spectral radius of $L_i^* L_i$ or its appropriate upper estimate

$$\mu_i^* \geq \max_{\lambda \in Sp(L_i^* L_i)} \lambda. \tag{4.205}$$

Then the parameters τ_l are chosen by means of the solution of optimization problem (4.25) with $d = \mu_i^*$. It gives us

$$\tau_l = (\mu_i^*)^{-1} \cos^{-2} \pi(2i+1)/2(2m+1), \qquad i = 0, 1, \dots, m-1. \tag{4.206}$$

Theorem 4.12 *For iterative procedure* (4.204) *with parameters* τ_l *from* (4.206), *the following estimate holds:*

$$\frac{1}{(\mu_i^*)^{1/2}} \|L_i J_i\|_i \leq \frac{1}{2m+1}, \qquad i = 1, \dots, k. \tag{4.207}$$

Proof. Let $v \in M_i$ be an arbitrary vector. Since $L_i^* L_i$ is self-adjoint and positive-definite, there exists a system of eigenvectors $g_1, \dots, g_{n_i}$ of operator $L_i^* L_i$ where n_i is dimension of M_i. Each g_i corresponds to some non-negative eigenvalue μ_j and this system is orthonormal in the inner product $(\cdot, \cdot)_i$. Let

$$v = \sum_{j=1}^{n_i} \alpha_j g_j \tag{4.208}$$

be decomposition of v in this system. Introduce the polinomial

$$N(\mu) = \prod_{l=0}^{m-1} (1 - \tau_l \mu) \tag{4.209}$$

with parameters (4.206). With this designation, we may describe the iterative operator as $J_i = N(L_i^* L_i)$. Then

$$\begin{aligned} \|v\|_i^2 &= \sum_{j=1}^{n_i} \alpha_j^2, \\ \|L_i J_i v\|_i^2 &= (J_i v, L_i^* L_i J_i v)_i = \sum_{j=1}^{n_i} \alpha_j^2 \mu_j N^2(\mu_j). \end{aligned} \tag{4.210}$$

From Theorem 4.4

$$\frac{\mu}{\mu_i^*}N^2(\mu) \leq 1/(2m+1)^2 \qquad \forall \mu \in [0, \mu_i^*]. \tag{4.211}$$

We use it in (4.210):

$$\begin{aligned}\frac{1}{\mu_i^*}\|L_iJ_iv\|_i^2 &\leq \sum_{j=1}^{n_i}\alpha_j\frac{\mu_j}{\mu_i^*}N^2(\mu_j) \leq \\ &\leq \frac{1}{(2m+1)^2}\sum_{j=1}^{n_i}\alpha_j^2 = \frac{1}{(2m+1)^2}\|v\|_i^2.\end{aligned} \tag{4.212}$$

Take square root, divide both sides by $\|v\|_i$ and take supremum. That gives (4.207). □

Ordinary situation for accuracy is characterized by the assumption

$$\|L_i^{-1} - I_{i-1}L_{i-1}^{-1}R_i\|_i \leq \frac{c_L}{(\mu_i^*)^{1/2}}, \qquad i = 1, \dots, k, \tag{4.213}$$

where c_L is independent of i. Combining (4.213) and (4.207) we come to inequality (4.194) with

$$\eta(m) = \frac{c_L}{2m+1}. \tag{4.214}$$

If we should use the usual trivial choice

$$\tau_l = 1/\mu_i^*,$$

then we have

$$\eta(m) = \frac{c_L}{\sqrt{2m+1}}\left(\frac{2m}{2m+1}\right)^m \approx \frac{c_L e^{-1/2}}{\sqrt{2m+1}}.$$

Of course, this value is worse than (4.214).

Remark 4.5.2 *The combination of iterative processes* (4.204), (4.206) *and convergence results of Theorem* 4.11 *is of interest for self-adjoint sign-indefinite operators L_i too, in spite of the special realization of the MG_k-algorithm for self-adjoint matrices in section* 4.4. *Here the convergence is proved in initial norm $\|\cdot\|_i$ in opposite to section* 4.4 *where it did in energy norm $[\![\cdot]\!]_i$. In practice both type of estimates are need.*

In this connection we again return to self-adjoint positive-definite operators to obtain convergence in the initial norm $\|\cdot\|_i$. For this purpose, we again use the smoothing procedure (4.97) with the iterative parameters

$$\tau_l = \frac{1+\cos\alpha}{\lambda_i^*(\cos\alpha - \cos(2l+3)\alpha)}, \qquad l = 0, \dots, m-1 \tag{4.215}$$

where $\alpha = \pi/(2m+2)$ and λ_i^* is the appropriate upper bound of largest eigenvalue of L_i (s.f. (4.179)).

Theorem 4.13 *Let* (4.69) *be valid and iterative parameters* τ_l *in the process* (4.97) *be chosen by means of* (4.215). *Then estimate holds*

$$\frac{1}{\lambda_i^*}\|L_iJ_i\|_i \leq \frac{\operatorname{tg}\alpha/2}{m+1}, \qquad \alpha = \frac{\pi}{2m+2}, \quad i = 1,\dots,k. \tag{4.216}$$

Proof. Let $v \in M_i$ be arbitrary vector. Take decomposition (4.110) with respect to eigenfunctions g_j of operator L_i:

$$v = \sum_{j=1}^{n_i} \alpha_j g_j. \tag{4.217}$$

Introduce polinomial

$$N(\lambda) = \prod_{l=0}^{m-1}(1-\tau_l\lambda) \tag{4.218}$$

with parameters (4.215). Then $J_i = N(L_i)$. System $\{g_j\}$ is orthonormal in norm $\|\cdot\|_i$ therefore

$$\|L_iJ_iv\|_i^2 = \sum_{j=1}^{n_i}\alpha_j^2\lambda_j^2N^2(\lambda_j). \tag{4.219}$$

From Theorem 4.1 we have

$$\frac{\lambda}{\lambda_i^*}N(\lambda) \leq \frac{\operatorname{tg}\alpha/2}{m+1} \qquad \forall\lambda \in [0,\lambda_i^*]. \tag{4.220}$$

Use it in (4.219):

$$\frac{1}{\lambda_i^*}\|L_iJ_iv\|_i \leq \Big(\sum_{j=1}^{n_i}\alpha_j^2\Big(\frac{\lambda_j}{\lambda_i^*}N(\lambda_j)\Big)^2\Big)^{1/2} \leq \frac{\operatorname{tg}\alpha/2}{m+1}\|v\|_i. \tag{4.221}$$

Divide both side by $\|v\|_i$ and take supremum. That gives (4.216). □

Ordinary situation for accuracy in terms of λ_i^* is characterized by the assumption (compaire with (4.213))

$$\|L_i^{-1} - I_{i-1}L_{i-1}^{-1}R_i\|_i \leq \frac{c_L}{\lambda_i^*} \tag{4.222}$$

where c_L is independent of i. Combining (4.222) and (4.216) we reach inequality (4.194) with

$$\eta\,(m) = \frac{c_L\operatorname{tg}\alpha/2}{m+1} \approx \frac{c_L\,\pi}{4(m+1)^2}. \tag{4.223}$$

If we use the usual trivial choice

$$\tau_l = 1/\lambda_i^*$$

we have

$$\eta(m) = \frac{c_L}{m+1}\left(\frac{m}{m+1}\right)^m \approx \frac{c_L e^{-1}}{m+1}.$$

Obviously, this value is worse than (4.223).

If we compaire (4.223) and (4.109), we see that the order of suppression multiplier with respect to m is the same, i. e., $O(m^{-2})$ but in different norms: $\|B_i\|_i$ and $[\![B_i]\!]_i$. Nevertheless the MG-algorithm in section 4.3 (or may be its proof) has one advantage before MG-algorithm in this section. The variant in section 4.3 converges for any positive m; i. e., $[\![B_i]\!]_i < 1$ for any $m = 1, 2, \ldots$. Theorem 4.11 in this section gives the convergence $\|B_i\|_i < 1$ only for m large enough and does not guarantee convergence for little m. But in computational practice, we do not have examples of disconvergence for little m.

4.6 The formulation of the convergence conditions for the Lagrange finite elements

In this section, we adapt the convergence conditions formulated above to the natural demands of the finite-element method for second-order elliptic equations. We begin with symmetric positive-definite bilinear form, then we consider only symmetric one, and finally, we stay on asymmetric one.

To develop the results, we use some definitions of section 1.2.

4.6.1 A symmetric positive-definite bilinear form

Let us apply the above results for solving the following problem: *find a solution* $u \in H_A \subset W_2^1(\Omega)$ *satisfying the equality*

$$\mathcal{L}(u, v) = f(v) \qquad \forall v \in H_A, \tag{4.224}$$

where bilinear form $\mathcal{L}$ is symmetric, bounded, and positive definite on $H_A \times H_A$; linear functional f is bounded on H_A.

Assume that there exists a set of $k+1$ parameters

$$c_1 = h_0 > h_1 > \ldots > h_k > 0, \tag{4.225}$$

satisfying the condition

$$h_i/h_{i+1} \leq c_2, \qquad i = 0, 1, \ldots, k-1. \tag{4.226}$$

For each, we construct the grid $\Omega_{h_i} \subset \bar{\Omega}$ and assume that Ω_{h_0} involves a rather small finite number of points (no more than c_3).

As in section 1.2, for each level i we introduce a set of basis functions $\varphi_y^{h_i}(x)$ and formulate the problem of constructing an approximate solution of the Bubnov-Galerkin method

$$w^{h_i}(x) = \sum_{y \in \Omega_{h_i}} \alpha_y^{h_i} \varphi_y^{h_i}(x) \qquad \text{on } \bar{\Omega} \tag{4.227}$$

with weights determined from the system

$$\sum_{y\in\Omega_{h_i}} \alpha_y^{h_i}\mathcal{L}(\varphi_y^{h_i},\varphi_z^{h_i}) = f(\varphi_z^{h_i}), \qquad z\in\Omega_{h_i}. \tag{4.228}$$

Let the following properties be satisfied for parameters h_i and basis functions $\varphi_y^{h_i}$.

C o n d i t i o n **G**. *For each* $i = 0,1,\dots,k-1$, *the basis functions* $\varphi_y^{h_i}$ *are linear combinations of a finite number (of no more than* c_4*) of basis functions of finer subdivision:*

$$\varphi_y^{h_i}(x) = \sum_{z\in\Omega_{h_{i+1}}} \beta_z^y\varphi_z^{h_{i+1}}(x) \qquad \forall y\in\Omega_{h_i}. \tag{4.229}$$

The coefficients β_z^y differ on each level. But for the sake of simplicity we do not mark these by an additional index i or $i+1$. Denote by H^{h_i} the linear span of the set $\{\varphi_y^{h_i}\}$, $y\in\Omega_{h_i}$. Then from (4.229) it follows that $H^{h_i}\subset H^{h_{i+1}}$.

Since in this section we want to construct a method for solving a systems of the form (4.228) rather than to analyse the convergence of an approximate solution, all what ensures convergence is reduced to one requirement. Moreover, we study the convergence rate of multigrid algorithms in L_2-norm first and therefore, we demand the convergence of the Bubnov-Galerkin method in the same norm.

C o n d i t i o n **H**. *For any functional* $f(v) = (g,v)$ *with function* g *from* $L_2(\Omega)$, *problem* (4.224) *has the unique solution* $u\in W_2^2(\Omega)$ *and the solution of the Bubnov-Galerkin method* (4.227), (4.228) *obeys the estimate*[1]

$$|u - w^{h_i}|_0 < c_5 h_i^2\,|g|_0.$$

For the trivial h-version, the parameters h_i may be taken as either the maximal size of cell edges or the maximal cell diameter. As we saw in Chapter 3, condition **H** has a natural form in this case. Under local refinement, h_i may have only indirect relation to the maximal size of cell edges or diameters because these values are unchanged from one level down to another whereas the accuracy becames better (i. e., h_i in condition **H** becames smaller). For p-version h_i may be taken as an inverse value of the power p of the trial polinomials. Finally, for hp-version we must consider both tendencies, i. e., h_i displays a behaviour of accuracy in dependence on the decrease of cell diameters on h-step and on the increase of power of trial polinomials on p-step.

For each vector W^{h_i} with components $W_y^{h_i}$, $y\in\Omega_{h_i}$, we put in correspondence the function

$$w^{h_i} = \sum_{y\in\Omega_{h_i}} W_y^{h_i}\varphi_y^{h_i}(x) \tag{4.230}$$

called the prolongation from H^{h_i} and introduce, by means of it, the vector norm

$$\|W^{h_i}\|_h = |w^{h_i}|_0. \tag{4.231}$$

Then we simplify system (4.228) to read:

$$L^{h_i}V^{h_i} = F^{h_i}. \tag{4.232}$$

[1]Here and below, we will write the norms $\|\cdot\|_{m,\Omega}$ and $|\cdot|_{m,\Omega}$ without index Ω where it is possible.

Here, L^{h_i} is a symmetric square matrix; V^{h_i}, F^{h_i} are vectors of unknowns and of the right-hand side of dimension N_i where N_i is the number of nodes in Ω_{h_i}.

Consider the grid Ω_{h_0}. For it, the system (4.232) has no more than c_3 unknowns and can be solved, for example, by means of a triangular decomposition with the number of arithmetical operations no more than $c_6 \approx 2c_3^2$.

Assume that there is some guess $V_0^{h_i}$ to solution of system (4.232) with index $i \geq 1$. Then, perform one step of the MG-algorithm formulated in section 4.2. On the basis of section 4.5, we recommend the W-cycle (i. e., $\gamma = 2$) with Jacobi-type pre-smoothing procedure (4.97) with parameters (4.215) and without post-smoothing one. Let us call this concrete kind of algorithm the $MG^{(1)}$.

Note that we have the nesting $H^{h_i} \subset H^{h_{i+1}}$ due to (4.229). Therefore, as we wrote already in subsection 3.1.3, on functional level, we may put the interpolation from H^{h_i} to $H^{h_{i+1}}$ to be identity. Here and below we fix this rule. Hence the explicit form of the operators I_i, R_i follows. Namely, take again a vector $W^{h_i} \in \mathbf{R}^{N_i}$ with the components $W_y^{h_i}$, $y \in \Omega_{h_i}$, and compute

$$W_z^{h_{i+1}} = \sum_{y \in \Omega_{h_i}} \beta_z^y W_y^{h_i} \qquad \forall z \in \Omega_{h_{i+1}}. \tag{4.233}$$

We take the obtained vector $W^{h_{i+1}} \in \mathbf{R}^{N_{i+1}}$ with these components as a result of the interpolation $I_i : W^{h_i} \to W^{h_{i+1}}$. Then the restriction operator $R_{i+1} : W^{h_{i+1}} \to W^{h_i}$ is defined by formula for components:

$$W_y^{h_i} = \sum_{z \in \Omega_{h_{i+1}}} \beta_z^y W_z^{h_{i+1}} \qquad \forall y \in \Omega_{h_i}. \tag{4.234}$$

Note that these operators are mutually ajoint in the Euclidian space with weighted norm

$$\|W^{h_i}\|_E = \Big(\sum_{y \in \Omega_{h_i}} (W_y^{h_i})^2 h_i^n \Big)^{1/2} \tag{4.235}$$

and that n is a dimensionality of the space $\mathbf{R}^n$ the domain Ω is taken from. We assume that this norm is equivalent to the norm (4.231) introduced earlier

$$c_7 \, \|W^{h_i}\|_E \leq \|W^{h_i}\|_h \leq c_8 \, \|W^{h_i}\|_E. \tag{4.236}$$

Now we can formulate the convergence conditions for the $MG^{(1)}$-algorithm in this notation.

Theorem 4.14 *Assume that conditions* **G**, **H**, (4.225), (4.226), (4.236) *are satisfied for* (4.224) *with $i = 0, \ldots, k$ and with symmetric positive-definite bilinear form $\mathcal{L}$ and for the Bubnov-Galerkin systems* (4.228)*; let the eigenvalues λ_j of matrices L^{h_i} be bounded in the following sense:*

$$0 < \lambda_j \leq \lambda_i^* \leq c_9 \, h_i^{n-2}, \qquad j = 1, \ldots, N_i, \quad i = 1, \ldots, k. \tag{4.237}$$

Assume also that we perform one step of the $MG^{(1)}$-algorithm. Then for any $\varepsilon \in (0, 1)$, there exists m_0 independent of h_i, f and such that $\forall m \geq m_0$ the error of result $V_1^{h_i}$ diminishes by a factor ε in comparison with the initial guess $V_0^{h_i}$:

$$\|V_1^{h_i} - V^{h_i}\|_E \leq \varepsilon \|V_0^{h_i} - V^{h_i}\|_E. \tag{4.238}$$

Proof. We show that the convergence conditions of Theorem 4.11 apply. To this end, we need to transform our assumptions. This gives two results formulated as lemmas.

Examine the system

$$L^{h_i} W^{h_i} = G^{h_i}. \tag{4.239}$$

Lemma 4.6.1 *If conditions* **G** *and* (4.236) *are satisfied, any vector* G^{h_i} *is associated with a function* $g \in H^{h_i}$ *such that* (4.239) *is the system of the Bubnov-Galerkin method for the problem*

$$\mathcal{L}(w, v) = (g, v) \qquad \forall v \in H_A, \tag{4.240}$$

where

$$|g|_0 \le \frac{h_i^{-n}}{c_7} \|G^{h_i}\|_E. \tag{4.241}$$

Proof. Let us consider the system of equations

$$\sum_{x \in \Omega_{h_i}} g(x) \gamma_x^y = G_y^{h_i}, \qquad y \in \Omega_{h_i}, \tag{4.242}$$

where $\gamma_x^y = (\varphi_x^{h_i}, \varphi_y^{h_i})$. First, suppose that some solution does exist and find an a priori estimate for it. Multiply (4.242) by $g(y)$ and take a sum over all the nodes of Ω_{h_i}:

$$\sum_{x,y \in \Omega_{h_i}} g(x) g(y) \gamma_x^y = \sum_{y \in \Omega_{h_i}} G_y^{h_i} g(y). \tag{4.243}$$

Let us introduce a function $g \in H^{h_i}$:

$$g(y) = \sum_{x \in \Omega_{h_i}} g(x) \varphi_x^{h_i}(y). \tag{4.244}$$

The left-hand side of (4.243) is then written as $|g|_0^2$. Applying the Cauchy-Bunyakovsky inequality and the equivalence of the norms of (4.236) to the right-hand side, we have

$$|g|_0^2 \le h_i^{-n} \|G^{h_i}\|_E \Big(\sum_{y \in \Omega_{h_i}} g^2(y) h_i^n \Big)^{1/2} \le c_7^{-1} h_i^{-n} \|G^{h_i}\|_E |g|_0^2.$$

From this inequality, (4.241) follows. It tells that there exists only the trivial solution for a uniform system of the form (4.242). The nonuniform system (4.242) therefore has a unique solution, which is used for defining function (4.244) satisfying estimate (4.241).

According to (4.242) and (4.244),

$$G_y^{h_i} = \sum_{x \in \Omega_{h_i}} g(x) (\varphi_x^{h_i}, \varphi_y^{h_i}) = (g, \varphi_y^{h_i}) \qquad \forall y \in \Omega_{h_i},$$

i. e., the vector G^{h_i} can be obtained as the right-hand side of the system of the Bubnov-Galerkin method with the function g. On the basis of construction of (4.239), the matrix L^{h_i} is also consistent with this method. □

Now construct the Bubnov-Galerkin system on the grid Ω_{h_i}:

$$L^{h_{i-1}} W^{h_{i-1}} = G^{h_{i-1}}, \tag{4.245}$$

where $G_y^{h_{i-1}} = (g, \varphi_y^{h_{i-1}})\ \forall y \in \Omega_{h_{i-1}}$. From the condition **G** it follows that $G^{h_{i-1}}$ and G^{h_i} are related by R_i, i. e., $G^{h_{i-1}} = R_i G^{h_i}$.

Lemma 4.6.2 *Assume that $w^{h_{i-1}}$, w^{h_i} are prolongations in $H^{h_{i-1}}$, H^{h_i} of the solutions $W^{h_{i-1}}$, W^{h_i} of* (4.239) *and* (4.245). *Then, when conditions* **G**, **H** *and* (4.236) *are satisfied the estimate*

$$|w^{h_i} - w^{h_{i-1}}|_0 \le c_5(1 + c_2^2)c_7^{-1} h_i^{2-n} \|G^{h_i}\|_E \tag{4.246}$$

holds.

Proof. condition **H** and (4.241) tell that the estimate

$$|w - w^{h_i}|_0 \le c_5 h_i^2 |g|_0 \le \frac{c_5 h_i^{2-n}}{c_7} \|G^{h_i}\|_E \tag{4.247}$$

holds, where w is a solution of (4.240).

Similarly, the estimate

$$|w - w^{h_{i-1}}|_0 \le c_5 h_{i-1}^2 |g|_0 \le \frac{c_2^2 c_5 h_i^{2-n}}{c_7} \|G^{h_i}\|_E \tag{4.248}$$

holds, by virtue of **H**, (4.241), and (4.226). Combining it and (4.247), we obtain (4.246). □

Now, let us continue proof of Theorem 4.14. Let us put the scalar product $(V, W)_i$ in section 4.5 to be equal to $\sum_{y \in \Omega_{h_i}} V_y W_y h_i^n$ for vectors V, W with components V_y, W_y, $y \in \Omega_{h_i}$. Then $\|V\|_i = \|V\|_E$. In this scalar product, we indeed have equality (4.70): $I_{i+1}^* = R_i$. Since the basis $\{\varphi_y^{h_i}\}$ is linearly independent, the matrix L^{h_i} is positive-definite and inversible. From symmetry of bilinear form $\mathcal{L}$, the symmetry of L^{h_i} follows.

On the basis of (4.11), the condition (4.192) follows:

$$\|J_i\|_E \le 1 \qquad \forall i = 1, \dots, k. \tag{4.249}$$

Now again take a vector $W^{h_i} \in \mathbf{R}^{N_i}$ and its prolongation w^{h_i} from (4.230). Compute the vector $W^{h_{i+1}} = I_i W^{h_i}$ and form its prolongation $w^{h_{i+1}}$. In this case $w^{h_{i+1}} = w^{h_i}$. Therefore, on the basis of (4.236), (4.231), we have

$$\begin{aligned} \|W^{h_i}\|_E &\le \frac{1}{c_7}\|W^{h_i}\|_h = \frac{1}{c_7}|w^{h_{i+1}}|_0 \le \frac{c_8}{c_7}\|W^{h_{i+1}}\|_E = \frac{c_8}{c_7}\|I_i W^{h_i}\|_E, \\ \|W^{h_i}\|_E &\ge \frac{1}{c_8}\|W^{h_i}\|_h = \frac{1}{c_8}|w^{h_{i+1}}|_0 \ge \frac{c_7}{c_8}\|W^{h_{i+1}}\|_E = \frac{c_7}{c_8}\|I_i W^{h_i}\|_E. \end{aligned}$$

So (4.193) holds as well.

Now let us show the validity of inequality (4.222). Take any vector G^{h_i}. Then from (4.239), (4.245) it follows that

$$((L^{h_i})^{-1} - I_{i-1}(L^{h_{i-1}})^{-1}R_i)G^{h_i} = W^{h_i} - I_{i-1}W^{h_{i-1}}. \tag{4.250}$$

Take a norm of both sides and pass to prolongations. Due to (4.236), (4.231), (4.246)

$$\|W^{h_i} - I_{i-1}W^{h_{i-1}}\|_E \leq \frac{1}{c_7}|w^{h_i} - w^{h_{i-1}}|_0 \leq c_5(1+c_2^2)c_7^{-2}h_i^{2-n}\|G^{h_i}\|_E. \tag{4.251}$$

Since G^{h_i} is arbitrary vector then

$$\|(L^{h_i})^{-1} - I_{i-1}(L^{h_{i-1}})^{-1}R_i\|_E \leq c_L/\lambda_i^* \tag{4.252}$$

which proves (4.222) with constant $c_L = c_5(1+c_2^2)c_9c_7^{-2}$. Combining this estimate with (4.216), we come to inequality (4.194) with function (4.223).

So, all assumptions of Theorem 4.11 hold. Therefore (4.195) holds which gives statement of Theorem 4.14. □

Note that in this case on the basis of (4.203), (4.223) we have next dependence of factor ε in (4.238) on the number m of iterations:

$$\varepsilon = O((m+1)^{-2}). \tag{4.253}$$

Now we use the FMG-algorithm from subsection 4.2.1 for solving the whole sequence of discrete problems (4.232) for $i = 0, 1, \ldots, k$. Suppose that functional $f(v)$ in (4.224) ensures the fulfilment of estimate analogous with condition **H**:

$$|u - w^{h_i}|_0 \leq c_{11}h_i^2 \tag{4.254}$$

where c_{11} is dependent on f and independent of h_i. Let also all assumptions of Theorem 4.14 valid. Take m to be such that $\varepsilon < 1$ in (4.238). Then we may choose an integer t

$$\varepsilon^t \leq c_8^{-1}c_7c_2^{-2}. \tag{4.255}$$

Note that ε and t is independent of f and h_i.

Theorem 4.15 *Let all assumptions of Theorem* 4.14 *be valid and let* (4.254), (4.255) *hold. Then application of the FMG-algorithm gives a sequence of approximate solutions $\tilde{V}^{h_i}$ of the problems* (4.232) *which satisfy the inequality*

$$\|\tilde{V}^{h_i} - V^{h_i}\|_E \leq c_{11}h_i^2 \cdot (1+\rho)/c_8(1-\rho), \quad \rho \equiv \varepsilon^t c_7^{-1}c_8c_2^2 < 1, \tag{4.256}$$

and their prolongations $\tilde{v}^{h_i}$ in H^{h_i} satisfy the estimates

$$|\tilde{v}^{h_i} - u|_0 \leq c_{11}h_i^2 \cdot 2/(1-\rho), \quad i = 1, 2, \ldots, k. \tag{4.257}$$

Proof. Apply induction. When $i = 0$ the FMG-algorithm gives the exact solution of (4.232), i. e., $\tilde{V}^{h_0} = V^{h_0}$, $\tilde{v}^{h_0} = w^{h_0}$. Therefore, the estimate (4.256) holds with right-hand side equal to 0 and (4.257) follows from (4.254). Now suppose that the estimate holds

$$|\tilde{v}^{h_{i-1}} - u|_0 \leq c_{11}h_{i-1}^2\sigma, \tag{4.258}$$

where

$$\alpha = 1 + \varepsilon^t c_8 c_7^{-1}, \qquad \sigma = \alpha/(1-\rho). \tag{4.259}$$

This estimate is obviously valid for $i = 1$. Prove it for any level i. To this end, we evaluate error of the initial guess $V_0^{h_i} = I_{i-1}\widetilde{V}^{h_{i-1}}$. Due to (4.236), (4.231), (4.258), (4.254) we have

$$\|V_0^{h_i} - V^{h_i}\|_E \le c_7^{-1}\|V_0^{h_i} - V^{h_i}\|_h \le$$
$$\le c_7^{-1}(|\tilde{v}^{h_{i-1}} - u|_0 + |u - w^{h_i}|_0) \le c_{11}h_i^2 c_7^{-1}(1 + c_2^2\sigma).$$

After performing t W-cycles on the level i, we have the result $\widetilde{V}^{h_i}$ with prolongation $\tilde{v}^{h_i}$ in H^{h_i}. On the basis of (4.238)

$$\|\widetilde{V}^{h_i} - V^{h_i}\|_E \le c_{11}h_i^2\varepsilon^t c_7^{-1}(1 + c_2^2\sigma). \tag{4.260}$$

Due to (4.254), (4.260) we have

$$|\tilde{v}^{h_i} - u|_0 \le |\tilde{v}^{h_i} - w^{h_i}|_0 + |w^{h_i} - u|_0 \le$$
$$\le c_8\|\widetilde{V}^{h_i} - V^{h_i}\|_E + c_{11}h_i^2 \le c_{11}h_i^2(\alpha + \rho\sigma) = c_{11}h_i^2\sigma.$$

Thus (4.258) is proved.

It follows from (4.259) that

$$\alpha \le 2, \qquad \sigma \le 2/(1-\rho). \tag{4.261}$$

This and (4.258) imply (4.257). Combining (4.260), (4.261) we get (4.256):

$$\|\widetilde{V}^{h_i} - V^{h_i}\|_E \le c_{11}h_i^2 c_8^{-1}(\alpha - 1 + \rho\sigma) \le c_{11}h_i^2 c_8^{-1}(1+\rho)/(1-\rho).\square$$

Remark 4.6.1 *In the constant ρ and the estimate* (4.255) *the multiplier $c_8^{-1}c_7$ is caused by implementation of standard estimate* (4.254) *in L_2-norm. In principle, we may get an analogous estimate directly in grid norm $\|\cdot\|_h$, put the condition $\varepsilon^t \le c_2^{-2}$ instead of* (4.255), *and take $\rho = \varepsilon^t c_2^2$ in* (4.256), (4.257).

Now pass to the convergence rate of the multigrid MG-algorithm in energy norm. Therefore we need to formulate a convergence condition of the Bubnov-Galerkin method in the same norm.

To do this into $H_A \subset W_2^1(\Omega)$ we introduce the energy norm

$$[\![w]\!] = \{\mathcal{L}(w,w)\}^{1/2} \tag{4.262}$$

and the corresponding vector norms. Let again W^{h_i} be an arbitrary vector with components $W_y^{h_i}$, $y \in \Omega_{h_i}$. Make the prolongation w^{h_i} from H^{h_i} corresponding to it and define the vector norm

$$\|W^{h_i}\|_h^{(1)} = [\![w^{h_i}]\!]. \tag{4.263}$$

The definitions of the prolongation w^{h_i}, the matrix L^{h_i} and the norms (4.262), (4.235) tell that

$$\|W^{h_i}\|_h^{(1)} = ((W^{h_i})^T L^{h_i} W^{h_i})^{1/2} = h_i^{-n/2}\|(L^{h_i})^{1/2}W^{h_i}\|_E. \tag{4.264}$$

The following assumptions will be applied below.

Condition **I**. *For any functional $f(v) = (g, v)$ with function $g \in L_2(\Omega)$, problem (4.224) has unique solution $u \in W_2^2(\Omega)$; the solution w^{h_i} of the Bubnov-Galerkin method (4.227), (4.228) satisfies the estimate*

$$[\![u - w^{h_i}]\!] \leq c_{11} h_i |g|_0. \tag{4.265}$$

As we saw in sections 4.3–4.5, the symmetric V-cycle is of the best quality in energy norm. So let us consider the V-cycle (i. e., $\gamma = 1$) of the MG-algorithm formulated in section 4.2 with Jacobi-type pre-smoothing and post-smoothing procedures (4.97), (4.98) with parameters (4.99). Let us call this concrete kind the $MG^{(2)}$-algorithm.

Now we can prove the convergence of the MG-algorithm in the energy norm for any m.

Theorem 4.16 *Let the conditions* **G, I,** (4.225), (4.226), (4.236), (4.237) *for the problem* (4.224) *and the Bubnov-Galerkin system* (4.228) *or* (4.232) *with symmetric positive-definite bilinear form $\mathcal{L}$ be satisfied. Assume also that we perform one step of the $MG^{(2)}$-algorithm. Then for any number m of iterations, the error of result $V_1^{h_i}$ diminishes by a factor ε for any initial guess $V_0^{h_i}$:*

$$\|V_1^{h_i} - V^{h_i}\|_h^{(1)} \leq \varepsilon \|V_0^{h_i} - V^{h_i}\|_h^{(1)} \tag{4.266}$$

where

$$\varepsilon = 1/(1 + c_c \text{ctg}^2(\pi/2(2m+1))) \tag{4.267}$$

with a constant c_c independent of m, h_i, f, $V_0^{h_i}$.

Proof. We show that the convergence conditions of Lemma 4.3.2 hold. To this end, we need again to transform our assumptions. We introduce the inner product $(\cdot,\cdot)_i$. Hence, we have

$$[\![W^{h_i}]\!]_i = h_i^{n/2} \|W^{h_i}\|_h^{(1)} \tag{4.268}$$

with the norm (4.75) from subsection 4.3.1.

Instead of Lemma 4.6.2, we use the analogous result in energy norm.

Lemma 4.6.3 *Let $w^{h_{i-1}}$, w^{h_i} be the prolongations in $H^{h_{i-1}}$, H^{h_i} of the solutions $W^{h_{i-1}}$, W^{h_i} of* (4.239) *and* (4.245)*. Then under conditions* **G, I,** (4.236)*, the estimate*

$$[\![w^{h_i} - w^{h_{i-1}}]\!] \leq c_{11}(1 + c_2) c_7^{-1} h_i^{1-n} \|G^{h_i}\|_E \tag{4.269}$$

holds.

Proof. Lemma 4.6.1 remains true under these conditions. Let w be a solution of (4.240). Then from condition **I** and (4.241), we have

$$[\![w - w^{h_i}]\!] \leq c_{11} h_i |g|_0 \leq c_{11} c_7^{-1} h_i^{1-n} \|G^{h_i}\|_E.$$

Using (4.226), we find

$$[\![w - w^{h_{i-1}}]\!] \le c_{11} h_{i-1} |g|_0 \le c_{11} c_2 c_7^{-1} h_i^{1-n} \|G^{h_i}\|_E.$$

Combining these two inequalities, we obtain (4.269). □

Let us continue the proof of Theorem 4.16 and use again equalities (4.239), (4.245) for arbitrary vector W^{h_i} and the corresponding right-hand sides G^{h_i}, $G^{h_{i-1}} = R_i G^{h_i}$. On the basis of (4.78)

$$[\![Q_i W^{h_i}]\!]_i = [\![(I - I_{i-1}(L^{h_{i-1}})^{-1} R_i L^{h_i}) W^{h_i}]\!]_i = [\![W^{h_i} - I_{i-1} W^{h_{i-1}}]\!]_i.$$

Hence, with the help of (4.268), (4.269), (4.263), we have

$$[\![Q_i W^{h_i}]\!]_i = h_i^{n/2} \|W^{h_i} - I_{i-1} W^{h_{i-1}}\|_h^{(1)} =$$

$$= h_i^{n/2} [\![w^{h_i} - w^{h_{i-1}}]\!] \le c_{11}(1 + c_2) c_7^{-1} h_i^{1-n/2} \|G^{h_i}\|_E.$$

Due to (4.237) and the equality $\|G^{h_i}\|_i = \|G^{h_i}\|_E$, we have

$$[\![Q_i W^{h_i}]\!]_i^2 \le c_q (\lambda_i^*)^{-1} \|L^{h_i} W^{h_i}\|_i^2$$

with constant $c_q = c_9 c_{11}^2 (1 + c_2)^2 c_7^{-2}$. Then the condition (4.89) holds with constant $c_1 = c_q$. Condition (4.90) is true on the basis of Theorem 4.6. Then Theorem 4.5 is valid with constant $c_c = c_q^{-1}$ and gives us (4.266) with (4.267). □

Now let us consider the implementation of the FMG-algorithm from subsection 4.2.1 with the $MG^{(2)}$-algorithm. Suppose that the functional $f(v)$ in (4.224) ensures the estimate analogous to condition **I**:

$$[\![u - w^{h_i}]\!] \le c_{12} h_i \tag{4.270}$$

where c_{12} is dependent on f and independent of h_i. Let also all assumptions of Theorem 4.16 be valid. Now the V-cycle converges for any m, i. e., (4.266) is valid with some $\varepsilon(m) < 1$. So fix some $m \ge 1$ and choose integer t thus:

$$\varepsilon^t \le c_2^{-1}. \tag{4.271}$$

Of course, ε and t are independent of f, h_i.

Theorem 4.17 *Let all assumptions of Theorem* 4.16 *be valid and let* (4.270), (4.271) *hold. Then application of the* FMG*-algorithm gives a sequence of approximate solutions* $\widetilde{V}^{h_i}$ *of the problems* (4.232) *which satisfy the inequality*

$$\|\widetilde{V}^{h_i} - V^{h_i}\|_h^{(1)} \le c_{12} h_i \cdot (1 + \rho)/(1 - \rho), \qquad \rho \equiv \varepsilon^t c_2 < 1, \tag{4.272}$$

and their prolongations $\tilde{v}^{h_i}$ *in* H^{h_i} *satisfy the estimates*

$$[\![\tilde{v}^{h_i} - u]\!] \le c_{12} h_i \cdot 2/(1 - \rho), \qquad i = 1, \dots, k. \tag{4.273}$$

Proof. Use induction. When $i = 0$, the FMG-algorithm gives the exact solution of (4.232), i. e., $\widetilde{V}^{h_0} = V^{h_0}$, $\tilde{v}^{h_0} = w^{h_0}$. Therefore, the estimate (4.272) holds with right-hand side equal to 0, and (4.273) follows from (4.270). Now suppose that the estimate

$$[\![\tilde{v}^{h_{i-1}} - u]\!] \leq c_{12} h_{i-1} \sigma \tag{4.274}$$

holds where

$$\alpha = 1 + \varepsilon^t, \qquad \sigma = \alpha/(1-\rho). \tag{4.275}$$

This estimate is valid for $i = 1$. Prove it for any level i. First we evaluate error of initial guess $V_0^{h_i} = I_{i-1}\widetilde{V}^{h_{i-1}}$. Due to (4.263), (4.274), (4.270), we get

$$\|V_0^{h_i} - V^{h_i}\|_h^{(1)} \leq [\![\tilde{v}^{h_{i-1}} - u]\!] + [\![u - w^{h_i}]\!] \leq c_{12} h_i (1 + c_2 \sigma).$$

After performing t V-cycles on the level i, we have the result $\widetilde{V}^{h_i}$ with prolongation $\tilde{v}^{h_i}$ in H^{h_i}. On the basis of (4.266), we have

$$\|\widetilde{V}^{h_i} - V^{h_i}\|_h^{(1)} = [\![\tilde{v}^{h_i} - w^{h_i}]\!] \leq c_{12} h_i \varepsilon^t (1 + c_2 \sigma). \tag{4.276}$$

Due to (4.270), (4.276), we have

$$[\![\tilde{v}^{h_i} - u]\!] \leq [\![\tilde{v}^{h_i} - w^{h_i}]\!] + [\![w^{h_i} - u]\!] \leq c_{12} h_i (\alpha + \rho\sigma) = c_{12} h_i \sigma.$$

Thus, (4.274) is proved.

It follows from (4.259) that

$$\alpha \leq 2, \qquad \sigma \leq 2/(1-\rho). \tag{4.277}$$

The last and (4.272) imply (4.273). Combining (4.276), (4.277), we get (4.272):

$$\|\widetilde{V}^{h_i} - V^{h_i}\|_h^{(1)} \leq c_{12} h_i (\alpha - 1 + \rho\sigma) \leq c_{12} h_i (1+\rho)/(1-\rho). \square$$

4.6.2 Symmetric sign-indefinite bilinear form

We continue studying the problem (4.224) with a symmetric bounded bilinear form $\mathcal{L}$. Now we discard the positive-definiteness of $\mathcal{L}$. First, in contrast with the previous case, the Bubnov-Galerkin problems (4.228) may be solvable only for h_i small enough. So we need to construct systems (4.228), (4.232) subject to this and take h_0 small enough. Second, in this case, we should use another smoothing procedure than in subsection 4.6.1. Of course, in practice, we have a worse rate of convergence of multigrid algorithms than for positive-definite $\mathcal{L}$.

Again we start with a convergence in L_2-norm. On the basis of sections 4.4, 4.5, we again use the W-cycle ($\gamma = 2$) without a post-smoothing procedure. The pre-smoothing procedure is taken in the form (4.180) with parameters (4.206), where $\mu_i^* = (\lambda_i^*)^2$. We call this concrete combination the $MG^{(3)}$-algorithm.

Theorem 4.18 *Assume that conditions* **G**, (4.225), (4.226), (4.236) *are satisfied for* (4.224) *and the systems* (4.228), (4.232) *with symmetric bilinear form* $\mathcal{L}$. *Moreover, let condition* **H** *be valid for systems* (4.232) *with* $i = 0, 1, \ldots, k$ *(perhaps with* h_0 *small enough); let eigenvalues* λ_j *of matrices* L^{h_i} *be bounded in absolute value:*

$$0 < |\lambda_j| \leq \lambda_i^* \leq c_9 h_i^{n-2}, \qquad j = 1, \ldots, N_i. \tag{4.278}$$

Assume also that we perform one step of the $MG^{(3)}$*-algorithm. Then for any* $\varepsilon \in (0,1)$ *there exists* m_0, *independent of* h_i, f, *and such that* $\forall m \geq m_0$ *the error of result* V_1^i *diminishes by the factor* ε *for any initial guess (i. e.,* (4.238) *is valid).*

Proof. We show that again the convergence conditions of Theorem 4.11 hold. To this end, we put $\|V\|_i = \|V\|_E$ for $V \in \mathbf{R}^{N_i}$. Note that Lemma 4.6.1 is valid and Lemma 4.6.2 holds under assumption that h_0 is small enough. As a result, we again reach the estimate (4.238) of Theorem 4.14. Combining this estimate with (4.207), we come to inequality (4.194) with function (4.214).

Other assumptions (4.192), (4.193) of Theorem 4.11 are verified as in Theorem 4.14. Therefore on the basis of Theorem 4.11, the required statement is valid. □

Remark 4.6.2 *In this case, on the basis of* (4.203), (4.214) *we have the following dependence of the factor* ε *in inequality* (4.238) *on number* m *of iterations:*

$$\varepsilon = O((m+1)^{-1}). \tag{4.279}$$

The power is twice worse than in (4.253). *This is the cost of the absence of positive definiteness of* $\mathcal{L}$.

Later we demonstrate three other applications of multigrid algorithm for symmetric case without positive definiteness for singular, spectral, and mixed problems.

The implementation of the FMG-algorithm with such $MG^{(3)}$-algorithm is a subject to the same conditions as in subsection 4.6.1 for L_2-norm. So we present the result without proof which coincides with that in Theorem 4.15.

Theorem 4.19 *Let all assumptions of Theorem* 4.18 *be valid and let* (4.254), (4.255) *hold. Then application of the* FMG*-algorithms with the* $MG^{(3)}$*-algorithm gives a sequence of approximate solutions* $\widetilde{V}^{h_i}$ *of problems* (4.232) *with prolongations* $\tilde{v}^{h_i}$ *in* H^{h_i} *which satisfy the estimates* (4.256), (4.257).

4.6.3 An asymmetric sign-indefinite bilinear form

Let us consider the case where the bilinear form $\mathcal{L}$ in (4.224) is not necessarily positive definite. So is the matrix L^{h_i} of (4.232). Bearing this in mind, we use W-cycle from section 4.2 which converges in L_2-norm. On the basis of section 4.5, we take the pre-smoothing procedure (4.204) with the parameters (4.206) and no post-smoothing one. We call such combination the $MG^{(4)}$-algorithm. Note that the solvability of problems (4.232) holds perhaps only for h_i small enough.

Theorem 4.20 *Assume that conditions* **G**, (4.225), (4.226), (4.236) *are satisfied for* (4.224) *and the systems* (4.232) *with a (asymmetric sign-indefinite) bilinear form* $\mathcal{L}$. *Let also condition* **H** *be valid for systems* (4.232) *with* $i = 0, 1, \dots, k$ *(perhaps with* h_0 *small enough); let the eigenvalues* μ_j *of symmetric matrices* $(L^{h_i})^T L^{h_i}$ *be bounded:*

$$0 < \mu_j \le \mu_i^* = c_{13} h_i^{2n-4}, \qquad j = 1, \dots, N_i, \quad i = 1, \dots, k. \tag{4.280}$$

Assume also that we perform one step of the $MG^{(4)}$*-algorithm. Then, for any* $\varepsilon \in (0,1)$, *there exists* m_0 *independent of* h_i, f *and such that* (4.238) *is valid.*

Proof. First we make sure that assumptions of Theorem 4.11 are fulfiled in the norm $\|V\|_i = \|V\|_E$. For this purpose we again use Lemma 4.6.1 and Lemma 4.6.2 which is valid for h_0 small enough. In analogy with Theorem 4.14, we come to inequality (4.213). Combining this estimate with (4.207), we achieve inequality (4.194) with function (4.214).

Other assumptions (4.192), (4.193) of Theorem 4.11 are verified as in Theorem 4.14. Therefore on the basis of Theorem 4.11, we get the required statement of Theorem 4.20. □

Remark 4.6.3 *In this case we again have the same dependence* (4.279) *of factor* ε *in* (4.238) *on number* m *of iterations.*

Let us show how to define in practice the upper bound of eigenvalues μ_j of the matrix $(L^{h_i})^T L^{h_i}$. For the matrix L^{h_i}, two quantities

$$\delta_1^{h_i} = \max_{1 \le k \le N_i} \sum_{l=1}^{N_i} |L_{kl}^{h_i}| \quad \text{and} \quad \delta_2^{h_i} = \max_{1 \le l \le N_i} \sum_{k=1}^{N_i} |L_{kl}^{h_i}|$$

are easy to define; here $L_{kl}^{h_i}$ are elements of the matrix L^{h_i}. Then, by virtue of Gerschgorin disks, it is easy to see that

$$|\mu_j| \le \delta_1^{h_i} \delta_2^{h_i} \qquad \forall j = 1, \dots, N_i.$$

The implementation of the FMG-algorithm with the described multigrid $MG^{(4)}$-algorithm is subject to the same conditions as those in subsection 4.6.1 for L_2-norm. So we present the main result without proof which coincides with that of Theorem 4.20.

Theorem 4.21 *Let all assumptions of Theorem* 4.20 *be valid and let* (4.254), (4.255) *hold. Then application of the* FMG*-algorithms with the* $MG^{(4)}$*-algorithm gives the sequence of approximate solutions* $\widetilde{V}^{h_i}$ *of problems* (4.232) *with prolongations* $\tilde{v}^{h_i}$ *in* H^{h_i} *which satisfy estimates* (4.256), (4.257).

4.7 A simultaneous application of the multigrid algorithms and the Richardson extrapolation

Both algorithms provided in sections 4.4, 3.5, developed by R.P. Fedorenko and L. Richardson, use a solution of the sequence of difference problems of the same kind on several grids. The algorithm to be constructed below relies on their simultaneous application. It has advantages of both algorithms — it yields the approximate solution of an improved accuracy using simple approximations, and, as we will see later, the number of arithmetical operations is proportional to the number of unknowns.

Let us first formulate an algorithm giving improved accuracy in the energy norm (4.262) for the case (4.224) with symmetric positive-definite form $\mathcal{L}$. Take the norm $[\![u]\!]$ and use the construction of section 3.5. In particular, together with usual interpolation operator I_{i-1} denoted in subsection 3.1.3 $I^{h_i}_{h_{i-1}}$, we will use one more interpolation operator $\widetilde{I}_{i-1}$ which is introduced in section 3.5 as $\widetilde{I}^{h_i}_{h_{i-1}}$.

In this section we will use the h-version only; therefore, h_i is a characteristic size of the triangulation $\mathcal{T}_i$. As usual, for the Richardson extrapolation [123], it is necessary to strengthen the assumption (4.225) about mesh sizes. Together with (4.226) that gives the inequalities

$$1 + c_l \leq h_i/h_{i+1} \leq c_r \qquad i = 0, 1, \dots, k-1. \tag{4.281}$$

Let us consider the $RFMG$-algorithm (Richardson full multigrid algorithm) for finding the sequence of approximate solutions $\widetilde{V}^{h_i}$ of systems (4.232) for $i = 0, 1, \dots, k$.

1. Set $\widetilde{V}^{h_0} = V^{h_0} = (L^{h_0})^{-1}F^{h_0}$; $\widetilde{V}^{h_1} = V^{h_1} = (L^{h_1})^{-1}F^{h_1}$.

2. For $i = 2, \dots, k$ do

   2.1 set

$$\widetilde{V}^{h_i} = \rho_i \widetilde{I}_{i-1} \widetilde{V}^{h_{i-1}} + \sigma_i \widetilde{I}_{i-1} \widetilde{I}_{i-2} \widetilde{V}^{h_{i-2}}, \tag{4.282}$$

   where weights are defined from the system

$$\sigma_i + \rho_i = 1, \qquad \sigma_i h^2_{i-2} + \rho_i h^2_{i-1} = h^2_i; \tag{4.283}$$

   2.2 repeat the MG_i-algorithm t times:

$$\widetilde{V}^{h_i} = MG_i(\widetilde{V}^{h_i}, F^{h_i}).$$

3. With k steps done, we have the solution $\widetilde{V}^{h_k}$. Use besides the solution $\widetilde{V}^{h_{k-1}}$. For these, we construct smooth prolongations $\tilde{v}^{h_k} \in \widetilde{H}^{h_k}$, $\tilde{v}^{h_{k-1}} \in \widetilde{H}^{h_{k-1}}$ and find the linear combination

$$v^H = \gamma_{k-1}\tilde{v}^{h_{k-1}} + \gamma_k \tilde{v}^{h_k} \tag{4.284}$$

   with weights defined from the system

$$\gamma_{k-1} + \gamma_k = 1, \qquad \gamma_{k-1} h^2_{k-1} + \gamma_k h^2_k = 0. \tag{4.285}$$

4.7.1 Convergence in energy norm

Now we prove that the approximate solution v^H will have accuracy of order h^3 under assumption (3.112). Namely, assume that the expansion

$$w^{h_i} = u_i^I + h_i^2 v_i^I + \eta^{h_i} \tag{4.286}$$

holds for the solutions w^{h_i} of the Bubnov-Galerkin method (4.227), (4.228) on each of the grid Ω_{h_i}, $i = 0, 1, \ldots, k$. Here u_i^I, v_i^I are interpolants in H^{h_i} of the solution $u \in W_2^4(\Omega)$ and the function $v \in W_2^2(\Omega)$ is independent of h_i; η^{h_i} is bounded

$$[\![\eta^{h_i}]\!] \leq c_1 h_i^3. \tag{4.287}$$

Under assumption (4.281), from the explicit form of weights we can find two constants c_e, c_f independent of h_i and such that

$$|\rho_i| h_{i-1}^3 + |\sigma_i| h_{i-2}^3 \;\leq\; c_e h_i^3, \qquad i = 2, \ldots, k; \tag{4.288}$$
$$|\gamma_{k-1}| h_{k-1}^3 + |\gamma_k| h_k^3 \;\leq\; c_f h_k^3. \tag{4.289}$$

We need some estimates for norms of piecewise linear and piecewise cubic prolongations of the same vector $W^{h_i} \in \mathbf{R}^{N_i}$.

Lemma 4.7.1 *Let $\hat{w}$, $\tilde{w}$ be the prolongations of vector W^{h_i} in H^{h_i} and $\tilde{H}^{h_i}$. Then*

$$c_I [\![\hat{w}]\!] \leq [\![\tilde{w}]\!] \leq c_c [\![\hat{w}]\!] \tag{4.290}$$

with positive constants independent of W^{h_i}.

Proof. On the basis of the theory of interpolation by linear elements, the estimate

$$[\![\hat{w} - \tilde{w}]\!]_T^2 \leq c_3^2 \, \|\tilde{w}\|_{1,T}^2 \leq c_4^2 \, [\![\tilde{w}]\!]_T^2$$

holds for any triangle T of subdivision $\mathcal{T}_{3h}$. Summing it over all $T \in \mathcal{T}_{3h}$, we get the inequality

$$[\![\hat{w} - \tilde{w}]\!] \leq c_4 [\![\tilde{w}]\!].$$

Applying it to the triangle inequality, we arrive at the left-hand side of (4.290):

$$[\![\hat{w}]\!] \leq [\![\hat{w} - \tilde{w}]\!] + [\![\tilde{w}]\!] \leq (1 + c_4) [\![\tilde{w}]\!].$$

The right-hand side of (4.290) follows in the same way from the theory of interpolation by cubic elements. □

To simplify the presentation, we are dwelling on a symmetric positive-definite bilinear form $\mathcal{L}$. So we may implement the symmetric V-cycle described in subsection 4.6.2 as a particular $MG^{(2)}$-algorithm. This V-cycle converges for any m, i. e., (4.266) is valid with some $\varepsilon(m) < 1$. So we fix some $m \geq 1$ and choose integer t:

$$\varepsilon^t \leq c_e c_I^{-1} c_c. \tag{4.291}$$

Theorem 4.22 *Assume that conditions of Theorem* 4.16 *and expansion* (4.286) *with estimates* (4.287)–(4.289) *are satisfied. Then implementation of the RFMG-algorithm with the $MG^{(2)}$-algorithm gives sequence of approximate solutions $\widetilde{V}^{h_i}$ of problems* (4.232) *which satisfy the inequality*

$$\|\widetilde{V}^{h_i} - V^{h_i}\|_h^{(1)} \leq c_R h_i^3 \qquad \forall i = 0, 1, \dots, k. \tag{4.292}$$

The extrapolated solution v^H satisfies estimate

$$[\![v^H - u]\!] \leq c_H h_k^3. \tag{4.293}$$

Proof. Let $\tilde{u}_i^I$, $\tilde{v}_i^I$ be interpolants in $\tilde{H}^{h_i}$ of u, v. Then on the basis of interpolating properties of cubic elements

$$[\![u - \tilde{u}_i^I]\!] \leq c_3 h_i^3 \|u\|_4, \tag{4.294}$$
$$[\![v - \tilde{v}_i^I]\!] \leq c_4 h_i \|v\|_2. \tag{4.295}$$

Set

$$c_5 = c_1 c_c + c_3\|u\|_4 + c_4\|v\|_2$$

and prove the inequality

$$\|\widetilde{V}^{h_i} - V^{h_i}\|_h^{(1)} \leq \sigma_i h_i^3 \tag{4.296}$$

with constants

$$\sigma_i = \alpha \sum_{j=0}^{i-2} \rho^j, \qquad \rho = \varepsilon^t c_I^{-1} c_e c_c, \qquad \alpha = 2c_5 \varepsilon^t c_I^{-1} c_e \tag{4.297}$$

with the help of induction. When $i = 0, 1$, the *RFMG*-algorithm gives the exact solutions of (4.232), i. e., $\widetilde{V}^{h_0} = V^{h_0}$, $\widetilde{V}^{h_1} = V^{h_1}$. Therefore, the estimate (4.296) holds with right-hand side equal to 0. Suppose that it is satisfied for $i-1$, i. The function w^{h_i} is a prolongation in H^{h_i} of the vector V^{h_i}. Now, from (4.286), for prolongation $\hat{v}^{h_i} \in H^{h_i}$ of the vector $\widetilde{V}^{h_i}$, we find the following expansion

$$\hat{v}^{h_i} = u_i^I + h_i^2 v_i^I + \hat{\xi}^{h_i}, \tag{4.298}$$

where, by virtue of (4.287) and (4.296),

$$[\![\hat{\xi}^{h_i}]\!] \leq (\sigma_i + c_1) h_i^3. \tag{4.299}$$

Construct now a smooth prolongation $\tilde{v}^{h_i} \in \tilde{H}^{h_i}$ of the vector $\widetilde{V}^{h_i}$. The functions u, v coincide with their interpolants u_i^I, v_i^I at the nodes of the grid Ω_{h_i}. Therefore, the smooth interpolants $\tilde{u}_i^I$, $\tilde{v}_i^I \in \tilde{H}^{h_i}$ constructed by u, v and u_i^I, v_i^I are identical. Reffering to (4.298), we have

$$\tilde{v}^{h_i} = \tilde{u}_i^I + h_i^2 \tilde{v}_i^I + \tilde{\xi}^{h_i}. \tag{4.300}$$

On the basis of (4.290)

$$[\![\tilde{\xi}^{h_i}]\!] \leq c_c [\![\hat{\xi}^{h_i}]\!] \leq c_c(\sigma_i + c_1) h_i^3. \tag{4.301}$$

Now employ (4.294), (4.295) to (4.300). As a result, we have

$$\tilde{v}^{h_i} = u + h_i^2 v + \xi^{h_i}, \tag{4.302}$$

where

$$[\![\xi^{h_i}]\!] \leq (c_5 + c_c\sigma_i)h_i^3. \tag{4.303}$$

The same relations are found on the grid $\Omega_{h_{i-1}}$. Adding them together as in (4.282), we arrive at the function

$$\tilde{w}^{h_{i+1}} \equiv \sigma_i \tilde{v}^{h_{i-1}} + \rho_i \tilde{v}^{h_i} = u + h_{i+1}^2 v + \tilde{\xi}^{h_{i+1}}, \tag{4.304}$$

with the remainder term

$$[\![\tilde{\xi}^{h_{i+1}}]\!] \leq c_6 h_{i+1}^3, \qquad c_6 = c_e(c_5 + c_c\sigma_i). \tag{4.305}$$

Consider now the function $\tilde{u}^{h_{i+1}}$, a smooth interpolant in $\tilde{H}^{h_{i+1}}$ of the solution $w^{h_{i+1}}$ of (4.232) on grid $\Omega_{h_{i+1}}$. By virtue of calculations similar to (4.294)–(4.302), we have the expansion

$$\tilde{u}^{h_{i+1}} = u + h_{i+1}^2 v + r^{h_{i+1}} \tag{4.306}$$

with the estimate of the remainder term

$$[\![r^{h_{i+1}}]\!] \leq c_5 c_e h_{i+1}^3. \tag{4.307}$$

Subtract (4.306) from (4.304) and apply (4.305) and (4.307). We get

$$[\![\tilde{w}^{h_{i+1}} - \tilde{u}^{h_{i+1}}]\!] \leq (c_5 c_e + c_6)h_{i+1}^3. \tag{4.308}$$

Thus we obtained the estimate of the function being a smooth prolongation in $\tilde{H}^{h_{i+1}}$ of the vector $\tilde{W}^{h_{i+1}} - V^{h_{i+1}}$.

By definition of introduced norms and the estimates (4.290) and (4.308),

$$\|\tilde{W}^{h_{i+1}} - V^{h_{i+1}}\|_h^{(1)} \leq c_I^{-1}(c_5 c_e + c_6)h_{i+1}^3. \tag{4.309}$$

Hence, application of formula (4.282) yields the initial guess to vector $V^{h_{i+1}}$ of an improved accuracy. On the basis of Theorem 4.16, it follows that after t applications of the $MG^{(2)}$-algorithm we have

$$\|\tilde{V}^{h_{i+1}} - V^{h_{i+1}}\|_h^{(1)} \leq \varepsilon^t \, \|\tilde{W}^{h_{i+1}} - V^{h_{i+1}}\|_h^{(1)} \leq \varepsilon^t c_I^{-1} c_e(2c_5 + c_c\sigma_i)h_{i+1}^3. \tag{4.310}$$

Using the explicit form of constants σ_i, α, ρ, we find the inequality

$$\|\tilde{V}^{h_{i+1}} - V^{h_{i+1}}\|_h^{(1)} \leq (\rho\sigma_i + \alpha)h_{i+1}^3 = \sigma_{i+1}h_{i+1}^3. \tag{4.311}$$

Thus, (4.296) is proved. On the basis of (4.291), $\rho < 1$. Therefore, $\sigma_i \leq \alpha/(1-\rho)$. Thus the estimate (4.292) is attained for all $i = 0, 1, \ldots, k$.

Use now estimate (4.302) for $i = k-1, k$. Summing them as in (4.284), we get the equality

$$v^H = u + \tilde{r}^{h_k}.$$

From (4.289), the inequality

$$[\![r^{h_k}]\!] \le c_H h_k^3$$

equivalent to (4.293) follows. □

In principle, we may implement the improved (cubic) interpolation $\widetilde{I}_{i-1}$ instead of I_{i-1} in the MG-algorithm not only in the $RFMG$-algorithm. But in this case, we violate the condition (4.72) since $L^{h_{i-1}} \neq \widetilde{I}_{i-1}^{*} L^{h_i} \widetilde{I}_{i-1}$. So we can use only the results of section 4.5 where this condition is not necessary. We will not repeat our reasoning for this modification of the $MG^{(2)}$-algorithm and pass to convergence in L_2-norm.

4.7.2 Convergence in L_2-norm

As a rule, the accuracy order of approximate solutions in L_2-norm is higher. For instance, assume that the remainder term in (4.286) is estimated as follows:

$$|r^{h_i}|_0 \le c_7 h_i^4. \tag{4.312}$$

Then, convergence in L_2-norm is accelerated:

$$\|\widetilde{V}^{h_i} - V^{h_i}\|_h \le c_R' h_i^4. \tag{4.313}$$

Since proofs of this and other facts are very similar to those presented above, we quote only results without proving them. For example, instead of (4.288), (4.289), we have

$$|\rho_i| h_{i-1}^4 + |\sigma_i| h_{i-2}^4 \le c_e' h_i^4, \qquad i = 2, \ldots, k; \tag{4.314}$$

$$|\gamma_{k-1}| h_{k-1}^4 + |\gamma_k| h_k^4 \le c_f' h_k^4. \tag{4.315}$$

Lemma 4.7.2 *Let $\hat{w}$, $\tilde{w}$ be prolongations of the vector W^{h_i} in H^{h_i} and $\tilde{H}^{h_i}$. Then*

$$c_I' |\hat{w}|_0 \le |\tilde{w}|_0 \le c_c' |\hat{w}|_0. \tag{4.316}$$

Although we continue to study the positive-definite bilinear form $\mathcal{L}$, we should use the W-cycle described in subsection 4.6.3 as the $MG^{(1)}$-algorithm with parameters (4.215) in the pre-smoothing procedure (4.97) and without a post-smoothing one. Let us fix some $\varepsilon \in (0,1)$ and take m_0 such that (4.238) is valid $\forall m \ge m_0$. It is possible on the basis of Theorem 4.14. After that we choose integer t:

$$\varepsilon^t \le c_e' c_c' / c_I'. \tag{4.317}$$

Theorem 4.23 *Assume that conditions of Theorem* 4.14 *and expansion* (4.286) *with estimates* (4.312), (4.314), (4.315) *are satisfied. Then implementation of the $RFMG$-algorithm with the $MG^{(1)}$-algorithm gives a sequence of approximate solutions $\widetilde{V}^{h_i}$ of the problems* (4.232) *which satisfy inequality* (4.313) $\forall i = 0, 1, \ldots, k$.

Proof of this theorem is very similar to one of Theorem 4.22 and distinquished by the norm of remainder. Therefore we do not present it.

4.8 Solving the singular problems

In this section, we treat the case where the initial differential problem is singular. It arises, for example, during the solving K.G. Neumann's boundary value problem and the spectral problem. In these cases, we will look for *the normal solution* [186], i. e., a pseudo-solution with minimal norm. To implement our search, we also succeed in synthezing a multigrid algorithm which uses the vectors approximately characterizing the null space of the initial differential problem.

We will again use the notation of section 4.6. Consider the spectral problem of defining the eigenvalues λ and the corresponding eigenfunctions $u \in H_A \subset L_2(\Omega)$ satisfying the identity

$$\mathcal{L}(u,v) = \lambda(u,v) \qquad \forall v \in H_A \tag{4.318}$$

where (u,v) is the inner product in $L_2(\Omega)$; the bilinear form $\mathcal{L}(u,v)$ is bounded in $H_A \times H_A$, positive definite, and symmetric. Assume that λ_0 is some fixed s-tuple eigenvalue associated with the set of eigenfunctions $v_1, \dots, v_s \in H_A$ orthonormed in $L_2(\Omega)$. Denote its linear span by $\mathcal{B}$.

Our problem is to find a solution $u \in H_A$ satisfying the identity

$$\mathcal{L}(u,v) - \lambda_0(u,v) = (f,v) \qquad \forall v \in H_A \tag{4.319}$$

where $f \in L_2(\Omega)$ is a given function. Under such conditions, the usual solution may not exist or may not be unique. We will therefore look for the normal solution, i. e., the function $u_H \in H_A$ orthogonal in $L_2(\Omega)$ to vectors $v_1, \dots, v_s$ and satisfying the identity

$$\mathcal{L}(u_H,v) - \lambda_0(u_H,v) = (f_H,v) \qquad \forall v \in H_A \tag{4.320}$$

where the function $f_H \in L_2(\Omega)$ is obtained by orthogonalizing f to the null space $\mathcal{B}$ in $L_2(\Omega)$.

Let us consider an approximate method for calculating the normal solution to (4.319). To this end, we introduce parameters h_i satisfying (4.225) and (4.226). For each of them, we construct a grid Ω_{h_i} and basis functions $\varphi_y^{h_i}$ $\forall y \in \Omega_{h_i}$ satisfying condition **G**. Suppose that we have some guess $\lambda_0^{h_i}$ for eigenvalue λ_0.

We first formulate the Bubnov-Galerkin system for problem (4.318). An approximate solution is to be in the form

$$w^{h_i}(x) = \sum_{y\in\Omega_{h_i}} \alpha_y^{h_i} \varphi_y^{h_i}(x). \tag{4.321}$$

The weights $\alpha_y^{h_i}$ are defined from the system

$$\sum_{y\in\Omega_{h_i}} \alpha_y^{h_i} \mathcal{L}(\varphi_y^{h_i}, \varphi_z^{h_i}) = \lambda^{h_i} \sum_{y\in\Omega_{h_i}} \alpha_y^{h_i} (\varphi_y^{h_i}, \varphi_z^{h_i}), \quad z \in \Omega_{h_i}. \tag{4.322}$$

Performing the vectorial-matric re-notation as in (4.232), we have

$$L^{h_i} V^{h_i} = \lambda^{h_i} M^{h_i} V^{h_i} \tag{4.323}$$

where λ^{h_i} is an eigenvalue; V^{h_i} is the corresponding eigenvector; L^{h_i} and M^{h_i} are the $N_i \times N_i$ symmetric matrices with elements $\mathcal{L}(\varphi_y^{h_i}, \varphi_z^{h_i})$ and $(\varphi_y^{h_i}, \varphi_z^{h_i})$, respectively.

For further characterization of eigenvectors, we introduce a scalar product by the formula

$$(U, V)_i \equiv (u, v) = U^T M^{h_i} V, \tag{4.324}$$

where u, v are the prolongations in H^{h_i} of vectors $U, V \in \mathbf{R}^{N_i}$. Now the total system of the eigenvectors of problem (4.323) can be orthonormed in this scalar product.

Assume now that the eigenvalues and vectors of (4.323) can be divided into 2 groups. One group of the s eigenvalues falls into the class of approximations of λ_0. Denote these by $\lambda_1^{h_i}, \dots, \lambda_s^{h_i}$. They are associated with eigenvectors $V_1^{h_i}, \dots, V_s^{h_i}$ for which we know the approximating system of vectors $\widetilde{V}_1^{h_i}, \dots, \widetilde{V}_s^{h_i}$ orthonormed in the scalar product $(\cdot, \cdot)_i$.

To characterize the closeness of this vectorial systems, we introduce linear spans

$$\begin{aligned} \mathcal{V}^{h_i} &= \operatorname{span}\{V_1^{h_i}, \dots, V_s^{h_i}\}, \\ \widetilde{\mathcal{V}}^{h_i} &= \operatorname{span}\{\widetilde{V}_1^{h_i}, \dots, \widetilde{V}_s^{h_i}\}, \end{aligned}$$

and define *the opening* $\Theta_h(\mathcal{V}^{h_i}, \widetilde{\mathcal{V}}^{h_i})$ of subspaces $\mathcal{V}^{h_i}, \widetilde{\mathcal{V}}^{h_i} \subset H^{h_i}$. To this end, we designate

$$\operatorname{dis}_h(F, \widetilde{\mathcal{V}}^{h_i}) = \inf_{G \in \widetilde{\mathcal{V}}^{h_i}} \|F - G\|_h \tag{4.325}$$

as the distance from a vector F to a subspace $\mathcal{V}^{h_i}$ and analogously do for $\widetilde{\mathcal{V}}^{h_i}$. Then we put [2]

$$\Theta_h(\mathcal{V}^{h_i}, \widetilde{\mathcal{V}}^{h_i}) \equiv \max\{ \sup_{F \in \mathcal{V}^{h_i}, \|F\|_h = 1} \operatorname{dis}_h(F, \widetilde{\mathcal{V}}^{h_i}), \sup_{G \in \widetilde{\mathcal{V}}^{h_i}, \|G\|_h = 1} \operatorname{dis}_h(G, \mathcal{V}^{h_i})\}. \tag{4.326}$$

Since we deal with Hilbert space, the opening can be written in other terms. Let P_h, $\widetilde{P}_h$ be orthogonal projectors from H^{h_i} to $\mathcal{V}^{h_i}$, $\widetilde{\mathcal{V}}^{h_i}$ respectively. Then (4.326) is equivalent to another definition [2], [87]:

$$\Theta_h(\mathcal{V}^{h_i}, \widetilde{\mathcal{V}}^{h_i}) = \|P_h - \widetilde{P}_h\|_h. \tag{4.327}$$

Note that magnitude of the opening depends on chosen norm. In principle, we may use the norm $\|\cdot\|_E$ instead of $\|\cdot\|_h$ but we should have another value of Θ_h.

In these terms we may determine the closeness of two systems by inequality

$$\Theta_h(\mathcal{V}^{h_i}, \widetilde{\mathcal{V}}^{h_i}) \le c_{11} h_i^2, \qquad i = 1, 2, \dots . \tag{4.328}$$

As for the rest of the eigenvalues (numbered $s+1, \dots, N_i$), we assume that they are separated from $\lambda_0^{h_i}$ which we take as known approximate value of λ_0:

$$|\lambda_j^{h_i} - \lambda_0^{h_i}| \ge c_9, \qquad j = s+1, \dots, N_i. \tag{4.329}$$

Problem (4.319) is also associated with the Bubnov-Galerkin system with this approximate value of λ_0:

$$(L^{h_i} - \lambda_0^{h_i} M^{h_i}) W^{h_i} = F^{h_i}, \tag{4.330}$$

where F^{h_i} is the N_i-vector with components $(f, \varphi_z^{h_i})$. The matrix of this system

$$P^{h_i} = L^{h_i} - \lambda_0^{h_i} M^{h_i}$$

is either singular or close to such one. Its usual solution is therefore unstable. We reformulate this problem as follows. Orthogonalize the right-hand side F^{h_i} to vectors $V_1^{h_i}, \dots, V_s^{h_i}$ in the following sense. Construct the vector

$$\bar{F}^{h_i} = F^{h_i} + \sum_{j=1}^{s} \alpha_j M^{h_i} V_j^{h_i} \tag{4.331}$$

with weights α_j determined from the system

$$\sum_{j=1}^{s} \alpha_j (V_j^{h_i}, V_k^{h_i})_i = -(F^{h_i})^T V_k^{h_i}, \qquad k = 1, \dots, s. \tag{4.332}$$

Since $\{V_j^{h_i}\}$ are linearly independent, the system has a unique solution. As a result, we get a vector $\bar{F}^{h_i}$ for which $(\bar{F}^{h_i})^T V_j^{h_i} = 0$ $(j = 1, \dots, s)$. For the problem

$$P^{h_i} W_H^{h_i} = \bar{F}^{h_i}, \tag{4.333}$$

find the normal solution, i. e., a vector satisfying (4.333) and orthogonal to $\mathcal{V}^{h_i}$ in scalar product $(\cdot, \cdot)_i$. Actually, we define the desired *quasi-solution of the Bubnov-Galerkin system* (4.330). Denote its prolongation in H^{h_i} by $w_H^{h_i}$. The following condition is supposed to be satisfied for it.

C o n d i t i o n **J**. *For any function* $f \in L_2(\Omega)$, *problem* (4.319) *has a unique normal solution* $u_H \in H_A$; *and the Bubnov-Galerkin system* (4.330) *has a unique quasi-solution* $W_H^{h_i}$ *which prolongation* $w_H^{h_i} \in H^{h_i}$ *obeys the estimate*

$$|u_H - w_H^{h_i}|_0 \leq c_{10} h_i^2 |f|_0. \tag{4.334}$$

Let us develop *the* $MG^{(5)}$*-algorithm* to calculate the approximate quasi-solution of (4.330) in the form of a procedure $MG_i^{(5)}(W_0, F^{h_i})$ with an initial guess W_0. Consider first the grid Ω_{h_0}. System (4.330) has a rather small number of unknowns on it. The eigenvectors $V_1^{h_0}, \dots, V_s^{h_0}$ can therefore be considered known exactly. The first level of the $MG^{(5)}$-algorithm is then to define the quasi-solution of (4.330) directly using the orthogonalizing. So we have $W_H^{h_0} = MG_0^{(5)}(W_0, F^{h_0})$ as a result of procedure within the small number of arithmetical operations. Initial guess W_0 is of no importance at this level.

Continue recurrently. Assume that there exists some guess $W_0^{h_i}$ for the quasi-solution of system (4.330) with index $i \geq 1$. Then procedure $MG_i^{(5)}(W_0^{h_i}, F^{h_i})$ permitting to reduce the error norm of the approximate quasi-solution involves 5 stages.

$\mathbf{A}_1^{(5)}$. Orthogonalize vector F^{h_i} to the set of vectors $\widetilde{V}_j^{h_i}$ $(j = 1, \dots, s)$ by the same way as (4.331), (4.332) where $V_j^{h_i}$ substituted by $\widetilde{V}_j^{h_i}$. Denote the obtained vector by $\widetilde{F}^{h_i}$.

$\mathbf{A}_2^{(5)}$. Execute m iterations by the formula

$$U_{l+1} = U_l - \tau_l (P^{h_i} U_l - \widetilde{F}^{h_i}), \qquad l = 0, 1, \dots, m-1, \tag{4.335}$$

with the initial guess $U_0 = W_0^{h_i}$ and the parameters τ_l to be chosen by formula (4.215) with constant λ_i^* equal to the upper bound of eigenvalues μ of the problem $P^{h_i}V = \mu V$. We get U_m and the residual

$$G^{h_i} = P^{h_i}U_m - \tilde{F}^{h_i}. \tag{4.336}$$

$\mathbf{A}_3^{(5)}$. Put $G^{h_{i-1}} = R_i G^{h_i}$.
$\mathbf{A}_4^{(5)}$. Take vector $G^{h_{i-1}}$ as the right-hand side of the system

$$P^{h_{i-1}}W^{h_{i-1}} = G^{h_{i-1}}. \tag{4.337}$$

To calculate its approximate quasi-solution, use the procedure $MG_{i-1}^{(5)}$ twice:

$$Z = MG_{i-1}^{(5)}(0, G^{h_{i-1}}), \qquad \tilde{W}^{h_{i-1}} = MG_{i-1}^{(5)}(Z, G^{h_{i-1}}).$$

$\mathbf{A}_5^{(5)}$. Calculate vector $U_m - I_{i-1}\tilde{W}^{h_{i-1}}$ and orthogonalize it to vectors $\tilde{V}_1^{h_i}, \dots, \tilde{V}_s^{h_i}$ in *the scalar product* $(\cdot,\cdot)_i$. Denote the obtained vector by $W_1^{h_i}$ and regard it as the result: $W_1^{h_i} = MG_i^{(5)}(W_0^{h_i}, F^{h_i})$.

Let us consider the conditions under which the $MG^{(5)}$-algorithm converges.

Theorem 4.24 *Assume that conditions* **G**, **J**, (4.225), (4.226), (4.236), (4.328), (4.329) *are satisfied for* (4.319) *and the Bubnov-Galerkin systems* (4.330) *at levels* $i = 0, 1, \dots, k$; *let also the eigenvalues* μ *of matrices* P^{h_i} *(i. e.,* $P^{h_i}V = \mu V$*) be bounded:*

$$-c_{12}h_i^n \le \mu \le \lambda_i^* \le c_{13}h_i^{n-2}, \qquad i = 1, \dots, k. \tag{4.338}$$

Then for any $\varepsilon \in (0,1)$ *one can find an integer* m_0 *independent of* h_i, f *and such that* $\forall m \ge m_0$ *for sufficiently small* h_1, *the accomplishment of the* $MG^{(5)}$*-algorithm reduces the error of the approximate quasi-solution:*

$$\|W_1^{h_i} - W_H^{h_i}\|_h \le \varepsilon\|W_0^{h_i} - W_H^{h_i}\|_h + c_{14}h_i^2|f|_0 \tag{4.339}$$

where

$$c_{14} = c_{11}(0.26c_7^2/c_{12} + 5/c_9). \tag{4.340}$$

Proof. Put

$$\begin{aligned} \varepsilon_1 &= \min\{\varepsilon, c_7/2c_8q_1\}, && (4.341)\\ c_{15} &\equiv 2(c_{10}(1+c_2^2) + c_2^2c_{14})/c_7, && (4.342)\\ c_{16} &\equiv c_{15} + 1.68c_8c_{11}q_1/c_{12} && (4.343)\end{aligned}$$

with constants from (4.10), (4.226), (4.236), (4.329), (4.334), (4.328). As m increases, the left-hand side of the inequality

$$\frac{c_{13}}{m+1}\mathrm{tg}\frac{\pi}{4(m+1)} \le \frac{\varepsilon_1 c_7}{2c_{16}} \tag{4.344}$$

decreases monotonically. Therefore there exists m_0 such that (4.344) is valid $\forall m \geq m_0$. From the definition of λ_i^* and (4.4), (4.338), (4.344), the inequality follows

$$h_i^{2-n} q_0 = \frac{h_i^{2-n}\lambda_i^*}{m+1}\mathrm{tg}\frac{\pi}{4(m+1)} \leq \frac{\varepsilon_1 c_7}{2c_{16}}. \tag{4.345}$$

Let us fix some $m \geq m_0$. While h_i decreases, the right-hand side of the inequality

$$c_{12} h_i^n \leq \lambda_i^* \mathrm{tg}^2 \frac{\pi}{4(m+1)} \tag{4.346}$$

is the value of order $O(h_i^{n-2}) \sim c_{13} h_i^{n-2}$. Therefore there exists h_e such that (4.346) is valid $\forall h_i \leq h_e$. Below we demand that

$$h_1 \leq h_e. \tag{4.347}$$

It implies $h_i \leq h_e$ and correctness of (4.346). Combine (4.346), (4.345):

$$c_{12} h_i^n \leq (m+1)\mathrm{tg}\frac{\pi}{4(m+1)} \frac{\varepsilon_1 c_7}{2c_{16}} h_i^{n-2}.$$

Divide both sides by $c_{12} h_i^{n-2}$ and use the inequality $\mathrm{tg}x/x \leq 1.05$ on $[0, \pi/8]$:

$$h_i^2 \leq \frac{\varepsilon_1 c_7 \pi}{8 c_{16} c_{12}} (\mathrm{tg}\frac{\pi}{4(m+1)} \cdot \frac{4(m+1)}{\pi}) \leq 0.42 \frac{\varepsilon_1 c_7}{c_{16} c_{12}}. \tag{4.348}$$

From (4.346) on the basis of (4.15), the useful inequality follows:

$$q_2 \leq 0.28 / c_{12} h_i^n. \tag{4.349}$$

We prove inequality (4.339) using induction in i but with the multiplier ε_1 instead of ε. For $i = 0$, (4.339) follows from the assumption that quasi-solutions of the problem on the grid Ω_{h_0} can be computed exactly. Assume that this inequality has also been proved for $i-1$ with multiplier ε_1.

Consider the first stage $\mathbf{A}_1^{(5)}$. Vector $\widetilde{F}^{h_i}$ is obtained by orthogonalizing F^{h_i} to vectors $\widetilde{V}_1^{h_i}, \ldots, \widetilde{V}_s^{h_i}$; and $\bar{F}^{h_i}$ is done to vectors $V_1^{h_i}, \ldots, V_s^{h_i}$. For each of vectors $V_j^{h_i}$, $\widetilde{V}_j^{h_i}$, we put in correspondence their prolongations $v_j^{h_i}$, $\tilde{v}_j^{h_i}$ in H^{h_i} by usual way. Denote spans of these functions as

$$\begin{aligned} \mathcal{B}^{h_i} &= \mathrm{span}\{v_1^{h_i}, \ldots, v_s^{h_i}\}, \\ \widetilde{\mathcal{B}}^{h_i} &= \mathrm{span}\{\tilde{v}_1^{h_i}, \ldots, \tilde{v}_s^{h_i}\}. \end{aligned}$$

For these subspaces we also introduce the *opening in* $L_2(\Omega)$:

$$\Theta(\mathcal{B}^{h_i}, \widetilde{\mathcal{B}}^{h_i}) \equiv \max\{ \sup_{f \in \mathcal{B}^{h_i}, |f|_0 = 1} \mathrm{dis}(f, \widetilde{\mathcal{B}}^{h_i}), \sup_{g \in \widetilde{\mathcal{B}}^{h_i}, |g|_0 = 1} \mathrm{dis}(g, \mathcal{B}^{h_i})\} \tag{4.350}$$

with distance

$$\mathrm{dis}(f, \widetilde{\mathcal{B}}^{h_i}) = \inf_{g \in \widetilde{\mathcal{B}}^{h_i}} |f - g|_0. \tag{4.351}$$

On the basis of the one-to-one correspondence between vectors and their prolongations, it follows

$$\Theta_h(\mathcal{V}^{h_i}, \widetilde{\mathcal{V}}^{h_i}) = \Theta(\mathcal{B}^{h_i}, \widetilde{\mathcal{B}}^{h_i}). \tag{4.352}$$

Let $\bar{P}$, $\widetilde{P}$ be the orthogonal projectors from $L_2(\Omega)$ into $\mathcal{B}^{h_i}$, $\widetilde{\mathcal{B}}^{h_i}$ correspondingly. Put $\bar{f} = (I - \bar{P})f$, $\tilde{f} = (I - \widetilde{P})f$ and prove for components of vectors $\bar{F}^{h_i}$, $\widetilde{F}^{h_i}$ the formulae

$$\bar{F}_y^{h_i} = (\bar{f}, \varphi_y^{h_i}) \tag{4.353}$$

$$\widetilde{F}_y^{h_i} = (\tilde{f}, \varphi_y^{h_i}), \qquad y \in \Omega_{h_i}. \tag{4.354}$$

Indeed, separate in f the part $\bar{f}$ orthogonal to $\mathcal{B}^{h_i}$. That may be made in the form of linear combination

$$\bar{f} = f + \sum_{j=1}^{s} \alpha_j v_j^{h_i} \tag{4.355}$$

with weights defined from system

$$\sum_{j=1}^{s} \alpha_j (v_j^{h_i}, v_k^{h_i}) = -(f, v_k^{h_i}), \qquad k = 1, \ldots, s. \tag{4.356}$$

This system is another representation of (4.332); therefore, their solutions α_j coincide. Multiply (4.355) by $\varphi_y^{h_i}$ in inner product of $L_2(\Omega)$ and use the explicit form of elements of matrix M^{h_i} in (4.331). As a result, we come to (4.353). Analogously, (4.354) is proved.

For the opening Θ, the property analogous to (4.327) is valid [2], [87]:

$$\Theta(\mathcal{B}^{h_i}, \widetilde{\mathcal{B}}^{h_i}) = |\bar{P} - \widetilde{P}|_0. \tag{4.357}$$

Consider the vector $Y = \widetilde{F}^{h_i} - \bar{F}^{h_i}$ and the function $f^* = \tilde{f} - \bar{f}$. By definition of functions $\bar{f}$, $\tilde{f}$ with the help (4.352), (4.357), (4.328), we have

$$|f^*|_0 = |(I - \widetilde{P})f - (I - \bar{P})f|_0 \leq |\widetilde{P} - \bar{P}|_0 |f|_0 \leq c_{11} h_i^2 |f|_0. \tag{4.358}$$

On the basis of (4.353), (4.354), the components of vector Y are equal to

$$Y_y = (f^*, \varphi_y^{h_i}), \qquad y \in \Omega_{h_i}. \tag{4.359}$$

Hence

$$\|Y\|_E^2 = \sum_{y \in \Omega_{h_i}} (f^*, \varphi_y^{h_i})^2 h_i^n = (f^*, \sum_{y \in \Omega_{h_i}} (f^*, \varphi_y^{h_i}) \varphi_y^{h_i}) h_i^n.$$

Note that in the last inner product, the second argument is a prolongation of vector Y in H^{h_i}. Therefore, with the help of the Cauchy-Bunyakovski inequality and (4.236), (4.358), we have

$$\|Y\|_E^2 \leq |f^*|_0 \|Y\|_h h_i^n \leq c_8 c_{11} h_i^{n+2} |f|_0 \|Y\|_E.$$

Dividing both parts by $\|Y\|_E$, we come to inequality

$$\|Y\|_E \leq c_8 c_{11} h_i^{n+2} |f|_0. \tag{4.360}$$

Denote $E_j = W_H^{h_i} - U_j$. The relation

$$E_{j+1} = E_j - \tau_j(P^{h_i}E_j + Y), \qquad j = 0, 1, \dots, m-1, \tag{4.361}$$

holds by virtue of (4.333) and (4.335). Using (4.333), (4.336) and induction, we get

$$G^{h_i} = -(\prod_{j=0}^{m-1}(I - \tau_j P^{h_i}))(Y + P^{h_i}E_0), \tag{4.362}$$

where I is the $N_i \times N_i$ identity matrix. The matrix P^{h_i} is symmetric and so the inequality

$$\|G^{h_i}\|_E \le \frac{q_0}{c_7}\|E_0\|_h + q_1\|Y\|_E \tag{4.363}$$

follows from the definition of polynomials P_{m+1}, Q_m in section 4.1 and estimates (4.7), (4.10), (4.236). Besides, from (4.361), the definition of polynomials Q_m, S_{m-1}, and estimates (4.10),(4.15), (4.236), using induction we have

$$\|E_m\|_h \le q_1\frac{c_8}{c_7}\|E_0\|_h + q_2c_8\|Y\|_E. \tag{4.364}$$

In view of orthogonality of $W_H^{h_i}$ to $\mathcal{V}^{h_i}$, we have

$$W_H^{h_i} = \sum_{j=s+1}^{N_i} \beta_j V_j^{h_i} \quad \text{with weights} \quad \beta_j = (V_j^{h_i})^T M^{h_i} W_H^{h_i}. \tag{4.365}$$

Multiply (4.333) from the left by $(V_j^{h_i})^T$ and use (4.353):

$$\beta_j(\lambda_j^{h_i} - \lambda_0^{h_i}) = (V_j^{h_i})^T P^{h_i} W_H^{h_i} = (V_j^{h_i})^T \bar{F}^{h_i} = (\bar{f}, v_j^{h_i}), \qquad j \ge s+1. \tag{4.366}$$

Hence, with the help of the Bessel inequality [2] and (4.329), we have

$$\|W_H^{h_i}\|_h^2 = \sum_{j=s+1}^{N_j} \beta_j^2 \le c_9^{-2} \sum_{j=s+1}^{N_i} (\bar{f}, v_j^{h_i})^2 \le c_9^{-2}|\bar{f}|_0^2. \tag{4.367}$$

Taking into consideration the relation between f and $\bar{f}$, we come to the inequality

$$\|W_H^{h_i}\|_h \le c_9^{-1}|f|_0. \tag{4.368}$$

From this and the equality $E_m = W_H^{h_i} - U_m$, the estimate

$$\|U_m\|_h \le \|E_m\|_h + c_9^{-1}|f|_0 \tag{4.369}$$

follows. Consider the quasi-solutions of the systems

$$P^{h_i}Z^{h_i} = G^{h_i}, \tag{4.370}$$

$$P^{h_{i-1}}Z^{h_{i-1}} = G^{h_{i-1}}, \tag{4.371}$$

where $G^{h_{i-1}}$ has been obtained in $\mathbf{A}_3^{(5)}$. Denote the prolongations in $H^{h_{i-1}}$, H^{h_i} of quasi-solutions $Z_H^{h_{i-1}}$, $Z_H^{h_i}$ by $z_H^{h_{i-1}}$, $z_H^{h_i}$.

Lemma 4.8.1 . *Let conditions* **G**, **J**, (4.236) *be satisfied at levels* $i-1$, i; *then the following estimate holds:*

$$|z_H^{h_i} - z_H^{h_{i-1}}|_0 \leq h_i^{2-n} c_{10}(1 + c_2^2)c_7^{-1}\|G^{h_i}\|_E. \tag{4.372}$$

Proof. From Lemma 4.6.1, we can find a function $g \in H^{h_i}$ such that the equalities (4.370), (4.371) become the systems of the Bubnov-Galerkin method (4.330) on grids Ω_{h_i}, $\Omega_{h_{i-1}}$ for the singular differential problem

$$\mathcal{L}(z,v) - \lambda_0(z,v) = (g,v) \qquad \forall v \in H_A. \tag{4.373}$$

Let z_H be the normal solution of this problem. Then from condition **J**, it follows that

$$|z_H - z_H^{h_i}|_0 \leq c_{10}h_i^2|g|_0, \tag{4.374}$$

$$|z_H - z_H^{h_{i-1}}|_0 \leq c_{10}h_{i-1}^2|g|_0. \tag{4.375}$$

Combining these estimates and (4.241), (4.226), we get the statement of the lemma. □

Continue proving the Theorem 4.22.

At the stage $\mathbf{A}_4^{(5)}$ we find, using $MG_{i-1}^{(5)}$ on grid $\Omega_{h_{i-1}}$ twice, the vector $\tilde{W}^{h_{i-1}}$ instead of quasi-solution $Z_H^{h_{i-1}}$. From inequality (4.339) valid on the grid $\Omega_{h_{i-1}}$ due to induction assumption with multiplier ε_1, it follows that

$$\|Z_H^{h_{i-1}} - \tilde{W}^{h_{i-1}}\|_h \leq \varepsilon_1^2\|Z_H^{h_{i-1}}\|_h + 2c_{14}h_{i-1}^2|g|_0 \tag{4.376}$$

with constant c_{14} from (4.372). From (4.372),

$$\|Z_H^{h_{i-1}}\|_h \leq \|Z_H^{h_i}\|_h + c_7^{-1}c_{10}(1 + c_2^2)h_i^{2-n}\|G^{h_i}\|_E \tag{4.377}$$

follows. We combine the last two relations, (4.241), (4.372) and use the designation $\tilde{W}^{h_i} = I_{i-1}\tilde{W}^{h_{i-1}}$. As a result, we have the estimate

$$\|Z_H^{h_i} - \tilde{W}^{h_i}\|_h \leq \varepsilon_1^2\|Z_H^{h_i}\|_h + c_{15}h_i^{2-n}\|G^{h_i}\|_E \tag{4.378}$$

where c_{15} is defined by (4.342).

Orthogonalize $Z_H^{h_i}$ and $\tilde{W}^{h_i}$ to approximate eigenvectors $\tilde{V}_1^{h_i}, \ldots, \tilde{V}_s^{h_i}$ in the scalar product $(\cdot,\cdot)_h$. We get $\bar{Z}_H^{h_i}$ and $\bar{W}^{h_i}$. Under orthogonalizing, a corresponding norm decreases and so

$$\|\bar{Z}_H^{h_i} - \bar{W}^{h_i}\|_h \leq \|Z_H^{h_i} - \tilde{W}^{h_i}\|_h. \tag{4.379}$$

The vector $Z_H^{h_i}$ is orthogonal to exact eigenvectors $V_1^{h_i}, \ldots, V_s^{h_i}$. Therefore from (4.327), (4.328), the estimate

$$\|Z_H^{h_i} - \bar{Z}_H^{h_i}\|_h = \|(I - P_h)Z_H^{h_i} - (I - \tilde{P}_h)Z_H^{h_i}\|_h = \|(\tilde{P}_h - P_h)Z_H^{h_i}\|_h \leq c_{11}h_i^2\|Z_H^{h_i}\|_h$$

follows. We use also the rougher estimate:

$$\|Z_H^{h_i} - \bar{Z}_H^{h_i}\|_h \leq (\|\tilde{P}_h\|_h + \|P_h\|_h)\|Z_H^{h_i}\|_h = 2\|Z_H^{h_i}\|_h.$$

In total, this gives

$$\|Z_H^{h_i} - \bar{Z}_H^{h_i}\|_h \leq \min\{c_{11}h_i^2, 2\}\|Z_H^{h_i}\|_h.$$

Taking the last estimate and (4.379), (4.378) together, we come to the inequality

$$\|Z_H^{h_i} - \bar{W}^{h_i}\|_h \leq (\varepsilon_1^2 + \min\{c_{11}h_i^2, 2\})\|Z_H^{h_i}\|_h + c_{15}h_i^{2-n}\|G^{h_i}\|_E. \tag{4.380}$$

Introduce vector $Q_H^{h_i}$ as a quasi-solution of the problem

$$P^{h_i}Q_H^{h_i} = \widetilde{F}^{h_i}.$$

Noting that the vector $W_H^{h_i}$ satisfies (4.333), we get, for the difference of these quasi-solutions by analogy with (4.364)–(4.367), the estimates

$$\|Q_H^{h_i} - W_H^{h_i}\|_h^2 \leq c_9^{-2} \sum_{j=s+1}^{N_i} (f^*, v_j^{h_i})^2 \leq c_9^{-2}|f^*|_0^2.$$

From this, on the basis of (4.358), the inequality

$$\|Q_H^{h_i} - W_H^{h_i}\|_h \leq c_9^{-1}c_{11}h_i^2|f|_0 \tag{4.381}$$

follows. The vector U_m satisfies the equality $P^{h_i}U_m = G^{h_i} + \widetilde{F}^{h_i}$ from (4.336). The difference $U_m - Q_H^{h_i} - Z_H^{h_i}$ is therefore linear combination of vectors $V_1^{h_i}, \ldots, V_s^{h_i}$. $Q_H^{h_i}$, $Z_H^{h_i}$ are orthogonal to these in the scalar product $(\cdot,\cdot)_h$. Here we have two corollaries. First,

$$\begin{aligned}\|Z_H^{h_i}\|_h = \|(I - P_h)(U_m &- Q_H^{h_i})\|_h \leq \|U_m - Q_H^{h_i}\|_h \leq \\ &\leq \|E_m\|_h + \|Q_H^{h_i} - W_H^{h_i}\|_h\end{aligned} \tag{4.382}$$

Second, orthogonalization to the vectors $V_1^{h_i}, \ldots, V_s^{h_i}$ transforms the difference $U_m - Q_H^{h_i} - Z_H^{h_i}$ into zero. Note that during this procedure, only vector U_m changes; it becomes $\bar{U}_m$ and so we have

$$\bar{U}_m = Q_H^{h_i} + Z_H^{h_i}. \tag{4.383}$$

But orthogonalizing U_m to approximate eigenvectors $\widetilde{V}_1^{h_i}, \ldots, \widetilde{V}_s^{h_i}$, one gets the vector $\widetilde{U}_m$ obeying, in view of (4.327), (4.328), the estimate

$$\|\bar{U}_m - \widetilde{U}_m\|_h = \|(\widetilde{P}_h - P_h)U_m\|_h \leq c_{11}h_i^2\|U_m\|_h. \tag{4.384}$$

From the method used to obtain the vector $W_1^{h_i}$, it follows that $W_1^{h_i} = \widetilde{U}_m - \bar{W}^{h_i}$. Therefore, the inequality

$$\begin{aligned}\|W_1^{h_i} - W_H^{h_i}\|_h &\leq \|Z_H^{h_i} - \bar{W}^{h_i}\|_h + \|\widetilde{U}_m - \bar{U}_m\|_h + \\ &+ \|\bar{U}_m - Q_H^{h_i} - Z_H^{h_i}\|_h + \|Q_H^{h_i} - W_H^{h_i}\|_h\end{aligned}$$

is valid. To estimate the terms on the right-hand side, we apply first (4.380), (4.384), (4.383), then (4.369), (4.382), (4.381). As a result,

$$\|W_1^{h_i} - W_H^{h_i}\|_h \leq (\varepsilon_1^2 + 2c_{11}h_i^2)\|E_m\|_h + c_{15}h_i^{2-n}\|G^{h_i}\|_E + 5c_{11}c_9^{-1}h_i^2|f|_0.$$

Now use (4.364), (4.363), then (4.360). After grouping the like terms, we have the estimate

$$\|W_1^{h_i} - W_H^{h_i}\|_h \leq q_\varepsilon\|E_0\|_h + c_{11}h_i^2\{q_\varepsilon' + 5c_9^{-1}\}|f|_0 \tag{4.385}$$

where

$$q_\varepsilon \equiv q_1 c_8(\varepsilon_1^2 + 2c_{11}h_i^2)/c_7 + c_{15}h_i^{2-n}q_0/c_7, \tag{4.386}$$

$$q'_\varepsilon \equiv q_2 h_i^n c_8^2(\varepsilon_1^2 + 2c_{11}h_i^2) + c_8 c_{15} h_i^2 q_1. \tag{4.387}$$

On the basis of (4.341), (4.348), (4.345), (4.343), we come to the estimates

$$q_\varepsilon \leq \varepsilon_1/2 + \varepsilon_1(1.68 q_1 c_{11}/c_{12} + c_{15})/2c_{16} \leq \varepsilon_1. \tag{4.388}$$

Applying also (4.349), (4.348), (4.343), (4.341), we have

$$\begin{aligned} q'_\varepsilon &\leq 0.07\, c_7^2/c_{12}q_1^2 + c_8 q_1 h_i^2(c_{15} + 0.56\, c_8 c_{11}/c_{12}q_1) \leq \\ &\leq 0.043\, c_7^2/c_{12} + 0.42\,\varepsilon_1 c_8 q_1 c_7/c_{12} \leq 0.26 c_7^2/c_{12}. \end{aligned} \tag{4.389}$$

Assembling (4.385), (4.388), (4.389), we obtain the inequality

$$\|W_1^{h_i} - W_H^{h_i}\|_h \leq \varepsilon_1 \|E_0\|_h + c_{14}h_i^2|f|_0. \tag{4.390}$$

On the basis of (4.341), the estimate (4.339) follows from (4.390). □

Remark 4.8.1 *Let us investigate the situation for large m. First, from (4.344), it follows that $\varepsilon = O((m+1)^{-2})$. It is usually a good characteristic of convergence. Second, from (4.348), it follows that $h_1 = O((m+1)^{-1})$. For convergence, we can begin our multigrid algorithm only with h_1 small enough, i. e., on the grid Ω_{h_1} with a large number of nodes and a great dimension of algebraic system. This is a case for a large ordinal number of eigenvalue λ_0.*

To get round this difficulty, we may implement another smoothing procedure on the lower levels. Instead of (4.335), at stage $\mathbf{A}_2^{(5)}$, we can use

$$U_{l+1} = U_l - \tau_l P^{h_i}(P^{h_i}U_l - \widetilde{F}^{h_i}), \qquad l = 0, \ldots, m-1, \tag{4.391}$$

with parameters τ_l from formula (4.206) with the constant μ_i^* equal to the upper bound of the squared eigenvalues μ of the problem $P^{h_i}V = \mu V$. With such pre-smoothing procedure, we can discard a restriction analogous to (4.347). It gives us an opportunity to use the multigrid algorithm for moderate values of h_1. In fact, on the basis of section 4.5, we have $\varepsilon = O((m+1)^{-1})$ only. It takes rather more iterations m in (4.391) than in (4.335). Therefore, we recommend (4.391) for moderate values h_1 only where large m does not involve an essential contribution to computational time.

One can not entirely avoid some restrictions of h_1, for example, with a large ordinal number of eigenvalue λ_0. In this situation we need at most a good guess of λ_0 which is reached at h_0, h_1 small enough.

Let us show how to seek the quasi-solution of system (4.330) on the most fine grid, when $i = k$. It results from the following $FMG^{(2)}$-algorithm.

1. Set $\tilde{W}^{h_0} = W_H^{h_0}$ is the exact quasi-solution of system (4.330) for $i = 0$.
2. For $i = 1, \ldots, k$ do
   (a) set $\tilde{W}^{h_i} = I_{i-1}\tilde{W}^{h_{i-1}}$;

(b) repeat the procedure $MG_i^{(5)}$ t times:

$$\tilde{W}^{h_i} := MG_i^{(5)}(\tilde{W}^{h_i}, F^{h_i}).$$

3. Having made k steps, we come to the quasi-solution $\tilde{W}^{h_k}$. Using this vector we construct the prolongation $\tilde{w}^{h_k}$ from H^{h_k} which is result of the $FMG^{(2)}$-algorithm.

Let the assumptions of Theorem 4.22 hold. Take m such that $\varepsilon < 1$ in (4.339) and choose integer t:

$$\varepsilon^t \leq c_2^{-2} \tag{4.392}$$

with constant c_2 from (4.226).

Theorem 4.25 *Let the assumptions of Theorem 4.24 be valid and let (4.392) hold. Then application of the $FMG^{(2)}$-algorithm gives a sequence of vectors $\tilde{W}^{h_i}$ which approximate the quasi-solutions $W_H^{h_i}$ in following sense:*

$$\|\tilde{W}^{h_i} - W_H^{h_i}\|_h \leq \sigma h_i^2 |f|_0 \tag{4.393}$$

with the constants

$$\sigma = \{(1 + c_2^{-2})c_{10} + c_{14}/(1-\varepsilon)\}/(1-\rho),$$

$$\rho = c_2^2 \varepsilon^t < 1$$

independent of i, f. Their prolongations $\tilde{w}^{h_i}$ in H^{h_i} satisfy inequalities

$$|\tilde{w}^{h_i} - u_H|_0 \leq (\sigma + c_{10}) h_i^2 |f|_0, \qquad i = 1, 2, \dots, k, \tag{4.394}$$

with the normal solution u_H of the problem (4.320).

Proof. Apply induction. When $i = 0$, the $FMG^{(2)}$-algorithm gives the exact quasi-solution of (4.330), i. e., $\tilde{W}^{h_0} = W_H^{h_0}$, $\tilde{w}^{h_0} = w_H^{h_0}$. Therefore, the estimate (4.393) holds with right-hand side equal to 0 and (4.394) follows from condition **J**. Now suppose that the estimate (4.393) holds for some level $i - 1 \geq 0$ and derive it for the level i. To this end, we first evaluate the error of initial guess $W_0^{h_i} = I_{i-1}\tilde{W}^{h_{i-1}}$ for procedure $MG_i^{(5)}(W_0^{h_i}, F^{h_i})$. Due to definitions of I_{i-1}, the norm $\|\cdot\|_h$ and estimates (4.334), (4.226), (4.393) for level $i - 1$, we have

$$\|W_0^{h_i} - W_H^{h_i}\|_h = |\tilde{w}^{h_{i-1}} - w_H^{h_i}|_0 \leq$$
$$\leq \|\tilde{W}^{h_{i-1}} - W_H^{h_{i-1}}\|_h + |w_H^{h_{i-1}} - u_H|_0 + |u_H - w_H^{h_i}|_0 \leq \{(1 + c_2^2)c_{10} + c_2^2\sigma\} h_i^2 |f|_0.$$

On the basis of (4.339), (4.392), we come after performance of t applications of procedure $MG^{(5)}$ to the inequality

$$\|\tilde{W}^{h_i} - W_H^{h_i}\|_h \leq \{\varepsilon^t (1 + c_2^2)c_{10} + \sigma\rho + c_{14}/(1+\varepsilon)\} h_i^2 |f|_0 = \sigma h_i^2 |f|_0.$$

It proves (4.393). (4.394) follows from it and (4.334). □

4.9 Solving the spectral problems

In this section, we will describe the algorithm of approximate solution of the spectral finite-dimensional problem obtained from discretization of the spectral problem for elliptic equations by the Bubnov-Galerkin method. The algorithm uses the method of computing an approximate quasi-solution of systems on a sequence of the grids discussed in the preceding section.

We want to solve the spectral problem of determination of several eigenvalues λ and corresponding eigenfunctions $u \in H_A$ satisfying the identity

$$\mathcal{L}(u,v) = \lambda(u,v) \qquad \forall v \in H_A, \tag{4.395}$$

where (u,v) is the inner product in $L_2(\Omega)$; bilinear form $\mathcal{L}$ is bounded, symmetric and positive-definite in H_A. The eigenfucntions will be considered normed:

$$|u|_0 = 1, \qquad |u|_0^2 = (u,u). \tag{4.396}$$

Let the problem (4.395) have an infinite set of the eigenvalues $0 < \lambda_1 \leq \lambda_2 \leq \dots$; $\lambda_n \to \infty$ when $n \to \infty$. Every eigenvalue λ_n corresponds to only eigenfunction v_n; in total, they form a system orthonormed in $L_2(\Omega)$.

Assume that we are looking for the r-th eigenvalue and the corresponding eigenfunction of (4.395); here two situations arise. First, this number is isolated from the other numbers

$$\dots \leq \lambda_{r-1} < \lambda_r < \lambda_{r+1} \leq \dots . \tag{4.397}$$

Then the eigenfunction v_r is uniquely defined (excepting a sign) by conditions (4.396). Second, this number may have algebraic multiplicity greater than 1:

$$\lambda_{l-1} < \lambda_l = \lambda_{l+1} = \dots = \lambda_k < \lambda_{k+1}, \qquad l \leq r \leq k. \tag{4.398}$$

The signs of strict inequality signify that λ_k, λ_l are separated from λ_{k+1}, λ_{l-1}:

$$\lambda_{k+1} - \lambda_k \geq c_{20} > 0, \qquad \lambda_l - \lambda_{l-1} \geq c_{20} > 0. \tag{4.399}$$

Then, the whole subspace $\mathcal{B}$ of eigenfunctions with dimension $k - l + 1$ corresponds to this eigenvalue. In terms of above introduced functions v_i, this subspace $\mathcal{B}$ is a linear span of the functions $v_l, \dots, v_k$:

$$\mathcal{B} \equiv \operatorname{span}\{v_l, \dots, v_k\}. \tag{4.400}$$

In this situation, it is expedient to find not one accidental representative of $\mathcal{B}$ but its basis. The first situation with the simple eigenvalue is a particular case of the second one at $l = r = k$. Therefore we consider only the second situation.

To construct the spectral discrete problem, introduce parameters h_i satisfying inequalities (4.225) and (4.226). For each parameter h_i, we build the grid Ω_{h_i} and on it we form the basis functions $\varphi_y^{h_i}$ $\forall y \in \Omega_{h_i}$ satisfying condition **G**.

In the preceding section, we constructed the algebraic spectral problem

$$L^{h_i} V^{h_i} = \lambda^{h_i} M^{h_i} V^{h_i}. \tag{4.401}$$

Recall that it has N_i eigenvalues $0 < \lambda_1 \leq \ldots \leq \lambda_{N_i}$ which are associated with the orthonormal eigenvectors $V_j^{h_i}$:

$$(V_j^{h_i}, V_k^{h_i})_i = (V_j^{h_i})^T M^{h_i} V_k^{h_i} = \delta_{j,k}, \quad j,k = 1, \ldots, N_i. \tag{4.402}$$

On the basis of subsection 3.2.2, we get the following result.

Condition **K**. *The inequality*

$$|\lambda_j^{h_i} - \lambda_j| \leq c_{18} h_i^2, \qquad j = l-1, \ldots, k+1, \tag{4.403}$$

is satisfied for the eigenvalues of problems (4.395) *and* (4.401).

Note that the algebraic multiplicities of discrete and exact eigenvalues with the same ordinal number may not coincide. It obviously happens at rough grid where discrete and exact eigenvalues may be essentially different. But this is the case when $h \to \infty$ too. For example, $\lambda_l^{h_i}, \ldots, \lambda_k^{h_i}$ may be simple but tend to the same eigenvalue λ_r with multiplicity $k - l + 1$. This is once more an argument for the search of approximation of whole $\mathcal{B}$ and not its accidental representatives.

Therefore, let us introduce prolongations $v_j^{h_i} \in H^{h_i}$ of vectors $V_j^{h_i}$ and the linear span

$$\mathcal{B}^{h_i} = \text{span}\{v_l^{h_i}, \ldots, v_k^{h_i}\}. \tag{4.404}$$

To characterize the convergence of eigensubspaces, we use the definition of the opening introduced in the previous section [87], [2].

Condition **L**. *The opening of above formulated eigensubspaces is bounded:*

$$\Theta(\mathcal{B}, \mathcal{B}^{h_i}) \leq c_{19} h_i^2. \tag{4.405}$$

The constants c_{18}, c_{19} are independent of h_i but depend on number r of the eigenvalue (usually they increase with increasing r).

For simple eigenvalue λ_r, the convergence is usually formulated in other terms [192].

Condition **L′**. *We may take such sign before* v_r *that*

$$|v_r^{h_i} - v_r|_0 \leq c'_{19} h_i^2. \tag{4.406}$$

This condition is equivalent to the previous one for a simple eigenvalue. In particular, condition **L** follows from **L′** with $c_{19} \leq c'_{19}$ and **L′** does from **L** with $c'_{19} \leq 2c_{19}$.

Let us describe the $FMG^{(3)}$-algorithm which gives approximate eigenvalues $\lambda_j^{h_i}$ and eigenfunctions $V_j^{h_i}$ for $j = l, \ldots, k$ at levels $0, 1, 2, \ldots, q$.

1. First we consider the initial level $i = 0$ on the grid Ω_{h_0}. We take Ω_{h_0} to involve a rather small number of points (but not less than k). For the problem (4.401) with $i = 0$, find eigenvalues $\lambda_j^{h_0}$ and eigenvectors $V_j^{h_0}$ $(j = l, \ldots, k)$. This can be done practically exactly, in view of the fact that the problem is of rather small dimension.

2. Then for $i = 1, 2, \ldots, q$, we describe the constructing the approximate solutions $\tilde{\lambda}_r^{h_i}$, $\tilde{V}_r^{h_i}$ $(l \leq r \leq k)$ of problem (4.401). Before we begin computations at the level i, on all lower levels $s = 0, 1, \ldots, i-1$, the approximate eigenvalues $\tilde{\lambda}_r^{h_s}$ and eigenfunctions $\tilde{V}_r^{h_s}$ of (4.401) are considered known $\forall r = l, \ldots, k$. Moreover, on each of the grids Ω_{h_s}, the approximate eigenvectors are orthonormed in the scalar product $(\cdot, \cdot)_i$.

2.1 For $r = l, \dots, k$ the determination of approximate eigenvalue $\tilde{\lambda}_r^{h_i}$ involves 6 stages.

B$_1^{(3)}$. Put $\bar{V}_r^{h_i} = I_{i-1}\widetilde{V}_r^{h_{i-1}}$.

B$_2^{(3)}$. Execute m iterations by the formula

$$U_{j+1} = U_j - \tau_j(L^{h_i} - \tilde{\lambda}_r^{h_{i-1}} M^{h_i})U_j, \qquad j = 0, 1, \dots, m-1, \quad (4.407)$$

with the initial guess $U_0 = \bar{V}_r^{h_i}$ and the parameters τ_j to be chosen by formula (4.215) with the constant λ_i^* equal to the upper bound of eigenvalues μ of the problem $L^{h_i}V = \mu V$. Using vector U_m, we compute the residual

$$G^{h_i} = (L^{h_i} - \tilde{\lambda}_r^{h_{i-1}} M^{h_i})U_m. \quad (4.408)$$

B$_3^{(3)}$. Put $G^{h_{i-1}} = R_i G^{h_i}$.

B$_4^{(3)}$. Take this vector as the right-hand side of the system

$$(L^{h_{i-1}} - \tilde{\lambda}_r^{h_{i-1}} M^{h_{i-1}})W^{h_{i-1}} = G^{h_{i-1}} \quad (4.409)$$

and find its approximate quasi-solution $\tilde{W}^{h_{i-1}}$ by applying the $MG_{i-1}^{(5)}$-algorithm from section 4.8:

$$\tilde{W}^{h_{i-1}} = MG_{i-1}^{(5)}(0, G^{h_{i-1}}).$$

This time, we take iterative parameters in (4.335) by formula (4.215) with λ_i^* defined above by means of L^{h_i} but not P^{h_i}.

B$_5^{(3)}$. The vector

$$\approx{V}_r^{h_i} = U_m - I_{i-1}\tilde{W}^{h_{i-1}} \quad (4.410)$$

is taken as a new approximation to the eigenvector $V_r^{h_i}$ of spectral problem (4.401).

B$_6^{(3)}$. A new approximation for the eigenvalue is calculated by the formula

$$\tilde{\lambda}_r^{h_i} = (\approx{V}_r^{h_i})^T L^{h_i}\, \approx{V}_r^{h_i} / (\approx{V}_r^{h_i})^T M^{h_i}\, \approx{V}_r^{h_i}. \quad (4.411)$$

2.2 Having system $\{\approx{V}_l^{h_i}, \dots, \approx{V}_k^{h_i}\}$, we perform J.P.Gram's – E.Schmidt's orthogonalization [193] in scalar product $(\cdot,\cdot)_i$ and put an orthonormed system $\{\widetilde{V}_l^{h_i}, \dots, \widetilde{V}_k^{h_i}\}$. In the particular case of simple eigenvalue λ_l, when $k = l$, the orthogonalization consists in normalization $\widetilde{V}_l^{h_i} = \approx{V}_l^{h_i} / \| \approx{V}_l^{h_i} \|_h$.

3. Algorithm stops when we find $\tilde{\lambda}_r^{h_q}$, $\widetilde{V}_r^{h_q}$ $(l \le r \le k)$ at the highest level q.

It is convinient to formulate the closeness of obtained vectors in the terms not of individual representatives but for the whole subspaces

$$\mathcal{V}^{h_i} = \operatorname{span}\{V_l^{h_i}, \dots, V_k^{h_i}\}, \qquad \widetilde{\mathcal{V}}^{h_i} = \operatorname{span}\{\widetilde{V}_l^{h_i}, \dots, \widetilde{V}_k^{h_i}\}.$$

Note that the orthogonalization process does not change the linear span of system, therefore

$$\widetilde{\mathcal{V}}^{h_i} = \mathrm{span}\{\overset{\approx}{V}{}_l^{h_i}, \dots, \overset{\approx}{V}{}_k^{h_i}\}.$$

Let us show one useful estimate.

Let G be Gram's matrix of a linearly independent system of vectors $\{\overset{\approx}{V}{}_l^{h_i}, \dots, \overset{\approx}{V}{}_k^{h_i}\}$, i. e., the elements of matrix G are computed by the formula

$$g_{rj} = (\overset{\approx}{V}{}_r^{h_i}, \overset{\approx}{V}{}_j^{h_i})_i, \qquad r, j = l, \dots, k. \tag{4.412}$$

Assume that the system $\{\overset{\approx}{V}{}_l^{h_i}, \dots, \overset{\approx}{V}{}_k^{h_i}\}$ is close to the orthonormed one in the sense that G is close to the unit matrix I, i. e., elements s_{rj} of the matrix $S = I - G$ is uniformly bounded by a small value δ:

$$|s_{rj}| \le \delta \le 1/2(k - l + 1), \qquad r, j = l, \dots, k. \tag{4.413}$$

Lemma 4.9.1 *Let condition* (4.413) *hold. Then the dimension of* $\widetilde{\mathcal{V}}^{h_i}$ *equals* $(k-l+1)$, *and any vector* $V \in \widetilde{\mathcal{V}}^{h_i}$ *has the unique representation*

$$V = \sum_{r=l}^{k} \gamma_r \overset{\approx}{V}{}_r^{h_i} \tag{4.414}$$

with the following weights:

$$\sum_{r=l}^{k} |\gamma_r| \le \sqrt{2(k - l + 1)} \|V\|_h. \tag{4.415}$$

Proof. From (4.413), we have

$$g_{jj} - \sum_{\substack{r=l \\ r \ne j}}^{k} |g_{jr}| \ge 1/2 \qquad \forall j = l, \dots, k.$$

Therefore because of Gershgorin's theorem,

$$\lambda_{\min} = \min_{\lambda \in \mathrm{Sp}(G)} \lambda \ge 1/2. \tag{4.416}$$

Hence, matrix G is non-singular. From this, the dimension of $\widetilde{\mathcal{V}}^{h_i}$ equals $(k-l+1)$ and system $\{\overset{\approx}{V}{}_l^{h_i}, \dots, \overset{\approx}{V}{}_k^{h_i}\}$ is the basis of $\widetilde{\mathcal{V}}^{h_i}$. Therefore any vector $V \in \widetilde{\mathcal{V}}^{h_i}$ has the unique representation (4.414). Let us square both sides of it and denote $\Gamma = (\gamma_l, \dots, \gamma_k)^T$:

$$\|V\|_h^2 = \sum_{r=l}^{k} \sum_{j=l}^{k} \gamma_r \gamma_j (\overset{\approx}{V}{}_r^{h_i}, \overset{\approx}{V}{}_j^{h_i})_i = \Gamma^T G \Gamma.$$

Then we use (4.416) and the evident inequality (e. g., following from the Cauchy-Bunyakovski one):

$$\left(\sum_{r=l}^{k} |\gamma_r|\right)^2 \le (k - l + 1)\Gamma^T \Gamma.$$

We get

$$\Gamma^T G \Gamma \geq 1/2\, \Gamma^T \Gamma \geq (\sum_{r=l}^{k} |\gamma_r|)^2/2(k-l+1)$$

which is equivalent to (4.415). □

To prove the convergence, we need condition **J** for several values of $\lambda_0^{h_i}$. Let us reformulate it in notation of this section.

C o n d i t i o n **J′**. *For any integer $r \in [l,k]$ and any function $f \in L_2(\Omega)$, the problem* (4.319) *with parameter $\lambda_0 = \lambda_r$ has a unique normal solution $u_H \in H_A$. Moreover, on each level $i = 1,\ldots,q$, the corresponding Bubnov-Galerkin system* (4.330) *for each of parameters $\lambda_0^{h_i} = \tilde{\lambda}_r^{h_{i-1}}$ or $\lambda_0^{h_i} = \tilde{\lambda}_r^{h_i}$ has a unique quasi-solution $W_H^{h_i}$ which prolongation $w_H^{h_i} \in H^{h_i}$ obeys the estimate* (4.334), *i. e.,*

$$|u_H - w_H^{h_i}|_0 \leq c_{10} h_i^2 |f|_0. \tag{4.417}$$

On the level $i = 0$, this assumption holds for parameter $\lambda_0^{h_i} = \lambda_r^{h_i}$.

Now we prove the main result on the convergence of the $FMG^{(3)}$-algorithm.

Theorem 4.26 *Let conditions* **G, J′, K, L,** (4.225), (4.226), (4.236), (4.398), (4.399) *be satisfied for the differential problems* (4.395), (4.319) *and the algebraic problems* (4.401), (4.330) *at levels $i = 0,1,\ldots,q$. Let also the inequality*

$$\mu \leq \lambda_i^* \leq c_{13} h_i^{n-2}, \qquad i = 1,\ldots,q, \tag{4.418}$$

hold for all eigenvalues of problem $L^{h_i} V = \mu V$. Then for any $\varepsilon \in (0,1)$ one can find an integer m_0 independent of h_i and such that $\forall m \geq m_0$ under sufficiently small h_0, the accomplishment of $FMG^{(3)}$-algorithm gives a sequence of the approximate eigenvalues $\tilde{\lambda}_j^{h_i}$ and the eigensubspace $\tilde{\mathcal{V}}^{h_i}$ which obey the estimates

$$\lambda_l^{h_i} - \varepsilon^2 h_i^2 \leq \tilde{\lambda}_j^{h_i} \leq \lambda_k^{h_i} + \varepsilon^2 h_i^2, \qquad j = l,\ldots,k; \tag{4.419}$$

$$\Theta_h(\tilde{\mathcal{V}}^{h_i}, \mathcal{V}^{h_i}) \leq \varepsilon h_i^2, \qquad i = 1,2,\ldots,q. \tag{4.420}$$

Proof. Put

$$c'_{12} = c_8(\lambda_k + 1), \tag{4.421}$$
$$c'_{14} = 0.26 c_7^2/c'_{12} + 10/c_{20}, \tag{4.422}$$
$$c'_{15} = 2(c_{10}(c_2^2+1) + c_2^2 c'_{14})/c_7, \tag{4.423}$$
$$c'_{16} = c'_{15} + 1.68 c_8 q_1/c'_{12}, \tag{4.424}$$
$$c''_{15} = 2c_{10}(c_2^2+1) + c_2^2 c'_{14}, \tag{4.425}$$
$$c_{21} = c_2^2 + c_{18}(c_2^2+1), \tag{4.426}$$
$$c_{22} = 2(c_2^2 + c_{19}(c_2^2+1)), \tag{4.427}$$
$$c_{23} = c_7^{-1} c_{22}(c_8 q_1 + c''_{15}/2c'_{16}) + c_{21}(0.28 c_8 + 0.42 c''_{15} q_1/c'_{16})/(\lambda_k+1), \tag{4.428}$$
$$c_{24} = \sqrt{2(k-l+1)}, \tag{4.429}$$
$$c_{25} = (2(\lambda_k+1)/(c_{18}+1) + 2c_{13}/c_7^2)^{1/2}, \tag{4.430}$$
$$\varepsilon_1 = \min\{c_7/2c_8 q_1, \varepsilon/c_{23}c_{24}, \varepsilon/c_{23}c_{25}\} \tag{4.431}$$

with the constants from (4.10), (4.226), (4.236), (4.398), (4.399), (4.334), (4.418), (4.403), (4.405). By analogy with the beginning of Theorem 4.24, let us take an integer m_0 such that

$$\frac{c_{13}}{m+1}\mathrm{tg}\frac{\pi}{4(m+1)} \leq \frac{\varepsilon_1 c_7}{2c'_{16}} \qquad \forall m \geq m_0. \tag{4.432}$$

Then similarly to (4.345), we get

$$h_i^{2-n} q_0 \leq \frac{\varepsilon_1 c_7}{2c'_{16}}. \tag{4.433}$$

Fix some $m \geq m_0$ and take a small h_e such that

$$c'_{12} h_i^n \leq \lambda_i^* \mathrm{tg}^2 \frac{\pi}{4(m+1)} \qquad \forall h_i \leq h_e \tag{4.434}$$

holds similarly to (4.346). From this, the inequalities

$$\begin{aligned} h_i^2 &\leq 0.42\varepsilon_1 c_7 / c'_{16} c'_{12}, \\ q_2 &\leq 0.28 / c'_{12} h_i^n \end{aligned} \tag{4.435}$$

follow similarly to (4.348), (4.349). Below we assume that

$$h_0 \leq \min\{h_e, (c_{20}/2c_{21})^{1/2}, (c_{18}+1)^{-1/2}\}. \tag{4.436}$$

It implies $h_i \leq h_e$ and, hence, (4.434) holds at levels $1, 2, \ldots, q$.

Now use induction on i. As we assumed, at the grid Ω_{h_0} all computations are performed exactly. Therefore $\tilde{\lambda}_j^{h_0} = \lambda_j^{h_0}$, $\tilde{\mathcal{V}}^{h_0} = \mathcal{V}^{h_0}$, and estimates (4.419), (4.420) hold for any $\varepsilon > 0$. Now suppose that the estimates (4.419), (4.420) are proved for $i-1$. Take an integer r such that $l \leq r \leq k$. Consider stage $\mathbf{B}_1^{(3)}$. On the basis of (4.420) for the vector $\tilde{V}_r^{h_{i-1}}$, the representative $V_r^{h_{i-1}} \in \mathcal{V}^{h_{i-1}}$ exists such that

$$\|\tilde{V}_r^{h_{i-1}} - V_r^{h_{i-1}}\|_h = |\tilde{v}_r^{h_{i-1}} - v_r^{h_{i-1}}|_0 \leq \varepsilon h_{i-1}^2 \tag{4.437}$$

where $\tilde{v}_r^{h_{i-1}}$, $v_r^{h_{i-1}}$ are the corresponding prolongations. Norm of $v_r^{h_{i-1}}$ is not equal to 1 in general. Normalizing it, we obtain the prolongation $\hat{v}_r^{h_{i-1}} = v_r^{h_{i-1}}/|v_r^{h_{i-1}}|_0$ with the estimate

$$\begin{aligned} |\tilde{v}_r^{h_{i-1}} - \hat{v}_r^{h_{i-1}}|_0 &\leq |\tilde{v}_r^{h_{i-1}} - v_r^{h_{i-1}}|_0 + |v_r^{h_{i-1}} - \hat{v}_r^{h_{i-1}}|_0 = \\ &= |\tilde{v}_r^{h_{i-1}} - v_r^{h_{i-1}}|_0 + |\,|v_r^{h_{i-1}}|_0 - 1| \leq 2|v_r^{h_{i-1}} - \tilde{v}_r^{h_{i-1}}|_0 \leq 2\varepsilon h_{i-1}^2. \end{aligned} \tag{4.438}$$

Analogously, for $v_r^{h_{i-1}}$ on the basis of (4.405), the representative $w_r \in \mathcal{B}$ exists with unit norm:

$$|\hat{v}_r^{h_{i-1}} - w_r|_0 \leq 2c_{19} h_{i-1}^2. \tag{4.439}$$

Finally, for w_r on the basis of (4.405) again, the vector $W_r^{h_i} \in \mathcal{V}^{h_i}$ exists with unit norm and the prolongation $w_r^{h_i}$ such that

$$|w_r - w_r^{h_i}|_0 \leq 2c_{19} h_i^2. \tag{4.440}$$

Summation of estimates (4.438)–(4.440) with employment of (4.226) gives us the inequality

$$\|\bar{V}_r^{h_i} - W_r^{h_i}\|_h = |\tilde{v}_r^{h_{i-1}} - w_r^{h_i}|_0 \leq$$
$$\leq |\hat{v}_r^{h_{i-1}} - \hat{v}_r^{h_{i-1}}|_0 + |\hat{v}_r^{h_{i-1}} - w_r|_0 + |w_r - w_r^{h_i}|_0 \leq c_{22}h_i^2. \tag{4.441}$$

Analogously, on the basis of (4.419), (4.403), (4.226), we acquire the inequality

$$|\tilde{\lambda}_r^{h_{i-1}} - \lambda_r^{h_i}| \leq |\tilde{\lambda}_r^{h_{i-1}} - \lambda_r^{h_{i-1}}| + |\lambda_r^{h_{i-1}} - \lambda_r| + |\lambda_r - \lambda_r^{h_i}| \leq c_{21}h_i^2. \tag{4.442}$$

Put $S^{h_i} = L^{h_i} - \tilde{\lambda}_r^{h_{i-1}} M^{h_i}$. The relation

$$S^{h_i} W_r^{h_i} = Y, \quad \text{where} \quad Y = (\lambda_r^{h_i} - \tilde{\lambda}_r^{h_{i-1}}) M^{h_i} W_r^{h_i},$$

holds for vector $W_r^{h_i}$. Use the explicit form $(\varphi_y^{h_i}, \varphi_z^{h_i})$, $y, z \in \Omega_{h_i}$, of the elements of matrix M^{h_i} and denote by $\tilde{\tilde{w}}_r^{h_i}$ the prolongation of the vector $M^{h_i} W_r^{h_i}$ with components $(\varphi_y^{h_i}, w_r^{h_i})$, $y \in \Omega_{h_i}$, in H^{h_i}:

$$\|M^{h_i} W_r^{h_i}\|_E^2 = \sum_{y \in \Omega_{h_i}} (\varphi_y^{h_i}, w_r^{h_i})^2 h_i^n = (\sum_{y \in \Omega_{h_i}} (\varphi_y^{h_i}, w_r^{h_i}) \varphi_y^{h_i}, w_r^{h_i}) h_i^n = (\tilde{\tilde{w}}_r^{h_i}, w_r^{h_i}) h_i^n.$$

Then use the Cauchy-Bunyakovski inequality, the equality $|w_r^{h_i}|_0 = 1$, the definition of the norm $\|\cdot\|_h$, and (4.236):

$$\|M^{h_i} W_r^{h_i}\|_E^2 \leq h_i^n |\tilde{\tilde{w}}_r^{h_i}|_0 |w_r^{h_i}|_0 = h_i^n \|M^{h_i} W_r^{h_i}\|_h \leq c_8 h_i^n \|M^{h_i} W_r^{h_i}\|_E.$$

Dividing both sides by $\|M^{h_i} W_r^{h_i}\|_E$, we have

$$\|M^{h_i} W_r^{h_i}\|_E \leq c_8 h_i^n.$$

With the help of this inequality and (4.442), we get

$$\|Y\|_E \leq c_{21} c_8 h_i^{n+2}. \tag{4.443}$$

Now introduce the designation $E_j = W_r^{h_i} - U_j$. Specifically,

$$E_0 = W_r^{h_i} - \bar{V}_r^{h_i}. \tag{4.444}$$

Then from (4.407), the equality

$$E_{j+1} = E_j - \tau_j (S^{h_i} E_j - Y), \qquad j = 0, 1, \ldots, m-1, \tag{4.445}$$

follows. Using (4.408), (4.445), and induction, we have

$$G^{h_i} = Y - S^{h_i} E_m = (\prod_{j=0}^{m-1} (I - \tau_j S^{h_i}))(Y - S^{h_i} E_0) \tag{4.446}$$

where I is the $N_i \times N_i$ identity matrix. Consider the eigenvalues σ_j of symmetric matrix S^{h_i} and the corresponding eigenvectors Ψ_j (i. e., $S^{h_i} \Psi_j = \sigma_j \Psi_j$) orthonormed in the Euclidean scalar product. Let us show that

$$\sigma_j \in [-\lambda_i^* \text{tg}^2 \pi / 4(m+1),\ \lambda_i^*]. \tag{4.447}$$

First, matrices $L^{h_{i-1}}$, $M^{h_{i-1}}$ are positive-definite, therefore $\tilde{\lambda}_r^{h_{i-1}}$ computed by (4.411) is positive for $i \geq 2$. When $i = 1$, the equality (4.411) holds with exact vectors $\tilde{\tilde{V}}_r^{h_0} = V_r^{h_0}$ and gives the same:

$$\tilde{\lambda}_r^{h_{i-1}} > 0. \tag{4.448}$$

Second, due to the previous facts and the left-hand inequality in (4.417), we get

$$V^T S^{h_i} V \leq V^T L^{h_i} V \leq \lambda_i^* V^T V \qquad \forall V \in \mathbf{R}^{N_i}.$$

Let us take here $V = \Psi_j$ and come to the inequality

$$\sigma_j \leq \lambda_i^* \qquad \forall j = 1, \ldots, N_i.$$

Third, the inequality

$$h_i^2 \leq (1 + c_{18})^{-1} \tag{4.449}$$

follows from (4.436). Together with (4.419), (4.403), it gives

$$\tilde{\lambda}_r^{h_{i-1}} \leq \lambda_k + \varepsilon h_{i-1}^2 + c_{18} h_{i-1}^2 \leq \lambda_k + 1. \tag{4.450}$$

Fourth, the right-hand inequality in (4.236) is equivalent to the following:

$$V^T M^{h_i} V \leq c_8 h_i^n V^T V \qquad \forall V \in \mathbf{R}^{N_i}.$$

Therefore we have

$$V^T S^{h_i} V \geq -c_8(\lambda_k + 1) h_i^n V^T V.$$

Let us take here $V = \Psi_j$ and use (4.421), (4.434):

$$\sigma_j \geq -c_{12}' h_i^n \geq -\lambda_i^* \mathrm{tg}^2 \pi / 4(m+1). \tag{4.451}$$

Expand vectors E_0, Y, G^{h_i}, E_m in terms of Ψ_j. Using these expansions, from (4.446) and the definition of polynomials P_{m+1}, Q_m (estimates (4.7), (4.10) hold due to (4.447)), we get the inequality

$$\|G^{h_i}\|_E \leq \frac{q_0}{c_7} \|E_0\|_h + q_1 \|Y\|_E. \tag{4.452}$$

Moreover, using (4.445) and the definition of polynomials Q_m, S_{m-1}, by induction and (4.236) (estimate (4.15) holds due to (4.447)), we have the inequality

$$\|E_m\|_h \leq q_1 \frac{c_8}{c_7} \|E_0\|_h + q_2 c_8 \|Y\|_E. \tag{4.453}$$

Let us consider the normal solution $w_H \in H_A$ of the problem

$$\mathcal{L}(w, \varphi) - \lambda_r(w, \varphi) = (g, \varphi) \qquad \forall \varphi \in H_A \tag{4.454}$$

with the right-hand side $g \in H^{h_i}$. We define its values at nodes of Ω_{h_i} from the system of linear algebraic equations

$$\sum_{x \in \Omega_{h_i}} (\varphi_x^{h_i}, \varphi_y^{h_i}) g(x) = G_y^{h_i}, \qquad y \in \Omega_{h_i}.$$

Its unique solvability and the estimate

$$|g|_0 \leq \frac{h_i^{-n}}{c_7}\|G^{h_i}\|_E \tag{4.455}$$

follow from Lemma 4.6.1. The problem (4.454) on grid Ω_{h_i} is associated with the Bubnov-Galerkin system with an approximate value of λ_r

$$(L^{h_i} - \tilde{\lambda}_r^{h_{i-1}} M^{h_i})W^{h_i} = G^{h_i}. \tag{4.456}$$

For the prolongation $w_H^{h_i}$ from H^{h_i} of the quasi-solution $W_H^{h_i}$ of this system, condition $\mathbf{J}'$ at level i with approximate value $\lambda_0^{h_i} = \tilde{\lambda}_r^{h_{i-1}}$ tells the estimate

$$|w_H - w_H^{h_i}|_0 \leq c_{10} h_i^2 |g|_0. \tag{4.457}$$

Consider system (4.456) and the Bubnov-Galerkin system on the grid $\Omega_{h_{i-1}}$:

$$(L^{h_{i-1}} - \tilde{\lambda}_r^{h_{i-1}} M^{h_{i-1}})W^{h_{i-1}} = G^{h_{i-1}}, \tag{4.458}$$

where $G_y^{h_{i-1}} = (g, \varphi_y^{h_{i-1}})\ \forall y \in \Omega_{h_{i-1}}$. This system coincides with (4.409) due to restriction $\mathbf{B}_3^{(3)}$. Denote the prolongation from $H^{h_{i-1}}$ of the quasi-solution $W_H^{h_{i-1}}$ of this system by $w_H^{h_{i-1}}$. Then, from (4.457), (4.226), condition $\mathbf{J}'$ at level $i-1$ with approximate value $\lambda_0^{h_{i-1}} = \tilde{\lambda}_r^{h_{i-1}}$, we get the inequality

$$|w_H^{h_i} - w_H^{h_{i-1}}|_0 \leq c_{10}(1 + c_2^2) h_i^2 |g|_0. \tag{4.459}$$

Now we need an estimate analogous to (4.339) of Theorem 4.24.

Lemma 4.9.2 *Let all assumptions of Theorem 4.26 be satisfied and let (4.419), (4.420) hold for levels $1, 2, \ldots, i-1$. Then for $m \geq m_0$ and $h_1 \leq h_e$ chosen on the ground of (4.432), (4.434), the accomplishment of $MG^{(5)}$-algorithm reduces the error of the approximate quasi-solution in the following way:*

$$\|W_1^{h_{i-1}} - W_H^{h_{i-1}}\|_h \leq \varepsilon_1 \|W_0^{h_{i-1}} - W_H^{h_{i-1}}\|_h + c'_{14} h_{i-1}^2 |g|_0 \tag{4.460}$$

where $W_1^{h_{i-1}} = MG_{i-1}^{(5)}(W_0^{h_{i-1}}, G^{h_{i-1}})$.

Proof. Let us verify the assumptions of Theorem 4.24 for levels $1, 2, \ldots, i-1$. Excepting (4.328), (4.329), (4.338), they are listed in conditions of Theorem 4.26. Now we show that (4.329) holds. Indeed, from (4.436), it follows that

$$h_{i-1}^2 \leq c_{20}/2c_{21} \tag{4.461}$$

with the constant c_{21} from (4.426). Then on the basis of (4.399), (4.403), (4.419), we have

$$|\lambda_{k+1}^{h_{i-1}} - \tilde{\lambda}_r^{h_{i-2}}| \geq |\lambda_{k+1}^{h_{i-1}} - \tilde{\lambda}_k^{h_{i-2}}| \geq |\lambda_{k+1} - \lambda_k| - |\lambda_{k+1}^{h_{i-1}} - \lambda_{k+1}| -$$
$$-|\lambda_k - \lambda_k^{h_{i-2}}| - |\lambda_k^{h_{i-2}} - \tilde{\lambda}_k^{h_{i-2}}| \geq c_{20} - c_{21} h_{i-1}^2 \geq c_{20}/2.$$

Analogously,

$$|\lambda_{l-1}^{h_{i-1}} - \tilde{\lambda}_r^{h_{i-2}}| \geq c_{20}/2.$$

Therefore, supposing that $c_9 = c_{20}/2$, we get (4.329).

Since $\varepsilon \leq 1$, the inequality

$$\Theta_h(\tilde{\mathcal{V}}^{h_{i-1}}, \mathcal{V}^{h_{i-1}}) \leq \varepsilon h_{i-1}^2 \leq h_{i-1}^2 \tag{4.462}$$

follows from (4.420). Therefore, assumption (4.328) holds with the constant $c_{11} = 1$.

It remains only to prove inequalities (4.338). These proof is similar in detail with justification of (4.447), and we do not reproduce it.

So, all assumptions of Theorem 4.24 are valid. Let us show that m and h_1 chosen in the proof of Theorem 4.26 satisfy conditions guaranteeing (4.339). We see from (4.341) that one can put $\varepsilon_1 = \varepsilon$ in the proof of Theorem 4.24 if ε is small enough: $\varepsilon \leq c_7/2c_8q_1$. We have namely such situation due to (4.431). Then constants c'_{12}, c'_{14}–c'_{16} coincide with constants c_{12}, c_{14}–c_{16} to within the substitution of 1, $c_{20}/2$ for c_{11}, c_9. Therefore, the choice of m and h_e is the same in both theorems. Hence, a validity of condition (4.347) follows from (4.436). So, we get (4.339) which has the form (4.460) in the notation of Theorem 4.26. □

Let us continue to prove Theorem 4.26. At the stage $\mathbf{B}_4^{(3)}$ in accord with (4.460), we have

$$\|\tilde{W}^{h_{i-1}} - W_H^{h_{i-1}}\|_h \leq \varepsilon_1 \|W_H^{h_{i-1}}\|_h + c'_{14} h_{i-1}^2 |g|_0. \tag{4.463}$$

For $W_H^{h_{i-1}}$ from (4.459), the estimate

$$\|W_H^{h_{i-1}}\|_h \leq \|W_H^{h_i}\|_h + c_{10}(1 + c_2^2) h_i^2 |g|_0$$

follows. Combining the last two inequalities with (4.459) and denoting $\tilde{W}^{h_i} = I_{i-1}\tilde{W}^{h_{i-1}}$ at stage $\mathbf{B}_5^{(3)}$, we get

$$\|\tilde{W}^{h_i} - W_H^{h_i}\|_h \leq \varepsilon_1 \|W_H^{h_i}\|_h + c''_{15} h_i^2 |g|_0 \tag{4.464}$$

with the constant c''_{15} from (4.425). By virtue of (4.408), (4.456), and the definition of quasi-solution $W_H^{h_i}$, we come to the equality

$$W_H^{h_i} = (I - P_h) U_m \tag{4.465}$$

with orthogonal projector P_h from (4.327). In view of the fact that $(I - P_h) W_r^{h_i} = 0$, (4.465) tells the inequality

$$\|W_H^{h_i}\|_h = \|(I - P_h)(U_m - W_r^{h_i})\|_h \leq \|U_m - W_r^{h_i}\|_h = \|E_m\|_h. \tag{4.466}$$

From (4.453), (4.443), (4.441), and (4.349), its right-hand side is estimated as follows:

$$\begin{aligned} \|E_m\|_h \leq q_1 c_8 c_7^{-1} c_{22} h_i^2 \; &+ \; q_2 c_8^2 c_{21} h_i^{n+2} \leq \alpha \equiv \\ &\equiv \; (q_1 c_8 c_{22}/c_7 + 0.28 c_8^2 c_{21}/c'_{12}) h_i^2. \end{aligned} \tag{4.467}$$

The definition of vector $\overset{\approx}{V}{}_r^{h_i} = U_m - \tilde{W}^{h_i}$ at stage $\mathbf{B}_5^{(3)}$ and (4.464), (4.465) tell the inequality

$$\|\overset{\approx}{V}{}_r^{h_i} - P_h U_m\|_h = \|W_H^{h_i} - \tilde{W}^{h_i}\|_h \leq \varepsilon_1 \|W_H^{h_i}\|_h + c''_{15} h_i^2 |g|_0. \tag{4.468}$$

Apply the estimates (4.466), (4.453), (4.455), (4.452) to the terms in the right-hand side. As a result, we have

$$\|\tilde{W}^{h_i} - W_H^{h_i}\|_h \leq \beta \equiv \varepsilon_1 c_7^{-1} a_\varepsilon \|E_0\|_h + \varepsilon_1 b_\varepsilon \|Y\|_E \tag{4.469}$$

where

$$a_\varepsilon = q_1 c_8 + c_{15}'' h_i^{2-n} q_0/\varepsilon_1 c_7, \qquad b_\varepsilon = q_2 c_8 + c_{15}'' h_i^{2-n} q_1/\varepsilon_1 c_7.$$

From estimates (4.345), (4.348), (4.349), (4.441), (4.443), and relation (4.444), we find

$$a_\varepsilon \leq q_1 c_8 + c_{15}''/2c_{16}', \qquad b_\varepsilon \leq q_2 c_8 + c_{15}'' h_i^{2-n} c_7^{-1} q_1, \qquad \beta \leq \varepsilon_1 h_i^2 c_{23} \tag{4.470}$$

with the constant c_{23} from (4.428). Now take $Z_r = P_h \, \tilde{\tilde{V}}_r^{h_i}$ and $S_r = (I - P_h) \, \tilde{\tilde{V}}_r^{h_i}$. Hence, with the help of (4.468), (4.469) and properties of projector P_h, we come to inequalities

$$\|S_r\|_h = \|(I - P_h)(\tilde{\tilde{V}}_r^{h_i} - P_h U_m)\|_h \leq \| \, \tilde{\tilde{V}}_r^{h_i} - P_h U_m\|_h \leq \beta. \tag{4.471}$$

The vectors S_r and Z_r are orthogonal in both scalar products: $S_r^T L^{h_i} Z_r = 0$ and $S_r^T M^{h_i} Z_r = 0$. Therefore, (4.411) can be calculated by the formula

$$\tilde{\lambda}_r^{h_i} = (Z_r^T L^{h_i} Z_r + S_r^T L^{h_i} S_r)/(Z_r^T M^{h_i} Z_r + S_r^T M^{h_i} S_r).$$

Consider the quantity

$$\tilde{\tilde{\lambda}}_r^{h_i} = Z_r^T L^{h_i} Z_r / Z_r^T M^{h_i} Z_r.$$

Take the difference $\tilde{\tilde{\lambda}}_r^{h_i} - \tilde{\lambda}_r^{h_i}$ and allow for positive definiteness of matrices L^{h_i}, M^{h_i}. We get

$$|\tilde{\lambda}_r^{h_i} - \tilde{\tilde{\lambda}}_r^{h_i}| \leq (S_r^T L^{h_i} S_r + \tilde{\tilde{\lambda}}_r^{h_i} \|S_r\|_h^2)/\| \, \tilde{\tilde{V}}_r^{h_i}\|_h^2. \tag{4.472}$$

To estimate the denominator, prove that the norm of vector $\tilde{\tilde{V}}_r^{h_i}$ is close to unit. Use the following representation of the vector $\tilde{\tilde{V}}_r^{h_i}$:

$$\tilde{\tilde{V}}_r^{h_i} = W_r^{h_i} - \Xi_r \quad \text{where} \quad \Xi_r = E_m + (\tilde{W}^{h_i} - W_H^{h_i}) + W_H^{h_i}. \tag{4.473}$$

Subtract $W_r^{h_i}$ from both sides of this equality and take the norm. Using estimates (4.467), (4.469), (4.466), we get

$$|\|W_r^{h_i}\|_h - \| \, \tilde{\tilde{V}}_r^{h_i}\|_h| \leq \|\Xi_r\|_h \leq \beta + 2\alpha. \tag{4.474}$$

We see from estimates (4.467), (4.470) that α and β can be such small as desired only due to h_i. Make it so sufficiently small that the right-hand side in (4.474) does not exceed 1/2. Since $\|W_r^{h_i}\|_h = 1$, by virtue of (4.474) we have

$$\| \, \tilde{\tilde{V}}_r^{h_i}\|_h \geq 1/2. \tag{4.475}$$

The first summand in the numerator of (4.472) is estimated by means of (4.418), (4.471), (4.236):

$$S_r^T L^{h_i} S_r \leq \lambda_i^* h_i^{-n} \|S_r\|_E^2 \leq c_{13} h_i^{-2} c_7^{-2} \beta^2. \tag{4.476}$$

In the addend of numerator in (4.472), we have

$$\approx{\lambda}_r^{h_i} \in [\lambda_l^{h_i}, \lambda_k^{h_i}]. \tag{4.477}$$

So, from condition **K** and (4.449), we get

$$\approx{\lambda}_r^{h_i} \leq \lambda_k + c_{18}h_i^2 \leq \lambda_k + 1. \tag{4.478}$$

Then (4.472), (4.476), (4.478), (4.471), (4.475) lead to the inequality

$$|\tilde{\lambda}_r^{h_i} - \approx{\lambda}_r^{h_i}| \leq 2\beta^2(1 + \lambda_k + c_{13}h_i^{-2}c_7^{-2}).$$

Now use (4.470), (4.449), (4.430), (4.431):

$$|\tilde{\lambda}_r^{h_i} - \approx{\lambda}_r^{h_i}| \leq 2\varepsilon_1^2 h_i^2 c_{23}^2((1 + \lambda_k)/(1 + c_{18}) + c_{13}c_7^{-2}) = \varepsilon_1^2 c_{23}^2 c_{25}^2 h_i^2 \leq \varepsilon^2 h_i^2. \tag{4.479}$$

Due to (4.477), the required estimate (4.419) follows from here.

Now assume that we already find $\{\approx{V}_l^{h_i}, \dots , \approx{V}_k^{h_i}\}$ and let us proceed to the proof of estimate (4.420). Consider Gram's matrix G of the system of vectors $\approx{V}_j^{h_i}$ $(j = l, \dots , k)$ in the scalar product $(\cdot, \cdot)_i$ from (4.324). Let us first evaluate an arbitrary off-diagonal element. Let $r \neq j$. Transform $(\approx{V}_r^{h_i}, \approx{V}_j^{h_i})_i$, representing both cofactors in the form of (4.473). From (4.474), the Cauchy-Bunyakovski inequakity, and unit norm of vectors $W_r^{h_i}$, $W_j^{h_i}$, we have

$$|(\approx{V}_r^{h_i}, \approx{V}_j^{h_i})_i| \leq |(W_r^{h_i}, W_j^{h_i})_i| + (\beta + 2\alpha)(2 + \beta + 2\alpha). \tag{4.480}$$

As stated, α and β can be made as small as we please when $h_i \to 0$. Let us consider the first term on the right-hand side of (4.480) at length. Represent its cofactors as follows: $W_r^{h_i} = \bar{V}_r^{h_i} + W_r^{h_i} - \bar{V}_r^{h_i}$. The vectors $\bar{V}_r^{h_i}$ and $\bar{V}_j^{h_i}$ are orthogonal at $r \neq j$ since

$$(\bar{V}_r^{h_i}, \bar{V}_j^{h_i})_i = (\tilde{v}_r^{h_i}, \tilde{v}_j^{h_i}) = (\tilde{V}_r^{h_{i-1}}, \tilde{V}_j^{h_{i-1}})_{i-1} = 0.$$

Therefore, from (4.441), the Cauchy-Bunyakovski inequality, and unit norm of vectors $\bar{V}_r^{h_i}$, $\bar{V}_j^{h_i}$, we get

$$|(W_r^{h_i}, W_j^{h_i})_i| \leq c_{22}h_i^2(2 + c_{22}h_i^2). \tag{4.481}$$

From (4.480) and (4.481), we see that each off-diagonal element is such small as desired when $h_i \to 0$. Let us then consider an arbitrary diagonal element of matrix G. Since $\|W_r^{h_i}\|_h = 1$, on the basis of (4.474),

$$|1 - \| \approx{V}_r^{h_i}\|_h^2| \leq (\beta + 2\alpha)(2 + \beta + 2\alpha). \tag{4.482}$$

So, each diagonal element is such close to 1 as desired. Thus, the matrix G tends to the identity matrix when $h_i \to 0$. Take a sufficiently small h_G such that (4.413) holds for any

$$h_i \leq h_G. \tag{4.483}$$

Due to Lemma 4.9.1, the system $\{\tilde{\tilde{V}}_j^{h_i}\}$, $j = l, \ldots, k$, is a basis of $\tilde{\mathcal{V}}^{h_i}$.

Now let us take an arbitrary vector $\tilde{V} \in \tilde{\mathcal{V}}^{h_i}$ with unit norm. Decompose it into the basis $\tilde{\tilde{V}}_j^{h_i}$ and use the representation $\tilde{\tilde{V}}_r^{h_i} = Z_r + S_r$ defined before (4.471):

$$\tilde{V} = \sum_{r=l}^{k} \gamma_r \tilde{\tilde{V}}_r^{h_i} = \tilde{Z} + \tilde{S} \quad \text{where} \quad \tilde{Z} = \sum_{r=l}^{k} \gamma_r Z_r, \quad \tilde{S} = \sum_{r=l}^{k} \gamma_r S_r. \tag{4.484}$$

The vector $\tilde{Z}$ belongs to $\mathcal{V}^{h_i}$, therefore

$$\text{dis}_h(\tilde{V}, \mathcal{V}^{h_i}) \leq \|\tilde{V} - \tilde{Z}\|_h = \|\tilde{S}\|_h.$$

From (4.415), (4.471), we get

$$\|\tilde{S}\|_h \leq \sum_{r=l}^{k} \gamma_r \|S_r\|_h \leq \beta\sqrt{2(k-l+1)}. \tag{4.485}$$

Hence, due to arbitrariness of $\tilde{V}$,

$$\sup_{\tilde{V} \in \tilde{\mathcal{V}}^{h_i}, \|\tilde{V}\|_h = 1} \text{dis}_h(\tilde{V}, \mathcal{V}^{h_i}) \leq \beta\sqrt{2(k-l+1)}. \tag{4.486}$$

Instead of proving the symmetric estimate for an arbitrary vector $V \in \mathcal{V}^{h_i}$, we use the result from [48, p. 215, Lemma 3]. In our notation, it asserts that when dimensions of $\mathcal{V}^{h_i}$ and $\tilde{\mathcal{V}}^{h_i}$ are finite and coincide, both suprema in braces at (4.326) coincide too. Therefore due to (4.486), we have

$$\Theta_h(\mathcal{V}^{h_i}, \tilde{\mathcal{V}}^{h_i}) \leq \beta\sqrt{2(k-l+1)}. \tag{4.487}$$

Now use (4.470), (4.429), (4.431):

$$\Theta_h(\mathcal{V}^{h_i}, \tilde{\mathcal{V}}^{h_i}) \leq \varepsilon_1 c_{23} c_{24} h_i^2 \leq \varepsilon h_i^2.$$

This completes the proof of Theorem 4.26. □

In the proof, we repeatedly restrict h_0, h_1. At first sight, it might lead to such bounds that we have to solve the algebraic spectral problems on grids Ω_{h_0}, Ω_{h_1} using too many nodes. Indeed, all introduced restraints on mesh width except one are satisfied automatically or they are not a factor. We will see this from examples of Chapter 5. Only one constraint does appear to be a factor. At level 0, we have to take a grid Ω_{h_0} with number of nodes $N_0 \geq k$ to get k-th approximate eigenvalue $\lambda_k^{h_0}$. At level 1, eigenvalues of matrices $S^{h_i} = L^{h_i} - \lambda_r^{h_{i-1}} M^{h_i}$, $P^{h_i} = L^{h_i} - \tilde{\lambda}_r^{h_i} M^{h_i}$ must belong to the interval $[-\lambda_i^* \text{tg}^2 \pi/4(m+1), \lambda_i^*]$. This was already mentioned in Remark 4.8.1. Namely, these constraints lead in practice to too fine initial grids Ω_{h_0}, Ω_{h_1} for higher eigenvalues. So to define these on rough grids, one should use another smoothing procedure (4.391) with a better interval of convergence but a worse rate of it.

4.10 The algorithm in the symmetrized case

In this section, we consider a general case where, first, finite elements can be both Lagrangian and Hermitean; second, scaling the system is used to improve conditionality; and third, the algorithm is applied to equations of order $2s$ with $s \geq 1$. In contrast to section 4.6 we study only the case of symmetric positive-definite bilinear form $\mathcal{L}$. The asymmetric or sign-indefinite cases are analized analogously as projection of notation and results of this section onto the corresponding subsection of 4.6.

Thus let us study the problem: find a solution $u \in H_A \subset W_2^s(\Omega)$ satisfying the equality

$$\mathcal{L}(u, v) = f(v) \qquad \forall v \in H_A, \tag{4.488}$$

where bilinear form $\mathcal{L}$ is symmetric, bounded, positive-definite on $H_A \times H_A$; and linear functional f is bounded on H_A.

Assume that we have grids Ω_{h_i} for which conditions (4.225)–(4.226) hold. On each grid Ω_{h_i}, introduce a set of basis functions $\varphi_j^{h_i}(x)$, $j = 1, \ldots, N_i$. Denote its linear span by H^{h_i}, as before. This time, however, several basis functions can correspond to one grid node, and so N_i does not equal the number of the nodes of grid Ω_{h_i}. An approximate solution is found in the form

$$w^{h_i}(x) = \sum_{j=1}^{N_i} \alpha_j^{h_i} \varphi_j^{h_i}(x) \tag{4.489}$$

where the weights $\alpha_j^{h_i}$ are determined from the Bubnov-Galerkin system

$$\sum_{j=1}^{N_i} \alpha_j^{h_i} \mathcal{L}(\varphi_j^{h_i}, \varphi_l^{h_i}) = f(\varphi_l^{h_i}), \qquad l = 1, \ldots, N_i. \tag{4.490}$$

Let the following condition similar to **G** be satisfied for the basis functions.

C o n d i t i o n **G′**. *For each $i = 0, \ldots, k-1$, basis function $\varphi_j^{h_i}$ is a linear conbination of a finite number of the basis functions on a finer grid:*

$$\varphi_j^{h_i}(x) = \sum_{l=1}^{N_{i+1}} \beta_l^j \varphi_l^{h_{i+1}}(x), \qquad j = 1, \ldots, N_i. \tag{4.491}$$

From (4.491) it follows that $H^{h_i} \subset H^{h_{i+1}}$. For the convergence of w^h to u, some requirement should hold.

4.10.1 Convergence in L_2-norm

First, we study the convergence in the norm $|\cdot|_0$.

C o n d i t i o n **H′**. *For any functional $f(v) = (g, v)$ with a function $g \in L_2(\Omega)$, problem* (4.488) *has a unique solution $u \in W_2^{2s}(\Omega)$; and the solution of the Bubnov-Galerkin method* (4.489), (4.490) *satisfies the estimate*

$$|u - w^{h_i}|_0 \leq c_5 h_i^{2s} |g|_0.$$

As we showed already in section 4.6, the parameters h_i may be not only the maximal diameter of a cell in corresponding triangulation (as in the h-version) but they also may be some total indicators of both the size of triangulation and the power of finite element (as in the hp-version).

Let each vector W^{h_i} with components $W_j^{h_i}$ ($j = 1, \dots, N_i$) correspond to prolongation from H^{h_i}, i. e., to the function

$$w^{h_i}(x) = \sum_{j=1}^{N_i} W_j^{h_i} \varphi_j^{h_i}(x). \tag{4.492}$$

Introduce, using it, the vector norm

$$\|W^{h_i}\|_h = |w^{h_i}|_0. \tag{4.493}$$

Recast the system (4.490)

$$L^{h_i} V^{h_i} = F^{h_i} \tag{4.494}$$

where L^{h_i} is a symmetric square matrix with the elements $L_{jl}^{h_i}$ ($j, l = 1, \dots, N_i$); V^{h_i} and F^{h_i} are the vectors of unknowns and right-hand sides of dimension N_i.

For each $i \geq 1$, assume that there exists a diagonal matrix $\mathcal{D}^{h_i} = \operatorname{diag}(d_1^{h_i}, \dots, d_{N_i}^{h_i})$ with positive $d_j^{h_i}$ and the following properties:

1. norm (4.493) is equivalent to the Euclidean norm

$$\|W^{h_i}\|_{\mathcal{D}} = \Big(\sum_{j=1}^{N_i} (W_j^{h_i})^2 (d_j^{h_i})^{-1} h_i^n\Big)^{1/2} = \|(\mathcal{D}^{h_i})^{-1/2} W^{h_i}\|_E, \tag{4.495}$$

i. e.,

$$c_7 \|W^{h_i}\|_{\mathcal{D}} \leq \|W^{h_i}\|_h \leq c_8 \|W^{h_i}\|_{\mathcal{D}}; \tag{4.496}$$

2. the eigenvalues of matrix $\mathcal{D}^{h_i} L^{h_i}$ are bounded:

$$0 < \lambda(\mathcal{D}^{h_i} L^{h_i}) \leq \lambda_i^* \leq c_6 h_i^{n-2s}. \tag{4.497}$$

In section 4.6 we fixed the rule that, on the functional level, the operator of interpolation from H^{h_i} to $H^{h_{i+1}}$ is identity. From this rule, the explicit form of interpolation and restriction operators follows in vector spaces. For example, take again the vector $W^{h_i} \in \mathbf{R}^{N_i}$ and compute

$$W_l^{h_{i+1}} = \sum_{j=1}^{N_i} \beta_l^j W_j^{h_i}, \qquad l = 1, \dots, N_{i+1}. \tag{4.498}$$

We put the vector $W^{h_{i+1}} \in \mathbf{R}^{N_{i+1}}$ with these components as the result of interpolation $I_i : W^{h_i} \to W^{h_{i+1}}$. The restriction operator $R_{i+1} : W^{h_{i+1}} \to W^{h_i}$ is defined by formula for components

$$W_j^{h_i} = \sum_{l=1}^{N_{i+1}} \beta_l^j W_l^{h_{i+1}}, \qquad j = 1, \dots, N_i. \tag{4.499}$$

These operators are mutually ajoint in Euclidian vector space with the norm (4.495).

Take the grid Ω_{h_0}. For it, system (4.494) has no more than c_3 unknowns and can be solved without any preconditioning.

Let some approximation $V_0^{h_i}$ be given for solution of system (4.494) with $i \geq 1$. Then perform one step of the MG-algorithm formulated in section 4.2. On the basis of section 4.5, we recommend W-cycle (i. e., $\gamma = 2$) without post-smoothing procedure (i. e., $m_2 = 0$ and the step $\mathbf{A}_5$ is absent). In the pre-smoothing procedure $\mathbf{A}_1$, we use Jacobi-type scaled iterations

$$U_{l+1} = U_l - \tau_l \mathcal{D}^{h_i}(L^{h_i}U_l - F^{h_i}), \qquad l = 0, 1, \ldots, m-1, \tag{4.500}$$

with an initial guess $V_0^{h_i}$ and the parameters τ_l from the formula (4.215). Call this concrete kind of the MG-algorithm the $MG^{(7)}$-algorithm.

Theorem 4.27 *Assume that conditions* $\mathbf{G}'$, $\mathbf{H}'$, (4.225), (4.226), (4.496), *and* (4.497) *are satisfied for the problem* (4.488) *and the Bubnov-Galerkin system* (4.490). *Then for any* $\varepsilon \in (0,1)$, *one can find integer* m_0 *independent of* h_i, f *and such that* $\forall m \geq m_0$ *the error of an initial guess* $V_0^{h_i}$ *at one step of the* $MG^{(7)}$*-algorithm reduces by a factor* ε*:*

$$\|V_1^{h_i} - V^{h_i}\|_{\mathcal{D}} \leq \varepsilon \|V_0^{h_i} - V^{h_i}\|_{\mathcal{D}} \quad \textit{where} \quad V_1^{h_i} = MG_i^{(7)}(V_0^{h_i}, F^{h_i}). \tag{4.501}$$

Proof. Consider a symmetric matrix

$$S^{h_i} = (\mathcal{D}^{h_i})^{1/2} L^{h_i} (\mathcal{D}^{h_i})^{1/2}. \tag{4.502}$$

It has the same eigenvalues as $\mathcal{D}^{h_i} L^{h_i}$ but other eigenvectors. This follows from comparing the relations

$$(\mathcal{D}^{h_i})^{1/2} L^{h_i} (\mathcal{D}^{h_i})^{1/2} U = \lambda U \qquad \text{and} \qquad \mathcal{D}^{h_i} L^{h_i} V = \lambda V,$$

where we can put $V = (\mathcal{D}^{h_i})^{1/2} U$. For the eigenvalues of matrix S^{h_i}, the following inequality like (4.497) is therefore satisfied:

$$0 < \lambda(S^{h_i}) \leq \lambda_i^* \leq c_6 h_i^{n-2s}. \tag{4.503}$$

Now show that we are under convergence condition of Theorem 4.11. To this end, we transform our assumptions to others by application of two lemmata.

First consider the system

$$L^{h_i} W^{h_i} = G^{h_i}. \tag{4.504}$$

Lemma 4.10.1 . *When conditions* $\mathbf{G}'$ *and* (4.496) *are satisfied, any vector* G^{h_i} *is associated with a function* $g \in H^{h_i}$ *such that equality* (4.504) *is the Bubnov-Galerkin system for the problem*

$$\mathcal{L}(w, v) = (g, v) \qquad \forall v \in H_A. \tag{4.505}$$

Here

$$|g|_0 \leq c_7^{-1} h_i^{-n} \|\mathcal{D}^{h_i} G^{h_i}\|_{\mathcal{D}}. \tag{4.506}$$

Proof. Take the system

$$\sum_{j=1}^{N_i} g_i \gamma_j^l = G_l^{h_i}, \qquad l = 1, \dots, N_i, \tag{4.507}$$

where $\gamma_j^l = (\varphi_j^{h_i}, \varphi_l^{h_i})$. We first suppose that it has some solution and seek to find an a priori estimate for it. Multiply each equation in (4.507) by g_l and sum over l:

$$\sum_{j,l=1}^{N_i} g_j g_l \gamma_j^l = \sum_{l=1}^{N_i} g_l G_l^{h_i}. \tag{4.508}$$

Introduce the function $g \in H^{h_i}$ by the formula

$$g(x) = \sum_{j=1}^{N_i} g_j \varphi_j^{h_i}(x). \tag{4.509}$$

The left-hand side of (4.508) is then brought to the form $|g|_0^2$. Apply the Cauchy-Bunyakovski inequality, the definition of norm (4.495), and inequality (4.496) to the right-hand side of (4.508):

$$|g|_0^2 \le (\sum_{l=1}^{N_i} (G_l^{h_i})^2 d_l^{h_i})^{1/2} \cdot (\sum_{l=1}^{N_i} g_l^2 (d_l^{h_i})^{-1})^{1/2} \le c_7^{-1} \|\mathcal{D}^{h_i} G^{h_i}\|_{\mathcal{D}} |g|_0 h_i^{-n}.$$

The above dictates inequality (4.506). For system like (4.507) with zero right-hand side, this inequality dictates that the trivial solution is unique. Non-uniform system (4.507) has therefore a unique solution for any vector G^{h_i}.

From (4.509) and system (4.507), it follows that

$$G_l^{h_i} = (g, \varphi_l^{h_i}), \qquad l = 1, \dots, N_i.$$

Hence, G^{h_i} is the right-hand side of the Bubnov-Galerkin method for the problem (4.505) with right-hand side g. From the construction of system (4.494), in turn, it follows that matrix L^{h_i} is also consistent with this method. □

Along with system (4.504) on the grid Ω_{h_i}, let us formulate a system of the Bubnov-Galerkin method on the grid $\Omega_{h_{i-1}}$ for problem (4.505). It has the form

$$L^{h_{i-1}} W^{h_{i-1}} = G^{h_{i-1}} \quad \text{where} \quad G^{h_{i-1}} = R_i G^{h_i}. \tag{4.510}$$

Lemma 4.10.2 *Let $w^{h_{i-1}}$, w^{h_i} be prolongations in $H^{h_{i-1}}$, H^{h_i} of solutions $W^{h_{i-1}}$, W^{h_i} of systems* (4.510), (4.504). *Then under conditions* **G′**, **H′**, *and* (4.496), *the estimate*

$$|w^{h_i} - w^{h_{i-1}}|_0 \le c_9 h_i^{2s-n} \|\mathcal{D}^{h_i} G^{h_i}\|_{\mathcal{D}} \tag{4.511}$$

holds, where $c_9 = c_5(1 + c_2^{2s})/c_7$.

Proof. condition **H′** and inequalities (4.506), (4.226) yield the estimates

$$|w - w^{h_i}|_0 \le c_5 h_i^{2s} |g|_0 \le c_5 h_i^{2s-n} c_7^{-1} \|\mathcal{D}^{h_i} G^{h_i}\|_{\mathcal{D}},$$

$$|w - w^{h_{i-1}}|_0 \le c_5 h_{i-1}^{2s} |g|_0 \le c_5 c_2^{2s} c_7^{-1} h_i^{2s-n} \|\mathcal{D}^{h_i} G^{h_i}\|_{\mathcal{D}}.$$

Taking these together, we get the inequality (4.511). □

Now continue to prove Theorem 4.27. For direct application of Theorem 4.11, we rewrite the $MG^{(7)}$-algorithm in other terms. For each system (4.494), we put in correspondence the equivalent one

$$\bar{L}_i V^{h_i} = \bar{F}_i \tag{4.512}$$

with the matrix $\bar{L}_i = \mathcal{D}^{h_i} L^{h_i}$ and the right-hand side

$$\bar{F}_i = \mathcal{D}^{h_i} F^{h_i}. \tag{4.513}$$

Introduce also the operators of interpolation and restriction

$$\bar{I}_i = I_i \qquad \text{and} \qquad \bar{R}_i = \mathcal{D}^{h_{i-1}} R_i (\mathcal{D}^{h_i})^{-1}. \tag{4.514}$$

Finally, we may rewrite pre-smoothing procedure (4.500) in the form

$$U_{l+1} = U_l - \tau_l(\bar{L}_i U_l - \bar{F}_i), \qquad l = 0, 1, \dots, m-1, \tag{4.515}$$

with the iterative operator

$$\bar{J}_i = (I - \tau_{m-1}\bar{L}_i) \cdots (I - \tau_0 \bar{L}_i). \tag{4.516}$$

So, we transform the $MG^{(7)}$-algorithm in equivalent form with another operators. We call this form the $\overline{MG}^{(7)}$-algorithm. Let us introduce the scalar product $(V, W)_i$ in section 4.5 equal to

$$(V, W)_i = \sum_{j=1}^{N_i} V_j W_j (d_j^{h_i})^{-1} h_i^n \tag{4.517}$$

for vectors $V, W \in \mathbf{R}^{N_i}$. Then $\|V\|_i = \|V\|_{\mathcal{D}}$. It is easy to verify that in this scalar product:

1. operator $\bar{L}_i$ is self-ajoint and positive-definite; (4.518)
2. $\bar{I}_{i-1} = \bar{R}_i^*$; (4.519)
3. $\bar{L}_{i-1} = \bar{R}_i \bar{L}_i \bar{I}_{i-1}$; (4.520)
4. $\bar{J}_i \bar{L}_i = \bar{L}_i \bar{J}_i$, (4.521)

i. e., properties (4.69), (4.70), (4.72), (4.73) are valid. On the basis of (4.503), (4.11), the condition (4.192) follows:

$$\|\bar{J}_i\|_{\mathcal{D}} \le 1 \qquad \forall i = 1, \dots, k.$$

Now again take vector $W^{h_i} \in \mathbf{R}^{N_i}$ and its prolongation w^{h_i} from (4.492). Compute vector $W^{h_{i+1}} = \bar{I}_i W^{h_i} = I_i W^{h_i}$ and form its prolongation $w^{h_{i+1}}$. Then $w^{h_{i+1}} = w^{h_i}$. On the basis of (4.496), (4.493) we have

$$\begin{aligned}
\|W^{h_i}\|_{\mathcal{D}} &\le c_7^{-1} \|W^{h_i}\|_h = c_7^{-1} |w^{h_{i+1}}|_0 \le c_8 c_7^{-1} \|W^{h_{i+1}}\|_{\mathcal{D}} = c_8 c_7^{-1} \|\bar{I}_i W^{h_i}\|_{\mathcal{D}}, \\
\|W^{h_i}\|_{\mathcal{D}} &\ge c_8^{-1} \|W^{h_i}\|_h = c_8^{-1} |w^{h_{i+1}}|_0 \ge c_7 c_8^{-1} \|W^{h_{i+1}}\|_{\mathcal{D}} = c_7 c_8^{-1} \|\bar{I}_i W^{h_i}\|_{\mathcal{D}}.
\end{aligned}$$

So, (4.193) is true. Now let us show the validity of inequality (4.194). Take any vector G^{h_i} and put $\bar{G}_i = \mathcal{D}^{h_i} G^{h_i}$. Then from (4.504), (4.510), it follows that

$$\begin{aligned}(\bar{L}_i^{-1} \quad &- \quad \bar{I}_{i-1}\bar{L}_{i-1}^{-1}\bar{R}_i)\bar{G}_i = ((L^{h_i})^{-1} - I_{i-1}(L^{h_{i-1}})^{-1}R_i)G^{h_i} = \\ &= \quad W^{h_i} - I_{i-1}W^{h_{i-1}} = W^{h_i} - \bar{I}_{i-1}W^{h_{i-1}}.\end{aligned} \tag{4.522}$$

Due to (4.496), (4.493), (4.511), we have

$$\|W^{h_i} - \bar{I}_{i-1}W^{h_{i-1}}\|_{\mathcal{D}} \le c_7^{-1}|w^{h_i} - w^{h_{i-1}}|_0 \le c_9 c_7^{-1} h_i^{2s-n}\|\bar{G}_i\|_{\mathcal{D}}. \tag{4.523}$$

Since $\bar{G}_i$ is an arbitrary vector, we get

$$\|\bar{L}_i^{-1} - \bar{I}_{i-1}\bar{L}_{i-1}^{-1}\bar{R}_i\|_{\mathcal{D}} \le c_L/\lambda_i^* \tag{4.524}$$

which proves (4.222) with the constant $c_L = c_9 c_7^{-1} c_6$. Combining this estimate with (4.216), we come to inequality (4.194) with function (4.223).

So, all assumptions of Theorem 4.11 are valid for the $\overline{MG}^{(7)}$-algorithm. Therefore, (4.195) holds which gives statement (4.501). □

Note that in this case on the basis of (4.203), (4.223), we have such dependence of factor ε in (4.501) on the number m of iterations:

$$\varepsilon = O((m+1)^{-2}). \tag{4.525}$$

Now we use the FMG-algorithm from subsection 4.2.1 for solving the whole sequence of discrete problems (4.494) for $i = 0, 1, \ldots, k$. Suppose that functional $f(v)$ in (4.488) ensures the estimate

$$|u - w^{h_i}|_0 \le c_{11} h_i^{2s} \tag{4.526}$$

where c_{11} is dependent on f and independent of h_i. Take any m in Theorem 4.27 such that $\varepsilon < 1$ in (4.501). Then we may choose integer t:

$$\varepsilon^t \le c_8^{-1} c_7 c_2^{-2s}. \tag{4.527}$$

Theorem 4.28 *Let all assumptions of Theorem 4.27 be valid and (4.526), (4.527) hold. Then application of the FMG-algorithm gives sequence of approximate solutions $\widetilde{V}^{h_i}$ of problems (4.494) which satisfy the inequality*

$$\|\widetilde{V}^{h_i} - V^{h_i}\|_{\mathcal{D}} \le c_{11} h_i^{2s}(1+\rho)/c_8(1-\rho), \qquad \rho \equiv \varepsilon^t c_7^{-1} c_8 c_2^{2s} < 1, \tag{4.528}$$

and their prolongations $\tilde{v}^{h_i}$ in H^{h_i} satisfy the estimates

$$|\tilde{v}^{h_i} - u|_0 \le 2c_{11} h_i^{2s}/(1-\rho), \qquad i = 1, 2, \ldots, k. \tag{4.529}$$

The proof is like one of Theorem 4.15 and is omitted.

4.10.2 Convergence in energy norm

Now we pass to the convergence rate of the MG-algorithm in energy norm. Therefore we need to formulate the convergence condition of the Bubnov-Galerkin method in the same norm.

To do this, we introduce into $H_A \subset W_2^s$ the energy norm

$$[\![w]\!] = \{\mathcal{L}(w, w)\}^{1/2}. \tag{4.530}$$

Let again $W^{h_i} \in \mathbf{R}^{N_i}$ be an arbitrary vector and w^{h_i} is its prolongation from H^{h_i}. Then put

$$\|W^{h_i}\|_h^{(1)} = [\![w^{h_i}]\!]. \tag{4.531}$$

The definitions of prolongation w^{h_i}, matrices L^{h_i}, $\bar{L}_i$ and norms (4.495), (4.530), (4.531) dictate that

$$\|W^{h_i}\|_h^{(1)} = (W^{h_i})^T L^{h_i} W^{h_i} = h_i^{-n/2}\|(L^{h_i})^{1/2} W^{h_i}\|_E = h_i^{-n/2}\|\bar{L}_i^{1/2} W^{h_i}\|_{\mathcal{D}}. \tag{4.532}$$

Below we use the following assumption.

C o n d i t i o n **I′**. *For any functional $f(v) = (g, v)$ with a function $g \in L_2(\Omega)$, the problem* (4.488) *has a unique solution $u \in W_2^{2s}$; the solution w^{h_i} of the Bubnov-Galerkin method* (4.489), (4.490) *satisfies the estimate*

$$[\![u - w^{h_i}]\!] \le c_{12} h_i^s |g|_0. \tag{4.533}$$

On the basis of sections 4.3–4.5, we consider V-cycle (i. e. $\gamma = 1$) of MG-algorithm from section 4.2 because namely V-cycle gives the best effectiveness in energy norm. Moreover, we use Jacobi-type pre-smoothing and post-smoothing procedures (4.500) and

$$Y_{l+1} = Y_l - \tau_l \mathcal{D}^{h_i}(L^{h_i} Y_l - F^{h_i}), \qquad l = 0, 1, \ldots, m-1, \tag{4.534}$$

with parameters (4.99) and constant λ_i^* from (4.497). Let us call this concrete kind of algorithm the $MG^{(8)}$-algorithm.

Theorem 4.29 *Let conditions* **G′**, **I′**, (4.225), (4.226), (4.496), (4.497) *be satisfied for the problem* (4.488) *and the Bubnov-Galerkin system* (4.490), (4.494) *with a symmetric positive-definite bilinear form $\mathcal{L}$. Assume also that we perform one step of the $MG^{(8)}$-algorithm. Then for any number m of iterations, the error of result $V_1^{h_i}$ diminishes by a factor ε for any initial guess $V_0^{h_i}$:*

$$\|V_1^{h_i} - V^{h_i}\|_h^{(1)} \le \varepsilon \|V_0^{h_i} - V^{h_i}\|_h^{(1)} \tag{4.535}$$

where

$$\varepsilon = 1/(1 + c_c \mathrm{ctg}^2 \pi/2(2m+1)) \tag{4.536}$$

with constant c_c independent of m, h_i, f, $V_0^{h_i}$.

Proof. We show that the convergence conditions of Lemma 4.3.2 hold. To this end, we again introduce scalar product (4.517). Then we have properties (4.518)–(4.521). Since operator $\bar{L}_i$ is self-ajoint and positive-definite, the norm $\|\cdot\|_h^{(1)}$ is indeed the energy norm with respect to $\bar{L}_i$. Hence, we have connection

$$[\![W^{h_i}]\!]_i = h_i^{n/2}\|W^{h_i}\|_h^{(1)} \tag{4.537}$$

with norm (4.75) from subsection 4.3.1.

Note that Lemma 4.10.1 remains true. With the help of this lemma and (4.533), we transform Lemma 4.10.2 in another one.

Lemma 4.10.3 *Let $w^{h_{i-1}}$, w^{h_i} be the prolongations in $H^{h_{i-1}}$, H^{h_i} of the solutions $W^{h_{i-1}}$, W^{h_i} of* (4.504), (4.510). *Then under conditions* **G′**, **I′**, (4.496), *the estimate*

$$[\![w^{h_i} - w^{h_{i-1}}]\!] \le c_{11}(1 + c_2^s)c_7^{-1}h_i^{s-n}\|\mathcal{D}^{h_i}G^{h_i}\|_{\mathcal{D}} \tag{4.538}$$

holds.

We omit the standard proof of this lemma and continue the proof of Theorem 4.29. Use equalities (4.504), (4.510) for arbitrary vector W^{h_i} and corresponding right-hand sides G^{h_i} and $G^{h_{i-1}}$. On the basis of (4.78),

$$[\![Q_iW^{h_i}]\!]_i = [\![(I - \bar{I}_{i-1}\bar{L}_{i-1}^{-1}\bar{R}_i\bar{L}_i)W^{h_i}]\!]_i = [\![W^{h_i} - \bar{I}_{i-1}W^{h_{i-1}}]\!]_i.$$

Therefore, with the help of (4.537), (4.538), (4.531), we obtain the inequality

$$\begin{aligned}[\![Q_iW^{h_i}]\!]_i &= h_i^{n/2}[\![W^{h_i} - \bar{I}_{i-1}W^{h_{i-1}}]\!]_h^{(1)} = \\ &= h_i^{n/2}[\![w^{h_i} - w^{h_{i-1}}]\!] \le c_{11}(1 + c_2^s)c_7^{-1}h_i^{s-n/2}\|\mathcal{D}^{h_i}G^{h_i}\|_{\mathcal{D}}.\end{aligned}$$

Due to (4.497) and equality $\mathcal{D}^{h_i}G^{h_i} = \bar{L}_iW^{h_i}$, we have

$$[\![Q_iW^{h_i}]\!]_i^2 \le c_q(\lambda_i^*)^{-1}\|\bar{L}_iW^{h_i}\|_i^2$$

with constant $c_q = c_6c_{11}^2(1+c_2^s)^2c_7^{-2}$. Then condition (4.89) holds with constant $c_1 = c_q$. Condition (4.90) is valid on the basis of Theorem 4.6. Then Theorem 4.5 is valid with constant $c_c = c_q^{-1}$ and gives us (4.535), (4.536). □

Now let us implement the FMG-algorithm from subsection 4.2.1 with the $MG^{(8)}$-algorithm. Suppose that the functional $f(v)$ in (4.488) ensures the estimate

$$[\![u - w^{h_i}]\!] \le c_{12}h_i^s \tag{4.539}$$

where c_{12} is dependent on f and independent of h_i. Let also assumptions of Theorem 4.29 be valid. So, fix *any* $m \ge 1$ and choose integer t:

$$\varepsilon^t \le c_2^{-s}. \tag{4.540}$$

Theorem 4.30 *Let all assumptions of Theorem* 4.29 *be valid and* (4.539), (4.540) *hold. Then application of the FMG-algorithm gives a sequence of approximate solutions $\widetilde{V}^{h_i}$ of problems* (4.494) *which satisfy the inequality*

$$\|\widetilde{V}^{h_i} - V^{h_i}\|_h^{(1)} \le c_{12}h_i^s(1 + \rho)/(1 - \rho), \qquad \rho = \varepsilon^t c_2^s < 1, \tag{4.541}$$

and their prolongations $\tilde{v}^{h_i}$ in H^{h_i} satisfy the estimates

$$[\![\tilde{v}^{h_i} - u]\!] \le c_{12}h_i^s \cdot 2/(1 - \rho), \qquad i = 0, \dots, k. \tag{4.542}$$

The proof of this theorem is very similar to standard proof of Theorem 4.17 and is omitted.

4.11 The algorithm for the mixed method

In this section, we deal with an algorithm applied for the system of second-order equations in the mixed method. It differs from the algorithm given in section 4.10 by iterative parameters and another operators of interpolation and restriction.

Let us study the following problem: *find a solution* $(u, v) \in U \times V$ *satisfying the relations*

$$a(u, \xi) + b(\xi, v) = f(\xi) \qquad \forall \xi \in U, \tag{4.543}$$

$$b(u, \psi) = g(\psi) \qquad \forall \psi \in V. \tag{4.544}$$

The meaning of the notation was explained in subsection 1.2.3. Recall that U and V are the spaces of the functions defined on Ω and Ω', respectively. Assume that for each of these sets we have sequences of grids Ω_{h_i} and Ω'_{h_i} with parameters h_i satisfying conditions (4.225), (4.226). Note that Ω_{h_0}, Ω'_{h_0} involve a rather small number of nodes.

For each parameter h_i, we introduce finite-dimensional sets of basis functions $\xi_j^{h_i} \in U$ $(j = 1, \ldots, n_i)$ and $\psi_j^{h_i} \in V$ $(j = 1, \ldots, r_i)$. Denote the linear spans of these basis functions by U^{h_i} and V^{h_i}. Put $N_i = n_i + r_i$ and define $H^{h_i} = U^{h_i} \times V^{h_i}$.

We will seek two functions $w^{h_i} = (u^{h_i}, v^{h_i}) \in H^{h_i}$ of the form

$$u^{h_i}(x) = \sum_{j=1}^{n_i} \alpha_j^{h_i} \xi_j^{h_i}(x), \qquad x \in \Omega, \tag{4.545}$$

$$v^{h_i}(x) = \sum_{j=1}^{r_i} \gamma_j^{h_i} \psi_j^{h_i}(x), \qquad x \in \Omega' \tag{4.546}$$

as an approximate solution. The weights $\alpha_j^{h_i}$ and $\gamma_j^{h_i}$ are obtained from the system of the Bubnov-Galerkin method:

$$\sum_{j=1}^{n_i} \alpha_j^{h_i} a(\xi_j^{h_i}, \xi_l^{h_i}) + \sum_{j=1}^{r_i} \gamma_j^{h_i} b(\xi_l^{h_i}, \psi_j^{h_i}) = f(\xi_l^{h_i}), \quad l = 1, \ldots, n_i, \tag{4.547}$$

$$\sum_{j=1}^{n_i} \alpha_j^{h_i} b(\xi_j^{h_i}, \psi_l^{h_i}) = g(\psi_l^{h_i}), \quad l = 1, \ldots, r_i. \tag{4.548}$$

Let us number the basis functions as follows:

$$\varphi_j^{h_i} = \begin{cases} \xi_j^{h_i}, & j = 1, \ldots, n_i, \\ \psi_{j-n_i}^{h_i}, & j = n_{i+1}, \ldots, N_i. \end{cases}$$

Assume that condition $\mathbf{G}'$ is satisfied for $\varphi_j^{h_i}$, therefore $H^{h_i} \subset H^{h_{i+1}}$.

4.11.1 Convergence in L_2-norm

Let us reduce the conditions of convergence of u^h, v^h to u, v to the following requirement.

C o n d i t i o n **D**. *For functionals of the form* $f(\xi) = (\tilde{f}, \xi)_\Omega$, $g(\psi) = (\tilde{g}, \psi)_{\Omega'}$ *with functions* $\tilde{f} \in L_2(\Omega) \cap U^{h_i}$, $\tilde{g} \in L_2(\Omega') \cap V^{h_i}$ *the problem* (4.543), (4.544) *has a unique solution* $u \in U$, $v \in V$; *and the solution of the Bubnov-Galerkin method* u^{h_i}, v^{h_i} *satisfies the estimate*

$$|u - u^{h_i}|_{0,\Omega} + h_i^\sigma |v - v^{h_i}|_{0,\Omega'} \le c_5 h_i^2 (|\tilde{f}|_{0,\Omega} + h_i^{-\sigma} |\tilde{g}|_{0,\Omega'}) \tag{4.549}$$

with a certain σ *(which can be both positive and negative in different problems).*

Every vector W^{h_i} with components $W_j^{h_i}$ ($j = 1, \dots, N_i$) is associated with the prolongation $w^{h_i} = (\tilde{u}^{h_i}, \tilde{v}^{h_i})$ from H^{h_i}, i. e., two functions

$$\begin{aligned} \tilde{u}^{h_i}(x) &= \sum_{j=1}^{n_i} W_j^{h_i} \xi_j^{h_i}(x), \qquad x \in \Omega, \\ \tilde{v}^{h_i}(x) &= \sum_{j=1}^{r_i} W_{j+n_i}^{h_i} \psi_j^{h_i}(x), \qquad x \in \Omega'. \end{aligned} \tag{4.550}$$

Using these functions, introduce the vector norm

$$\|W^{h_i}\|_h = |\tilde{u}^{h_i}|_{0,\Omega} + h_i^\sigma |\tilde{v}^{h_i}|_{0,\Omega'}. \tag{4.551}$$

Rewrite system (4.547), (4.548) in a more compact form

$$L^{h_i} V^{h_i} = F^{h_i}. \tag{4.552}$$

Here L^{h_i} is an $N_i \times N_i$ symmetric square matrix; and V^{h_i}, F^{h_i} are the vectors of unknowns and right-hand sides of dimension N_i, the ordering being made in accordance with numbers of basis functions $\varphi_j^{h_i}$.

For every $i \ge 1$, introduce the matrix $\mathcal{D}^{h_i} = \operatorname{diag}\{d_1^{h_i}, \dots, d_{N_i}^{h_i}\}$ with the elements

$$d_j^{h_i} = \begin{cases} 1, & j = 1, \dots, n_i, \\ h_i^{2\sigma} & j = n_i + 1, \dots, N_i. \end{cases} \tag{4.553}$$

We now assume that the following conditions hold:

1. the norm (4.551) is equivalent to the Euclidean weighted norm

$$\|W^{h_i}\|_E = \Big(\sum_{j=1}^{n_i} (W_j^{h_i})^2 h_i^n + \sum_{j=1}^{r_i} (W_{j+n_i}^{h_i})^2 h_i^{r-2\sigma}\Big)^{1/2} \tag{4.554}$$

with integers $n = \dim \Omega$, $r = \dim \Omega'$, i. e.,

$$c_7 \|W^{h_i}\|_E \le \|W^{h_i}\|_h \le c_8 \|W^{h_i}\|_E; \tag{4.555}$$

2. the eigenvalues of matrix $\mathcal{D}^{h_i} L^{h_i}$ are bounded:

$$|\lambda(\mathcal{D}^{h_i} L^{h_i})| \le \lambda_i^* \le c_6 h_i^{n-2}. \tag{4.556}$$

Remark 4.11.1 *The above inequality does not demand sign-definiteness of the spectrum, which is very often the case in the mixed method.*

Since condition $\mathbf{G}'$ is valid, we can introduce operators of interpolation I_i by the formula (4.498) and restriction R_{i+1} by (4.499).

On the basis of section 4.5, for convergence in L_2-norm, we recommend W-cycle ($\gamma = 2$) without post-smoothing iterations ($m_2 = 0$ and $\mathbf{A_5}$ is absent). In the pre-smoothing procedure $\mathbf{A_1}$, we use iterations

$$U_{l+1} = U_l - \tau_l \mathcal{D}^{h_i} L^{h_i} \mathcal{D}^{h_i} (L^{h_i} U_l - F^{h_i}), \qquad l = 0, \dots, m-1, \tag{4.557}$$

with parameters τ_l from formula (4.206) with $\mu_i^* = (\lambda_i^*)^2$.

We call this concrete kind of the MG-algorithm the $MG^{(9)}$-algorithm.

As usual, at the level h_0 the system (4.552) and any other with the matrix L^{h_0} has a few unknowns and can be solved directly without any preconditioning. Now let some approximation $V_0^{h_i}$ be given for solution of system (4.552) at level h_i with $i \geq 1$.

Theorem 4.31 *Let conditions* $\mathbf{D}$, $\mathbf{G}'$, (4.225), (4.226), (4.555), *and* (4.556) *be satisfied for problem* (4.543), (4.544) *and the Bubnov-Galerkin system* (4.552). *Then for any* $\varepsilon \in (0,1)$, *one can find integer* m_0 *independent of* h_i, f *and such that* $\forall m \geq m_0$ *the error of an initial guess* $V_0^{h_i}$ *at one step of the* $MG^{(9)}$*-algorithm reduces by a factor* ε, *i. e.,*

$$\|V_1^{h_i} - V^{h_i}\|_E \leq \varepsilon \|V_0^{h_i} - V^{h_i}\|_E, \quad \textit{where} \quad V_1^{h_i} = MG_i^{(9)}(V_0^{h_i}, F^{h_i}). \tag{4.558}$$

Proof. Let us rewrite the $MG^{(9)}$-algorithm in terms (4.512)–(4.514) and put

$$U_{l+1} = U_l - \tau_l \bar{L}_i (\bar{L}_i U_l - \bar{F}_i), \qquad l = 0, 1, \dots, m-1, \tag{4.559}$$

so that

$$\bar{J}_i = (I - \tau_{m-1} \bar{L}_i^2) \cdots (I - \tau_0 \bar{L}_i^2). \tag{4.560}$$

As result, we put equivalent form of algorithm which we call $\overline{MG}^{(9)}$.

The unique distinction of consiquent justification from the proof of Theorem 4.27 consists in proving the criterium (4.213) instead of (4.222) and using the estimate (4.207) instead of (4.216). Combining (4.213) with (4.207), we come to inequality (4.194) with function (4.214).

So for the $\overline{MG}^{(9)}$-algorithm, all assumptions of Theorem 4.11 are valid. Therefore, (4.195) holds which gives statement (4.558). □

Note that on the basis of (4.203), (4.214) we have such dependence of factor ε in (4.558) on the number m of iterations:

$$\varepsilon = O((2m+1)^{-1}). \tag{4.561}$$

To solve the whole sequence of discrete problems (4.552) for $i = 0, 1, \dots, k$, we use the FMG-algorithm from subsection 4.2.1 with $MG^{(8)}$. Suppose that functionals $f(\xi)$, $g(\psi)$ in (4.543), (4.544) ensures satisfaction of the estimate

$$|u - u^{h_i}|_{0,\Omega} + h_i^{\sigma} |v - v^{h_i}|_{0,\Omega'} \leq c_{11} h_i^2 \tag{4.562}$$

with a constant c_{11} independent of h_i. Take any m in Theorem 4.31 to attain the inequality $\varepsilon < 1$ and choose integer t:

$$\varepsilon^t \leq c_8^{-1} c_7 c_2^{-2}. \tag{4.563}$$

Theorem 4.32 *Let all assumptions of Theorem* 4.31 *be valid and* (4.562), (4.563) *hold. Then application of the FMG-algorithm with the $MG^{(9)}$-algorithm gives a sequence of approximate solutions $\widetilde{V}^{h_i}$ of problems* (4.552) *which satisfy the inequality*

$$\|\widetilde{V}^{h_i} - V^{h_i}\|_E \leq c_{11} h_i^2 (1+\rho)/c_8(1-\rho), \qquad \rho \equiv \varepsilon^t c_7^{-1} c_8 c_2^2 < 1, \tag{4.564}$$

and their prolongations $\tilde{w}^{h_i} = (\tilde{u}^{h_i}, \tilde{v}^{h_i}) \in H^{h_i}$ satisfy the estimates

$$\begin{aligned} |u - \tilde{u}^{h_i}|_{0,\Omega} &\leq 2c_{11} h_i^2/(1-\rho), \\ |v - \tilde{v}^{h_i}|_{0,\Omega'} &\leq 2c_{11} h_i^{2-\sigma}/(1-\rho), \qquad i = 0, 1, \ldots, k. \end{aligned} \tag{4.565}$$

The proof is very similar to one of Theorem 4.15 with the norm of elements $\tilde{w}^{h_i} = (\tilde{u}^{h_i}, \tilde{v}^{h_i}) \in U^{h_i} \times V^{h_i} = H^{h_i}$ defined by the formula

$$|\tilde{w}^{h_i}|_0 \equiv |\tilde{u}^{h_i}|_{0,\Omega} + h_i^\sigma |\tilde{v}^{h_i}|_{0,\Omega'}.$$

Therefore it is omitted.

4.11.2 Convergence in "energy" norm

Now we consider the convergence rate of multigrid algorithm in a special norm which is similar to energy norm but is not such in strong sense because the operator of problem is not positive-definite.

Pay attention that operator $L_i = \mathcal{D}^{h_i} L^{h_i}$ is self-ajoint in the vector space M_i with the scalar product

$$(U, V)_i = U^T (\mathcal{D}^{h_i})^{-1} V, \qquad U, V \in \mathbf{R}^{N_i}, \tag{4.566}$$

and the norm (4.554). Therefore, we can introduce operator Λ_i by the rule (4.154) in the subsection 4.4.1. It gives Λ_i-inner product (4.156) and "energy" norm (4.157).

Using the prolongations (4.550) of vector W^{h_i}, let us introduce the functional norm in H^{h_i}:

$$\|w^{h_i}\|_{H_i} \equiv \|\tilde{u}^{h_i}, \tilde{v}^{h_i}\|_{H_i} = \|W^{h_i}\|_{U_i}. \tag{4.567}$$

In contrast to usual energy norm this one depends on the level i. For the same function $w^{h_i} \in H^{h_{i-1}} \subset H^{h_i}$ the norm $\|w^{h_i}\|_{H_i}$, $\|w^{h_i}\|_{H_{i-1}}$ are different. Therefore their relationship is important. Fortunately, for problems studied below this requirement is natural:

$$\|w^{h_i}\|_{H_{i-1}} \leq c_I \|w^{h_i}\|_{H_i} \qquad \forall w \in H^{h_{i-1}} \subset H^{h_i}. \tag{4.568}$$

In these terms, let us formulate the convergence of Bubnov-Galerkin method.

C o n d i t i o n **D′**. *For functionals of the form* $f(\xi) = (\tilde{f}, \xi)_\Omega$, $g(\psi) = (\tilde{g}, \psi)_{\Omega'}$ *with functions* $\tilde{f} \in L_2(\Omega) \cap U^{h_i}$, $\tilde{g} \in L_2(\Omega') \cap V^{h_i}$, *the problem* (4.543), (4.544) *has a unique solution* $w = (u, v) \in U \times V$ *and the solution of the Bubnov-Galerkin method* $w^{h_i} = (u^{h_i}, v^{h_i})$ *satisfies the estimate*

$$\|w - w^{h_i}\|_{H_i} = \|u - u^{h_i}, v - v^{h_i}\|_{H_i} \leq c_5' h_i(|\tilde{f}|_{0,\Omega} + h_i^{-\sigma} |\tilde{g}|_{0,\Omega'}). \qquad (4.569)$$

Above we introduced the operators of interpolation I_i and restriction R_{i+1}. On the basis of section 4.4, for convergence in "energy" norm, we recommend W-cycle ($\gamma = 2$) with both pre-smoothing iterations (4.557) and the same post-smoothing iterations

$$Y_{l+1} = Y_l - \tau_l \mathcal{D}^{h_i} L^{h_i} \mathcal{D}^{h_i} (L^{h_i} Y_l - F^{h_i}), \qquad l = 0, \ldots, m-1, \qquad (4.570)$$

with parameters τ_l from the formula (4.182) with λ_i^* from (4.556).

We call this concrete kind of the MG-algorithm the $MG^{(10)}$-algorithm. As usual, at the level h_0, any system (4.552) is solved by direct method. Assume that we have some initial guess $V_0^{h_i}$ for the solution V^{h_i} of the system (4.552) at the level $i \geq 1$.

Theorem 4.33 *Let conditions* **D′**, **G′**, (4.225), (4.226), (4.555), (4.556) *be satisfied for the problem* (4.543), (4.544) *and the Bubnov-Galerkin system* (4.552). *Then for any* $\varepsilon \in (0, 1)$, *one can find an integer* m_0 *independent of* h_i, f *and such that* $\forall m \geq m_0$ *the error of an initial guess* $V_0^{h_i}$ *at one step of the* $MG^{(10)}$*-algorithm reduces by a factor* ε:

$$\|V_1^{h_i} - V^{h_i}\|_{U_i} \leq \varepsilon \|V_0^{h_i} - V^{h_i}\|_{U_i} \qquad (4.571)$$

where $V_1^{h_i}$ *is the result of* $MG^{(10)}$.

Proof. The main purpose consists in justification of the assumptions of Theorem 4.9. To this end, we introduce the notation (4.512)–(4.514), (4.560). Then (4.159) follows from (4.42); (4.160) does from (4.568); (4.161) follows from (4.183) and standard reasoning which gives (4.178). On the basis of Theorem 4.9, (4.571) follows. □

Note that on the basis of (4.176) and (4.188), we have such dependence of factor ε in (4.571) on the number m:

$$\varepsilon = O((m+1)^{-1}). \qquad (4.572)$$

First this algorithm was studied in the paper [148] by P. Peisker for the concrete problem where the convergence rate was examined in other norm. Also, in this paper the question was arised about an optimization of iterative parameters τ_l.

To solve the whole sequence of discrete problems (4.552) for $i = 0, 1, \ldots, k$, we use the FMG-algorithms from subsection 4.2.1 with $MG^{(10)}$. Suppose that functionals $f(\xi)$, $g(\psi)$ in (4.543), (4.544) ensures satisfaction of the estimate

$$\|w - w^{h_i}\|_{H_i} \leq \|u - u^{h_i}, v - v^{h_i}\|_{H_i} \leq c_{11} h_i. \qquad (4.573)$$

Take any m in Theorem 4.33 to attain the inequality $\varepsilon < 1$ and choose integer t:

$$\varepsilon^t \leq c_I^{-1} c_2^{-1}. \qquad (4.574)$$

Theorem 4.34 *Let all assumptions of Theorem* 4.33 *be valid and* (4.573), (4.574) *hold. Then application of the FMG-algorithm with the $MG^{(10)}$-algorithm gives a sequence of approximate solutions $\widetilde{V}^{h_i}$ of problems* (4.552) *which satisfy the inequality*

$$\|\widetilde{V}^{h_i} - V^{h_i}\|_{U_i} \leq c_{11} h_i (1+\rho)/(1-\rho), \qquad \rho \equiv \varepsilon^t c_I c_2 < 1, \tag{4.575}$$

and their prolongations $\tilde{w}^{h_i} = (\tilde{u}^{h_i}, \tilde{v}^{h_i}) \in H^{h_i}$ satisfy the estimate

$$\|w - \tilde{w}^{h_i}\|_{H_i} = \|u - \tilde{u}^{h_i}, v - \tilde{v}^{h_i}\|_{H_i} \leq 2c_{11} h_i/(1-\rho). \tag{4.576}$$

The proof is very similar to one of Theorem 4.17 and is omitted.

Chapter 5

Realization of the algorithms for second-order equations

In this chapter, we treat specific applications of the multigrid inerative algorithms proposed in Chapter 4 to linear second-order equations. The main theoretical result is justification (for a wide range of differential problems) of two facts. First one is convergence of multigrid algorithms. Second is finite number of arithmetic operations per one unknown for attainment of accuracy stipulated by discretization.

In section 5.1, we consider some modifications of these algorithms illustrated by the two-dimensional Dirichlet problem on a convex polygon, and perform calculation of the number of arithmetic operations needed to obtain the required accuracy.

One of the methods used to take account of curvilinear boundaries for second-order equations is provided in section 5.2. It uses the breaking algorithm for obtaining the nested triangulations and differs from known methods by a simpler and more economical structure. This time, auxiliary systems of lesser order are obtained algorithmically by summing lines and columns of an initial system rather than as independent Bubnov-Galerkin systems on more rough triangulations.

In section 5.3, we deal with a boundary value problem having a singularity in the angle on the boundary. In order to prevent the order accuracy from reducing, refining triangulation in the neighboorhood of this angle are used. It is shown that pre-conditionality using a diagonal matrix leaves the multigrid algorithms as effective as they are on a uniform grid for problems with smooth data.

In section 5.4, we show how to apply these algorithms to the three-dimensional Dirichlet problem. In essence, in this section we show that there is no basic difference in application, justification of efficiency, and convergence between two-dimensional and three-dimensional problems.

In section 5.5, we show how to apply the multigrid algorithm to the general spectral problem $Au = \lambda Bu$. Note that both matrix A and matrix B obtained in the Bubnov-Galerkin method are not diagonal. The iterative algorithm yields an eigenvalue and the corresponding eigenfunction or an eigenspace (if the eigenvalue is multiple).

In section 5.6, we treat applications of the multigrid algorithms to the boundary value problems of second and third kind. A separate investigation of the Neuman problem having a singular operator presents specially modified algorithms. Two approaches to the construction of the Bubnov-Galerkin system are compared for a uniform rectangular grid and for a non-uniform triangulation subordinate to the boundary.

5.1 The two-dimensional Dirichlet problem

In this section, we treat the two-dimensional Dirichlet problem for a second-order elliptic equation. As in section 3.5, the Bubnov-Galerkin method with piecewise linear basis functions on triangles is used to discretize the problem. The algorithms from section 4.6 are used to solve approximately the obtained system of linear algebraic equations. They yield an approximate solution of the initial differential problem with accuracy $O(h^2)$ in the norm $L_2(\Omega)$ and accuracy $O(h)$ in the energy norm within $O(N)$ arithmetic operations; here h is the characteristic linear cell-size of the grid, and N is the number of its nodes.

5.1.1 Properties of a differential and a difference problems

Let us first consider the Dirichlet problem on a *convex* polygon Ω with a boundary Γ

$$-\sum_{i,j=1}^{2} \partial_i(a_{ij}\partial_j u) + au = f \quad \text{in} \quad \Omega, \tag{5.1}$$

$$u = 0 \quad \text{on} \quad \Gamma. \tag{5.2}$$

The coefficients and the right-hand side of (5.1) satisfy the conditions

$$\begin{aligned} &\partial_k a_{ij} \in L_q(\Omega), \quad q > 2, \quad i,j,k = 1,2; \qquad a_{12} = a_{21} \quad \text{on} \quad \bar{\Omega}; \\ &\mu\sum_{i=1}^{2}\xi_i^2 \leq \sum_{i,j=1}^{2} a_{ij}\xi_i\xi_j \leq \nu\sum_{i=1}^{2}\xi_i^2 \quad \text{on} \quad \bar{\Omega} \quad \forall\xi_i \in \mathbf{R}, \quad \nu \geq \mu > 0; \\ &a, f \in L_2(\Omega), \qquad a \geq 0 \qquad \text{on convex} \quad \bar{\Omega}. \end{aligned} \tag{5.3}$$

These conditions are sufficient [94, p.272] to solve the problem (5.1), (5.2) in the class $W_2^2(\Omega)$ uniquely and for the estimate

$$\|u\|_2 \leq c_1|f|_0 \tag{5.4}$$

with constant c_1 independent of f. This problem can be reduced to the general formulation (1.20) with a bilinear form $\mathcal{L}$.

To construct a finite element scheme, we use the notation of section 3.5. We first divide the initial polygon Ω into a small number of closed triangles (zones) so that this triangulation $\mathcal{T}_0$ is concordant. Denote the maximal length of the triangles sides by l_0. Put $n_i = 2^i$, $h_i = l_0/n_i$; and for all $i = 0, 1, \ldots, p$, divide every initial triangle into n_i^2 equal triangles. Denote the union of all vertices of the obtained concordant triangulation $\mathcal{T}_i$ by $\bar{\Omega}_{h_i}$ and introduce $\Omega_{h_i} = \bar{\Omega}_{h_i} \bigcap \Omega$ and the number N_i of points of the set Ω_{h_i}. For every point $y \in \Omega_{h_i}$, let's introduce the piecewise linear basis function $\varphi_y^{h_i} \in \overset{\circ}{W}{}_2^1(\Omega)$, likewise in section 3.5, and denote the linear span of this system by H^{h_i}.

For realizing the algorithms below, it is necessary that set Ω_{h_0} should have at least one point. Otherwise, the subdivision should be taken as Ω_{h_0} which is obtained from the initial one by segmentation of the triangles sides into 2 or 3 parts so that at least one point is in the interior of Ω. Denote the maximum number of triangles meeting in one node of Ω_{h_i} by k_1.

Note that each triangle of subdivision $\bar{\Omega}_{h_i}$ involves 4 triangles of subdivision $\bar{\Omega}_{h_{i+1}}$, and so condition **G** of section 4.6 holds, viz., each basis function of the i-th subdivision is a linear combination of a finite amount ($c_4 \leq \max\{7, k_1\}$) of basis functions of the $(i+1)$-th subdivision.

Let us introduce the bilinear form

$$\mathcal{L}(u,v) = \int_\Omega (\sum_{i,j=1}^{2} a_{ij}\partial_j u \partial_i v + auv)dx$$

and for each $i = 0, 1, \dots, p$ construct the system of linear algebraic equations of the Bubnov-Galerkin method

$$\sum_{y\in\Omega_{h_i}} \alpha_y \mathcal{L}(\varphi_y^{h_i}, \varphi_z^{h_i}) = (f, \varphi_z^{h_i}) \qquad \forall z \in \Omega_{h_i}. \tag{5.5}$$

Use its solution to form the function

$$u^{h_i}(x) = \sum_{y\in\Omega_{h_i}} \alpha_y \varphi_y^{h_i}(x)$$

which is an approximate solution of problem (5.1), (5.2).

The convergence of u^{h_i} to the exact solution was dealt within a number of papers. Not listing all of them, we refer the reader to [146, p.118, 148] and [115, p.186], where the following estimates were formulated.

Lemma 5.1.1 *If conditions* (5.3) *and* (5.4) *are satisfied, the approximate solution* u^{h_i} *obeys the estimates*

$$|u - u^{h_i}|_0 \leq c_2 h_i^2 |f|_0,$$

$$[\![u - u^{h_i}]\!] \leq c_3 h_i |f|_0. \tag{5.6}$$

Hence, conditions **H** and **I** of section 4.6 are satisfied. We make a piecewise linear prolongation from H^{h_i}; the function

$$w^{h_i}(x) = \sum_{y\in\Omega_{h_i}} W_y^{h_i} \varphi_y^{h_i}(x) \quad \text{on} \quad \bar{\Omega} \tag{5.7}$$

corresponds to each vector W^{h_i} with components $W_y^{h_i}$, $y \in \Omega_{h_i}$; and we introduce two norms

$$\|W^{h_i}\|_h = |w^{h_i}|_0, \tag{5.8}$$

$$\|W^{h_i}\|_E = (\sum_{y\in\Omega_{h_i}} (W_y^{h_i})^2 h_i^2)^{1/2}. \tag{5.9}$$

It is easy to show [146, p.73] (see also Theorem 3.13 that these norms are equivalent:

$$c_7 \|W^{h_i}\|_E \leq \|W^{h_i}\|_h \leq c_8 \|W^{h_i}\|_E. \tag{5.10}$$

Write system (5.5) in the form

$$L^{h_i} V^{h_i} = F^{h_i} \tag{5.11}$$

where V^{h_i}, F^{h_i} are the vectors of unknowns and the right-hand side with components $V_y^{h_i} = \alpha_y$, $F_z^{h_i} = (f, \varphi_z^{h_i})$; and L^{h_i} is $N_i \times N_i$ symmetric matrix. It obeys the following assertion [146, p.120] (see also Theorem 3.14).

Lemma 5.1.2 *Under assumptions* (5.3), *eigenvalues* λ *of matrix* L^{h_i} *satisfy the inequality*

$$0 < \lambda \leq c_5. \tag{5.12}$$

Hence, the assumption of Theorems 4.14, 4.15 and 4.16, 4.17 are satisfied both for $MG^{(1)}$-algorithm from section 4.6 in L_2-norm and $MG^{(2)}$-algorithm in the energy norm. The estimates (4.238), (4.256), (4.257), (4.266), (4.272), and (4.273) hold true, therefore.

5.1.2 A calculation of the number of arithmetic operations

Let us take first $MG^{(1)}$-algorithm from section 4.6 to estimate the number of arithmetic operations required to solve our problem. Denote by $\Phi_i(m)$ the number of arithmetic operators in $MG_i^{(1)}$-algorithm with m iterations in pre-smoothing procedure (4.97).

At the first stage A_1', the iterative process (4.97) of section 4.3 calls for $2m(c_4+2)N_i$ arithmetic operations. The second stage $\mathbf{A_2}$, the restricting (4.51) of section 4.2 calls for $2(c_4+1)N_i$ operations to find the residual and $2N_i$ arithmetic operations for restriction R_i since a value in each point of the set Ω_{h_i} is exploited no more than 2 times. At the third stage $\mathbf{A_3}$, the coarse grid solving (4.52) in section 4.2 takes $2\Phi_{i-1}(m)$ arithmetic operations since $\gamma = 2$. The fourth stage $\mathbf{A_4}$, the correcting (4.53) takes no more than $3N_i$ operations for interpolation I_{i-1} and N_i for addition of vectors. The fifth stage $\mathbf{A_5}$, the post-smoothing (4.54) is absent in $MG^{(2)}$-algorithm, i. e., in (4.55) $w_1 = y_{m_2} = y_0$. As a result,

$$\Phi_i(m) \leq c_6 N_i + 2\Phi_{i-1}(m) \quad \text{where} \quad c_6 = 2(m+1)(c_4+2)+3. \tag{5.13}$$

At $i = 0$ system (5.11) is solved directly during Φ_0 arithmetic operations, where Φ_0 is independent of m.

Lemma 5.1.3 *For any integer* $m \geq 1$ *in* $MG^{(2)}$*-algorithm, we have the estimate*

$$\Phi_i(m) \leq c_{11} N_i, \qquad i = 1, \ldots, p, \tag{5.14}$$

where c_{11} *is independent of* N_i *but linearly depends on* m.

Proof. Let T_i be the number of triangles of the i-th subdivision. Then

$$T_{i+1} \geq 4T_i. \tag{5.15}$$

Each node of subdivision Ω_{h_i} enters in no more than c_4 triangles and so

$$T_i \leq c_4 N_i. \tag{5.16}$$

Every triangle has three vertices; nodes of Ω_{h_i} and $\bar{\Omega}_{h_i}/\Omega_{h_i}$ are among them. Each node of Ω_{h_i} appears in no less than 3 triangles. Therefore,

$$N_i \leq T_i. \tag{5.17}$$

(5.13) is then recast as

$$\Phi_i(m) \le c_6 T_i + 2\Phi_{i-1}(m). \tag{5.18}$$

Let us prove that

$$\Phi_i(m) \le 2(c_6 + \Phi_0/2)T_i. \tag{5.19}$$

Use induction. It is obvious that

$$\Phi_0 \le 2(c_6 + \Phi_0/2)T_0.$$

Let us suppose that (5.19) is satisfied and consider $\Phi_{i+1}(m)$. Using (5.15), we get the sequence of inequalities

$$\Phi_{i+1}(m) \le c_6 T_{i+1} + 4(c_6 + \Phi_0/2)T_i \le 2(c_6 + \Phi_0/2)T_{i+1}.$$

(5.19) is thus proved. From this, by virtue of (5.16), the estimate (5.14) follows with the constant $c_{11} = (2c_6 + \Phi_0)c_4$. □

Besides of guaranteeing upper estimate, the principle part of $\Phi_i(m)$ can be used to define the largeness order of $\Phi_i(m)$. Let us calculate it for sufficiently large m and i, assuming that breaking the triangles proceeds in 4 parts at higher levels. Recall that most part of points of Ω_{h_i} are vertices of six triangles, and for relatively finer grids

$$N_i = 4N_{i-1} + o(N_{i-1}). \tag{5.20}$$

Then a calculation of the number of arithmetic operations similar to (5.13) yields the asymptotical equality

$$\Phi_i(m) = 16(m+1)N_i + 2\Phi_{i-1}(m) + 9N_i/4 + o(N_i).$$

Summing, we come to the relation

$$\Phi_i(m) \approx (16(m+1) + 9/4)N_i + o(N_i). \tag{5.21}$$

The summand $2^i\Phi_0$ is discarded because it is of smaller order $O(\sqrt{N_i})$.

In principle, we may use $MG^{(2)}$-algorithm independently without any additional approaches. For example, at the level p we may take the initial guess $V_0^{h_p} = 0$ and repeat $MG^{(2)}$-algorithm t times:

$$\tilde{V}_l^{h_p} = MG_p^{(2)}(\tilde{V}_{l-1}^{h_p}, F^{h_p}), \qquad l = 1, 2, \dots, t. \tag{5.22}$$

Due to the estimate (4.238) of Theorem 4.14, we come to inequality

$$\|\tilde{V}_t^{h_p} - V^{h_p}\|_E \le \varepsilon^t \|V^{h_p}\|_E. \tag{5.23}$$

It is natural that error in a right-hand side would have the same order of smallness as discretization error. Indeed, let (5.6) hold. Due to (5.10) the discretization error in norm $\|\cdot\|_E$ has the same order h_p^2. Owing to (4.238), (4.223), (4.203) we have the asymptotic equality

$$\varepsilon \approx \frac{c_L \pi}{4(m+1)^2}. \tag{5.24}$$

Then from assumption $\varepsilon^t \approx c_0 h_p^2$, the equality follows

$$m + 1 = O(h_p^{-1/t}). \tag{5.25}$$

Substituting this value in (5.21), we come to dependence of number

$$\varphi_u \equiv \Phi_p(m)/N_p \tag{5.26}$$

on h_p, i. e.,

$$\varphi_u = O(h_p^{-1/t}). \tag{5.27}$$

This number is a measure of the number of arithmetic operations per one known; and its dependence on h_p is a bad feature of direct employment of $MG^{(2)}$-algorithm. Of course, we may use some additional techniques such as conjugate-gradient method [31]. This somewhat improves the dependence of φ_u on h_p but does not exclude it entirely: $O(h_p^{-1/2t})$. Complete independence of φ_u is attained in FMG-algorithm of subsection 4.2.1.

Consider now this algorithm to find the solution $\widetilde{V}^{h_p}$ on the finest grid Ω_{h_p}.

Lemma 5.1.4 *Under assumptions* (5.3), *FMG-algorithm in combination with $MG^{(2)}$-algorithm take no more than $n_u N_p$ arithmetic operations with constant n_u independent of h_p, N_p to attain accuracy of $\widetilde{V}^{h_p}$ coinsiding with discretization error, i. e., for its prolongation $\tilde{v}^{h_p}$ we have estimates*

$$|u^{h_p} - \tilde{v}^{h_p}|_0 \le c_2 h_p^2 |f|_0, \tag{5.28}$$

$$|u - \tilde{v}^{h_p}|_0 \le 2c_2 h_p^2 |f|_0. \tag{5.29}$$

Proof. Fix an integer $i \in [1,p]$. The stage 2 in FMG-algorithm takes $3N_i$ arithmetic operations for interpolations I_{i-1} and $t\Phi_i(m)$ operations for employment of $MG_i^{(2)}$-algorithm t times. Using estimate (5.14), we conclude that the number of arithmetic operations needed to go from $\widetilde{V}^{h_i}$ to $\widetilde{V}^{h_{i+1}}$ is bounded above by $(3+tc_{11})N_{i+1}$. Since a similar estimate holds for lesser indices, we get the following result: no more than

$$(3 + tc_{11})(N_0 + N_1 + \ldots + N_{i+1}) \le \frac{4}{3}(3 + tc_{11})T_{i+1}$$

arithmetic operations are required for the whole chain

$$\widetilde{V}^{h_0} \to \widetilde{V}^{h_1} \to \ldots \to \widetilde{V}^{h_{i+1}}$$

where T_{i+1} is the number of the triangles of the $i+1$-th subdivision. We used here the estimate (5.17). Applying (5.16) to the obtained equality, we get upper estimation

$$n_u \le 4(1 + tc_{11}/3)c_4. \tag{5.30}$$

Show how to make constant c_{11} to be independent of h_p, N_p. Take $t = 1$ and $\varepsilon = c_7^{-1} c_8/(1 + 2c_2^2)$. For this ε on the basis of Theorem 4.14, there exists m_0 such that

(4.238) holds. Take an integer $m \in [m_0, 2m_0]$. All assumptions of Theorem 4.15 are valid. Owing to (4.260) we have

$$|\tilde{v}^{h_p} - u^{h_p}|_0 \leq c_2 h_p^2(\sigma - 1)|f|_0. \tag{5.31}$$

From definitions of ε and (4.259), the estimate (5.28) follows. Then (5.28) with (5.6) give (5.29). Since ε is independent of h_p, N_p; m_0 is the same. Thus on the basis of (5.13)

$$c_{11} = (2c_6 + \Phi_0)c_4 \leq (4(2m_0 + 1)(c_4 + 2) + 6 + \Phi_0)c_4,$$

i. e., the constant c_{11} and, consequently, n_u are bounded by constants independent of h_p, N_p. □

In the previous proof, we put $t = 1$. In principle, we should be able take $t = 2$ or $t = 3$. For the same multiplier of error suppression, it gives us possibility to increase ε and decrease m. When we get a gain? To answer this question, perform $MG^{(2)}$-algorithm two times with $m = m'$ and one time with $m = 2m' + 1$. On a basis of (5.21), (5.24)

$$2\Phi_p(m') \approx (32(m' + 1) + 9/2)N_p, \qquad \varepsilon^2(m') \approx (\frac{c_L\pi}{4(m + 1)^2})^2;$$

$$\Phi_p(2m' + 1) \approx (32(m' + 1) + 9/4)N_p, \qquad \varepsilon(2m' + 1) \approx \frac{c_L\pi}{16(m + 1)^2}. \tag{5.32}$$

In the first situation, the quantity of arithmetic operations is somewhat greater. Consider when first multiplier is less:

$$\varepsilon^2(m') \leq \varepsilon(2m' + 1).$$

Let square both sides of this inequality and carry out the reduction in view of numerical values (5.32). As a result, we get (approximate) inequality

$$\varepsilon^2(m') \leq 1/16. \tag{5.33}$$

In real computations this variant is not case as a rule. Usually, it is sufficient to suppress the error in 4–5 times at breaking the triangles into 4 parts and in 9–11 times at breaking into 9 parts.

Thus the strategy $t = 1$ is more effective in non-symmetric W-cycle ($MG^{(2)}$-algorithm). This multiplier would be useful in hp-version at powers $p \geq 2$. But in this situation we have another asymptotic behaviour of ε with respect to m and again strategy $t = 1$ is more preferable.

So, we treat the non-symmetric W-cycle for convergence in L_2-norm. Now examine the symmetric V-cycle for convergence in energy norm ($MG^{(1)}$-algorithm of section 4.6). We cite main results without proof because of their close analogy. First, denote by $\Phi'_i(m)$ the quantity of arithmetic operations in $MG_i^{(1)}$-algorithm. The count analogous to (5.13) gives

$$\Phi'_i(m) \leq c'_6 N_i + \Phi'_{i-1}(m), \quad \text{where} \quad c'_6 = (4m + 1)(c_4 + 2)N_i + 3N_i. \tag{5.34}$$

Lemma 5.1.5 *For any integer $m \geq 1$ in $MG_i^{(1)}$-algorithm, we have the estimate*

$$\Phi'_i(m) \leq c'_{11} N_i, \qquad i = 1, \dots, p, \tag{5.35}$$

with constant $c'_{11} = (4c'_6/3 + \Phi_0)c_4$ independent of N_i.

Lemma 5.1.6 *Under assumptions* (5.9), *FMG-algorithm in combination with $MG^{(1)}$ take no more than $n'_u N_p$ arithmetic operations with constant n'_u independent of h_p, N_p to attain the estimates*

$$[\![u^{h_p} - \tilde{v}^{h_p}]\!] \leq c_3 h_p |f|_0,$$

$$[\![u - \tilde{v}^{h_p}]\!] \leq 2c_3 h_p |f|_0$$

for prolongation $\tilde{v}^{h_p}$ of vector $\widetilde{V}^{h_p}$ — the result performance of FMG-algorithm.

5.1.3 A numerical experiment

In corroboration of these calculation, we give the results of numerical experiment on solving the following differential problem. Let Ω be a square $(0,1) \times (0,1)$ with a boundary Γ. Seek to determine the function u which is a solution of the problem

$$\begin{aligned} -\Delta u &= f \quad \text{in} \quad \Omega, \\ u &= 0 \quad \text{on} \quad \Gamma. \end{aligned} \tag{5.36}$$

The right-hand side

$$f = -(2 - 12x^2)y(1-y) + 2x^2(1-x^2)$$

corresponds to the solution

$$u = x^2(1-x^2)y(1-y).$$

The initial triangulation is constructed by drawing the diagonal of square from point $(0,0)$. Then every triangle is divided into 4 parts. As a result, we obtain a grid Ω_{h_0} consisting of one node $(1/2, 1/2)$. Then every triangle is again divided into four parts etc. Finally, we obtain grids Ω_{h_i} having $N_i = (2^{i+1} - 1)^2$ nodes for $i = 1, \dots, 6$. The last grid has 16129 nodes (127 x 127). On each of seven grids, systems of the Bubnov-Galerkin method (5.11) are formed, and then approximate solutions are found using FMG-algorithm in combination with $MG^{(2)}$ from section 4.2 with different m.

The errors of the obtained solutions and the computation time on the computer EC–1052[1] are provided in Table 5.1. To estimate the convergence acceleration effect owing to the τ_l parameters optimization, the data are provided, in the end of Table 5.1, when the choice of the parameters $\tau_l = 1/\lambda_i^*$ is stationary, λ_i^* is taken from section 4.6.

In Column 2, the number of interior grid nodes is given, i. e., the number of the Bubnov-Galerkin system unknowns. In Columns from 3 to 5, the grid norms of errors are given. Column 3 involves the values of $\|U^{h_i} - V^{h_i}\|_h$ showing the difference between the vector U^{h_i} of exact values and solution V^{h_i} of the Bubnov-Galerkin system . Column 4 involves the values of $\|V^{h_i} - \widetilde{V}^{h_i}\|_h$ showing the difference between the solution V^{h_i} of the Bubnov-Galerkin system and the approximate solution $\widetilde{V}^{h_i}$ of the above-cited multigrid algirithm. The full error of the approximate solution $\|U^{h_i} - \widetilde{V}^{h_i}\|_h$ is given in Column 5.

[1]This computer of United Series gives approximately the same speed of computations as IBM 386 SX with 25 MHz-processor and without co-processor.

Table 5.1: For $m = 2, 4, 6$ we use Algorithm FMG in combination with $MG^{(2)}$. For $m = 9^*$ we employ the trivial choice $\tau = 1/\lambda_i^*$ in Algorithm MG.

m	Grid	The error norm			Computer time	
					a, sec	b, $msec$
1	2	3	4	5	6	7
	3×3	$7.6 \cdot 10^{-4}$	$2.8 \cdot 10^{-3}$	$3.1 \cdot 10^{-3}$	–	–
	7×7	$2.1 \cdot 10^{-4}$	$1.2 \cdot 10^{-3}$	$1.3 \cdot 10^{-3}$	0.04	0.82
2	15×15	$5.3 \cdot 10^{-5}$	$3.3 \cdot 10^{-4}$	$3.6 \cdot 10^{-4}$	0.30	1.33
	31×31	$1.3 \cdot 10^{-5}$	$6.8 \cdot 10^{-5}$	$7.3 \cdot 10^{-5}$	1.28	1.34
	63×63	$3.3 \cdot 10^{-6}$	$1.3 \cdot 10^{-5}$	$1.4 \cdot 10^{-5}$	5.32	1.34
	127×127	$8.3 \cdot 10^{-7}$	$2.5 \cdot 10^{-6}$	$2.7 \cdot 10^{-6}$	21.72	1.35
	3×3	$7.6 \cdot 10^{-4}$	$1.3 \cdot 10^{-3}$	$1.2 \cdot 10^{-3}$	–	–
	7×7	$2.1 \cdot 10^{-4}$	$3.4 \cdot 10^{-4}$	$4.5 \cdot 10^{-4}$	0.08	1.63
4	15×15	$5.3 \cdot 10^{-5}$	$9.0 \cdot 10^{-5}$	$1.3 \cdot 10^{-4}$	0.42	1.87
	31×31	$1.3 \cdot 10^{-5}$	$1.4 \cdot 10^{-5}$	$2.4 \cdot 10^{-5}$	2.02	2.10
	63×63	$3.3 \cdot 10^{-6}$	$2.3 \cdot 10^{-6}$	$4.7 \cdot 10^{-6}$	8.68	2.19
	127×127	$8.3 \cdot 10^{-7}$	$4.3 \cdot 10^{-7}$	$1.1 \cdot 10^{-6}$	36.50	2.26
	3×3	$7.6 \cdot 10^{-4}$	$5.0 \cdot 10^{-4}$	$1.1 \cdot 10^{-3}$	–	–
	7×7	$2.1 \cdot 10^{-4}$	$1.3 \cdot 10^{-4}$	$2.7 \cdot 10^{-4}$	0.08	1.63
6	15×15	$5.3 \cdot 10^{-5}$	$5.3 \cdot 10^{-5}$	$9.6 \cdot 10^{-5}$	0.54	2.40
	31×31	$1.3 \cdot 10^{-5}$	$9.3 \cdot 10^{-6}$	$1.9 \cdot 10^{-5}$	2.76	2.87
	63×63	$3.3 \cdot 10^{-6}$	$1.5 \cdot 10^{-6}$	$3.9 \cdot 10^{-6}$	12.08	3.04
	127×127	$8.3 \cdot 10^{-7}$	$2.7 \cdot 10^{-7}$	$9.0 \cdot 10^{-7}$	51.30	3.18
	3×3	$7.6 \cdot 10^{-4}$	$6.5 \cdot 10^{-4}$	$1.0 \cdot 10^{-3}$	–	–
	7×7	$2.1 \cdot 10^{-4}$	$4.8 \cdot 10^{-4}$	$6.4 \cdot 10^{-4}$	0.12	2.45
9*	15×15	$5.3 \cdot 10^{-5}$	$1.3 \cdot 10^{-4}$	$1.7 \cdot 10^{-4}$	0.74	3.29
	31×31	$1.3 \cdot 10^{-5}$	$2.1 \cdot 10^{-5}$	$3.0 \cdot 10^{-5}$	3.86	4.02
	63×63	$3.3 \cdot 10^{-6}$	$3.6 \cdot 10^{-6}$	$5.4 \cdot 10^{-6}$	17.18	4.33
	127×127	$8.3 \cdot 10^{-7}$	$6.2 \cdot 10^{-7}$	$1.1 \cdot 10^{-6}$	73.48	4.56

The time (a) in seconds was taken to compute the solution $\widetilde{V}^{h_i}$ is given in Column 6. Column 7 presents the calculation time (b) in milliseconds related to one unknown. The time was noted up to $0.02 sec$, and the calculations were performed with the double mantissa with 32 bits.

The calculations obtained earlier by analyzing the main terms agree with the numerical experiment.

5.1.4 Some statements for the other situations

In the case when other Lagrange elements are used (of degree $2, 3, \ldots$ on triangles and serendipity ones of degree $1, 2, 3, \ldots$ on quadrangles), the main statements of this section remain valid. Moreover, if the smoothness of the solution u guarantees greater order convergence than linear elements do, this results in increasing corresponding

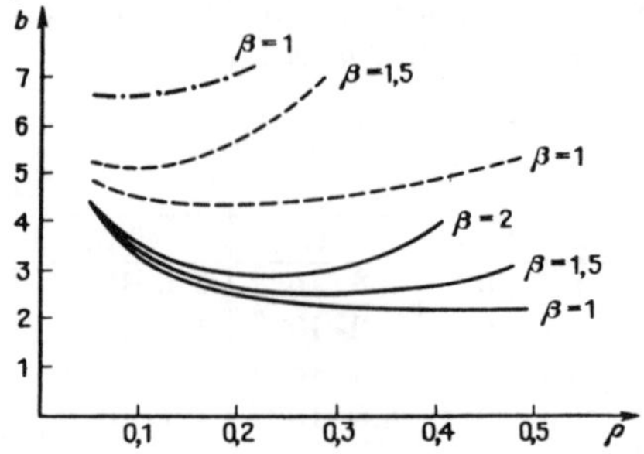

Figure 5.1: Reccurent representation of various realizations of MG-algorithm. a — symmetric V-cycle; b — symmetric W-cycle; c — non-symmetric W-cycle; d — non-symmetric V-cycle. **A** — MG_i-algorithm at the corresponding level i; **S** — smoothness procedure; ↘ — restriction; ↗ — interpolation; → — data transfer.

power of h_p in (5.6).

One important peculiarity should be noted which is related to application of high degrees elements. Referring to the justification of the algorithms of Chapter 4, we see that at lower layers of $MG^{(1)}$-algorithm it is sufficient to use piecewise linear elements on triangles and bilinear elements on quadrangles. Their accuracy is quite adequate to satisfy conditions **H** and **I**. The number of nonzero elements of the obtained matrices is largely less, the procedures of interpolation and restriction are simpler, which improves the efficiency of the algorithm.

Moreover, it is possible to apply MG-algorithm, to other finite elements on different grids, for instance, for the Clough-Tocher elements in subsection 2.2.1. As for the nestedness of the space of linear elements from a more rough grid, this is always available.

One more remark concerning Hermitean elements is in order here. Without correspondingly normalizing the matrix, MG-algorithm converges gradually. It is necessary, therefore, to apply the algorithm having diagonal normalization from section 4.10.

If the function a in (5.1) changes the sign, the positive definiteness of the bilinear form $\mathcal{L}$ fails. In this case, one should not use $MG^{(3)}$-algorithm instead of $MG^{(1)}$. This leads to both complicating the iterative process and increasing the number of iterations m. One should instead make other iterative parameters τ_l viz according to Remark 4.5.2 about $MG^{(1)}$-algorithm.

When introducing non-self-adjoint terms $a_i\partial_i u$ into the equation (5.1), the convergence of algorithms $MG^{(1)}$ and $MG^{(2)}$ greatly decreases or fails, especially when higher coefficients a_{ij} are close to $h_k|a_i|$ on sparse (rough) grids. In this case, one should use $MG^{(4)}$-algorithm to solve non-self-adjoint problems. A calculation of arithmetic operators is here different in that the iteration at the first stage becomes twice as tedious.

5.1.5 Graphic representation of algorithms

Represented graphically, the initial version of the multigrid algorithm in the bas study by R.P.Fedorenko [53] has the form of letter V (Fig. 5.1, a) and so was named as (symmetric) V-cycle. The initial iterations suppress the high-frequency component in the error of an approximate solution. The final iterations, in turn, suppress the high-frequency component of the interpolation error from a rough grid to a finer one.

When it was found that in some situations (for example, for non-positive-definite operators), one transition to a lower level can take too many iterations (their number was taken equal along all levels), a version of non-symmetric W-cycle came to light [137] (see Fig. 5.1, *b*). To be exact, at first, there was a need for a multiple $(2, 3, \dots)$ use of V-cycle. Then practice should that the double use, i. e., W-loop, is most optimal in some situations. Subsequent works by R.P. Fedorenko [54] and N.S. Bakhvalov [19] present a version of non-symmetric W-cycle. It is described in section 4.5 and section 5.1 and represented graphically in Fig. 5.1, *c*. Note that the non-symmetric W-cycles are not always considered to be a special class; in many papers they are regarded as variants of W-cycle and called correspondingly W-cycles.

It is easy to see that in the V-cycle an alternative is available for executing a different number of initial and final iterations. For example, all iterations can be executed at the beginning, which is the case in Fig. 5.1, *d*. We will call this situation non-symmetric V-cycle. On the one hand, we lose the procedure for smoothing the interpolation error. On the other hand, however, we diminish the error of the first stage to such a degree that the interpolation error itself will be small.

We have completely proved the convergence of the algorithms in three cases: where all iterations are executed at the beginning (non-symmetric W-cycle, section 4.5) and where the iterative process at the beginning is identical with that at the end, i. e., their numbers of iterations and their iterative parameters coincide (sections 4.3, 4.4). We will call the last variants symmetric V- and W-cycles correspondingly.

Numerical computations show that the V-cycles are usually more efficient than the W-cycles in cases they are both suitable. Moreover, the *V-cycles are easier to make parallel.* But the *W-cycles have a wider field of application*: they are applicable to non-self-adjoint problems, to problems with non-positive definite operators. For instance, applied to the Helmholtz equation (5.1) with complex coefficient a, they displayed adaquate efficiency.

Therefore, when the applicability is verified for both kinds of cycles, symmetric V-cycle is usually more effective than symmetric and non-symmetric W-cycles.

Namely with this purpose, the symmetric V-cycle was presented with non-stationary number of iterations in smoothing procedures [31].

5.2 A modified algorithm for domains with a curvilinear boundary

We continue discussing the two-dimensional Dirichlet problem (see section 5.1). Now we dwell upon investigation of a domain having a curvilinear boundary. Suppose that it consists of several curves of class C^2.

For multigrid algorithms, of value is the "nestedness" of finite elements, i. e., possibility of expressing the basis functions on sparse grids as linear combinations of several ones on finer grids (see (4.229) in section 4.6). This works well, say, on polygonal domains Ω yielding simple rules for interpolation and restriction of functions from one grid to another.

Further, the nestedness of elements permits one to form, using matrix L^{h_p} of the Bubnov-Galerkin method on the finest grid, auxiliary matrices L^{h_s} with indices $r < p$ on more sparse grids by only summing lines and columns. Indeed, from (4.229) of section 4.6, the elements of matrix $L^{h_{i-1}}$ are expressed as linear combinations of elements of matrix L^{h_i}, i. e., $L^{h_{i-1}} = R_i L^{h_i} I_{i-1}$:

$$L^{h_{i-1}}_{y_1,y_2} = \mathcal{L}(\varphi^{h_{i-1}}_{y_1}, \varphi^{h_{i-1}}_{y_2}) = \sum_{z_1,z_2\in\Omega_{h_i}} \beta^{y_1}_{z_1}\beta^{y_2}_{z_2}\mathcal{L}(\varphi^{h_i}_{z_1}, \varphi^{h_i}_{z_2}) =$$

$$= \sum_{z_1,z_2\in\Omega_{h_i}} \beta^{y_1}_{z_1}\beta^{y_2}_{z_2} L^{h_i}_{z_1,z_2} \qquad \forall y_1, y_2 \in \Omega_{h_{i-1}}. \tag{5.37}$$

This gives some ease of implementing the algorithms on a computer.

With the curvilinear boundary, when refining triangulation, the usual approximation of boundary results in that usual piecewise linear elements do not possess the nestedness property near the boundary.

As it was shown in [84], an application of the multigrid algorithms gets complicated just due to operations of interpolation and restriction. In [7], nestedness is available, and extrapolation of basis functions outside the domain is used to improve approximation of the boundary. In this case, the matrix of the Bubnov-Galerkin method differs from the usual one and that does not permit the routine software to be used.

To insure nestedness, we begin with the following procedure of triangulation [84]. Divide an initial domain into a not great number of triangles which can have one or two curvilinear sides. All boundary angular points, if any, must be the vertices of triangles; subdivision must be concordant. Denote by h_0 the maximum distance between vertices of one triangle and by θ_0 the smallest of the angles included between lines connecting the vertices of the triangle. Introduce the additional nodes on the sides of triangles; they will be used for segmentation. As these nodes, we take on the straight side its midpoint; on the curvilinear side, the point where this side is cut with the perpendicular from the midpoint of the chord connecting the ends of the side (Fig. 5.2). Transition from one triangulation to another (more fine one) proceeds by connecting three additional nodes by straight lines in every triangle. The number of triangles eventually becomes quadrupled. It is clear that this procedure may be repeated over and over again. We want this to be done p times. As before, denote by $\bar{\Omega}_{h_i}$ the union of all vertices available after splitting the triangles i times and determine $\Omega_{h_i} = \bar{\Omega}_{h_i} \bigcap \Omega$, $h_i = h_0/2^i$. Let N_i be, as before, the number of nodes of the set Ω_{h_i}. Rectilinear triangles with chords instead of curvilinear sides, resulting from the p-th division will be called elementary.

For definiteness suppose that the domain Ω is *convex*.

For every point $y \in \Omega_{h_p}$, we introduce a usual piecewise linear function $\varphi^{h_p}_y(x)$ equal to 1 at $x = y$ and to 0 at the other nodes of $\bar{\Omega}_{h_p}$, linear on every elementary triangle and being zero on the rest of $\bar{\Omega}$. Obviously, $\varphi^{h_p}_y \in \overset{\circ}{W}{}^1_2(\Omega)$. Basis functions on other grids will be formed as linear combinations of basis functions on finer grids. Suppose that we already have basis functions $\varphi^{h_{i+1}}_y$ for all $y \in \Omega_{h_{i+1}}$. Take an arbitrary node $y \in \Omega_{h_i}$. Several straight sides of triangles emanate from it; their midpoints are nodes

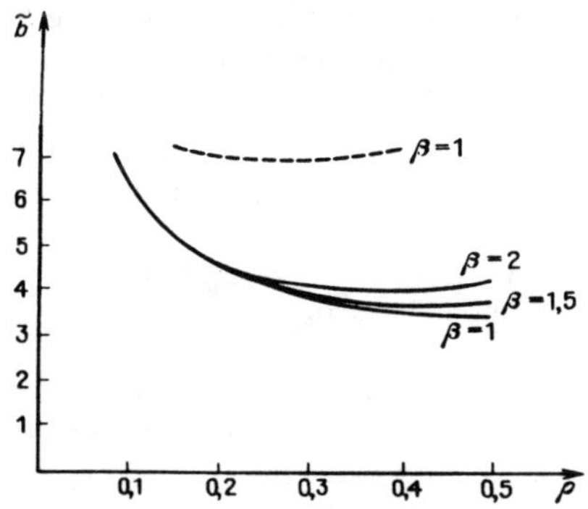

Figure 5.2: Breaking the triangle ABC with curvilinear side BEC.

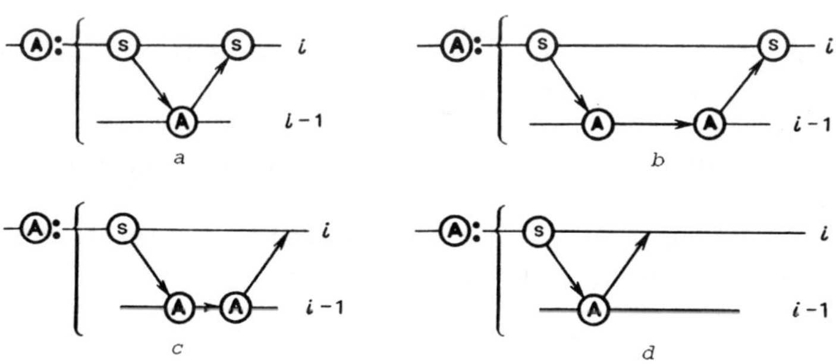

Figure 5.3: The basis function of $(p-2)$-th division near the boundary.

of $i+1$-triangulation $y_1, \dots, y_m$. Assume

$$\varphi_y^{h_i}(x) = \varphi_y^{h_{i+1}}(x) + \frac{1}{2}\sum_{j=1}^{m} \varphi_{y_j}^{h_{i+1}}(x). \tag{5.38}$$

Note that these functions are linear on rectilinear triangles of the i-th triangulation; and on triangles having curvilinear sides contiguous with the boundary, they are either equal to zero or composed of pieces of functions linear only on each elementary triangle (Fig. 5.3). Denote the linear span of functions $\varphi_y^{h_i}$ by H^{h_i}.

For each $i = 0, \dots, p$, we construct the system of linear algebraic equations (5.5) of the Bubnov-Galerkin method. Solve it to get the function

$$u^{h_i}(x) = \sum_{y \in \Omega_{h_i}} \alpha_y \varphi_y^{h_i}(x), \tag{5.39}$$

which is just the approximate solution of differential problem (5.1), (5.2).

In the long run, of interest for us will be u^{h_p} on the finest grid. On it, basis functions look as usual and from results of many studies we infer the convergence to the exact solution. However, justification of multigrid algorithms calls for estimation of accuracy (condition **H**) on all intermediate grids.

Theorem 5.1 *If conditions* (5.3) *and* (5.4) *are satisfied, approximate solutions* (5.39) *obey the estimates*

$$|u - u^{h_i}|_0 \le c_2 h_i^2 |f|_0, \tag{5.40}$$

$$[\![u - u^{h_i}]\!] \le c_2 h_i |f|_0 \tag{5.41}$$

on each of the grids Ω_{h_i} $(i = 0, 1, \dots, p)$.

Proof. Dividing a rectilinear triangle as above gives 4 triangles similar to the initial, i. e., they have the same set of angles and the same proportions of the sides' lengths. On triangles having curvilinear sides, these values are not retained. Show that they are only slightly different from initial triangles, no matter how many times the breaking algorithm was applied.

Consider the triangle in Fig. 5.2. Let the slopes of line segments AB, AC, BC to the axis Ox_1 be equal to θ_1, θ_2, θ_3; and their lengths — to l_1, l_2, l_3. According to the definition of belonging Γ to class C^2, specify local coordinates at point E (the tangent plus the normal) [94, p.31]. In these, the boundary portion BEC is described by a twice continuously differentiable function. Expanding it in Taylor's series, we can see that deviation of points B and C from the tangent line to Γ at point E does not exceed $c_3 l_3^2$. The length of straight segment GE is not over this value as well. Then, the lengths of new line segments DE, BE, FE, EC are not greater than, respectively, $l_2/2$, $l_3/2$, $l_1/2$, $l_3/2$ plus $c_3 l_3^2$. Hence, the estimate of possible decrease in lengths of the sides contiguous with the boundary is bounded by the inequality

$$a_i \le a_{i-1}/2 + c_3 a_{i-1}^2, \qquad i = 1, 2, \dots . \tag{5.42}$$

Here, a_i is the length of the chord subtending the curvilinear side in a triangle of the i-th subdivision. Let the initial subdivision of the domain obeys the condition

$$h_0 \leq 3c_3/64. \tag{5.43}$$

Then from (5.42), it follows that the maximal distance between vertices of one triangle of the i-th subdivision does not exceed $2h_i$.

Note that maximum-minimum ratio of distances between vertices of every initial triangle is governed by constant $1/\sin\theta_0$, according to the theorem of sines. On subsequent subdivisions, therefore, it can be come not greater than $2/\sin\theta_0$.

Consider now the angle EDG in Fig. 5.2. From the theorem of sines, and the above-cited facts as well, it follows that

$$|\sin\angle EDG| \leq 2c_3l_3^2/l_2 \leq 4c_3l_3/\sin\theta_0. \tag{5.44}$$

The same applies to turning angles of the other sides of triangles in Fig. 5.2. Summing these changes over all breakings, we come to inequality

$$\sin\mu \leq 12c_3h_0/\sin\theta_0$$

where μ is total change of any angle. Assume that in the initial subdivision

$$12c_3h_0/\sin\theta_0 \leq \frac{1}{4}\sin\theta_0. \tag{5.45}$$

Then on all subsequent subdivisions, the smallest θ_i of the angles contained by lines connecting vertices of one triangle satisfies the inequality

$$\sin\theta_i \geq \frac{1}{2}\sin\theta_0. \tag{5.46}$$

Now consider the interpolant in H^{h_i} for exact solution u

$$\hat{u}^{h_i}(x) = \sum_{y\in\Omega_{h_i}} u(y)\varphi_y^{h_i}(x)$$

and and prove the estimate

$$\|\hat{u}^{h_i} - u\|_1 \leq c_4h_i\|u\|_2. \tag{5.47}$$

For Ω_{h_p}, this follows from results of Chapter 3. Now find it for an arbitrary subdivision with index $i < p$.

On the most part Ω' of domain Ω composed of rectilinear triangles of the i-th subdivision, the required estimate is also obtained according to Chapter 3:

$$\|\hat{u}^{h_i} - u\|_{1,\Omega'}^2 \leq c_5h_i^2\|u\|_2^2. \tag{5.48}$$

In a strip ω_δ lying between the union of all elementary triangles and boundary Γ, we apply an inequality from [146, p.24]:

$$\int_{\omega_\delta} v^2dx \leq c_6\delta\|v\|_1^2. \tag{5.49}$$

Here, δ is the maximal width of the strip ω_δ, and v is an arbitrary function from $W_2^1(\Omega)$. Bear in mind that

$$\hat{u}^{h_i} = 0 \quad \text{in} \quad \omega_\delta \qquad \text{and} \qquad \delta \leq c_7 h_i^2.$$

Then from (5.49), the inequality

$$\|u - \hat{u}^{h_i}\|_{1,\omega_\delta}^2 \leq c_8 h_i^2 \|u\|_2 \tag{5.50}$$

follows.

It remains only to estimate the difference $u - \hat{u}^{h_i}$ in curvilinear triangles except for ω_δ. Consider an arbitrary curvilinear triangle Δ of the i-th subdivision, say, ΔABC in Fig. 5.2. Denote by $\Delta' = \Delta \setminus \omega_\delta$ the set of all elementary triangles involved in Δ. Form on Δ a linear function u^l by three values of function u at vertices of Δ. Then, from usual considerations [115, p.145],

$$\|u - u^l\|_{1,\Delta'}^2 \leq c_9 h_i^2 \|u\|_{2,\Delta'}^2. \tag{5.51}$$

On ΔADF function $\hat{u}^{h_i}$ coincides with u^l. Estimate the derivatives of their difference on the other triangles included in Δ'. Take ΔDEF as an example. Make the convention that $\partial v/\partial ED$ is the derivative in the direction from E to D, and $\angle DEx_1$ is the value of the angle contained by axis Ox_1 and the ray from E to D. Then on ΔDEF

$$\frac{\partial \hat{u}^{h_i}}{\partial x_1} = \frac{u(A)}{2}\left(\frac{\cos\angle DEx_1}{|DE|} + \frac{\cos\angle FEx_1}{|FE|}\right). \tag{5.52}$$

Similarly, on ΔDEF, as on the all Δ,

$$\frac{\partial u^l}{\partial x_1} = -u(A)\left(\frac{\cos\angle CAx_1}{|CA|} + \frac{\cos\angle BAx_1}{|BA|}\right). \tag{5.53}$$

According to considerations at the beginning of the proof,

$$\left|\frac{\cos\angle DFx_1}{2|DE|} - \frac{\cos\angle ACx_1}{|AC|}\right| \leq \frac{6c_3 l_3^2}{l_2^2} \leq \frac{6c_3}{\sin^2\theta_0}. \tag{5.54}$$

A similar inequality holds also for the addends in (5.52), (5.53). Therefore,

$$\int_{\Delta DEF} |\partial_1(u^l - \hat{u}^{h_i})|^2 dx \leq c_{10} u^2(A) \mathrm{mes}(\Delta DEF). \tag{5.55}$$

On the other smaller triangles, this difference is estimated in a similar way; note that constant c_{10} may be chosen common. According to the theorem of embedding $W_2^2(\Omega)$ into $C^{1/2}(\bar{\Omega})$ and the definition of the norm in $C^{1/2}(\bar{\Omega})$

$$|u(A)|^2 \leq c_{11} h_i \|u\|_2^2. \tag{5.56}$$

Apply this inequality to the sum of inequalities like (5.55) over all rectilinear triangles involded in Δ'. As a result we have the estimate

$$\int_{\Delta'} |\partial_1(u^l - \hat{u}^{h_i})|^2 dx \leq c_{10} c_{11} h_i \mathrm{mes}\,\Delta' \|u\|_2^2. \tag{5.57}$$

As the triangle Δ is arbitrary, this inequality holds for any curvilinear triangle near the boundary. The overall area of such triangles is bounded by $c_{12}h_i$. Moreover, the same inequality applies to the derivative with respect to x_2. In view of (5.51), we eventually get

$$\|u - \hat{u}^{h_i}\|^2_{1,\Omega\setminus(\Omega'\cup\omega_\delta)} \leq c_{13}h_i^2\|u\|_2^2. \tag{5.58}$$

Taking (5.48), (5.50), and (5.58) together, we have the estimate which is valid over the whole domain:

$$\|u - \hat{u}^{h_i}\|_1^2 \leq c_{14}h_i^2\|u\|_2^2.$$

With this estimate, inequalities (5.41), then (5.40) are derived in the usual way. □

Another important factor is boundedness of the matrix eigenvalues of the Bubnov-Galerkin system, i. e., satisfaction of the condition (4.237) of section 4.6. For it to be proved, system (5.5) is put into vector form (5.11):

$$L^{h_i}V^{h_i} = F^{h_i}. \tag{5.59}$$

Theorem 5.2 *Under assumptions* (5.3), *eigenvalues* λ *of matrix* L^{h_i} *satisfy the inequality*

$$0 \leq \lambda \leq c_{15}. \tag{5.60}$$

Proof. Take an arbitrary vector U with components U_x, $x \in \Omega_{h_i}$, define it to be zero at nodes Ω_{h_i} lying on Γ, and construct the prolongation $\hat{u}$ in H^{h_i}. Now we have the equality

$$\sum_{x\in\Omega_{h_i}} (L^{h_i}U)_x U_x = \mathcal{L}(\hat{u}, \hat{u}). \tag{5.61}$$

Using (5.3), we get

$$\mathcal{L}(\hat{u}, \hat{u}) \leq c_{16}\|\hat{u}\|_1^2. \tag{5.62}$$

Like in the proof of Theorem 5.1, divide domain Ω into 3 parts: Ω', ω_δ and $\Omega \setminus (\Omega' \bigcup \omega_\delta)$. On rectilinear triangles of the i-th subdivision, calculations such as ones in [168, p.16–17] yield the inequality

$$\|\hat{u}\|^2_{1,\Omega'} \leq c_{17} \sum_{x\in\Omega_{h_i}} U_x^2. \tag{5.63}$$

Now consider the rest $\Omega \setminus \Omega'$. Take an arbitrary curvilinear triangle of the i-th subdivision, for instance, ΔABC in Fig. 5.2. Then according to (5.53), on ΔADF

$$\partial_1\hat{u} = -\hat{u}(A)\left(\frac{\cos\angle CAx_1}{|CA|} + \frac{\cos\angle BAx_1}{|BA|}\right). \tag{5.64}$$

Hence,

$$\int_{\Delta ADF} (\partial_1\hat{u})^2 dx \leq \hat{u}^2(A)\frac{4}{|CA||BA|}\text{mes}(\Delta ADF). \tag{5.65}$$

Similar estimates (with c_{18} instead of 4) hold for all subsequent triangles appearing in Δ'. Sum these estimates over Δ' allowing for the fact that the interpolant equals zero on $\Delta \setminus \Delta'$. As a result, we get the inequality

$$\int_{\Delta} (\partial_1 \hat{u})^2 dx \leq c_{18} \hat{u}^2(A).$$

The derivative with respect to x_2 obeys this inequality as well. Sum then over all set $\Omega \setminus \Omega'$ allowing for the fact that every node is a vertex of only a few triangles:

$$\|\hat{u}\|^2_{1,\Omega\setminus\Omega'} \leq c_{19} \sum_{x\in\Omega_{h_i}} U_x^2.$$

Add this with (5.63) and multiply by c_{16}. We get the inequality which, together with (5.61) and (5.62), yields the estimate

$$\sum_{x\in\Omega_{h_i}} (L^{h_i}U)_x U_x \leq c_{16}(c_{17} + c_{19}) \sum_{x\in\Omega_{h_i}} U_x^2.$$

Since the matrix L^{h_i} is symmetric, from the above the estimate $\lambda \leq c_{15} = c_{16}(c_{17} + c_{19})$ follows by virtue of the Rayleigh ratio. The lower estimate follows immediately from properties of bilinear form $\mathcal{L}$. □

Thus, we verified satisfying all assumptions of section 4.6. So, all the results on multigrid algorithms obtained in sections 4.6, 5.1, 5.2 are valid for the solution of the Bubnov-Galerkin system

$$L^{h_p} V^{h_p} = F^{h_p}. \tag{5.66}$$

Recall that matrix L^{h_p} is formed in the standard way since the p-th subdivision is associated with usual piecewise linear basis functions. The other matrices are obtained in the recurrent way, one from the other, by summing lines and columns, as was stated at the beginning of the section. Thus, complex form of basis functions on more rough subdivisions does not influence the complexity of realization as well as the number of arithmetic operations.

In the final analysis, we have all assumptions of section 4.6 to be valid including the condition **G**. Therefore, we may use FMG-algorithm in combination with $MG^{(1)}$, $MG^{(2)}$ for which results of section 4.6 and Lemmata 5.1.4, 5.1.6 are fully true.

Remark 5.2.1 . *Another way to construct intermediate systems is provided in* [84] *where they are formed independently as the Bubnov-Galerkin problems on corresponding grids. This way seems to be less efficient. First, to form the Bubnov-Galerkin problems is more difficult than to add together a matrix elements on finer grids. Second, the procedure of interpolation becomes complicated. Third, theoretic justification gets also complicated due to the additional analysis of errors from an interpolation and a restriction since H^{2h} is not nested in H^h.*

5.3 The problem with a pointwise singularity

We continue discussing the two-dimensional Dirichlet problem and consider a situation when the domain Ω has interior angles greater than π. Their existence results in

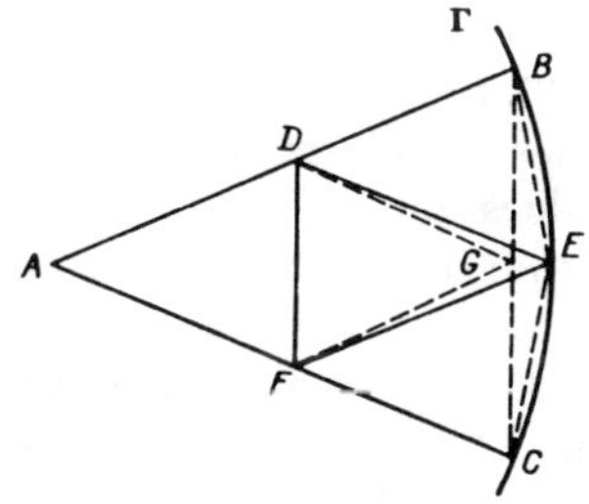

Figure 5.4: The breaking a triangle with a vertex at a singular point.

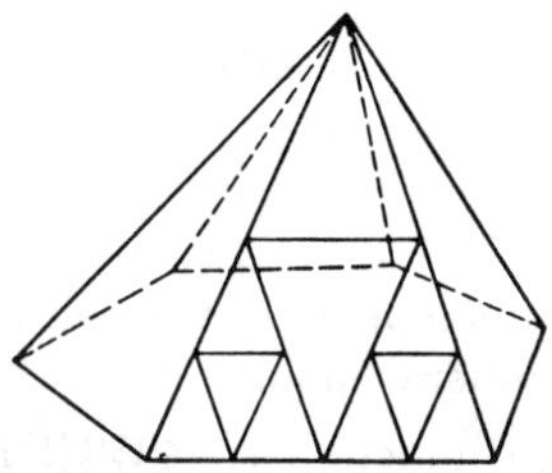

Figure 5.5: The triangulation of an initial triangle with index $\rho = 2$.

decrease of smoothness of a differential problem solution which, generally speaking, will not belong to $W_2^2(\Omega)$. Therefore, usual methods of triangulation and construction yield lesser order accuracy of an approximate solution [146, p.265].

The literature on this subject presents three ways out of the situation permitting one to obtain the usual order of accuracy. First, in [10], [146] it is suggested that one or several functions describing a solution behaviour near angles should be added to the ordinary basis functions. These functions have large area of support, which greatly complicates algorithms for forming and solving linear algebraic systems of the Bubnov-Galerkin method. Second, [167] suggests using norms whose weights degenerate into zero in singular points. In such a norm, accuracy remains unchanged. However, because the weight is degenerated, the accuracy of the approximate solution near a singular point is worse than that far from it. Third, in [167], [146, p.273] it is suggested that near a singular point, one should refine triangulation in a special way. This refinement can be performed in such a way that the total number of nodes of a difference grid is of the same order as usual. Some increase in the number of nodes (and corespondingly of unknowns) still takes place unlike the ordinary case, but stages of automatization do not change. It is technique that we will consider to show that the algorithms given in Chapter 4 may be extended also to this case without loss of efficiency.

In order to simulate a singular point, we take a polygon Ω whose interior angles are all less than π except for one at the origin of coordinates. Denote its value by θ (Fig. 5.4).

In the domain Ω with a boundary Γ, let us consider problem (5.1), (5.2) with conditions (5.3).

In developing a discrete problem of finite element method, we exploit the notation and the terms of section 5.1. We first perform the concordant breaking of the polygon

$\bar{\Omega}$ into a small number of closed triangles. Denote the maximal length of the triangles sides by l_0 and assume that $n_i = 2^i$, $h_i = l_0/n_i$ $(i = 0, 1, \ldots, p)$. Every initial triangle is further divided into more fine ones as follows. We introduce *a refinement index* $\rho \geq 1$. If a triangle of i-th subdivision does not touch to the origin of coordinates, it is being broken into 4 equal triangles of the $(i+1)$-th subdivision by connecting midpoints of its sides. Consider now some triangle of the i-th subdivision having vertex $(0,0)$, for example, ΔABC in Fig. 5.4. Denote by b the length of the height from A to the opposite side of an initial triangle. To construct triangles of the $(i+1)$-th subdivision, we then draw, at a distance $bn_i^{-\rho}$ from A, a straight line $B'C'$ parallel to BC. Denote the midpoint of BC by A'. Joining the points A', B', C' by straight lines gives 4 finer triangles of the $(i+1)$-th subdivision. Proportion $|AB'|/|AC| = |AC'|/|AB| = n_i^{-\rho}$ ensures a concordant segmentation of sides for another triangles with vertex $(0,0)$.

By breaking in the same way consistently for $i = 1, \ldots, p$, we get concordant subdivisions. An example of this triangulation is provided in Fig. 5.5. When splitted, one initial triangle gives only 4 kinds of triangles similar to ones of the first subdivision. Therefore the obtained triangles will not yield singular angles.

As before, denote by $\bar{\Omega}_{h_i}$ the union of all vertices of the i-th subdivision and assume that $\Omega_{h_i} = \bar{\Omega}_{h_i} \bigcap \Omega$, N_i is the number of points of set Ω_{h_i}. For each point $y \in \Omega_{h_i}$, we introduce the piecewise linear basis function $\varphi_y^{h_i} \in \overset{\circ}{W}{}_2^1(\Omega)$, as in section 5.1, and denote the linear span of this system by H^{h_i}.

For each $i = 0, 1, \ldots, p$, we construct a system of linear algebraic equations of the Bubnov-Galerkin method (5.5) and write it down in the form

$$L^{h_i} V^{h_i} = F^{h_i} \tag{5.67}$$

where V^{h_i}, F^{h_i} are the vectors of unknowns and the right-hand side with components $V_y^{h_i} = \alpha_y$, $F_z^{h_i} = (f, \varphi_z^{h_i})$, and L^{h_i} is an $N_i \times N_i$ symmetric matrix with elements $\mathcal{L}(\varphi_y^{h_i}, \varphi_z^{h_i})$.

Piecewise linear prolongations in H^{h_i} for vectors will be constructed like in (5.7); we introduce also norm (5.8). Recall that the prolongation in H^{h_i} of vector V^{h_i} is the function u^{h_i}, an approximate solution by the Bubnov-Galerkin method. For this the following result is valid.

Theorem 5.3 *Let conditions* (5.3) *be satisfied for problem* (5.1), (5.2). *Then for the solution* u^{h_i} *of the Bubnov-Galerkin method, we can choose the refinement index* ρ *such that the estimates hold*

$$[\![u - u^{h_i}]\!] \leq c_1 h_i |f|_0, \tag{5.68}$$
$$|u - u^{h_i}|_0 \leq c_2 h_i^2 |f|_0. \tag{5.69}$$

Proof. First we consider how to choose ρ. Make the substitution of variables in the plane x:

$$y_1 = \alpha_1 x_1 + \alpha_2 x_2, \quad y_2 = \beta_2 x_2.$$

Choose the parameters α_i, β_2 in such a way that after substitution, the principal part of equation (5.1) in point $(0,0)$ has the form

$$-\frac{\partial^2 u}{\partial y_1^2} - \frac{\partial^2 u}{\partial y_2^2}.$$

The initial angle of vertex $(0,0)$ changes into another one whose value $\theta_1 > \pi$. Let us assume that

$$\rho > \theta_1/\pi. \tag{5.70}$$

Note that the obtained triangulation satisfies conditions of paper [146, p.273] with index $\rho = 1/\mu$ on each level $i = 0, 1, \ldots, p$. This paper gives (using explicit functions of the singularity) the required estimate (5.68). The estimate (5.69) follows from (5.68) in the usual way likewise in Theorem 3.7. But we have to take $v^h \in H_A$ as the solution of the Bubnov-Galerkin problem

$$\mathcal{L}(v, v^h) = (u - u^h, v) \qquad \forall v \in H_A.$$

Because of [146, p.273], we get

$$[\![w - v^h]\!] \le ch|u - u^h|_{0,\Omega},$$

$$[\![u - u^h]\!] \le ch|f|_{0,\Omega}$$

instead of (3.52), (3.53). Hence,

$$|u - u^h|^2_{0,\Omega} \le ch^2|f|_{0,\Omega}|u - u^h|_{0,\Omega},$$

which gives (5.69). □

Note that due to refining the grid, equivalence (5.10) is not valid for auxiliary norm (5.9) in sections 4.6, 5.1. Therefore, let us modify this norm. Each node $y \in \Omega_{h_i}$ corresponds to the value $s_y^{h_i}$, a total area of triangles of the i-th subdivision with vertex y. Let us construct the diagonal matrix $\mathcal{D}^{h_i} = \mathrm{diag}\{d_y^{h_i}\}$, $y \in \Omega_{h_i}$, with the elements $d_y^{h_i} = (s_y^{h_i})^{-1}h_i^2$. Instead of (5.9), we introduce the norm (4.510):

$$\|W^{h_i}\|_{\mathcal{D}} = \Big(\sum_{y \in \Omega_{h_i}} (W_y^{h_i})^2 (d_y^{h_i})^{-1} h_i^2 \Big)^{1/2}.$$

The estimates (4.511) are valid for it with constants $c_7 = 1/2\sqrt{3}$ and $c_8 = 1/\sqrt{3}$.

The values $s_y^{h_i}$ are evaluated from below by the minimal area of a triangle of the i-th triangulation. Therefore

$$s_y^{h_i} \ge s_1 l_0^2 n_i^{-2\rho} \ge c_{13} h_i^{2\rho}$$

where s_1 is the least sine of a triangle in the first (not zeroth) triangulation. Hence we have

$$d_y^{h_i} \le c_{14} h_i^{2-2\rho}.$$

Because of Theorem 3.14, we get the estimate

$$\lambda(\mathcal{D}^{h_i} L^{h_i}) \le \lambda_i^* \le c_6 h_i^{2-2\rho}. \tag{5.71}$$

If we would try to enlist the results of subsection 4.10.2, we see that the exponent $2 - 2\rho$ is worse than $n - 2s = 0$ which we need in estimate (4.512). Therefore we have the non-regular case described in subsection 4.3.3. If we would not apply the refinement of cells near the angle, we get the non-regular case all the same. But the order of convergence would be worse.

In the framework of subsection 4.3.3, we need to enlist the V-cycle with nonstationary choice $m = m(i)$ of an amount of iterations at each level i. For this purpose we use modified $MG^{(8)}$-algorithm from subsection 4.10.2 in which the amount of iterations equals

$$m(i) = \bar{m} \cdot \sigma^{p-i}, \qquad \sigma \in (1,2), \tag{5.72}$$

at levels $i = 1, 2, \dots, p$. For any value $\sigma \in (1,2)$, the order of convergence rate and the order of amount of arithmetic operations remain the same.

We call this modification the $MMG^{(8)}$-algorithm.

Theorem 5.4 *Let $MMG^{(8)}$ and FMG-algorithms be used to solve system* (5.67) *at $i = p$. Then no more than $c_3 N_p$ arithmetic operations is adequate to find an approximate solution $\widetilde{V}^{h_p}$ satisfying the estimate*

$$\|\widetilde{V}^{h_p} - V^{h_p}\|_h^{(1)} = [\![\tilde{v}^{h_p} - u^{h_p}]\!] \le c_1 h_p |f|_0. \tag{5.73}$$

Here c_3 is independent of f, h_i, p; c_1 is the same as in (5.68)*; $\tilde{v}^{h_p}$ is the piecewise linear prolongation of vector $\widetilde{V}^{h_p}$; and u^{h_p} is the piecewise linear solution of the Bubnov-Galerkin method.*

Proof. We employ the notation of sections 4.3, 4.10. In particular, we introduce the matrices

$$\bar{L}_i = \mathcal{D}^{h_i} L^{h_i}, \qquad \bar{I}_i = I_i, \qquad \bar{R}_i = \mathcal{D}^{h_{i-1}} R_i (\mathcal{D}^{h_i})^{-1} \tag{5.74}$$

as in (4.527)–(4.529). Let us justify the assumptions of Theorem 4.7. The conditions (4.69)–(4.73) for matrices (5.74) was verified in (4.533)–(4.536). We need to verify only one of criteria (4.113) or (4.114). We decide on (4.114) because its justification is simpler.

We rewrite this criterion in the notation of section 4.10. Let $W^{h_i} \in \mathbf{R}^{N_i}$. Then (4.114) is equivalent to the relation

$$[\![Q_i W^{h_i}]\!]_i^2 \le \frac{c_4}{(\lambda_i^*)^\alpha} \|\bar{L}_i W^{h_i}\|_i^{2\alpha} [\![W^{h_i}]\!]_i^{2(1-\alpha)}. \tag{5.75}$$

Due to Lemma 4.10.3, we have

$$[\![Q_i W^{h_i}]\!]_i = h_i [\![w^{h_i} - w^{h_{i-1}}]\!] \le c_{15} \|\bar{L}_i W^{h_i}\|_i, \tag{5.76}$$

where w^{h_i} is the prolongation in H^{h_i} of vector W^{h_i}; $w^{h_{i-1}} \in H^{h_{i-1}}$ is a solution of the Bubnov-Galerkin problem

$$\mathcal{L}(w^{h_{i-1}}, v) = \mathcal{L}(w^{h_i}, v) \qquad \forall v \in H^{h_{i-1}}. \tag{5.77}$$

First, because of (5.76), we have

$$[\![Q_i W^{h_i}]\!]_i^{2\alpha} \le c_{15}^{2\alpha} \|\bar{L}_i W^{h_i}\|_i^{2\alpha}. \tag{5.78}$$

Second, due to (5.77),

$$\mathcal{L}(w^{h_i} - w^{h_{i-1}}, w^{h_{i-1}}) = 0.$$

Therefore, owing to the Cauchy-Bunyakovski inequality, we get

$$[\![w^{h_i} - w^{h_{i-1}}]\!]^2 = \mathcal{L}(w^{h_i} - w^{h_{i-1}}, w^{h_i} - w^{h_{i-1}}) =$$
$$= \mathcal{L}(w^{h_i} - w^{h_{i-1}}, w^{h_i}) \leq [\![w^{h_i} - w^{h_{i-1}}]\!][\![w^{h_i}]\!]$$

and

$$[\![w^{h_i} - w^{h_{i-1}}]\!] \leq [\![w^{h_i}]\!].$$

Because of (5.76), (4.546), (4.552), we have

$$[\![Q_i W^{h_i}]\!]_i = h_i[\![w^{h_i} - w^{h_{i-1}}]\!] \leq h_i[\![W^{h_i}]\!]_i.$$

Let us raise both sides of it to the power $2(1-\alpha)$:

$$[\![Q_i W^{h_i}]\!]_i^{2(1-\alpha)} \leq h_i^{2(1-\alpha)}[\![W^{h_i}]\!]_i^{2(1-\alpha)}.$$

Multiplying left- and right-hand sides of this inequality and (5.78), we get

$$[\![Q_i W^{h_i}]\!]_i^2 \leq c_{15}^{2\alpha} h_i^{2(1-\alpha)} \|\bar{L}_i W^{h_i}\|_i^{2\alpha} [\![W^{h_i}]\!]_i^{2(1-\alpha)}. \tag{5.79}$$

Due to (5.71), we have

$$h_i \leq (c_6/\lambda_i^*)^{1/2(\rho-1)}.$$

Let us put

$$\alpha = 1/\rho, \tag{5.80}$$

then

$$h_i^{2(1-\alpha)} \leq (c_6/\lambda_i^*)^{\alpha}.$$

Employing it in (5.79), we get (5.75) with the constant $c_4 = c_6^{\alpha} c_{15}^{2\alpha}$.

Thus, all assumptions of Theorem 4.7 are valid and we have the convergence of $MMG^{(8)}$-algorithm with the rate characterized by (4.116)–(4.119). The rest proof of (5.73) follows from Theorem 4.30. Namely, there exists an integer $\bar{m}$ in (5.72) such that the estimate

$$\|\widetilde{V}^{h_i} - V^{h_i}\|_h^{(1)} \leq c_1 h_i |f|_0 \tag{5.81}$$

holds at each level $i = 1, 2, \ldots, p$. This $\bar{m}$ is independent of i, h_i, f.

The calculation of an amount of arithmetic operations is performed likewise in Lemma 5.1.3. Let Φ_i be the amount of arithmetic operations in $MMG^{(8)}$-algorithm with the numbers of iterations from (5.72). Then instead of (5.13) and (5.18), we have

$$\Phi_i \leq c_{16}\sigma^{p-i}\bar{m}N_i + 2\Phi_{i-1},$$
$$\Phi_i \leq c_{16}\sigma^{p-i}\bar{m}T_i + 2\Phi_{i-1}.$$

Using induction, we get

$$\Phi_i \leq \frac{2}{2-\sigma}\sigma^{p-i}\bar{m}c_{16}T_i + 2^i\Phi_0.$$

The rest calculations of the amount of arithmetic operations coincides with the proof of Lemma 5.1.4. □

Remark 5.3.1 *Inspite of worse regularity, we may implement $MG^{(7)}$-algorithm with the same m at each level i. Of course, the rate of convergence becomes worse than in regular case. Namely, instead of the contraction multiplier $O((m+1)^{-2})$ in (4.516), we get $O((m+1)^{-2\alpha})$, $\alpha \in (0,1)$. But the results of Theorem 4.28 remain the same.*

Remark 5.3.2 *Normalization of matrix L^{h_i} using a diagonal matrix shows to good advantage also in solving problems whose coefficients largely change in value in different zones. Such a situation occurs, for example, when solving the stationary heat equation for a medium composed of different thermal conductivity materials. In this connection, note that the line of discontinuity, when it intersects the boundary, can also produce singularities of the solution. The same applies to a case where different kinds of boundary-value conditions come in contact. To avoid after-effects of these singularities, the grid can also be refined with required ρ [146, p.273]. FMG-algorithm plus $MG^{(7)}$ or $MMG^{(8)}$ will then produce the same effect likewise in Theorem 5.4.*

5.4 The three-dimensional Dirichlet problem

In this section, we deal with the three-dimensional Dirichlet problem for a second-order elliptic equation. The Bubnov-Galerkin method with piecewise linear basis functions on tetrahedra is used for discretizing the problem. Algorithms synthesized in section 4.6 are used to approximately solve the system of linear algebraic equations obtained. They produce an approximate solution of the initial differential problem with accuracy $O(h^2)$ in norm $L_2(\Omega)$ using $O(N)$ arithmetic operations, where h is the characteristic linear size of spatial triangulation, and N is the number of its nodes.

Let us consider the Dirichlet problem on a *convex* polyhedron $\Omega \subset \mathbf{R}^3$ with a boundary Γ:

$$-\sum_{i,j=1}^{3} \partial_i(a_{ij}\partial_j u) + au = f \quad \text{in} \quad \Omega, \tag{5.82}$$

$$u = 0 \quad \text{on} \quad \Gamma. \tag{5.83}$$

The coefficients and the right-hand side of the equation satisfy the conditions

$$\partial_k a_{ij} \in L_3(\Omega), \qquad a_{ij} = a_{ji} \quad \text{on} \quad \bar{\Omega}, \qquad i,j,k = 1,2,3;$$

$$\mu \sum_{i=1}^{3} \xi_i^2 \le \sum_{i,j=1}^{3} a_{ij}\xi_i\xi_j \le \nu \sum_{i=1}^{3} \xi_i^2 \quad \text{on} \quad \bar{\Omega} \quad \forall \xi_i \subset \mathbf{R}, \quad \nu \ge \mu > 0; \tag{5.84}$$

$$a, f \in L_2(\Omega), \qquad a \ge 0 \quad \text{on convex } \bar{\Omega}.$$

These conditions are sufficient [94, p.230] for problem (5.82), (5.83) to be uniquely solvable in class $W_2^2(\Omega)$ and the estimate

$$\|u\|_2 \le c_1 |f|_0 \tag{5.85}$$

to be satisfied with constant c_1 independent of f.

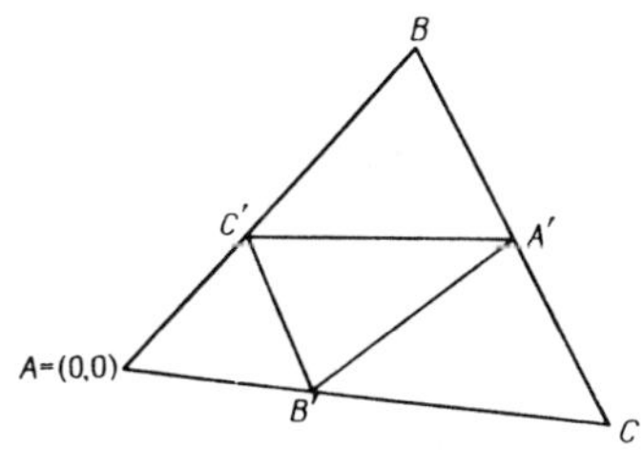

Figure 5.6: The complement of tetrahedron $ABCD$ upto prism.

Construct spatial triangulation of polyhedron Ω. First we divide it into a small number of closed regular tetrahedra (zones). We call this subdivision concordant if two any tetrahedra are mutually disjointed or have either one common vertex, or common entire edge, or common entire face. Denote the maximal length of the edges by l_0. Put $n_i = 2^i$, and for all $i = 0, 1, \dots, p$ divide every initial tetrahedron into n_i^3 equivolumed tetrahedra. For this purpose, complete every initial tetrahedron with two tetrahedra of the same volume to obtain a trihedral prism (Fig. 5.6). Divide its every edge into n_i equal parts and pass, through the obtained point, 4 families of planes parallel to the edges. As a result, we get n_i^3 prisms similar to the initial one with coefficient $1/n_i$. Each of these is further divided into 3 tetrahedra, just like the initial prism. Of $3n_i^3$ tetrahedra obtained, we retain only n_i^3 tetrahedra forming the initial tetrahedron. Finally, we have 3 kinds of tetrahedra of equal volume but with different lengths of edges.

Assume that the initial subdivision is concordant. Then, when divided, every initial tetrahedron again yields a concordant subdivision, the maximal edge length being not over $h_i = \sqrt{2}l_0/n_i$. Denote by $\bar{\Omega}_{h_i}$ the union of all vertices of tetrahedra obtained by dividing the edges of the initial tetrahedra into n_i parts and assume that $\Omega_{h_i} = \bar{\Omega}_{h_i} \bigcap \Omega$. We introduce in every point $y \in \Omega_{h_i}$ the basis function $\varphi_y^{h_i} \in \overset{\circ}{W}{}_2^1(\Omega)$ equal to 1 at node y, 0 at the other nodes of $\bar{\Omega}_{h_i}$ and linear on each tetrahedron of the i-th subdivision. Denote the linear span of this system of functions by H^{h_i}.

Introduce k_1 as the maximal number of tetrahedra edges meeting at one node $y \in \Omega_{h_0}$. Note that every tetrahedron of subdivision $\bar{\Omega}_{h_i}$ involves 8 tetrahedra of subdivision $\bar{\Omega}_{h_{i+1}}$, and so condition **G** of section 4.6 is valid about representation of the basis function of i-th subdivision by a linear combination of the finite number $c_4 = \max\{15, k_1\}$ of basis functions of the $(i+1)$-th subdivision.

Let us introduce the bilinear form

$$\mathcal{L}(u, v) = \int_\Omega (\sum_{i,j=1}^{3} a_{ij}\partial_j u \partial_i v + auv)dx.$$

According to the Bubnov-Galerkin method, we will seek the approximate solution $u^{h_i} \in H^{h_i}$ in the following form:

$$u^{h_i}(x) = \sum_{y \in \Omega_{h_i}} \alpha_y \varphi_y^{h_i}(x) \qquad (5.86)$$

where $\{\alpha_y\}$ are certain constants defined from the system of linear algebraic equations

$$\sum_{y\in\Omega_{h_i}} \alpha_y \mathcal{L}(\varphi_y^{h_i}, \varphi_z^{h_i}), \quad z \in \Omega_{h_i}. \tag{5.87}$$

The convergence of u^{h_i} to the exact solution is characterized by the following estimates (see Chapter 3):

$$|u - u^{h_i}|_0 \le c_2 h_i^2 |f|_0, \tag{5.88}$$

$$[\![u - u^{h_i}]\!] \le c_3 h_i |f|_0. \tag{5.89}$$

Thus, conditions **H** and **I** of section 4.6 are satisfied.

For vector W^{h_i} with components $W_y^{h_i}$, $y \in \Omega_{h_i}$, the piecewise linear prolongation is constructed by the formula

$$w^{h_i}(x) = \sum_{y\in\Omega_{h_i}} W_y^{h_i} \varphi_y^{h_i}(x).$$

Introduce the vector norm

$$\|W^{h_i}\|_h = |w^{h_i}|_0 \tag{5.90}$$

equivalent (on the ground of Theorem 3.13 of section 3.6) to the norm

$$\|W^{h_i}\|_E = (\sum_{y\in\Omega_{h_i}} (W_y^{h_i})^2 h_i^3)^{1/2},$$

i. e., condition **G** of section 4.6 is satisfied.

Put system (5.87) into vector-matrix form:

$$L^{h_i} V^{h_i} = F^{h_i}. \tag{5.91}$$

Here V^{h_i}, F^{h_i} are vectors of unknowns and the right-hand side with components $V_y^{h_i} = \alpha_y$, $F_z^{h_i} = (f, \varphi_z^{h_i})$; and L^{h_i} is an $N_i \times N_i$ symmetric matrix. For it, Theorem 3.14 of section 3.6 yields the following statement.

Lemma 5.4.1 *Under assumptions* (5.84), *eigenvalues* λ *of matrix* L^{h_i} *satisfy the inequality*

$$0 < \lambda \le c_5 h_i. \tag{5.92}$$

Thus, the assumptions of Theorems 4.14–4.17 of Chapter 4 are satisfied for both combinations of FMG-algorithm with $MG^{(1)}$ or $MG^{(2)}$.

Let us estimate the efficiency of $MG^{(2)}$-algorithm in three-dimensional case. We would remind that $\Phi_i(m)$ denotes the number of arithmetic operations in $MG^{(2)}$-algorithm with m iterations in pre-smoothing procedure (4.97). The computations analogous with Lemma 5.1.3 give the following result.

Lemma 5.4.2 *For* $MG^{(2)}$*-algorithm with any integer* $m \ge 1$, *we have estimate* (5.14).

Besides of this quarantee upper estimate, we are interested in the principle part of $\Phi_i(m)$ which gives the order of largness. We calculate it for sufficiently large m and i, assuming two facts: 14 edges of triangulation emanate from most of the points of Ω_{h_i}; and for relatively fine grids,

$$N_i = 8N_{i-1} + o(N_{i-1}). \tag{5.93}$$

Then, a calculation of arithmetic operations in the case of the double strategy ($\gamma = 2$) yields the equality

$$\Phi_i(m) = (32(m+1) + 21/8)N_i + 2\Phi_{i-1}(m) + 21N_i/8 + o(N_i).$$

The summation finally gives

$$\Phi_i(m) = (32(m+1) + 21/8)4N_i/3. \tag{5.94}$$

A result for combination of FMG-algorithm with $MG^{(2)}$ is not distinguish from Lemma 5.1.4. Again strategy $t = 1$ in FMG-algorithm is more effective than $t > 1$.

If we need the convergence in energy norm, then we have to use combination of FMG and $MG^{(1)}$-algorithms. For it in the three-dimensional case, the results of Lemmata 5.1.5, 5.1.6 remain valid.

5.5 The spectral problem

In this section, we deal with the spectral problem for a second-order elliptic differential equation. The Bubnov-Galerkin method with piecewise linear basis functions on triangles is used to discretize the problem as in section 5.1. The algorithms from sections 4.8 and 4.9 are used to solve approximately the obtained algebraic spectral problem. They give simple and multiple eigenvalues with accuracy $O(h^2)$ and corresponding eigenfunctions of the initial differential problem with the same accuracy in norm of $L_2(\Omega)$. To achieve this accuracy, it is necessary to perform $O(k^2N)$ arithmetic operations where k is the multiplicity of the eigenvalue of a differential problem, N is the number of nodes of a difference grid.

Let Ω be a convex polygon in $\mathbf{R}^2$ with a boundary Γ. Consider the spectral problem

$$-\sum_{i,j=1}^{2} \partial_i(a_{ij}\partial_j u) + au = \lambda u \quad \text{in} \quad \Omega, \tag{5.95}$$

$$u = 0 \quad \text{on} \quad \Gamma. \tag{5.96}$$

Let the coefficients satisfy conditions (5.3) and

$$0 \le a \le c_1 \quad \text{on} \quad \bar{\Omega}. \tag{5.97}$$

We want to calculate approximately the r-th eigenvalue λ_r and the r-th eigenfunction v_r normed as follows:

$$|v_r|_0 = 1. \tag{5.98}$$

Let λ_r be multiple:

$$\lambda_{l-1} < \lambda_l = \lambda_{l+1} = \ldots = \lambda_k < \lambda_{k+1}, \qquad l \le r \le k. \tag{5.99}$$

Therefore the whole subspace $\mathcal{B}$ of eigenfunctions with dimension $k-l+1$ corresponds to eigenvalues $\lambda_l = \ldots = \lambda_k$. We already wrote that it is expedient to find not one representative of the subspace $\mathcal{B}$ but its basis.

To construct an algebraic spectral problem, we will use the notation and the terms of section 5.1. First we divide the initial polygon Ω into a small number of closed triangles so that this subdivision is concordant. Then for $i = 0, 1, \ldots, q$ we construct grids Ω_{h_i} by dividing every initial triangle into 4^i equal parts. Afterwards we introduce piecewise linear basis functions $\varphi_y^{h_i}$ and denote their linear span by H^{h_i}.

According to the Bubnov-Galerkin method, approximate eigenfunctions will be sought in the following form:

$$u^{h_i}(x) = \sum_{y \in \Omega_{h_i}} \alpha_y \varphi_y^{h_i}(x) \tag{5.100}$$

where $\{\alpha_y\}$ are certain constants defined from algebraic spectral problem (4.322) of section 4.8. Let us label the nodes of set Ω_{h_i} consistently from 1 to N_i and write this problem in matrix form:

$$L^{h_i} V^{h_i} = \lambda^{h_i} M^{h_i} V^{h_i} \tag{5.101}$$

where L^{h_i}, M^{h_i} are symmetric positive-definite $N_i \times N_i$-matrices with elements $\mathcal{L}(\varphi_y^{h_i}, \varphi_z^{h_i})$, $(\varphi_y^{h_i}, \varphi_z^{h_i})$ in the notation of sections 5.1, 4.8; λ^{h_i} is an eigenvalue; V^{h_i} is an eigenvector.

A piecewise linear prolongation w^{h_i} from H^{h_i} is assigned by formula (5.7) to each vector W^{h_i}, and vector norms are introduced by (5.8), (5.9). We introduce also the vector scalar product

$$(V^{h_i}, W^{h_i})_i = (v^{h_i}, w^{h_i}) \tag{5.102}$$

where v^{h_i} is the prolongation of vector $V^{h_i} \in \mathbf{R}^{N_i}$ in H^{h_i}. Using matrix M^{h_i}, this scalar product is written as follows:

$$(V^{h_i}, W^{h_i})_i = (V^{h_i})^T M^{h_i} W^{h_i}. \tag{5.103}$$

Note that $\lambda_l^{h_i}, \ldots, \lambda_k^{h_i}$ may be not equal in algebraic problem (5.101). Nevertheless we will find the whole subspace $\mathcal{V}^{h_i}$ of eigenvectors with dimension $k-l+1$ corresponding to all these eigenvalues. To describe the convergence, let us introduce also the space $\mathcal{B}^{h_i}$ of prolongations v^{h_i} in H^{h_i} of all elements $V^{h_i} \in \mathcal{V}^{h_i}$. Due to linearity of isomorphism introduced by (5.7), (5.8) between $\mathbf{R}^{N_i}$ and H^{h_i}, this definition coincides with (4.404).

The convergence of solutions of the algebraic spectral problem (5.101) is characterized by properties cited in subsection 1.2.2 and section 4.9. Conditions **K** and **L**, e. g., follow from [48], [192]:

$$|\lambda_j^{h_i} - \lambda_j| \le c_{18} h_i^2, \qquad j = l, \ldots, k, \tag{5.104}$$

$$\Theta(\mathcal{B}, \mathcal{B}^{h_i}) \le c_{19} h_i^2, \tag{5.105}$$

where Θ is the opening defined by (4.350).

For the numerical solution of formulated problem, consider first an initial triangulation and assume that the set Ω_{h_0} involves no less than k nodes. For the spectral problem (5.101) on this grid, we find practically exact eigenvalues $\lambda_j^{h_0}$ and eigenvectors $V_j^{h_0}$ with $j = l, \dots, k$ orthonormed in scalar product $(\cdot,\cdot)_i$. Their accuracy is characterized by (5.104), (5.105) at $i = 0$.

On subsequent grids $\Omega_{h_1}, \dots, \Omega_{h_p}$, approximate eigenvalues and vectors are constructed using the $FMG^{(3)}$-algorithm discussed in section 4.9. To use the results of this section, the condition $\mathbf{J}'$ is necessary to be satisfied. It applies to the following problem:

$$-\sum_{i,j=1}^{2} \partial_i(a_{ij}\partial_j u) + au - \lambda_r u = f \quad \text{in} \quad \Omega, \tag{5.106}$$

$$u = 0 \quad \text{on} \quad \Gamma. \tag{5.107}$$

Since the problem is singular, its 'solution' will be understood as a normal solution like u_H in section 4.8. On each grid Ω_{h_i}, this problem will be juxtaposed with the Bubnov-Galerkin system which has the form

$$(L^{h_i} - \lambda_0^{h_i} M^{h_i})W^{h_i} = F^{h_i} \tag{5.108}$$

with the right-hand side

$$F_z^{h_i} = (f, \varphi_z^{h_i}), \qquad z \in \Omega_{h_i},$$

and approximate eigenvalue $\lambda_0^{h_i}$ which may take values $\tilde{\lambda}_r^{h_{i-1}}$, $\tilde{\lambda}_r^{h_i}$, $\lambda_r^{h_i}$ depending on situation. As a 'solution' of problem (5.108), we consider the quasi-solution $W_H^{h_i}$ defined in section 4.8. Denote its piecewise linear prolongation in H^{h_i} by $w_H^{h_i}$. Now we have to prove the estimate (4.417).

Theorem 5.5 *Let conditions* (5.97), (5.3), (5.99), (5.104), (5.105) *be satisfied. Let also the approximate value* $\lambda_0^{h_i}$ *satisfy the estimates*

$$|\lambda_j^{h_i} - \lambda_0^{h_i}| \geq c_9 \qquad \forall j \notin [l, k], \tag{5.109}$$

$$|\lambda_r - \lambda_0^{h_i}| \leq c_2^2(c_{18} + 1)h_i^2 \tag{5.110}$$

with constant c_2 *from* (4.226)*; and let* h_i *be sufficiently small:*

$$h_i \leq (c_{18} + 1)^{-1/2}. \tag{5.111}$$

Then the normal solution u_H *of problem* (5.106), (5.107) *and the prolongation* $w_H^{h_i}$ *of quasi-solution of problem* (5.108) *obey the estimate*

$$|u_H - w_H^{h_i}|_0 \leq c_6 h_i^2 |f|_0. \tag{5.112}$$

Proof. Let us first show that $u_H \in W_2^2(\Omega)$. Consider the infinite system $\{v_1, v_2, \dots\}$ of eigenfunctions v_j corresponding to eigenvalues λ_j. This system is complete and is supposed to be orthonormed in $L_2(\Omega)$, therefore

$$f = \sum_{j=1}^{\infty} \alpha_j v_j \qquad \text{where} \qquad \alpha_j = (f, v_j). \tag{5.113}$$

By definition, the normal solution is described by formula

$$u_H = \sum_{\substack{j=1 \\ j\notin[l,k]}}^{\infty} \frac{\alpha_j}{\lambda_j - \lambda_r} v_j. \tag{5.114}$$

Since $\lambda_l, \dots, \lambda_k$ are separated from other eigenvalues on the ground of (5.99), the estimate (4.399) is valid. Use it with (5.114):

$$|u_H|_0^2 \le c_{20}^{-2} \sum_{j=1}^{\infty} \alpha_j^2 = c_{20}^{-2} |f|_0^2;$$

hence,

$$|u_H|_0 \le c_{20}^{-1} |f|_0 \tag{5.115}$$

and $u_H \in L_2(\Omega)$. Let $f_H = (I - P)f$ with the orthogonal projector P from $L_2(\Omega)$ into $\mathcal{B}$. Then

$$|f_H|_0 \le |f|_0, \tag{5.116}$$

and we can rewrite the simbolic equation (5.106) into the real equality

$$-\sum_{i,j=1}^{2} \partial_i(a_{ij}\partial_j u) + au = f_H + \lambda_r u_H \quad \text{in} \quad \Omega. \tag{5.117}$$

On the ground of well-known results from [94], the problem (5.117), (5.107) has a unique solution coincident with u_H, and the following estimate holds on convex domain Ω:

$$\|u_H\|_2 \le c|f_H + \lambda_r u_H|_0.$$

Using (5.115), (5.116), we get

$$\|u_H\|_2 \le c(1 + c_{20}^{-1}\lambda_r)|f|_0 \le c|f|_0, \tag{5.118}$$

i. e., $u_H \in W_2^2(\Omega)$. During this proof, we denote by letter c the different constants independent of h_i, f for the sake of simplicity.

Second, let us consider system (5.108). Decompose F^{h_i} into the orthonormed system $\{V_1^{h_i}, \dots, V_{N_i}^{h_i}\}$ of eigenvectors $V_j^{h_i}$ of spectral problem (5.101):

$$F^{h_i} = M^{h_i} \sum_{j=1}^{N_i} \beta_j V_j^{h_i} \quad \text{where} \quad \beta_j = (F^{h_i})^T V_j^{h_i}. \tag{5.119}$$

By definition of quasi-solution,

$$W_H^{h_i} = \sum_{\substack{j=1 \\ j\notin[l,k]}}^{N_i} \frac{\beta_j}{\lambda_j^{h_i} - \lambda_0^{h_i}} V_j^{h_i}. \tag{5.120}$$

Moreover, we can rewrite the symbolic system (5.108) into the real equality

$$(L^{h_i} - \lambda_0^{h_i} M^{h_i}) W_H^{h_i} = \bar{F}^{h_i} \tag{5.121}$$

with the vector

$$\bar{F}^{h_i} = M^{h_i} \sum_{\substack{j=1 \\ j \notin [l,k]}}^{N_i} \beta_j V_j^{h_i}. \tag{5.122}$$

On the ground of (4.353), components of this vector equal

$$\bar{F}_y^{h_i} = (\bar{f}, \varphi_y^{h_i}), \qquad y \in \Omega_{h_i}, \tag{5.123}$$

where $\bar{f} = (I - \bar{P})f$ with the orthogonal projector $\bar{P}$ from $L_2(\Omega)$ into $\mathcal{B}^{h_i}$.

For any $x \in \mathbf{R}$ such that $|x - \lambda_0^{h_i}| \geq c_9$, we have

$$|x/(x - \lambda_0^{h_i})| \leq 1 + \lambda_0^{h_i}/c_9. \tag{5.124}$$

On the ground of (5.110), (5.111), we get

$$\lambda_0^{h_i} \leq \lambda_r + c_2^2(c_{18} + 1)h_i^2 \leq \lambda_k + c_2^2. \tag{5.125}$$

Hence, the right-hand side of (5.124) is bounded:

$$|x/(x - \lambda_0^{h_i})| \leq c_{25} = 1 + (\lambda_k + c_2^2)/c_9. \tag{5.126}$$

From this, (5.109), (4.324), (5.120), we obtain

$$\|W_H^{h_i}\|_h^2 = (W_H^{h_i}, W_H^{h_i})_i = \sum_{\substack{j=1 \\ j \notin [l,k]}}^{N_i} \beta_j^2 (\lambda_j^{h_i} - \lambda_0^{h_i})^{-2} \leq c_{25}^2 \sum_{j=1}^{N_i} \beta_j^2 (\lambda_j^{h_i})^{-2}. \tag{5.127}$$

There is the estimate

$$\sum_{j=1}^{N_i} \beta_j^2 (\lambda_j^{h_i})^{-2} \leq \sup_{\gamma_j} \{(\sum_{j=1}^{N_i} \beta_j \gamma_j)^2 / \sum_{j=1}^{N_i} (\lambda_j^{h_i})^2 \gamma_j^2\} \tag{5.128}$$

because the expression in braces of the right-hand side equals the left-hand side when $\gamma_j = \beta_j / \lambda_j^{h_i}$. The set $\{\gamma_1, \ldots, \gamma_{N_i}\}$ one-to-one corresponds to vector

$$\Psi = \sum_{j=1}^{N_i} \gamma_j V_j^{h_i}. \tag{5.129}$$

Since $V_j^{h_i}$ are orthonormed in scalar product $(\cdot, \cdot)_i$, the right-hand side of (5.128) equals

$$\sup_{\Psi \in \mathbf{R}^{N_i}} \{(F^{h_i})^T \Psi / \|\Psi\|_h^{(2)}\}^2$$

where

$$\|\Psi\|_h^{(2)} = \|(M^{h_i})^{-1} L^{h_i} \Psi\|_h. \tag{5.130}$$

Let us combine (5.127) with last four relations and extract the square root:

$$\|W_H^{h_i}\|_h \leq c_{25} \sup_{\Psi \in \mathbf{R}^{N_i}} \{(F^{h_i})^T \Psi / \|\Psi\|_h^{(2)}\}. \tag{5.131}$$

Let us introduce the interpolant $u_H^I \in H^{h_i}$ of u_H by the formula

$$u_H^I = \sum_{y\in\Omega_{h_i}} u_H(y)\varphi_y \tag{5.132}$$

and the vector U_H^I with components $U_{H,y}^I = u_H(y)$. On the ground of Theorem 3.3 and (5.118), we get

$$|u_H - u_H^I|_0 \le ch_i^2\|u_H\|_2 \le ch_i^2|f|_0. \tag{5.133}$$

Consider the problem: find a quasi-solution of the system

$$(L^{h_i} - \lambda_0^{h_i}M^{h_i})Z^{h_i} = \bar{F}^{h_i} - (L^{h_i} - \lambda_0^{h_i}M^{h_i})U_H^I. \tag{5.134}$$

The vector $W_H^{h_i} - U_H^I$ satisfies this equality due to (5.121). Therefore the vector $V^{h_i} = (I-P_h)(W_H^{h_i} - U_H^I)$ is the quasi-solution of (5.134), where P_h is the orthogonal projector from $\mathbf{R}^{N_i}$ into $\mathcal{V}^{h_i}$ in the scalar product $(\cdot,\cdot)_i$. It follows also from comparison of weights in the decomposition of vectors U_H^I, $W_H^{h_i}$ into the basis $\{V_j^{h_i}\}$. For the quasi-solution of problem (5.134), we have the estimate like (5.131):

$$\|V^{h_i}\|_h \le c_{25} \sup_{\Psi\in\mathbf{R}^{N_i}} \{(\bar{F}^{h_i} - (L^{h_i} - \lambda_0^{h_i}M^{h_i})U_H^I)^T\Psi/\|\Psi\|_h^{(2)}\}. \tag{5.135}$$

Let us introduce the prolongation $\psi \in H^{h_i}$ of vector $\Psi \in \mathbf{R}^{N_i}$ and transform the numerator in braces with the help of (5.117) and explicit form of elements of matrices L^{h_i}, M^{h_i}:

$$(\bar{F}^{h_i} - (L^{h_i} - \lambda_0^{h_i}M^{h_i})U_H^I)^T\Psi = (\bar{f},\psi) - \mathcal{L}(u_H^I,\psi) - \lambda_0^{h_i}(u_H^I,\psi) =$$

$$= (f_H,\psi) + (\bar{f} - f_H,\psi) - \mathcal{L}(u_H^I,\psi) - \lambda_0^{h_i}(u_H^I,\psi) = \tag{5.136}$$

$$= \mathcal{L}(u_H - u_H^I,\psi) - (\lambda_r - \lambda_0^{h_i})(u_H,\psi) - \lambda_0^{h_i}(u_H - u_H^I,\psi) + ((\bar{P} - P)f,\psi).$$

Let us evaluate each term in the right-hand side. For the first term, we introduce the function $\hat{u}_H \in H^{h_i}$ which is a usual solution of the Bubnov-Galerkin problem

$$\mathcal{L}(\hat{u}_H, v) = \mathcal{L}(u_H, v) \qquad \forall v \in H^{h_i}. \tag{5.137}$$

Since $u_H \in W_2^2(\Omega)$, we get $\mathcal{L}(u_H, v) = (g, v)\ \ \forall v \in \overset{\circ}{W}{}_2^1(\Omega)$ with the function

$$g = -\sum_{i,j=1}^{2} \partial_i(a_{ij}\partial_j u_H) + au_H \in L_2(\Omega).$$

Therefore, the usual considerations (e. g., Theorem 3.7) together with (5.118) give

$$|\hat{u}_H - u_H|_0 \le ch_i^2\|u_H\|_2 \le ch_i^2|f|_0. \tag{5.138}$$

Denote by $\hat{U}_H$ the vector with components $\hat{U}_{H,y} = \hat{u}_H(y)$. Let us use (5.137) and the explicit form of matrices M^{h_i}, L^{h_i}:

$$\mathcal{L}(u_H - u_H^I,\psi) = \mathcal{L}(\hat{u}_H - u_H^I,\psi) = (\hat{U}_H - U_H^I)^T L^{h_i}\Psi =$$

$$((M^{h_i})^{1/2}(\hat{U}_H - U_H^I))^T (M^{h_i})^{1/2}(M^{h_i})^{-1}L^{h_i}\Psi.$$

Then we apply the algebraic Cauchy-Bunyakovski inequality and definitions (5.130), (4.231), (4.324):

$$|\mathcal{L}(u_H - u_H^I, \psi)| \leq \|\hat{U}_H - U_H^I\|_h \cdot \|(M^{h_i})^{-1}L^{h_i}\Psi\|_h = |\hat{u}_H - u_H^I|_0 \cdot \|\Psi\|_h^{(2)}.$$

On the ground of (5.138) and (5.133), we have

$$|\hat{u}_H - u_H^I|_0 \leq |\hat{u}_H - u_H|_0 + |u_H - u_H^I|_0 \leq ch_i^2|f|_0.$$

Combining three last relations, we get

$$|\mathcal{L}(u_H - u_H^I, \psi)| \leq ch_i^2|f|_0\|\Psi\|_h^{(2)}. \tag{5.139}$$

To evaluate the second term in the right-hand side of (5.136), we use (5.110), (5.118), the Cauchy-Bunyakovski inequality:

$$|(\lambda_r - \lambda_0^{h_i})(u_H, \psi)| \leq ch_i^2|u_H|_0|\psi|_0 \leq ch_i^2|f|_0\|\Psi\|_h. \tag{5.140}$$

Now we prove the inequality

$$\|\Psi\|_h \leq \lambda_1^{-1}\|\Psi\|_h^{(2)}. \tag{5.141}$$

Indeed, let us use the decomposition (5.129). Then

$$\|\Psi\|_h^2 = \sum_{j=1}^{N_i} \gamma_j^2, \tag{5.142}$$

$$(\|\Psi\|_h^{(2)})^2 = (L^{h_i}\Psi)^T(M^{h_i})^{-1}L^{h_i}\Psi = \sum_{j=1}^{N_i}(\lambda_j^{h_i}\gamma_j)^2.$$

Owing to the minimum principle [132], [192],

$$\lambda_j^{h_i} \geq \lambda_j \qquad \forall j = 1, \ldots, N_i.$$

Since $\mathcal{L}$ is positive-definite and the sequence λ_j is monotone, we have

$$\lambda_j^{h_i} \geq \lambda_j \geq \lambda_1 > 0.$$

Therefore

$$\lambda_1^2 \sum_{j=1}^{N_i} \gamma_j^2 \leq \sum_{j=1}^{N_i}(\lambda_j^{h_i}\gamma_j)^2,$$

that proves (5.141) on the ground of (5.142). Combining (5.140) with (5.141), we get

$$|(\lambda_r - \lambda_0^{h_i})(u_H, \psi)| \leq ch_i^2|f|_0\|\Psi\|_h^{(2)}. \tag{5.143}$$

To evaluate the third term in the right-hand side of (5.136), we apply (5.133), (5.125), (5.118), (5.141), the Cauchy-Bunyakovski inequality:

$$|\lambda_0^{h_i}(u_H - u_H^I, \psi)| \leq (\lambda_k + c_2^2)|u_H - u_H^I|_0|\psi|_0 \leq ch_i^2|f|_0\|\Psi\|_h^{(2)}. \tag{5.144}$$

For the fourth term in (5.136), we use the Cauchy-Bunyakovski and Cauchy inequalities, (5.141), (5.105), the equality

$$\Theta(\mathcal{B},\mathcal{B}^{h_i}) = |P - \bar{P}|_0. \tag{5.145}$$

As a result, we have

$$((\bar{P} - P)f,\psi) \le |(\bar{P} - P)f|_0|\psi|_0 \le ch_i^2|f|_0\|\Psi\|_h^{(2)}. \tag{5.146}$$

Let us combine (5.135), (5.136), (5.139), (5.143), (5.144), (5.146):

$$\|V^{h_i}\|_h \le ch_i^2|f|_0. \tag{5.147}$$

The isomorphism introduced by (5.7), (5.8) between normed spaces $\mathbf{R}^{N_i}$ and H^{h_i} gives correspondences $\mathcal{V}^{h_i} \leftrightarrow \mathcal{B}^{h_i}$, $P_h \leftrightarrow \bar{P}$. Therefore, by definition of V^{h_i}, we get

$$\|V^{h_i}\|_h = \|(I - P_h)(W_H^{h_i} - U_H^I)\|_h = |(I - \bar{P})(w_H^{h_i} - u_H^I)|_0 \le ch_i^2|f|_0. \tag{5.148}$$

Moreover, from the method of definition, it follows that

$$u_H = (I - P)u_H, \qquad w_H^{h_i} = (I - \bar{P})w_H^{h_i}.$$

Hence,

$$|w_H^{h_i} - u_H|_0 = |(I - \bar{P})w_H^{h_i} - (I - P)u_H|_0 \le$$

$$\le |(I - \bar{P})(w_H^{h_i} - u_H^I)|_0 + |(P - \bar{P})u_H^I|_0 + |(I - P)(u_H^I - u_H)|_0.$$

Operator $I - P$ is an orthogonal projector in $L_2(\Omega)$, therefore

$$|I - P|_0 \le 1.$$

Then we use (5.133), (5.118), (5.111):

$$|u_H^I|_0 \le |u_H|_0 + |u_H^I - u_H|_0 \le c|f|_0 + ch_i^2|f|_0 \le c|f|_0.$$

Combining three last inequalities with (5.145), (5.105), we get (5.112). □

Let us show that assumptions of Theorem 5.5 are satisfied under conditions of Theorem 4.26. We have 3 situations for use of condition $\mathbf{J}'$, i. e., estimate (5.112).

First situation happens at stage $\mathbf{B}_4^{(3)}$ with $i \ge 2$, where $\lambda_0^{h_i} = \tilde{\lambda}_r^{h_{i-1}}$. Then the estimate (4.434) is supposed to be already proved for $i-1$, and we can use it with (4.226), (4.403):

$$|\lambda_r - \tilde{\lambda}_r^{h_{i-1}}| \le |\lambda_r - \lambda_r^{h_{i-1}}| + |\lambda_r^{h_{i-1}} - \tilde{\lambda}_r^{h_{i-1}}| \le c_{18}h_{i-1}^2 + \varepsilon h_{i-1}^2 \le c_2^2(c_{18}+1)h_i^2.$$

Thus, (5.110) is proved. Let us use it for $r = k$ together with (4.399) and (4.403) for $j = k+1$:

$$\lambda_{k+1}^{h_i} - \tilde{\lambda}_r^{h_{i-1}} \ge \lambda_{k+1}^{h_i} - \tilde{\lambda}_k^{h_{i-1}} \ge$$

$$\ge (\lambda_{k+1} - \lambda_k) - |\lambda_k - \tilde{\lambda}_k^{h_{i-1}}| - |\lambda_{k+1} - \lambda_{k+1}^{h_i}| \ge$$

$$\geq c_{20} - c_2^2(c_{18}+1)h_i^2 - c_{18}h_i^2.$$

Now we use the constant c_{21} defined by (4.430) and the inequality

$$h_i^2 \leq c_{20}/2c_{21} \tag{5.149}$$

following from (4.440). As a result, we have

$$\lambda_{k+1}^{h_i} - \tilde{\lambda}_r^{h_{i-1}} \geq c_{20}/2.$$

Analogously,

$$\tilde{\lambda}_r^{h_{i-1}} - \lambda_{l-1}^{h_i} \geq c_{20}/2.$$

Therefore, (5.109) is proved with $c_9 = c_{20}/2$.

Second situation happens again at stage $\mathbf{B}_4^{(3)}$ but with $i = 1$, where $\lambda_0^{h_i} = \lambda_r^{h_0}$. Then the previous evaluation is simplified. Indeed, on the ground of (4.403), (4.226), we have

$$|\lambda_r - \lambda_r^{h_0}| \leq c_{18}h_0^2 \leq c_2^2(c_{18}+1)h_1^2.$$

The consequent steps are the same.

Third situation happens at stage $\mathbf{A}_4^{(5)}$ where $\lambda_0^{h_i} = \tilde{\lambda}_r^{h_i}$. We need to take into consideration the replacement of $i-1$ by i for the sake of uniformity of all three situations. With this replacement, the estimate (4.434) is supposed to be already proved for i, and we can use it with (4.403):

$$|\lambda_r - \tilde{\lambda}_r^{h_i}| \leq |\lambda_r - \lambda_r^{h_i}| + |\lambda_r^{h_i} - \tilde{\lambda}_r^{h_i}| \leq c_{18}h_i^2 + \varepsilon h_i^2 \leq c_2^2(c_{18}+1)h_i^2.$$

Since (5.110) is proved, let us use it for $r = k$ together with (4.399) and (4.403) for $j = k+1$:

$$\lambda_{k+1} - \tilde{\lambda}_r^{h_i} \geq \lambda_{k+1}^{h_i} - \tilde{\lambda}_k^{h_i} \geq$$

$$(\lambda_{k+1} - \lambda_k) - |\lambda_k - \lambda_k^{h_i}| - |\lambda_{k+1} - \lambda_{k+1}^{h_i}| \geq c_{20} - c_{21}h_i^2 \geq c_{20}/2.$$

We again apply (4.430) and (5.149). Analogously,

$$\tilde{\lambda}_r^{h_i} - \lambda_{l-1}^{h_i} \geq c_{20}/2,$$

and (5.109) is proved with $c_9 = c_{20}/2$.

So, all three situations are treated, and (5.109), (5.110) are proved. The remaining inequality (5.111) coincides with (4.449) following from (4.440).

As a result, we have the estimates (4.424), (4.425) for eigenvalues $\tilde{\lambda}_r^{h_i}$ and eigensubspace $\tilde{\mathcal{V}}^{h_i}$ computed by the $FMG^{(3)}$-algorithm. In the framework of mensioned isomorphism between $\mathbf{R}^{N_i}$ and H^{h_i}, the subspace $\tilde{\mathcal{V}}^{h_i}$ corresponds to the subspace $\tilde{\mathcal{B}}^{h_i} = \text{span}\{\tilde{v}_l^{h_i}, \ldots, \tilde{v}_k^{h_i}\}$ of prolongations for all vectors from $\tilde{\mathcal{V}}^{h_i}$. Thus,

$$\Theta(\tilde{\mathcal{B}}^{h_i}, \mathcal{B}^{h_i}) = \Theta_h(\tilde{\mathcal{V}}^{h_i}, \mathcal{V}^{h_i}) \leq \varepsilon h_i^2, \qquad i = 1, \ldots, q.$$

The amount of arithmetic operations are counted in the same way as in section 5.1. The only difference consists in the amount of operations for orthogonalization. Therefore we omit the proof of the following

Table 5.2:

m	Grid	$\lvert\lambda_1 - \tilde{\lambda}_1^h\rvert$	$\lvert\lambda_2 - \tilde{\lambda}_2^h\rvert$	$\lvert\lambda_3 - \tilde{\lambda}_3^h\rvert$	Computer time a, *sec*	Computer time b, *msec*
1	2	3	4	5	6	7
2	3×3	3.1	13.2	22.2	0.20	22.22
	7×7	0.80	3.53	5.61	0.30	6.12
	15×15	$2.0 \cdot 10^{-1}$	0.89	1.39	0.88	3.91
	31×31	$4.9 \cdot 10^{-2}$	$2.1 \cdot 10^{-1}$	$3.3 \cdot 10^{-1}$	3.42	3.56
	63×63	$1.3 \cdot 10^{-2}$	$5.2 \cdot 10^{-2}$	$8.1 \cdot 10^{-2}$	13.98	3.52
	127×127	$3.0 \cdot 10^{-2}$	$1.3 \cdot 10^{-2}$	$2.0 \cdot 10^{-2}$	56.88	3.53
4	3×3	3.1	13.2	22.2	0.20	22.22
	7×7	$7.7 \cdot 10^{-1}$	3.30	5.30	0.32	6.53
	15×15	$1.9 \cdot 10^{-1}$	0.82	1.29	1.02	4.53
	31×31	$4.8 \cdot 10^{-2}$	$2.1 \cdot 10^{-1}$	$3.2 \cdot 10^{-1}$	4.20	4.37
	63×63	$1.2 \cdot 10^{-2}$	$5.1 \cdot 10^{-2}$	$8.0 \cdot 10^{-2}$	17.69	4.46
	127×127	$3.0 \cdot 10^{-3}$	$1.3 \cdot 10^{-2}$	$2.0 \cdot 10^{-2}$	73.00	4.53
6	3×3	3.1	13.2	22.2	0.20	22.22
	7×7	$7.7 \cdot 10^{-1}$	3.29	5.27	0.34	6.94
	15×15	$1.9 \cdot 10^{-2}$	$8.2 \cdot 10^{-1}$	1.29	1.14	5.07
	31×31	$4.8 \cdot 10^{-2}$	$2.0 \cdot 10^{-1}$	$3.2 \cdot 10^{-1}$	4.96	5.16
	63×63	$1.2 \cdot 10^{-2}$	$5.1 \cdot 10^{-2}$	$8.0 \cdot 10^{-2}$	21.62	5.45
	127×127	$3.0 \cdot 10^{-3}$	$1.3 \cdot 10^{-2}$	$2.0 \cdot 10^{-2}$	89.34	5.54

Theorem 5.6 *Let* (5.3), (5.97), (5.99) *be satisfied. Then for any* $\varepsilon \in (0,1)$, *the* $FMG^{(3)}$*-algorithm gives approximate eigenvalues* $\tilde{\lambda}_r^{h_q}$, $r = l, \dots, k$, *and approximate eigensubspace* $\tilde{\mathcal{B}}^{h_q}$ *with accuracy*

$$|\tilde{\lambda}_r^{h_q} - \lambda_r^{h_q}| \le \varepsilon^2 h_q^2,$$

$$\Theta(\tilde{\mathcal{B}}^{h_q}, \mathcal{B}^{h_q}) \le \varepsilon h_q^2.$$

It takes an amount of arithmetic operations less than $cN_q(k-l+1)^2$, *where* N_q *is the amount of nodes in* Ω_{h_q}, $k-l+1$ *is the multiplicity of eigenvalue* λ_r.

To illustrate these conclusions, we give numerical experiments on solving the following spectral problem. Let Ω be square $(0,1) \times (0,1)$ with boundary Γ. It is necessary to find eigenvalues and eigenfunctions of the spectral problem

$$-\Delta u = \lambda u \quad \text{in} \quad \Omega, \tag{5.150}$$

$$u = 0 \quad \text{on} \quad \Gamma. \tag{5.151}$$

The triangulation of Ω and grids Ω_{h_i} are constructed in the same way, as in section 5.1. Table 5.2 gives the data on the accuracy of three first approximate eigenvalues of the algebraic spectral problem (5.101) which are determined by $FMG^{(3)}$-algorithm

Table 5.3:

m	Grid	$\Vert U^h - \widetilde{V}_1^h \Vert_h$	$\Vert U^h - \widetilde{V}_2^h \Vert_h$	$\Vert U^h - \widetilde{V}_3^h \Vert_h$	Computer time	
					a, *sec*	b, *msec*
1	2	3	4	5	6	7
2	3×3	$9.6 \cdot 10^{-2}$	$1.9 \cdot 10^{-1}$	$2.4 \cdot 10^{-1}$	0.80	22.22
	7×7	$3.1 \cdot 10^{-2}$	$7.2 \cdot 10^{-2}$	$8.7 \cdot 10^{-2}$	0.37	7.55
	15×15	$9.1 \cdot 10^{-3}$	$2.4 \cdot 10^{-2}$	$3.0 \cdot 10^{-2}$	1.27	5.64
	31×31	$2.0 \cdot 10^{-3}$	$5.6 \cdot 10^{-3}$	$7.1 \cdot 10^{-3}$	5.80	6.04
	63×63	$4.4 \cdot 10^{-4}$	$1.1 \cdot 10^{-3}$	$1.3 \cdot 10^{-3}$	26.18	6.60
	127×127	$1.1 \cdot 10^{-4}$	$2.4 \cdot 10^{-4}$	$3.0 \cdot 10^{-4}$	112.95	7.00
4	3×3	$9.6 \cdot 10^{-2}$	$1.9 \cdot 10^{-1}$	$2.4 \cdot 10^{-1}$	0.20	22.22
	7×7	$2.6 \cdot 10^{-2}$	$5.6 \cdot 10^{-2}$	$7.3 \cdot 10^{-2}$	0.40	8.16
	15×15	$7.1 \cdot 10^{-3}$	$1.6 \cdot 10^{-2}$	$2.0 \cdot 10^{-2}$	1.66	7.38
	31×31	$1.7 \cdot 10^{-3}$	$4.0 \cdot 10^{-3}$	$5.2 \cdot 10^{-3}$	7.69	8.00
	63×63	$4.2 \cdot 10^{-4}$	$9.5 \cdot 10^{-4}$	$1.2 \cdot 10^{-3}$	34.12	8.60
	127×127	$1.0 \cdot 10^{-4}$	$2.3 \cdot 10^{-4}$	$3.0 \cdot 10^{-4}$	142.48	8.83
6	3×3	$9.6 \cdot 10^{-2}$	$1.9 \cdot 10^{-1}$	$2.4 \cdot 10^{-1}$	0.20	22.22
	7×7	$2.6 \cdot 10^{-2}$	$5.5 \cdot 10^{-2}$	$7.2 \cdot 10^{-2}$	0.48	9.80
	15×15	$6.8 \cdot 10^{-3}$	$1.5 \cdot 10^{-2}$	$2.0 \cdot 10^{-2}$	2.19	9.73
	31×31	$1.7 \cdot 10^{-3}$	$3.9 \cdot 10^{-3}$	$5.0 \cdot 10^{-3}$	9.83	10.23
	63×63	$4.2 \cdot 10^{-4}$	$9.4 \cdot 10^{-4}$	$1.2 \cdot 10^{-3}$	42.41	10.68
	127×127	$1.0 \cdot 10^{-4}$	$2.3 \cdot 10^{-4}$	$3.0 \cdot 10^{-4}$	175.16	10.86

for $m = 2, 4, 6$. Analogous data on the accuracy of the approximate eigenvectors corresponding to them are provided in Table 5.3.

In column 2, the number of interior nodes of the grid is given. In Columns 3 to 5 of Table 5.2, the errors of three first eigenvalues are provided. Column 6 shows the time (a) in seconds to compute the first eigenvalue and eigenfunction. Column 7 gives the same time (b) in milliseconds related to one node of the grid.

In Columns 3 to 5 of Table 5.3, the error norm of three first eigenfunctions compared to the exact vector U^h is given. Column 6 gives the overall time (a) in seconds of computing the second and third eigenvalues and eigenfunctions. In Column 7, this time (b) in milliseconds is related to one node of the grid.

Analyzing the tables, we can note that when refinding the grid, the number of arithmetic operations per one node really tends to its finite limit. Moreover, comparing the multiplicities of defined eigenvalues, one can note that the number of operations depends, inconsiderably though, on increasing multiplicity from 1 to 2.

5.6 The boundary value problems of second and third kind

In this section, we deal with the boundary value problems of second and third kinds for a second-order elliptic differential equation. Discretization is effected by the Bubnov-

Galerkin method. Multigrid algorithms from Chapter 4 are used for the solution of the system produced. Note that in the case of third boundary value problem, the assertains that the Bubnov-Galerkin system is solvable are supported by subsection 1.1.4; and second boundary value problem will use, in view of singularity of the system, the results of subsection 1.1.5. Similar results for the third boundary value problem are first obtained in [3].

5.6.1 The third boundary value problem on a subordinate triangulation

Let Ω be a *convex* polygon in $\mathbf{R}^2$ with boundary Γ. Again consider equation (5.1), the boundary value condition being as follows:

$$\partial_c u + \sigma u = g \quad \text{on} \quad \Gamma. \tag{5.152}$$

Here $\partial_c u$ is a derivative with respect to the conormal:

$$\partial_c u = \sum_{i,j=1}^{2} a_{ij} \partial_j u \cos(n, x_i) \quad \text{on} \quad \Gamma$$

where $\cos(n, x_i)$ is the cosine of the angle contained by the external normal to Γ and the axis Ox_i. The problem data are supposed to satisfy conditions (5.3) and

$$g \in L_2(\Gamma), \quad 0 \le c_0 \le \sigma(x) \le c_1 \quad \text{on} \quad \Gamma. \tag{5.153}$$

In order to synthesize a discrete problem, we divide polygon Ω into a system of triangles, as in section 5.1, and retain the notation Ω_{h_i}, $\bar{\Omega}_{h_i}$. This time we introduce piecewise linear basis functions $\varphi_y^{h_i} \in W_2^1(\Omega)$ for all $y \in \bar{\Omega}_{h_i}$, i. e., for boundary nodes as well. Denote the linear span of this system by $\bar{H}^{h_i}$ and the number of nodes of set $\bar{\Omega}_{h_i}$ by $\bar{N}_i$.

Note that condition **G** in section 4.6 remains valid about the representation of each basis function of the i-th subdivision via a linear conbination of a finite amount ($c_4 = \max\{7, k_1 + 2\}$) of basis functions of the $(i+1)$-th subdivision .

For each $i = 0, \dots, p$, we construct a system of linear algebraic equations of the Bubnov-Galerkin method:

$$\sum_{y \in \bar{\Omega}_{h_i}} \alpha_y \mathcal{L}(\varphi_y^{h_i}, \varphi_z^{h_i}) = (f, \varphi_z^{h_i}) + \int_\Gamma g \varphi_z^{h_i} d\gamma \qquad \forall z \in \bar{\Omega}_{h_i}. \tag{5.154}$$

Here the bilinear form $\mathcal{L}$ is defined as follows:

$$\mathcal{L}(u, v) = \int_\Omega (\sum_{i,j=1}^{2} a_{ij} \partial_j u \partial_i v + a u v) dx + \int_\Gamma \sigma u v d\gamma.$$

The solution of system (5.154) (or its quasi-solution if this system is singular) yields the function

$$u^{h_i}(x) = \sum_{y \in \bar{\Omega}_{h_i}} \alpha_y \varphi_y^{h_i}(x) \tag{5.155}$$

which will be called the approximate solution of the Bubnov-Galerkin method of problem (5.1), (5.152).

Recast this system abridged:

$$L^{h_i} V^{h_i} = F^{h_i} \tag{5.156}$$

where L^{h_i} is an $\bar{N}_i \times \bar{N}_i$ symmetric matrix; V^{h_i} is a vector of unknowns with components $V_y^{h_i} = \alpha_y$ $(y \in \bar{\Omega}_{h_i})$; a right-hand side F^{h_i} is known. Prolongation in $\bar{H}^{h_i}$ will be constructed as follows: the function

$$v^{h_i}(x) = \sum_{y \in \bar{\Omega}_{h_i}} V_y^{h_i} \varphi_y^{h_i}(x) \quad \text{on} \quad \bar{\Omega} \tag{5.157}$$

will be assigned to vector V^{h_i}.

Continue for the second and third problems individually. First we suppose that in condition (5.153)

$$c_0 > 0. \tag{5.158}$$

Then

$$[\![u]\!] = \mathcal{L}^{1/2}(u, u)$$

is the norm in $W_2^1(\Omega)$ [133]. According to [94, p.170], system (5.156) is uniquely solvable and the approximate solution (5.155) obeys the estimate

$$[\![u - v^{h_i}]\!] \leq c_2 h_i(|f|_0 + |g|_{0,\Gamma}) \tag{5.159}$$

whence, in the usual way [115, p.175],

$$|u - v^{h_i}|_0 \leq c_3 h_i^2(|f|_0 + |g|_{0,\Gamma}). \tag{5.160}$$

Moreover, from Theorem 3.14 of section 3.6 it follows that eigenvalues λ of matrix L^{h_i} obey the estimate

$$0 \leq \lambda \leq c_4 \tag{5.161}$$

with the constant independent of h_i. Thus, all conditions of Theorems 4.14, 4.15 in section 4.6 are satisfied about application of FMG-algorithm and $MG^{(2)}$-algorithm described in the same section. We come to results similar to the ones of section 5.1.

Theorem 5.7 *Let the combination of FMG and $MG^{(2)}$-algorithms of subsection* 4.2.1 *be used to solve system* (5.156) *when $i = p$. Then $c_5 \bar{N}_p$ arithmetic operations are adequate to produce the approximate solition $\widetilde{V}^{h_p}$ satisfying the estimate*

$$\|\widetilde{V}^{h_p} - V^{h_p}\|_h \equiv |\tilde{v}^{h_p} - v^{h_p}|_0 \leq c_3 h_p^2(|f|_0 + |g|_{0,\Gamma}). \tag{5.162}$$

Here $\tilde{v}^{h_p}$ is the prolongation in $\bar{H}^{h_p}$ of vector $\widetilde{V}^{h_p}$; constant c_5 is independent of f, g, h_i; $\bar{N}_p$ is the number of unknows of system (5.156) *when $i = p$; c_3 is the same as in* (5.160).

If we use the combination of FMG and $MG^{(1)}$-algorithms then the similar statement holds for energy norm:

$$\|\widetilde{V}^{h_p} - V^{h_p}\|_h^{(1)} \equiv [\![\tilde{v}^{h_p} - v^{h_p}]\!] \leq c_2 h_i(|f|_0 + |g|_{0,\Gamma})$$

with c_2 from (5.159).

The proof is analogous to that of Lemmata 5.1.3–5.1.6 from section 5.1.

5.6.2 The Neumann problem

Let us now proceed to the second boundary value problem, the Neumann one:

$$\sum_{i,j=1}^{2} \partial_i(a_{ij}\partial_j u) = f \quad \text{on} \quad \Gamma, \tag{5.163}$$

$$\partial_c u = 0 \quad \text{on} \quad \Gamma. \tag{5.164}$$

Here the operator is singular. Consider the corresponding spectral problem

$$\sum_{i,j=1}^{2} \partial_i(a_{ij}\partial_j u) = \lambda u \quad \text{on} \quad \Omega \tag{5.165}$$

with the condition (5.164). Obviously, it has zero eigenvalue corresponding to the eigenfunction identically equal to 1 on $\bar{\Omega}$. The multiplicity of the zero eigenvalue is 1, the other eigenvalues are positive [133, p.336]. We introduce the subspace $\widetilde{L}_2(\Omega)$ of space $L_2(\Omega)$ which is orthogonal to unit. In it, the problem operator is positive definite and there exists a unique solution [133, p.320] which coincides with the normal solution u_H introduced in section 4.8. Therefore, we will consider function f orthogonal to unit in $L_2(\Omega)$.

The system of the Bubnov-Galerkin method

$$\sum_{y\in\bar{\Omega}_{h_i}} \alpha_y \mathcal{L}(\varphi_y^{h_i}, \varphi_z^{h_i}) = (f, \varphi_z^{h_i}) \qquad \forall z \in \bar{\Omega}_{h_i} \tag{5.166}$$

also proves to be singular. This follows from the fact that the bilinear form

$$\mathcal{L}(u,v) = \int_\Omega \sum_{i,j=1}^{2} a_{ij}\partial_i v \partial_j u dx \tag{5.167}$$

becomes zero on functions u or v equal to the constant.

Consider a suitable algebraic spectral problem following from (5.165), (5.164) according to the Bubnov-Galerkin method:

$$\sum_{y\in\bar{\Omega}_{h_i}} \alpha_y \mathcal{L}(\varphi_y^{h_i}, \varphi_z^{h_i}) = \lambda^{h_i} \sum_{y\in\bar{\Omega}_{h_i}} (\varphi_y^{h_i}, \varphi_z^{h_i}) \quad \forall z \in \bar{\Omega}_{h_i}. \tag{5.168}$$

Its eigenvalues λ^{h_i} approximate the corresponding eigenvalues λ of differential problem (5.165), (5.124) [132, p.340]. The zero eigenvalue λ^{h_i} is simple; the other eigenvalues are strictly positive:

$$\lambda_1^{h_i} = 0, \quad 0 < c_6 \le \lambda_2^{h_i} \le \lambda_3^{h_i} \le \ldots \le \lambda_{N_i}^{h_i}. \tag{5.169}$$

Thus, the assumption (4.329) of section 4.8 is satisfied. We can therefore use the definition of a quasi-solution introduced in section 4.8. Denote the quasi-solution of system (5.166) by W^{h_i}, and its prolongation in $\bar{H}^{h_i}$ by w^{h_i}.

To show convergence of w^{h_i} to w_H, we consider the Bubnov-Galerkin method in space $\widetilde{L}_2(\Omega)$. System (5.166) is here retained entirely; and w^{h_i} is kept in space $\widetilde{L}_2(\Omega)$ due to the requirement that $(w^{h_i}, 1) = 0$. In the present situation, therefore, finding

w^{h_i} is none other than the Bubnov-Galerkin method for problem (5.165), (5.164) in subspace $\widetilde{L}_2(\Omega)$. In this subspace, $\mathcal{L}^{1/2}(u,u)$ is a norm [133, p.323]. The ordinary reasoning, therefore, leads to the estimate

$$\|w_H - w^{h_i}\|_1 \le c_7 h_i |f|_0. \tag{5.170}$$

It yields, as usual, the root-mean-square convergence

$$|w_H - w^{h_i}|_0 \le c_8 h_i^2 |f|_0. \tag{5.171}$$

That is to say, condition **J** of section 4.8 is satisfied.

Thus, all conditions of section 4.8 is verified. Therefore, FMG- and $MG^{(5)}$-algorithms described in section 4.8 may be used to search a quasi-solution of system (5.166).

Theorem 5.8 *Let the combination of $FMG^{(2)}$- and $MG^{(5)}$-algorithms from section 4.8 be used to solve system* (5.166) *when $i = p$. Then, $c_9\bar{N}_p$ arithmetic operations is sufficient to obtain the approximate solution $\widetilde{W}^{h_p}$ satisfying the estimate*

$$\|\widetilde{W}^{h_p} - W^{h_p}\|_h = |\tilde{w}^{h_p} - w^{h_p}|_0 \le c_8 h_p^2 |f|_0. \tag{5.172}$$

Here $\tilde{w}^{h_p}$ is the prolongation in $\bar{H}^{h_p}$ of the vector $\widetilde{W}^{h_p}$; constant c_9 is independent of f, h_i; $\bar{N}_p$ is the number of unknowns of system (5.166) *when $i = p$; c_8 is the same like in* (5.171).

Proof. In view of the fact that we use an exact eigenvector of algebraic spectral problem (5.168) in $FMG^{(2)}$-algorithm, the constant c_{11} equals zero in condition (4.328) of section 4.8, constant c_{14} also becomes zero, and restrictions (4.347) on mesh-size h_i are lifted. As a result, the estimate (4.339) takes a simpler form, likewise in Theorem 4.14 of section 4.6. Using it and the fact that the orthogonalization takes additional arithmetic operations, we come to (5.172), likewise in the justification of Lemmata 5.1.3–5.1.4. □

5.6.3 The third boundary value problem on regular grids

To apply the algorithms of this section to the second and third boundary value problems in domains with a piecewise smooth boundary, one can first use geometrical constructions of section 5.2 and then put corresponding changes into justification of the results. Theorems 5.7 and 5.8 will hold also for problems like these, as a result.

At the same time, the other technique may be realized on uniform grids [146]. The description of curvilinear boundary Γ being convenient, it will present some advantages in the two-dimensional case, and these will show a sharp rise in the three-dimensional case.

In treating it, we redefine the notation $\bar{\Omega}_h$ and $\bar{H}^h$. Let us partition the plane of variables (x_1, x_2) by straight lines $x_1 = ih$, $x_2 = jh$, where $i, j = 0, \pm 1, \pm 2, \dots$, into squares $\Pi_{ij} = \{ih \le x_1 \le (i+1)h;\ jh \le x_2 \le (j+1)h\}$ which we call the grid cells. Denote by Π_h the smallest union of the grid cells having a common part with Ω (see Fig. 5.7). Points $(ih, jh) \in \Pi_h$ will be called the nodes. Denote their set by $\bar{\Omega}_h$.

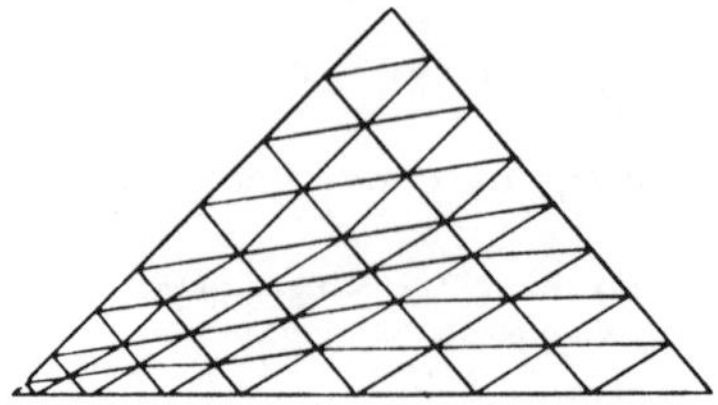

Figure 5.7: Uniform non-subordinate triangulation of domain.

For each node $y \in \bar{\Omega}_h$, we introduce a basis function $\varphi_y(x)$ bilinear on each cell $\Pi \subset \Pi_h$, equal to 1 in y and 0 in the other nodes of $\bar{\Omega}_h$. As earlier, denote the linear span of these functions by $\bar{H}^h$.

In this notation, the Bubnov-Galerkin problem again reduces to the formulation (5.154) with a solution like (5.155). This time, however, a few points $y \in \bar{\Omega}_h$ is located outside the domain $\bar{\Omega}$. The general theory of approximation given in Chapter 3 dictates the estimates (5.159) and (5.160).

The only disadvantage (often noted) is a poor conditionality of the matrix of system (5.154). Indeed, as it is shown in detail in [146], if the intersection area of the square Π_{ij} and domain Ω is slight then elements of matrix can be arbitrary small on line corresponding to a node outside Ω. Such a situation is illustrated in Fig. 5.7 for node z.

This situation does, in fact, degrades convergence in multigrid algorithms. We show how to improve the matter using a diagonal preconditioning.

Let us label all nodes of set $\bar{\Omega}_h$ from 1 to $\bar{N}$ and put system (5.154) into the form

$$L^h V^h = F^h \tag{5.173}$$

with the symmetric $N \times N$-matrix and the vector V^h of unknowns with components $V_y^h = \alpha_y^h$ $(y \in \bar{\Omega}_h)$. Prolongations of vectors in $\bar{H}^h$ are constructed like (5.157). Using these, define the vector norms

$$\|V^h\|_h \equiv |v^h|_{0,\Omega}, \qquad \|V^h\|_h^{(1)} = [\![v^h]\!]. \tag{5.174}$$

On the ground of [146], we have the estimates (5.119), (5.120).

Let us introduce a diagonal matrix $\mathcal{D}^h = \mathrm{diag}\{d_y^h\}$, $y \in \bar{\Omega}_h$, with the elements

$$d_y^h = 4h^2 \left(\sum_{\Pi \ni y} \mathrm{mes}(\Pi \bigcap \Omega) \right)^{-1} \tag{5.175}$$

where the summation is taken over 4 cells $\Pi \subset \Pi^h$ which contain node y. Instead of the exact area of curvilinear figures $\Pi \bigcap \Omega$, we can use the areas of polygons obtained by replacing curvilinear boundary arcs with their chords.

Instead of (5.9), let us introduce the norm

$$\|V^h\|_{\mathcal{D}} = \left(\sum_{y \in \bar{\Omega}_h} (V_y^h)^2 (d_y^h)^{-1} \right)^{1/2}.$$

The estimates (4.511) are valid for it. From the proof of Theorem 3.14 of section 3.6 and its one-dimensional analogue, it follows that eigenvalues λ of matrix $\mathcal{D}^h L^h$ satisfy the inequality

$$0 < \lambda(\mathcal{D}^h L^h) \leq c_{11}. \tag{5.176}$$

They are real-valued due to coincidence with eigenvalues of the symmetric matrix $(\mathcal{D}^h)^{1/2} L^h (\mathcal{D}^h)^{1/2}$. Therefore we have the usual regular case studied in subsection 4.10.2.

Assume that we constructed a sequence of grids $\bar{\Omega}_h$ and problems (5.173) with parameters $h = h_0, h_1, \dots, h_p$; let ratio h_i/h_{i+1} is equal to 2 or 3. Then we can use the combinations of FMG-algorithm with both $MG^{(7)}$ or $MG^{(8)}$.

Note that $\Pi_{h_{i+1}}$ may differ from Π_{h_i} but $\Pi_{h_{i+1}} \subset \Pi_{h_i}$ since h_i is multiple of h_{i+1}. Therefore, interpolation from grid $\bar{\Omega}_{h_i}$ to grid $\bar{\Omega}_{h_{i+1}}$ does not present any difficulties, and $\bar{H}^{h_i} \subset \bar{H}^{h_{i+1}}$ when constricting the domain of definition from Π_{h_i} to $\Pi_{h_{i+1}}$. As far as (4.491) is concerned, it always contains 9 nonzeroth coefficients β_l^j. At the same time, a few of them can refer to points z which are not nodes of $\Pi_{h_{i+1}}$ because all four cells containing z do not intersect with Ω. In this situation, one should exclude from (4.491) corresponding components for such z.

Theorem 5.9 *Let the combination of FMG and $MG^{(7)}$-algorithms of section 4.10 be used for the solution of system (5.173) when $h = h_p$. Then $c_{12} N_p$ arithmetic operations suffice to obtain the approximate solution $\widetilde{V}^{h_p}$ satisfying the estimate*

$$\|\widetilde{V}^{h_p} - V^{h_p}\|_h = |\tilde{v}^{h_p} - v^{h_p}|_0 \leq c_3 h_p^2 |f|_0. \tag{5.177}$$

Here $\tilde{v}^{h_p}$ is the prolongation in $\bar{H}^{h_p}$ of vector $\widetilde{V}^{h_p}$; constant c_{12} is independent of f, g, h_i; $\bar{N}_p$ is the number of unknowns of system (5.173); c_3 is the same as in (5.120).

If we use the combination of FMG and $MG^{(8)}$-algorithms then the same statement holds for the energy norm:

$$\|\widetilde{V}^{h_p} - V^{h_p}\|_h^{(1)} = [\![\tilde{v}^{h_p} - v^{h_p}]\!] \leq c_2 h_i |f|_0$$

with c_2 from (5.119).

The proof consists in verification of conditions of Theorems 4.28 and 4.30 of section 4.10 and implementation of Lemmata 5.1.3–5.1.6.

Chapter 6

Solving nonlinear problems and systems of equations

In this chapter, we deal with various generalizations of iterative algorithms of Chapter 5, firstly, to quasi-linear problems and, secondly, to wider classes of equations. In section 6.1, we present a general formulation of boundary value problems for a quasi-linear second-order equation with an operator of monotone type and formulate general results on the solvability of the Bubnov-Galerkin method. In section 6.2, we deal with two particular problems having such operators and different kinds of non-linearity: in the right-hand side and in coefficients of the equation. In section 6.3, we treat Lame's equations system of the elasticity. From the theoretic standpoint, the algorithm here synthesized is a simple (vector) generalization of results of Chapter 5. A numerical experiment shows a high efficiency of this algorithm.

In section 6.4, the biharmonic equation is dealt with. Of several ways to solve it, the mixed one is here considered which determines not only the solution u but also the vortex Δu. This gives rise to an opportunity for solving, instead of a fourth-order equation, a system of two second-order equations. The requirement that basis functions belong to class $W_2^2(\Omega)$ is lifted, which offers a feasible application of simple basis functions.

In section 6.5, the Bubnov-Galerkin mixed method is applied to the stationary Stokes problem. A modified multigrid algorithm is also efficient to solve the discrete problem obtained in spite of the matrix singularity and the spectrum with alternating signs. In section 6.6, the stationary Navier-Stokes problem is studied. A combination of the modified multigrid algorithm and the Newton method for non-linearity is here realized, which gives the optimal amount of arithmetic operators per one unknown needed to insure the required accuracy.

6.1 Nonlinear problems with an operator of monotone type

Nonlinear equations exhibit a greater variety than linear equations. In terms of the finite element method, problems with operators of monotone type are best studied [192], [40], [144]. We also consider such operators having a divergent principle part for second-order equations [94]. Namely: consider the equation

$$-\sum_{i=1}^{n} \frac{\partial}{\partial x_i} a_i(x, u, \nabla u) + a_0(x, u, \nabla u) = 0 \quad \text{in} \quad \Omega \tag{6.1}$$

where Ω is a bounded domain in $\mathbf{R}^n$. On boundary Γ, add to (6.1) the first boundary value condition

$$u = 0 \quad \text{on} \quad \Gamma. \tag{6.2}$$

The case of the third boundary-value condition is studied in [144]. The problem (6.1), (6.2) is a certain generalization of a linear boundary value problem. Introduce a definition of a generalized solution.

Definition 6.1 *The function* $u \in \overset{\circ}{W}{}_2^1(\Omega)$ *is called the generalized solution of problem* (6.1), (6.2) *if it satisfies the integral equality*

$$\mathcal{L}(u,v) \equiv \int_\Omega \{\sum_{i=1}^n a_i(x,u,\nabla u)\partial_i v + a_0(x,u,\nabla u)v\}dx = 0 \qquad \forall v \in \overset{\circ}{W}{}_2^1(\Omega). \tag{6.3}$$

This time, the form $\mathcal{L}(u,v)$ is linear only in the second argument. Remind that for justifying the convergence of the finite elements method, we used the ellipticity and the continuity of the form $\mathcal{L}$. Let us show generalizations of these properties to the nonlinear case.

Definition 6.2 *The form* $\mathcal{L}(\cdot,\cdot)$ *is called strong-monotone if*

$$\mathcal{L}(u,u-v) - \mathcal{L}(v,u-v) \geq c_0\|u-v\|_1^2. \tag{6.4}$$

Definition 6.3 *We call the form* $\mathcal{L}(\cdot,\cdot)$ *Lipschitz-continuous if*

$$|\mathcal{L}(u,w) - \mathcal{L}(v,w)| \leq c_1\|u-v\|_1\|w\|_1 \qquad \forall u,v,w \in \overset{\circ}{W}{}_2^1(\Omega). \tag{6.5}$$

Obviously, these two estimates are sufficient for a number of useful properties of linear problems to be generalized. For instance, from strong monotonicity it follows that the generalized solution is unique. Indeed, let u_1, u_2 be two solutions of problem (6.3). Then from (6.4):

$$0 = \mathcal{L}(u_1,u_1-u_2) - \mathcal{L}(u_2,u_1-u_2) \geq c_0\|u_1-u_2\|_1^2, \tag{6.6}$$

i. e., $u_1 = u_2$.

Other, more general definitions of the monotonicity and the continuity of operators and of the form $\mathcal{L}$ are provided in [40], [105], [84].

Consider an approximation of (6.3) in finite-dimensional space $H^h \subset \overset{\circ}{W}{}_2^1(\Omega)$: *find the function* $u^h \in H^h$ *such that*

$$\mathcal{L}(u^h,v) = 0 \qquad \forall v \in H^h. \tag{6.7}$$

Assume that the basis of H^h consists of functions φ_i $(i = 1,\dots,N)$. Then this problem is equivalent to the solution of the system of nonlinear algebraic equations:

$$\mathcal{L}(\sum_{i=1}^N \alpha_i\varphi_i,\varphi_j) = 0, \qquad j = 1,\dots,N, \tag{6.8}$$

where

$$u^h(x) = \sum_{i=1}^{N} \alpha_i \varphi_i(x) \quad \text{on} \quad \Omega. \tag{6.9}$$

Prove that system (6.8) and problem (6.7) are solvable in terms of the known lemma by J.L. Lions [105]. Preliminary, fix a certain scalar product $(\cdot,\cdot)_{\mathbf{R}^N}$ and the norm $|\xi|_{\mathbf{R}^N} = (\xi,\xi)_{\mathbf{R}^N}^{1/2}$ in $\mathbf{R}^N$.

Lemma 6.1.1 *Let $\xi \to P(\xi)$ be a continuous mapping $\mathbf{R}^N$ in itself such that for a suitable $\rho > 0$*

$$(P(\xi),\xi)_{\mathbf{R}^N} > 0 \qquad \forall \xi : \ |\xi|_{\mathbf{R}^N} = \rho. \tag{6.10}$$

Then we can find an ξ from the ball $|\xi|_{\mathbf{R}^N} \leq \rho$ such that $P(\xi) = 0$.

To be exact, note that the formulation in [105] contains a specific Euclidian scalar product, but the proof is valid for an arbitrary one. The next result follows from this lemma and is similar to that obtained in [144].

Theorem 6.1 *Assume that the form $\mathcal{L}$ is strong-monotone, Lipschitz-continuous, and besides bounded at zero in the second argument* [1]

$$|\mathcal{L}(0,v)| \leq c_2\|v\|_1 \qquad \forall v \in \overset{\circ}{W}{}_2^1(\Omega). \tag{6.11}$$

Then the problem (6.7) has a unique solution u^h satisfying the estimate

$$\|u^h\|_1 \leq c_2/c_0.$$

Proof. Consider the inequality

$$|\mathcal{L}(u,u)| \geq |\mathcal{L}(u,u) - \mathcal{L}(0,u)| - |\mathcal{L}(0,u)|, \qquad u \in H^h.$$

Owing to strong-monotonisity of (6.4),

$$\mathcal{L}(u,u) - \mathcal{L}(0,u) \geq c_0\|u\|_1^2.$$

Combining the last three inequalities, we get the estimate

$$|\mathcal{L}(u,u)| \geq c_0\|u\|_1^2 - c_2\|u\|_1. \tag{6.12}$$

Each vector $V \in \mathbf{R}^N$ with components V_i can be associated with the prolongation $v^h \in H^h$ by the rule:

$$v^h(x) = \sum_{i=1}^{N} V_i \varphi_i(x).$$

Using the prolongations, let us concretize the scalar product and the norm in $\mathbf{R}^N$:

$$(V,W)_{\mathbf{R}^N} = \int_\Omega (\nabla v^h \cdot \nabla w^h + v^h \cdot w^h)dx, \quad \|V\|_{\mathbf{R}^N} = \|v^h\|_1.$$

[1] In linear problems, this condition is equivalent to boundedness of the linear functional of right-hand side $f(v)$.

Then for every vector $W \subset \mathbf{R}^N$, the expression $\mathcal{L}(w^h, v^h)$ defines the linear functional with respect to v^h.

Let us prove its boundedness. Consider the inequality

$$|\mathcal{L}(w^h, v^h)| \leq |\mathcal{L}(w^h, v^h) - \mathcal{L}(0, v^h)| + |\mathcal{L}(0, v^h)|.$$

Apply estimate (6.11) and Lipschitz-continuity (6.5):

$$|\mathcal{L}(w^h, v^h)| \leq c_1 \|w^h\|_1 \, \|v^h\|_1 + c_2 \|v^h\|_1 = (c_1 \|W\|_{\mathbf{R}^N} + c_2) \|V\|_{\mathbf{R}^N}.$$

The boundedness follows just from the above. Therefore, from the F. Riesz theorem (see, e.g., [99]), it follows that there exists a vector $P(W)$ defining this functional:

$$(P(W), V)_{\mathbf{R}^N} = \mathcal{L}(w^h, v^h). \tag{6.13}$$

The operator $P(W) : \mathbf{R}^N \to \mathbf{R}^N$ is given thereby.

Let us prove its continuity. Indeed, consider the expression

$$(P(W) - P(U), V)_{\mathbf{R}^N} = \mathcal{L}(w^h, v^h) - \mathcal{L}(u^h, v^h).$$

From the Lipschitz-continuity of the form $\mathcal{L}$, it follows that

$$|(P(W) - P(U), V)_{\mathbf{R}^N}| \leq c_1 \|w^h - u^h\|_1 \|v^h\|_1 = c_1 \|W - U\|_{\mathbf{R}^N} \|V\|_{\mathbf{R}^N}.$$

Put here $V = P(W) - P(U)$ and cancel $\|V\|_{\mathbf{R}^N}$. We obtain the estimate

$$\|P(W) - P(U)\|_{\mathbf{R}^N} \leq c_1 \|W - U\|_{\mathbf{R}^N}$$

which confirms the continuity of the operator P.

Assume that $\rho = c_2/c_0$. Then for any $V \in \mathbf{R}^N$ such that $\|V\|_{\mathbf{R}^N} = \rho$, by virtue of (6.13), (6.12), we have

$$(P(V), V)_{\mathbf{R}^N} = \mathcal{L}(v^h, v^h) \geq c_0 \rho^2 - c_2 \rho = 0.$$

Thus, we obtain the conditions of Lemma 6.1.1. From this lemma, it follows that there exists a solution of the system

$$P(U) = 0,$$

the estimate

$$\|U\|_{\mathbf{R}^N} = \|u^h\|_1 \leq c_2/c_0 \tag{6.14}$$

being valid for it. Subject to (6.13),

$$(P(U), V)_{\mathbf{R}^N} = \mathcal{L}(u^h, v^h) = 0 \qquad \forall v^h \in H^h.$$

Thus, u^h is really the solution of problem (6.7) and U is the solution of system (6.8).

The uniqueness of the solution u^h follows from the strong monotonicity condition, as in (6.6). □

The proof of the convergence is analogous with the justification for linear problems [144].

Theorem 6.2 *Let the form $\mathcal{L}$ be strong-monotone, Lipschitz-continuous and let* (6.11) *be satisfied. Then the estimate*

$$\|u - u^h\|_1 \leq \frac{c_1}{c_0} \inf_{v \in H^h} \|u - v\|_1 \tag{6.15}$$

is valid for the solution of problem (6.7).

Proof. From equalities (6.3) and (6.7), it follows that

$$\mathcal{L}(u, w) - \mathcal{L}(u^h, w) = 0 \qquad \forall w \in H^h.$$

Put here $w = (u - u^h) - (u - v)$ where v is an arbitrary function from H^h. Taking into account linearity in the second coefficient , we get

$$\mathcal{L}(u, u - u^h) - \mathcal{L}(u^h, u - u^h) = \mathcal{L}(u, u - v) - \mathcal{L}(u^h, u - v).$$

Use strong monotonicity in the left-hand side and Lipschitz-continuity in the right-hand side. Then

$$c_0\|u - u^h\|_1^2 \leq c_1\|u - u^h\|_1 \, \|u - v\|_1.$$

Reduce the expression by $c_0\|u - u^h\|_1$ and take infimum with respect to v for both sides. We obtain (6.15). □

Thus, the question of the accuracy of u^h is reduced to possible accuracy of approximation. Last question was at length studied in Chapter 3.

6.2 Solution of quasi-linear equations of order 2

Instead of considering a variety of general cases, we examine two simple but typical problems. One of them occurs in nonlinear mechanics (in magnetic hydrodynamics, elasticity theory), ecology and is characterized by the dependence of the right-hand side of equation on the solution rather than on its derivatives. The second problem often occurs in magnetostatic computations [72], [60]. In it, the equation coefficients depend on the solution derivatives. This distinction affects both the choice of algorithms and their justification.

6.2.1 The equation with a weak nonlinearity

Let $\Omega \subset \mathbf{R}^2$ be a *convex* polygon with a boundary Γ. Consider the problem of defining the function $u(x)$:

$$\Delta u = f(x, u) \quad \text{in} \quad \Omega, \tag{6.16}$$

$$u = 0 \quad \text{on} \quad \Gamma. \tag{6.17}$$

The function $f(x, v) \in C(\bar{\Omega} \times \mathbf{R})$ has a non-negative partial derivative in second argument:

$$0 \leq \frac{\partial f}{\partial v}(x, v) \leq c_3 \qquad \forall x \in \Omega, \quad \forall v \in \mathbf{R}. \tag{6.18}$$

This condition ensures that the problem (6.16), (6.17) is uniquely solvable in class $W_2^2(\Omega)$ [94].

Remark 6.2.1 *The upper estimate* (6.18) *often fails for rather simple functions, e.g.,* $f(x,u) = -e^{-u}$ *or* $f(x,u) = u^3$. *At the same time, it is known that the problem has the bounded solution*

$$|u| \le c_6. \tag{6.19}$$

Using the cutoff function, we can then form a function $\tilde{f}(x,v)$ *such that*

$$\tilde{f}(x,v) = f(x,v) \qquad \forall x \in \Omega, \quad \forall v \in [-c_6, c_6].$$

Now the upper estimate in (6.18) *is satisfied. The new problem with a right-hand side* $\tilde{f}$ *is equivalent to the initial problem in the following sense: both have the same bounded solution* u. *The new problem will, true, lose unbounded solution (if any).*

Now proceed from (6.16), (6.17) to a weak formulation, namely: *find* $u \in \overset{\circ}{W}{}_2^1(\Omega)$ *satisfying the relation*

$$\mathcal{L}(u,v) = 0 \qquad \forall v \in \overset{\circ}{W}{}_2^1(\Omega) \tag{6.20}$$

where

$$\mathcal{L}(u,v) = \int_\Omega \{\nabla u \cdot \nabla v + f(x,u)v\} dx.$$

Strong monotonicity and Lipschitz-continuity are valid for this problem. Indeed, consider the expression

$$\mathcal{L}(u,u-v) - \mathcal{L}(v,u-v) =$$

$$= \int_\Omega \{\nabla(u-v)\cdot\nabla(u-v) + (f(x,u)-f(x,v))(u-v)\} dx. \tag{6.21}$$

Because of the Lagrange theorem,

$$f(x,u) - f(x,v) = (u-v)\frac{\partial f}{\partial v}(x,\xi) \tag{6.22}$$

where ξ is between u and v. Therefore, by virtue of (6.18),

$$(f(x,u)-f(x,v))(u-v) \ge 0.$$

From the Friedrichs inequality (1.1), the estimate

$$\int_\Omega \nabla(u-v)\cdot\nabla(u-v)dx = |u-v|_1^2 \ge c_0'\|u-v\|_1^2$$

follows. Combining the last two inequalities and (6.21), we get

$$\mathcal{L}(u,u-v) - \mathcal{L}(v,u-v) \ge c_0'\|u-v\|_1^2$$

which proves strong monotonicity.

Now consider

$$|\mathcal{L}(u,w) - \mathcal{L}(v,w)| = |\int_\Omega \{\nabla(u-v)\cdot\nabla w + (f(x,u)-f(x,v))w\} dx|.$$

From (6.22) and (6.18), it follows that

$$|(f(x,u)-f(x,v))w| \leq c_0|u-v|\cdot|w|.$$

Therefore, using the Cauchy-Bunyakovski inequality, we have

$$|\mathcal{L}(u,w)-\mathcal{L}(v,w)| \leq$$

$$\leq |u-v|_1|w|_1 + c_0|u-v|_0|w|_0 \leq (1+c_0)\|u-v\|_1\|w\|_1.$$

Thus Lipschitz-continuity is also proved.

From the strong monotonicity, the uniquiness of the solution (6.20) follows in the usual way.

To construct a discrete problem, we apply piecewise linear elements, constructions and notation from section 5.1. As a result, we have the problem: *find* $u^h \in H^h$ *satisfying the equality*

$$\mathcal{L}(u^h, v) = 0 \qquad \forall v \in H^h. \tag{6.23}$$

It is equivalent to the system of algebraic nonlinear equations

$$\mathcal{L}(\sum_{y\in\Omega_y} \alpha_y \varphi_y^h, \varphi_z^h) = 0 \qquad \forall z \in \Omega_h. \tag{6.24}$$

The solution of (6.23) is related to this system by formula

$$u^h(x) = \sum_{y\in\Omega_h} \alpha_y \varphi_y^h(x). \tag{6.25}$$

The unique solvability of system (6.24) and the convergence of u^h to u are supported by the results of the preciding subsection.

Lemma 6.2.1 *When conditions* (6.18), (3.9) *are satisfied, the approximate solution* (6.25) *of problem* (6.23) *is defined uniquely and the following estimate holds:*

$$\|u-u^h\|_1 \leq c_4 h\|u\|_2. \tag{6.26}$$

Proof. Verify the condition (6.11) of boundedness at zero. Apply the Cauchy-Bunyakovski inequality to the expression

$$|\mathcal{L}(0,v)| - |\int_\Omega f(x,0)v dx| \leq |v|_0|f(x,0)|_0.$$

Since $f(x,0) \in C(\bar{\Omega})$, the value $|f(x,0)|_0$ is bounded and therefore

$$|\mathcal{L}(0,v)| \leq c|v|_0.$$

Thus, from Theorem 6.1, the problem (6.23) has a unique solution u^h. Theorem 6.2 dictates the estimates

$$\|u-u^h\| \leq c \inf_{v\in H^h} \|u-v\|_1 \leq c\|u-u_I^h\|_1,$$

where u_I^h is the interpolant in H^h of function u. According to [94], $u \in W_2^2(\Omega)$ and, hence, by Theorem 3.3

$$\|u - u_I^h\|_1 \leq ch\|u\|_2.$$

Combining the last two inequalities, we get (6.26). □

To obtain the convergence estimate in the root-mean-square norm, we modify the usual representation of the error norm by putting it into bilinear form.

Lemma 6.2.2 *When conditions* (6.18), (3.9) *are satisfied, the following estimate holds*

$$|u - u^h|_0 \leq c_5 h^2 \|u\|_2. \tag{6.27}$$

Proof. Introduce the function

$$a(x) = \begin{cases} \partial f(x)/\partial u, & \text{if } \ u(x) = u^h(x), \\ (f(x,u) - f(x,u^h))/(u - u^h), & \text{otherwise.} \end{cases}$$

Note that it is non-negative by virtue of the Lagrange theorem and the condition (6.18).

Consider solving the problem: *find a function* $w \in \overset{\circ}{W}{}_2^1(\Omega)$ *such that*

$$\int_\Omega (\nabla w \cdot \nabla v + awv)dx = (u - u^h, v) \qquad \forall v \in \overset{\circ}{W}{}_2^1(\Omega). \tag{6.28}$$

This problem is linear and $u - u^h$ belongs to $L_2(\Omega)$. Therefore, according to [94], $w \in W_2^2(\Omega)$. Consider also its finite elements approximation being the solution of the following problem: *find* $w^h \in H^h$ *such that*

$$\int_\Omega (\nabla w^h \cdot \nabla v + aw^h v)dx = (u - u^h, v) \qquad \forall v \in H^h. \tag{6.29}$$

Then, from results of Chapter 3,

$$|w - w^h|_1 \leq c_6 h |u^h - u|_0. \tag{6.30}$$

Put $v = u - u^h$ into (6.28):

$$|u - u^h|_0^2 = \mathcal{L}(u, w) - \mathcal{L}(u^h, w). \tag{6.31}$$

By virtue of the definition of u and u^h,

$$\mathcal{L}(u, w^h) - \mathcal{L}(u^h, w^h) = 0.$$

Subtracting this from (6.31), we get the following estimates allowing for Lipschitz-continuity (6.5):

$$|u - u^h|_0^2 = \mathcal{L}(u, w - w^h) - \mathcal{L}(u^h, w - w^h) \leq c_1 \|u - u^h\|_1 \cdot \|w - w^h\|_1.$$

Using (6.26) and (6.30), we get:

$$|u - u^h|_0^2 \leq c_5 h^2 \|u\|_2 |u - u^h|_0$$

which leads to (6.27). □

6.2.2 The Newton method and the multigrid algorithm

To solve problem (6.20), we use the Newton method where the initial guess is taken from a more rough grid. Consider one iteration of this method with the initial guess $u_0 \in H^h$ in the following form: *find $u_1 \in H^h$ satisfying the relation*

$$\mathcal{L}_1(u_1, v; u_0) = f_1(v; u_0) \qquad \forall v \in H^h \tag{6.32}$$

where

$$\begin{aligned} \mathcal{L}_1(u_1, v; u_0) &= \int_\Omega \left(\nabla u_1 \cdot \nabla v + \frac{\partial f}{\partial u}(x, u_0) u_1 v \right) dx, \\ f_1(v; u_0) &= \int_\Omega \left(f(x, u_0) v + \frac{\partial f}{\partial u}(x, u_0) u_0 v \right) dx. \end{aligned} \tag{6.33}$$

This problem is equivalent to the system of linear algebraic equations relative to degrees of freedom β_ν defining function u_1:

$$\sum_{y \in \Omega_h} \beta_y \mathcal{L}_1(\varphi_y^h, \varphi_z^h; u_0) = f_1(\varphi_z^h; u_0), \qquad z \in \Omega_h, \tag{6.34}$$

where

$$u_1(x) = \sum_{y \in \Omega_h} \beta_y \varphi_y^h(x).$$

This method exhibits the quadratic convergence in norm $|\cdot|_0$ with a factor weakly dependent on h.

Theorem 6.3 *When the restriction*

$$\left| \frac{\partial^2 f}{\partial u^2} \right| \le c_{17} \qquad on \quad \Omega \times \mathbf{R} \tag{6.35}$$

and (3.9) *are satisfied, for any $u_0 \in H^h$ the solution u_1 of problem* (6.32) *is defined uniquely and the estimate*

$$|u^h - u_1|_0 \le c_{18} |\ln h|^{1/2} |u^h - u_0|^2 \tag{6.36}$$

is valid.

Proof. Take the Taylor series of the function f:

$$f(x, u^h) = f(x, u_0) + (u^h - u_0) \frac{\partial f}{\partial u}(x, u_0) + \frac{1}{2}(u^h - u_0)^2 \frac{\partial^2 f}{\partial u^2}(x, \xi)$$

where $\xi(x)$ is a certain function whose values in every x are found in the interval from u_0 to u^h. (6.23) is then equivalent to the equality

$$\mathcal{L}_1(u^h, v; u_0) = f_1(v; u_0) + \frac{1}{2} \int_\Omega \frac{\partial^2 f}{\partial u^2}(x, \xi)(u^h - u_0)^2 v dx.$$

Subtract (6.32) from it and put $v = u^h - u_1$:

$$\mathcal{L}_1(u^h - u_1, u^h - u_1; u_0) = \frac{1}{2}\int_\Omega \frac{\partial^2 f}{\partial u^2}(x,\xi)(u^h - u_0)^2(u^h - u_1)dx.$$

Allowing for estimates (6.18) and (6.35), we come to the inequality

$$|u^h - u_1|_1^2 \le \frac{1}{2}c_{17}\int_\Omega (u^h - u_0)^2|u^h - u_1|dx. \tag{6.37}$$

In the two-dimensional case, piecewise linear Courant elements obey the following estimate [146]:

$$\max_{\bar\Omega}|v| \le c_9|\ln h|^{1/2}|v|_1 \qquad \forall v \in H^h. \tag{6.38}$$

Applying it to the right-hand side of (6.37) for $|u^h - u_1|$, we get

$$|u^h - u_1|_1 \le \frac{1}{2}c_{17}c_9|\ln h|^{1/2}|u^h - u_0|_0^2.$$

Finally, applying the Friedrichs inequality (1.1), we obtain (6.36). □

Let us describe now $FMG^{(5)}$-algorithm which gives a sequence of approximate solutions $\tilde u^{h_i} \in H^{h_i}$ $(i = 0, 1, \dots, p)$ satisfying the estimate

$$|\tilde u^{h_i} - u^{h_i}|_0 \le \varepsilon h_i^2\|u\|_2 \tag{6.39}$$

with an arbitrary fixed $\varepsilon > 0$.

On the zeroth level h_0, the system of nonlinear algebraic equations (6.24) has a rather small number of unknowns. Therefore, its solution does not present great difficulties and can be effected with an arbitrary accuracy controlled only by rounding-off errors.

Let us continue in the recurrent way. Suppose that we have a solution $\tilde u^{h_{i-1}}$ on level h_{i-1} with the vector of components $\tilde U^{h_{i-1}} \in \mathbf{R}^{N_{i-1}}$. The transition to the next level involves two stages.

$\mathbf{B_1^{(5)}}$. Since spaces H^h are nested, $\tilde u^{h_{i-1}} \in H^{h_i}$. To get the corresponding vector in $\mathbf{R}^{N_i}$, make vector $W^{h_i} = I_{i-1}\tilde U^{h_{i-1}}$.

$\mathbf{B_2^{(5)}}$. Form the approximate system of the Newton method (6.34). Solve then this system approximately, using $MG^{(1)}$ or $MG^{(2)}$-algorithm of section 4.6 with the initial guess $V_0 = W^{h_i}$. The obtained vector V_1 corresponds to the interpolant $\tilde u^{h_i}$ in H^{h_i} which we consider as a result.

Thus, passing from one level to another one by $FMG^{(5)}$-algorithm, we get the approximate solution on the finest grid Ω_{h_p}.

Theorem 6.4 *Assume that $u \in W_2^2(\Omega)$ and conditions* **G**, (3.9), (4.225), (4.226), (4.236), (6.18), (6.35) *are valid for problems* (6.16), (6.17) *and* (6.24). *Realizing $MG^{(1)}$-algorithm, for any $\varepsilon \in (0,1)$ we can choose an integer $m \ge 1$ and h_0 small enough such that $FMG^{(5)}$-algorithm produces an approximate solution $\tilde u^{h_p} \in H^{h_p}$ satisfying*

$$|u^{h_p} - \tilde u^{h_p}|_0 \le \varepsilon h_p^2\|u\|_2, \tag{6.40}$$

$$|u - \tilde u^{h_p}|_0 \le (\varepsilon + c_5)h_p^2\|u\|_2, \tag{6.41}$$

where u^{h_p} is the solution of the discretized nonlinear Bubnov-Galerkin problem (6.23) on grid Ω_{h_p}. Here, the number of arithmetic operations is not over $c_{12}N_p$ where N_p is the number of unknowns of system (6.24).

With $MG^{(2)}$-algorithm applied instead of $MG^{(1)}$, the corresponding estimates have the form

$$|u^{h_p} - \tilde{u}^{h_p}|_1 \leq \varepsilon h_p \|u\|_2,$$

$$|u - \tilde{u}^{h_p}|_1 \leq (c_4 + \varepsilon) h_p \|u\|_2.$$

Proof. We use induction. On the zeroth level, the system (6.24) is also nonlinear, and so we have to apply some linearizing method [147]. The obtained systems of linear algebraic equations are solved directly. As a result, the finite number of arithmetic operations is used at this level to insure the accuracy (6.40) (when h_0 is fixed).

Let us introduce

$$c_{11} = c_5 + (c_5 + 1)c_2^2, \tag{6.42}$$

$$\varepsilon_1 = \frac{\varepsilon c_7}{2c_8 c_{11}} \tag{6.43}$$

with constants from (6.27), (4.226), (4.236). The left-hand side of the inequality

$$h_i^2 |\ln h_i|^{1/2} \leq \frac{\varepsilon}{(2c_{11} + 1)c_{11}c_{18}\|u\|_2} \tag{6.44}$$

tends to 0 when $h_i \to 0$. Therefore, there exists a constant h_e such that (6.44) holds $\forall h_i \leq h_e$. Below we demand that

$$h_1 \leq h_e. \tag{6.45}$$

Let us now verify that the assumptions of Theorem 4.14 from section 4.6 are satisfied uniformly for all possible linear systems (6.34). The first point is condition **H**. Consider the problem: find $w \in \overset{\circ}{W}{}_2^1(\Omega)$ such that

$$\mathcal{L}_1(w, v; u_0) = (g, v) \qquad \forall v \in \overset{\circ}{W}{}_2^1(\Omega) \tag{6.46}$$

with some given functions $u_0 \in \overset{\circ}{W}{}_2^1(\Omega)$, $g \in L_2(\Omega)$. Since $\partial f(x, u_0)/\partial v \in L_\infty(\Omega)$, the solution w on the ground of [94] belongs to $W_2^2(\Omega)$. We want to get the uniform estimate

$$\|w\|_2 \leq c_{12}|g|_0 \tag{6.47}$$

with constant c_{12} independent of u_0. For this purpose let us substitute w for v in (6.46) and use (6.18) with the Friedrichs and the Cauchy-Bunyakovski inequalities (1.1):

$$|w|_0^2 \leq c^2(\Omega)|w|_1^2 \leq c^2(\Omega)|g|_0|w|_0.$$

Hence,

$$|w|_0 \leq c^2(\Omega)|g|_0. \tag{6.48}$$

Let us transfer the differentiation-free term in (6.46) from the left-hand side into the right-hand one and go over to the problem: find $w \in \overset{\circ}{W}{}_2^1(\Omega)$ such that

$$\int_\Omega \nabla w \cdot \nabla v dx = (g_1, v) \qquad \forall v \in \overset{\circ}{W}{}_2^1(\Omega), \tag{6.49}$$

where

$$g_1(x) = g(x) - w(x)\partial f(x, u_0)/\partial v.$$

Due to (6.48) and (6.18), the function g_1 is bounded:

$$|g_1|_0 \leq (1 + c^2(\Omega)c_3)|g|_0.$$

The operator of problem (6.49) is independent of u_0. Therefore on the ground of [94], we come to (6.47).

Now consider the discretized problem: find $w^{h_i} \in H^{h_i}$ such that

$$\mathcal{L}_1(w^{h_i}, v; u_0) = (g, v) \qquad \forall v \in H^{h_i}. \tag{6.50}$$

Let us repeat shortly the usual way to prove the inequality

$$|w - w^{h_i}|_0 \leq c_{13} h_i^2 |g|_0 \tag{6.51}$$

with a constant c_{13} independent of u_0. Let w_I be interpolant in H^{h_i} of function w. Then due to (6.47), (6.18) and Theorem 3.3, we have

$$[\![w - w_I]\!]_1 \leq |w - w_I|_1 + c_3|w - w_I|_0 \leq ch_i\|w\|_2 \leq ch_i|g|_0, \tag{6.52}$$

where we put

$$[\![v]\!]_1 = \mathcal{L}_1^{1/2}(v, v; u_0), \qquad v \in \overset{\circ}{W}{}_2^1(\Omega).$$

From (6.46), (6.50) and the Cauchy-Bunyakovski inequality, we get

$$[\![w - w^{h_i}]\!]_1^2 = \mathcal{L}_1(w - w^{h_i}, w - w^{h_i}; u_0) =$$

$$\mathcal{L}_1(w - w^{h_i}, w - w_I) \leq [\![w - w^{h_i}]\!]_1 \, [\![w - w_I]\!]_1.$$

Together with (6.52), it gives the estimate

$$[\![w - w^{h_i}]\!]_1 \leq c_{14} h_i |g|_0 \tag{6.53}$$

with the constant c_{14} independent of u_0.

Let us introduce the auxiliary problem: find a function $z \in \overset{\circ}{W}{}_2^1(\Omega)$ such that

$$\mathcal{L}_1(z, v; u_0) = (w - w^{h_i}, v) \qquad \forall v \in \overset{\circ}{W}{}_2^1(\Omega). \tag{6.54}$$

Denote the interpolant of z in H^{h_i} by z_I. By analogy with (6.52),

$$[\![z - z_I]\!]_1 \leq ch_i|w - w^{h_i}|_0. \tag{6.55}$$

Putting $v = w - w^{h_i}$ in (6.54), we have due to symmetry of $\mathcal{L}_1$:

$$|w - w^{h_i}|_0^2 = \mathcal{L}_1(z, w - w^{h_i}; u_0) = \mathcal{L}_1(w - w^{h_i}, z; u_0).$$

From (6.46) and (6.50), we get

$$\mathcal{L}_1(w - w^{h_i}, z_I; u_0) = 0.$$

Therefore, on the ground of the Cauchy-Bunyakovski inequality, we have

$$|w - w^{h_i}|_0^2 = \mathcal{L}_1(w - w^{h_i}, z - z_I; u_0) \le [\![w - w^{h_i}]\!]_1 \, [\![z - z_I]\!]_1.$$

Taking (6.55) and (6.53), we get the required inequality:

$$|w - w^{h_i}|_0 \le c_{15} h_i^2 |g|_0. \tag{6.56}$$

Thus, condition **H** is satisfied with the constant c_{15} independent of u_0.

The second point of the assumptions of Theorem 4.14 is estimate (4.237). Due to (6.18), the linear form $\mathcal{L}_1(u, v; u_0)$ is positive-definite. Therefore the left-hand side of this estimate is proved. The right-hand side was proved in Theorem 3.14 of section 3.6 where one can take the constant c_9 to be independent of u_0.

So, all assumptions of Theorem 4.14 are valid with constants independent of u_0. Therefore for ε_1 there exists m_0 such that $\forall m \ge m_0$ the error is suppressed by $MG^{(1)}$-algorithm with the factor ε_1 for any $u_0 \in H^{h_i}$. Let us fix namely such m.

Let now we have an approximate solution $\tilde{u}^{h_{i-1}}$ satisfying (6.40) at level h_{i-1}. Consider stage $\mathbf{B}_1^{(5)}$. Let us determine the accuracy with that $\tilde{u}^{h_{i-1}}$ approximates the exact solution u^{h_i} of problem (6.23). From (6.39) at level $i-1$, (6.42), (4.226), (6.27), it follows that

$$\begin{aligned} |u^{h_i} - \tilde{u}^{h_{i-1}}|_0 &\le |u^{h_i} - u|_0 + |u - \tilde{u}^{h_{i-1}}|_0 \le \\ &\le (c_5 h_i^2 + (c_5 + \varepsilon) h_{i-1}^2) \|u\|_2 \le c_{11} h_i^2 \|u\|_2. \end{aligned} \tag{6.57}$$

Let us proceed to stage $\mathbf{B}_2^{(5)}$. We use Theorem 6.3. Putting $u_0 = \tilde{u}^{h_{i-1}}$, we come to the inequality

$$|u^{h_i} - u_1|_0 \le c_{18} |\ln h_i|^{1/2} |u^{h_i} - \tilde{u}^{h_{i-1}}|_0^2.$$

This inequality, (6.44) and (6.57) yield the estimate

$$|u^{h_i} - u_1|_0 \le c_{18} c_{11}^2 |\ln h_i|^{1/2} h_i^4 \|u\|_2^2 \le \frac{\varepsilon c_{11} h_i^2}{2c_{11} + 1} \|u\|_2. \tag{6.58}$$

Instead of the exact solution u_1 of problem (6.32), we get the approximation $\tilde{u}^{h_i}$ as a result of applying $MG^{(1)}$-algorithm to system (6.34). Using Theorem 4.14 and (4.236), we come to the inequality

$$|u_1 - \tilde{u}^{h_i}|_0 \le \varepsilon_1 c_8 c_7^{-1} |u_1 - \tilde{u}^{h_{i-1}}|_0. \tag{6.59}$$

Let us evaluate the right-hand side of this inequality, using (6.58), (6.57):

$$|u_1 - \tilde{u}^{h_{i-1}}|_0 \le |u_1 - u^{h_i}|_0 + |u^{h_i} - \tilde{u}^{h_{i-1}}|_0 \le \frac{2c_{11}(c_{11} + 1)}{2c_{11} + 1} h_i^2 \|u\|_2.$$

From this, (6.43), (6.59), it follows that

$$|u_1 - \tilde{u}^{h_i}|_0 \le \frac{\varepsilon(c_{11} + 1)}{2c_{11} + 1} h_i^2 \|u\|_2.$$

From this and (6.58), we get the inequality

$$|u^{h_i} - \tilde{u}^{h_i}|_0 \le |u^{h_i} - u_1|_0 + |u_1 - \tilde{u}^{h_i}|_0 \le \varepsilon h_i^2 \|u\|_2.$$

Thus estimate (6.40) is proved, and (6.41) follows from it with the help of (6.27).

The calculation of the number of arithmetic operations is identical with calculations of section 5.1.

The estimates for $MG^{(2)}$-algorithm are proved analogously, they are somewhat easier to prove. Instead of (6.36), the following estimate should be used:

$$|u^h - u_1|_1 \le c_{16}|u^h - u_0|_1^2$$

which arises from (6.37) by virtue of the Cauchy-Bunyakovski and Friedrichs inequalities and the estimate of the norms embedded from $\overset{\circ}{W}{}_2^1(\Omega)$ in $L_4(\Omega)$. □

6.2.3 The magnetostatic problem

Let $\Omega \subset \mathbf{R}^2$ be, as before, a convex polygon with a boundary Γ. Consider a function $\nu(t) \in C^1(0,\infty)$ hereafter called *the magnetic resistance* and having the following properties:

$$0 < \nu_1 \le \nu(t) \le \nu_2 < \infty, \tag{6.60}$$

$$0 \le t\nu'(t) \le \nu_3 \qquad \forall t \in (0,\infty). \tag{6.61}$$

Instead of these, one property is often formulated which includes no derivatives:

$$\nu_1(t-s) \le t\nu(t^2) - s\nu(s^2) \le \nu_4(t-s) \qquad \forall t \ge s \ge 0. \tag{6.62}$$

For continuously differentiable function ν, (6.62) follows from (6.60), (6.61) because, by virtue of the Lagrange theorem,

$$\nu_1(t-s) \le t\nu(t^2) - s\nu(s^2) = (t-s)(\nu(\xi^2) + 2\xi^2\nu^1(\xi^2)) \le (\nu_2 + 2\nu_3)(t-s)$$

where ξ is found between t and s.

Let it be required to solve the problem

$$-\mathrm{div}(\nu(|\nabla u|^2)\,\mathrm{grad} u) = f \quad \text{in} \quad \Omega, \tag{6.63}$$

$$u = 0 \quad \text{on} \quad \Gamma \tag{6.64}$$

with a known right-hand side $f \in L_2(\Omega)$. Pass from this problem to the generalized formulation: *find* $u \in \overset{\circ}{W}{}_2^1(\Omega)$ *satisfying the equality*

$$\mathcal{L}(u,v) = 0 \qquad \forall v \in \overset{\circ}{W}{}_2^1(\Omega) \tag{6.65}$$

where

$$\mathcal{L}(u,v) = \int_\Omega \{\nu(|\nabla u|^2)(\nabla u \cdot \nabla v) + fv\}dx. \tag{6.66}$$

Let us prove that form $\mathcal{L}$ satisfies the conditions of Theorem 6.1. Note, that in this problem it is more convenient to deal with norm $|\cdot|_1$ in $\overset{\circ}{W}{}_2^1(\Omega)$.

Lemma 6.2.3 *When conditions* (6.60) *and* (6.61) *or* (6.62) *are satisfied, the form* (6.66) *is strong-monotone, Lipschitz-continuous and bounded at zero in the second argument, i. e.,* (6.4), (6.5), *and* (6.11) *are satisfied in norm* $|\cdot|_1$.

Proof. In order to abbreviate the notation, we introduce $\tilde{\nu}(u) = \nu(|\nabla u|^2)$ and treat the following transformations using the Cauchy-Bunyakovski inequality (likewise in [57]):

$$\mathcal{L}(u, u-v) - \mathcal{L}(v, u-v) =$$

$$= \int_\Omega \{(\tilde{\nu}(u) - \nu_1)(\nabla u \cdot \nabla(u-v)) - (\tilde{\nu}(v) - \nu_1)(\nabla v \cdot \nabla(u-v))\}dx +$$

$$+\nu_1 \int_\Omega \nabla(u-v) \cdot \nabla(u-v) dx \geq$$

$$\geq \int_\Omega \{(\tilde{\nu}(u) - \nu_1)(|\nabla u|^2 - |\nabla u||\nabla v|) - (\tilde{\nu}(v) - \nu_1)(|\nabla u||\nabla v| - |\nabla v|^2)\}dx +$$

$$+\nu_1 |u-v|_1^2 =$$

$$= \int_\Omega \{(\tilde{\nu}(u) - \nu_1)|\nabla u| - (\tilde{\nu}(v) - \nu_1)|\nabla v|\}(|\nabla u| - |\nabla v|)dx + \nu_1 |u-v|_1^2.$$

Now from the left-hand inequality in (6.62), the non-negativeness of the integrand follows by virtue of the inequality

$$(\nu(t^2) - \nu_1)t - (\nu(s^2) - \nu_1)s \geq 0 \qquad \forall t \geq s \geq 0.$$

Indeed, where $|\nabla u| \geq |\nabla v|$, the expression in braces is non-negative; and where $|\nabla u| < |\nabla v|$, it is non-positive. Hence

$$\mathcal{L}(u, u-v) - \mathcal{L}(v, u-v) \geq \nu_1 |u-v|_1^2.$$

Strong monotonicity is thus proved.

Now consider the inequalities

$$|\mathcal{L}(u, w) - \mathcal{L}(v, w)| \leq \int_\Omega |\tilde{\nu}(u)\nabla u \cdot \nabla w - \tilde{\nu}(v)\nabla v \cdot \nabla w| dx \leq$$

$$\leq \int_\Omega \tilde{\nu}(u)|\nabla(u-v) \cdot \nabla w| dx + \int_\Omega |\tilde{\nu}(u) - \tilde{\nu}(v)||\nabla v \cdot \nabla w| dx.$$

Apply to the augent first the algebraic Cauchy inequality then the integral one:

$$\int_\Omega \tilde{\nu}(u)|\nabla(u-v) \cdot \nabla w| dx \leq \nu_4 |u-v|_1 |w|_1.$$

In the addend, we also use the Cauchy-Bunyakovski inequalities and perform some manipulations in view of inequality (6.62):

$$\int_\Omega |\tilde{\nu}(u) - \tilde{\nu}(v)||\nabla v \cdot \nabla w| dx \leq \int_\Omega |\tilde{\nu}(u) - \tilde{\nu}(v)||\nabla v||\nabla w| dx \leq$$

$$\leq \int_\Omega \{\tilde{\nu}(u)||\nabla v| - |\nabla u|| + |\tilde{\nu}(u)|\nabla u| - \tilde{\nu}(v)|\nabla v||\}|\nabla w| dx \leq$$

$$\leq \int_\Omega 2\nu_4 ||\nabla v| - |\nabla u|| \cdot |\nabla w| dx \leq 2\nu_4 \int_\Omega |\nabla(v-u)||\nabla w| dx \leq$$

$$\leq 2\nu_4 |u-v|_1 |w|_1.$$

Combining all the three inequalities, we get

$$|\mathcal{L}(u,w) - \mathcal{L}(v,w)| \leq 3\nu_4 |u-v|_1 |w|_1.$$

Thus Lipschitz-continuity is also proved.

It remains to show that (6.11) is satisfied. Application of the Cauchy-Bunyakovski and the Friedrichs inequalities yields

$$|\mathcal{L}(0,v)| = |\int_\Omega fv dx| \leq |f|_0 |v|_0 \leq |f|_0 |v|_1. \quad \square$$

Note that according to [94], problem (6.63), (6.64) and consequently problem (6.65) are solvable, their solution belongs to $W_2^2(\Omega)$. It is the same and unique subject to strong monotonicity.

Remark 6.2.2 *When conditions* (6.60), (6.61) *are satisfied only in some interval containing the values of* $|\nabla u|^2$, *the function* ν *should be corrected using the cutoff function, likewise in Remark* 6.2.1.

To construct a discrete problem, we use piecewise linear elements, constructions and notation of section 5.1. Finally, we get the problem: *find a function* $u^h \in H^h$ *satisfying the relation*

$$\mathcal{L}(u^h, v) = 0 \qquad \forall v \in H^h \tag{6.67}$$

which is equivalent to the system of non-linear algebraic equations

$$\mathcal{L}(\sum_{y\in\Omega_h} \alpha_y \varphi_y^h, \varphi_z^h) = 0, \qquad z \in \Omega_h. \tag{6.68}$$

The solution of (6.67) is defined from this system in the following way:

$$u^h(x) = \sum_{y\in\Omega_h} \alpha_y \varphi_y^h(x). \tag{6.69}$$

The unique solvability of system (6.68) and the convergence of u^h to the exact solution follow from Theorems 6.1, 6.2.

Lemma 6.2.4 *Under conditions* (6.62) *and* (3.9), *approximate solution* (6.69) *is defined from the system* (6.68) *in the unique way and the following estimate holds:*

$$|u - u^h|_1 \leq c_{10} h \|u\|_2. \tag{6.70}$$

6.2.4 The simplest two-stage iterative process

We first consider the linearized iterative process from [86]. Introduce the designation

$$\mathcal{L}_\Delta(u,v) = \int_\Omega \nabla u \cdot \nabla v dx.$$

Then the process is written as follows: *with known $u^k \in H^h$, find $u^{k+1} \in H^h$ satisfying the equality*

$$\mathcal{L}_\Delta(u^{k+1},v) = \mathcal{L}_\Delta(u^k,v) - \omega\mathcal{L}(u^k,v) \qquad \forall v \in H^h. \tag{6.71}$$

Note that every step of this implicit iterative process contains the solution of the discrete Poisson equation. Applying here multigrid iterative algorithms, we get a two-stage method permitting to find a sequence of approximate solutions $\tilde{u}^{h_i} \in H^{h_i}$ ($i = 0,1,\dots,p$) satisfying the estimate

$$|\tilde{u}^{h_i} - u^{h_i}|_1 \leq \varepsilon h_i \|u\|_2 \tag{6.72}$$

with an arbitrary fixed $\varepsilon > 0$.

Describe this method called the $FMG^{(6)}$-algorithm. On the lower level $h = h_0$, problem (6.67) is associated with the system of non-linear equations having a rather small number of unknowns. Due to this fact, its solution does not require any special effort and can be effected with an arbitrary accuracy.

Now assume that we have an approximate solution $\tilde{u}^{h_{i-1}}$ on level h_{i-1} satisfying (6.72). The transition to the next level involves 2 stages.

$\mathbf{B}_1^{(6)}$. In view of the nestedness of spaces H^h, we have $\tilde{u}^{h_{i-1}} \in H^{h_i}$. In algorithmic sense, we compute some deficient degrees of freedom, using linear interpolation.

$\mathbf{B}_2^{(6)}$. Assume that $w^0 = \tilde{u}^{h_{i-1}}$ and execute r loops for $k = 0,\dots,r-1$. First we formulate the problem: find $u^{k+1} \in H^{h_i}$ such that

$$\mathcal{L}_\Delta(u^{k+1},v) = \mathcal{L}_\Delta(w^k,v) - \omega\mathcal{L}(w^k,v) \qquad \forall v \in H^{h_i}. \tag{6.73}$$

Then the obtained system of linear equations

$$\sum_{y\in\Omega_h} \gamma_y \mathcal{L}_\Delta(\varphi_y^{h_i},\varphi_z^{h_i}) = f_2(\varphi_z^{h_i}), \qquad z \in \Omega_{h_i}, \tag{6.74}$$

where

$$f_2(\varphi_z^{h_i}) = \mathcal{L}_\Delta(w^k,\varphi_z^{h_i}) - \omega\mathcal{L}(w^k,\varphi_z^{h_i}),$$

is solved approximately using $MG^{(2)}$-algorithm from section 4.6. Therefore, instead of the exact solution

$$u^{k+1} = \sum_{y\in\Omega_{h_i}} \gamma_y \varphi_y^{h_i}(x)$$

of problem (6.73), we get an approximate solution we denote by w^{k+1}.

With r loops executed, we have function w^r as a result, which is denoted by $\tilde{u}^{h_i}$.

In going from one level to other, we get the approximate solution $\tilde{u}^{h_i}$ on the finest grid Ω_{h_p}.

Before proving the convergence of $FMG^{(6)}$-algorithm, we establish the convergence of iterative process (6.71) and show how to choose parameter ω in the optimal way.

Lemma 6.2.5 *Let conditions* (3.9), (6.62) *be valid and* $\omega \in (0, 2c_0/c_1^2)$ *with constants of strong monotonicity* $c_0 = \nu_1$ *and Lipschitz-continuity* $c_1 = 3\nu_4$ *because of Lemma 6.2.3. Then iterative process* (6.71) *converges and obeys the estimate*

$$|u^h - u^{k+1}|_1 \leq q|u^h - u^k|_1 \tag{6.75}$$

with the multiplier

$$q = (1 - 2\omega c_0 + \omega^2 c_1^2)^{1/2}. \tag{6.76}$$

Proof. Show that the formula (6.71) gives the contractive operator $S: u^k \to u^{k+1}$ under some restriction of ω. Take two arbitrary functions $y, z \in H^h$ and consider their images $\bar{y} = S(y)$, $\bar{z} = S(z)$. From (6.71), they satisfy the equalities

$$\begin{aligned} \mathcal{L}_\Delta(\bar{y}, v) &= \mathcal{L}_\Delta(y, v) - \omega\mathcal{L}(y, v), \\ \mathcal{L}_\Delta(\bar{z}, v) &= \mathcal{L}_\Delta(z, v) - \omega\mathcal{L}(z, v), \qquad \forall v \in H^h. \end{aligned}$$

Subtracting one equality from the other, we get the relation

$$\mathcal{L}_\Delta(\bar{y} - \bar{z}, v) = \mathcal{L}_\Delta(y - z, v) - \omega(\mathcal{L}(y, v) - \mathcal{L}(z, v)) \quad \forall v \in H^h. \tag{6.77}$$

First we put $v = \tilde{v} \equiv (\bar{y} - \bar{z}) - (y - z)$ in it. By virtue of Lipschitz-continuity,

$$|\tilde{v}|_1^2 = -\omega(\mathcal{L}(y, \tilde{v}) - \mathcal{L}(z, \tilde{v})) \leq \omega c_1 |y - z|_1 |\tilde{v}|_1.$$

Hence

$$|\tilde{v}|_1 \leq \omega c_1 |y - z|_1. \tag{6.78}$$

Putting then $v = \bar{v} \equiv (\bar{y} - \bar{z}) + (y - z)$ and using (6.77), we get after simple manipulations:

$$|\bar{y} - \bar{z}|_1^2 = |y - z|_1^2 - 2\omega(\mathcal{L}(y, y - z) - \mathcal{L}(z, y - z) - \omega(\mathcal{L}(y, \tilde{v}) - \mathcal{L}(z, \tilde{v})).$$

Let us evaluate the last two summands using strong monotonicity and the Lipschitz-continuity:

$$|\bar{y} - \bar{z}|_1^2 = |y - z|_1^2 - 2\omega c_0 |y - z|_1^2 + \omega c_1 |y - z|_1 |\tilde{v}|_1.$$

Allowing for (6.78), we come to the inequality

$$|\bar{y} - \bar{z}|_1^2 \leq (1 - 2\omega c_0 + \omega^2 c_1^2)|y - z|_1^2. \tag{6.79}$$

It shows that when $0 < \omega < 2c_0/c_1^2$, the formula (6.71) really sets the contractive operator in norm $|\cdot|_1$. The point $u^h \in H^h$ is stationary, which is easy to prove by substitution into (6.71). Therefore, putting $y = u^h$, $z = u^k$ in (6.79), we obtain (6.75). □

Minimizing q in terms of ω yields

$$\omega_{opt} = c_0/c_1^2, \qquad q_{opt} = (1 - c_0^2/c_1^2)^{1/2}. \tag{6.80}$$

Now let us prove the convergence of $FMG^{(6)}$-algorithm.

Theorem 6.5 *Let conditions (3.9), (6.62) be valid. Then for any $\varepsilon \in (0,1)$, we can choose ω, integers m and r in algorithms $MG^{(2)}$ and $FMG^{(6)}$ such that the approximate solution $\tilde{u}^{h_p}$ satisfies the estimates*

$$|u^{h_p} - \tilde{u}^{h_p}|_1 \leq \varepsilon h_p \|u\|_2,$$
$$|u - \tilde{u}^{h_p}|_1 \leq (\varepsilon + c_{10})\|u\|_2,$$

where u, u^{h_p} are solutions of problems (6.65) and (6.67) with the parameter $h = h_p$. The amount of arithmetic operations does not exceed $c_{11}N_p$ where N_p is the number of unknowns of system (6.68) at level h_p.

Proof. Let us put

$$\begin{aligned} c_{11} &= c_{10} + c_2(c_{10} + 1), \\ \omega &= \omega_{opt} = c_0/c_1^2, \\ q &= q_{opt} = (1 - c_0^2/c_1^2)^{1/2}, \\ \varepsilon_1 &= (1-q)/10, \\ q_0 &= q + \varepsilon_1 + \varepsilon_1 q \end{aligned}$$

with constants of strong monotonicity $c_0 = \nu_1$ and Lipschitz-continuity $c_1 = 3\nu_4$ because of Lemma 6.2.3. Since $q \in (0,1)$, one can easily show that $q_0 \in (0,1)$.

Let us use induction. At the level h_0, the statement of the theorem is obvious, since the approximate solution can be found for an arbitrary small ε using a small amount of operations.

Suppose now that we have an approximate solution $\tilde{u}^{h_{i-1}}$ satisfying the inequality

$$|\tilde{u}^{h_{i-1}} - u^{h_{i-1}}|_1 \leq \varepsilon h_{i-1}\|u\|_2. \tag{6.81}$$

Consider stage $\mathbf{B}_1^{(6)}$ and evaluate how $\tilde{u}^{h_{i-1}}$ approximates u^{h_i}. From (6.70) and (6.81),

$$\begin{aligned} |u^{h_i} - \tilde{u}^{h_{i-1}}|_1 &\leq |u^{h_i} - u|_1 + |u - u^{h_{i+1}}|_1 + |u^{h_{i-1}} - \tilde{u}^{h_{i-1}}|_1 \leq \\ &\leq (c_{10}h_i + c_{10}h_{i-1} + \varepsilon h_{i-1})\|u\|_2. \end{aligned}$$

Using inequality (4.226), we get

$$|u^{h_i} - \tilde{u}^{h_{i-1}}|_1 \leq c_{11}h_i\|u\|_2. \tag{6.82}$$

Proceed to stage $\mathbf{B}_2^{(6)}$. According to Lemma 6.2.5,

$$|u^{h_i} \quad u^{k+1}|_1 \leq q|u^{h_i} - w^k|_1. \tag{6.83}$$

But instead of solution u^{k+1} we get w^{k+1}. In subsection 5.1.1, we verified the conditions of Theorem 4.16. In principle, one can take an integer m_0 such that for any number $m \geq m_0$ we have

$$1 + c_c \mathrm{ctg}^2(\pi/2(2m+1)) \geq 1/\varepsilon_1.$$

Let us fix namely such number m of iterations in $MG^{(2)}$-algorithm. Therefore, because of Theorem 4.16, we get

$$|u^{k+1} - w^{k+1}|_1 \leq \varepsilon_1 |u^{k+1} - w^k|_1. \tag{6.84}$$

Hence, subject to (6.83), (6.84)

$$|u^{h_i} - w^{k+1}|_1 \le |u^{h_i} - u^{k+1}|_1 + |u^{k+1} - w^{k+1}|_1 \le$$

$$\le |u^{h_i} - u^{k+1}|_1 + \varepsilon_1 |u^{k+1} - w^k|_1 \le (1+\varepsilon_1)|u^{h_i} - u^{k+1}|_1 + \varepsilon_1 |u^{h_i} - w^k|_1 \le \tag{6.85}$$

$$(q + \varepsilon_1 + \varepsilon_1 q)|u^{h_i} - w^k|_1 = q_0 |u^{h_i} - w^k|_1.$$

Since $q_0 < 1$, one can choose an integer r such that

$$q_0^r \le \varepsilon / c_{11}. \tag{6.86}$$

Then, from (6.82), (6.85),

$$|u^{h_i} - \tilde{u}^{h_i}|_1 = |u^{h_i} - w^r|_1 \le q_0^r |u^{h_i} - w^0|_1 =$$

$$= q_0^r |u^{h_i} - \tilde{u}^{h_{i-1}}|_1 \le c_{11} q_0^r h_i \|u\|_2 \le \varepsilon h_i \|u\|_2. \quad \square \tag{6.87}$$

6.2.5 Other linearizations

In actual problems where values of magnetic resistance ν are greatly different, the iterative process (6.71) and correspondingly $FMG^{(6)}$-algorithm converge very slowly. It is especially due to disproportion of the values: $c_0/c_1 \ll 1$.

This drawback is rectified to a large measure by applying another iterative process

$$\mathcal{L}_{\tilde{\Delta}}(u^{k+1}, v; u^k) = \mathcal{L}_{\tilde{\Delta}}(u^k, v; u^k) - \omega \mathcal{L}(u^k, v) \qquad \forall v \in H^h,$$

$$k = 0, 1, \ldots, r-1, \tag{6.88}$$

where

$$\mathcal{L}_{\tilde{\Delta}}(u, v; w) = \int_\Omega \nu(|\nabla w|^2) \nabla u \cdot \nabla v dx.$$

It converges much quicker than (6.71), especially in zones of saturation, where magnetic resistance is almost independent of the change of solution gradient.

Theoretically, it is accounted for the following. Introduce the norm

$$\|v\|_{\tilde{1}} = \{\mathcal{L}_{\tilde{\Delta}}(v, v; u)\}^{1/2},$$

where u is the exact solution of problem (6.65). Assume that $u \in C^1(\bar{\Omega})$ and put into consideration some elements from H^h lying inside a sphere B with radius $c_{12}h^\alpha$, $\alpha > 0$, and center u:

$$B = \{v \in H^h;\ \sup_\Omega \text{vrai}|\nabla(u - v)| \le c_{12} h^\alpha\}.$$

Now the calculations of Lemma 6.2.3 show that under the conditions of strong monotonicity and Lipschitz-continuity, constants c_0 and c_1 are quantities like $1 - c_{13}h^\alpha$ and $1 + c_{14}h^\alpha$. Moreover, the family of norms

$$\{\mathcal{L}_{\tilde{\Delta}}(v, v; w)\}^{1/2} \tag{6.89}$$

is equivalent $\forall w \in B$ with constants $1 \pm c_{15}h^{\alpha}$. All three properties allow to prove the variant of Lemma 6.2.5 for iterative process (6.88) with the parameter $\omega = 1$ and the factor

$$q = c_{16}h^{\alpha/2}. \tag{6.90}$$

Thus, when h are small, $FMG^{(6)}$-algorithm can use one iteration of process (6.88) instead of r iterations of process (6.71). This follows from the fact that q_0 can be sufficiently small due to m and (6.90), i. e., the estimate (6.86) can be achieved at $r = 1$.

The question arises about the gradient convergence in the uniform norm to insure the belonging the approximate solutions to the sphere B. Note that the root-mean-square convergence with the first order does not lead to the convergence in the C-norm, because functions $v \in H^h$ are estimated as follows [146]:

$$\max_{\bar{\Omega}} |\nabla v| \leq ch^{-1}|v|_1 \qquad \text{in} \quad \Omega \subset \mathbf{R}^2. \tag{6.91}$$

Therefore the requirement of belonging the approximate solution u^h to the sphere B is really additional. In some cases, it is nevertheless valid.

I. When the right-hand side f is somewhat smoother, convergence will occur in more strong norm. Indeed, according to [40],

$$\|u - u^h\|_{1,p,\Omega} \leq ch\|f\|_{0,p,\Omega}, \qquad p > 2.$$

This estimate permits to keep the approximate solutions in sphere B, since [40]

$$\max_{\bar{\Omega}} |\nabla v| \leq ch^{-2/p}\|v\|_{1,p,\Omega}$$

and so α can be taken equal to $1 - 2/p$.

II. When finite elements are employed with degree higher than 1 for the more smooth u, the convergence will be of order higher than 1:

$$|u - u^h|_1 \leq c(u)h^{1+\alpha}, \qquad \alpha > 0.$$

Due to (6.91) $u^h \in B$, i. e., the uniform convergence of gradient takes place with degree α.

III. Now let us especially concern finite elements of degree 1. In section 3.5, the superconvergence of solution gradient at some particular knots was discussed. Choose these knots as numerical quadrature nodes when assemble systems of linear algebraic equations following from (6.88). Then we have discrete analogues of the conditions of strong monotonicity and the norm family (6.89) with constants like $1 + O(h^{\alpha})$. Here, α will be much greater than in the case of an arbitrary choice of the quadrature nodes.

Now discuss application of the Newton method. Consider it in following form: *find* $u^{k+1} \in H^h$ *such that*

$$\mathcal{L}_2(u^{k+1}, v; u^k) = f_2(v; u^k) \qquad \forall v \in H^h \tag{6.92}$$

where

$$\mathcal{L}_2(u, v; w) = \int_{\Omega} \{\nu(|\nabla w|^2)(\nabla u \cdot \nabla v) + 2\nu'(|\nabla w|^2)(\nabla u \cdot \nabla w)(\nabla v \cdot \nabla w)\}dx,$$

$$f_2(v;w) = \int_\Omega \{fv + 2\nu'(|\nabla w|^2)|\nabla w|^2(\nabla v \cdot \nabla w)\}dx.$$

This problem is equivalent to the system of linear algebraic equations for degrees of freedom γ_y of function u^{k+1}:

$$\sum_{y\in\Omega_h} \gamma_y \mathcal{L}_2(\varphi_y, \varphi_z; u^k) = f_2(\varphi_z^h; u^k), \qquad z \in \Omega_h, \tag{6.93}$$

where

$$u^{k+1}(x) = \sum_{y\in\Omega_h} \gamma_y \varphi_y(x).$$

Note that the structure of the system matrix became more complicated in comparison with the proceeding linearization method. To clear up a form of additional terms, one can write the Euler differential equation corresponding to problem (6.92) in $\overset{\circ}{W}{}_2^2(\Omega)$. It is easy to see that mixed derivatives appear in it.

Therefore, despite a higher quadratic order of convergence, the Newton method is sometimes less efficient than (6.88). Indeed, when h is small, only one iteration each of both methods is used. But the construction of systems of linear algebraic equations of the Newton method is more complex. That is just why the iterations (6.88) may be more efficient.

6.3 Solving the elasticity problem

The material of this section is simple generalization of section 5.1 from one equation to a system of second-order elliptic equations. Theoretical consideration is compact, therefore. At the end of the section, a numerical illustration and possible generalizations are provided.

6.3.1 The elasticity plane problem

Let Ω be a convex polygon in $\mathbf{R}^2$ with a boundary Γ. Consider Lame's equations in vector form:

$$\mu\Delta\vec{u} + (\lambda+\mu)\nabla(\nabla\cdot\vec{u}) = -\vec{f} \qquad \text{in} \quad \Omega, \tag{6.94}$$

$$\vec{u} = 0 \qquad \text{on} \quad \Gamma \tag{6.95}$$

where λ, μ are Lame's constants,

$$\vec{u} = \begin{bmatrix} u_1 \\ u_2 \end{bmatrix}, \vec{f} = \begin{bmatrix} f_1 \\ f_2 \end{bmatrix}.$$

For two-dimensional vector functions, introduce the scalar product, the norm, and the bilinear form:

$$(\vec{u},\vec{f}) = \int_\Omega \vec{u}\cdot\vec{f}dx, \qquad |\vec{u}|_{0,\Omega} = (\vec{u},\vec{u})^{1/2},$$

$$\mathcal{L}(\vec{u},\vec{f}) = \mathcal{L}(u_1,u_2;f_1,f_2) =$$

$$= \int_\Omega \{2\mu(\partial_1 u_1\cdot\partial_1 f_1 + \partial_2 u_2\cdot\partial_2 f_2) + \lambda(\partial_1 u_1 + \partial_2 u_2)(\partial_1 f_1 + \partial_2 f_2) +$$

$$+\mu(\partial_2 u_1 + \partial_1 u_2)(\partial_2 f_1 + \partial_1 f_2)\}dx. \tag{6.96}$$

Let $f_1, f_2 \in L_2(\Omega)$, then from [94] it follows that there exists a unique solution of problem (6.94), (6.95) for which $u_1, u_2 \in W_2^2(\Omega)$.

In subsection 1.1.6, transition to a generalized formulation has been made. In the notation of (6.96), it has the form: *find* $\vec{u} \in (\overset{\circ}{W}{}_2^1(\Omega))^2$ *satisfying the equality*

$$\mathcal{L}(\vec{u}, \vec{v}) - (\vec{f}, \vec{v}) \qquad \forall \vec{v} \in (\overset{\circ}{W}{}_2^1(\Omega))^2. \tag{6.97}$$

As was stated in subsection 1.1.6, this problem also has a unique solution which coincides with that of problem (6.94), (6.95) for $\vec{u}$ smooth enough.

6.3.2 Projective-difference problem

Triangulate a polygon in the same way like in section 5.1, keeping the notation $\bar{\Omega}_h$, Ω_h for grid domains and φ_y^h, for piecewise linear basis functions of space H^h. An approximate solution of problem (6.97) on grid Ω_h will be sought in the form:

$$\vec{u}^h = \begin{bmatrix} u_1^h \\ u_2^h \end{bmatrix} = \sum_{y \in \Omega_h} \begin{bmatrix} \alpha_{1y}^h \\ \alpha_{2y}^h \end{bmatrix} \varphi_y^h \tag{6.98}$$

where α_{1y}^h, α_{2y}^h are defined from the system of linear algebraic equations of the Bubnov-Galerkin method

$$\begin{aligned} \mathcal{L}(u_1^h, u_2^h; \varphi_y^h, 0) &= (f_1, \varphi_y^h), \qquad y \in \Omega_h, \\ \mathcal{L}(u_1^h, u_2^h; 0, \varphi_y^h) &= (f_2, \varphi_y^h), \qquad y \in \Omega_h. \end{aligned} \tag{6.99}$$

In the usual way, using the approximating properties of linear finite elements, we get the estimates

$$\begin{aligned} |\vec{u} - \vec{u}^h|_{0,\Omega} &\le c_1 h^2 |\vec{f}|_{0,\Omega}, \\ |\vec{u} - \vec{u}^h|_{1,\Omega} &\le c_2 h |\vec{f}|_{0,\Omega}. \end{aligned} \tag{6.100}$$

Let us label the nodes of set Ω_h from 1 to N. In compact matrix notation, system (6.99) looks thus:

$$L^h V^h = F^h \tag{6.101}$$

where L^h is a $2N \times 2N$ nonsingular square matrix, V^h is a $2N$-vector of unknowns; the first N vector conponents are the values of u_1^h at the nodes of Ω_h, the other N coordinates are the values of u_2^h.

An arbitrary $2N$-vector W^h is associated with an prolongation from $\vec{H}^h = (H^h)^2$ — the vector-function

$$w^h(x) = \sum_{y \in \Omega_h} \begin{bmatrix} W_{1y}^h \\ W_{2y}^h \end{bmatrix} \varphi_y^h(x) \tag{6.102}$$

where W_{1y}^h are the first N components, and W_{2y}^h the later N components of vector W^h arranged according to the enumeration of nodes $y \in \Omega_h$. Using w^h, we introduce the vector norm

$$\|W^h\|_h = |w^h|_{0,\Omega}. \tag{6.103}$$

6.3.3 The multigrid iterative algorithm

According to Theorem 3.14, eigenvalues of the symmetric matrix L^h are bounded:

$$\lambda(L^h) \le c_2. \qquad (6.104)$$

To solve system (6.101) on a sequence of grids Ω_h with parameters $h = h_0, h_1, \dots, h_p$ (decreasing twice or thrice), we use generalization of $MG^{(1)}$-algorithm from section 4.6 with the iterative parameters chosen by formula (4.215). Generalization is here expressed in that the vector prolongations are taken in $\vec{H}^h$ instead of H^h and restriction of the residual G^h is effected individually for two components. Stage $\mathbf{A_2}$ is modified as follows.

$\mathbf{A_2'}$. The residual G^{h_i} with components $G^{h_i}_{jz}$, $z \in \Omega_{h_i}$ $(j = 1, 2)$ numbered like in (6.102) will be restricted by the rule

$$G^{h_{i-1}}_{jy} = \sum_{z\in\Omega_{h_i}} \beta^y_z G^{h_i}_{jz} \qquad \forall y \in \Omega_{h_{i-1}}, \quad j = 1, 2 \qquad (6.105)$$

into a space of dimension $2N_{i-1}$. The coefficients β^y_z are the same like in (4.233). As a result, we have vector $G^{h_{i-1}} = R_i G^{h_i}$ of dimension $2N_{i-1}$.

Applying FMG-algorithm in combination with this vector $\overrightarrow{MG}^{(1)}$-algorithm, we get the following result.

Theorem 6.6 *For any $\varepsilon > 0$, the application of FMG-algorithm with vector $\overrightarrow{MG}^{(1)}$-algorithm to system (6.101) on a sequence of nested grids with $h = h_0, \dots, h_p$ (decreasing twice or thrice) yields the approximate solution $\widetilde{V}^{h_p}$ satisfying the estimate*

$$\|V^{h_p} - \widetilde{V}^{h_p}\|_h \le \varepsilon h_p^2 |\vec{f}|_{0,\Omega}, \qquad (6.106)$$

the amount of arithmetic operations is not over than $c_3 N_p$ with constant c_3 independent of $\vec{f}$, h.

Denoting the vector of prolongation of $\widetilde{V}^{h_p}$ in $\vec{H}^{h_p}$ by $\tilde{\vec{v}}^{h_p}$, we get the estimate

$$|\vec{u} - \tilde{\vec{v}}^{h_p}|_{0,\Omega} \le (c_1 + \varepsilon) h_p^2 |\vec{f}|_{0,\Omega}. \qquad (6.107)$$

With algorithms FMG and $\overrightarrow{MG}^{(2)}$ (with modified stage $\vec{\mathbf{A}}_2$), we have corresponding estimates in the $\overset{\circ}{W}{}^1_2(\Omega)$ norm:

$$\|V^{h_p} - \widetilde{V}^{h_p}\|^{(1)}_h \le \varepsilon h_p |\vec{f}|_{0,\Omega},$$
$$|u - \tilde{\vec{v}}^{h_p}|_{1,\Omega} \le (c_2 + \varepsilon) h_p |f|_{0,\Omega}.$$

6.3.4 The numerical experiment

To illustrate Theorem 6.6, we consider a numerical solution of problem (6.94), (6.95) in unit square $(0, 1)^2$ with the coefficients $\mu = 1.5$, $\lambda = 1.0$ and the right-hand side

$$f_1 = 2.5\pi^2 \cos \pi x \ \cos \pi y + 8y^2 - 8y + 3x^2 - 3x,$$

Table 6.1:

h	N	$m = 4$		$m = 6$	
		$\|\vec{u} - \tilde{v}^h\|_0$	$\|\vec{u} - v^h\|_1$	$\|\vec{u} - \tilde{v}^h\|_0$	$\|\vec{u} - v^h\|_1$
1/2	1×1	0.2175	1.268	0.2175	1.268
1/4	3×3	0.0769	0.879	0.0476	0.434
1/8	7×7	0.0160	0.217	0.0124	0.111
1/16	15×15	0.0042	0.097	0.0032	0.040
1/32	31×31	0.0009	0.026	0.0008	0.014
1/64	63×63	0.0002	0.010	0.0002	0.006

$$f_2 = -5.5\pi^2 \sin \pi x \, \sin \pi y + 10xy - 5x - 5y + 2.5.$$

The exact solution of this problem is the functions

$$u_1 = xy(x-1)(y-1),$$

$$u_2 = \sin \pi x \, \sin \pi y.$$

To calculate the right-hand side of the Bubnov-Galerkin system, we used a quadrature formula such that system (6.101) coincides with the difference scheme up to the factor. The estimates (6.100) remains here valid.

To solve system (6.101), we used the FMG-algorithm and vector $\overrightarrow{MG}^{(1)}$-algorithm with the amount of iterations $m = 4, 6$ and optimal parameters τ_i chosen by formula (4.215).

In Table 6.1, the errors are given of the solutions $\tilde{v}^{h_i}$ obtained on a sequence of grids.

If m increases further, the errors in L_2-norm remain unchanged. This testifies that the error of the algorithm became much less than the approximation error of the Bubnov-Galerkin method given in Table at $m = 6$.

When algorithms FMG and $\overrightarrow{MG}^{(2)}$ are used in the form of V-cycle with optimal parameters (4.99), the error norm is almost the same for m half as less, equal to 2 and 3, respectively.

6.3.5 Possible generalizations

In principle, Chapter 5 involves the main stages for necessary generalizations. Problems of curvilinear boundaries are treated in section 5.2, possible decrease in smoothness near angles greater than π is used in section 5.3. The second and third boundary value problems for Lame's equations are formulated in a different way (see subsection 1.1.6), but two approaches explained in section 5.6 are easy to modify also for such formulation.

Transition to three-dimensional problems can be effected on the basis of section 5.4. At least, various cases of nonlinear dependence of coefficients and right-hand sides can be studied on the basis of section 6.2.

6.4 The biharmonic equation

In this section, we deal with the mixed formulation of the finite element method including the unknown solution u as well as the vortex $-\Delta u$ (see subsection 1.1.9). This formulation allows to bypass the requirement of the initial formulation of subsection 1.1.7 that the approximate solution should belong to class $C^1(\bar{\Omega})$. The ordinary Lagrange elements of class $C(\bar{\Omega})$ can be used here, as a result.

The matrix of the discrete problem has a spectrum with alternating signs. To solve this problem, we use multigrid algorithms given in Chapter 4 for symmetric sign-indefinite operators.

An analogous multigrid algorithm was examined in the paper [148]. Here we use a different smoothing procedure with the simpler explicit iterations in contrast with [148] where the implicit iterations were employed. Becides, we use the special iterative parameters which essentially increase the rate of convergence. True, the possibility of these modifications was predicted in [148]. Here we give the complete proof.

6.4.1 The mixed formulation

Let $\Omega \subset \mathbf{R}^2$ be a convex polygon with a boundary Γ. Consider the Dirichlet problem for the biharmonic equation

$$\Delta^2 u = f \qquad \text{in} \quad \Omega, \tag{6.108}$$

$$u = \partial_\nu u = 0 \qquad \text{on} \quad \Gamma. \tag{6.109}$$

Let also

$$f \in W_2^{-1}(\Omega). \tag{6.110}$$

According to [80], $u \in W_2^3(\Omega)$. But, broadly speaking, $u \notin W_2^4(\Omega)$ even if $f \in L_2(\Omega)$ because of angular singularities.

Introduce the notation

$$a(v,\psi) = \int_\Omega v\psi dx, \qquad b(u,\varphi) = -\int_\Omega \nabla u \cdot \nabla \varphi dx,$$

$$l(\varphi) = -\langle f, \varphi\rangle_\Omega.$$

Now the mixed formulation of subsection 1.1.9 can be read as follows: *find* $v \in W_2^1(\Omega)$, $u \in \overset{\circ}{W}{}_2^1(\Omega)$ *satisfying the equalities*

$$a(v,\psi) \;+\; b(u,\psi) = 0 \qquad \forall \psi \in W_2^1(\Omega), \tag{6.111}$$

$$b(\varphi, v) \;=\; l(\varphi) \qquad \forall \varphi \in \overset{\circ}{W}{}_2^1(\Omega). \tag{6.112}$$

Remark 6.4.1 *For the chosen spaces, this mixed formulation does not satisfy the Brezzi conditions in norms* $\|\cdot\|_1$, $|\cdot|_1$. *Hence, we cannot conclude anything on the stability. We should have a stable formulation if we transform the bilinear form* b *into*

$$b_1(u,\psi) = \int_\Omega \Delta u \cdot \psi \, dx \tag{6.113}$$

and find the solution $v \in L_2(\Omega)$, $u \in \overset{\circ}{W}{}_2^2(\Omega)$ *satisfying the equalities*

$$a(v,\psi) \;+\; b_1(u,\psi) = 0 \qquad \forall \psi \in L_2(\Omega), \tag{6.114}$$

$$b_1(\varphi, v) \;=\; l(\varphi) \qquad \forall \varphi \in \overset{\circ}{W}{}_2^2(\Omega). \tag{6.115}$$

Indeed, this formulation satisfies the Brezzi conditions (1.14)–(1.16) *in norms* $|\cdot|_0$, $|\cdot|_2$. *But for discretization, it again requires the basis functions belonging to* $C^1(\bar{\Omega})$.

Note that

$$b(u,\psi) = b_1(u,\psi) \tag{6.116}$$

if $u \in \overset{\circ}{W}{}_2^2(\Omega)$, $\psi \in W_2^1(\Omega)$ because of Green's formula

$$\int_\Omega \nabla u \cdot \nabla \psi \, dx = -\int_\Omega \Delta u \cdot \psi \, dx + \int_\Gamma \psi \cdot \partial_\nu u \, d\gamma. \tag{6.117}$$

Hence, under sufficiently smooth solution u of the initial problem (6.108)–(6.109), we have the same unique pair v, u in both formulations (6.111)–(6.112) and (6.114)–(6.115) due to Theorems 1.3 and 1.6. In principle, we can use the first formulation to find the solution and the second one to justificate its properties.

To construct a discrete problem, we use the Lagrange elements of degree 2 on triangles. To this end, we take the notation and the rule of triangulation from section 5.1. Besides the principal triangulation $\mathcal{T}_h$ with nodes $\bar{\Omega}_h$, we also introduce the set $\bar{\Omega}_h'$ as a collection of nodes of quadratic elements being, in fact, the set $\bar{\Omega}_{h/2}$. Also introduce sets $\Omega_h' = \bar{\Omega}_h' \cap \Omega$ and $\Gamma_h' = \bar{\Omega}_h' \cap \Gamma$. Denote the number of nodes in $\bar{\Omega}_h'$ and Ω_h' by N_h' and n_h' respectively.

Introduce operations of prolongation of the vectors and projecting the functions onto a grid. Suppose that the vector W^h of dimension N_h' has components W_y^h where $y \in \bar{\Omega}_h'$. It is associated with a prolongation $w^h \in C(\bar{\Omega})$ being a complete polynomial of degree 2 on every triangle of $\mathcal{T}_h$ and satisfying the equality

$$w^h(y) = W_y^h \qquad \text{on} \quad \bar{\Omega}_h'. \tag{6.118}$$

The set of such prolongations forms a linear finite-dimensional space H_h'. Taking one of the components W_y^h equal to 1 and the other components of W^h to zero, we get, as a prolongation, the basis function $\varphi_y^h(x)$.

Projecting the function $w^h \in C(\bar{\Omega})$ onto the grid $\bar{\Omega}_h'$ yields vector W^h of dimension N_h' with components defined by equalities (6.118).

Prolongation $v^h \in C(\bar{\Omega})$ of vector V^h of dimension n_h' with components V_y^h where $y \in \Omega_h'$ is introduced in the similar way. Instead of (6.118), we now assume that

$$v^h(y) \;=\; V_y^h \qquad \text{on} \qquad \Omega_h', \tag{6.119}$$

$$v^h(y) \;=\; 0 \qquad \text{on} \qquad \Gamma_h'. \tag{6.120}$$

The set of such prolongations also forms a linear finite-dimensional space $\overset{\circ}{H}{}_h'$ being a subspace of $\overset{\circ}{W}{}_2^1(\Omega)$. The function $v^h \in C(\bar{\Omega})$ projected onto the grid $\bar{\Omega}_h'$ yields n_h'-vector

V^h with components defined by equalities (6.119). Introduce $H^h = H'_h \times \overset{\circ}{H}{}'_h$. Let $N = N' + n'$. The correspondences (6.118) and (6.119)–(6.120) define the isomorphism of linear spaces $H^h \leftrightarrow \mathbf{R}^N$.

According to the Bubnov-Galerkin method, the approximate solution $u^h = (u_1^h, u_2^h) \in H^h$ is sought in the form:

$$u_1^h(x) = \sum_{y \in \bar{\Omega}'_h} \alpha_{y1}^h \varphi_y^h(x) \quad \text{on} \quad \bar{\Omega}, \tag{6.121}$$

$$u_2^h(x) = \sum_{y \in \Omega'_h} \alpha_{y2}^h \varphi_y^h(x) \quad \text{on} \quad \bar{\Omega}, \tag{6.122}$$

where α_{yi}^h are parameters defined from the system of equations

$$a(u_1^h, \psi) + b(u_2^h, \psi) = 0, \qquad \psi \in H'_h, \tag{6.123}$$

$$b(\varphi, u_1^h) = l(\varphi), \qquad \varphi \in \overset{\circ}{H}{}'_h. \tag{6.124}$$

Let us label nodes $y \in \Omega'_h$ from 1 to n' and nodes $y \in \bar{\Omega}'_h \setminus \Omega'_h$ from $n' + 1$ to N'. Now problem (6.123), (6.124) is equivalent to the system of linear algebraic equations

$$L^{h_i} V^{h_i} = F^{h_i}. \tag{6.125}$$

The matrix L^{h_i} is symmetric and has the following form:

$$L^{h_i} = \begin{bmatrix} \left[a(\varphi_k^h, \varphi_j^h)\right]_{k=1,\dots,N'}^{j=1,\dots,N'} & \left[b(\varphi_k^h, \varphi_j^h)\right]_{k=1,\dots,n'}^{j=1,\dots,N'} \\ \left[b(\varphi_j^h, \varphi_k^h)\right]_{k=1,\dots,N'}^{j=1,\dots,n'} & [0]_{k=1,\dots,n'}^{j=1,\dots,n'} \end{bmatrix} \tag{6.126}$$

where the superscript denotes the line number and the subscript, the column number. Accordingly,

$$V^h = \begin{bmatrix} \left[\alpha_{k,1}^h\right]^{k=1,\dots,N'} \\ \left[\alpha_{k,2}^h\right]^{k=1,\dots,n'} \end{bmatrix}, \quad F^h = \begin{bmatrix} [0]^{k=1,\dots,N'} \\ \left[l(\varphi_k^h)\right]^{k=1,\dots,n'} \end{bmatrix}. \tag{6.127}$$

Let us investigate a solvability of problem (6.123)–(6.124). Again, likewise in differential case, the Brezzi conditions are not satisfied in norms $\|\cdot\|_1$, $|\cdot|_1$ or in their discrete analogues. Therefore, we transform the bilinear form b by analogy with (6.113) to get a stable formulation. This time, Green's formula (6.117) is not applicable due to a discontinuity of the first derivatives of functions from $\overset{\circ}{H}{}'_h$ along interior edges of triangulation $\mathcal{T}_h$. Instead of it, we use its local version on each triangle $T \in \mathcal{T}_h$ with a boundary ∂T:

$$\int_T \nabla u \cdot \nabla \psi \, dx = -\int_T \Delta u \cdot \psi \, dx + \int_{\partial T} \psi \cdot \partial_\nu u \, d\gamma. \tag{6.128}$$

Let us denote the set of all edges of triangulation $\mathcal{T}_h$ by

$$\mathcal{E}_h = \bigcup_{T \in \mathcal{T}_h} \partial T$$

and introduce the jump of normal derivative

$$J(\partial_\nu u)|_e = \partial_\nu u$$

on the boundary edge $e \in \mathcal{E}_h$ and

$$J(\partial_\nu u)|_e = \partial_{\nu_1} u + \partial_{\nu_2} u$$

on the interior edge $e = \partial T_1 \cap \partial T_2$ of two triangles $T_1, T_2 \in \mathcal{T}_h$, where ν_i are the unit normals to e exterior to T_i. Then, summing equalities (6.128) over all triangles, we get

$$\int_\Omega \nabla u \cdot \nabla \psi \, dx = - \sum_{T \in \mathcal{T}_h} \int_T \Delta u \cdot \psi \, dx + \int_{\mathcal{E}_h} \psi \cdot J(\partial_\nu u) d\gamma. \tag{6.129}$$

We define the new bilinear form [15]

$$b_2(u, \psi) = \sum_{T \in \mathcal{T}_h} \int_T \Delta u \cdot \psi \, dx - \int_{\mathcal{E}_h} \psi \cdot J(\partial_\nu u) \, d\gamma \tag{6.130}$$

and a semi-discrete analogue of $W_2^2(\Omega) \cap \overset{\circ}{W}{}_2^1(\Omega)$, the space

$$H_h^2 = \{u \in \overset{\circ}{W}{}_2^1(\Omega) : \quad u \in W_2^2(T) \quad \text{on each} \quad T \in \mathcal{T}_h\}$$

with the norm

$$\|u\|_{2,h} = (\sum_{T \in \mathcal{T}_h} \|u\|_{2,T}^2 + h^{-1} \int_{\mathcal{E}_h} J^2(\partial_\nu u) \, d\gamma)^{1/2}. \tag{6.131}$$

Then on $W_2^1(\Omega)$ we define the norm

$$\|u\|_{0,h} = (|u|_{0,\Omega}^2 + h \int_{\mathcal{E}_h} u^2 d\gamma)^{1/2} \tag{6.132}$$

and put the space H_h^0 as the completion of $W_2^1(\Omega)$ with respect to norm $\| \cdot \|_{0,h}$. In this notation, let us go over to the I.Babuška–J.Osborn–J.Pitkäranta formulation: *find* $v \in H_h^0$, $u \in H_h^2$ *satisfying the equalities*

$$a(v, \psi) \; + \; b_2(u, \psi) = 0 \qquad \forall \psi \in H_h^0, \tag{6.133}$$

$$b_2(\varphi, v) \; = \; l(\varphi) \qquad \forall \varphi \in H_h^2. \tag{6.134}$$

It is proved in [15] that this formulation satisfies the Brezzi conditions (1.14)–(1.16). Moreover, if $u \in \overset{\circ}{W}{}_2^2(\Omega)$, $\psi \in W_2^1(\Omega)$ then

$$b_2(u, \psi) = b(u, \psi). \tag{6.135}$$

Again, under sufficiently smooth solution u of the initial problem (6.108)–(6.109), we have the same unique pair v, u in both formulations (6.111)–(6.112) and (6.133)–(6.134) owing to Theorems 1.3 and 1.6.

Note that $H'_h \subset H^0_h$, $\overset{\circ}{H}'_h \subset H^2_h$. According to the Bubnov-Galerkin method, let us find the approximate solution $u^h = (u^h_1, u^h_2) \in H^h$ in the form (6.121)–(6.122) with parameters α^h_{yi} from the system of equations

$$a(u^h_1, \psi) + b_2(u^h_2, \psi) = 0, \qquad \psi \in H'_h, \tag{6.136}$$

$$b_2(\varphi, u^h_1) = l(\varphi), \qquad \varphi \in \overset{\circ}{H}'_h. \tag{6.137}$$

Again, this formulation satisfies the Brezzi conditions (1.149)–(1.151) [15] and the estimate of Theorem 1.15:

$$\|\Delta u + u^h_1\|_{0,h} + \|u - u^h_2\|_{2,h} \leq c\,(\inf_{\psi \in H'_h} \|\Delta u - \psi\|_{0,h} + \inf_{\varphi \in \overset{\circ}{H}'_h} \|u - \varphi\|_{2,h}). \tag{6.138}$$

Because of (6.110), Lemmata 3, 4 of [15] on approximation and the equivalence of the norms $\|\cdot\|_{0,h}$ and $|\cdot|_0$, we have

$$|\Delta u + u^h_1|_0 + \|u - u^h_2\|_{2,h} \leq ch\|u\|_{3,\Omega} \leq ch\|f\|_{-1,\Omega}. \tag{6.139}$$

But for functions $v \in H'_h$ and $u \in \overset{\circ}{H}'_h$, we have (6.135). Therefore, we get the same algebraic system (6.125). So, we executed a loop in proof over formulation (6.133)–(6.134) with the unique purpose: to justificate such specific choice of norms (6.131), (6.132).

Let us take an arbitrary vector $W^h \in \mathbf{R}^N$ and introduce the vector norm

$$\|W^h\|^{(2)}_h = (|w^h_1|^2_0 + \|w^h_2\|^2_{2,h})^{1/2} \tag{6.140}$$

with the help of its isomorphic image $w^h = (w^h_1, w^h_2) \in H^h$.

6.4.2 The multigrid algorithm

Let us introduce the diagonal matrix $\mathcal{D}^h = \mathrm{diag}\{d^h_1, \dots, d^h_N\}$ with the elements

$$d^h_j = \begin{cases} h^{-4}, & j = 1, \dots, N', \\ 1, & j = N'+1, \dots, N. \end{cases}$$

Consider the symmetric matrix

$$S^h = (\mathcal{D}^h)^{1/2} L^h (\mathcal{D}^h)^{1/2}.$$

Due to (6.126), this matrix also has four blocks. Let us employ the standard estimate (3.143) to find the upper bound λ^* of the maximal modulus of eigenvalues. To examine the elements of S^h in each blocks, we apply equality (6.135) and the evaluation like the consideration of Theorem 3.14. As a result, we get the estimate

$$|\lambda_{max}(S^h)| \leq \lambda^* \leq c_4 h^{-4}. \tag{6.141}$$

Note that matrix $\mathcal{D}^h L^h$ has the same eigenvalues and another complete system of eigenvectors. Therefore, estimate (6.141) is valid for $\mathcal{D}^h L^h$ too.

To solve system (6.125) on a sequence of triangulations $\mathcal{T}_0, \mathcal{T}_1, \dots, \mathcal{T}_p$, we use $MG^{(10)}$-algorithm from section 4.11 with the upper bound λ_i^*.defined for each matrix $\mathcal{D}^{h_i} L^{h_i}$ as above.

Let us introduce the interpolation operator $I_{h_{i+1}}^{h_i} : \mathbf{R}^{N_i} \to \mathbf{R}^{N_{i+1}}$ as in the subsection 3.1.3. Namely, let us take an arbitrary vector $V^{h_i} \in \mathbf{R}^{N_i}$. Put V^{h_i} in isomorphic correspondence with a vector-function $v^{h_i} = (v_1^{h_i}, v_2^{h_i}) \in H^{h_i}$. Note that $H^{h_i} \subset H^{h_{i+1}}$. Therefore we can put v^{h_i} as the element of $H^{h_{i+1}}$ in isomorphic correspondence with vector $V^{h_{i+1}} \in \mathbf{R}^{N_{i+1}}$. Finally, we take this vector as the result of interpolation: $V^{h_{i+1}} = I_{h_{i+1}}^{h_i} V^{h_i}$. Practically, this operator is defined by formula (2.7) of quadratic interpolation which is simplified along sides of triangles. Operator $I_{h_{i+1}}^{h_i}$ defines a rectangular matrix which we denote by the same symbol. The restriction matrix $R_{h_i}^{h_{i+1}}$ is introduced by the formula $R_{h_i}^{h_{i+1}} = (I_{h_{i+1}}^{h_i})^T$. Thus, we defined the restriction operator $R_{h_i}^{h_{i+1}} : \mathbf{R}^{N_{i+1}} \to \mathbf{R}^{N_i}$.

Theorem 6.7 *Let* (6.110) *hold. Then for any* $\varepsilon \in (0,1)$, *one can find an integer* m_0 *independent of* h_i, f *and such that* $\forall m \geq m_0$ *the error of an initial guess* $V_0^{h_i}$ *at one step of the* $MG^{(10)}$*-algorithm reduces by a factor* ε:

$$\|V_1^{h_i} - V^{h_i}\|_h^{(2)} \leq \varepsilon \|V_0^{h_i} - V^{h_i}\|_h^{(2)} \quad where\, V_1^{h_i} = MG^{(10)}(V_0^{h_i}, F^{h_i}). \tag{6.142}$$

Proof. In comparison with subsection 4.11.2, we have a deficient regularity of solution and can not use the results of this section. Therefore we need to turn immediately to the Theorem 4.9 of subsection 4.4.1. To that end, we employ the following notation:

$$L_i = \mathcal{D}^{h_i} L^{h_i}, \qquad I_i = I_{h_{i+1}}^{h_i}, \qquad R_i = \mathcal{D}^{h_{i-1}} R_{h_{i-1}}^{h_i} (\mathcal{D}^{h_i})^{-1}.$$

The system (6.125) is equivalent to

$$L_i V^{h_i} = F_i \tag{6.143}$$

with the right-hand side $F_i = \mathcal{D}^{h_i} F^{h_i}$. Then we can rewrite smoothing procedures (4.557) and (4.570) in $MG^{(10)}$-algorithm in the form

$$\begin{aligned} U_{l+1} &= U_l - \tau_l L_i (L_i U_l - F_i), \\ Y_{l+1} &= Y_l - \tau_l L_i (L_i Y_l - F_i), \qquad l = 0, 1, \dots, m-1, \end{aligned}$$

with the iterative operator

$$J_i = (I \quad \tau_{m-1} L_i^2) \dots (I - \tau_0 L_i^2).$$

Finally, we introduce the scalar product

$$(U, V)_i = U^T (\mathcal{D}^{h_i})^{-1} V, \qquad U, V \in \mathbf{R}^{N_i}, \tag{6.144}$$

and the corresponding norm

$$\|U\|_i = (U, U)_i, \qquad U \in \mathbf{R}^{N_i}.$$

We denote the space $\mathbf{R}^{N_i}$ with such scalar product by M_i.

Note that operator L_i is self-adjoint in M_i and has the full system $g_1, \dots, g_{N_i}$ of eigenvectors orthonormal in this scalar product. Let $V \in \mathbf{R}^{N_i}$ be an arbitrary vector and let

$$V = \sum_{j=1}^{N_i} \alpha_j g_j \tag{6.145}$$

be the decomposition into the system $\{g_j\}$. Then

$$L_i V = \sum_{j=1}^{N_i} \alpha_j \lambda_j g_j. \tag{6.146}$$

Now we introduce the operator $\Lambda_i : \mathbf{R}^{N_i} \to \mathbf{R}^{N_i}$ by the formula

$$\Lambda_i V = \sum_{j=1}^{N_i} \alpha_j |\lambda_j| g_j. \tag{6.147}$$

Since Λ_i is self-adjoint and positive-definite in M_i, we can introduce the fractional powers of it, for example,

$$\Lambda_i^{-1/2} V = \sum_{j=1}^{N_i} \alpha_j |\lambda_j|^{-1/2} g_j. \tag{6.148}$$

Note that any power of Λ_i commutes with L_i. With the help of these operators, we define the norms

$$\|V\|_{U_i} = (\Lambda_i V, V)_i^{1/2}, \tag{6.149}$$

$$\|V\|_{\mathcal{F}_i} = (\Lambda_i^{-1/2} V, V)_i^{1/2}, \qquad V \in \mathbf{R}^{N_i}. \tag{6.150}$$

Now let us check the assumptions of Theorem 4.9. It is easy to verify the properties (4.153), (4.70), (4.72), (4.73):

1. operator L_i is self-adjoint and inversible;
2. $I_{i-1} = R_i^*$;
3. $L_{i-1} = R_i L_i I_{i-1}$;
4. $J_i L_i = L_i J_i$.

To verify the inequality (4.159), let us take an arbitrary vector $V \in M_i$ and employ the decomposition (6.145). Due to the orthogonality of system $\{g_j\}$, we get

$$\|J_i V\|_{U_i}^2 = \sum_{j=1}^{N_i} \alpha_j^2 N^2(\lambda_j^2) |\lambda_j|.$$

Here $N(x)$ is the polinomial

$$N(x) = (1 - \tau_{m-1} x) \dots (1 - \tau_0 x).$$

Due to (4.42), we have

$$|N(x)| \le 1 \qquad \forall x \in [0, (\lambda_i^*)^2].$$

Therefore,

$$\|J_iV\|_{U_i}^2 \le \sum_{j=1}^{N_i} \alpha_j^2|\lambda_j| = \|V\|_{U_i}^2$$

and (4.159) is valid with the constant $c_J = 1$.

To verify the inequality (4.160), we need the additional result.

Lemma 6.4.1 *The norms* (6.140) *and* (6.149) *are equivalent, i. e., there exist the constants* c_9, c_{10} *which are independent of* i, h_i *and such that*

$$c_9\|V\|_{U_i} \le \|V\|_h^{(2)} \le c_{10}\|V\|_{U_i} \qquad \forall V \in \mathbf{R}^{N_i}. \tag{6.151}$$

Proof. We employ the results of paper [148]. In Remark 3.5 of this paper, the case is discussed in which namely the scalar product (6.144) is used with the multiplier h^2.

Let us compair two spectral problems. The first one is algebraic:

$$L_iV = \lambda V, \qquad V \in \mathbf{R}^{N_i}. \tag{6.152}$$

The second problem arises from mentioned Remark 3.5: find $(v_1, v_2) \in H^{h_i}$ such that $\forall(w_1, w_2) \in H^{h_i}$

$$\begin{aligned} a(v_1, w_1) + b(v_2, w_1) &= \tilde{\lambda} h^4 \sum_{x\in\bar{\Omega}'_{h_i}} v_1(x)w_1(x)h_i^2, \\ b(w_2, v_1) &= \tilde{\lambda} \sum_{x\in\Omega'_{h_i}} v_2(x)w_2(x)h_i^2. \end{aligned} \tag{6.153}$$

Note that we have

$$\begin{aligned} &(L_iV, W)_i = a(v_1, w_1) + b(v_2, w_1) + b(w_2, v_1), \qquad \forall V, W \in \mathbf{R}^{N_i}, \\ &(V, W)_i = h^4 \sum_{x\in\bar{\Omega}'_{h_i}} v_1(x)w_1(x) + \sum_{x\in\Omega'_{h_i}} v_2(x)w_2(x) \end{aligned}$$

for isomorphic pairs $V \leftrightarrow (v_1, v_2) \in H^{h_i}$, $W \leftrightarrow (w_1, w_2) \in H^{h_i}$. Therefore, (6.152) is equivalent to the spectral problem which differs from (6.153) only by the last multipliers h_i^2 in both equations. In consequence, we get the equality

$$\lambda_j = h_i^2\tilde{\lambda}_j, \qquad j = 1, \dots, N_i, \tag{6.154}$$

between j-th eigenvalues λ_j and $\tilde{\lambda}_j$ of problems (6.152) and (6.153). The j-th eigenvector $V_j \in \mathbf{R}^{N_i}$ are connected with the j-th eigenvector-function $v_j = (v_{1,j}, v_{2,j}) \in H^{h_i}$ by the mentioned isomorphism $V_j \leftrightarrow h_iv_j$. The multiplier h_i appears because of different multipliers in normalization conditions. Taking these relations into consideration, we come to the correspondences

$$\|V\|_i = h_i^{-1}|||(v_1, v_2)|||_{0,M}, \tag{6.155}$$

$$\|V\|_{U_i} = |||(v_1, v_2)|||_{1,M}, \tag{6.156}$$

$$(\Lambda_i^{3/2}V, V)_i^{1/2} = h_i^{1/2}|||(v_1, v_2)|||_{3/2,M} \tag{6.157}$$

for any isomorphic pair $V \leftrightarrow (v_1, v_2) \in H^{h_i}$ between the notations of this subsection and paper [148]. Then we employ the final consideration in Remark 3.5 about the equivalence of the norms $|||\cdot|||_{s,M}$ and $|||\cdot|||_s$ for $0 \leq s \leq 2$ and use the results of Theorem 3.3 and Lemma 3.4 of this paper. In consequence, we have the equivalence (6.151). □

We continue to prove Theorem 6.7. Let us take an arbitrary vector $V \in \mathbf{R}^{N_i}$ with the isomorphic image $v = (v_1, v_2) \in H^{h_i}$. Then

$$\|v_2\|^2_{2,h_i} = \sum_{T \in \mathcal{T}_{h_{i+1}}} \|v_2\|^2_{2,T} + (2h_{i+1})^{-1} \int_{\mathcal{E}_{h_{i+1}}} J^2(\partial_\nu v_2) d\gamma \leq \|v_2\|^2_{2,h_{i+1}}. \quad (6.158)$$

Note that vector $I_i V \in \mathbf{R}^{N_{i+1}}$ has the same isomorphic image $v \in H^{h_i} \subset H^{h_{i+1}}$. Therefore

$$\|V\|_h^{(2)} \leq \|I_i V\|_h^{(2)}.$$

With the help of (6.151), we arrive at the inequality

$$\|V\|_{U_i} \leq c_{10} c_9^{-1} \|I_i V\|_{U_{i+1}}, \qquad V \in M_i, \quad (6.159)$$

which is equivalent to (4.160).

Now one need to prove the inequality (4.161). Again let us take an arbitrary vector $V \in \mathbf{R}^{N_i}$ and employ the decomposition (6.145). Then

$$\|L_i J_i V\|^2_{\mathcal{F}_i} = \sum_{j=1}^{N_i} \alpha_j^2 |\lambda_j|^{3/2} N^2(\lambda_j^2).$$

Due to (4.41), we have

$$|\lambda_j|^{1/2} N^2(\lambda_j^2) \leq \sqrt{\lambda_i^*}/\sqrt{2m+1}.$$

Therefore

$$\|L_i J_i V\|^2_{\mathcal{F}_i} \leq \frac{\sqrt{\lambda_i^*}}{\sqrt{2m+1}} \|V\|^2_{U_i} \qquad \forall V \in \mathbf{R}^{N_i},$$

and

$$\|L_i J_i\|_{\mathcal{F}_i \leftarrow U_i} \leq (\lambda_i^*/(2m+1))^{1/4}. \quad (6.160)$$

To evaluate the first multiplier in (4.161), we take an arbitrary vector $F \in \mathbf{R}^{N_i}$ and examine the algebraic system

$$L_i W^{h_i} = F. \quad (6.161)$$

The solution W^{h_i} is isomorphic to a vector-function $(w_1^{h_i}, w_2^{h_i}) \in H^{h_i}$. Let us formulate the problem: find $z_1 \in H^0_{h_i}$, $z_2 \in H^2_{h_i}$ such that

$$\begin{aligned} a(z_1, \psi) + b_2(z_2, \psi) &= a(w_1^{h_i}, \psi) + b_2(w_2^{h_i}, \psi) \qquad \forall \psi \in H^0_{h_i}. \\ b_2(\varphi, z_1) &= b_2(\varphi, w_1^{h_i}) \qquad \forall \varphi \in H^2_{h_i}. \end{aligned} \quad (6.162)$$

The bilinear forms in the right-hand sides are bounded functionals of ψ and φ in corresponding spaces. Therefore, problem (6.162) has the unique solution $w_1^{h_i}$, $w_2^{h_i}$. Note that the Bubnov-Galerkin systems for this problem have the form

$$L^{h_i} W^{h_i} = G^{h_i} \quad \text{in} \quad H^{h_i}$$

and

$$L^{h_{i-1}} W^{h_{i-1}} = G^{h_{i-1}} \quad \text{in} \quad H^{h_{i-1}}$$

where

$$G^{h_{i-1}} = R^{h_i}_{h_{i-1}} G^{h_i}, \qquad F = \mathcal{D}^{h_i} G^{h_i}.$$

Due to our notation, we have

$$(L_i^{-1} - I_{i-1} L_{i-1}^{-1} R_i) F = W^{h_i} - I_{i-1} W^{h_{i-1}}. \tag{6.163}$$

Let $W^{h_{i-1}}$ be isomorphic to a vector-function $(w_1^{h_{i-1}}, w_2^{h_{i-1}}) \in H^{h_{i-1}}$. Because of (6.151), (6.140), (6.158), we get

$$\|W^{h_i} - I_{i-1} W^{h_{i-1}}\|_{U_i} \le c_9^{-1} (|w_1^{h_i} - w_1^{h_{i-1}}|_0^2 + \|w_2^{h_i} - w_2^{h_{i-1}}\|_{2,h_i})^{1/2}. \tag{6.164}$$

Now we employ the estimate (4.6) from [148]. Considering our notation and the equivalence of norms $|||(w_1^{h_i}, w_2^{h_i})|||_{3/2}$ and $|||(w_1^{h_i}, w_2^{h_i})|||_{3/2,M} = \|L_i^{3/4} W^{h_i}\|_i$, we can write this estimate in the form

$$|w_1^{h_i} - w_1^{h_{i-1}}|_0 + \|w_2^{h_i} - w_2^{h_{i-1}}\|_{2,h_i} \le c_{11} h_i \|L_i^{3/4} W^{h_i}\|_i. \tag{6.165}$$

Employing (6.161), we have

$$\|L_i^{3/4} W^{h_i}\|_i = \|F\|_{\mathcal{F}_i}. \tag{6.166}$$

Since $(a^2 + b^2)^{1/2} \le a + b$ for $a, b \ge 0$, we can combine (6.163)–(6.166):

$$\|(L_i^{-1} - I_{i-1} L_{i-1}^{-1} R_i) F\|_{U_i} \le c_9^{-1} c_{11} h_i \|F\|_{\mathcal{F}_i}.$$

From the arbitrariness of F, we get

$$\|L_i^{-1} - I_{i-1} L_{i-1}^{-1} R_i\|_{U_i \leftarrow \mathcal{F}_i} \le c_9^{-1} c_{11} h_i.$$

Combining this inequality with (6.160) and (6.141), we obtain (4.161) with

$$\eta(m) = c_9^{-1} c_{11} \left(\frac{c_4}{2m+1} \right)^{1/4}. \tag{6.167}$$

Thus, all assumptions of Theorem 4.9 are valid and we get the inequality (4.164). Employing (6.151), we have (6.142) with

$$\varepsilon = c_9^{-1} c_{10} \xi. \tag{6.168}$$

Therefore, we can choose an integer m_0 in accordance with considerations (4.165)–(4.167). □

For a large m, we have

$$\varepsilon \leq c/\sqrt{2m+1} \tag{6.169}$$

because of (6.168), (6.167), (4.176). This rate of convergence indeed is squared in comparison with Theorem 4.1 in [148] as it was predicted at the final conclusion of this paper.

Then, application of FMG-algorithm of section 4.2 leads to the following result. The proof is very similar to one of Theorem 4.17 and is omitted.

Theorem 6.8 *Let* (6.110) *hold. Then for any* $\varepsilon > 0$, *to compute the approximate solution* $\widetilde{V}^{h_p}$ *of system* (6.125), *FMG-algorithm with* $MG^{(10)}$*-algorithm on a sequence of nested triangulations* $\mathcal{T}_0, \dots, \mathcal{T}_p$ *(decreasing twice) needs less than* $c_5 N_p$ *arithmetic operations to achive the estimate*

$$\|V^{h_p} - \widetilde{V}^{h_p}\|_h^{(2)} \leq \varepsilon h_p \|f\|_{-1,\Omega} \tag{6.170}$$

where the constant $c_5(\varepsilon)$ *is independent of* f, h_i.

Denote the prolongation of vector $\widetilde{V}^{h_p}$ in H^{h_p} by $\tilde{v}^{h_p} = (\tilde{v}_1^{h_p}, \tilde{v}_2^{h_p})$. Then from (6.170) and (6.139), the estimates follow

$$\begin{aligned} \|u - \tilde{v}_2^{h_p}\|_{2,h} &\leq (c+\varepsilon) h_p \|f\|_{-1,\Omega}, \\ |\Delta u + \tilde{v}_1^{h_p}|_{0,\Omega} &\leq (c+\varepsilon) h_p \|f\|_{-1,\Omega}. \end{aligned} \tag{6.171}$$

6.4.3 Another approach

In principle, it is possible to use algorithms for the generalized formulation in $\overset{\circ}{W}{}_2^2(\Omega)$ likewise in subsection 1.1.7 [46]. The Hermitian elements of degree 3 on rectangles are suitable. The triangular J.H.Argyris's, K.Bell's, R.W.Clough–J.L.Tocher's elements are less usefull for algorithms on a sequence of grids, since they are not nested on different grids, which leads to complex operations of interpolation and restriction [84].

In the above algorithm, the problem of the curvilinear boundary Γ is resolved using isoparametric elements on the finest grid with subsequent convolution of systems and finite elements onto more rough grids by the rules cited in section 5.2.

For the smooth boundary Γ and the right-hand side f, the solutiuon also shows greater smoothness. Application of higher degrees elements is possible, therefore. For example, the justification of convergence of the mixed method for elements of degree 3 and higher is provided in [6].

Another way which seems perspective is the applirationn of the initial generalized formulation of subsection 1.1.7 and additional functions — the Lagrange multipliers, likewise in subsection 3.4.3. Namely: consider the generalized formulation: *find three functions* $u \in W_2^2(\Omega)$, $v_1 \in W_2^{-3/2}(\Gamma)$, $v_2 \in W_2^{-1/2}(\Gamma)$ *satisfying the relations*

$$\begin{aligned} &\int_\Omega \Delta u \cdot \Delta v dx + \int_\Gamma v_1 v d\gamma + \int_\Gamma v_2 \partial_\nu v d\gamma = \langle f, v\rangle \qquad \forall v \in W_2^2(\Omega), \\ &\int_\Gamma \varphi_1 u d\gamma = \int_\Gamma g_1 \varphi_1 d\gamma \qquad \forall \varphi_1 \in W_2^{-3/2}(\Gamma), \\ &\int_\Gamma \varphi_2 \partial_\nu u d\gamma = \int_\Gamma g_2 \varphi_2 d\gamma \qquad \forall \varphi_2 \in W_2^{-1/2}(\Gamma). \end{aligned} \tag{6.172}$$

The simplest way to define the mentioned spaces with the fractional indices consists in the following. Let

$$W_2^{1/2}(\Gamma) = \{r \in L_2(\Gamma): \quad \exists v \in W_2^1(\Omega); \quad \operatorname{tr} v = r\},$$
$$W_2^{3/2}(\Gamma) = \{r \in L_2(\Gamma): \quad \exists v \in W_2^2(\Omega); \quad \operatorname{tr} v = r\},$$

where tr is the trace operator [106]. The norms in these spaces are introduced by formulae [40]

$$\|r\|_{1/2,\Gamma} = \inf_{\substack{v \in W_2^1(\Omega) \\ tr\ v=r}} \|v\|_{1,\Omega},$$
$$\|r\|_{3/2,\Gamma} = \inf_{\substack{v \in W_2^2(\Omega) \\ tr\ v=r}} \|v\|_{2,\Omega}.$$

Then $W_2^{-3/2}(\Gamma)$, $W_2^{-1/2}(\Gamma)$ are the space dual of $W_2^{3/2}(\Gamma)$, $W_2^{1/2}(\Gamma)$ respectively. Let us introduce the relationship of duality $\langle \cdot, \cdot \rangle_\Gamma$ between the pair of elements in $W_2^{-1/2}(\Gamma)$, $W_2^{1/2}(\Gamma)$ or $W_2^{-3/2}(\Gamma)$, $W_2^{3/2}(\Gamma)$. Then the norms in the spaces with a negative index are defined as in dual ones by formulae

$$\|r\|_{-3/2,\Gamma} = \sup_{s \in W_2^{3/2}(\Gamma)} \frac{\langle r, s\rangle_\Gamma}{\|s\|_{3/2,\Gamma}},$$
$$\|r\|_{-1/2,\Gamma} = \sup_{s \in W_2^{1/2}(\Gamma)} \frac{\langle r, s\rangle_\Gamma}{\|s\|_{1/2,\Gamma}}.$$

This definition gives the same spaces like $H^\sigma(\Gamma)$ in [106] with corresponding index σ, but it is more convenient for our purposes.

Let u be the solution of the Dirichlet problem

$$\Delta^2 u = f \quad \text{in} \quad \Omega, \qquad u = g_1 \quad \text{on} \quad \Gamma, \qquad \partial_\nu u = g_2 \quad \text{on} \quad \Gamma, \tag{6.173}$$
$$\text{where} \quad v_1 = \partial_\nu \Delta u, \qquad v_2 = \Delta u \qquad \text{on} \quad \Gamma. \tag{6.174}$$

Then the triplet u, v_1, v_2 will be the solution of problem (6.172). To discretize problem (6.172) with respect to u, one can use the Hermitian elements of degree 3 on a regular rectangular grid covering the domain Ω, which insures belonging the basis functions to class $C^1(\bar{\Omega})$. To insure the same (second) order approximation for functions v_1 and v_2 on Γ, it suffices to use piecewise linear elements on a regular subdivision with respect to γ. For the Brezzi stability condition (1.14), every elementary interval with respect to variable γ (the arc of boundary Γ) must cover one (as a minimum) rectangular mesh in variables (x_1, x_2).

In the case $u \in W_2^4(\Omega)$, this discretization ensures the following estimate for the approximate solution of the Bubnov-Galerkin method:

$$|u - u^h|_{2,\Omega} + \|v_1 - v_1^h\|_{-3/2,\Gamma} + \|v_2 - v_2^h\|_{-1/2,\Gamma} \leq$$
$$\leq c_7 h^2 (|f|_{0,\Omega} + \|g_1\|_{3/2,\Gamma} + \|g_2\|_{1/2,\Gamma}). \tag{6.175}$$

Application of inverse inequalities and the dual argument technique yield the estimates:

$$|u - u^h|_{1,\Omega} \leq ch^3 F, \qquad |u - u^h|_{0,\Omega} \leq ch^4 F,$$

$$|\Delta u - v_2^h|_{0,\Gamma} \leq ch^{3/2} F, \qquad |\partial_\nu \Delta u - v_1^h|_{0,\Gamma} \leq ch^{1/2} F,$$

where

$$F = |f|_{0,\Omega} + \|g_1\|_{3/2,\Gamma} + \|g_2\|_{1/2,\Gamma}.$$

Note, that this method is rather convenient, firstly, for realizing on a sequence of grids (with respect to both x and γ) due to the nestedness property of finite elements on different grids; secondly, it is closed to the traditional technique of finite differences due to a regular grid inside the domain. This technique is related to paper [7], where the correction of equations near the boundary is effected using another method, namely: extrapolating the solution to the outside of Ω.

The justification of these methods calls for a rather large body of theoretic material, nontraditional as well, and is therefore not provided here.

6.5 The stationary Stokes problem

In this section, we deal with the stationary Stokes problem of viscous incompressible fluid. At present, two generalized formulations of this problem have been widely used. One of these has been worked out at length in the sense of theory by O.A. Ladyženskaja [92] and in terms of the finite elements method by R. Temam [185]. It gives an elliptic formulation of both the differential and the discrete problems but in special function spaces satisfying some additional differential equalities (the solenoidity). This leads to a number of inconveniences when choosing the Ritz method spaces.

The second generalized formulation is related to the mixed method [47], [25] and yields a hyperbolic-like formulation of the discrete problem. This time, the basis functions obey no differential equations, though some geometric conditions must be satisfied which are, generally speaking, weak but rather unexpected. Naturally, the Ritz method is not applicable and the application of finite elements is based on the Bubnov-Galerkin method for determining a stationary point of functional.

6.5.1 The formulation of the differential problem

Let Ω be a two-dimensional bounded convex poligonal domain with a boundary Γ. Our problem is to determine function p and vector-function $u = (u_1, u_2)$ provided the right-hand sides $f = (f_1, f_2)$, g are known:

$$-\nu\Delta u + \nabla p = f \quad \text{in} \quad \Omega, \tag{6.176}$$

$$\operatorname{div} u = g \quad \text{in} \quad \Omega, \tag{6.177}$$

$$u = 0 \quad \text{on} \quad \Gamma. \tag{6.178}$$

Here, $\nu > 0$ is the kinematic viscocity coefficient, p is the pressure, u_1, u_2 are components of the velocity vector.

It is obvious that the function p satisfies equation (6.176) up to the constant term $c = \text{const}$. So there is sense in separating one solution from this set such that

$$\int_\Omega p\,dx = 0. \tag{6.179}$$

On the other hand, due to Stokes formula (1.112), we have

$$\int_\Omega \operatorname{div} u\; dx = 0. \tag{6.180}$$

Because of (6.177), we are compelled to demand

$$\int_\Omega g\,dx = 0. \tag{6.181}$$

Introduce spaces $\mathbf{U} \equiv (\overset{\circ}{W}{}_2^1(\Omega))^2$ with the norm

$$|u|_1 = (|u_1|_1^2 + |u_2|_1^2)^{1/2}$$

and $\mathbf{V} = \widetilde{L}_2(\Omega)$ being an orthogonal complement to unit in space $L_2(\Omega)$ with norm $|\cdot|_0$, i. e., the set of functions from $L_2(\Omega)$ satisfying (6.179).

To pass to the generalized formulation, we take the scalar product of vector-function $v = (v_1, v_2) \in \mathbf{U}$ and equation (6.176) and integrate over Ω:

$$-\nu \int_\Omega \Delta u \cdot v\,dx + \int_\Omega \nabla p \cdot v\,dx = \int_\Omega f \cdot v\,dx.$$

Integrating by parts in the first two integrals likewise in subsection 1.1.10, we get the formula

$$\mathcal{L}(u, v) + l(p, v) = f(v)$$

where

$$\mathcal{L}(u, v) = \nu \sum_{i=1}^{2} \int_\Omega \nabla u_i \cdot \nabla v_i\,dx, \tag{6.182}$$

$$l(p, v) = -\int_\Omega p \operatorname{div} v\,dx, \tag{6.183}$$

$$f(v) = \int_\Omega f \cdot v\,dx. \tag{6.184}$$

Take now an arbitrary function $q \in L_2(\Omega)$, multiply equation (6.177) by it and also integrate over Ω. Now

$$l(q, u) = g(q) \equiv -\int_\Omega gq\,dx.$$

We have got the generalized (mixed) formulation of the stationary Stokes problem: *find a vector-function $u \in \mathbf{U}$ and a function $p \in \mathbf{V}$ satisfying the equalities*

$$\mathcal{L}(u, v) + l(p, v) = f(v) \qquad \forall v \in \mathbf{U}, \tag{6.185}$$

$$l(q, u) = g(q) \qquad \forall q \in \mathbf{V}. \tag{6.186}$$

All conditions (excepting one) of unique solvability of this problem can be easy to verify: the positive definiteness and the boundedness of bilinear form $\mathcal{L}(\cdot,\cdot)$, the boundedness of bilinear form $l(\cdot,\cdot)$ and functionals $f(v)$, $g(q)$ in corresponding spaces. We made above these considerations many times and so we will not repeat them. But one condition calls for particular consideration, namely: the satisfaction of inequality (1.149). In the notation introduced here, it has the form:

$$\sup_{v\in U} |l(q,v)|/|v|_1 \geq c_0|q|_0 \qquad \forall q \in \mathbf{V}. \tag{6.187}$$

With different requirements for the boundary, it has been proved, for example, in [47], [78]. Then, all conditions of Theorem 1.9 are satisfied and the generalized Stokes problem is uniquely solvable for

$$f \in (W_2^{-1}(\Omega))^2, \qquad g \in \widetilde{L}_2(\Omega). \tag{6.188}$$

In our further considerations, we will treat the problem with smoother right-hand sides:

$$f \in (L_\alpha(\Omega))^2, \qquad g \in W_\alpha^1(\Omega)\bigcap \widetilde{L}_2(\Omega), \qquad \alpha \in (1,2]. \tag{6.189}$$

For a domain Ω with a smooth boundary $\Gamma \subset C^2$, we have immediately [185, proposition 2.3 of chapter 1]:

$$u \in (W_\alpha^2(\Omega))^2, \qquad p \in W_\alpha^1(\Omega)\bigcap \widetilde{L}_2(\Omega). \tag{6.190}$$

But for a poligonal domain (even convex) this result is known only for $g = 0$ [58]. Therefore we need to prove it.

Theorem 6.9 *Let Ω be a convex bounded poligon and let* (6.189) *hold for the problem* (6.176)–(6.178). *Then there exists a unique solution u, p satisfying* (6.190).

Proof. Let us take a convex bounded domain $\widetilde{\Omega} \supset \Omega$ with a smooth boundary $\widetilde{\Gamma} \subset C^4$ and construct an expansion $\tilde{g} \in W_\alpha^1(\widetilde{\Omega})$ by the technique from [146, §3 of chapter 1]. It gives us

$$\tilde{g} = g \quad \text{on} \quad \Omega \qquad \text{and} \qquad \|\tilde{g}\|_{1,\alpha,\widetilde{\Omega}} \leq c\,\|g\|_{1,\alpha,\Omega}. \tag{6.191}$$

Then we inroduce a vector-funcion $\sigma\,\vec{\nu}$ with the unit external normal $\vec{\nu} = (\nu_1,\nu_2)^T$ and the constant

$$\sigma = \int_{\widetilde{\Omega}} \tilde{g}\,dx \Bigg/ \int_\Gamma d\gamma\,. \tag{6.192}$$

Consider the first problem:

$$-\vec{\nu}\Delta\tilde{u} + \operatorname{grad}\tilde{p} = 0 \quad \text{in} \quad \widetilde{\Omega}, \tag{6.193}$$

$$\operatorname{div}\tilde{u} = \tilde{g} \quad \text{in} \quad \widetilde{\Omega}, \tag{6.194}$$

$$\tilde{u} = \sigma\vec{\nu} \quad \text{on} \quad \widetilde{\Gamma}. \tag{6.195}$$

Because of [185, proposition 2.3 of chapter 1], we have

$$\tilde{u} \in (W_\alpha^2(\widetilde{\Omega}))^2, \qquad \tilde{p} \in W_\alpha^1(\widetilde{\Omega}). \tag{6.196}$$

Besides, due to imbedding theorem [185],

$$\bar{r} = \text{tr}_\Gamma \tilde{u} \in (W_\alpha^{3/2}(\Gamma))^2 \tag{6.197}$$

where

$$W_\alpha^{3/2}(\Gamma) = \{r \in L_\alpha(\Gamma) : \quad \exists v \in W_\alpha^2(\Omega);\ \text{tr}_\Gamma v = r\}.$$

Owing to (6.191) and the Stokes formula,

$$\int_\Gamma \bar{r} \cdot \vec{\nu}\, d\gamma = \int_\Omega \text{div}\, \tilde{g}\, dx = \int_\Omega \text{div}\, g\, dx. \tag{6.198}$$

Consider the second problem:

$$-\vec{\nu}\Delta\bar{u} + \text{grad}\,\bar{p} = f \quad \text{in} \quad \Omega, \tag{6.199}$$

$$\text{div}\,\bar{u} = 0 \quad \text{in} \quad \Omega, \tag{6.200}$$

$$\bar{u} = -\bar{r} \quad \text{on} \quad \Gamma. \tag{6.201}$$

Because of [59, remark 5.6 of chapter 1], we have

$$\bar{u} \in (W_\alpha^2(\Omega))^2, \qquad \bar{p} \in W_\alpha^1(\Omega) \cap \widetilde{L}_2(\Omega). \tag{6.202}$$

Now let us put

$$\hat{u} = \tilde{u} + \bar{u}, \qquad \hat{p} = \tilde{p} + \bar{p} - \rho \qquad \text{where} \quad \rho = \int_\Omega \tilde{p}\, dx. \tag{6.203}$$

Functions $\hat{u}$, $\hat{p}$ satisfy (6.176)–(6.178) and are the unique solution of this problem. Because of (6.196) and (6.202), we have (6.190). □

In particular, we assume in this section that

$$f \in (L_2(\Omega))^2, \qquad g \in \tilde{W}_2^1(\Omega) \tag{6.204}$$

where $\tilde{W}_2^1(\Omega) = \overset{\circ}{W}{}_2^1(\Omega) \cap \widetilde{L}_2(\Omega)$. Then from Theorem 6.9 we have $u \in (W_2^2(\Omega))^2$, $p \in \tilde{W}_2^1(\Omega)$ and the following estimate holds:

$$\|u\|_2 + \|p\|_1 \leq c_1\,(|f|_0 + \|g\|_1). \tag{6.205}$$

6.5.2 The discrete problem

To construct a discrete problem, we use a sequence of nested grids and spaces H^{h_i} introduced in section 5.1 for subdivisions of multiplicity of 2. Introduce the designation $\mathbf{U}^{h_i} \equiv (H^{h_i})^2$ and the space of functions $\mathbf{V}^{h_i}$ being constant on every elementary triangle $T_j^{h_{i-1}}$ of grid $\Omega_{h_{i-1}}$. The basis functions $\psi_j^{h_i}$ $(j = 1, \ldots, m_i)$ coincide with characteristic functions of triangles $T_j^{h_{i-1}}$. Refer them to the centers of these triangles as to the nodes (Fig. 6.1) and denote the set of these nodes by Ω'_{h_i}. Then, the nestedness

$$\Omega'_{h_{i-1}} \subset \Omega'_{h_i}, \qquad \mathbf{V}^{h_{i-1}} \subset \mathbf{V}^{h_i} \tag{6.206}$$

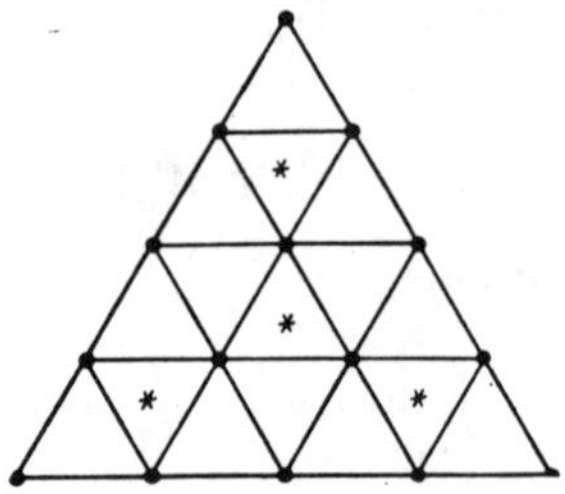

Figure 6.1: A fragment of grids Ω_h, Ω'_h: sign • marks a node of piecewise linear elements for velocities u_1, u_2; sign $*$ marks a node of piecewise constant element for pressure p.

are valid for these grids and spaces. Also denote

$$\tilde{\mathbf{V}}^{h_i} = \{q \in \mathbf{V}^{h_i}; \int_\Omega q dx = 0\}. \tag{6.207}$$

The approximate solution will be sought by the Bubnov-Galerkin method: *in the form of functions* $u^{h_i} = (u_1^{h_i}, u_2^{h_i}) \in \mathbf{U}^{h_i}$, $p^{h_i} \in \tilde{\mathbf{V}}^{h_i}$ *satisfying the relations*

$$\mathcal{L}(u^{h_i}, v) + l(p^{h_i}, v) = f(v) \qquad \forall v \in \mathbf{U}^{h_i}, \tag{6.208}$$

$$l(q, u^{h_i}) = g(q) \qquad \forall q \in \tilde{\mathbf{V}}^{h_i}. \tag{6.209}$$

Consider the solvability of this discrete problem. Again, likewise in the differential case, all conditions of Theorem 1.10 are easy to verify except for a discrete analogue of inequality (6.187). We succeded in proving it due to the chosen relation between the basis functions supports of spaces H^{h_i} and $\mathbf{V}^{h_i}$.

Remark 6.5.1 *An attempt to improve the approximation of the function* p *using the same triangles for* u^h *and* p^h *results in an ill-conditioned system from which* u^{h_i} *and* p^{h_i} *are defined with an unsatisfactory accuracy.*

Lemma 6.5.1 [47] *The constructed spaces* $\mathbf{U}^{h_i}$, $\tilde{\mathbf{V}}^{h_i}$ *obey the inequality*

$$\sup_{v \in \mathbf{U}^{h_i}} |l(q, v)|/|v|_1 \geq c_2 |q|_0 \qquad \forall q \in \tilde{\mathbf{V}}^{h_i}. \tag{6.210}$$

Thus, all conditions of Theorem 1.10 are satisfied. Therefore, discrete problem (6.208), (6.209) is uniquely solvable and the estimates

$$|u - u^{h_i}|_1 \leq c_3 h_i (|f|_0 + \|g\|_1), \tag{6.211}$$

$$|u - u^{h_i}|_0 \leq c_4 h_i^2 (|f|_0 + \|g\|_1), \tag{6.212}$$

$$|p - p^{h_i}|_0 \leq c_5 h_i (|f|_0 + \|g\|_1) \tag{6.213}$$

are valid. Recall that the estimate (6.212) is obtained by a standard duality technique [59, remark 1.6 of chapter II] and the estimate (6.213) is valid for functions satisfying condition (6.179). In this connection, interpolation in space $\widetilde{L}_2(\Omega)$ should be mentioned. For arbitrary $q \in \widetilde{L}_2(\Omega)$, it is necessary that interpolant $q^I \in \tilde{\mathbf{V}}^{h_i}$ satisfying the estimate

$$|q - q^I|_0 \leq c_6 h_i \|q\|_1 \tag{6.214}$$

should exist. To insure this, we take the interpolant in the form:

$$q^I(x) = \text{mes}^{-1}(T_j^{h_i-1}) \int_{T_j^{h_i-1}} q(y)dy, \qquad x \in T_j^{h_i-1}. \tag{6.215}$$

Now

$$\int_\Omega q^I(x)dx = \int_\Omega q(x)dx = 0,$$

and, according to [115], the estimate (6.214) is satisfied.

Note that when going from (6.208), (6.209) to a system of algebraic equations in the usual way, we have to introduce the special basis into $\widetilde{L}_2(\Omega)$ since the mentioned basis functions $\psi_j^{h_i}$ are not orthogonal to unit. Orthogonalizing $\psi_j^{h_i}$ would largely increase supports of these functions and the construction of a system of algebraic equations would become a very tedious procedure. Pass instead to a singular problem on space $\mathbf{U}^{h_i} \times \mathbf{V}^{h_i}$ by analogy with the Neuman problem. *Seek to determine functions $u^{h_i} \in \mathbf{U}^{h_i}$, $p^{h_i} \in \mathbf{V}^{h_i}$ satisfying the equalities*

$$\mathcal{L}(u^{h_i}, v) + l(p^{h_i}, v) = f(v) \qquad \forall v \in \mathbf{U}^{h_i}, \tag{6.216}$$

$$l(q, u^{h_i}) = g(q) \qquad \forall q \in \mathbf{V}^{h_i}. \tag{6.217}$$

Let us label the basis functions as follows:

$$\xi_j^{h_i} = \begin{cases} (\varphi_j^{h_i}, 0), & 1 \leq j \leq N_i, \\ (0, \varphi_{j-N_i}^{h_i}), & N_i + 1 \leq j \leq 2N_i, \\ \psi_{j-2N_i}^{h_i}, & 2N_i + 1 \leq j \leq 2N_i + m_i. \end{cases} \tag{6.218}$$

According to this enumeration, we construct the system of linear algebraic equations

$$L^{h_i} U^{h_i} = F^{h_i}. \tag{6.219}$$

The matrix L^{h_i} is symmetric and has the following form:

$$L^{h_i} = \begin{bmatrix} \left[\mathcal{L}(\xi_k^{h_i}, \xi_j^{h_i})\right]_{k=1,\dots,2N_i}^{j=1,\dots,2N_i} & \left[l(\psi_k^{h_i}, \xi_j^{h_i})\right]_{k=1,\dots,m_i}^{j=1,\dots,2N_i} \\ \left[l(\psi_j^{h_i}, \xi_k^{h_i})\right]_{k-1,\dots,2N_i}^{j=1,\dots,m_i} & [0]_{k=1,\dots,m_i}^{j=1,\dots,m_i} \end{bmatrix}, \tag{6.220}$$

where the superscript points to a line number in the block; the subscript points to a column number.

Note that the matrix of the system is singular. Indeed, let us take the vector

$$Z^{h_i} = (\underbrace{0, \dots, 0}_{2N_i}, \underbrace{1, \dots, 1}_{m_i})^T \tag{6.221}$$

and multiply it by matrix L^{h_i}. Due to the form of matrix and the enumeration of the basis functions, the last m_i components of vector $L^{h_i} Z^{h_i}$ as well as the first $2N_i$

components of Z^{h_i} become zero. When $j = 1, \dots, 2N_i$, $[L^{h_i}Z^{h_i}]_j = (1, \text{div}\xi_j^{h_i}) = 0$ as a result of integration by parts. Thus, $L^{h_i}Z^{h_i} = 0$. In the null space of the matrix L^{h_i}, there are no other linear independent vectors since its rank less than its dimension by 1. If we add to this system the equality

$$\int_\Omega p^{h_i}\,dx = 0, \tag{6.222}$$

then we get a set of equations being equivalent to the nonsingular problem (6.208), (6.209). System (6.219) is compatible since the right-hand side F^{h_i} is orthogonal to vector Z^{h_i}.

Let us introduce the isomorphism between vectors and functional triplets. We put the prolongation $(w^{h_i}, r^{h_i}) = (w_1^{h_i}, w_2^{h_i}, r^{h_i})$ from $\mathbf{U}^{h_i} \times \mathbf{V}^{h_i}$ as three functions

$$\begin{aligned} w_k^{h_i}(x) &= \sum_{j=1}^{N_i} W_{j+(k-1)N_i}^{h_i}\varphi_j^{h_i}(x), \quad x \in \Omega, \quad k = 1, 2, \\ r^{h_i}(x) &= \sum_{j=1}^{m_i} W_{j+2N_i}^{h_i}\psi_j^{h_i}(x), \quad x \in \Omega, \end{aligned} \tag{6.223}$$

one-to-one corresponding to the arbitrary vector W^{h_i} with components $W_j^{h_i}$ ($j = 1, \dots, 2N_i + m_i$) and introduce the vector norm:

$$\|W^{h_i}\|_h = (|w_1^{h_i}|_0^2 + |w_2^{h_i}|_0^2 + h_i^2|r^{h_i}|_0^2)^{1/2}. \tag{6.224}$$

By virtue of Theorem 3.13, it is equivalent to the simpler weighted Euclidean norm

$$\|W^{h_i}\|_E = \left(\sum_{j=1}^{2N_i}(W_j^{h_i})^2 h_i^2 + \sum_{j=1}^{m_i}(W_{j+2N_i}^{h_i})^2 h_i^4\right)^{1/2}, \tag{6.225}$$

i. e.,

$$c_7\|W^{h_i}\|_E \le \|W^{h_i}\|_h \le c_8\|W^{h_i}\|_E. \tag{6.226}$$

Remark 6.5.2 *The orthogonality of function $\tilde{p}^{h_i}$ in space $L_2(\Omega)$ to unit is equivalent to the orthogonality of W^{h_i} to vector Z^{h_i}.*

Let us define the operators of interpolation $I_{h_i}^{h_{i-1}}$ and restriction $R_{h_{i-1}}^{h_i}$. Let $W^{h_{i-1}}$ be an arbitrary vector of dimension $2N_{i-1} + m_{i-1}$ with an isomorphic pair $(w^{h_{i-1}}, r^{h_{i-1}}) \in \mathbf{U}^{h_{i-1}} \times \mathbf{V}^{h_{i-1}}$. Since $\mathbf{U}^{h_{i-1}} \subset \mathbf{U}^{h_i}$ and $\mathbf{V}^{h_{i-1}} \subset \mathbf{V}^{h_i}$, we have $(w^{h_{i-1}}, r^{h_{i-1}}) \in \mathbf{U}^{h_i} \times \mathbf{V}^{h_i}$. Now this pair isomorphically corresponds to a vector W^{h_i} of dimension $2N_i + m_i$. Thus, we have defined the correspondence $I_{h_i}^{h_{i-1}} : W^{h_{i-1}} \to W^{h_i}$. This linear correspondence can be represented by a rectangular matrix which we denote by $I_{h_i}^{h_{i-1}}$ too. Finally, we introduce the restriction matrix by transposition: $R_{h_{i-1}}^{h_i} = (I_{h_i}^{h_{i-1}})^T$.

6.5.3 The multigrid algorithm

Introduce the diagonal matrix $\mathcal{D}^{h_i} = \operatorname{diag}\{d_1^{h_i}, \dots, d_{2N_i+m_i}^{h_i}\}$ with the elements

$$d_j^{h_i} = \begin{cases} 1, & j = 1, \dots, 2N_i, \\ h_i^{-2}, & j = 2N_i + 1, \dots, 2N_i + m_i. \end{cases}$$

To evaluate the eigenvalues of symmetric matrix $(\mathcal{D}^{h_i})^{1/2} L^{h_i} (\mathcal{D}^{h_i})^{1/2}$, we employ Gerschgorin's Lemma 3.6.1 in combination with considerations from the proof of Theorem 3.14 with reference to the elements $\mathcal{L}(\xi_k^{h_i}, \xi_j^{h_i})$, $h_i^{-1} l(\psi_k^{h_i}, \xi_j^{h_i})$ of this matrix (in the notation of (6.220)). In the result, these eigenvalues are bounded in magnitude by a constant c_9. Since the eigenvalues of matrix $\mathcal{D}^{h_i} L^{h_i}$ coincide with the eigenvalues of the preceding matrix, the estimate

$$|\lambda(\mathcal{D}^{h_i} L^{h_i})| \le \lambda_i^* \le c_9 \tag{6.227}$$

is valid.

To solve system (6.219), we use $MG^{(9)}$-algorithm described in section 4.11. On the zeroth level, i. e., on grids Ω_{h_0}, Ω'_{h_0}, we seek a normal solution of singular systems using a direct method with orthogonalization. Denote an initial guess to the normal solution U^{h_i} of system (6.219) by $V_0^{h_i}$ and the result of the application of $MG^{(9)}$-algorithm on grids with the parameter h_i by $V_1^{h_i}$.

Theorem 6.10 *Let Ω be a convex polygon and (6.204) hold. Then for any $\varepsilon \in (0,1)$ we can choose an integer m_0 independent of h_i, f and such that $\forall m \ge m_0$ $MG^{(9)}$-algorithm reduces the error of the approximate normal solution by a factor ε, i. e.,*

$$\|V_1^{h_i} - U^{h_i}\|_h \le \varepsilon \|V_0^{h_i} - U^{h_i}\|_h, \tag{6.228}$$

where an initial guess $V_0^{h_i}$ must be orthogonal to vector Z^{h_i}.

Proof. Let us show that we are under conditions of Theorem 4.11. To this end, we rewrite $MG^{(9)}$-algorithm in other terms. First, we introduce the linear subspace $\mathbf{E}^{h_i}$ of $2N_i + m_i$-vectors orthogonal to vector Z^{h_i}. Second, we define the operator L_i as the constriction of operator $\mathcal{D}^{h_i} L^{h_i}$ in (invariant) subspace $\mathbf{E}^{h_i}$. Similarly we put $I_{i-1} : \mathbf{E}^{h_{i-1}} \to \mathbf{E}^{h_i}$ and $R_i : \mathbf{E}^{h_i} \to \mathbf{E}^{h_{i-1}}$ as the constrictions of operators $I_{h_{i-1}}^{h_i}$ and $\mathcal{D}^{h_{i-1}} R_{h_i}^{h_{i-1}} \mathcal{D}^{h_i}$ in $\mathbf{E}^{h_{i-1}}$ and $\mathbf{E}^{h_i}$ respectively.

Note that system (6.219) is equivalent to the operator equation

$$L_i U^{h_i} = F_i \tag{6.229}$$

with the right-hand side $F_i = \mathcal{D}^{h_i} F^{h_i}$. Next, we can rewrite pre-smoothing procedure (4.557) in the form

$$U_{l+1} = U_l - \tau_l L_i (L_i U_l - F_i), \qquad l = 0, 1, \dots, m-1, \tag{6.230}$$

with the iterative operator

$$J_i = (I - \tau_{m-1} L_i^2) \dots (I - \tau_0 L_i^2). \tag{6.231}$$

Finally, we introduce the scalar product $(V, W)_i$ in section 4.5 equal to

$$(V, W)_i = \sum_{j=1}^{2N_i+m_i} V_j W_j (d_j^{h_i})^{-1} h_i^2 \tag{6.232}$$

for vectors $V, W \in \mathbf{R}^{2N_i+m_i}$. Then $\|V\|_i = \|V\|_E$.

Let us verify that all intermediate vectors do not leave the corresponding subspaces and we are able to rewrite $MG^{(9)}$-algorithm in the form of another algorithm $\overline{MG}^{(9)}$ using terms L_i, I_{i-1}, R_i, J_i only.

On the zeroth level this assertion is valid for both the right-hand side F_0 due to (6.181) and the normal solution U^{h_0} obtained.

Now suppose that $V_0^{h_i}$ is orthogonal to Z^{h_i}. Consider stage $\mathbf{A_1}$. Multiplication by matrices L^{h_i}, $\mathcal{D}^{h_i}$ and subtraction of vector F^{h_i} do not withdraw the result from subspace $\mathbf{E}^{h_i}$. Therefore, due to iteration (4.557) both the obtained vector U_m and its residual will belong to $\mathbf{E}^{h_i}$. At stage $\mathbf{A_2}$, restriction of the residual does not disturb orthogonalization as well due to the rule of addition of the last components in groups of 4 components. At stage $\mathbf{A_3}$, orthogonalization is maintained subject to the induction assumption for rough grids. Subject to Remark 6.5.2, at stage $\mathbf{A_4}$ $\tilde{W}^{h_i}$ does not fall outside the subspace $\mathbf{E}^{h_i}$ as well. At last, $\mathbf{A_5}$ consists in computing a linear combination of the vectors from $\mathbf{E}^{h_i}$. Thus, at all stages of $MG^{(9)}$-algorithm, the computed vectors are in subspaces $\mathbf{E}^{h_i}$ orthogonal to Z^{h_i}.

It is easy to verify that properties (4.153), (4.70), (4.72), (4.73) are valid in scalar product (6.232). Because of (6.227) and (4.42), the condition (4.192) follows. Due to (6.226), we have (4.193).

Now let us show the validity of inequality (4.194). Take an arbitrary vector $G_i \in \mathbf{E}^{h_i}$ and consider the systems

$$L^{h_i} W^{h_i} = G^{h_i}, \qquad L^{h_{i-1}} W^{h_{i-1}} = G^{h_{i-1}} \tag{6.233}$$

with the right-hand sides

$$G^{h_i} = (\mathcal{D}^{h_i})^{-1} G_i, \qquad G^{h_{i-1}} = R_{h_i}^{h_{i-1}} G^{h_i}. \tag{6.234}$$

Let us introduce the symmetric bilinear form

$$\mathcal{B}(u, p; v, q) = \mathcal{L}(u, v) + l(p, v) + l(q, u) \tag{6.235}$$

in $\mathbf{U}^{h_i} \times \tilde{\mathbf{V}}^{h_i}$, i. e., $u, v \in \mathbf{U}^{h_i}$, $p, q \in \tilde{\mathbf{V}}^{h_i}$. Vectors W^{h_i} and $W^{h_{i-1}}$ are isomorphic to pairs w^{h_i}, r^{h_i} and $w^{h_{i-1}}$, $r^{h_{i-1}}$. Due to (6.233), the prolongation $w^{h_{i-1}}$, $r^{h_{i-1}}$ is the solution of problem: for given w^{h_i} and r^{h_i}, find $w^{h_{i-1}} \in \mathbf{U}^{h_{i-1}}$, $p^{h_{i-1}} \in \tilde{\mathbf{V}}^{h_{i-1}}$ such that

$$\mathcal{B}(w^{h_{i-1}}, r^{h_{i-1}}; v, q) = \mathcal{B}(w^{h_i}, r^{h_i}; v, q) \qquad \forall v \in \mathbf{U}^{h_{i-1}},\ q \in \tilde{\mathbf{V}}^{h_{i-1}}. \tag{6.236}$$

The Babuška conditions are equivalent to the Brezzi conditions for a mixed formulation. Therefore, due to (1.154), there exists a pair $v^{h_i} \in \mathbf{U}^{h_i}$, $q^{h_i} \in \tilde{\mathbf{V}}^{h_i}$ such that

$$\begin{aligned} & c\left(|w^{h_i} - w^{h_{i-1}}|_1 + |r^{h_i} - r^{h_{i-1}}|_0\right) \le \\ & \le \mathcal{B}(w^{h_i} - w^{h_{i-1}}, r^{h_i} - r^{h_{i-1}};\ v^{h_i}, q^{h_i}) / (|v^{h_i}|_1 + |q^{h_i}|_0). \end{aligned} \tag{6.237}$$

Due to the standard dual technique, we get

$$|w^{h_i} - w^{h_{i-1}}|_0 + h_i|r^{h_i} - r^{h_{i-1}}|_0 \leq \\ \leq ch_{i-1}(\inf_{v \in \mathbf{U}^{h_{i-1}}} |w^{h_i} - v|_1 + \inf_{q \in \tilde{\mathbf{V}}^{h_{i-1}}} |r^{h_i} - q|_0). \tag{6.238}$$

Because of (6.226), (6.233), (6.234) and definition of operators, we have

$$\|(L_i^{-1} - I_{i-1}L_{i-1}^{-1}R_i)G_i\|_E = \\ = \|W^{h_i} - I_{i-1}W^{h_{i-1}}\|_E \leq c_7^{-1}\|W^{h_i} - I_{i-1}W^{h_{i-1}}\|_h = \\ = c_7^{-1}(|w^{h_i} - w^{h_{i-1}}|_0^2 + h_i^2|r^{h_i} - r^{h_{i-1}}|_0^2)^{1/2}. \tag{6.239}$$

Combining (6.237)–(6.239), we get

$$\|(L_i^{-1} - I_{i-1}L_{i-1}^{-1}R_i)G_i\|_E \leq \\ \leq ch_i\mathcal{B}(w^{h_i} - w^{h_{i-1}}, r^{h_i} - r^{h_{i-1}};\ v^{h_i}, q^{h_i})/(|v^{h_i}|_1 + |q^{h_i}|_0). \tag{6.240}$$

Let us put the problem: for given v^{h_i} and q^{h_i}, find $v^{h_{i-1}} \in \mathbf{U}^{h_{i-1}}$, $q^{h_{i-1}} \in \tilde{\mathbf{V}}^{h_{i-1}}$ such that

$$\mathcal{B}(v^{h_{i-1}}, q^{h_{i-1}};\ w, r) = \mathcal{B}(v^{h_i}, q^{h_i};\ w, r) \qquad \forall w \in \mathbf{U}^{h_{i-1}}, r \in \tilde{\mathbf{V}}^{h_{i-1}}. \tag{6.241}$$

Because of Theorem 1.15 and the standard dual technique

$$|v^{h_i} - v^{h_{i-1}}|_0 + h_i|q^{h_i} - q^{h_{i-1}}|_0 \ \leq \ ch_i(\inf_{v \in \mathbf{U}^{h_{i-1}}} |v^{h_i} - v|_1 + \\ + \inf_{q \in \tilde{\mathbf{V}}^{h_{i-1}}} |q^{h_i} - q|_0) \ \leq \ ch_i(|v^{h_i}|_1 + |q^{h_i}|_0). \tag{6.242}$$

From the formulation of problems (6.236) and (6.241), it follows that

$$\mathcal{B}(w^{h_i} - w^{h_{i-1}}, r^{h_i} - r^{h_{i-1}};\ v^{h_i}, q^{h_i}) = \\ = \mathcal{B}(w^{h_i}, r^{h_i};\ v^{h_i} - v^{h_{i-1}}, q^{h_i} - q^{h_{i-1}}). \tag{6.243}$$

Pairs v^{h_i}, q^{h_i} and $v^{h_{i-1}}$, $q^{h_{i-1}}$ isomorphically corresponds to vectors $V^{h_i} \in \mathbf{E}^{h_i}$ and $V^{h_{i-1}} \in \mathbf{E}^{h_{i-1}}$. Therefore we can rewrite the right-hand side of (6.243) in the vector form

$$\mathcal{B}(w^{h_i}, r^{h_i};\ v^{h_i} - v^{h_{i-1}}, q^{h_i} - q^{h_{i-1}}) = \\ = (L^{h_i}W^{h_i})^T(V^{h_i} - I_{i-1}V^{h_{i-1}}) = \\ = ((\mathcal{D}^{h_i})^{-1/2}L_iW^{h_i})^T(\mathcal{D}^{h_i})^{-1/2}(V^{h_i} - I_{i-1}V^{h_{i-1}}). \tag{6.244}$$

Because of the algebraic Cauchy-Bunyakovski inequality and definition (6.225), we get

$$((\mathcal{D}^{h_i})^{-1/2}L_iW^{h_i})^T(\mathcal{D}^{h_i})^{-1/2}(V^{h_i} - I_{i-1}V^{h_{i-1}}) = \\ = h_i^{-2}(L_iW^{h_i}, V^{h_i} - I_{i-1}V^{h_{i-1}})_i \leq \\ \leq h_i^{-2}\|L_iW^{h_i}\|_E\ \|V^{h_i} - I_{i-1}V^{h_{i-1}}\|_E. \tag{6.245}$$

We transform the right-hand side with the help of (6.226), (6.233), (6.234), (6.224):

$$h_i^{-2}\|L_iW^{h_i}\|_E\|V^{h_i}-I_{i-1}V^{h_{i-1}}\|_E \le c_7^{-1}h_i^{-2}\|G_i\|_E\|V^{h_i}-I_{i-1}V^{h_{i-1}}\|_h \le$$
$$\le c_7^{-1}h_i^{-2}\|G_i\|_E(|v^{h_i}-v^{h_{i-1}}|_0^2+h_i^2|q^{h_i}-q^{h_{i-1}}|_0^2)^{1/2}. \quad (6.246)$$

Combining (6.242)–(6.246), we have

$$\mathcal{B}(w^{h_i}-w^{h_{i-1}}, r^{h_i}-r^{h_{i-1}};\ v^{h_i}, q^{h_i}) \le ch_i^{-1}\|G_i\|_E(|v^{h_i}|_1+|q^{h_i}|_0).$$

This inequality with (6.240) gives us

$$\|(L_i^{-1}-I_{i-1}L_{i-1}^{-1}R_i)G_i\|_E \le c_{10}\|G_i\|_E.$$

Due to (6.227) and the arbitrariness of G_i, we get

$$\|L_i^{-1}-I_{i-1}L_{i-1}^{-1}R_i\|_E \le c_{10}c_9/\lambda_i^*. \quad (6.247)$$

Theorem 4.12 gives us the second part of the required assertion:

$$\|L_iJ_i\|_E \le \lambda_i^*/(2m+1). \quad (6.248)$$

Combining two last inequalities, we have (4.194).

Thus, all assumptions of Theorem 4.11 are valid and we get

$$\|V_1^{h_i}-U^{h_i}\|_E \le \frac{c_L}{2m+1}\|V_0^{h_i}-U^{h_i}\|_E.$$

Because of (6.226), we have

$$\|V_1^{h_i}-U^{h_i}\|_h \le \frac{c_Lc_8}{c_7(2m+1)}\|V_0^{h_i}-U^{h_i}\|_h. \quad (6.249)$$

Taking m_0 such that $c_Lc_8/c_7(2m_0+1) \le \varepsilon$, we finish the proof. □

Remark 6.5.3 *If we should use the continuous elements for pressure from $W_2^1(\Omega)$, we can implement the usual estimate following* (6.212) *and* (6.213)*:*

$$|u-u^{h_i}|_0+h_i|p-p^{h_i}|_0 \le c_5h_i^2(|f|_0+\|g\|_1).$$

Besides, for a function $g\in\mathbf{V}^{h_i}\cap W_2^1(\Omega)$ we have the inverse inequality (3.58)*:*

$$\|g\|_1 \le ch_i^{-1}|g|_0.$$

Both inequalities give condition **D** *of subsection* 4.11*. It allows us to implement Theorem* 4.31 *directly.*

In our case a piecewise constant $g\in\mathbf{V}^{h_i}$ does not belong to $W_2^1(\Omega)$ and the expression $\|g\|_1$ has no sense. Therefore we need to prove inequality (6.247) *by more complex way.*

From the computational standpoint, the rounding errors will, though slightly, remove the vectors from subspace $\mathbf{E}^{h_i}$. What will happen in actual fact? Show that these errors remain on the initial level. Indeed, the greatest source of rounding errors is the multiplication by matrix L^{h_i}. But this sends an arbitrary vector into subspace $\mathbf{E}^{h_i}$. In formula (4.557), therefore, rounding errors will actually be accumulated at worst linearly in m. The rules of interpolation and restriction retain rounding errors unchanged. As a result, when m is not great, the influence of rounding errors is slight. But if the number of iterations increases from one level to another one, like in dynamic V-cycle, an appreciable error can be accumulated, as a result. To avoid this, at stage $\mathbf{A}_5$ it is sufficient to orthogonalize vector $U_m - \widetilde{W}^{h_i}$ to Z^{h_i}.

Now consider FMG-algorithm from section 4.2 with $MG^{(9)}$. Let a sequence of grids with the parameters $h_0, h_1, \ldots, h_r$ be given.

Theorem 6.11 *To produce the approximate normal solution $\widetilde{V}^{h_r}$ of system* (6.219) *satisfying the estimate*

$$\|U^{h_r} - \widetilde{V}^{h_r}\|_h \leq \varepsilon h_r^2(|f|_0 + \|g\|_1), \tag{6.250}$$

the FMG-algorithm with the above-cited realization of $MG^{(9)}$-algorithm needs no more than $c_{11}(2N_r + m_r)$ arithmetic operations where the constant $c(\varepsilon)$ is independent of f, g, h_i, r.

Proof. First we make sure of the validity of this conbination of algorithms when used to find the normal solution of system (6.219). Let us use induction. It is obvious that on level h_0 the normal solution of system (6.219) will belong to $\mathbf{E}^{h_0}$. Suppose now that approximate normal solution $\widetilde{V}^{h_i}$ of system (6.219) belongs to $\mathbf{E}^{h_i}$. At first stage, its prolongation $\tilde{v}^{h_i}$, $\tilde{q}^{h_i}$ in $\mathbf{U}^{h_i} \times \mathbf{V}^{h_i}$ belongs to subspace $\mathbf{U}^{h_i} \times \tilde{\mathbf{V}}^{h_i}$ subject to Remark 6.5.2. Since the vector $W^{h_{i+1}}$ has the same prolongation $\tilde{v}^{h_i}$, $\tilde{q}^{h_i}$ in $\mathbf{U}^{h_{i+1}} \times \tilde{\mathbf{V}}^{h_{i+1}}$, it also belongs to $\mathbf{E}^{h_{i+1}}$. At second stage, therefore, the initial guess $W^{h_{i+1}}$ satisfies the requirements of Theorem 6.10 and the estimate is valid owing to the induction assumption (6.250) for level h_i:

$$\|U^{h_{i+1}} - W^{h_{i+1}}\|_h \leq \varepsilon c_2 h_{i+1}^2(|f|_0 + \|g\|_1). \tag{6.251}$$

Let integer m be sufficiently large. Then, using Theorem 6.10, we infer that $MG^{(9)}$-algorithm with the initial guess $W^{h_{i+1}}$ yields the approximate normal solution $\widetilde{V}^{h_{i+1}}$ obeying the estimate

$$\|U^{h_{i+1}} - \widetilde{V}^{h_{i+1}}\|_h \leq \varepsilon h_{i+1}^2(|f|_0 + \|g\|_1). \tag{6.252}$$

Thus, both the validity of the algorithms and the estimate (6.250) are proved.

Arithmetic operations are counted up in the usual fashion, likewise in section 5.1. If an orthogonalization to Z^{h_i} is carried out at stage $\mathbf{A}_5$, a corresponding number of operations must be added. □

Corollary 6.5.1 *For prolongation $\tilde{v}^{h_r}$, $\tilde{q}^{h_r}$ of vector $\widetilde{V}^{h_r}$ the estimate* (6.250) *can be transformed:*

$$\begin{aligned} |u - \tilde{v}^{h_r}|_0 &\leq (c_4 + \varepsilon)h_r^2(|f|_0 + \|g\|_1), \\ |p - \tilde{q}^{h_r}|_0 &\leq (c_5 + \varepsilon)h_r(|f|_0 + \|g\|_1). \end{aligned} \tag{6.253}$$

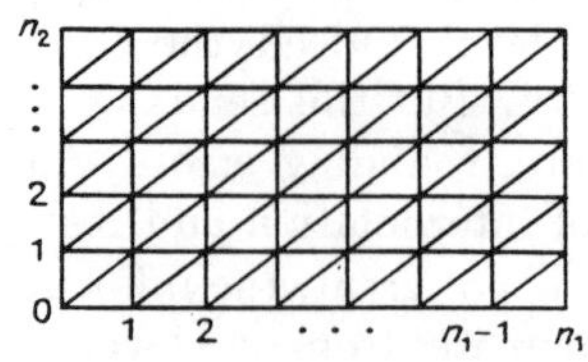

Figure 6.2: A uniform triangulation of a rectangle

Remark 6.5.4 *In principle, we can apply $MG^{(10)}$-algorithm as symmetric W-cycle. The convergence can be proved in another vector norm:*

$$\|W^h\|_h^{(1)} = (|\tilde{u}_1^h|_1^2 + |\tilde{u}_2^h|_1^2 + |\tilde{p}^h|_0^2)^{1/2}.$$

Results analogous to Theorems 6.10 *and* 6.11 *and Corollary* 6.5.1 *are valid for W-cycle with the following estimates instead of* (6.228), (6.250), (6.253) (*see also* [152]):

$$\begin{aligned}
\|V_1^{h_i} - U^{h_i}\|_h^{(1)} &\leq \varepsilon\|V_0^{h_i} - U^{h_i}\|_h^{(1)}, \quad \text{where } V_1^{h_i} = MG_i^{(10)}(V_0^{h_i}, F^{h_i}),\\
\|U^{h_r} - \tilde{V}^{h_r}\|_h^{(1)} &\leq \varepsilon h_r(|f|_0 + \|g\|_1),\\
|u^{h_r} - \tilde{u}^{h_r}|_1 &\leq \varepsilon h_r(|f|_0 + \|g\|_1),\\
|u - \tilde{u}^{h_r}|_1 &\leq (c_3 + \varepsilon)h_r(|f|_0 + \|g\|_1).
\end{aligned}$$

6.5.4 Other combinations of finite elements

It should be noted that not every combination of finite elements approximating velocity and pressure yields optimal orders of convergence following from approximating properties. We often get an ill-conditioned system even in space $\mathbf{U}^{h_i} \times \tilde{\mathbf{V}}^{h_i}$.

One simple rule cuts off a number of poor combinations: *the number of degrees of freedom for elements approximating u_1, u_2 must not be less by unit than the number of degrees of freedom for elements approximating p, i. e.,* $2N_i \geq m_i - 1$ $(i = 0, 1, \ldots, p)$. Indeed, consider system (6.216), (6.217) and suppose u^{h_i} to have been found. Then the only way to determine p^{h_i} is to solve the system following from the identity:

$$l(p^{h_i}, v) = f(v) - \mathcal{L}(u^{h_i}, v) \qquad \forall v \in \mathbf{U}^{h_i}. \tag{6.254}$$

Since p^{h_i} is determined up to the constant term, the rank of matrix of this system must be $m_i - 1$, whence it follows that the dimension of $\mathbf{U}^{h_i}$ must not be less than $m_i - 1$.

It is clear that this condition is necessary but insufficient (some of the sufficient conditions are given in [180], [47]). Nevertheless, it is sufficient for some frequently used combinations to be cut off. For instance, to illustrate Remark 6.5.1, we consider the rectangular triangulation in Fig. 6.2. Piecewise linear Courant elements when used for approximating u yield $2(n_1-1)(n_2-1)$ degrees of freedom including boundary value conditions. On the same triangles, the number of piecewise constant basis functions for approximating p is $2n_1n_2$. Hence, the rule is not satisfied and the system is ill-conditioned, which is just the case in practice.

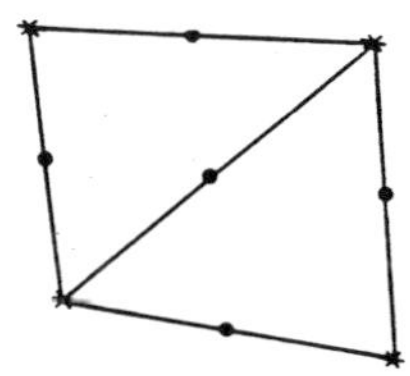

Figure 6.3: The stable combination of finite elements: $*$ and $\bullet$ mark nodes of quadratic elements for velocities; $*$ marks also nodes of continuous linear elements for pressure.

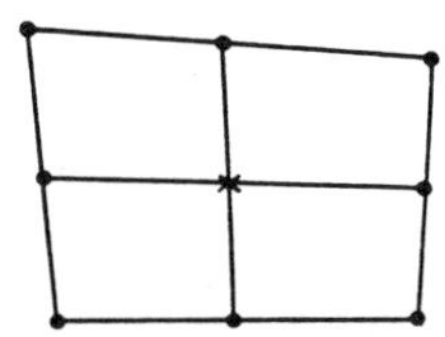

Figure 6.4: The stable combination of finite elements on quadrangles: $*$ and $\bullet$ mark nodes of bilinear elements for velocities; $*$ marks also node of constant element for pressure.

Consider some other simple examples of stable combinations of finite elements.

On triangular meshes, the following combination is also possible. We can [63] use quadratic elements for approximating u and continuous linear elements for approximating p (Fig. 6.3). The estimates (6.210)–(6.213), (6.253) and Theorems 6.10 and 6.11 are valid for this combination of finite elements with degree of h unit greater.

With a domain divided into quadrangles, one of the simplest combinations is as follows. Let $\mathcal{T}^h$ be a concordant triangulation of polygon Ω into quadrangles. Also construct the triangulation $\mathcal{T}^{h/2}$ by drawing lines joining the sides midpoints in every quadrangle (see Fig. 6.4). Then we can use bilinear elements on $\mathcal{T}^{h/2}$ for approximating u and piecewise-constant elements on $\mathcal{T}^h$ for approximating p. The estimates (6.210)–(6.213), (6.253) and Theorems 6.10 and 6.11 are also valid for this combination of finite elements.

A number of stable combinations of higher degrees elements satisfying (6.210) is given in [112], [45], [113], [180], [187], [177], for three-dimensional problems as well.

6.6 The stationary Navier-Stokes problem

In this section we treat the stationary Navier-Stokes problem of viscous incompressible fluid as well as continue studying the generalized formulation related to the mixed method by analogy with the preceding section. But unlike the proceding, the discrete problem obtained is nonlinear. One of the stages of its solution is therefore the Newton method. Moreover, the matrices of the Newton method systems are nonsymmetric, and so we have to use some other modifications of the multigrid algorithms.

6.6.1 The formulation of a differential problem

Let Ω be a convex bounded poligon with a boundary Γ. Our problem is to define a function p and a vector-function $u = (u_1, u_2)$ if $f = (f_1, f_2)$ is known:

$$\begin{aligned} -\nu\Delta u + (u\cdot\nabla)u + \nabla p &= f \quad \text{in} \quad \Omega, && (6.255)\\ \operatorname{div} u &= 0 \quad \text{in} \quad \Omega, && (6.256)\\ u &= 0 \quad \text{on} \quad \Gamma. && (6.257) \end{aligned}$$

To pass to a generalized formulation, we take arbitrary functions $q \in \mathbf{V} = \widetilde{L}_2(\Omega)$, $v = (v_1, v_2) \in \mathbf{U} = (\overset{\circ}{W}{}_2^1(\Omega))^2$ and perform the integration by parts as in the preceding section. We come to the formulae:

$$\mathcal{L}(u,v) + a_1(u,u,v) + l(p,v) = f(v) \qquad \forall v \in \mathbf{U}, \tag{6.258}$$

$$l(q,u) = 0 \qquad \forall q \in \mathbf{V}. \tag{6.259}$$

Here and further, the notation is like one in the previous section excepting the trilinear form

$$a_1(w,u,v) = \frac{1}{2}\left(\int_\Omega (w\cdot\nabla)u\cdot v dx - \int_\Omega (w\cdot\nabla)v\cdot u dx\right). \tag{6.260}$$

Note its skew symmetric properties [185]:

$$\begin{aligned} a_1(w,u,v) &= -a_1(w,v,u)\\ a_1(w,u,u) &= 0, \qquad u,v,w \in \mathbf{U}. \end{aligned} \tag{6.261}$$

Besides, the paper [59] guarantees the existence of a constant N such that

$$|a_1(w,u,v)| \le N|w|_1|u|_1|v|_1 \qquad \forall w,u,v \in \mathbf{U}. \tag{6.262}$$

Note also that (6.187) holds again for bilinear form l.

A solvability of the problem (6.258), (6.259) is not evident. The following assumption is usually supposed for it:

$$f \in (W_2^{-1}(\Omega))^2, \qquad \|f\|_{-1} < \nu^2/N. \tag{6.263}$$

Theorem 6.12 [185] *Let Ω be a convex bounded poligon and* (6.263) *hold; then the solution of problem* (6.258), (6.259) *exists and is unique in $\mathbf{U}\times\mathbf{V}$; the estimate*

$$|u|_1 < \|f\|_{-1}/\nu \tag{6.264}$$

is valid. Moreover, if

$$f \in (L_2(\Omega))^2, \tag{6.265}$$

then $u \in (W_2^2(\Omega))^2$, $p \in W_2^1(\Omega)$ and

$$\|u\|_2 + \|p\|_1 \le c|f|_0. \tag{6.266}$$

6.6.2 The discrete problem

To construct a difference problem, we use a sequence of nested grids Ω_{h_i}, Ω'_{h_i} and spaces $\mathbf{U}^{h_i}$, $\mathbf{V}^{h_i}$, $\tilde{\mathbf{V}}^{h_i}$ introduced in the preceding section. The approximate solution will be sought using the Bubnov-Galerkin method: *in the form of functions* $u^{h_i} = (u_1^{h_i}, u_2^{h_i}) \in \mathbf{U}^{h_i}$, $p \in \tilde{\mathbf{V}}^{h_i}$ *satisfying the equalities*

$$\begin{aligned}\mathcal{L}(u^{h_i}, v) + a_1(u^{h_i}, u^{h_i}, v) + l(p^{h_i}, v) &= f(v) \qquad \forall v \in \mathbf{U}^{h_i}, &(6.267)\\ l(q, u^{h_i}) &= 0 \qquad \forall q \in \tilde{\mathbf{V}}^{h_i}. &(6.268)\end{aligned}$$

The solvability of this nonlinear problem is rather difficult to prove.

Theorem 6.13 [63] *Let* (6.263) *and* (6.265) *be valid. Then for the chosen spaces* $\mathbf{U}^{h_i}$, $\tilde{\mathbf{V}}^{h_i}$ *on a convex bounded polygon* Ω, *the problem* (6.267), (6.268) *is uniquely solvable and the following estimates hold:*

$$\begin{aligned}|u - u^{h_i}|_1 &\le c_3 h_i |f|_0, &(6.269)\\ |u - u^{h_i}|_0 &\le c_4 h_i^2 |f|_0, &(6.270)\\ |p - p^{h_i}|_0 &\le c_5 h_i |f|_0. &(6.271)\end{aligned}$$

6.6.3 The Newton method and the multigrid algorithm

To solve problem (6.267), (6.268), we use the Newton method in which the initial guess is taken from a more rough grid. Consider one iteration of the Newton method with the initial guess $u_0 \in \mathbf{U}^{h_i}$ in the following form: *find* $u_1 \in \mathbf{U}^{h_i}$, $p_1 \in \tilde{\mathbf{V}}^{h_i}$ *satisfying the relations*

$$\begin{aligned}&\mathcal{L}(u_1, v) + a_1(u_1, u_0, v) + a_1(u_0, u_1, v) + l(p_1, v) =\\ &\qquad = f(v) + a_1(u_0, u_0, v) \qquad \forall v \in \mathbf{U}^{h_i}, &(6.272)\\ &\qquad l(q, u_1) = 0 \qquad \forall q \in \tilde{\mathbf{V}}^{h_i}. &(6.273)\end{aligned}$$

Given certain conditions, the Newton method exhibits the quadratic convergence.

Theorem 6.14 [63], [58] *Positive constants* c_6, c_7 *exist such that for* $u_0 \in U^{h_i}$ *satisfying*

$$|u_0 - u^{h_i}|_1 \le c_6, \tag{6.274}$$

the functions $u_1 \in \mathbf{U}^{h_i}$, $p_1 \in \tilde{\mathbf{V}}^{h_i}$ *are uniquely defined from* (6.272), (6.273) *and*

$$\begin{aligned}|u^{h_i} - u_1|_1 &\le c_6^{-1} |u^{h_i} - u_0|_1^2, &(6.275)\\ |p^{h_i} - p_1|_0 &\le c_7 |u^{h_i} - u_0|_1^2. &(6.276)\end{aligned}$$

The constant c_6 *can be constructed in terms of the data of problems* (6.258), (6.259) *and* (6.267), (6.268).

From the algorithmic standpoint, instead of this problem, another one is more suitable which has a solution defined all over $\mathbf{V}^{h_i}$. Namely: *find* $u_1 \in \mathbf{U}^{h_i}$, $p_1 \in \mathbf{V}^{h_i}$ *satisfying the relations* (6.272) *and*

$$l(q, u_1) = 0 \qquad \forall q \in \mathbf{V}^{h_i}. \tag{6.277}$$

Problem (6.272), (6.277) is linear with respect to u_1, p_1 and can be written as a system of linear algebraic equations

$$L^{h_i}(u_0) W^{h_i} = F^{h_i}(u_0). \tag{6.278}$$

The matrix $L^{h_i}(u_0)$ linearly depends on u_0, and W^{h_i}, $F^{h_i}(u_0)$ are vectors of unknowns and the right-hand side. As it was already stated in the preceding section, the matrix $L^{h_i}(u_0)$ is singular and its null space basis consists of one vector Z^{h_i} (see (6.221)) if ν is not very small.

On the zeroth level h_0, the system of nonlinear algebraic equations following from (6.267), (6.268) has a rather small number of unknowns. Its solution does not present essential difficulties, therefore, and can be effected to an arbitrary accuracy controlled in practice only by rounding errors. Now we describe $FMG^{(4)}$-algorithm permitting to find a sequence of approximate solutions $\tilde{u}^{h_i} \in \mathbf{U}^{h_i}$, $\tilde{p}^{h_i} \in \tilde{\mathbf{V}}^{h_i}$ $(i = 1, \dots, r)$. We use induction. Let us suppose that we already have the solution $\tilde{u}^{h_{i-1}} \in \mathbf{U}^{h_{i-1}}$, $\tilde{p}^{h_{i-1}} \in \tilde{\mathbf{V}}^{h_{i-1}}$.

$\mathbf{B}_1^{(4)}$. In view of the nestedness $\mathbf{U}^{h_{i-1}} \subset \mathbf{U}^{h_i}$, $\tilde{\mathbf{V}}^{h_{i-1}} \subset \tilde{\mathbf{V}}^{h_i}$, the vector-function $\tilde{u}^{h_{i-1}}$ belongs to $\mathbf{U}^{h_i}$ and $\tilde{p}^{h_{i-1}}$ belongs to $\tilde{\mathbf{V}}^{h_i}$. Using the definition of prolongations (6.223), we get an isomorphic vector W^{h_i}.

$\mathbf{B}_2^{(4)}$. Using the initial guess $u_0 = \tilde{u}^{h_{i-1}}$, we carry out two iterations of the Newton method by formulae (6.272), (6.277). Note that the approximate solution of system (6.278) is computed using $MG^{(11)}$-algorithm described below. As a result, we get functions $\tilde{u}^{h_i} \in \mathbf{U}^{h_i}$, $\tilde{p}^{h_i} \in \mathbf{V}^{h_i}$.

In passing from one level to other by means of $FMG^{(4)}$-algorithm, with r steps executed, we get an approximate solution on the finest grid.

Now describe $MG^{(11)}$-algorithm. It differs from $MG^{(9)}$-algorithm given in section 4.11 only in the pre-smoothing iterations at the first stage. Describe it dropping argument u_0 of matrix L^{h_i} and right-hand side F^{h_i} in system (6.278). Denote the initial guess and the result of the application of $MG^{(11)}$-algorithm by $W_0^{h_i}$ and $W_1^{h_i}$, i. e., $W_1^{h_i} = MG^{(11)}(W_0^{h_i}, F^{h_i})$.

$\mathbf{A}_1^{(5)}$. Execute m iterations by formula

$$U_{l+1} = U_l - \tau_l \mathcal{D}^{h_i} (L^{h_i})^T \mathcal{D}^{h_i} (L^{h_i} U_l - F^{h_i}), \qquad l = 0, 1, \dots, m-1, \tag{6.279}$$

with the initial guess $W_0^{h_i}$ and the parameters τ_l chosen by formula (4.206) with the constant μ_i^* from the condition

$$\lambda((\mathcal{D}^{h_i})^{1/2} (L^{h_i})^T \mathcal{D}^{h_i} L^{h_i} (\mathcal{D}^{h_i})^{1/2}) \le \mu_i^* \le c_9. \tag{6.280}$$

The existence of constant c_9 independent of h_i follows from the proof of Theorem 3.14. As a result of the iterative process, we have U_m and the residual

$$G^{h_i} = L^{h_i} U_m - F^{h_i}. \tag{6.281}$$

Note that components of G^{h_i} corresponding to the pressure are *not zero*. Therefore we need to study the following auxiliary *linear* problem. Let

$$w \in \mathbf{U}, \quad f \in (L_2(\Omega))^2, \quad g \in \tilde{W}_2^1(\Omega) \tag{6.282}$$

be given, *find* $u \in \mathbf{U}$, $p \in \tilde{\mathbf{V}}$ *such that*

$$\begin{aligned} \mathcal{L}(u,v) + a_1(w,u,v) + a_1(u,w,v) + l(p,v) &= (f,v) \quad \forall v \in \mathbf{U}, & (6.283)\\ l(q,u) &= (g,q) \quad \forall q \in \tilde{\mathbf{V}}. & (6.284) \end{aligned}$$

This time, equation (6.284) is inhomogeneous even if (6.259) are homogeneous in the initial problem. Therefore we lose almost all well-known sources of information about such problem and are compelled to give at least short proofs of standard results.

Theorem 6.15 *Let* (6.282) *hold and*

$$|w|_1 < \nu/N \tag{6.285}$$

with the constant N *from* (6.262). *Then the problem* (6.283)–(6.284) *has a unique solution* $u \in (W_2^2(\Omega))^2$, $p \in W_2^1(\Omega)$.

Proof. Let us use Theorem 1.3. To this end, define

$$\begin{aligned} a(u,v) &= \mathcal{L}(u,v) + a_1(w,u,v) + a_1(u,w,v),\\ b(u,\psi) &= l(u,\psi). \end{aligned}$$

Then (1.14) is equivalent to (6.187). Because of (6.261), (6.262) and (6.285), we have

$$\begin{aligned} a(u,u) &= \mathcal{L}(u,u) + a_1(u,w,u) \geq\\ &\geq \nu|u|_1^2 - N|w|_1\,|u|_1^2 \geq \gamma|u|_1^2 \qquad \forall u \in \mathbf{U} \end{aligned} \tag{6.286}$$

with a constant $\gamma > 0$. Hence,

$$\sup_{u\in Z\setminus\{0\}} a(u,v)/|u|_1 \geq \gamma|v|_1 \qquad \forall v \in Z \subset \mathbf{U}$$

and

$$\sup_{v\in Z\setminus\{0\}} a(u,v)/|v|_1 \geq \gamma|u|_1 \qquad \forall u \in Z \subset \mathbf{U}.$$

Thus, all assumptions of Theorem 1.3 are valid and we have a unique solution $u \in \mathbf{U}$, $p \in \tilde{\mathbf{V}}$.

Let us rewrite (6.283)–(6.284) in a form of the Stokes problem

$$\begin{aligned} -\nu\Delta u + \operatorname{grad} p &= \bar{f} \quad \text{in } \Omega,\\ \operatorname{div} u &= -g \quad \text{in } \Omega,\\ u &= 0 \quad \text{on } \Gamma, \end{aligned}$$

with the right-hand side

$$\bar{f} = f - (w\cdot\nabla)u - (u\cdot\nabla)w - u \operatorname{div} w/2 - w \operatorname{div} u/2.$$

Because of the imbedding theorem [94], [185],

$$u, w \in (L_\beta(\Omega))^2 \qquad \forall \beta \in (1, \infty). \tag{6.287}$$

Let us fix a constant $\alpha \in (1, 2)$. Due to the Hölder inequality,

$$u_i \partial_j w_k,\ w_i \partial_j u_k \ \in L_\alpha(\Omega)$$

for any i, j, k equal to 1, 2. Hence,

$$\bar{f} \in (L_\alpha(\Omega))^2, \qquad g \in W_\alpha^1(\Omega).$$

Owing to Theorem 6.9, we have

$$u \in (W_\alpha^2(\Omega))^2.$$

Because of imbedding theorems [94], [185],

$$u_i \in L_\infty(\Omega),\ \partial_j u_k \in L_q(\Omega) \qquad \forall q \in (2, 2\alpha/(2-\alpha)).$$

Together with (6.287) and the Hölder inequality, it gives

$$u_i \partial_j w_k,\ w_i \partial_j u_k \ \in L_2(\Omega)$$

for any i, j, k equal to 1, 2. Therefore

$$\bar{f} \in (L_2(\Omega))^2.$$

Owing to Theorem 6.9 again, we have

$$u \in (W_2^2(\Omega))^2, \qquad p \in W_2^1(\Omega). \qquad \square$$

Remark 6.6.1 *Note that the problem ajoint of* (6.283)–(6.284) *has the form: find* $u \in \mathbf{U}$ *and* $v \in \tilde{\mathbf{V}}$ *such that*

$$\mathcal{L}(u, v) + a_1(w, v, u) + a_1(v, w, u) + l(p, v) \ = \ (f, v) \qquad \forall v \in \mathbf{U}, \tag{6.288}$$

$$l(q, u) \ = \ (g, q) \qquad \forall q \in \tilde{\mathbf{V}}. \tag{6.289}$$

The statement of Theorem 6.15 *is valid for it too.*

Denote the normal solution of system (6.278) by $W_H^{h_i}$.

Theorem 6.16 *Let* Ω *be a convex polygon and let* $W_0^{h_i} \in \mathbf{E}^{h_i}$,

$$|u_0|_1 < \nu/N. \tag{6.290}$$

Then for any $\varepsilon \in (0, 1)$ *we can choose an integer* m_0 *independent of* h_i, F^{h_i} *and such that* $\forall m \geq m_0$ $MG^{(11)}$*-algorithm reduces the error of the approximate normal solution* $W_1^{h_i} \in \mathbf{E}^{h_i}$ *by a factor* ε:

$$\|W_1^{h_i} - W_H^{h_i}\|_h \leq \varepsilon \|W_0^{h_i} - W_H^{h_i}\|_h \quad \text{where} \quad W_1^{h_i} = MG^{(11)}(W_0^{h_i}, F^{h_i}). \tag{6.291}$$

Proof. First, likewise in proving Theorem 6.10, we establish that the vectors do not leave the subspace $\mathbf{E}^{h_i}$ at all stages of $MG^{(11)}$-algorithm.

Further considerations literally coincide with the proof of Theorem 6.8 with some unprincipal distinctions. First, pre-smoothing procedure (6.279) transforms into

$$U_{l+1} = U_l - \tau_l L_i^T (L_i U_l - F_i), \qquad l = 0, 1, \dots, m-1,$$

with the iterative operator

$$J_i = (I - \tau_{m-1} L_i^T L_i) \dots (I - \tau_0 L_i^T L_i)$$

instead of (6.230), (6.231). Second, we introduce the form

$$\mathcal{B}(u,p;\ v,q) = \mathcal{L}(u,v) + a_1(w,u,v) + a_1(u,w,v) + l(p,v) + l(q,u)$$

instead of (6.235). Since this form is not symmetric, we have to solve an ajoint problem in analogue of (6.241):

$$\mathcal{B}(w,r;\ v^{h_{i-1}}, q^{h_{i-1}}) = \mathcal{B}(w,r;\ v^{h_i}, q^{h_i}) \qquad \forall w \in \mathbf{U}^{h_{i-1}}, v \in \tilde{\mathbf{V}}^{h_{i-1}}. \tag{6.292}$$

Finally, comparing (6.280) and (6.227), we have to change λ_i^* by $\sqrt{\mu_i^*}$ in (6.247) and (6.248):

$$\|L_i^{-1} - I_{i-1} L_{i-1}^{-1} R_i\|_E \le c/\sqrt{\mu_i^*},$$

$$\|L_i J_i\|_E \le \sqrt{\mu_i^*}/(2m+1). \quad \square$$

6.6.4 The main result

Theorem 6.17 *Let* (6.263) *and* (6.265) *hold. Then for any* $\varepsilon \in (0,1)$, *we can choose an integer* m_0 *and* h_0 *small enough such that* $\forall m \ge m_0$ $FMG^{(4)}$*-algorithm gives the approximate solution* $\tilde{u}^{h_r} \in \mathbf{U}^{h_r}$, $\tilde{p}^{h_r} \in \tilde{\mathbf{V}}^{h_r}$ *with the estimates*

$$|u^{h_r} - \tilde{u}^{h_r}|_0 \le \varepsilon h_r^2 |f|_0, \tag{6.293}$$
$$|p^{h_r} - \tilde{p}^{h_r}|_0 \le \varepsilon h_r |f|_0 \tag{6.294}$$

where u^{h_r}, p^{h_r} *are exact solutions of the discrete problem* (6.272), (6.273) *on the finest grid. The number of arithmetic operations is not over* $c_8(2N_r + m_r)$ *where the constant* $c_8(\varepsilon)$ *is independent of* f, h_i, r.

Proof. Let us use the inverse inequality (3.58) and the Friedrichs one (1.1) in the vectoral form

$$|v|_1 \le c_1 h_i^{-1} |v|_0 \qquad \forall v \in \mathbf{U}^{h_i}, \tag{6.295}$$
$$|v|_0 \le c_{11} |v|_1 \qquad \forall v \in \mathbf{U}. \tag{6.296}$$

Then we put

$$\begin{aligned}
c_9 &= 5\,c_4 + 4, && (6.297)\\
c_{10} &= 3\,c_5 + 2, && (6.298)\\
c_{12} &= ((c_1^2 c_6^{-1} c_9 c_{11}|f|_0 + c_9)^2 + (c_1 c_6 c_7 c_9 + c_{10})^2)^{1/2}, && (6.299)\\
c_{13} &= c_1(c_9 + c_{12}), && (6.300)\\
c_{14} &= c_1^2 c_6^{-1} c_9^2 c_{11}|f|_0 + c_{12}, && (6.301)\\
c_{15} &= c_1 c_6 c_7 c_9 + c_{12}, && (6.302)\\
c_{16} &= ((c_{14} + c_6^{-1} c_{11} c_{13}|f|_0)^2 + (c_6 c_7 c_{13} + c_{15})^2)^{1/2}, && (6.303)\\
\varepsilon_1 &= \varepsilon \min\{1, 4c_1^2/c_{13}^2, 1/2c_{16}, c_6/2c_{11}c_{13}^2|f|_0, 1/2c_6c_7c_{13}\} && (6.304)
\end{aligned}$$

with the constants from (6.295), (6.270), (6.271), (6.274), (6.276), (6.296). To ensure the convergence of Newton method and the solvability of nonlinear problem, we assume that

$$h_0 < \min\{2\sqrt{\varepsilon_1}c_6/c_1c_9|f|_0,\ 2c_6/c_{13}|f|_0,\ (\nu - N|u|_1)/N(c_1 + c_3)|f|_0\} \quad (6.305)$$

with the additional constants from (6.269) and (6.262). In particular,

$$h_1 \le \min\{\sqrt{\varepsilon_1}c_6/c_1c_9|f|_0,\ c_6/c_{13}|f|_0\}. \quad (6.306)$$

Due to (6.263) and (6.264), the constant $\nu - N|u|_1$ is positive and the right-hand part of (6.305) is positive too.

Then we choose an integer m_0 such that the statement (6.291) of Theorem 6.16 is valid with constant ε_1 and take an integer $m \ge m_0$ in the pre-smoothing procedure (6.279).

Further we use induction. On the zeroth level, because of non-linearity, we do not manage to obtain the exact solution of problem (6.267), (6.268) or, what is the same, the exact normal solution of a nonlinear system like (6.278). So there is sense in applying variuos linearizing methods already on this level: we can use the Newton method, chords, simple iteration etc. [63], [58]. Unlike other levels, linear systems like (6.278) are solved directly since the number of unknowns is small. We leave this question to be open assuming that zeroth level calls for the finite number of arithmetic operations (since h_0 is fixed).

Now we assume that we already have the approximate solution $\tilde{u}^{h_{i-1}}$, $\tilde{p}^{h_{i-1}}$ at the level h_{i-1} with the estimates

$$\begin{aligned}
|u^{h_{i-1}} - \tilde{u}^{h_{i-1}}|_0 &\le \varepsilon h_{i-1}^2|f|_0, && (6.307)\\
|p^{h_{i-1}} - \tilde{p}^{h_{i-1}}|_0 &\le \varepsilon h_{i-1}|f|_0. && (6.308)
\end{aligned}$$

Our purpose is to prove these estimates at the level h_i. Consider stage $\mathbf{B}_1^{(4)}$. Let us see how $\tilde{u}^{h_{i-1}}$ approximates the exact solution u^{h_i} of problem (6.267), (6.268) at level h_i. From (6.270), (6.307), it follows that

$$|u^{h_i} - \tilde{u}^{h_{i-1}}|_0 \le |u^{h_i} - u|_0 + |u - \tilde{u}^{h_{i-1}}|_0 \le (c_4 h_i^2 + (c_4 + \varepsilon)h_{i-1}^2)|f|_0.$$

Further we use inverse inequality (6.295). Then

$$|u^{h_i} - \tilde{u}^{h_{i-1}}|_0 \leq c_9 h_i^2 |f|_0, \tag{6.309}$$
$$|u^{h_i} - \tilde{u}^{h_{i-1}}|_1 \leq c_1 c_9 h_i |f|_0. \tag{6.310}$$

Evaluate the error of pressure in the similar way using inequalities (6.271) and (6.308):

$$|p^{h_i} - \tilde{p}^{h_{i-1}}|_0 \leq |p^{h_i} - p|_0 + |p - \tilde{p}^{h_{i-1}}|_0 \leq$$

$$\leq c_5 h_i |f|_0 + (c_5 + \varepsilon) h_{i-1} |f|_0 \leq c_{10} h_i |f|_0. \tag{6.311}$$

Let us pass to stage $\mathbf{B}_2^{(4)}$. Take Theorem 6.14 on the quadratic convergence of the Newton method. Put in it $u_0 = \tilde{u}^{h_{i-1}}$. Because of (6.306) and (6.310), we have the inequalities

$$|u^{h_i} - u_0|_1 \leq c_1 c_9 h_1 |f|_0 \leq c_6,$$

which coincides with (6.274) and ensures the convergence of the Newton method. Due to Theorem 6.14 we get

$$|u^{h_i} - u_1|_1 \leq c_6^{-1} |u^{h_i} - \tilde{u}^{h_{i-1}}|_1^2,$$
$$|p^{h_i} - p_1|_0 \leq c_7 |u^{h_i} - \tilde{u}^{h_{i-1}}|_1^2.$$

From this and (6.310)

$$|u^{h_i} - u_1|_1 \leq c_1^2 c_6^{-1} c_9^2 h_i^2 |f|_0^2, \tag{6.312}$$
$$|p^{h_i} - p_1|_0 \leq c_1^2 c_7 c_9^2 h_i^2 |f|_0^2. \tag{6.313}$$

Instead of the exact solution u_1, p_1 of problem (6.272), (6.273), we get the approximate solution $\tilde{u}_1$, $\tilde{p}_1$ in view of the application of $MG^{(11)}$-algorithm to the solution of system (6.278). Because of (6.305), (6.307), (6.295), (6.296) we have

$$|u_0|_1 \leq |u|_1 + |\tilde{u}^{h_{i-1}} - u|_1 \leq |u|_1 + (c_1 + c_3) h_0 |f|_0 < \nu/N.$$

Thus, all assumptions of Theorem 6.16 are valid. Using this Theorem and (6.224), we come to the inequality

$$|u_1 - \tilde{u}_1|_0 \leq \varepsilon_1 (|u_1 - \tilde{u}^{h_{i-1}}|_0^2 + h_i^2 |p_1 - \tilde{p}^{h_{i-1}}|_0^2)^{1/2}. \tag{6.314}$$

Evaluate its right-hand side because of (6.296), (6.312), (6.309):

$$|u_1 - \tilde{u}^{h_{i-1}}|_0 \leq |u_1 - u^{h_i}|_0 + |u^{h_i} - \tilde{u}^{h_{i-1}}|_0 \leq$$
$$\leq c_{11} |u_1 - u^{h_i}|_1 + c_9 h_i^2 |f|_0 \leq (c_1^2 c_6^{-1} c_9^2 c_{11} |f|_0 + c_9) h_i^2 |f|_0. \tag{6.315}$$

Similarly, using (6.311), (6.313), we get

$$|p_1 - \tilde{p}^{h_{i-1}}|_0 \leq |p_1 - p^{h_i}|_0 + |p^{h_i} - \tilde{p}^{h_{i-1}}|_0 \leq c_1^2 c_7 c_9^2 h_i^2 |f|_0^2 + c_{10} h_i |f|_0. \tag{6.316}$$

Combining (6.314), (6.315), (6.316), (6.306), we obtain the inequality

$$|u_1 - \tilde{u}_1|_0 \leq \varepsilon_1 c_{12} h_i^2 |f|_0. \tag{6.317}$$

From this and inverse inequality (6.295)

$$|u_1 - \tilde{u}_1|_1 \le \varepsilon_1 c_1 c_{12} h_i |f|_0. \tag{6.318}$$

Use the above, (6.306) and (6.312) simultaneously:

$$|u^{h_i} - \tilde{u}_1|_1 \le |u^{h_i} - u_1|_1 + |u_1 - \tilde{u}_1|_1 \le \sqrt{\varepsilon_1} c_{13} h_i |f|_0. \tag{6.319}$$

Now use inequality (6.317) together with (6.312) and (6.296):

$$|u^{h_i} - \tilde{u}_1|_0 \le |u^{h_i} - u_1|_0 + |u_1 - \tilde{u}_1|_0 \le c_{14} h_i^2 |f|_0. \tag{6.320}$$

The error of computed pressure is estimated analogously. From Theorem 6.16,

$$|p_1 - \tilde{p}_1|_0 \le h_i^{-1} \varepsilon_1 (|u_1 - \tilde{u}^{h_{i-1}}|_0^2 + h_i^2 |p_1 - \tilde{p}^{h_{i-1}}|_0^2)^{1/2}.$$

Since the expression in parentheses has already been estimated in (6.314) and (6.317), we have

$$|p_1 - \tilde{p}_1|_0 \le \varepsilon_1 c_{12} h_i |f|_0. \tag{6.321}$$

Using the last inequality, (6.306) and (6.313) simultaneously, we get

$$|p^{h_i} - \tilde{p}_1|_0 \le |p^{h_i} - p_1|_0 + |p_1 - \tilde{p}_1|_0 \le c_{15} h_i |f|_0. \tag{6.322}$$

Put $u_0 = \tilde{u}_1$ in (6.272), (6.273) and denote the exact solution of the obtained problem by u_2, p_2. Because of (6.306) and (6.319), we have the inequalities

$$|u^{h_i} - \tilde{u}_1|_1 \le c_{13} h_1 |f|_0 \le c_6,$$

which ensures (6.274) and the convergence of the Newton method for this iteration. Then, by virtue of Theorem 6.14,

$$|u^{h_i} - u_2|_1 \le c_6^{-1} |u^{h_i} - \tilde{u}_1|_1^2. \tag{6.323}$$

Apply (6.319) to the right-hand side and (6.296) to the left-hand side :

$$|u^{h_i} - u_2|_0 \le \varepsilon_1 c_6^{-1} c_{11} c_{13}^2 h_i^2 |f|_0^2. \tag{6.324}$$

Moreover, the estimate

$$|p^{h_i} - p_2|_0 \le c_7 \, |u^{h_i} - \tilde{u}_1|_1^2 \le \varepsilon_1 c_7 c_{13}^2 h_i^2 |f|_0^2 \tag{6.325}$$

follows from (6.319) and Theorem 6.14 for p_2.

Instead of the exact solution u_2, p_2 of problem (6.272), (6.273), we obtain the approximate solution $\tilde{u}_2$, $\tilde{p}_2$, by application of $MG^{(11)}$-algorithm to the solution of system (6.278) with $u_0 = \tilde{u}_1$. Because of (6.269) and (6.319), we get

$$\begin{aligned} |\tilde{u}_1|_1 &\le |u|_1 + |\tilde{u}_1 - u^{h_i}|_1 + |u^{h_i} - u|_1 \le \\ &\le |u|_1 + \sqrt{\varepsilon_1} c_{13} h_i |f|_0 + c_3 h_i |f|_0. \end{aligned}$$

Due to (6.304) and (6.305), we have

$$|\tilde{u}_1|_1 \leq |u|_1 + (c_1 + c_3/2)h_0|f|_0 \leq \nu/N.$$

Thus, all assumptions of Theorem 6.16 are valid. By virtue of this Theorem and (6.224),

$$|u_2 - \tilde{u}_2|_0 \leq \varepsilon_1 \left(|u_2 - \tilde{u}_1|_0^2 + h_i^2|p_2 - \tilde{p}_1|_0^2\right)^{1/2}. \tag{6.326}$$

Evaluate the terms of the right-hand side. From (6.320) and (6.324),

$$\begin{aligned} |u_2 - \tilde{u}_1|_0 &\leq |u_2 - u^{h_i}|_0 + |u^{h_i} - \tilde{u}_1|_0 \leq \\ &\leq (c_{14} + c_6^{-1}c_{11}c_{13}^2|f|_0)h_i^2|f|_0. \end{aligned} \tag{6.327}$$

Using (6.325), (6.322) and (6.306), we get

$$\begin{aligned} &|p_2 - \tilde{p}_1|_0 \leq |p_2 - p^{h_i}|_0 + |p^{h_i} - \tilde{p}_1|_0 \leq \\ &\leq (c_7c_{13}^2h_i|f|_0 + c_{15})h_i|f|_0 \leq (c_6c_7c_{13} + c_{15})h_i|f|_0. \end{aligned} \tag{6.328}$$

Combining (6.326)–(6.328), we obtain the estimate

$$|u_2 - \tilde{u}_2|_0 \leq \varepsilon_1 c_{16} h_i^2|f|_0. \tag{6.329}$$

The estimate

$$|p_2 - \tilde{p}_2|_0 \leq \varepsilon h_i^{-1}(|u_2 - \tilde{u}_1|_0^2 + h_i^2|p_2 - \tilde{p}_1|_0^2)^{1/2}$$

follows from Theorem 6.16 for pressure. Since the expression in parentheses has already been estimated in (6.326) and (6.329), we get the inequality

$$|p_2 - \tilde{p}_2|_0 \leq \varepsilon_1 c_{16} h_i|f|_0. \tag{6.330}$$

Use inequalities (6.329) and (6.324) with (6.304) simultaneously:

$$\begin{aligned} |u^{h_i} - \tilde{u}_2|_0 &\leq |u^{h_i} - u_2|_0 + |u_2 - \tilde{u}_2|_0 \leq \\ &\leq (\varepsilon_1 c_6^{-1}c_{11}c_{13}^2|f|_0 + \varepsilon_1 c_{16})h_i^2|f|_0 \leq \varepsilon h_i^2|f|_0. \end{aligned} \tag{6.331}$$

Thus, estimate (6.293) is proved.

Similarly for pressure as a result of (6.325), (6.330) and (6.304), we have

$$\begin{aligned} |p^{h_i} - \tilde{p}_2|_0 &\leq |p^{h_i} - p_2|_0 + |p_2 - \tilde{p}_2|_0 \leq \\ &\leq (\varepsilon_1 c_7 c_{13}^2 h_i|f|_0 + \varepsilon_1 c_{16})h_i|f|_0 \leq \varepsilon h_i|f|_0. \end{aligned} \tag{6.332}$$

Arithmetic operations are counted up in the usual way, likewise in section 5.1. □

Theorems 6.14 and 6.16 give a convergence in different norms. It complicate the proof of Theorem 6.17.

Here the assertions of subsection 6.5.4 are valid also about an application of other finite elements.

Bibliography

[1] Akhiezer N.I. Lectures on Approximation Theory. — Moscow: Nauka, 1965. **

[2] Akhiezer N.I., Glazman I.M. Theory of Linear Operators in Hilbert Space. Part 1. — Kharkov University, 1977. **

[3] Astrakhantsev G.P. An iterative method of solving elliptic net problems. — USSR Comput. Math. and Math. Phys., 1971, V. 11, No. 2, p. 171–182. *

[4] Astrakhantsev G.P. The iterative improvement of eigenvalues. — USSR Comput. Math. and Math. Phys., 1976, V. 16, No. 1, p. 123–132. *

[5] Astrakhantsev G.P. Reduction of problem on bending plate to system of second-order equations. — In: Variational Difference Methods in Mathematical Physics. Novosibirsk: Computing Center of Siberian Division of the USSR Academy of Sciences (below: Comp. Cen. Sib. Div. USSR Acad. Sci.), 1976, p. 62–72. **

[6] Astrakhantsev G.P. A method of approximate solution of Dirichlet problem for biharmonic eguation. — USSR Comput. Math. and Math. Phys., 1977, V. 17, No. 4, p. 980–998. **

[7] Astrakhantsev G.P., Rukhovets L.A. Fedorenko's method for variational difference schemes with extrapolation. — In: Variational Difference Methods in Mathematical Physics. Novosibirsk: Comp. Cen. Sib. Div. USSR Acad. Sci., 1981, p. 20–26. **

[8] Aubin J.P. Behavior of the error of the approximate solutions of boundary value problems for linear elliptic operators by Galerkin's and finite difference methods. — Ann. Scuola Norm. Sup.-Pisa, 1967., No. 21., p. 599–637.

[9] Axelsson O., Gustafsson I. Preconditioning and two-level multigrid methods of arbitrary degree of approximation. — Math. Comput., 1983., V. 40, No. 161., p. 219–242.

[10] Babuška I. Finite element method for domain with corners. — Computing., 1970., V. 6, No. 3, p. 264–273.

[11] Babuška I. Error-bounds for finite element method. — Numer. Math., 1971, V. 16, No. 2, p. 322–333.

*Published English Translation of Russian Journal.

**English translation of title of the work published in Russian.

[12] Babuška I. The finite element method with penalty. — Math. Comput., 1973, V. 27, No. 122, p. 221–228.

[13] Babuška I. The finite element method with Lagrangian multipliers. — Numer. Math., 1973, V. 20, No. 2, p. 179–192.

[14] Babuška I., Griebel M., Pitkäranta J. The problem of selecting the shape functions for a p–type finite element. — Inter. J. Numer. Meth. Engng., 1989, V. 28, p. 1891–1908.

[15] Babuška I., Osborn J., Pitkäranta J. Analysis of Mixed Methods Using mesh dependent Norms. — Math. Comput., 1980, V. 35, No. 152, p. 1039–1062.

[16] Babuška I., Suri M. The h–p version of the finite element method with quasiuniform meshes. — Math. Model. Numer. Anal., 1987, V. 21, p. 199–238.

[17] Bagaev B.M., Chaydourov V.V. Amélioration de la précision des schémas aux différences variationnelles pour les équations différentielles avec singularités. — Étude Numérique des Grands Systèmes. — Paris: Dunod, 1978, p. 110–123.

[18] Bajakovskii Yu.M., Ljakhovitskii B.A., Mikhailova T.N. GRAFOR: complex of graphics programs in FORTRAN. Triangulation and perspective projection of surfaces. — Moscow: Preprint No. 127 of Institute of Applied Mathematics of the USSR Acad. Sci., 1978. **

[19] Bakhvalov N.S. On the convergence of a relaxation method with natural constraints on the elliptic operator. — USSR Comput. Math. and Math. Phys., 1966, V. 6, No. 5, p. 101–135. *

[20] Bakhvalov N.S. Numerical methods. Second ed. — Moscow: Nauka, 1975. **

[21] Banerjee U., Suri M. The effect of numerical quadrature in the p-version of the finite element method. — Math. Comput., 1992, V. 59, No. 199, p. 1–20.

[22] Bank R.E., Douglas C.C. Sharp estimates for multigrid rates of convergence with general smoothing and acceleration. — SIAM J. Numer. Anal., 1985, V. 22, p. 617–633.

[23] Bank R.E., Dupont T.F. An optimal order process for solving elliptic finite element equations. — Math. Comput., 1981, V. 36, p. 35–51.

[24] Bercovier M., Pirnneau O. Error estimates for finite element solution of the Stokes problem in the primitive variables. — Numer. Math., 1979, V. 33, No. 2, p. 211–224.

[25] Berger A.E., Scott R., Strang G. Approximate boundary conditions in the finite element method. — Symposia Mathematica, 1972, V. X, p. 295–313.

[26] Boland J.M., Nicolaides R.A. Stability of finite elements under divergence constrains. — SIAM J. Numer. Anal., 1983, V. 20, No. 4, p. 722–731.

[27] Boland J.M., Nicolaides R.A. On the stability of bilinear-costant velocity-pressure finite element. — Numer. Math, 1984, V. 44, No. 2, p. 219–222.

[28] Boland J.M., Nicolaides R.A. Stable and semistable low order finite elements for viscous flows. — SIAM J. Numer. Anal., 1985, V. 22, No. 3, p. 474–492.

[29] Bowyer A. Computing Dirichlet tesselations. — Computer J., 1981, V. 24, No. 2, p. 162–166.

[30] Braess D., Hackbusch W. A new convergence proof for the Multigrid methods including the V-cycle. — SIAM J. Numer. Anal., 1983, V. 20, No. 5, p. 967–975.

[31] Bramble J.H., Pasciak J.E. New convergence estimates for multigrid algorithms. — Math. Comput., 1987, V. 49, No. 180, p. 311–329.

[32] Brandt A. Multilevel adaptive solutions to boundary-value problems. — Math. Comput., 1977, V. 31, No. 138, p. 333–390.

[33] Brandt A. Multigrid solvers on parallel computers. — In: Elliptic problem solvers. — N. Y.: Academic press, 1981, p. 39–84.

[34] Brandt A. Guide to multigrid development. — In: Lecture Notes Math., 1982, V. 960, p. 220–313.

[35] Brandt A., Dinar N. Multigrid Solutions to Elliptic Flow Problems. — In: Numerical Methods for Partial Different Equations. — N. Y.: Academic press, 1979, P. 53–148.

[36] Brezzi F. On the existence, uniqueness and approximation of saddle-point problems arising from Lagrangian multipliers. — RAIRO, 1974, R. 2, p. 129–151.

[37] Brostow W., Dissault J.P. Construction of Voronoi Polyhedra. — J. Comput. Physics., 1978, V. 29, No. 1, p. 81–92.

[38] Bungartz H., Griebel M., Rüde U. Extrapolation, combination and sparse grid techniques for elliptic boundary value problem. — Preprint No. 342/10/92A of Technische Universität, München, 1992.

[39] Cavendish J.C., Field D.A., Frey W.H. An approach to automatic to three-dimensional finite-element mesh generation. — Inter. J. Numer. Meth. Engng., 1985, V. 21. p. 329–347.

[40] Ciarlet P. The Finite Element Method for Elliptic Problems. — Amsterdam: North-Holland, 1978.

[41] Ciarlet P.G., Glowinski R. Dual iterative techniques for solving a finite element approximation of the biharmonic equation. — Comput. Methods Appl. Mech. Engng., 1975, p. 277–295.

[42] Ciarlet P.G., Raviart P.A. Interpolation theory over curved elements, with applications to finite element methods. — Comput. Methods Appl. Mech. Engr., 1972, V. 1, p. 217–249.

[43] Collatz L., Krabs W. Approximations Theorie. Tschebyscheffsche Approximation mit Anwendungen. — Stuttgart: Teubner, 1973.

[44] Creutziger J. The solution of systems of Fredholm integral equations of the second kind by a multigrid method. — In: [159], p. 18–35.

[45] Crouseix M., Raviart P.A. Conforming and nonconforming finite element methods for solving the stationary Stokes equations. — RAIRO, 1973, Ser. Rouge, V. 7, p. 33–76.

[46] D'jakonov E.G. Some classes of operators equivalent with respect to spectrum and their applications. — In: Variational Difference Methods in Math. Physics. — Novosibirsk: Comp. Cen. Sib. Div. USSR Acad. Sci., 1976, p. 49–61. **

[47] D'jakonov E.G. Evaluation of computational work for boundary-value problems with Stokes operator. — Proceedings of Institutes of Higher Education. Math., 1983, No. 7, p. 46–58. **

[48] D'jakonov E.G. Minimization of Computational Work. — Moscow: Nauka, 1989. **

[49] Dryja M., Widlund O. Multilevel additive methods for elliptic finite element problems. — In: Parallel Algorithms for Partial Differential Equations. Proceedings of the VI GAMM Seminar, Kiel, 1991, W. Hackbusch, ed., Braunschweig: Vieweg.

[50] Dunavant D. High degree efficient symmetrical Gaussian quadrature rules for the triangle. — Inter. J. Numer. Meth. Engng., 1985, V. 21, p. 1129–1148.

[51] Dunavant D. Economical symmetrical quadrature rules for complete polinomials over a square domain. — Inter. J. Numer. Meth. Engng., 1985, V. 21, p. 1777–1784.

[52] Faux I.D., Pratt M.J. Computational Geometry for Design and Manufacture. — New York: John Wiley, 1979.

[53] Fedorenko R.P. A relaxation method for solving elliptic difference equations. — USSR Comput. Math. and Math. Phys., 1961, V. 1, No. 5, p. 1092–1096. *

[54] Fedorenko R.P. The speed of convergence of one iterative process. — USSR Comput. Math. and Math. Phys., 1964, V. 4, No. 3, p. 227–235. *

[55] Fedorenko R.P. Iterative methods of solving the difference elliptic eqations. — USSR Successes of Math. Sciences, 1973, V. 28, issue 2, p. 121–182. **

[56] Fichera G. Existence Theorems in Elasticity. — Berlin: Springer, 1972.

[57] Gajewski H., Gröger K., Zacharias K. Nichtlineare operatorgleichungen und operatordifferentialgleichungen. — Berlin: Akademie-Verlag, 1974.

[58] Girault V., Raviart P.A. Finite element approximation of Navier-Stokes equations. — Lect. Notes in Math. — Berlin: Springer, 1979, V. 749.

[59] Girault V., Raviant P.A. Finite Element Methods for Navier-Stokes Equations. — Springer: Berlin, N. Y., 1987.

[60] Glowinski R., Marocco A. Analyse numerique du champ magnetique d'un alternateur par elements finis et sur-relaxation ponctuelle non lineaire. — Comput. Methods Appl. Engrg., 1974, V. 3, p. 55–85.

[61] Glowinski R., Pironneau O. Sur la resolution numerique du probleme de Dirichlet pour l'operateur biharmonique par une methode "quasi- directe". — C. R. Acad. Sci., Paris, Ser. A., 1976, V. 282, p. 223–226.

[62] Godunov S.K., Prokopov G.P. On calculations of conformal mapping and construction of difference grids. — USSR Comput. Math. and Math. Phys., V. 7, No. 5 (1967), p. 1031–1059. *

[63] Gunzburger M.D., Peterson J.S. On conforming finite element methods for the inhomogeneous stationary Navier-Stokes equations. — Numer. Math., 1983, V. 42, No. 2, p. 173–194.

[64] Hackbusch W. On the computation of approximate eigenvalues and eigenfunctions of elliptic operators by means of a multigrid method. — SIAM J. Numer. Anal., 1979, V. 16, No. 1, p. 201–215.

[65] Hackbusch W. On the fast solution of nonlinear elliptic equations. — Numer. Math., 1979, V. 32, No. 1, p. 83–95.

[66] Hackbusch W. On the fast solving of parabolic boundary control problems. — SIAM J. Control. Optim., 1979, V. 17, No. 1, p. 231–244.

[67] Hackbusch W. Multi-grid convergence for a singular perturbation problem. — Linear Algebra Appl., 1984, V. 58, No. 1, p. 125–145.

[68] Hackbusch W. Multi-Grid Methods and Applications. — Berlin, N. Y.: Springer-Verlag, 1985.

[69] Hart L., McCormick S. Asynchronous multilevel adaptive methods for solving partial differential equations on multiprocessors: Basis ideas. — Parallel Comput., 1989, No. 12, p. 131–144.

[70] Hermeline F. Triangulation automatique d'un polyedre en dimension N. — RAIRO, Analyse numerique, 1982, V. 16, No. 3, p. 211–242.

[71] Huang Hong-ci, E. Wei-nam, Mo Mo. Extrapolation combined with multigrid method for solving finite element equations. — J. Comput. Math., 1986, V. 4, No. 4, p. 362–367.

[72] Il'in V.P. Numerical Methods of Solving the Electrophysics Problems. — Moscow: Nauka, 1985. **

[73] Jonson C., Pitkäranta Ju. Analysis of some mixed finite element methods related to reduced integration. — Math. Comput., 1982, V. 38, No. 158, p. 375–400.

[74] Jung M. Convergence rates of multigrid methods for solving plane, linear elasticity problems. — In: [159], p. 88–102.

[75] Jung M. Finite element multi-grid package FEMGP (November 1985 version). — In: [159], p. 103–107.

[76] Jung M., Langer U. Projection-type multigrid methods for solving second-order elliptic boundary value problems in plane domains with curved boundaries. — In: [159], p. 63–87.

[77] Kantorovich L.V., Akilov G.P. Functional Analysis. Third ed. — Moscow: Nauka, 1984. **

[78] Kobel'kov G.M. On equivalent normalizations of subspace L_2. — Analysis Mathematics, 1977, No. 3, p. 177–186. **

[79] Kobel'kov G.M. On reduction of boundary-value problem for biharmonic equation to problem with Stokes operator. — Proceedings of Institutes of Higher Education. Math., 1985, No. 10, p. 39–46. **

[80] Kondrat'ev V.A. Boundary-value problems for elliptic equations in domains with conic and angular points. — Transactions of Moscow Math. Society, 1967, V. 16, p. 209–292. **

[81] Konovalov A.N. On construction method of iterative processes. — Proceedings of Siberian Division of the USSR Acad Sci. Ser. tech. sciences, 1967, No. 13, issue 3, p. 105–108. **

[82] Konovalov A.N. Numerical Solving the Problems of Elasticity Theory. — Novosibirsk State University, 1968. **

[83] Korn G.A., Korn T.M. Mathematical Handbook for Scientists and Engineers. — N. Y., London: McGraw-Hill, 1961.

[84] Korneev V.G. High-order accuracy schemes of finite element method. — Leningrad State University, 1977. **

[85] Korneev V.G. High-order accuracy schemes of finite element method for elliptic equations in three-dimensional domains. Part 1. — USSR Comput. Math. and Math. Phys., 1979, V. 19, No. 4, p. 937–949. *; Part 2. — USSR Comput. Math. and Math. Phys., 1979, V. 19, No. 5, p. 1141–1148. *

[86] Koshelev A.I. On convergence of successive approximation method for quasilinear elliptic equations. — Reports of the USSR Acad. Sci., 1962, V. 142, No. 5, p. 1007–1009. **

[87] Krasnosel'skii M.A. and others. Approximate Solving the Operator Equations. — Moscow: Nauka, 1969. **

[88] Kucherenko V.V. Numerical solving the elliptic problems by method of projection onto grid sequence. — Reports of the USSR Acad. Sci., 1986, V. 287, No. 4, p. 781-785. **

[89] Kuznetsov Yu.A. Algorithm of grid construction of finite element method for computation of stationary fields in three-dimensional domains. — In: Packages of Programs for Math. Physics Problems. — Novosibirsk: Comp. Cen. Sib. Div. USSR Acad. Sci., 1985, p. 67-81. **

[90] Kuznetsov Yu.A. Multigrid domain decomposition method for elliptic problems. — Proceedings 8 Int. Conf. on Comput. Meth. in Appl. Sciences and Engn. — Paris: INRIA, 1987, V. 2, p. 605–616.

[91] Kuznetsov Yu.A., Matsokin A.M., Shaidurov V.V. Fast iterative methods for solving the grid equation systems. — In: Urgent Problems of Computational Math. and Math. Modelling. Novosibirsk: Nauka, 1985, p. 207-228. **

[92] Ladyzenskaja O.A. Mathematical Questions of Dynamics of Viscous Incompressible Fluid. — Moscow: Nauka, 1970. **

[93] Ladyzenskaja O.A., Solonnikov V.A., Ural'tseva N.N. Linear and Quasilinear Equations of Parabolic Type. — Moscow: Nauka, 1967. **

[94] Ladyzenskaja O.A., Uraltseva N.N. Linear and Quasilinear Equations of Elliptic Type. — Moscow: Nauka, 1973. **

[95] Laevskii Yu.M., Shishkin S.A. On use of unconcordant grids in finite element method. — In: Finite Element Method in Some Problems of Numerical Analysis. — Novosibirsk: Comp. Cen. Sib. Div. USSR Acad. Sci., 1984, p. 55–72. **

[96] Langer U. On choice of iterative parameters in relaxation method on grid sequence. — USSR Comput. Math. and Math. Phys., 1982, V. 22, No. 6, p. 1118–1132. *

[97] Langmach H., Telschow G. On numerical simulation of semiconductor devices using multigrid methods. — In: [159], p. 1–17.

[98] Lebedev V.I., Agoshkov V.I. Poincare-Steklov operators and their applications in analysis. — Moscow: Computational Math. Department USSR Acad. Sci., 1983. **

[99] Lebedev V.I., Finogenov S.A. Solution of problem for ordering the parameters in Chebyshev iterative methods. — USSR Comput. Math. and Math. Phys., 1973, V. 13, No. 1, p. 18–33. *

[100] Lin Q. High accuracy from the linear elements. — Proceedings of the 1984 Beijing Symposium of Differential Geometry and Differential Equations. — Beijing, 1984.

[101] Lin Q., Lu T. Asymptotic expansions for finite element eigenvalues and finite element solution. — Proceedings 6 Int. Conf. on Comp. Meth. Appl. Sci. Eng. — Versailles, 1983.

[102] Lin Q., Lu T. Asymptotic expansions for finite element approximation of elliptic problem of polygonal domains. — Bonn. Math. Schrift, 1984.

[103] Lin Q., Wang J. Some expansions of the finite element approximation. — Research Report IMS-20. — Chengdu Branch of Academia Sinica, 1984.

[104] Lin Q., Zhu Q. Asymptotic expansion for the derivative of finite elements. — J. Comp. Math., 1984, V. 2, No. 4, p. 101–115.

[105] Lions J.-L. Quelques methodes de resolution des problemes aux limites non lineaires. — Paris: Dunod, 1969.

[106] Lions J.-L., Magenes E. Problemes aux limites non homogenes et applications. — Paris: Dunod, 1968.

[107] Lohner R., Morgan K. An unstructured multigrid method for elliptic problems. — Inter. J. Numer. Math. Engng., 1987, V. 24, p. 101–115.

[108] Maitre J.F., Musy F. Algebraic formalization of the multigrid method in the symmetric and positive-definite case. — a convergence estimation for the V-cycle. — In: Multigrid Methods of Integral and Differential Equations (D. J. Paddon and H. Holstein eds), Clarendon Press, Oxford, 1985.

[109] Maitre J.F., Musy F. Multigrid methods for symmetric variational problems: A general theory and convergence estimates for usual smooths. — Appl. Math. and Comput., 1987, V. 21, No. 1, p. 21–43.

[110] Mandel J. Multigrid convergence for nonsymmetric, indefinite variational problems and one smoothing step. — Applied Math. and Comput., 1986, No. 19, p. 201–216.

[111] Mandel J., McCormick S. and Ruge J. An algebraic theory for multigrid methods for variational problems. — SIAM J. Numer. Anal., 1988, V. 25, p. 91–110.

[112] Mansfield L. Finite element subspaces with optimal rates of convergence for the stationary Stokes problem. — RAIRO, Anal.Numer., 1982, V. 16, p. 49–66.

[113] Mansfield L. On finite element subspeces over quadrilateral and Hexahedral meshes for incompressible viscous flow problem. — Numer.Math, 1984, V. 45, No. 2, p. 165–172.

[114] Marchuk G.I. Methods of Computational Mathematics. — Moscow: Nauka, 1980. **

[115] Marchuk G.I., Agoshkov V.I. Introduction in Projective Grid Methods. — Moscow: Nauka, 1981. **

[116] Marchuk G.I., Lebedev V.I. Numerical Methods in Neutron Transport Theory. — Moscow: Atomizdat, 1981. **

[117] Marchouk G.I., Shaidurov V.V. Increasing accuracy of projective difference schemes. — Lecture Notes in Computer Science., 1974, V. 11, p. 120–141.

[118] Marchuk G.I., Shaidurov V.V. Increasing the accuracy of approximate problems. — Novosibirsk: Preprint of Comp. Cen. Sib. Div. USSR Acad. Sci., 1974, p. 3–12. **

[119] Marchuk G.I., Shaidurov V.V. On numerical solving the evolutional problem with bounded operator. — Reports of the USSR Acad. Sci., 1974, V. 216, No. 1, p. 749–751. **

[120] Marchouk G.I., Shaidurov V.V. Variational method for increasing the accuracy of the difference scheme. — Lecture Notes in Economics and Math. Systems., 1976, V. 134, p. 193–205.

[121] Marchuk G.I., Shaidurov V.V. Increasing the Accuracy of Difference Scheme Solutions. — Moscow: Nauka, 1979. **

[122] Marchouk G.I., Shaidurov V.V. Raffinement des solutions des schemas aux differences. — Moscow, Mir, 1983.

[123] Marchuk G.I., Shaidurov V.V. Difference Methods and Their Extrapolations. — N. Y.: Springer, 1983.

[124] Matsokin A.M. Automatization of triangulation of domain with smooth boundary when solving the equations of elliptic type. — Novosibirsk: Preprint No. 15 of Comp. Cen. Sib. Div. USSR Acad. Sci., 1975. **

[125] Matsokin A.M. On construction and methods of solving the system of variational difference equations. — Novosibirsk: Comp. Cen. Sib. Div. USSR Acad. Sci., Thesis of candidate in physical and math. sciences, 1975. **

[126] Matsokin A.M. Variational difference method of solving the elliptic equations in circle. — Novosibirsk: Preprint No. 13 of Comp. Cen. Sib. Div. USSR Acad. Sci., 1975. **

[127] McCormick S.F. Multigrid methods for variational problems: General theory for the V-cycle. — SIAM J. Numer. Anal., 1985, V. 22, p. 634–643.

[128] McCormick S.F. Multilevel Adaptive Methods for Partial Differential Equations. — SIAM: Philadelphia, 1989.

[129] McCormick S., Quinlan D. Asynchronous multilevel adaptive methods for solving partial differential equations on multiprocessors: Performance results. — Parallel Comput., 1989, No. 12, p. 145–156.

[130] McCormick S., Rüde U. On local refinement higher order methods for elliptic partial differential equations. — Int. J. High Speed Comput., 1990, No. 4, p. 311-334.

[131] McCormick S.F., Rüge J.W. Unigrid for multigrid simulation. — Math. Comput., 1983, V. 41, No. 163, p. 43–62.

[132] Mikhlin S.G. Variational Methods in Mathematical Physics. — Moscow: Nauka, 1970. **

[133] Mikhlin S.G. Linear Equations in Partial Derivatives. — Moscow: Vysshaya Shkola, 1977. **

[134] Mitchell A.R., Wait R. The Finite Element Method in Partial Differential Equations. — New York: John Wiley, 1977.

[135] Molchanov I.N. Numerical Methods of Solving Some Problems of Elasticity Theory. — Kiev: Naukova Dumka, 1979. **

[136] Mysovskikh I.P. Interpolation Quadrature Formulae. — Moscow: Nauka, 1981. **

[137] Nicolaides R.A. On the 1-convergence of an algorithm for solving finite element equations. — Math. Comput., 1977, V. 31, No. 140, p. 892–906.

[138] Nicolaides R.A. On some theoretical and practical aspects of Multigrid methods. — Math. Comput., 1979, V. 33, No. 147, p. 933–952.

[139] Nitsche J.A. Ein Kriterium fir die quasi-optimalitat des Ritzchen Verfahrens. — Nemer. Math., 1968, No. 11, p. 346–348.

[140] Nitsche J.A. Convergence of nonconforming methods. — Mathematical Aspects of finite Elements in Partial Differential Equations. — N. Y.: Academic Press, 1974, p. 15–53.

[141] Norrie D.H., de Vries G. A finite element biblography. — N. Y.: Plenum Press, 1976.

[142] Norrie D.H., de Vries G. An Introduction to Finite Element Analysis. — London: Academic Press, 1978.

[143] Oden J.T. Finite Elements of Nonlinear Continua. — New York: McGraw-Hill, 1972.

[144] Oganesjan L.A., Rivkind V.Ya., Rukhovets L.A. Variational difference methods of solving the elliptic equations. Part 2. — Transactions of seminar "Differential equations and their application". — Vilnius: Institute of Physics and Mathematics of Acad. Sci. of Lithuanian SSR, 1974. **

[145] Oganesjan L.A., Rukhovets L.A. Investigation of convergence rate of variational difference schemes for elliptic equations of second order in two-dimensional domain with smooth boundary. — USSR Comput. Math. and Math. Phys., 1969, V. 9, No. 9, p. 1102–1120. *

[146] Oganesjan L.A., Rukhovets L.A. Variational Difference Methods of Solving the Elliptic Equations. — Erevan: Acad. Sci of the Armenian SSR, 1979. **

[147] Ortega J.M., Rheinboldt W.C. Iterative Solution of Nonlinear Equations in Several Variables. — London: Academic Press, 1970.

[148] Peisker P. A miltilevel Algorithm for Bihanomic Problem. — Numer. Math., 1985, V. 46, No. 4, p. 623–634.

[149] Pissanetzky S. KUBIK: An automatic three dimesinal finite element mesh generator. — Inter. J. Numer. Meth. Engng., 1981, V. 17, p 255–269.

[150] Pitkäranta J. Local stability conditions for the Babuska method of Lagrange miltipliers. — Math. Comput., 1980, V. 35, No. 152, p. 1113–1130.

[151] Pitkäranta J. The finite element method with Lagrange multipliers for domains with corner. — Math. Comput., 1981, V. 37, No. 155, p. 13–30.

[152] Pitkäranta Ju., Saarinen T. A multigrid version of a simple finite element methods for the Stokes problem. — Math. Comput., 1985, V. 45, No. 171, p. 1–14.

[153] Pohl W. On the solution of three-dimensional nonlinear Poisson's equation for semiconductor devices. — In: [159], p. 36–44.

[154] Rüde U. Extrapolation and related techniques for solving elliptic equations. — Preprint No. 19135 of Technische Universität, München, 1991.

[155] Rukhovets L.A. On using the extrapolation for construction of VDS (variational difference scheme) on regular grid. — In: Variational-Difference Methods in Mathematical Physics. — Novosibirsk: Comp. Cen. Sib. Div. USSR Acad. Sci., 1976, p. 113–123. **

[156] Samarskii A.A., Nikolaev E.S. Methods of Solving the Grid Equations. — Moscow: Nauka, 1978. **

[157] Sapagovas M.P. Solving the quasilinear elliptic equations by finite difference method. — Lituvian Math. Transactions, 1965, V. 5, No. 2, p. 291–302. **

[158] Schieweck N. A multigrid convergence proof by a strengthened Cauchy inequalityfor symmetric eliptic boundary value problems. — In: [159], p. 49–62.

[159] Second multigrid seminar., ed. by G.Telschow. — Berlin: Institut fur mathematik, 1986.

[160] Segerlind L.J. Applied Finite Element Analysis. — New York: McGraw-Hill, 1976.

[161] Shaidurov V.V. On some method of increasing the accuracy of difference solutions. — Novosibirsk: Numerical Methods of Continuous Medium Mechanics, 1972, V. 3, No. 2, p. 96-104. **

[162] Shaidurov V.V. The continuation with respect to parameter in the regularization method. — In: Computational Methods of Linear Algebra. Novosibirsk: Comp. Cen. Sib. Div. USSR Acad. Sci., 1973, p. 77–85. **

[163] Shaidurov V.V. The Richardson extrapolation for the projective-difference Sturm-Liouville problem. — In: Variational Difference Methods in Mathematical Physics. — Novosibirsk: Comp. Cen. Sib. Div. USSR Acad. Sci., 1974, p. 116–125. **

[164] Shaidurov V.V. A regularization of systems with a symmetric matrix. — In: Computational Mathematics and Programing. Novosibirsk: Comp. Cen. Sib. Div. USSR Acad, Sci., 1974, p. 91–98. **

[165] Shaidurov V.V. Methods of increasing the accuracy of approximate problems. — Novosibirsk State University, 1977. **

[166] Shaidurov V.V. The solution extrapolation of problems containing an exponential boundary layer. — Novosibirsk: Preprint No. 53 of Comp. Cen. Sib. Div. USSR Acad. Sci., 1978. **

[167] Shaidurov V.V. Numerical solving the Dirichlet problem in a domain with angles. — In: Computational Methods in Applied Mathematics. Novosibirsk: Nauka, 1982, p. 173–188. **

[168] Shaidurov V.V. On solving the variational difference scheme on a grid sequence. — Novosibirsk: Preprint No. 92 of Comp. Cen. Sib. Div. USSR Acad. Sci., 1982. **

[169] Shaidurov V.V. On solving the spectral variational difference problem on a grid sequence. — Novosibirsk: Preprint No. 103 of Comp. Cen. Sib. Div. USSR Acad. Sci., 1983. **

[170] Shaidurov V.V. Projective grid schemes on a grid sequence. — In: Computational Methods of Linear Algebra. Moscow: Computational Mathematics Department of the USSR Acad. Sci., 1983, p. 238–246. **

[171] Shaidurov V.V. On solving the spectral variational difference problem on a grid sequence. — In: Variational Difference Methods in Mathematical Physics. Moscow: Computational Mathematics Department of the USSR Acad. Sci., 1984, p. 149–160. **

[172] Shaidurov V.V. An application of projective grid methods on a sequence of grids in problems of mathematical physics. — In: Application of Electronic Computers in Simulation of Math. Physics Problems. Krasnoyarsk: Comp. Cen. Sib. Div. USSR Acad, Sci., 1985, p. 145–157. **

[173] Shaidurov V.V. Computational methods on a grid sequence. — Krasnoyarsk: Comp. Cen. Sib. Div. USSR Acad. Sci., Thesis of doctor in physical and math. sciences, 1985.

[174] Shaidurov V.V. The theoretical aspects of multigrid methods / Vistas in Applied Mathematics. Numerical Analysis, atmospheric sciences, immunology. — N. Y.: Optimization software, 1986, p. 152-166.

[175] Shaidurov V.V. Multigrid iterative methods of solving the biharmonic equation. — In: Computational Processes and Systems. Moscow: Nauka, 1987, V. 5, p. 258–271.

[176] Shaidurov V.V. Multigrid methods of finite elements. — Nauka, Moscow, 1989. **

[177] Shaidurov N.N., Tobiska L. A survey of finite element spaces for an incompressible viscous flow satisfying the stability condition. I. — Siberian J. on Comp. Math., 1993, V. 1, No. 4.

[178] Sibson R. Locally equiangular triangulations. — Computer J., V. 21, No. 3, p. 243–245.

[179] Smirnov A.V., Shaidurov V.V. The projective-grid solving the Lame equations on a grid sequence. — Novosibirsk: Numerical Methods of Mechanics of Continua, 1986, V. 17, No. 1, p. 119–129. **

[180] Stenberg R. Analysis of Mixed Finite Element Methods for the Stokes Problem: A Unified Approach. — Math. Comput., 1984, V. 42, No. 165, p. 9–23.

[181] Stenberg R. On the construction of optimal mixed finite element methods for the linear elasticity problem. — Numer. Math., 1986, V 48, No. 4, p. 447–462.

[182] Strang G., Fix G.J. An Analysis of the Finite Element Method. — New Jersey: Englewood Cliffs Prentice-Hall, 1973.

[183] Stroud A.H. Approximate calculation of miltiple integrals. — Englewood Cliffs, New Jersey: Prentice-Hall, 1971.

[184] Thacker W.C. A brief review of techniques for generating irreqular computational grids. — Inter. J. Numer. Meth. Engng., 1990, V. 15, p. 1335–1341.

[185] Temam R. Navier-Stokes Equations. — Amsterdam: North-Holland, 1979.

[186] Tikhonov A.N., Arsenin V.Ya. Methods of Solving the Incorrect Problems. — Moscow: Nauka, 1979. **

[187] Tobiska L., Shaidurov V.V. A survey of finite element spaces for incompressible viscous flow satisfying the stability condition. I. — Novosibirsk, Modelling in Mechanics, 1992, V. 5, No. 3.

[188] Urvantsev A.L., Shaidurov V.V. Method of correction for one-dimensional quasilinear diffusion equation. — In: Computational Mathematics and Programing. Novosibirsk: Comp. Cen. Sib. Div. USSR Acad. Sci., 1974, p. 81–90. **

[189] Urvantsev A.L., Shaidurov V.V. Correction of approximate solution of quasilinear Poisson equation. — In: Variational Difference Methods in Mathematical Physics. Novosibirsk: Comp. Cen. Sib. Div. USSR Acad. Sci., 1976, p. 137–144. **

[190] Valedinskii V.D. A method of solving the difference Stokes problem. — Transactions of Xth All-Union school "Problems of viscous fluid dynamics", Novosibirsk, 1985, p. 56–59. **

[191] Valedinskii V.D., Kobel'kov G.M. On difference analogue of inequality $\|p\|_{L_2} \leq C \|\mathrm{grad}\, p\|_{W_2^{-1}}$. — Moscow: Preprint No. 67 of Computational Mathematics Department of the USSR Acad. Sci., 1983. **

[192] Varga R.S. Functional Analysis and Approximation Theory in Numerical Analysis. — Phila., Penn.: SIAM, 1971.

[193] Voevodin V.V. Computational Fundamentals of Linear Algebra. — Moscow: Nauka, 1977. **

[194] Volkov E.A. Differential properties of solutions of boundary-value problems for Laplace and Poisson equations on rectangle. — Transactions of Math. Inst. of the USSR Acad. Sci., 1965, V. 77, p. 89–112. **

[195] Volkov E.A. Approximate solution of Laplace and Poisson equations in weighted Holder spaces. — Transactions of Math. Inst of the USSR Acad Sci., 1972, V. 128, p. 76–112. **

[196] Volkov E.A. Numerical Methods. — Moscow: Nauka, 1982. **

[197] Warg Jin-xian, Huang Yu-xia, Gong-Jia-yao. Multigrid method for elasticity problems. — J. Comput. Math., 1986, V. 4, No. 2, p. 154–163.

[198] Watson D.F. Computing the n-dimensional Delauney tesselation with application to Voronoi Polytopes. — Computer J., 1981, V. 24, No. 2, p. 167–172.

[199] Zenisek A. A general theorem on triangular finite $C^{(m)}$-elements. — RAIRO, 1974, Analyse numerique, R2, p. 119–127.

[200] Zienkiewicz O.C. The Finite Element Method in Engineering Science. Second ed. — New York: McGraw-Hill, 1971.

Subject Index

Main references in *italics*

Other *Mathematics and Its Applications* titles of interest:

W.L. Miranker: *Numerical Methods for Stiff Equations and Singular Perturbation Problems*. 1980, 220 pp. ISBN 90-277-1107-0

K. Rektorys: *The Method of Discretization in Time and Partial Differential Equations*. 1982, 470 pp. ISBN 90-277-1342-1

L. Ixary: *Numerical Methods and Differential Equations and Applications.* 1984, 360 pp. ISBN 90-277-1597-1

B.S. Razumikhin: *Physical Models and Equilibrium Methods in Programming and Economics*. 1984, 368 pp. ISBN 90-277-1644-7

A. Marciniak: *Numerical Solutions of the N-Body Problem.* 1985, 256 pp. ISBN 90-277-2058-4

Y. Cherruault: *Mathematical Modelling in Biomedicine*. 1986, 276 pp. ISBN 90-277-2149-1

C. Cuvelier, A. Segal and A.A. van Steenhoven: *Finite Element Methods and Navier-Stokes Equations.* 1986, 500 pp. ISBN 90-277-2148-3

A. Cuyt (ed.): *Nonlinear Numerical Methods and Rational Approximation.* 1988, 480 pp. ISBN 90-277-2669-8

L. Keviczky, M. Hilger and J. Kolostori: *Mathematics and Control Engineering of Grinding Technology. Ball Mill Grinding*. 1989, 188 pp. ISBN 0-7923-0051-3

N. Bakhvalov and G. Panasenko: *Homogenisation: Averaging Processes in Periodic Media. Mathematical Problems in the Mechanics of Composite Materials.* 1989, 404 pp. ISBN 0-7923-0049-1

R. Spigler (ed.): *Applied and Industrial Mathematics*. Venice-1, 1989. 1991, 388 pp. ISBN 0-7923-0521-3

C.A. Marinov and P. Neittaanmaki: *Mathematical Models in Electrical Circuits. Theory and Applications*. 1991, 160 pp. ISBN 0-7923-1155-8

Z. Zlatev: *Iterative Improvement of Direct Solutions of Large and Sparse Problems*. 1991, 328 pp. ISBN 0-7923-1154-X

M. Vajtersic: *Algorithms for Elliptic Problems.* 1992, 352 pp. ISBN 0-7923-1918-4

V. Kolmanovskii and A. Myshkis: *Applied Theory of Functional Differential Equations*. 1992, 223 pp. ISBN 0-7923-2013-1

A.D. Egorov, P.I. Sobolevsky and L.A. Yanovich: *Functional Integrals: Approximate Evaluation and Applications.* 1993, 426 pp. ISBN 0-7923-2193-6

G.I. Marchuk: *Adjoint Equations and Analysis of Complex Systems*. 1994 ISBN 0-7923-3013-7

Other *Mathematics and Its Applications* titles of interest:

A. Bakushinsky and A. Goncharsky: *Ill-Posed Problems: Theory and Applications.* 1994, 256 pp. ISBN 0-7923-3073-0

G.N. Milstein: *Numerical Integration of Stochastic Differential Equations*. 1995, 170 pp. ISBN 0-7923-3213-X

V.V. Shaidurov: *Multigrid Methods for Finite Elements*. 1995, 331 pp. ISBN 0-7923-3290-3

Biomass and Remote Sensing of Biomass

Editor

Isak Olsen

scitus academics

Biomass and Remote Sensing of Biomass
Edited by **Isak Olsen**

ISBN: 978-1-68117-294-1
Library of Congress Control Number: 2016937479

SCITUS Academics LLC,
www.scitusacademics.com
Box No. 4766, 616 Corporate Way,
Suite 2, Valley Cottage,
NY 10989

Printed in United States of America on Acid Free Paper

Preface

Biomass is fuel that is developed from organic materials, a renewable and sustainable source of energy used to create electricity or other forms of power. Biomass is a renewable energy source not only because the energy in it comes from the sun, but also because biomass can re-grow over a relatively short period of time compared with the hundreds of millions of years that it took for fossil fuels to form. Through the process of photosynthesis, chlorophyll in plants captures the sun's energy by converting carbon dioxide from the air and water from the ground into carbohydrates—complex compounds composed of carbon, hydrogen, and oxygen. When these carbohydrates are burned, they turn back into carbon dioxide and water and release the energy they captured from the sun. Biomass can be converted to other usable forms of energy like methane gas or transportation fuels like ethanol and biodiesel. Rotting garbage, and agricultural and human waste, all release methane gas, also called landfill gas or biogas. Crops such as corn and sugarcane can be fermented to produce the transportation fuel ethanol. Biodiesel, another transportation fuel, can be produced from leftover food products like vegetable oils and animal fats. Also, biomass-to-liquids and cellulosic ethanol are still under research. Generally, the term biomass is used for all materials originating from photosynthesis. However, biomass can equally apply to animals. Conservation and management of biomass is very important. There are numerous methods and techniques for biomass evaluation. One of these methods is remote sensing. The book entitled Biomass and Remote Sensing of provides information about biomass, but also about biodiversity and environmental factors estimation over a wide area.

Table of Contents

CHAPTER 1

Biomass in Evolving World-Individual's Point of View

Biljana Stojković[1]

[1] University of Belgrade, Serbia

1. INTRODUCTION

For a long time, ecology has been criticized for being primarily descriptive science concentrated on the 'What' question rather than progressing further into the 'Why' and 'How' domains (O'Connor, 2000). Over the past few decades, however, ecology has moved toward dynamic mechanistic and more strongly predictive science (Kearney et al., 2010). It is becoming increasingly clear that to comprehend mechanisms underlying population dynamics, demography and ecological breadth it is necessary to regard the fact that discrete organisms, which constitute populations, might have different individual responses to ontogenetic and environmental cues (Begon et al., 1990). The challenge is, as noted by Kearney et al. (2010), "to derive an approach for studying penetrance of functional traits of individual organisms into higher, group-level phenomena".

Generally, the interdependency of population-level and individual-level processes is very complex. Although population is composed of individuals, it has emergent properties that are more than just the sum of the properties of individuals. Organisms come to life and die on particular days, but populations have birth and death rates. At any specific moment, individuals are of certain age, but populations have age structure which is very important for determining population growth. Individual characteristics, such as size, growth pattern, age at maturity, number of offspring and longevity, greatly influence population dynamics, but, on the other hand, physiology and patterns of growth and development of each organism depend both on its genotype and on population properties such as the number, sizes and spatial distribution of other individuals. Therefore, the relationship between organisms and their populations is reflexive; phenomena at one biological level are both the cause and the consequence of the phenomena on other.

This chapter is dealing with individual level processes – biomass allocation strategy, allometric growth and phenotypic plasticity. How these developmental processes may affect population dynamics will also be discussed.

2. INDIVIDUAL-LEVEL PHENOMENA

2.1. Allometry and Allocation Strategy

Allometry (Greek *allos*, "other", and *metron*, "measure"; Huxley, 1932) is the study of size-correlated variations in biological forms and processes. Niklas (1994) recognizes three conceptual and methodological meanings of this term: 1) the growth of one part of an organism in relation to the growth of the whole organism or some other part of it, 2) the study of the consequences of size on organic form or process, and 3) any departure from geometry and shape that is conserved among a series of objects differing in size. Literally, allometry means unequal growth of organs during development of an organism. The fundamental biological principle presumes that acquisition of external resources and metabolism, producing energy and materials for all biological processes, enable organisms to grow in size (i.e., enlarge biomass). However, in biological systems, increase in absolute size always goes along with modifications in relative sizes of organismal parts. In other words, by growing larger, individuals alter their shape; growth itself is size-dependent, i.e. allometric (Weiner, 2004). This process is a consequence of inherent continuous changes in directions of biomass allocation into different structures and activities during the course of development, and reflects alterations in priorities at any point of time of individual ontogenesis. For example, early in development, after germination and emergence of radicle (part of a plant embryo which develops in a root), plants have more roots than shoots. Later, as they grow, relative allocation into aboveground structures increases and results in more 'shooty' individuals. A late fetus has a larger head and shorter legs in relation to its body length than an adult human. Alteration in growth pattern during human ontogeny accounts for later changes in body part proportions. Metabolic rates and the heat produced by metabolism increase less rapidly than total body size.

From the ecological point of view, biomass allocation strategy plays a critical role in determining organismal ability to survive and reproduce (i.e., fitness). If an ideal organism would exist, it would be mature at birth, continuously produce a large number of high-quality offspring, and live forever. Such an organism, called 'Darwinian demon' (Law, 1979), would bedevil all other organisms. The same creature, named 'Hutchinsonian demon' in community ecology, would dominate in its habitat because it would be the best in colonizing new patches, utilizing all the resources, avoiding predators and resisting stresses (Kneitel & Chase, 2004), and, eventually, it would monopolize the life on Earth. In reality, however, the existence of such an organism is impossible because: 1) the amount of resources (i.e., nutrients and energy) that an organism can acquire is finite, and 2) a proportion of the resources allocated to one activity (for example to growth, that is to somatic maintenance and survival), decreases the amount of resources that can be allocated to another (e.g., to reproduction). As noted byStearns (1992), "allocation decisions between two or more processes that compete directly with one another for limited resources within a single individual" imply mutually exclusive allocation, or physiological trade-off.

If an increase in fitness due to a change in one trait is opposed by a decrease in fitness due to a concomitant change in the second trait, it is clear that adaptive growth strategy in one environment depends on optimal balance of biomass allocation between different organismal functions (Roff & Fairbairn, 2007). Individuals must allocate resources in a way that make the most of their chances for contributing offspring to the next generation while simultaneously maximizing their chance of surviving to reproduce (Gurevitch et al., 2002). Among characteristics that figure directly in reproduction and survival, and are often in trade-off between each other, Stearns (1992) indicated several principal life-history traits: size at birth, growth pattern, age at maturity, size at maturity, number, size and sex ratio of offspring, age- and size-specific reproductive investments, age- and size-specific mortality schedules, and length of life. Correlations between these traits may be positive or negative (trade-offs), but eventually they combine in many different ways to produce diverse schedules and durations of key events in an organism's lifetime. Logically, natural selection in one environment may prioritize some capabilities at the expense of others. As a consequence, different life-histories evolve.

2.2.1. The Evolution of Life-Histories

The developmental paths that describe changes in form ("ontogenetic trajectory"; Magwene, 2001) and life-history schedule are often considered to be genetically determined, i.e., species- or genotype-specific (Weiner, 2004), and/or the products of biomechanical and other physical constraints

(Givnish, 1986). These assertions have been brought into question by the well documented fact that allometry itself can be plastic and trade-offs may vary with environmental variations (e.g., Cheplick, 1995;Weiner, 2004), as well as because a significant degree of variability in life-histories can exist within populations. However, they still can serve as a starting point for understanding life-history evolution. Comparative biology has demonstrated a great variety of life-histories at the level of species and higher taxonomic groups. In plants, besides tremendous variation in life-cycle patterns, from annual semelparous forms to long-lived iteroparous woody perennials, interesting variations can be found in growth architecture of clonal plants with vegetative reproduction. Lovett Doust (1981) made characterization of these clonal forms on a continuum between ‘phalanx’, in which vegetative clones (ramets) of one parental plant are grouped tightly together, and ‘guerilla’ form, which is presented with ramets dispersed like guerilla forces. Vegetative reproduction makes an interesting case on the diversity of life-histories. For example, in quaking aspen (*Populus tremuloides*) individual trunks, which are genetically identical to their paternal plant, live for about 50 years, while the genotype composed of many individual plants, may live for more than 10 000 years. In animals, some species mature early and reproduce quickly, have small body size and a large number of eggs (e.g., many insects), whereas in other species maturation is delayed for several years, individuals are large and have a small number of offspring (e.g., some mammals). Between these extremes, a great variety of different combinations of life-history schedules and growth forms exists.

Although it is reasonable to presume that there is individual variability within each species, relations between life-history traits differ substantially more between higher taxonomic groups. Darwin elegantly explained this phenomenon – related species descended from a common ancestor and shared common evolutionary history for a long time. These ‘lineage-specific effects’ emphasize characteristics that are general for a group of related species or higher taxonomic levels. The comparative analyses of species, genera, families and classes demonstrate broad patterns of the evolution of allometry, trade-offs and life-history. The examples of how lineage-specific mode of growth affects metabolic and growth rates, and reproduction, can be found all over the living world. Major groups of ectothermal and endothermal organisms have different metabolisms and different growth rates per unit weight during growth, which is involved in determination of age at maturity and the cost of reproduction. For ectothermal organisms, about thirty times less energy supply is needed for the same growth rate as for endothermal (Peters, 1983). Organisms with determinate growth (e.g., annual plants, birds, mammals, and most insects) stop growing when mature, whereas allocation of energy between growth and reproduction continues through adult life for organisms with indeterminate growth, such as perennial plants, fish, amphibians, reptiles, etc. That means that ‘allocation decision’ between growth and reproduction is made only once for the first group, and many times for the second (Stearns, 1992). The analyses of more than 500 mammal species (Wootton, 1987) imply that body mass is positively correlated with age at first reproduction. Age at maturity is also positively correlated with adult lifespan within lineages of birds, mammals, some reptiles and fishes, although the relationships between the two life-history traits differ among these large groups. If corrected for body size, the data suggests that increase in longevity with delay of reproduction is the highest for birds and mammals (Charnov & Berrigan, 1990).

The results of comparative analyses of higher taxonomic groups imply that changes in life-histories are phylogenetically constrained in some degree, as a result of shared evolutionary history, genes and developmental pathways. However, it must be kept in mind that comparative biology provides information about boundary conditions on life-history evolution, but, within each lineage, populations and species differ and follow their own patterns of life-history adaptation to specific environment. Here, natural selection acts on life-histories to adjust biomass allocation in a way that maximizes total lifetime fitness. The genotypes (organisms) that have the ability to distribute their resources optimally for certain ecological conditions, will reach the highest fitness and their frequencies in next generations will rise. Those patterns of biomass allocation that present responses of populations to natural selection, Stearns (1992) defines as *microevolutionary trade-offs*. The relationship between individual-level (i.e., physiological trade-offs) and population-level (i.e., microevolutionary trade-offs) is inevitably complex. The physical division of limited materials and energy supply within an organism is a boundary condition on the evolutionary optimization of life-history strategy within a population inhabiting certain environment. However, the ability of organisms to optimally distribute their biomass and/or to alter the pattern of allocation in accordance with environmental change depends on evolutionary changes of genetic variation in a population. In other words, microevolutionary trade-offs set a trade-off structure that is a constraint for physiological trade-offs.

Intra-individual trade-offs depend on the amount of available resources and interactions between organisms, or in other words, they are plastic. To understand the nature of complex and dynamic relations between different types of trade-offs, which impose both constraints and a basis for their evolution, environmental influences on allometric patterns must be analyzed.

2.2.1.1. Plastic Allometry

It is a common knowledge that the fitness of an individual depends both on its genotype and its environment. When live in variable abiotic and biotic circumstances, organisms may achieve high fitness by changing their growth and life-histories so as to match the most fit trait values for each set of environmental conditions. This property of a genotype to express different phenotypes in distinct environments is called *phenotypic plasticity*, and the way that trait expression varies across a range of environments for a given genotype is called *its norm of reaction* (Bradshaw, 1965; West-Eberhard, 1989). From the allometric point of view, plasticity can be understood as a change in allometric growth/allocation patterns in response to the environment (Schmid & Weiner, 1993). According to the optimal allocation theory, organisms should allocate more resources to organs that capture the most limiting resource and less to organs that are involved in obtaining non-limiting resources. At the same time, as was previously noted, they must optimize biomass allocation into reproductive function in order to produce the highest possible number of quality offspring while limiting the losses for their own survival. The solution of this incredibly complex task depends on the characteristics of a population and physical environment. Besides variability in genetic background of their life-history strategies, individuals within a population may also differ significantly in their ability to cope with external conditions. Different genotypes may respond differently to the same environment, and this variability in reaction norm for allocation patterns accounts for the total phenotypic variation. As noted by Stearns (1992), microevolutionary trade-offs may evolve, or, in other words, population can respond to selection, if there is genetic variation for this reaction norm (i.e., for physiological trade-offs).

Before we explore some examples of relations between life-histories and their plasticity, several properties of phenotypic plasticity have to be explained. As a measure of change in genotype's trait value between different environments, plasticity need not always be adaptive. Some alterations in individual appearance and function are merely unavoidable consequences of organismal physiology (Sultan, 1995). Disadvantageous (maladaptive) plasticity may results from organismal inability to maintain a constant phenotype when faced with environmental circumstances despite fitness reduction due to variation (Alpert & Simms, 2002). For example, in low-quality environments, or under intense competition for resources, organisms are smaller compared with those in rich-environments; plants have yellow leaves when deprived of sufficient nitrogen, or have lower photosynthetic rate under low light intensity. In ecology, it is common to measure plasticity of a species as a range of ecological conditions that a species can grow in; this measure is also called species' niche (Grinell, 1917). Also, it is common to assign a species as generalist or specialist. However, it must be kept in mind that the niche of each species is determined by the sum of niches (i.e., reaction norms) of its members that may be plastic or nonplastic (Gurevitch, 2002). This is a very important remark for understanding life-history evolution – we can define life-history for each species, but its plastic responses to environmental changes give the opportunity for further evolution of life-histories.

Plasticity of trade-offs between life history traits have been demonstrated in a large number of studies and numerous taxa in laboratory and natural populations (e.g., Reznick, 1985; Sinervo & DeNardo, 1996; Zuk, 1996; Tucić et al. 1997, 1998; Tucić & Stojković 2001; Roff, 2002; Stojković et al. 2009). The number of possible relations between different life-history traits is great, and the ways in which they can change under various environmental conditions is, logically, much greater. Here, I present just a few examples to illustrate both the theoretical and empirical knowledge on life-history/allometry plasticity.

The allometry plasticity can be demonstrated with one of the best understood adaptive plastic systems in plants, generally termed as the 'shade avoidance' syndrome (Smith & Whitelam, 1997). Plants are able to detect low ratio of red to far-red radiation (R:FR) in ambient light as the first signal of future competitive interactions, well before mutual shading actually occurs (Ballaré et al., 1987, 1990). Because chlorophyll preferentially absorbs red light, radiation transmitted through or reflected from a leaf canopy exhibits lower R:FR ratio than does full sunlight (Smith et al., 1990). Therefore, the R:FR ratio can be seen as an environmental, external, cue of population density. It triggers a suite of photomorphogenic plastic responses (e.g., stem elongation, branching reduction, acceleration of flowering) that enables plants to minimize effects of mutual shading by neighbours and maximize the ability to deny light to proximal plants (Aarsen, 1995). The allometric shift in plant growth form is achieved through an increased shoot extension rate coupled with a strong apical dominance (main stem dominance). In crowded conditions this growth pattern enables plants to acquire more radiant energy for photosynthesis and improve their final performance. In uncrowded situations, however, elongation of stems has more costs than benefits. More resources must be allocated into support structures rather than to flowers and seeds. That is why elongated growth form of plants is adaptive only in dense environment. Many experiments on plants strongly corroborated the evolutionary ecological prediction that the shade avoidance phenotype is indeed an adaptation, likely moulded by natural selection from competition for light (Dudley & Schmitt, 1996; Schmitt,1997; Schwinning & Weiner, 1998; Tucić & Stojković, 2001).

In the study on perennial clonal species *Lamium maculatum*, Stojković et al. (2009) have shown that genotype by environment interaction could change the proportion of biomass allocated into reproductive function. The goal of the experiment was to analyze changes in biomass allocation patterns across genetically structured populations where plants are competing for access to light. Clonal replicates of 17 genotypes were grown under three regimes: 1) control (C; low level of competition), 2) intraclonal competition (S; competition between clones of the same genotype) and, 3) interclonal competition (M; competition between plants of different genotypes). It was shown that the growth of these plants was sensitive to genetic identity of competitors, and that the competition between genetically unrelated individuals was the most stressful environment for this plant species (the indices of competition intensity were the highest in this treatment, unpublished data). Analyses of allometric growth (mathematical procedure of this analysis will be explained later) revealed that in resource-rich, noncompetitive environment, where absolute fecundity is the highest, allocation to reproduction (flower weight - FW) is less determined by the size of plants than in competitive condition (insignificant correlation between flower weight and vegetative weight, $P = 0.720$, Table 1).

Table 1. Standardized major axis tests of the allometric relationship (log scaled variables) for reproductive effort (FW) and relative biomass investments to stems (SW), leaves (LW) and roots (RW) based on weight measures of *L. maculatum* plants grown in three experimental treatments (control - C, intraclonal - S and interclonal - M competition). Scaling slope α, R^2 and *P* values for correlations within treatments are reported. Results of pairwise slope comparisons between treatments (based on 1000 iteration in permutation testing) are presented as letters in superscript. If differences among slopes were insignificant, pairwise tests of shift in elevation were performed and results presented as letters in subscript [(e)-elevation]. Identical letters indicate insignificant difference of either slopes or elevation between treatments. Letter A points to the largest value. F statistics and*P* values of the test of differences between observed slope within treatments and α=1 are reported as statistics of isometry testing (Stojković et al., 2009).

Allometric relationship	Treatment	R^2	*P*	α	Test of isometry (Ho: α = 1) F	*P*
logFW: log(SW+LW+RW)	C	0.00	0.720	2.52^{A}	105.36	0.000
	S	0.10	0.003	1.99^{A}	52.39	0.000
	M	0.24	0.000	1.59^{B}	22.77	0.000
logSW: log(FW+LW+RW)	C	0.80	0.000	1.18^{A}	14.02	0.000
	S	0.89	0.000	1.07^{A}	3.37	0.070
	M	0.89	0.000	0.99^{B}	0.04	0.841
logLW: log(FW+SW+RW)	C	0.64	0.000	$0.82_{A(e)}$	10.92	0.001
	S	0.79	0.000	$0.80_{B(e)}$	22.37	0.000
	M	0.83	0.000	$0.78_{C(e)}$	33.75	0.000
logRW: log(FW+SW+LW)	C	0.68	0.000	$1.41_{B(e)}$	37.39	0.000
	S	0.75	0.000	$1.54_{A(e)}$	73.31	0.000
	M	0.86	0.000	$1.53_{A(e)}$	119.84	0.000

On the other hand, allocation patterns into reproductive function differed considerably between S and M treatments (Table 1). First, it was shown that relationship between weights of vegetative and reproduction modules was anisometric (slope of allometric relation significantly larger than 1), indicating that relative biomass allocation to reproductive effort was greater for larger plants in competition, which achieved higher reproductive outcome. As was shown in the analyses of two treatments with different genetic identity of competitors, small individuals in intense competition (interclonal) tended to allocate larger proportion of acquired resources to reproductive organs compared with small plants in less intense competition (intraclonal). The reverse is true for larger plants suggesting that successful, big individuals in severe asymmetric interaction can balance more productively between vegetative and reproductive fitness components than smaller plants. This conclusion was based on a significantly slighter allometric slope in interclonal competition (α = 1.59, $P < 0.000$ for M; α = 1.99, $P < 0.003$ for S; Table 1, Figure 1).

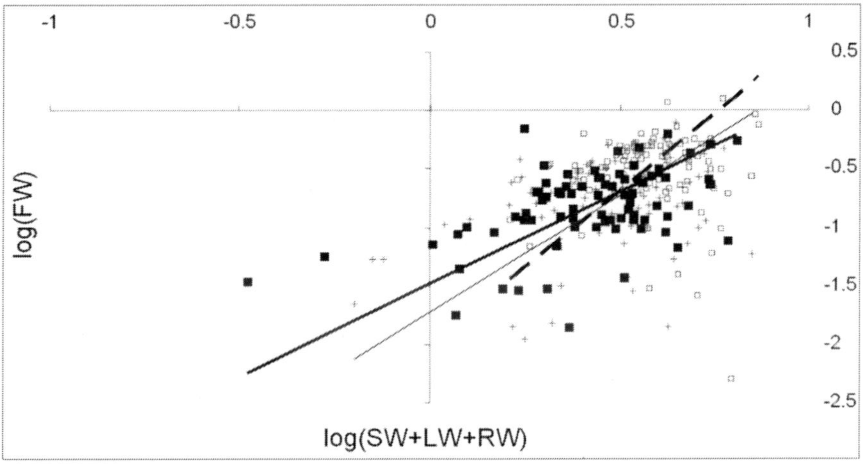

Figure 1. The allometric relationship (log scaled variables) between reproductive effort (flower weight; FW) and allocation to vegetative modules for *L. maculatum* grown in three experimental treatments (control, intraclonal and interclonal competition). The SMA allometric function plotted through the individuals in control treatment (dashed line), intraclonal competition (thin line) and interclonal competition (thick line). Symbols for individuals in control (□), intraclonal (+) and interclonal (■) competition (Stojković et al., 2009).

Allocation analyses between other plant organs (weight of flowers, stems, leaves and roots) also suggested that in *L. maculatum* specific allometry strategy of smaller plants in intense competition with unrelated individuals could reflect trade-offs in favor of reproductive effort, both directly via allocation to flowers and indirectly into stems (i.e., to new plant meristems which could be committed to reproductive function). Such investment to flowers may be beneficial for smaller individuals because allocation of limited acquired biomass to extensive vegetative growth (e.g., leaves) may leave insufficient time for successful reproduction before the end of growing season (Bonser & Aarssen, 2001). Many studies reported that plants grown in competitive environments invested relatively more in sexual reproduction (e.g., Prati & Schmid 2000; Van Kleunen et al., 2002).

Phenotypic plasticity of correlations between life-history traits has been confirmed in many insect species. In order to analyze trade-off between the size and number of eggs, Fox et al. (1997) performed a study on seed beetle *Stator limbatus*. These beetles develop completely inside seeds of over 50 different host plants, and emerge from seeds as adults. In their experiments, Fox and colleagues reared beetles on acacia (*Acacia greggii*) which is a good host, and a palo verde (*Cercidium floridum*) suboptimal host on which survival of larvae is less than 50%. Several presumptions from life-history theory were made: 1) there is a trade-off between size and number of offspring, i.e., the same amount of resources can be allocated into large number of small offspring, or into few big ones, 2) a probability of survival for any individual offspring is an increasing function of its size, and 3) the minimum size for offspring survival is smaller on the good host. If these assumptions are correct, females of *S. limbatus* should lay larger eggs on the poor host than on the good host. The study confirmed this hypothesis – females adjusted the size of eggs to the host on which they laid, and, also, these larger eggs came at cost of fewer egg produced over a lifetime. Additionally, it was shown that the production of larger eggs was adaptive. Survival of larvae hatching from small eggs was less than 1%, whereas 24% of the larvae hatching from large eggs survived to adulthood on suboptimal host. On the other hand, since the majority of larvae that developed on acacia seeds survive, higher lifetime reproductive success of females is achieved by producing more and smaller eggs. Berrigan (1991) performed meta-analysis of the relationship between egg size and number in three orders of insects and found negative correlations (i.e., trade-off) among these life-history traits.

One of the most important determinants of life-history evolution is 'age-specific selection' (Rose, 1991; Charlesworth, 1994) which is well described through several major trade-offs: between time schedules of reproduction and longevity, early and late fecundity, reproduction and growth, etc. Evolutionary changes in allocation strategy between different life-history traits have been continuously detected in laboratory evolution experiments on *Acanthoscelides obtectus* (Tucić et al., 1997, 1998). The methodology of experimental evolution is a valuable research tool for the study of basic mechanisms that shape individual life-history because it provides opportunity for testing direct and correlated responses to selection. In the laboratory of these researchers, seed beetle *A. obtectus* has been selected to reproduce either early (E selection line) or late in life (L selection line). About 200 generations of selection for early reproduction gave rise to beetles with enhanced fitness during early life, a short life span and small body size. On the other hand, adults of both sexes selected for late-reproduction are bigger, live longer, and have increased late fecundity and total fecundity compared with beetles from the E treatment. During the course of age-specific selection on *A. obtectus*, at least two trade-offs were experimentally documented: the trade-off between late fecundity and early fecundity and among early fecundity and longevity (Tucić et al., 1997).

Clearly, the complexity and dynamic relations between life-histories of organisms and their environments suggest that allometric patterns evolve in response to numerous selection pressures and constraints. But, how these processes can influence the 'behaviour' of populations? These problems will be discussed after a short description of mathematical procedures that are currently used in the analyses of allometry.

3. ALLOMETRY ANALYSIS

For the adequate empirical and analytical treatment of allometric phenomena in ecological studies it is important to estimate the relationship between two variables, or, in other words, to determine how one variable scales against another. Variables represent different measures of individuals in a sample, such as weight and length of some organismal parts (organs or modules), multivariate shape or size, number of specific modules (for example, leaves, stems, flowers, roots in plants), life-history traits (e.g. life span, fecundity, growth rate, age at first reproduction), metabolic rate (e.g. activity of enzymes, hormones), etc. The main goal of this approach is to understand the allocation patterns within certain species, populations and/or environments.

The general 'allometric equation' that describes relationship between two variables is

$$y = \gamma \cdot x^{\alpha} \tag{1}$$

where y and x are biological variables, γ is the 'scaling (proportionality) coefficient' and α is 'scaling exponent'. α and γ parameters describe the functional (mathematical) relation between x and y.

It can be converted into linear relationship between x and y if variables are log-transformed, so the above formula can be reexpressed as

$$\log(y) = \log(\gamma) + \alpha \log(x) \tag{2}$$

or

$$Y = \beta + \alpha X \tag{3}$$

where substitutions are made: Y=log(y), X=log(x) and β=log(γ). Now, β is the value of Y where it intercepts the vertical axis, and α is equal to the slope of linear function when plotted on logarithmic scale. The log transformation is useful for several reasons: 1) it allows the relationship between the two variables to be expressed as a linear relationship, 2) it puts the variables on a multiplicative or logarithmic scale, which tend to diminish differences among large numbers and accentuate differences among small numbers, 3) it may transform frequency distribution of the data into normal distribution, and 4) it reduces statistical problems resulting from a number of outlying data points.

There are several statistical procedures for finding the line of best fitting through a bivariate cloud of data – linear regression, major axis, standardized major axis and their modifications. Several authors (e.g. Niklas, 1994; Bonser & Aarssen, 2001, 2003; Warton et al., 2006) proposed standardized major axis (SMA) method (or reduced major axis, RMA) on log-transformed variables as the most appropriate for allometry analyses. Falster et al. (2003) developed statistical software, (S)MATR, for application of SMA method in studies of allometry patterns.

SMA methodology is appropriate where there is error in both the x and y variables of the regression models and when we are not interested in prediction but to estimate the line-of-best-fit relating two variables, which is the basic purpose of allometry estimates (Warton et al., 2006). A significant allometric relationship is indicated where the slope (α) of the relationship between logarithms of the two variables differs from isometry. An isometric relationship between biological variables (α = 1) implies that the relative biomass allocation to one organ or function is proportional to the allocation to other organ or function (Figure 2a). The best way to understand isometry and allometry is to imagine that one of the variables in the allocation analysis is some measure of the size of the whole organisms (for example, total weight or height). Then, isometry suggests that relative biomass allocation to specific organ or function is constant for all individual sizes. For example, the size of adult human heads would be several times greater than it is, if the growth of human fetus would proceed in isometric fashion. If the relative allocation to some organ or biological function is greater for larger individuals, than the scaling exponent, or slope of allometric relationships between the two variables is greater than one ($\alpha > 1$; Figure 2b). On the other hand, lower relative investment into one organ during the growth of an organism is detected as a value of scaling exponent that is less than one ($\alpha < 1$;Figure 2b). In the experiment on *Lamium maculatum* (Stojković et al., 2001), the biomass allocation into reproductive organs (flowers) and roots was generally greater for larger individuals, indicating that high ability of biomass acquisition was correlated with development of roots and, also, that these plants invested disproportionately high amount of energy and materials were into future offspring (Table 1, Figure 1). On the other hand, allocation of biomass into stems was shown to be isometric, i.e., directly proportional to the weight of other plant organs, whereas investment into leaves was greater for small plants (Table 1). These patterns of allocation suggested that when plants compete for the access to light, there was a difference in allometry strategy between different size classes of individuals – small plants invested more resources to organs that capture the most limiting resource (light) than larger plants. Allometry analysis gives the opportunity to answer some more questions about the nature of growth and differences between groups of organisms. For example, although the relative proportions of biomass allocated into one organ or biological function may be similar between groups (have a common allometric slope), two groups can differ in absolute values of biomass measures. Then, two groups can differ in elevation (i.e., intercepts) of their allometric function (Figure 2c), or they can diverge along a common axis (Figure 2d). In the study on *L. maculatum*, for plants with similar sum weights of flowers, roots and stems, the weights of leaves were significantly lower in competition, especially in the treatment with the most intense competition. This result indicated that plants in different competition treatment had different opportunities for acquiring resources. Although, as was noted above, an adaptive strategy of plants in competition for light (especially for small individuals) may be allocation into leaves, the difference in average absolute weights (C > S > M) resulted in observed shift in elevation (Table 1).

Negative value of slope of allometric relationship is particularly important for life-history studies because it indicates the trade-off between different functions of organisms, for example between developmental rate and life span, or between fertility and longevity.

4. INDIVIDUALS VERSUS POPULATIONS

Many ecological processes in populations and communities may be understood in terms of size and/or life-history allometric patterns. In other words, the way the individual growth and life-histories are shaped in certain environment could largely influence the demographic patterns of a population. For example, changes in life-history schedules of members of a population can change population demography parameters, such as rate of population growth and carrying capacity. The trade-off between seed size and seed number has been used as an explanation for difference in competition and colonization abilities of plant species. As suggested, competitive ability is enhanced by production of fewer, larger seeds, whereas colonization ability is improved by production of many small seeds (Turnbull et al., 1999; Levine & Rees, 2002). The members of natural populations often differ in size and relatedness to each other, which may affect the division of limited resources and have consequences on reproductive success, changes in the ratio of birth rate/mortality rate, and influence population growth in different ways (Aikio & Pakkasmaa, 2003).

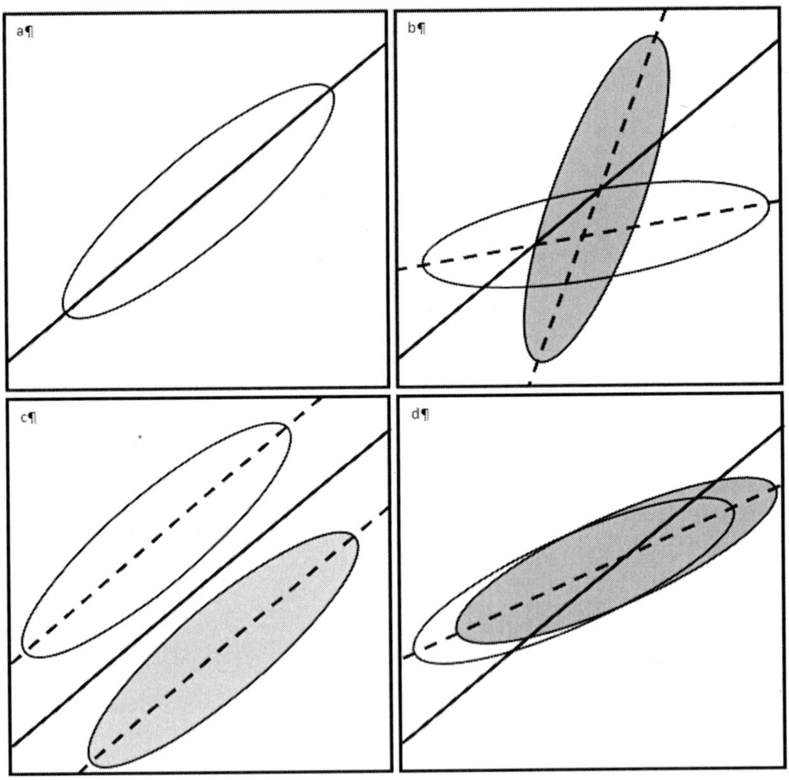

Figure 2. Illustration of different types of allometric analyses in (S)MATR statistical software (Falster et al., 2003): (a) test of the isometry (α = 1); (b) testing if slopes of allometric function are different between groups; (c) testing if elevations are different between groups; (d) testing for shift along the axis. (After Falster et al., 2003)

Here, we explore several theoretical deductions about the relationship between individual and population level responses to competition intensity, i.e. density.

4.1. The 'Rules' In Plant Ecology

"Plant growth is highly plastic, and the mass, height, number of leaves, and reproductive output of an individual plant can vary over orders of magnitude depending on growth conditions." (Gurevitch et al., 2002)

One of the regularities that were revealed in plant populations regarding competitive interaction was that the total final dry weight per unit area of all plants in a population is remarkably consistent over a wide range of densities. In other word, the average individual plant size became smaller as density increase, but this reduction is in linear relationship with increasing number of individuals per unit area (Kira et al., 1953). As a final result, total biomass will be the same for different population densities.

Regularity has been also found in the relationship between the size of a plant population (density), size of individual plant and mortality rate. For some time, this regularity has been considered as an ecological 'law' or 'first principle', and is known as '-3/2 self-thinning rule' (Yoda et al., 1963):

$$M = kN^{-3/2} \tag{4}$$

According to this rule, the average individual plant biomass (M) in a population is proportional to the -3/2 power of population density (N); k is a constant that differs among species. If N increases, M will decrease anisometrically as a consequence of density-dependent mortality, or 'self-thinning'. During the growth of seedlings, crowding becomes severe, and some individuals, usually the smallest and weakest ones, begin to die. The more plants are crowded the sooner and at smaller individual sizes mortality will begin. As a result, in less crowded plant populations, individuals may achieve larger sizes than in dense populations. Although this 'law' has been widely accepted until the 1980s, it has become clear that this scenario was not directly applicable to all populations and plants whose growth scaling is very complex. In other words, the 'law' neglects the plasticity of allocation strategy.Silvertown and Lovett Doust (1993) argued that this rule may be an upper limit of the relationship.

Another suite of empirical results and theoretical deductions comes from agronomy – the 'Law of Constant Final Yield'. This rule deals with size-dependent reproductive allocation in agricultural plant. Total crop biomass increases with density and then levels off, while reproductive output constantly decreases at higher densities. This is explained by the expected pattern according to which plants in competition allocate biomass more in competitive structures and less in reproduction.

All these rules, however, are based on the assumption that population mechanisms contribute to the maintenance of the *status quo* in population dynamics and demography. Numerous ecological and evolutionary models, nevertheless, explore circumstances and mechanisms by which populations do change. As noted by Gurevitch et al. (2002), mean plant size can be a misleading measurement in models because individual sizes in plants are generally extremely uneven as a consequence of plastic growth in asymmetric competition (Weiner, 1990; Schwinning & Fox, 1995). Largest individuals have disproportionate large negative effects on their small neighbors, since the relative amount of resources that small individuals can acquire is less than what could be expected by their biomass. Among a group of seedlings germinating together, a small advantage in size may confer a large benefit, i.e., progressively greater inequality in competitive abilities over time. Competitive asymmetry, which leads to increased individual variability in size, has been seen as one of the major processes that secure the existence of reproductive individuals, stabilize population dynamics and assure the persistence of populations (Aikio & Pakkasmaa, 2003). Under the assumption that there is a size-threshold for reproduction, asymmetry forces small individuals to decrease in size and to stay below the threshold. Therefore, in the presence of size-dependent mortality and reproduction, only large individuals remain in the population and reproduce, assuring population persistence. On the other hand, under symmetric competition, low variation of individual biomasses increases the possibility that either all individuals remain smaller than the size-threshold for reproduction or that all individuals exceed the threshold. This process may cause strong fluctuations in population size, destabilizes population dynamics (Lomnicki, 1988; Silvertown, 1991; Uchmanski, 2000) and increase the likelihood of extinction due to demographic stochasticity (Ripa & Lundberg 2000). One of the causes of symmetry in competition is genetic relatedness between neighboring individuals. Relatedness reduces size variations either because superior large individuals reduce their resource consumption as an altruistic act towards their smaller relatives, which, now, exceed the size-threshold for reproduction (kin selection; Hamilton, 1964; Maynard-Smith, 1964), or because relatives have similar environmental preferences and genetic uniformity, which result in similar growth rates (Jasienski, 1988; Tonsor, 1989).

All these models are strongly based on the premise that reproductive outcome is a linear function of plant size. Although it is basically true that larger individuals have more seeds, this premise does not allow for the possibility that plastic allometry may change the proportion of resources invested into reproduction. As shown in the study on *L.*

maculatum (Stojković et al., 2009), relative allocation to reproductive effort could be enhanced in competition, leading to the decreased effect of asymmetric competition on population dynamics. Also, it was revealed that *L. maculatum* plants grown with genetically identical individuals had higher fitness compared with plants in unrelated patches. It seems that these relations are common for clonal plants (Donohue, 2003). In these genetically structured populations, regulation of population dynamics may include advantageous kin effects. Although there is a possibility that some kin groups may stay bellow the size-threshold for reproduction, the persistence and stability of population size could be assured via selection between kin groups.

4.2. Life-History and Population Dynamics

Using the logistic model of population growth,

$$\frac{dN}{dt} = rN\left(\frac{K-N}{K}\right) \tag{5}$$

where *N* is the population size, *K* is the population's carrying capacity (i.e., the population size at which the per capita birth rate equals the per capita death rate), and *r* is intrinsic rate of population growth, MacArthur and Wilson (1967) established the '*r* / *K* selection theory'. This theoretical model, integrated with Pianka's concept of the evolution of life-history strategies (Pianka, 1970, 1974), proposed a relationship between density-dependent population regulation and life-history evolution. In spite of numerous critiques and limited empirical confirmations (see review in Reznick et al., 2002) this model remains one of the most influential theoretical frameworks for understanding life-history evolution. Undoubtedly, adaptive changes of life-history traits are related to the density-dependent adjustment and resource limitation that each population experience. As a consequence, under density-dependent *vs.* density-independent selection individual fitness must be associated with different traits (Boyce, 1984; Mueller, 1997) and evolved life-history strategies should differ between populations facing distinct densities. The organisms in dense populations (i.e., close to the carrying capacity, *K*) are exposed to intense competition and experience density-dependent mortality, which, according toPianka (1970), determine adaptive life-history changes toward slow development, delayed reproduction, high investment in biomass and greater competitive ability at the cost of low reproductive effort, low fecundity with large investment in each offspring, and high longevity. Contrary, in sparse populations (or populations inhabiting physically variable and unpredictable environments), where mortality factors are mainly density-independent, selection would favor individuals with rapid development, early maturity, high fecundity at the cost of investment in body size, low investment in each offspring, and shorter life span (Pianka, 1970). The later strategy, which is based on selection for traits that enhance population growth rate (*r*), is also expected in a resource-rich, noncompetitive environment.

Although well elaborated argument for life-history strategies as long-term adaptations to the environment in a continuum from pure *r*- to pure *K*-selection, this concept contradicts some basic assumptions about the short-term adaptive responses to competition. In other words, the plasticity of physiological trade-off may oppose long-term microevolutionary trade-offs in a population. For example, fast development is usually assumed to be associated with higher fitness because early hatching/germinated individuals benefit from more available resources compared with subsequent individuals. Also, due to higher possibilities for resource acquirement in a noncompetitive environment, one can expect overall individual performance, i.e., body mass, longevity and total fecundity, to be advanced compared with individuals in a dense population. The question is to what extent a long-term selection can limit the ability of single genotypes to plastically change their allometry strategy in response to environmental variation. Additionally, we may ask what is the consequence of these processes on population dynamics?

In the laboratory evolution experiments on *Acanthoscelides obtectus* two experimental lines were raised for 200 generations. The *r*- and *K*-selected lines were derived by rearing populations at persistently low and high densities, respectively. To test the possibility that plastic responses to the contrasting environmental conditions may oppose long-term life-history strategies established by density-dependent selection, the samples of beetles from both lines were reared for one generation either at their common environment (i.e., low density for the *r*- and high density for the *K*-line) or at the alternate environmental conditions (i.e., low density for the *K*- and high density for the *r*-line). Most of Pianka's predictions on the evolution of life-history strategies under different density conditions were confirmed in *A. obtectus* experimental lines (Stojković & Tucić, unpublished data; but see Tucić et al. (1997) for contrasting results on these experimental lines after only 73 generation of selection). However, preadult life-history traits (i.e., egg size, preadult viability and developmental time) were influenced by short-term density conditions. More importantly, these plastic changes induced by the novel environments (low density for the *K*- and high density for the *r*-line) were in opposite directions from the course of selection for life-history traits within experimental lines. Larval experience of *r*- females in dense conditions resulted in significant increase of investment into the egg dimension. This strategy may provide an advantage to offspring in competitive interactions. The short-term relaxation of competition in *K*-line enabled opportune investment into fast offspring development and increase of their viability. These plastic changes in allocation patterns in *K*-experimental line resulted in increase of demographic parameters - intrinsic rate of population growth (*r*) and net reproductive rate (*Ro*). It seems that amplification of per capita amount of resources at low density allowed the enlargement of carrying capacity in the *K*-line and, consequently, enhanced the opportunities for population growth. In population ecology it is well known that offspring born in early life-stages contribute more to the next generation (i.e., to the *r* parameter) than offspring born later. Fertility life tables of *K*-females raised for one generation at low density provided the evidence that the age-specific fecundity schedule was shifted toward earlier days of adulthood with narrow distribution of fecund days (Stojković & Tucić, unpublished data).

The experiment on rice weevil (*Calandra oryzae*) revealed that variations in temperature may change intrinsic rate of population growth (*r*) as a consequence of changes in rate of development, survival and fecundity (Birch, 1948).

Empirical data have provided excellent demonstration on how variation in survival and fecundity, as individuals vary in age, size, fecundity schedule or other life-history characteristics, affects dynamics in population demography.

5. CONCLUSIONS

In many ecological models populations are not perceived as being composed of individuals that vary in all aspects of their phenotype. Evolutionary biology is looking for the explanations of evolution and development of various organismal traits, but rarely explores the effects of evolutionary changes on dynamics of populations. The truth is that ecological processes provide the context for evolution, and, also, that changes in individual variability affect all population processes in a continuous feedback manner. Allometry, the study of size-correlated variations in biological form and function, may be seen as a discipline in which both theoretical programs can meet. Allometry investigates how allocation strategies evolved and how they can be changed in respect to the environment and characteristics of populations. Individuals must allocate resources in a way that make the most of their chances for contributing offspring to the next generation while simultaneously maximizing their chance of surviving to reproduce. How organisms manage to solve this complex task depends both on the evolutionary history of a population and on biotic and abiotic conditions at each point of time. Clearly, the dynamic relations between life-histories and growth architecture of organisms and their environments suggest that allometric patterns evolve in response to numerous selection pressures and constraints. At the same time, the way the individual growth and life-histories are shaped in certain environment could largely influence the demographic patterns of a population.

6. ACKNOWLEDGEMENTS

I gratefully acknowledge Nikola Tucić for helpful comments on the manuscript and Oliver Stojković for his help in graphic presentations. This study was supported by Ministry of Science and Technological Development of Serbia, project No. 173007.

REFERENCES

1. L. W. Aarssen, 1995 Hypotheses for the evolution of apical dominance in plants: implications for the interpretation of overcompensation. Oikos 74 149 156

2. S. Aikio, S. Pakkasmaa, 2003Relatedness and competitive asymmetry-implications for growth and population dynamics. Oikos 100 283 290

3. P. Alpert, E. L. Simms, 2002The relative advantages of plasticity and fixity in different environments: when is it good for a plant to adjust? Evolutionary Ecology 16 285 297

4. C. L. Ballaré, R. A. Sánchez, A. L. Scopel, J. J. Casal, C. M. Ghersa, 1987Early detection of neighbor plants by phytochrome perception of spectral changes in reflected sunlight. Plant Cell Environment 10 551 553

5. C. L. Ballare, A. L. Scopel, R. A. Sanchez, 1990Far-red radiation reflected from adjacent leaves: an early signal of competition in plant canopies. Science 247 329 332

6. M. Begon, J. L. Harper, C. R. Townsend, 1990Ecology: individuals, populations and communities. Blackwell, Boston, MA.

7. D. Berrigan, 1991The allometry of egg size and number in insects. Oikos 60 313 321

8. Birch, L.C 1948The intrinsic rate of natural increase of an insect population. Journal of Animal Ecology 17 15 26

9. S. P. Bonser, L. W. Aarssen, 2001Allometry and plasticity of meristem allocation throughout development ina Arabidopsis thaliana. Journal of Ecology 89 72 79

10. S. P. Bonser, L. W. Aarssen, 2003Allometry and development in herbaceous plants: functional responses of meristem allocation to light and nutrient availability. American Journal of Botany 90 404 412

11. M. S. Boyce, 1984Restitution of r- and K-selection as a model of density-dependent natural selection. Annual Review of Ecology and Systematics 15 427 447

12. A. D. Bradshaw, 1965Evolutionary significance of phenotypic plasticity in plants. Advances in Genetetics 13 115 155

13. B. Charlesworth, 1994Evolution in age-structured populations. 2nd edition, Cambridge University Press, Cambridge

14. E. L. Charnov, D. Berrigan, 1990Dimensionless numbers and life history evolution: age at maturity versus the adult lifespan. Evolutionary Ecology 4 273 275

15. G. P. Cheplick, 1995Genotypic variation and plasticity of clonal growth in relation to nutrient availability in Amphibromus scabrivalvis. Journal of Ecology 83 459 468

16. K. Donohue, 2003The influence of neighbor relatedness on multilevel selection in the Great Lakes sea rocket. American Naturalist 162 77 92

17. S. A. Dudley, J. Schmitt, 1996Testing the adaptive plasticity hypothesis: density dependent selection on manipulated stem length in Impatiens capensis. American Naturalist 147 445 465

18. D. S. Falster, D. I. Warton, I. J. Wright, 2003S)MATR: Standardised Major Axis Tests and Routines, Version 1.0.http://www.bio.mq.edu.au/ecology/SMATR.

19. C. W. Fox, M. S. Thakar, T. A. Mousseau, 1997Egg size plasticity in a seed beetle: An adaptive maternal effect. American Naturalist 149 149 163

20. T. J. Givnish, 1986Biomechanical constraints on self-thinning in plant populations. Journal of Theoretical Biology 119 139 146

21. J. Grinell, 1917The niche-relationships of the California thrasher. The Auk 34 427 433

22. J. Gurevitch, S. M. Scheiner, G. A. Fox, 2002The Ecology of Plants. Sinauer Associates Inc., Sunderland, MA

23. W. D. Hamilton, 1964The genetical evolution of social behaviour. I & II. Journal of Theoretical Biology 7 1 52

24. J. S. Huxley, 1932Problems of relative growth. MacVeagh, London.

25. M. Jasienski, 1988Kinship ecology of competition: size hiearchies in kin and non-kin laboratory cohorts of tadpoles. Oecologia 77 407 413

26. M. Kearney, S. J. Simpson, D. Raubenheimer, B. Helmuth, 2010Modelling the ecological niche from functional traits. Phil. Trans. R. Soc. B. 365 3469 3483

27. T. Kira, H. Ogawa, K. Sinozaki, 1953Intraspecific competition among higher plants. 1. Competition-density-yield interrelationships in regularly dispersed populations. Journal of Institute of Polytechnic. Osaka City University D4 1 16

28. J. M. Kneitel, J. M. Chase, 2004Trade-offs in community ecology: linking spatial scales and species coexistence. Ecology Letters 7 69 80

29. R. Law, 1979Ecological determinants in the evolution of life histories. In R. M. Anderson, B. D. Turner and L. R. Taylor, eds. Population Dynamics. Blackwell Scientific, Oxford, 81 103

30. J. M. Levine, M. Rees, 2002Coexistence and relative abundance in annual plant assemblages: the roles of competition and colonization. American Naturalist 160 452 67

31. A. Lomnicki, 1988Population Ecology of Individuals. Princeton Univ. Press.

32. Doust. L. Lovett, 1981Population dynamics and local specialization in a clonal perennial (Ranunculus repens). I. The dynamics of ramets in contrasting habitats. Journal of Ecology 69 743 755

33. Arthur. R. H. Mac, E. . Wilson, 1967The theory of island biogeography. Princeton Univ. Press, Princeton

34. P. M. Magwene, 2001Comparing ontogenetic trajectories using growth process data. System. Biology 50 640 656

35. Smith. J. Maynard, 1964Group selection and kin selection. Nature 201 1145 1147

36. L. D. Mueller, 1997Theoretical and empirical axamination of density-dependent selection. Annual Review of Ecology and Systematics 28 269 288

37. K. Niklas, 1994Plant allometry: the scaling of form and process. University of Chicago Press, Chicago.

38. R. J. O'Connor, 2000Why ecology lags behind biology. Scientist 14: 35.

39. R. H. Peters, 1983The ecological implications of body size. Cambridge University Press, Cambridge

40. E. R. Pianka, 1970On r- and K-Selection. American Naturalist 104 592 597

41. Pianka, E.R. (1974) Niche Overlap and Diffuse Competition. Proceedings of Natural Academy of Science, USA. 71: 2141-2145,

42. D. Prati, D. Schmid, 2000Genetic differentiation of life-history traits within populations of the clonal plant Ranunculus reptans. Oikos 90 442 456

43. D. Reznick, M. J. Bryant, F. Bashey, 2002r- and K-selection revisited: the role of population regulation in life-history evolution. Ecology 83 1509 1520

44. D. Reznick, 1985Cost of reproduction: an evolution of the empirical evidence. Oikos 44 257 267

45. J. Ripa, P. Lundberg, 2000The route to extinction in variable environments. Oikos 90 89 96

46. D. A. Roff, D. J. Fairbairn, 2007The evolution of trade-offs: where are we? Journal of Evolutionary Biology 20 433 447

47. D. A. Roff, 2002Life History Evolution. Sinauer Associates, Sunderland, MA.

48. M. R. Rose, 1991Evolutionary biology of aging. Oxford Univ. Press, Oxford

49. B. Schmid, J. Weiner, 1993Plastic relationships between reproductive and vegetative mass in Solidago altissima. Evolution 47 61 74

50. J. Schmitt, 1997Is photomorphogenic shade avoidance adaptive? Perspectives from population biology. Plant Cell Environment 20 826 830

51. S. Schwinning, G. A. Fox, 1995Population dynamic consequences of competitive symmetry in annual plants. Oikos 72 422 432

52. S. Schwinning, J. Weiner, 1998Mechanisms determing the degree of size asymmetry in competition among plants. Oecologia 113 447 455

53. J. W. Silvertown, Doust. L. Lovett, 1993Introduction to plant population biology. Blackwell, Oxford, UK.

54. J. W. Silvertown, 1991Modularity, reproductive tresholds and plant population dynamics. Functional Ecology 5 577 582

55. H. Smith, G. C. Whitelam, 1997The shade avoidance syndrome: multiple responses mediated by multiple phytochromes. Plant Cell Environment 20 849 844

56. H. Smith, J. J. Casal, G. M. Jackson, 1990Reflection signals and the perception by phytochrome of the proximity of neighbouring vegetation. Plant Cell Environment 13 73 78

57. S. C. Stearns, 1992The evolution of life histories. Oxford University Press, New York.

58. B. Stojković, N. Barišić-Klisarić, S. Avramov, A. Tarasjev, 2009Effect of genetic relatedness on the allometric relationship between biomass investment and sexual reproduction in clonal plant. Polish Journal of Ecology 57 371 375

59. S. E. Sultan, 1995Phenotypic plasticity and plant adaptation. Acta Botanica Neerl. 44 363 383

60. S. J. Tonsor, 1989Relatedness and intraspecific competition in Plantago lanceolata. American Naturalist 134 897 906

61. B. Tucić, B. Stojković, 2001Shade avoidance syndrome in Picea omorika seedlings: a growth-room experiment. Journal of Evolutionary Biology 14 444 455

62. N. Tucić, O. Stojković, I. Gliksman, D. Milanović, D. Šešlija, (1997, Laboratory Evolution of Life-History Traits in the Bean Weevil (Acanthoscelides obtectus): The Effects of Density-Dependent and Age-Specific Selection. Evolution 51 1896 1909

63. N. Tucić, I. Gliksman, D. Šešlija, O. Stojković, D. Milanović, 1998Laboratory Evolution of Life-History Traits in the Bean Weevil (Acanthoscelides obtectus): The Effects of Selection on Developmental

Time in Populations with Different Previous History. Evolution 52 1713 1725

64. J. Uchmanski, 2000Individual variability and population regulation: an individual-based approach. Oikos 90 539 548

65. M. van Kleunen, M. Fischer, B. Schmid, (2002, life-history. Experimental, selection. evolution, the. on, to. allocation, reproduction. sexual, plasticity. its, a. in, plant. clonal, Evolution 56 2168 2177

66. D. I. Warton, I. J. Wright, D. S. Falster, M. Westoby, 2006Bivariate line-fitting methods for allometry. Biological Review 81 259 291

67. J. Weiner, 1990Asymmetric competition in plant populations. Trends in Ecology and Evolution 5 360 364

68. J. Weiner, 2004Allocation, plasticity and allometry in plants. Perspectives Plant Ecol. Evol. Syst. 6 207 215

69. M. J. West-Eberhard, 1989Phenotypic plasticity and the origins of diversity. Annual Review in Ecology and Systematics 20 249 278

70. J. T. Wootton, 1987The effects of body mass, phylogeny, habitat, and trophic level on mammalian age at first reproduction. Evolution 41 732 749

71. K. Yoda, T. Kira, H. Ogawa, K. Hozumi, 1963Self-thinning in overcrowded pure stands under cultivated and natural conditions. Journal of Biology, Osaka City University, 14 107 129

72. M. Zuk, 1996Trade-offs in parasitology, evolution and behavior. Parasitology Today 12 46 47

CHAPTER 2

Biomass energy resources utilisation and waste management

Abdeen Mustafa Omer

Energy Research Institute (ERI), Ministry of Science and Technology, Khartoum, Sudan; abdeenomer2@yahoo.co.uk

ABSTRACT

This Article discusses a comprehensive review of biomass energy sources, environment and sustainable development. This includes all the biomass energy technologies, energy efficiency systems, energy conservation scenarios, energy savings and other mitigation measures necessary to reduce emissions. The current literature is reviewed regarding the ecological, social, cultural and economic impacts of biomass technology. This article gives an overview of present and future use of biomass as an industrial feedstock for production of fuels, chemicals and other materials. However, to be truly competitive in an open market situation, higher value products are required. Results suggest that biomass technology must be encouraged, promoted, invested, implemented, and demonstrated, but especially in remote rural areas.

KEYWORDS

biomass energy sources; resource utilisation; waste management

1. INTRODUCTION

There is strong scientific evidence that the average temperature of the earth's surface is rising. This was a result of the increased concentration of carbon dioxide (CO_2), and other greenhouse gases (GHGs) in the atmosphere as released by burning fossil fuels [1,2]. This global warming will eventually lead to substantial changes in the world's climate, which will, in turn, have a major impact on human life and the environment. Energy use can be achieved by minimising the energy demand, by rational energy use, by recovering heat and the use of more green energies. This will lead to fossil fuels emission reduction. This study was a step towards achieving this goal. The adoption of green or sustainable approaches to the way in which society is run is seen as an important strategy in finding a solution to the energy problem. The key factors to reducing and controlling CO_2, which is the major contributor to global warming, are the use of alternative approaches to energy generation and the exploration of how these alternatives are used today and may be used in the future as green energy sources. Even with modest assumptions about the availability of land, comprehensive fuel-wood farming programmes offer significant energy, economic and environmental benefits. These benefits would be dispersed in rural areas where they are greatly needed and can serve as linkages for further rural economic development. The nations as a whole would benefit from savings in foreign exchange, improved energy security, and socio-economic improvements. With a nine-fold increase in forest— plantation cover, the nation's resource base would be greatly improved. The international community would benefit from pollution reduction, climate change mitigation, and the increased trading opportunities that arise from new income sources. The non-technical issues, which have recently gained attention, include: 1) Environmental and ecological factors, e.g., carbon sequestration, reforestation and revegetation. 2) Renewables as a CO_2 neutral replacement for fossil fuels. 3) Greater recognition of the importance of renewable energy, particularly modern biomass energy carriers, at the policy and planning levels. 4) Greater recognition of the difficulties of gathering good and reliable biomass energy data, and efforts to improve it. 5) Studies on the detrimental health efforts of biomass energy particularly from traditional energy users. There is a need for some further development to suit local conditions, to minimise spares holdings, to maximise interchangeability both of engine parts and of the engine application. Emphasis should be placed on full local manufacture.

Energy is an essential factor in development since it stimulates, and supports economic growth and development. Fossil fuels, especially oil and natural gas, are finite in extent, and should be regarded as depleting assets, and efforts are oriented to search for new sources of energy. The clamour all over the world for the need to conserve energy and the environment has intensified as traditional energy resources continue to dwindle whilst the environment becomes increasingly degraded. Alternatively energy sources can potentially help fulfill the acute energy demand and sustain economic growth in many regions of the world. Bioenergy is beginning to gain importance in the global fight to prevent climate change. The scope for exploiting organic waste as a source of energy is not limited to direct incineration or burning refuse-derived fuels. Biogas, biofuels and woody biomass are other forms of energy sources that can be derived from organic waste materials. These biomass energy sources have significant potential in the fight against climate change.

The sources to alleviate the energy situation in the world are sufficient to supply all foreseeable needs. Conservation of energy and rationing in some form will however have to be practised by most countries, to reduce oil imports and redress balance of payments positions. Meanwhile development and application of nuclear power and some of the traditional solar, wind, biomass and water energy alternatives must be set in hand to supplement what remains of the fossil fuels. The encouragement of greater energy use is an essential component of development. In the short-term it requires mechanisms to enable the rapid increase in energy/capita, and in the long-term we should be working towards a way of life, which makes use of energy efficiency and without the impairment of the environment or of causing safety problems. Such a programme should as far as possible be based on renewable energy resources.

Large-scale, conventional, power plant such as hydropower has an important part to play in development. It does not, however, provide a complete solution. There is an important complementary role for the greater use of small-scale, rural based-power plants. Such plant can be used to assist development since it can be made locally using local resources, enabling a rapid built-up in total equipment to be made without a corresponding and unacceptably large demand on central funds. Renewable resources are particularly suitable for providing the energy for such equipment and its use is also compatible with the long-term aims.

In compiling energy consumption data one can categorise usage according to a number of different schemes:

- Traditional sector: industrial, transportation, etc.
- End-use: space heating, process steam, etc.
- Final demand: total energy consumption related to automobiles, to food, etc.
- Energy source: oil, coal, etc.
- Energy form at point of use: electric drive, low temperature heat, etc.

2. BIOENERGY DEVELOPMENT

Bioenergy is energy from the sun stored in materials of biological origin. This includes plant matter and animal waste, known as biomass. Plants store solar energy through photosynthesis in cellulose and lignin, whereas animals store energy as fats. When burned, these sugars break down and release energy exothermically, releasing carbon dioxide (CO_2), heat and steam. The by-products of this reaction can be captured and manipulated to create power, commonly called bioenergy. Biomass is considered renewable because the carbon (C) is taken out of the atmosphere and replenished more quickly than the millions of years required for fossil fuels to form. The use of biofuels to replace fossil fuels contributes to a reduction in the overall release of carbon dioxide into the atmosphere and hence helps to tackle global warming. The range of waste treatment technologies that are tailored to produce bioenergy is growing. There are a number of key areas of bioenergy from wastes including (but not limited to) biogas, biofuels and bioheat. When considering using bioenergy, it is important to take into account the overall emission of carbon in the process of electricity production.

The biomass energy resources are particularly suited for the provision of rural power supplies and a major advantage is that equipment such as flat plate solar driers, wind machines, etc., can be constructed using local resources and without the high capital cost of more conventional equipment. Further advantage results from the feasibility of local maintenance and the general encouragement such local manufacture gives to the build up of small-scale rural based industry. **Table 1** lists the energy sources available.

Currently the “non-commercial” fuels wood, crop residues and animal dung are used in large amounts in the rural areas of developing countries, principally for heating and cooking; the method of use is highly inefficient. **Table 2** presented some renewable applications. **Table 3** lists the most important of energy needs.

Table 4 listed methods of energy conversion.

Considerations when selecting power plant include the following:

- Power level-whether continuous or discontinuous.
- Cost-initial cost, total running cost including fuel, maintenance and capital amortised over life.
- Complexity of operation.
- Maintenance and availability of spares.
- Life.

- Suitability for local manufacture.

The internal combustion engine is a major contributor to rising CO_2 emissions worldwide and some pretty dramatic new thinking is needed if our planet is to counter the effects. With its use increasing in developing world economies, there is something to be said for the argument that the vehicles we use to help keep our inner-city environments free from waste, litter and grime should be at the forefront of developments in low-emissions technology. Materials handled by waste management companies are becoming increasingly valuable. Those responsible for the security of facilities that treat waste or manage scrap will testify to the precautions needed to fight an ongoing battle against unauthorised access by criminals and crucially, to prevent the damage they can cause through theft, vandalism or even arson. Of particular concern is the escalating level of metal theft, driven by various factors including the demand for metal in rapidly developing economies such as India and China.

Table 1. Sources of energy [3].

Energy source	Energy carrier	Energy end-use
Vegetation	Fuel-wood	Cooking Water heating Building materials Animal fodder preparation
Oil	Kerosene	Lighting Ignition fires
Dry cells	Dry cell batteries	Lighting Small appliances
Muscle power	Animal power	Transport Land preparation for farming Food preparation (threshing)
Muscle power	Human power	Transport Land preparation for farming Food preparation (threshing)

Table 2. Renewable applications [3].

Systems	Applications
Water supply	Rain collection, purification, storage and recycling
Wastes disposal	Anaerobic digestion (CH_4)
Cooking	Methane
Food	Cultivate the 1 hectare plot and greenhouse for four people
Electrical demands	Wind generator
Space heating	Solar collectors
Water heating	Solar collectors and excess wind energy
Control system	Ultimately hardware
Building fabric	Integration of subsystems to cut costs

Table 3. Energy needs in rural areas [3].

Transport, e.g., small vehicles and boats
Agricultural machinery, e.g., two-wheeled tractors
Crop processing, e.g., milling
Water pumping
Small industries, e.g., workshop equipment
Electricity generation, e.g., hospitals and schools
Domestic, e.g., cooking, heating, lighting

There is a need for greater attention to be devoted to this field in the development of new designs, the dissemination of information and the encouragement of its use. International and government bodies and independent organisations all have a role to play in biomass energy technologies. Environment has no precise limits because it is in fact a part of everything. Indeed, environment is, as anyone probably already knows, not only flowers blossoming or birds singing in the spring, or a lake surrounded by beautiful mountains. It is also human settlements, the places where people live, work, rest, the quality of the food we eat, the noise or silence of the street they live in. Environment is not only the fact that our cars consume a good deal of energy and pollute the air, but also, that we often need them to go to work and for holidays. Obviously man uses energy just as plants, bacteria, mushrooms, bees, fish and rats do (Figure 1). Man largely uses solar energy-food, hydropower, wood and thus participates harmoniously in the natural flow of energy through the environment. But man also uses oil, gas, coal and nuclear power. We always modify our environment with or without this source of energy.

Table 4. Methods of energy conversion [4].

Muscle power	Man, animals
Internal combustion engines	
Reciprocating	Petrol-spark ignition
	Diesel-compression ignition
	Humphrey water piston
Rotating	Gas turbines
Heat engines	
Vapour (Rankine)	
Reciprocating	Steam engine
Rotating	Steam turbine
Gas Stirling (Reciprocating)	Steam engine
Gas Brayton (Rotating)	Steam turbine
Electron gas	Thermionic, thermoelectric
Electromagnetic radiation	Photo devices
Hydraulic engines	Wheels, screws, buckets, turbines
Wind engines (wind machines)	Vertical axis, horizontal axis
Electrical/mechanical	Dynamo/alternator, motor

Economic importance of environmental issue is increasing, and new technologies are expected to reduce pollution derived both from productive processes and products, with costs that are still unknown. This is due to market uncertainty, weak appropriability regime, lack of a dominant design, and difficulties in reconfiguring organisational routines.. The degradation of the global environment is one of the most serious energy issues.

3. ENERGY USE AND THE ENVIRONMENT

Energy use is one of several essential components for every country:

- The overall situation and the implications of increased energy use in the future.
- The problem of the provision of power in rural areas, including the consideration of energy resources and energy conversion.

In addition to the drain on resources, such an increase in consumption consequences, together with the increased hazards of pollution and the safety problems associated with a large nuclear fission programmes. It would be equally unacceptable to suggest that the difference in energy between the developed and developing countries and prudent for the developed countries to move towards a way of life which, whilst maintaining or even increasing quality of life, reduce significantly the energy consumption per capita. Such savings can be achieved in a number of ways:

- Improved efficiency of energy use, for example environmental cost of thermal insulation must be taken into account, energy recovery, and total energy.
- Conservation of energy resources by design for long life and recycling rather than the short life throwaway product and systematic replanning of our way of life, for example in the field of transport.

Energy ratio is defined as the ratio of:

Energy content of the food product/Energy input to produce the food(1)

4. COMBINED HEAT AND POWER (CHP)

The atmospheric emissions of fossil fuelled installations are mostly aldehydes ($CH_3CH_2CH_2CHO$), carbon monoxide (CO), nitrogen oxides (NO_X), sulpher oxides (SOx) and particles (i.e., ash) as well as carbon dioxide. **Table 5** shows estimates include not only the releases occurring at the power plant itself but also cover fuel extraction and treatment, as well as the storage of wastes and the area of land required for operation (**Table 6**). A review of the potential range of recyclables is presented in **Table 7**.

Table 5. Annual GHG emissions from different types of power plants [5].

Primary source of energy	Emissions ($\times 10^3$ metric tons CO_2)		Waste ($\times 10^3$ metric tons CO_2)	Area (km^2)
	Atmosphere	Water		
Coal	380	7 - 41	60 - 3000	120
Oil	70 - 160	3 - 6	Negligible	70 - 84
Gas	24	1	-	84
Nuclear	6	21	2600	77

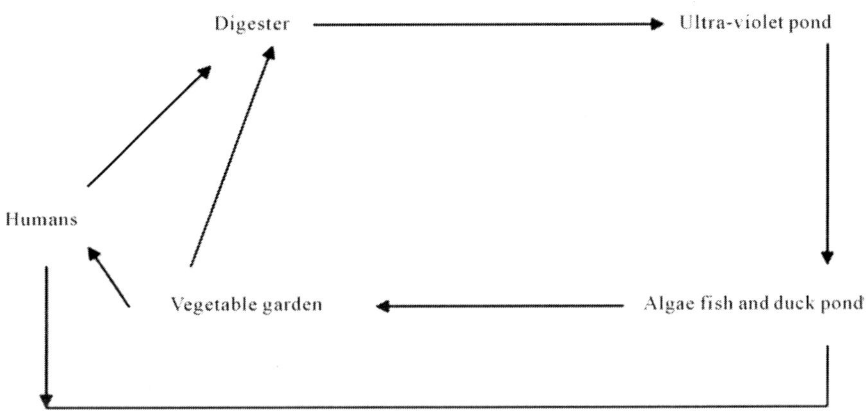

Figure 1. Biomass utilisation cycle concepts [7].

Combined heat and power (CHP) installations are quite common in greenhouses, which grow high-energy, input crops (e.g., salad vegetables, pot plants, etc.). Scientific assumptions for a short-term energy strategy suggest that the most economically efficient way to replace the thermal plants is to modernise existing power plants to increase their energy efficiency and to improve their environmental performance [6].

However, utilisation of wind power and the conversion of gas-fired CHP plants to biomass would significantly reduce the dependence on imported fossil fuels. Although a lack of generating capacity is forecasted in the long-term, utilisation of the existing renewable energy potential and the huge possibilities for increasing energy efficiency are sufficient to meet future energy demands in the short-term [7].

A total shift towards a sustainable energy system is a complex and long process, but is one that can be achieved within a period of about 20 years. Implementation will require initial investment, long-term national strategies and action plans. However, the changes will have a number of benefits including: a more stable energy supply than at present and major improvement in the environmental performance of the energy sector, and certain social benefits (**Figure 2**). A vision that used methodologies and calculations based on computer modelling can utilised:

- Data from existing governmental programmes.
- Potential renewable energy sources and energy efficiency improvements.
- Assumptions for future economy growth.
- Information from studies and surveys on the recent situation in the energy sector.

Table 6. Energy consumption per person [5].

Region	Population (millions)	Energy per person (Watt/m^2)
Africa	820	0.54
Asia	3780	2.74
Central America	180	1.44
North America	335	0.34
South America	475	0.52
Western Europe	445	2.24
Eastern Europe	130	2.57
Oceania	35	0.08
Russia	330	0.29

The main advantages are related to energy, agriculture and environment problems, are foreseeable both at national level and at worldwide level and can be summarised as follows:

- Reduction of dependence on import of energy and related products.
- Reduction of environmental impact of energy production (greenhouse effect, air pollution, and waste degradation).
- Substitution of food crops and reduction of food surpluses and of related economic burdens.

- Utilisation of marginal lands and of set aside lands and reduction of related socio-economic and environmental problems (soil erosion, urbanisation, landscape deterioration, etc.).

- Development of new know-how and production of technological innovation.

In some countries, a wide range of economic incentives and other measures are already helping to protect the environment. These include:

- Taxes and user charges that reflect the costs of using the environment, e.g., pollution taxes and waste disposal charges.

- Subsidies, credits and grants that encourage environmental protection.

- Deposit-refund systems that prevent pollution on resource misuse and promote product reuse or recycling.

- Financial enforcement incentives, e.g., fines for noncompliance with environmental regulations.

- Tradable permits for activities that harm the environment.

District Heating (DH), also known as community heating can be a key factor to achieve energy savings, reduce CO_2 emissions and at the same time provide consumers with a high quality heat supply at a competitive price. DH should generally only be considered for areas where the heat density is sufficiently high to make DH economical. In countries like Denmark DH may today be economical even to new developments with lower density areas due to the high level of taxation on oil and gas fuels combined with the efficient production of DH. To improve the opportunity for DH local councils can adapt the following plan:

- Analyse the options for heat supply during local planning stage.

- In areas where DH is the least cost solution it should be made part of the infrastructure just like for instance water and sewage connecting all existing and new buildings.

- Where possible all public buildings should be connected to DH.

- The government provides low interest loans or funding to minimise conversion costs for its citizens.

- Use other powers, for instance national legislation to ensure the most economical development of the heat supply and enable an obligation to connect buildings to a DH scheme.

Table 7. Summary of material recycling practices in the construction sector [7].

Construction and demolition material	Recycling technology options	Recycling product
Asphalt	Cold recycling; heat generation; Minnesota process; parallel drum process; elongated drum; microwave asphalt recycling system; finfalt; surface regeneration	Recycling asphalt; asphalt aggregate
Brick	Burn to ash, crush into aggregate	Slime burn ash; filling material; hardcore
Concrete	Crush into aggregate	Recycling aggregate; cement replacement; protection of levee; backfilling; filter
Ferrous metal	Melt; reuse directly	Recycled steel scrap
Glass	Reuse directly; grind to powder; polishing; crush into aggregate; burn to ash	Recycled window unit; glass fibre; filling material; tile; paving block; asphalt; recycled aggregate; cement replacement; manmade soil
Masonry	Crush into aggregate; heat to 900°C to ash	Thermal insulating concrete; traditional clay
Non-ferrous metal	Melt	Recycled metal
Paper and cardboard	Purification	Recycled paper
Plastic	Convert to powder by cryogenic milling; clopping; crush into aggregate; burn to ash	Panel; recycled plastic; plastic lumber; recycled aggregate; landfill drainage; asphalt; manmade soil
Timber	Reuse directly; cut into aggregate; blast furnace deoxidisation; gasification or pyrolysis; chipping; moulding by pressurising timber chip under steam and water	Whole timber; furniture and kitchen utensils; lightweight recycled aggregate; source of energy; chemical production; wood-based panel; plastic lumber; geofibre; insulation board

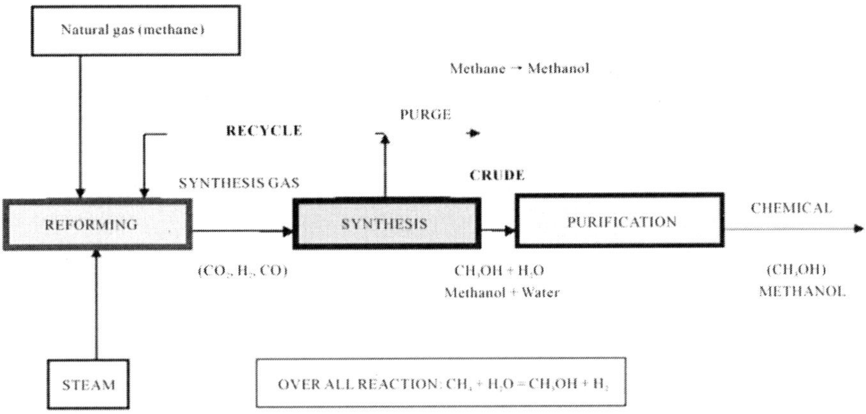

Figure 2. Schematic diagram shows methanol production [8].

Denmark has broadly seen three scales of CHP which where largely implemented in the following chronological order [9]:

- Large-scale CHP in cities (>50 MWe).
- Small (5 kWe - 5 MWe) and medium scale (5 - 50 MWe).
- Industrial and small-scale CHP.

Combined heat and power (CHP) installations are quite common in greenhouses, which grow high-energy, input crops (e.g., salad vegetables, pot plants, etc.). Most of the heat is produced by large CHP plants (gas-fired combined cycle plants using natural gas, biomass, waste or biogas). DH is energy efficient because of the way the heat is produced and the required temperature level is an important factor. Buildings can be heated to temperature of 21°C and domestic hot water (DHW) can be supplied with a temperature of 55°C using energy sources that are most efficient when producing low temperature levels (<95°C) for the DH water. Most of these heat sources are CO_2neutral or emit low levels. Only a few of these sources are available to small individual systems at a reasonably cost, whereas DH schemes because of the plant's size and location can have access to most of the heat sources and at a low cost. Low temperature DH, with return temperatures of around 30°C - 40°C can utilise the following heat sources:

- Efficient use of CHP by extracting heat at low calorific value (CV).
- Efficient use of biomass or gas boilers by condensing heat in economisers (**Table 8**).
- Efficient utilisation of geothermal energy.

- Direct utilisation of excess low temperature heat from industrial processes.
- Efficient use of large-scale solar heating plants.

Heat tariffs may include a number of components such as: a connection charge, a fixed charge and a variable energy charge. Also, consumers may be incentivised to lower the return temperature. Hence, it is difficult to generalise but the heat practice for any DH company no matter what the ownership structure can be highlighted as follows:

- To develop and maintain a development plan for the connection of new consumers.
- To evaluate the options for least cost production of heat.
- To implement the most competitive solutions by signing agreements with other companies or by implementing own investment projects.
- To monitor all internal costs and with the help of benchmarking, improve the efficiency of the company.
- To maintain a good relationship with the consumer and deliver heat supply services at a sufficient quality.

Installing DH should be pursued to meet the objectives for improving the environment through the improvement of energy efficiency in the heating sector. At the same time DH can serve the consumer with a reasonable quality of heat at the lowest possible cost. The variety of possible solutions combined with the collaboration between individual companies, the district heating association, the suppliers and consultants can, as it has been in Denmark, be the way forward for developing DH in the United Kingdom. Implementation will require initial investment, long-term national strategies and action plans. However, the changes will have a number of benefits including: a more stable energy supply than at present and major improvement in the environmental performance of the energy sector, and certain social benefits [10].

5. BIOMASS UTILISATION AND DEVELOPMENT OF CONVERSION TECHNOLOGIES

Sustainable energy is energy that, in its production or consumption, has minimal negative impacts on human health and the healthy functioning of vital ecological systems, including the global environment. It is an accepted fact that renewable energy is a sustainable form of energy, which has attracted more attention during recent years. A great amount of renewable energy potential, environmental interest, as well as economic consideration of fossil fuel consumption and high emphasis of sustainable development for the future will be needed. Explanations for the use of inefficient agricultural-environmental polices include: the high cost of information required to measure benefits on a site-specific basis, information asymmetries between government agencies and farm decision makers that result in high implementation costs, distribution effects and political considerations [11]. Achieving the aim of agric-environment schemes through:

- Sustain the beauty and diversity of the landscape.
- Improve and extend wildlife habitats.
- Conserve archaeological sites and historic features.
- Improve opportunities for countryside enjoyment.
- Restore neglected land or features, and
- Create new habitats and landscapes.
-

5.1. Efficient Bio-Energy Use and Improvement

The data required to perform the trade-off analysis simulation can be classified according to the divisions given in **Table 9**: the overall system or individual plants, and the existing situation or future development.

The effective economic utilisations of these resources are shown in **Table 10**, but their use is hindered by many problems such as those related to harvesting, collection, and transportation, besides the sanitary control regulations. Biomass energy is experiencing a surge in an interest stemming from a combination of factors, e.g., greater recognition of its current role and future potential contribution as a modern fuel, global environmental benefits, its development and entrepreneurial opportunities, etc. Possible routes of biomass energy development are shown in**Table 11**.

The key to successful future appears to lie with successful marketing of the treatment by products. There is also potential for using solid residue in the construction industry as a filling agent for concrete. Research suggests that the composition of the residue locks metals within the material, thus preventing their escape and any subsequent negative effect on the environment.

The use of biomass through direct combustion has long been, and still is, the most common mode of biomass utilisation as shown in Tables 9-11.

Examples for dry (thermo-chemical) conversion processes are charcoal making from wood (slow pyrolysis), gasification of forest and agricultural residues (fast pyrolysis – this is still in demonstration phase), and of course, direct combustion in stoves, furnaces, etc. Wet processes require substantial amount of water to be mixed with the biomass. Biomass technologies include:

- Briquetting.
- Improved stoves.
- Biogas.
- Improved charcoal.
- Carbonisation.
- Gasification.

Table 8. Final energy projections including biomass (Mtoe) [10].

Region	1995			
	Biomass	Conventional Energy	Total	Share of Biomass (%)
Africa	205	136	341	60
China	206	649	855	24
East Asia	106	316	422	25
Latin America	73	342	415	18
South Asia	235	188	423	56
Total developing countries	825	1632	2457	34
Other non-OECD* countries	24	1037	1061	2
Total non-OECD* countries	849	2669	3518	24
OECD countries	81	3044	3125	3
World	930	5713	6643	14
Region	**2020**			
	Biomass	Conventional Energy	Total	Share of Biomass (%)
Africa	371	266	637	59
China	224	1524	1748	13
East Asia	118	813	931	13
Latin America	81	706	787	10
South Asia	276	523	799	35
Total developing countries	1071	3825	4896	22
Other non-OECD* countries	26	1669	1695	2
Total non-OECD* countries	1097	5494	6591	17
OECD countries	96	3872	3968	2
World	1193	9365	10558	11

*Organisation for economic co-operation and development.

Table 9. Classifications of data requirements [12].

	Plant data	System data
Existing data	Size	Peak load
	Life	Load shape
	Cost (fixed and var. O and M)	Capital costs
	Forced outage	Fuel costs
	Maintenance	Depreciation
	Efficiency	Rate of return
	Fuel	Taxes
	Emissions	
Future data	All of above. plus	System lead growth
	Capital costs	Fuel price growth
	Construction trajectory	Fuel import limits
	Date in service	Inflation

Table 10. Agricultural residues routes for development [12].

Source	Process	Product	End use
Agricultural residues	Direct	Combustion	Rural poor
			Urban household
			Industrial use
	Processing	Briquettes	Industrial use
	Processing	Carbonisation (small scale)	Limited household use
		Briquettes	Rural household (self sufficiency)
	Carbonisation	Carbonised	Urban fuel
	Fermentation	Biogas	Energy services
			Household
			Industry
Agricultural. and animal residues	Direct	Combustion	(Save or less efficiency as wood)
	Briquettes	Direct combustion	(Similar end use devices or improved)
	Carbonisation	Carbonised	Use
	Carbonisation	Briquettes	Briquettes use
	Fermentation	Biogas	Use

Table 11. Effective biomass resource utilisation [13].

Subject	Tools	Constraints
Utilisation and land clearance for agriculture expansion	Stumpage fees	Policy
	Control	Fuel-wood planning
	Extension	Lack of extension
	Conversion	Institutional
	Technology	
Utilisation of agricultural residues	Briquetting	Capital
	Carbonisation	Pricing
	Carbonisation and briquetting	Policy and legislation
	Fermentation	Social acceptability
	Gasification	

The increased demand for gas and petroleum, food crops, fish and large sources of vegetative matter mean that the global harvesting of carbon has in turn intensified. It could be said that mankind is mining nearly everything except its waste piles. It is simply a matter of time until the significant carbon stream present in municipal solid waste is fully captured. In the meantime, the waste industry needs to continue on the pathway to increased awareness and better-optimised biowaste resources. Optimisation of waste carbon may require widespread regulatory drivers (including strict limits on the landfilling of organic materials), public acceptance of the benefits of waste carbon products for soil improvements/crop enhancements and more investment in capital facilities.

In short, a significant effort will be required in order to capture a greater portion of the carbon stream and put it to beneficial use. From the standpoint of waste practitioners, further research and pilot programmes are necessary before the available carbon in the waste stream can be extracted in sufficient quality and quantities to create the desired end products. Other details need to be ironed out too, including measurement methods, diversion calculations, sequestration values and determination of acceptance contamination thresholds.

5.1.1. Briquette

Charcoal stoves are very familiar to African society. As for the stove technology, the present charcoal stove can be used, and can be improved upon for better efficiency. This energy term will be of particular interest to both urban and rural households and all the income groups due to the simplicity, convenience, and lower air polluting characteristics. However, the market price of the fuel together with that of its end-use technology may not enhance its early high market penetration especially in the urban low income and rural households.

Briquetting is the formation of a charcoal (an energy-dense solid fuel source) from otherwise wasted agricultural and forestry residues. One of the disadvantages of wood fuel is that it is bulky with a low energy density and is therefore enquire to transport. Briquette formation allows for a more energy-dense fuel to be delivered, thus reducing the transportation cost and making the resource more competitive. It also adds some uniformity, which makes the fuel more compatible with systems that are sensitive to the specific fuel input.

5.1.2. Improved Cook Stoves

Traditional wood stoves can be classified into four types: three stone, metal cylindrical shaped, metal tripod and clay type. Another area in which rural energy availability could be secured where woody fuels have become scarce, are the improvements of traditional cookers and ovens to raise the efficiency of fuel saving. Also, by planting fast growing trees to provide a constant fuel supply. The rural development is essential and economically important since it will eventually lead to better standards of living, people's settlement, and self sufficient in the following:

- Food and water supplies.
- Better services in education and health care.
- Good communication modes.

5.1.3. Biogas

Biogas technology cannot only provide fuel, but is also important for comprehensive utilisation of biomass forestry, animal husbandry, fishery, agricultural economy, protecting the environment, realising agricultural recycling, as well as improving the sanitary conditions, in rural areas. The introduction of biogas technology on wide scale has implications for macro planning such as the allocation of government investment and effects on the balance of payments. Factors that determine the rate of acceptance of biogas plants, such as credit facilities and technical backup services, are likely to have to be planned as part of general macro-policy, as do the allocation of research and development funds [14].

Biogas is a generic term for gases generated from the decomposition of organic material. As the material breaks down, methane (CH_4) is produced as shown in **Figure 3**. Sources that generate biogas are numerous and varied. These include landfill sites, wastewater treatment plants and anaerobic digesters. Landfills and wastewater treatment plants emit biogas from decaying waste. To

date, the waste industry has focused on controlling these emissions to our environment and in some cases, tapping this potential source of fuel to power gas turbines, thus generating electricity. The primary components of landfill gas are methane (CH_4), carbon dioxide (CO_2), and nitrogen (N_2). The average concentration of methane is ~45%, CO_2 is ~36% and nitrogen is ~18%. Other components in the gas are oxygen (O_2), water vapour and trace amounts of a wide range of non-methane organic compounds (NMOCs).

For hot water and heating, renewables contributions come from biomass power and heat, geothermal direct heat, ground source heat pumps, and rooftop solar hot water and space heating systems. Solar assisted cooling makes a very small but growing contribution. When it comes to the installation of large amounts of PV, the cities have several important factors in common. These factors include:

- A strong local political commitment to the environment and sustainability.
- The presence of municipal departments or offices dedicated to the environment, sustainability or renewable energy.
- Information provision about the possibilities of renewables.
- Obligations that some or all buildings include renewable energy.

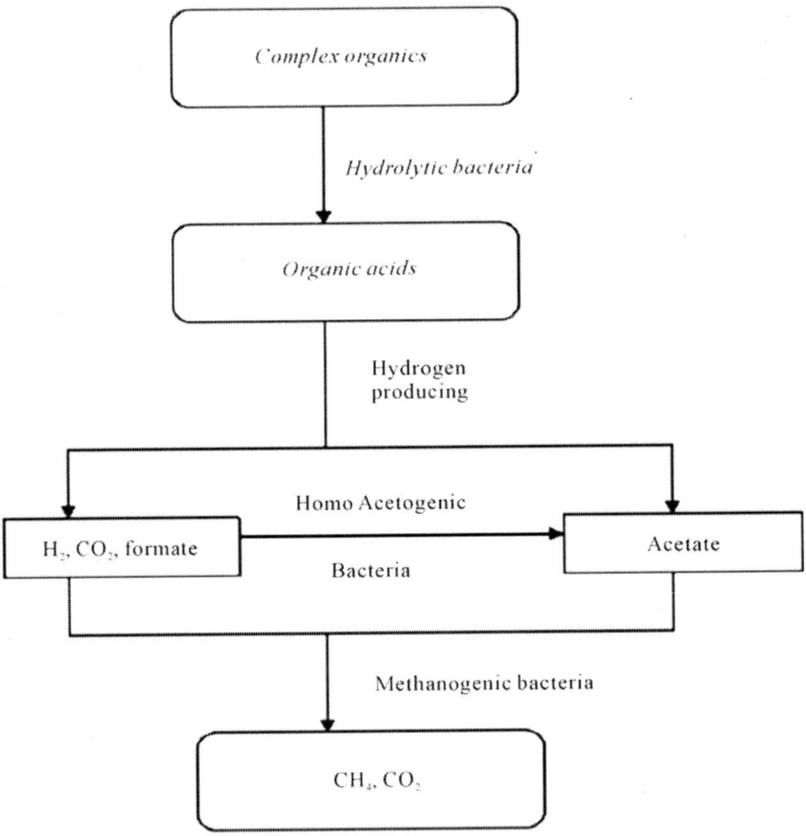

Figure 3. Biogas production process [15].

5.1.4. Improved Forest and Tree Management

Dry cell batteries are a practical but expensive form of mobile fuel that is used by rural people when moving around at night and for powering radios and other small appliances. The high cost of dry cell batteries is financially constraining for rural households, but their popularity gives a good indication of how valuable a versatile fuel like electricity is in rural area. Dry cell batteries can constitute an environmental hazard unless they are recycled in a proper fashion. Direct burning of fuel-wood and crop residues constitute the main usage of biomass, as is the case with many developing countries. However, the direct burning of biomass in an inefficient manner causes economic loss and adversely affects human health. In order to address the problem of inefficiency, research centres around the world have investigated the viability of converting the resource to a more useful form, namely solid briquettes and fuel gas (**Figure 4**). Biomass resources play a significant role in energy supply in all developing countries. Biomass resources should be divided into residues or dedicated resources, the latter including firewood and charcoal can also be produced from forest residues (**Table 12**).

Implementing measures for energy efficiency increase at the demand side and in the energy transformation sector. It is common practice to dispose of this waste wood in landfill where it slowly degraded and takes up valuable void space. This wood is a good source of energy and is an alternative to energy crops. Agricultural wastes are abundantly available globally and can be converted to energy and useful chemicals by a number of microorganisms. The success of promoting any technology depends on careful planning, management, implementation, training and monitoring. Main features of gasification project are:

- Networking and institutional development/strengthening.
- Promotion and extension.
- Construction of demonstration projects.
- Research and development, and training and monitoring.

Table 12. Biomass residues and current use [16].

Type of residue	Current use
Wood industry waste	Residues available
Vegetable crop residues	Animal feed
Food processing residue	Energy needs
Sorghum, millet, and wheat residues	Fodder, and building materials
Groundnut shells	Fodder, brick making, and direct fining oil mills
Cotton stalks	Domestic fuel considerable amounts available for short period
Sugar, bagasse, and molasses	Fodder, energy need, and ethanol production (surplus available)
Manure	Fertiliser, brick making, and plastering

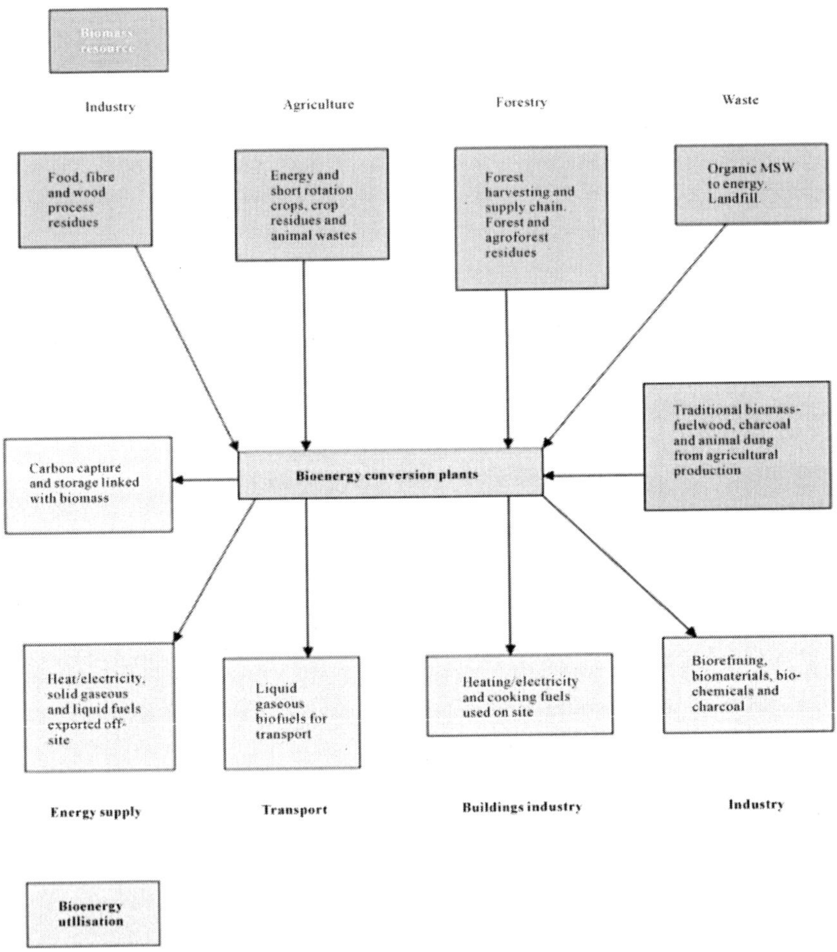

Figure 4. Biomass resources from several sources are converted into a range of products for use by transport, industry and building sectors [15].

5.1.5. Gasification

Gasification is based on the formation of a fuel gas (mostly CO and H_2) by partially oxidising raw solid fuel at high temperatures in the presence of steam or air. The technology can use wood chips, groundnut shells, sugar cane bagasse, and other similar fuels to generate capacities from 3 kW to 100 kW. Three types of gasifier designs have been developed to make use of the diversity of fuel inputs and to meet the requirements of the product gas output (degree of cleanliness, composition, heating value, etc.). The requirements of gas for various purposes, and a comparison between biogas and various commercial fuels in terms of calorific value, and thermal efficiency are presented in **Table 13**.

Sewage sludge is rich in nutrients such as nitrogen and phosphorous. It also contains valuable organic matter, useful for remediation of depleted or eroded soils. This is why untreated sludge has been used for many years as a soil fertiliser and for enhancing the organic matter of soil. A key concern is that treatment of sludge tends to concentrate heavy metals, poorly biodegradable trace organic compounds and potentially pathogenic organisms (viruses, bacteria and the like) present in wastewaters. These materials can pose a serious threat to the environment. When deposited in soils, heavy metals are passed through the food chain, first entering crops, and then animals that feed on the crops and eventually human beings, to whom they appear to be highly toxic. In addition they also leach from soils, getting into groundwater and further spreading contamination in an uncontrolled manner.

European and American markets aiming to transform various organic wastes (animal farm wastes, industrial and municipal wastes) into two main by-products:

- A solution of humic substances (a liquid oxidate).
- A solid residue.

Agricultural wastes are abundantly available globally and can be converted to energy and useful chemicals by a number of microorganisms. The organic matter was biodegradable to produce biogas and the variation show a normal methanogene bacteria activity and good working biological process as shown in Figures 5-7. The success of promoting any technology depends on careful planning, management, implementation, training and monitoring. Main features of gasification project are:

- Networking and institutional development/strengthening.

- Promotion and extension.
- Construction of demonstration projects.
- Research and development, and training and monitoring.

Table 13. Comparison of various fuels [16].

Fuel	Calorific value (kcal)	Burning mode	Thermal efficiency (%)
Electricity, kWh	880	Hot plate	70
Coal gas, kg	4004	Standard burner	60
Biogas, m^3	5373	Standard burner	60
Kerosene, l	9122	Pressure stove	50
Charcoal, kg	6930	Open stove	28
Soft coke, kg	6292	Open stove	28
Firewood, kg	3821	Open stove	17
Cow dung, kg	2092	Open stove	11

Biomass is a raw material that has been utilised for a wide variety of tasks since the dawn of civilisation. Important as a supply of fuel in the third world, biomass was also the first raw material in the production of textiles. The gasification of the carbon char with steam can make a large difference to the surface area of the carbon.

The corresponding stream gasification reactions are endothermic and demonstrate how the steam reacts with the carbon char [17].

$H_2O(g) + C_x(s) \rightarrow H_2(g) + CO(g) + C_{x-1}(s)$(2)

$CO(g) + H_2O(g) \rightarrow CO_2(g) + H_2(g)$(3)

$CO_2(g) + C_x(s) \rightarrow 2CO(g) + C_{x-1}(s)$(4)

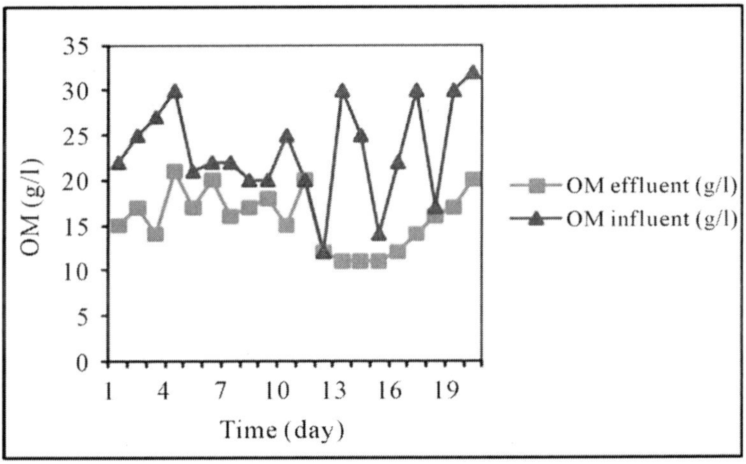

Figure 5. Organic matters before and after treatment in digester [18].

The encouragement of greater energy use is an essential component of development. In the short term it requires mechanisms to enable the rapid increase in energy/capita, and in the long term we should be working towards a way of life, which makes use of energy efficiency and without the impairment of the environment or of causing safety problems. Such a programme should as far as possible be based on renewable energy resources.

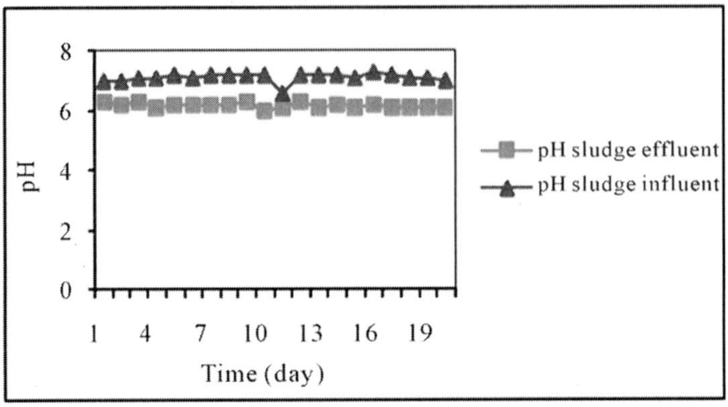

Figure 6. pH sludge before and after treatment in the digester [18].

The sources to alleviate the energy situation in the world are sufficient to supply all foreseeable needs. Conservation of energy and rationing in some form will however have to be practised by most countries, to reduce oil imports and redress balance of payments positions. Meanwhile development and application of nuclear power and some of the traditional solar, wind and water energy alternatives must be set in hand to supplement what remains of the fossil fuels.

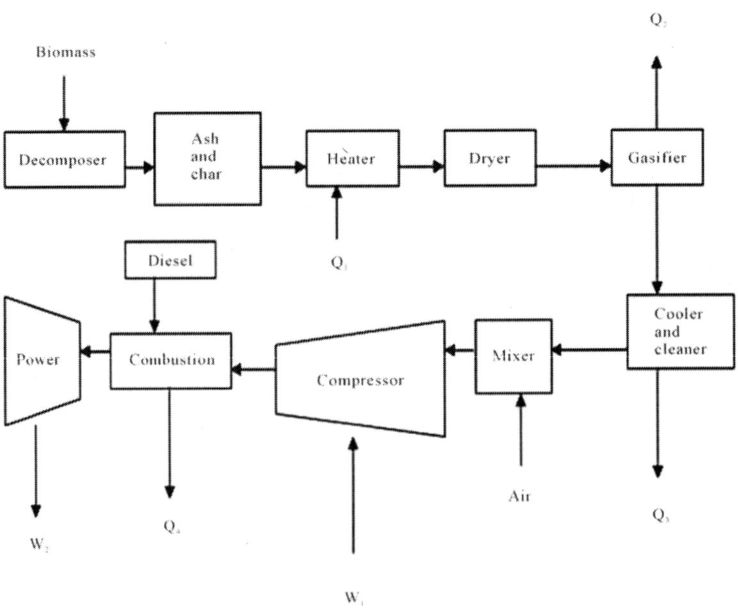

Figure 7. Advanced biomass power with diesel engine [19].

6. BIOHEAT

Bioenergy is a growing source of power that is playing an ever-increasing role in the provision of electricity. The potential contribution of the waste industry to bioenergy is huge and has the ability to account for a source of large amount of total bioenergy production. Woody biomass is usually converted into power through combustion or gasification. Biomass can be specially grown in the case of energy crops. Waste wood makes up a significant proportion of a variety of municipal, commercial and industrial waste streams. It is common practice to dispose of this waste wood in landfill where it slowly degraded and takes up valuable void space. This wood is a good source of energy and is an alternative to energy crops.

The biomass directly produced by cultivation can be transformed by different processes into gaseous, liquid or solid fuels (**Table 14**). The whole process of production of methyl or ethyl esters (biodiesel) is summarised in Figures 8 and 9.

6.1. Waste Policy in Context

In terms of solid waste management policy, many NGOs have changed drastically in the past ten years from a mass production and mass consumption society to "material-cycle society". In addition to national legislation, municipalities are legally obliged to develop a plan for handling the municipal solid waste (MSW) generated in administrative areas. Such plans contain:

- Estimates of future waste volume.
- Measures to reduce waste.
- Measures to encourage source separation.
- A framework for solid waste disposal and the construction and management of solid waste management facilities.

Landfilling is in the least referred tier of the hierarchy of waste management options: Waste minimisation, reuse and recycling, incineration with energy recovery, and optimised final disposal. The key elements are as follows: construction impacts, atmospheric emissions, noise, water quality, landscape, visual impacts, socio economics, ecological impacts, traffic, solid waste disposal and cultural heritage.

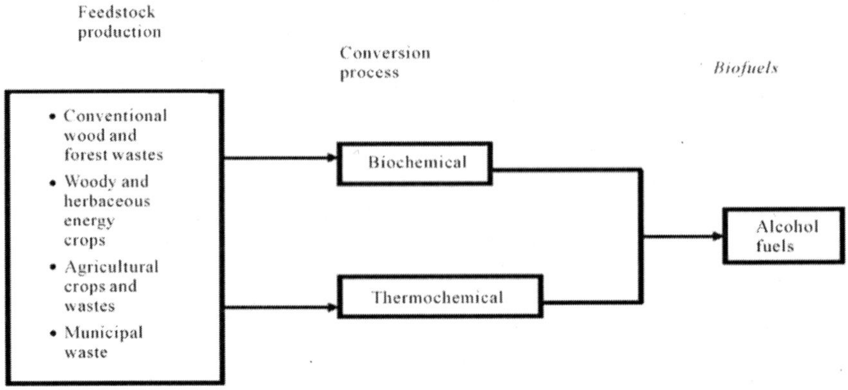

Figure 8. Biofuel pathways for renewable alcohol fuels [19].

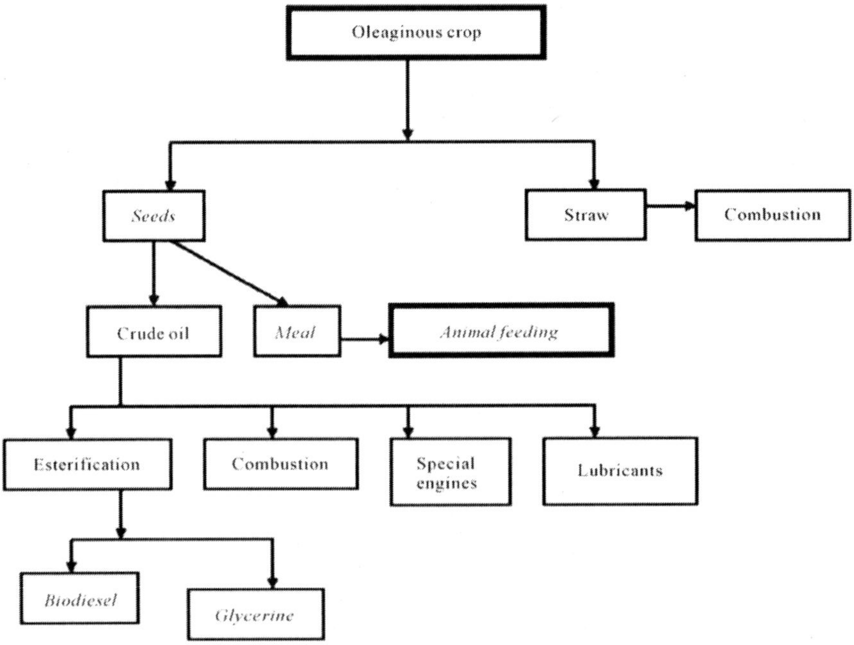

Figure 9. Flow chart of biodiesel production [20].

Table 14. Biomass conversions to energy [20].

Feedstock	Crops	Conversion process	End product
Wood-cellulosic biomass	Short rotation forest (poplar, willow), plant species (sorghum, mischantus, etc.), fibre-crops (cynara, kenaf, etc.)	Direct combustion Gasification Pyrolysis	Heat Methane Hydrogen Oil
Vegetable oils	Oleaginous crops (rapeseed, soybean, sunflower, etc.)	Direct combustion Esterification	Heat Biodiesel
Sugar/starch	Cereals, root and tuber crops, grape, topinambour, etc.	Fermentation	Ethanol

6.2. Energy from Agricultural Biomass

The main advantages are related to energy, agriculture and environment problems, are foreseeable both at regional level and at worldwide level and can be summarised as follows:

- Reduction of dependence on import of energy and related products.
- Reduction of environmental impact of energy production (greenhouse effect, air pollution, and waste degradation).
- Substitution of food crops and reduction of food surpluses and of related economic burdens.
- Utilisation of marginal lands and of set aside lands and reduction of related socio-economic and environmental problems (soil erosion, urbanisation, landscape deterioration, etc.).
- Development of new know-how and production of technological innovation.

A study [21] individuated on the basis of botanical, genetical, physiological, biochemical, agronomical and technological knowledge reported in literature some 150 species potentially exploitable divided as reported in **Table 15**.

7. ROLE OF CHEMICAL ENGINEERING

Turning to chemical engineering and the experience of the chemical process industry represents a wakening up but does not lead to an immediate solution to the problems. The traditional techniques are not very kind to biological products, which are controlled by difficulty and unique physico-chemical properties such as low mechanical, thermal and chemical stabilities. There is the question of selectivity. The fermentation broths resulting from microbial growth contain a bewildering mixture of many compounds closely related to the product of interests. By the standards of the process streams in chemical industry, fermenter is highly impure and extremely dilutes aqueous systems (**Table 16**).

The disadvantages of the fermentation media are as the following: mechanically fragile, temperature sensitive, rapidly deteriorating quality, harmful if escaping into the environment, corrosive (acids, chlorides, etc.), and troublesome (solids, theological, etc.), and expensive.

Thus, pilot plants for scale-up work must be flexible. In general, they should contain suitably interconnected equipment for: fermentation, primary separation, cell disruption fractionalises and clarifications, purification by means of high-resolution techniques and concentration and dry. The effects of the chlorofluorocarbons (CFCs) molecule can last for over a century.

Table 15. Plant species potentially exploitable for production of agricultural biomass for energy or industrial utilisations [21].

Groups of plants	Number of species
Plants cultivated for food purposes that can be reconverted to new uses	9
Plants cultivated in the past, but not in culture any more	46
Plants cultivated in other world areas	46
Wild species, both indigenous and exotic	47
Total	148

Plant product	Number of species
Biomass	8
Sugars and polysaccharides	38
Cellulose	17
Hydrocarbons	3
Polymeric hydrocarbons	5
Gums and resins	12
Tannins and phenolic compounds	3
Waxes	7
Vegetable oils	38
Total	131

Table 16. Typical product concentrations exiting fermenters [22].

Product	Concentration (kg/m^3)
Ethanol	70 - 120
Organic acids (e.g.. citric)	40 - 100
Vitamin B12	0.02
Interferon	50 - 70
Single-cell protein	30 - 50
Antibiotics (e.g.. Penicillin G)	10 - 30
Enzyme protein (e.g.. protease)	2 - 5

7.1. Fluidised Bed Drying

An important consideration for operators of wastewater treatment plants is how to handle the disposal of the residual sludge in a reliable, sustainable, legal and economical way. The benefits of drying sludge can be seen in two main treatment options:

- Use of the dewatered sludge as a fertiliser or in fertiliser blends.
- Incineration with energy recovery.

Use as a fertiliser takes advantage of the high organic content 40% - 70% of the dewatered sludge and its high levels of phosphorous and other nutrients. However, there are a number of concerns about this route including:

- The chemical composition of the sludge (e.g., heavy metals, hormones and other pharmaceutical residues).
- Pathogen risk (e.g., SALMOELLA, ESCHERICHIA COLI, prionic proteins, etc.).
- Potential accumulation of heavy metals and other chemicals in the soil.
- Sludge can be applied as a fertiliser in three forms: liquid sludge, wet cake blended into compost, and dried granules.
- The advantages of energy recovery sludge include:
- The use of dewatered sludge is a "sink" for pollutants such as heavy metals, toxic organic compounds and pharmaceutical residues. Thus,

offering a potential disposal route for these substances provided the combustion plant has adequate flue gas cleaning.

- The potential, under certain circumstances, to utilise the inorganic residue from sludge incineration (incinerator ash), such as in cement or gravel.
- The high calorific value (similar to lignite) of dewatered sludge.
- The use of dewatered sludge as a carbon dioxide neutral substitute for primary fuels such as oil, gas and coal.

7.2. Energy Efficiency

Energy efficiency is the most cost-effective way of cutting carbon dioxide emissions and improvements to households and businesses. It can also have many other additional social, economic and health benefits, such as warmer and healthier homes, lower fuel bills and company running costs and, indirectly, jobs. Britain wastes 20 per cent of its fossil fuel and electricity use in transportation. This implies that it would be cost-effective to cut £10 billion a year off the collective fuel bill and reduce CO_2 emissions by some 120 million tons CO_2. Yet, due to lack of good information and advice on energy saving, along with the capital to finance energy efficiency improvements, this huge potential for reducing energy demand is not being realised. Traditionally, energy utilities have been essentially fuel providers and the industry has pursued profits from increased volume of sales. Institutional and market arrangements have favoured energy consumption rather than conservation. However, energy is at the centre of the sustainable development paradigm as few activities affect the environment as much as the continually increasing use of energy. Most of the used energy depends on finite resources, such as coal, oil, gas and uranium. In addition, more than three quarters of the world's consumption of these fuels is used, often inefficiently, by only one quarter of the world's population. Without even addressing these inequities or the precious, finite nature of these resources, the scale of environmental damage will force the reduction of the usage of these fuels long before they run out.

Throughout the energy generation process there are impacts on the environment on local, national and international levels, from opencast mining and oil exploration to emissions of the potent greenhouse gas carbon dioxide in ever increasing concentration. Recently, the world's leading climate scientists reached an agreement that human activities, such as burning fossil fuels for energy and transport, are causing the world's temperature to rise. The Intergovernmental Panel on Climate Change has concluded that "the balance of evidence suggests a discernible human influence on global climate''. It predicts a rate of warming greater than any one seen in the last 10,000 years, in other words, throughout human history. The exact impact of climate change is difficult to predict and will vary regionally. It could, however, include sea level rise, disrupted agriculture and food supplies and the possibility of more freak weather events such as hurricanes and droughts. Indeed, people already are waking up to the financial and social, as well as the environmental, risks of unsustainable energy generation methods that represent the costs of the impacts of climate change, acid rain and oil spills. The insurance industry, for example, concerned about the billion dollar costs of hurricanes and floods, has joined sides with environmentalists to lobby for greenhouse gas emissions reduction. Friends of the earth are campaigning for a more sustainable energy policy, guided by the principal of environmental protection and with the objectives of sound natural resource management and long-term energy security. The key priorities of such an energy policy must be to reduce fossil fuel use, move away from nuclear power, improve the efficiency with which energy is used and increase the amount of energy obtainable from sustainable, renewable sources. Efficient energy use has never been more crucial than it is today, particularly with the prospect of the imminent introduction of the climate change levy (CCL). Establishing an energy use action plan is the essential foundation to the elimination of energy waste. A logical starting point is to carry out an energy audit that enables the assessment of the energy use and determine what actions to take. The actions are best categorised by splitting measures into the following three general groups:

1) High priority/low cost:

These are normally measures, which require minimal investment and can be implemented quickly. The followings are some examples of such measures:

- Good housekeeping, monitoring energy use and targeting waste-fuel practices.
- Adjusting controls to match requirements.
- Improved greenhouse space utilisation.
- Small capital item time switches, thermostats, etc.
- Carrying out minor maintenance and repairs.
- Staff education and training.
- Ensuring that energy is being purchased through the most suitable tariff or contract arrangements.

2) Medium priority/medium cost:

Measures, which, although involve little or no design, involve greater expenditure and can take longer to implement. Examples of such measures are listed below:

- New or replacement controls.
- Greenhouse component alteration, e.g., insulation, sealing glass joints, etc.
- Alternative equipment components, e.g., energy efficient lamps in light fittings, etc.

3) Long term/high cost:

These measures require detailed study and design. They can be best represented by the followings:

- Replacing or upgrading of plant and equipment.
- Fundamental redesign of systems, e.g., CHP installations.

This process can often be a complex experience and therefore the most cost-effective approach is to employ an energy specialist to help.

7.3. Policy Recommendations for a Sustainable Energy Future

Sustainability is regarded as a major consideration for both urban and rural development. People have been exploiting the natural resources with no consideration to the effects, both short-term (environmental) and longterm (resources crunch). It is also felt that knowledge and technology have not been used effectively in utilising energy resources. Energy is the vital input for economic and social development of any country. Its sustainability is an important factor to be considered. The urban areas depend, to a large extent, on commercial energy sources. The rural areas use non-commercial sources like firewood and agricultural wastes. With the present day trends for improving the quality of life and sustenance of mankind, environmental issues are considered highly important. In this context, the term energy loss has no significant technical meaning. Instead, the exergy loss has to be considered, as destruction of exergy is possible. Hence, exergy loss minimisation will help in sustainability. In the process of developing, there are two options to manage energy resources: 1) End use matching/demand side management, which focuses on the utilities. The mode of obtaining this is decided based on economic terms. It is, therefore, a quantitative approach. 2) Supply side management, which focuses on the renewable energy resource and methods of utilising it. This is decided based on thermodynamic consideration having the resource-user temperature or exergy destruction as the objective criteria. It is, therefore, a qualitative approach. The two options are explained schematically in **Figure 10**. The exergy-based energy, developed with supply side perspective is shown in **Figure 11**. The following policy measures had been identified:

- Clear environmental and social objectives for energy market liberalisation, including a commitment to energy efficiency and renewables.
- Economic, institutional and regulatory frameworks, which encourage the transition to total energy services.
- Economic measures to encourage utility investment in energy efficiency (e.g., levies on fuel bills).
- Incentives for demand side management, including grants for low-income households, expert advice and training, standards for appliances and buildings and tax incentives.
- Research and development funding for renewable energy technologies not yet commercially viable.
- Continued institutional support for new renewables (such as standard cost-reflective payments and obligation on utilities to buy).
- Ecological tax reform to internalise external environmental and social costs within energy prices.
- Planning for sensitive development and public acceptability for renewable energy.

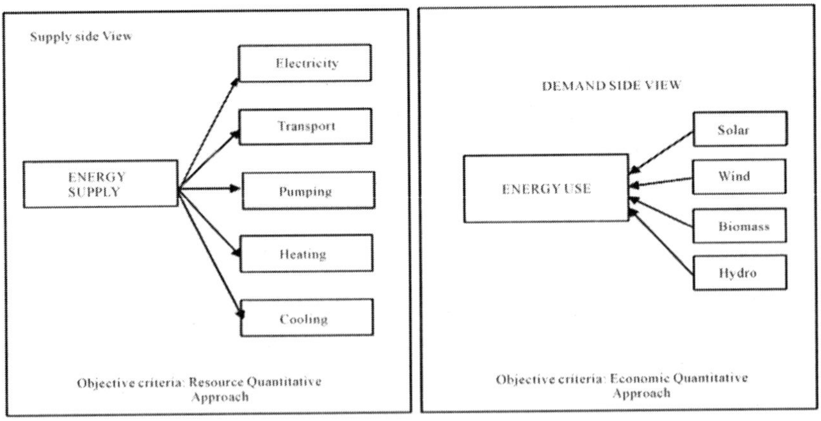

Figure 10. Supply side and demand side management approach for energy [23].

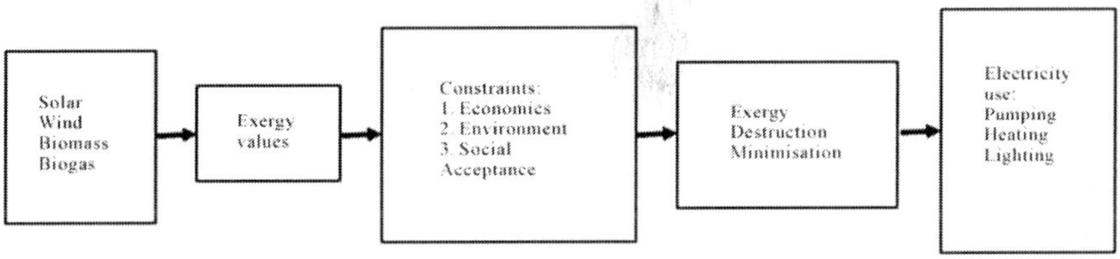

Figure 11. Exergy based optimal energy model [24].

Energy resources are needed for societal development. Their sustainable development requires a supply of energy resources that are sustainably available at a reasonable cost and can cause no negative societal impacts. Energy resources such as fossil fuels are finite and lack sustainability, while renewable energy sources are sustainable over a relatively longer term. Environmental concerns are also a major factor in sustainable development, as activities, which degrade the environment, are not sustainable. Hence, as much as environmental impact is associated with energy, sustainable development requires the use of energy resources, which cause as little environmental impact as possible. One way to reduce the resource depletion associated with cycling is to reduce the losses that accompany the transfer of exergy to consume resources by increasing the efficiency of exergy transfer between resources, i.e., increasing the fraction of exergy removed from one resource that is transferred to another [24].

As explained above, exergy efficiency may be thought of as a more accurate measure of energy efficiency that accounts for quantity and quality aspects of energy flows. Improved exergy efficiency leads to reduced exergy losses. Most efficiency improvements produce direct environmental benefits in two ways. First, operating energy input requirements are reduced per unit output, and pollutants generated are correspondingly reduced. Second, consideration of the entire life cycle for energy resources and technologies suggests that improved efficiency reduces environmental impact during most stages of the life cycle. Quite often, the main concept of sustainability, which often inspires local and national authorities to incorporate environmental consideration into setting up energy programmes have different meanings in different contexts though it usually embodies a long-term perspective. Future energy systems will largely be shaped by broad and powerful trends that have their roots in basic human needs. Combined with increasing world population, the need will become more apparent for successful implementation of sustainable development.

Heat has a lower exergy, or quality of energy, compared with work. Therefore, heat cannot be converted into work by 100% efficiency. Some examples of the difference between energy and exergy are shown in Table 17.

The terms used in **Table 17** have the following meanings:

Carnot Quality Factor (CQF) = $(1 - T_o/T_s)$(5)

Exergy = Energy (transferred) × CQF(6)

where T_o is the environment temperature (K) and T_s is the temperature of the stream (K).

Various parameters are essential to achieving sustainable development in a society. Some of them are as follows:

- Public awareness.
- Information.
- Environmental education and training.
- Innovative energy strategies.
- Renewable energy sources and cleaner technologies.
- Financing.
- Monitoring and evaluation tools.

The development of a renewable energy in a country depends on many factors. Those important to success are listed below:

1) Motivation of the population The population should be motivated towards awareness of high environmental issues, rational use of energy in order to reduce cost. Subsidy programme should be implemented as incentives to install biomass energy plants. In addition, image campaigns to raise awareness of renewable technology.

2) Technical product development To achieve technical development of biomass energy technologies the following should be addressed:

- Increasing the longevity and reliability of renewable technology.
- Adapting renewable technology to household technology (hot water supply).
- Integration of renewable technology in heating technology.
- Integration of renewable technology in architecture, e.g., in the roof or façade.
- Development of new applications, e.g., solar cooling.

- Cost reduction.

3) Distribution and sales Commercialisation of biomass energy technology requires:

- Inclusion of renewable technology in the product range of heating trades at all levels of the distribution process (wholesale, and retail).
- Building distribution nets for renewable technology.
- Training of personnel in distribution and sales, training of field sales force.

4) Consumer consultation and installation To encourage all sectors of the population to participate in adoption of biomass energy technologies, the following has to be realised:

- Acceptance by craftspeople, marketing by them.
- Technical training of craftspeople, initial and followup training programmes.
- Sales training for craftspeople.
- Information material to be made available to craftspeople for consumer consultation.

5) Projecting and planning Successful application of biomass technologies also require:

- Acceptance by decision makers in the building sector (architects, house technology planners, etc.).
- Integration of renewable technology in training.
- Demonstration projects/architecture competitions.
- Biomass energy project developers should prepare to participate in the carbon market by:

    Ensuring that renewable energy projects comply with Kyoto Protocol requirements.

    - Quantifying the expected avoided emissions.
    - Registering the project with the required offices.
    - Contractually allocating the right to this revenue stream.

- Other ecological measures employed on the development include:
    - Simplified building details.
    - Reduced number of materials.
    - Materials that can be recycled or reused.
    - Materials easily maintained and repaired.
    - Materials that do not have a bad influence on the indoor climate (i.e., non-toxic).
    - Local cleaning of grey water.
    - Collecting and use of rainwater for outdoor purposes and park elements.
    - Building volumes designed to give maximum access to neighbouring park areas.
    - All apartments have visual access to both backyard and park.

6) Energy saving measures The following energy saving measures should also be considered:

- Building integrated solar PV system.
- Day-lighting.
- Ecological insulation materials.
- Natural/hybrid ventilation.
- Passive cooling.
- Passive solar heating.
- Solar heating of domestic hot water.
- Utilisation of rainwater for flushing.

Improving access for rural and urban low-income areas in developing countries must be through energy efficiency and renewable energies. Sustainable energy is a prerequisite for development. Energy-based living standards in developing countries, however, are clearly below standards in developed countries. Low levels of access to affordable and environmentally sound energy in both rural and urban low-income areas are therefore a predominant issue in developing countries. In recent years many programmes for development aid or technical assistance have been focusing on improving access to sustainable energy, many of them with impressive results [26].

Table 17. Qualities of various energy sources [25].

Source	Energy (J)	Exergy (J)	CQF
Water at 80°C	100	16	0.16
Steam at 120°C	100	24	0.24
Natural gas	100	99	0.99
Electricity/work	100	100	1.00

Apart from success stories, however, experience also shows that positive appraisals of many projects evaporate after completion and vanishing of the implementation expert team. Altogether, the diffusion of sustainable technologies such as energy efficiency and renewable energies for cooking, heating, lighting, electrical appliances and building insulation in developing countries has been slow [27].

Energy efficiency and renewable energy programmes could be more sustainable and pilot studies more effective and pulse releasing if the entire policy and implementation process was considered and redesigned from the outset. New financing and implementation processes are needed which allow reallocating financial resources and thus enabling countries themselves to achieve a sustainable energy infrastructure. The links between the energy policy framework, financing and implementation of renewable energy and energy efficiency projects have to be strengthened and capacity building efforts are required.

8. CONCLUSIONS

Even with modest assumptions about the availability of land, comprehensive fuel-wood farming programmes offer significant energy, economic and environmental benefits. These benefits would be dispersed in rural areas where they are greatly needed and can serve as linkages for further rural economic development. The nations, as a whole would benefit from savings in foreign exchange, improved energy security, and socio-economic improvements. With a nine-fold increase in forest—plantation cover, the nation's resource base would be greatly improved. The international community would benefit from pollution reduction, climate mitigation, and the increased trading opportunities that arise from new income sources. The aim of any modern biomass energy systems must be:

- To maximise yields with minimum inputs.
- Utilisation and selection of adequate plant materials and processes.
- Optimum use of land, water, and fertiliser.
- Create an adequate infrastructure and strong R and D base.

Furthermore, investigating the potential to make use of more and more of its waste. Household waste, vegetable market waste, and waste from the cotton stalks, leather, and pulp; and paper industries can be used to produce useful energy either by direct incineration, gasification, digestion (biogas production), fermentation, or cogeneration. Therefore, effort has to be made to reduce fossil energy use and to promote green energies, particularly in the building sector. Energy use reductions can be achieved by minimising the energy demand, by rational energy use, by recovering heat and the use of more green energies. This study was a step towards achieving that goal. The adoption of green or sustainable approaches to the way in which society is run is seen as an important strategy in finding a solution to the energy problem. The key factors to reducing and controlling CO_2, which is the major contributor to global warming, are the use of alternative approaches to energy generation and the exploration of how these alternatives are used today and may be used in the future as green energy sources. Even with modest assumptions about the availability of land, comprehensive fuel-wood farming programmes offer significant energy, economic and environmental benefits. These benefits would be dispersed in rural areas where they are greatly needed and can serve as linkages for further rural economic development. The nations as a whole would benefit from savings in foreign exchange, improved energy security, and socio-economic improvements. With a nine-fold increase in forest—plantation cover, a nation's resource base would be greatly improved. The international community would benefit from pollution reduction, climate mitigation, and the increased trading opportunities that arise from new income sources. The non-technical issues, which have recently gained attention, include: 1) Environmental and ecological factors e.g., carbon sequestration, reforestation and revegetation. 2) Renewables as a CO_2 neutral replacement for fossil fuels. 3) Greater recognition of the importance of renewable energy, particularly modern biomass energy carriers, at the policy and planning levels. 4) Greater recognition of the difficulties of gathering good and reliable renewable energy data, and efforts to improve it. 5) Studies on the detrimental health efforts of biomass energy particularly from traditional energy users.

REFERENCES

1 Abdeen, M.O. (2008) Renewable building energy systems and passive human comfort solutions. Renewable and Sustainable Energy Reviews, 12, 1562-1587.

2 Abdeen, M.O. (2008) People, power and pollution. Renewable and Sustainable Energy Reviews, 12, 1864-1889.

3 Abdeen, M.O. (2008) Energy, environment and sustainable development. Renewable and Sustainable Energy Reviews, 12, 2265-2300.

4 Abdeen, M.O. (2008) Focus on low carbon technologies: The positive solution. Renewable and Sustainable Energy Reviews, 12, 2331-2357.

5 Abdeen, M.O. (2008) Chapter 10: Development of integrated bioenergy for improvement of quality of life of poor people in developing countries. In: Magnusson, F.L. and Bengtsson, O.W., Eds., Energy in Europe: Economics, Policy and Strategy, NOVA Science Publishers, New York, 341-373.

6 Abdeen, M.O. (2009) Environmental and socio-economic aspect of possible development in renewable energy use. Proceedings of the 4th International Symposium on Environment, Athens, 21-24 May 2009.

7 Abdeen, M.O. (2009) Energy use, environment and sustainable development. Proceedings of the 3rd International Conference on Sustainable Energy and Environmental Protection (SEEP 2009), Paper No. 1011, Dublin, 12-15 August 2009.

8 Abdeen, M.O. (2009) Energy use and environmental: Impacts: A general review. Journal of Renewable and Sustainable Energy, 1, 1-29.

9 Abdeen, M.O. (2009) Chapter 3: Energy use, environment and sustainable development. In: Mancuso, R.T., Ed., Environmental Cost Management, NOVA Science Publishers, New York, 129-166.

10 Aroyeun, S.O. (2009). Reduction of aflatoxin B1 and Ochratoxin A in cocoa beans infected with Aspergillus via Ergosterol Value. World Review of Science, Technology and Sustainable Development, 6, 75-90.

11 Bacaoui, A., Yaacoubi, A., Dahbi, C., Bennouna, J. and Mazet, A. (1998). Activated carbon production from Moroccan olive wastes-influence of some factors. Environmental Technology, 19, 1203-1212.

12 Barton A.L. (2007). Focus on sustainable development research advances. NOVA Science Publishers Inc., New York, 189-205.

13 Brain, G. and Mark, S. (2007) Garbage in, energy out: Landfill gas opportunities for CHP projects. Cogeneration and On-Site Power, 8, 37-45.

14 D'apote, S.L. (1998) IEA biomass energy analysis and projections. Proceedings of Biomass Energy Conference: Data, Analysis and Trends, Paris, 23-24 March 1998.

15 Erlich, P. (1991) Forward facing up to climate change. In: Wyman, R.C., Ed., Global Climate Change and Life on Earth, Chapman and Hall, London.

16 Hall O. and Scrase J. (1998) Will biomass be the environmentally friendly fuel of the future? Biomass and Bioenergy, 15, 357-367.

17 Jeremy, L. (2005) The energy crisis, global warming and the role of renewables. Energy World Magazine, 8, 21-30.

18 Levine, M. and Hirose, M. (2005) Energy efficiency improvement utilising high technology: An assessment of energy use in industry and buildings. Report and Case Studies, World Energy Council, London.

19 Omer, A.M. and Yemen, F. (2003) Biogas energy technology in Sudan. Renewable Energy, 28, 499-507.

20 Omer, A.M. (2006) Review: Organic waste treatment for power production and energy supply. Cells and Animal Biology, 1, 34-47.

21 Omer, A.M. (2008) Green energies and environment. Renewable and Sustainable Energy Reviews, 12, 1789- 1821.

22 Omer, A.M. (2007) Renewable energy resources for electricity generation in Sudan. Renewable and Sustainable Energy Reviews, 11, 1481-1497.

23 Pernille, M. (2004) Feature: Danish lessons on district heating. Energy Resource Sustainable Management and Environmental, March-April 2004, 16-17.

24 Robinson, G. (2007) Changes in construction waste management. Waste Management World, May-June 2007, 43-49.

25 Rossi, S., Arnone, S., Lai, A., Lapenta, E. and Sonnino, A. (1990) ENEA's activities for developing new crops for energy and industry. In: Grassi, G., Gosse, G. and dos Santos, G., Eds., Biomass for Energy and Industry, 1, Elsevier Applied Science, London and New York, 107-113.

26 Sims, R.H. (2007) Not too late: IPCC identifies renewable energy as a key measure to limit climate change. Renewable Energy World, 10, 31-39.

27 Wu, J. and Boggess, W. (1999). The optimal allocation of conservation funds. Journal of Environmental Economic Management, 38, 302-321.

CHAPTER 3

Forest Change and Its Effect on Biomass in Yok Don National Park in Central Highlands of Vietnam Using Ground Data and Geospatial Techniques

Nguyen Viet Luong[1], Ryutaro Tateishi[2], Nguyen Thanh Hoan[3], To Trong Tu[1]

[1]Space Technology Institute, Vietnam Academy of Science and Technology, Hanoi, Vietnam

[2]Center for Environmental Remote Sensing, Chiba University, Chiba, Japan

[3]Institute of Geography, Vietnam Academy of Science and Technology, Hanoi, Vietnam

ABSTRACT

This paper assesses the changes in forest cover in Yok Don National Park of Vietnam between 2004 and 2010, and the implications of such changes on the biomass stocks of this national park. Remote sensing and GIS tools along with the ground truth data collected from the field were employed for classifying the forest types of the study area from SPOT HRV satellite imagery for years 2004 and 2010. The total area considered in this study is 115.5 thousand ha. Five different categories of forests were identified. The results demonstrated that between 2004 and 2010, the Evergreen broad leaved rich quality forest decreased by 11.2 thousand ha (3.5 Mega tons of biomass) and the Dry open dipterocarps medium quality forest decreased by 15.3 thousand ha (2.5 Mega tons of biomass). In that time period, the Evergreen broad leaved medium quality forest increased by 3.2 thousand ha (0.8 Mega tons of biomass), the Evergreen broad leaved poor quality forest increased by 2.5 thousand ha (0.24 Mega tons of biomass), and the Dry open dipterocarps poor quality forest increased by 3.2 thousand ha (0.69 Mega tons of biomass). Total biomass of the study area decreased by 4.3 Mega tons.

KEYWORDS:

Satellite Data, SPOT HRV, Land Cover Change, Tropical Forest Biomass

1. INTRODUCTION

Nowadays, climate change is no longer a prediction but has become a threat and a serious challenge to humankind globally, including Vietnam. Climate change and its relation to CO_2 emissions are a matter of global concern. Forest ecosystem plays a very important role in the global carbon cycle; the CO_2 from the atmosphere is taken up by vegetation and stored as plant biomass. Biomass is defined as the total amount of aboveground living organic matter in trees expressed as oven-dry tons per unit area [1] and tropical forests hold large stores of carbon [2] . According to FAO (2010), the world's total forest area is just over 4 billion ha and covers 31 percent total land area and estimated store 289 Gt of carbon in their biomass alone. However, carbon stocks in forest biomass decreased by an estimated 0.5 Gt annually during the period 2005-2010, mainly because of a reduction in the global forest area [3]. In Southeast Asia region, total forest cover is estimated at 268 M ha in 1990, dropping to 236 M ha in 2010, with annual change rates of 1.75 M ha (~0.67%) and 1.45 M ha (~0.59%) for the periods 1990-2000 and 2000-2010, respectively [4] .

The quantifying of biomass and carbon sequestration in tropical forests is particularly relevant within the United Nations Framework Convention on Climate Change (UNFCC). Kyoto Protocol recognized the role of forests in carbon stock and pointed out forest as potential carbon storage in Articles 3.3 and 3.4 [5] of The Reducing Emission from Deforestation and Forest Degradation (REDD) program. In the effort towards mitigating global climate change, the initiative of reducing emission from deforestation and forest degradation (REDD) was proposed in COP 13 in Bali, Indonesia in 2007 and this initiative was formally adopted as a measure contributing to climate change mitigation, because, emission of GHGs from land use change, particularly the conversion of forestland to non-forestland, and unsustainable forest management, were claimed to contribute to as much as 20 percent of global GHG emissions [6] . The UN-REDD programs are being carried out in nine countries including Vietnam. Under the REDD mechanism, countries will need to measure and monitor the emissions of CO_2 resulting from deforestation and degradation within their borders. In other words, the countries participating in this program should have a system: "Measurement, Evaluation and Report" system (MRV) [6] . However, the majority of countries do not have time series data on growing stock, so the weaknesses in growing stock trend estimates is also directly translated into biomass [3] .

The remote sensing science and application communities have developed increasingly reliable and consistent [7] . A more comprehensive and reliable approach for estimating biomass change is to combine new field studies with analysis of high resolution remote sensing imagery [1] . The strengths of remote sensing come from its ability to provide spatially explicit information and repeated coverage including the possibility of covering large areas as well as remote areas that are difficult to access otherwise [8] . Remote sensing technologies can provide objective, practical and cost-effective solutions for developing and maintaining REDD+ monitoring systems [9] . Vietnam conducts a national forest survey every five years using optical satellite imagery from SPOT satellites and ground survey data. Hence, forest cover estimation has been periodically assessed. However, estimation of change in biomass due to changes in forest types has not been of research interest despite its importance in the face of climate change and applicability for REDD implementation. Therefore, this research aimed to fulfill an important research gap by estimating quantity and direction of change in forest types and its effects on biomass in tropical forests. The approach used in this study effectively applies ground truth data and geospatial techniques for estimating changes in forests and biomass and has potential to be adopted elsewhere.

2. STUDY AREA

The Yok Don National Park is located Dak Lak province in the Central Highlands, total area is 115.5 thousand ha. It is one of the largest nature conservation areas of Vietnam. The study area lies between; 12°45'N - 13°10'N Latitude and 107°29'E - 107°48'E Longitude (Figure 1). Most of the park lies at ~200 m elevation and the terrain is relatively flat. There are, however, several ranges of low hills within the national park, the highest point of which is the eponymous Mount Yok Don at 482 m in the south-eastern range [10] [11] .

Flora at Yok Don National Park is dominated by species of Dipterocarpaceae family, including Dipterocarpus tuberculatus, Dipterocarpus obtusifolius, Shorea obtuse, etc. However, the Anacardiaceae, Combretaceae, Fabaceae and Myrtaceae families are also well represented. The canopy of this forest type is open, and most trees have thick, fire-resistant bark [12] and tree canopies of predominant deciduous phenology during dry season [13] . Evergreen forests are distributed in higher elevations on the south-east slopes in the national park. These forest types are denser, and are dominated by the species from families as Fagaceae, Euphorbiaceae, Sapindaceae, Ebenaceae and Meliaceae [12] . According to Thin (2007), 854 vascular plant species belongs to 478 genera and 129 families, of which 28 are listed in the Red Data Book of Vietnam, have been recorded in the national park [14].

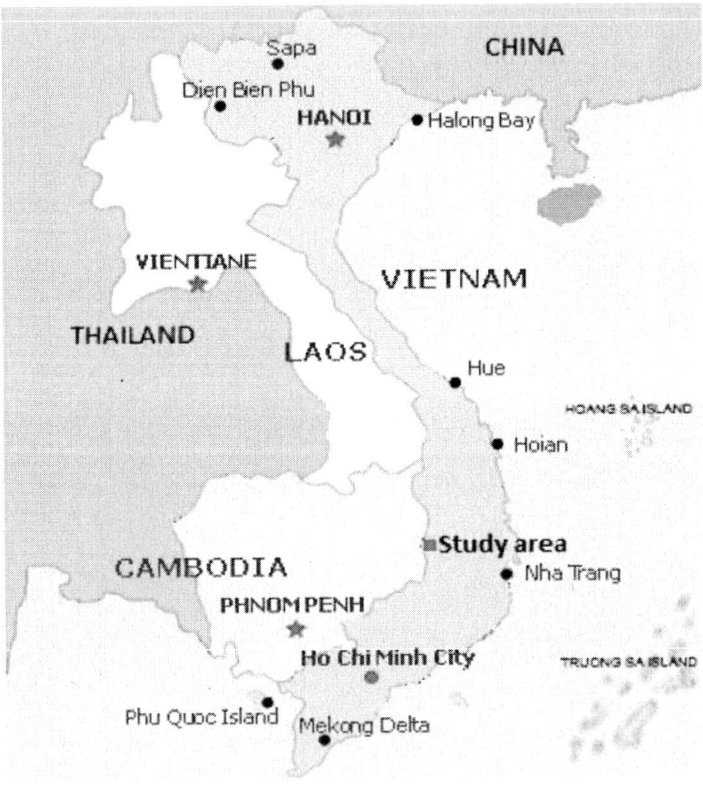

Figure 1. Local map of the study area.

3. DATA AND METHODOLOGY

3.1. Satellite Data

The use of satellite images for the change detection procedures should involve data acquired in the same sensor and also having same spatial resolution, spectral bands and viewing geometry. Especially, seasonal element in the deciduous forest region, because leaf shedding over the course of the dry season [15] . This study has used the SystèmeProbatoire de l'Observation de la Terre (SPOT) satellite data with 10 m spatial resolution SPOT-5 acquired in May 2004 and May 2010. The technical details of the satellite data used in the present study are given in Table 1 and Figure 2.

3.2. Satellite Image Processing

The method of satellite images processing in this study includes: Geometric correction, Image to map rectification by terrain map sheet on scale 1:50,000. Change detection analysis was used the Post classification comparison method (based on supervised classification) was adopted for change analysis.

3.3. Field Work

Fieldwork helps to collect and check most of the ground information required for the mapping purpose (Figure 2). Ground survey data are usually classified to provide estimates of the land cover and its corresponding area, and usually require ground survey data to provide an estimate of the classification accuracy [8] . The reconnaissance field survey was undertaken to get acquainted with the general patterns of vegetation types in the study area. Major vegetation types and few prime localities of characteristic types were recorded. The variation and tonal patterns were observed on existing images. Traverses along all main roads, trail roads inside forest, dry rivers were made for collecting ground truth between maps/images and on the ground. Various features were identified for establishing correlation with image element on FCC image (2010) and terrain map sheet on 1:50,000 scales. Correct GPS locations were obtained for various land cover types and land use categories. Ground truth data collection was conducted twice within the survey duration. Ground truth data were collected during the first survey and again independent samples were collected during second survey for checking the accuracy of the data.

Table 1. Details of satellite data used in the study.

No.	Satellite	Sensor	Date of pass	Total bands	Spectral bands used	Spatial resolution (m)
1	Spot 5	HRV	May 25, 2004	3	1, 2, 3	10
2	Spot 5	HRV	May 15, 2010	3	1, 2, 3	10

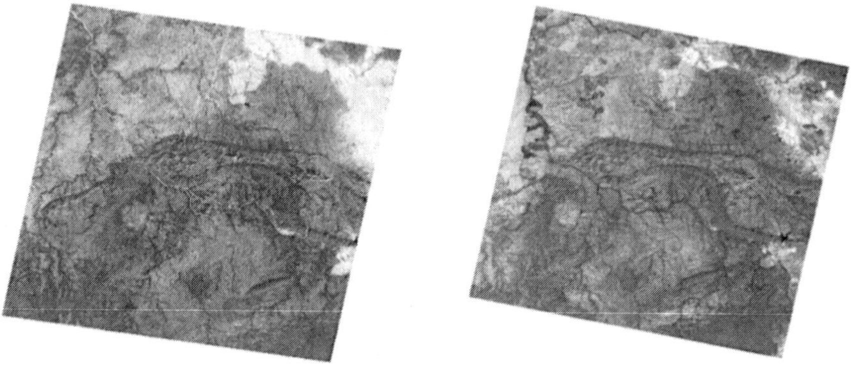

(a) (b)

Figure 2. SPOT HRV False Colour Composite (a) 2004, (b) 2010.

Sample plot establishment and measurement of parameter of structural forest cover based on of guidance of relevant previous research [1] [2] [16] - [19] . The size and shape of the sample plots is a trade-off between accuracy, precision, time, and cost of measurement. The establishment of sample plots needs to meet the following criteria: i) representativeness of the forest types being studied; ii) representativeness for topographic conditions; iii) covering a number of different trees sizes [19] . The most appropriate size and shape may also be dependent on the vegetation type and the type of satellite data used. In this study, a typical sample plot of 500 m^2 (25 m × 20 m) was used for Dry open dipterocarps and 1000 m^2 was used for Evergreen broad-leaved forest. At each sample plot various information on the individual woody trees such as the diameter at breast height (D_{13}) and height of trees and name of tree species (local and scientific names) were recorded.

3.4. Forest Cover Classification

Satellite imagery from SPOT 2004 and SPOT 2010 were employed for image classification. These data came from the same month (May). Therefore the advantage of these data is that they may yield higher accuracy in detecting change between two time periods. This classification schemes allows forest managers to easily identify different land cover types and use for management purpose. This study applied classification system of Trung (1973) [20] , Trung(1978) [21] and the results of the forest and vegetation cover classes mapped of Stibiget al (2004) [16] and was adopted classification criteria of the UNESSCO (1973) [22] for the classification into 2 main classes of forest coverare Evergreen broad leaved forest, Dry open dipterocarps forest and then use the Circular No. 34/TT-BNN [23] issued by Ministry of Agriculture and Rural Development (MARD) of Vietnamese government (2009) for the detailed classification into 6 classes of forest cover with the rich forest comprised a forest with a standing wood volume over 200 m^3/ha, the medium forest with 101 - 200 m^3/ha and the poor forest included the forest with 10 - 100 m^3/ha. Originally the forest in this ecosystem zone was classified in to 6 classes. However, as the results of this investigation, the forest vegetation of the study area has the 5 classes only as 1) Evergreen broad leaved rich forest (EB rich forest), 2) Evergreen broad leaved medium forest (EB medium forest), 3) Evergreen broad leaved poor forest (EB poor forest), 4) Dry open dipterocarps medium forest (DD medium forest) and 5) Dry open dipterocarps poor forest (DD poor forest), because Dry open dipterocarps rich forest does not exist in the study area.

Additionally, other land cover categories may be identified [22] as 6) Another land cover (mainly composed of woody tree from 0.5 to 5 m tall); scrubland, (most of the individual shrubs not touching each other, often with a grass stratum); Thicket (individual shrubs interlocked and barreland) and 7) Water body.

Stibiget al. (2004) [13], Trung (1973, 1978) [20] [21] and UNESSCO (1973) [22]	**Circular No. 34/TT-BNN issued by MARD (2009) [23]**
	1. EB rich forest
Evergreen broad-leaved forest (EB forest)	2. EB medium forest
	3. EB poor forest
	4. DD medium forest
Dry open Dipterocarps (DD forest)	5. DD poor forest
Another land cover	6. *Another land cover*
Water body	7. *Water body*

3.5. Method for Determining Forest Biomass

Above-ground biomass and changes can be derived in two ways [2] [24] , namely, i) directly by measuring sample tree attributes in the field, such as diameters and heights, and applying, species-specific allometric equations. (ii) indirectly by transforming available volume data from forest inventories.This study applied first way and the allometric equation developed for the estimate of above ground biomass of Evergreen broad-leaved and Dry open dipterocarps forest. These allometric equations for estimating biomass (correlation model) were developed by the UN-REDD program in 2012 [25] for the Highlands of Vietnam. The optimal equations for biomass estimation at tree level:

For Evergreen broad leaved forests, the optimal model for biomass estimation is:

$AGB = 0.0530*(D^2*H^{0.7})^{1.0072}$ (1)

For Dry open dipterocarps, the optimal model for biomass estimation is:

$AGB = 0.0154*(D^2*H^{0.7})^{1.1682}$ (2)

where:

AGB—Above ground tree biomass;

D—Diameter at breast height of tree;

H—Height of tree stand.

4. RESULTS

4.1. The Parameter of Structure and Biomass of Forest Cover

This study focuses on the current state of large biomass vegetation. The results from the sample plots were used to calculate the parameters of structure and biomass of forest cover at Yok Don National Park for the current state of five forest cover types include Evergreen broad-leaved rich forest (EB rich forest); Evergreen broad- leaved medium forest (EB medium forest); Evergreen broad-leaved poor forest (EB poor forest); Dry open dipterocarps medium forest (DD medium forest) and Dry open dipterocarps poor forest (DD poor forest). The parameters of structure of forest cover include the diameter of breast height at 1.3 m position ($D_{1.3} > 5$ cm), height at from bottom to top of wood tree (H_{vn}), height of wood tree under branch (H_{dc}), density of wood tree/ha (N/ha). The results are shown in Table 2 and Figure 3.

4.2. Land Cover Map of 2004

Land cover map based on supervised classification of SPOT 2004 is shown in Figure 4 and area analysis of land cover is shown in Histogram 1. The EB rich forest 23.7 thousand ha (20.53%), EB medium forest area is 21.2

thousand ha (18.35%), EB poor forest area is 9.3 thousand ha (8.03%), DD medium forest area is 53.2 thousand ha (46.05%), DD poor forest area is 7.2 thousand ha (6.21%), Another land cover area is 297 ha (0.26%) and Water body area is 676 thousand ha (0.59%).

Table 2. The parameters of the structure and biomass of forest cover.

No.	Class	$D_{1.3}$ (cm)	H_{vn} (m)	H_{dc} (m)	N/ha (tree)	Biomass (tons/ha)
1	EB rich forest	30.69	17.3	9.55	503	318.38
2	EB medium forest	26.6	12.07	8.61	545	249.98
3	EB poor forest	18.44	10.71	4.23	409	101.06
4	DD medium forest	21.98	13.09	8.08	615	163.87
5	DD poor forest	15.11	8.42	4.45	831	54.79

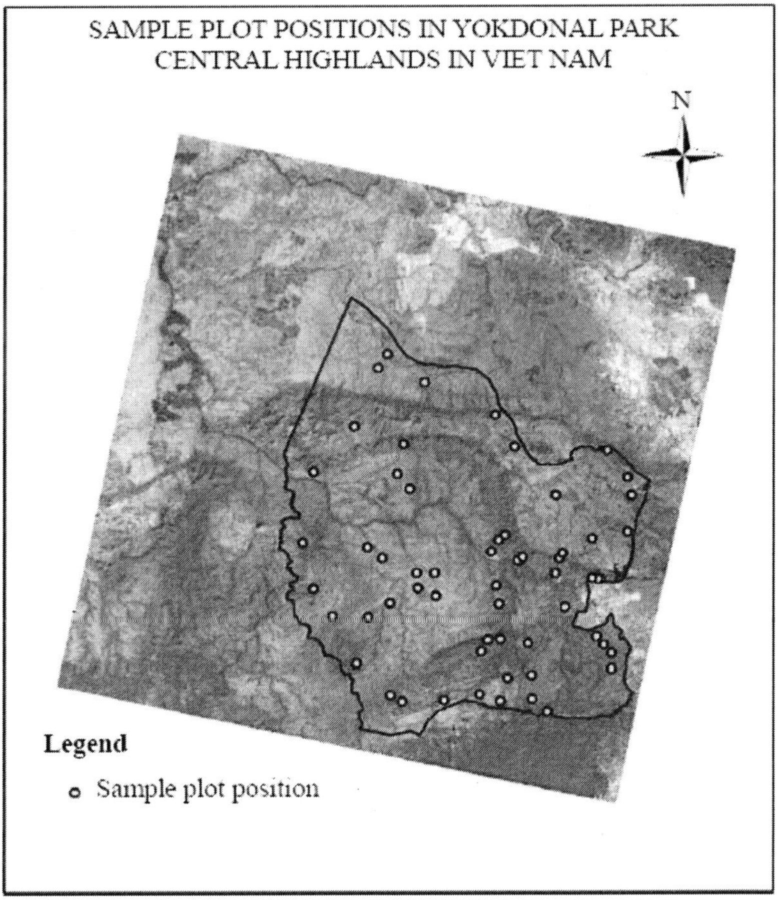

Figure 3. Sample plot positions in Yok Don National Park.

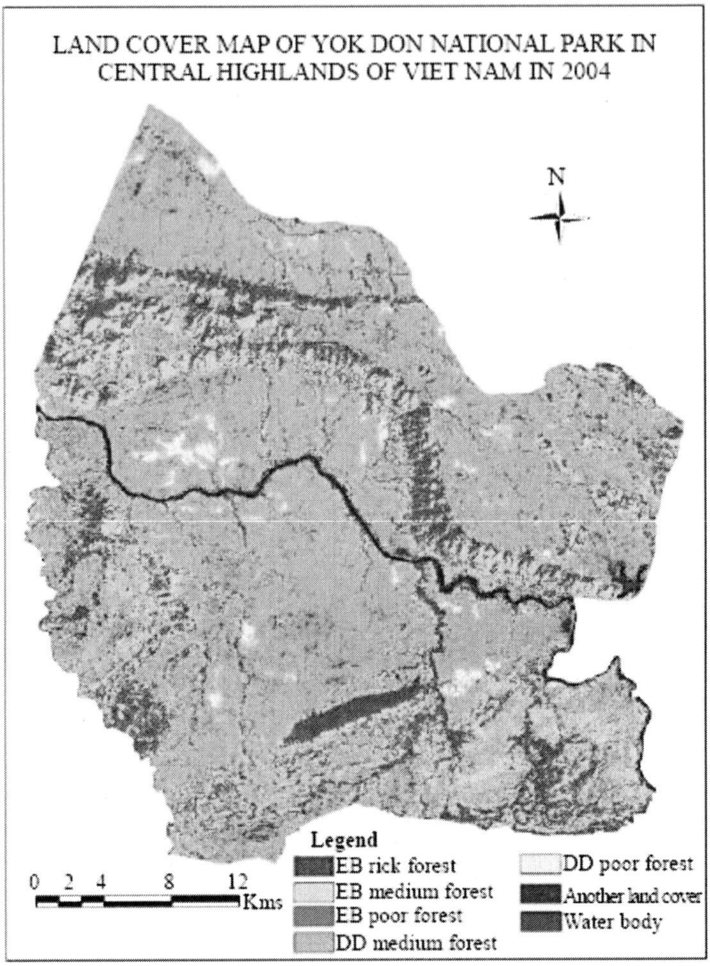

Figure 4. Land cover map in 2004.

The results of the assessment accuracy of the forest cover map of year 2004 are:84.3% as overall accuracy, 86.7% as producer accuracy and 84.3% as user accuracy.

4.3. Land Cover Area of 2010

The land cover map based on supervised classification for 2010 is shown in Figure 5 and the area statistics for land cover of 2010 is shown in Histogram 1. The EB rich forest area is 12.5 thousand ha (10.85%), EB medium forest area is 24.4 thousand ha (21.12%), EB poor forest area is 11.7 thousand ha (10.16%), DD medium forest area is 37.9 thousand ha (32.77%), DD poor forest area is 19.9 thousand ha (17.19%), Another land cover area is 6.2 thousand ha (5.9%) and Water body area is 2.9 thousand ha (2.55%).

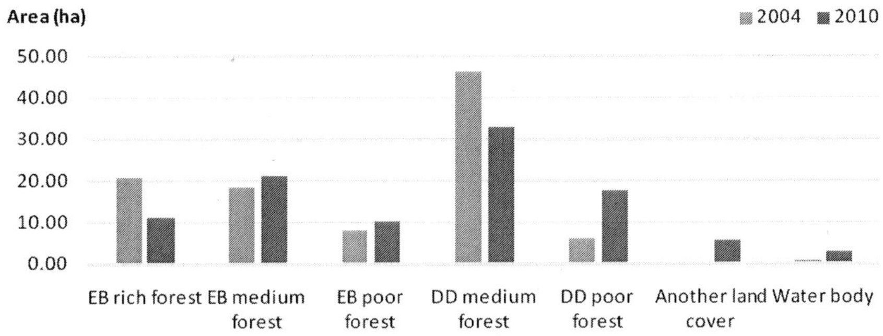

Histogram 1. Comparing the land cover area in 2004 and 2010.

The results of the assessment accuracy of the forest cover map of year 2010 are: 86.6% as overall accuracy, 87.3% as producer accuracy and 84.7% as user accuracy

4.4. Land Cover Change Map

The results of geospatial change maps from 2004 to 2010 based on post classification comparison method are shown in Histogram 1, Table 3, Table 4 and Figure 6. The analysis indicates that the EB medium quality forest increased by 3.2 thousand ha, EB poor quality forest increased by 2.5 ha and DD poor quality forest increased by 12.7 thousand ha. While the EB rich quality forest decreased by 11.2 thousand ha and DD medium quality forest decreased by 15.3 thousand ha. The analysis also indicate that another land cover increased by 5.9 thousand ha and water body increased by 2.3 thousand ha.

4.5. Estimates of Biomass and Biomass Change

The results of the estimation of biomass based on the data from the parameters of the structure and biomass of land cover are depicted in the Table 2 and land cover and land cover change area are presented in the Table 3 and the allometric Equation (1) and Equation (2) above for the years are found in (Table 5) depicting the change in biomass between 2004 and 2010.

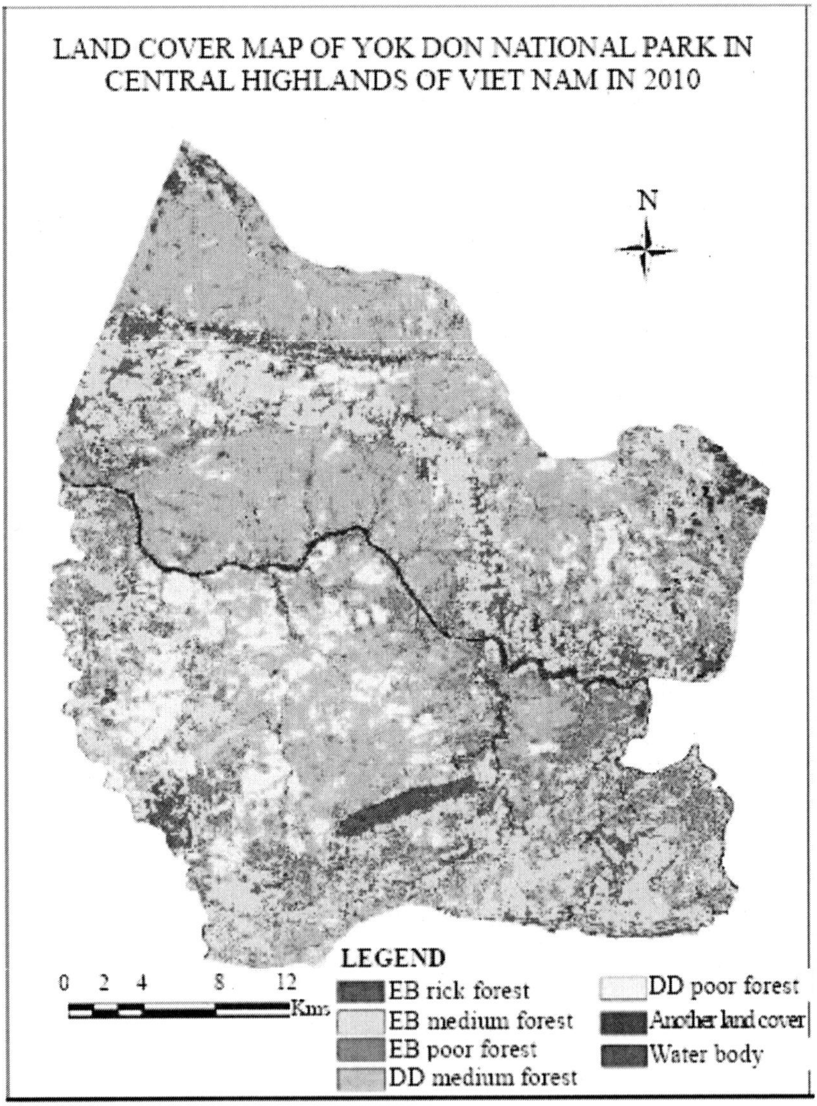

Figure 5. Land cover map in 2010.

Table 3. Area change matrix for the period 2004 to 2010 (units: ha).

2004/2010	EB rich forest	EB medium forest	EB poor forest	DD medium forest	DD poor forest	Another land cover	Water body	Total
EB rich forest	10354.85	9586.79	3034.23	50.74	50.55	414.77	226.62	23718.55
EB medium forest	1868.67	12797.10	5489.01	73.85	16.54	499.38	453.83	21198.38
EB poor forest	282.08	1982.24	3164.41	63.76	55.10	2584.91	1140.33	9272.83
DD medium forest	14.23	13.76	19.74	35999.50	14471.30	2258.05	428.88	53205.46
DD poor forest	7.46	10.26	14.69	1637.14	5212.82	231.26	62.59	7176.22
Another land cover	1.66	2.80	6.93	30.01	50.31	197.83	7.96	297.50
Water body	8.84	9.58	7.18	8.39	9.41	1.92	631.22	676.54
Total	12537.79	24402.53	11736.19	37863.39	19866.03	6188.12	2951.43	115545.48

Table 4. Area change distribution during 2004 and 2010.

No.	Class	Area (ha)	Percent (%)
1	Non change	68357.73	59.16
2	Positive change	5987.3	5.18
3	Negative change	41200.45	35.66
	Total	115545.48	100.00

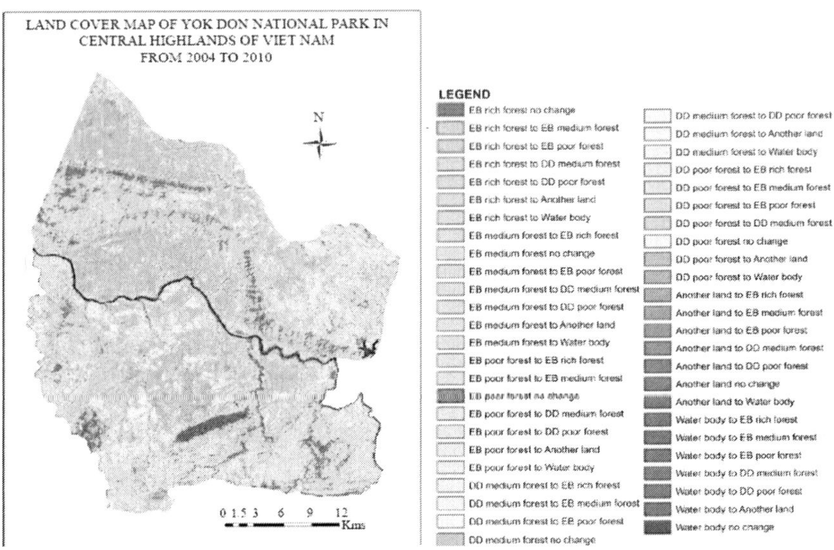

Figure 6. Land cover change map from 2004 to 2010.

Table 5. Biomass and biomass change in during 2004 and 2010.

No.	Class/Year	Biomass (tons)		Biomass change (tons)
		2004	2010	
1	EB rich forest	7551511.95	3991781.58	−3559730.37
2	EB medium forest	5299171.03	6100144.45	800973.42
3	EB poor forest	937112.20	1186059.36	248947.16
4	DD medium forest	8718778.73	6204673.72	−2514105.01
5	DD poor forest	393185.09	1088459.78	695274.69
	Total	22899759.01	18571118.89	−4328640.11

5. CONCLUSIONS

This study demonstrates the applicability of temporal data sets (2004 and 2010) from SPOT HRV satellite and the ground data for mapping forest types and analyzing the forest change. This method has been effectively employed for mapping of land cover in Yok Don National Park, Highlands of Vietnam with overall classification accuracy of 84.30% to 86.62%. The analysis indicated that during period 2004 and 2010, the EB rich quality forest decreased by 11.2 thousand ha, equivalent to 3.5 Mega tons of biomass; the DD medium quality forest decreased 15.3 thousand ha, equivalent to 2.5 Mega tons of biomass. In that time period, the EB medium quality forest increased by 3.2 thousand ha, equivalent to 0.8 Mega tons of biomass; the EB poor quality forest increased by 2.4 thousand ha, equivalent to 0.24 Mega tons of biomass; the DD poor quality forest increased by 12.68 thousand ha, equivalent to 0.69 Mega tons of biomass. The analysis of area change matrix indicated that the non-change area was 68.3 thousand ha (59.16%), the positive change area was 5.9 thousand ha (5.18%) and that the negative change area was 41.2 thousand ha (35.66%), where the much of these EB rich forest and DD medium forest got converted to EB medium forest and DD poor forest respectively. The total biomass of the study area decreased by 4.3 Mega tons. The analysis also indicated that another land cover increased by 5.9 thousand ha and that water body increased by 2.3 thousand ha. Based on the findings of this study, the following recommendations arise:

Ÿ Using satellite images with high resolution for preparing land cover map and land cover change map will aid in monitoring forest conditions. Combining this information with the field data can also be useful for estimating biomass stock and sequestered carbon aiding in the evaluation of the existing forest resources in terms of its ability to reduce carbon emissions. We recommend forest change analyses to be performed on a yearly base to monitor the forest's condition and the ecosystem services it may provide;

Ÿ Should be build a permanent sample plot network in the forested areas so that a consistent sample can be obtained for monitoring forest status annually;

Ÿ Should be development the use of radar data for structure of forest, as well as the directly calculation and monitoring of the forest biomass for in the study area.

ACKNOWLEDGEMENTS

The authors are highly grateful to the Presidents of Vietnam Academy of Science and Technology (VAST) and Japan Society for the Promotion of Science (JSPS) have supported, encouraged and provided funding for this study.

REFERENCES

1 Brown, S. (1997) Estimating Biomass and Biomass Change of Tropical Forests: A Primer. FAO Forestry Paper, 134, ISBN 92-5-103955-0.

2 Chave, J., Andalo, C., Brown, S., Cairns, M.A., et al. (2005) Tree Allometry and Improved Estimation of Carbon Stocks and Balance in Tropical Forests. Oecologia, 145, 87-99.

3 FAO (2010) Global Forest Resources Assessment 2010—Main Report. FAO Forestry Paper 163, Rome, 378 p.

4 Stibig, H.J., Achard, F., Carboni, S., Rasi, R. and Miettinen, J. (2014) Change in Tropical Forest Cover of Southeast Asia from 1990 to 2010. Biogeosciences, 11, 247-258.

5 United Nations (1998) Kyoto Protocol to the United Nations Framework Convention on Climate Change.

6 UN-REDD Vietnam Programme (2012) Guidelines on Destructive Measurement for Forest Biomass Estimation for Technical Staff Use, 35 p. (Version for Discussion)

7 Olofsson, P., Foody, G.M., Herold, M., Stehman, S.V., Woodcock, C.E. and Wulder, M.A. (2014) Good Practices for Estimating Area and Assessing Accuracy of Land Change. Remote Sensing of Environment, 148, 42-57.

8 IPCC (2003) Good Practice Guidance for Land Use, Land-Use Change and Forestry. IPCC National Greenhouse Gas Inventories Programme Technical Support Unit, Printed in Japan, ISBN 4-88788-003-0.

9 De Sy, V., et al. (2012) Synergies of Multiple Remote Sensing Data Sources for REDD+ Monitoring. Current Opinion in Environmental Sustainability, 4, 696-706.

10 Canh, N.X., et al. (2009) Report on Conservation Planning and Sustainable Development of Yok Don National Park in 2010-2020. Ministry of Agriculture and Rural Development (MARD), 140 p.

11 Luong, N.V. (2011) Essay to Use Remote Sensing Images to Estimate Biomass as a Basis for Calculating the Amount of CO_2 Sequestration by Vegetation Cover in Yokdon National Park, Highlands of Viet Nam. Proceedings of the Scientific Conference on Research, Development and Application of Space Technology, Hanoi, 10-14 October 2011, 9 p.

12 Anonymous (1998) The Investment Project to Expand the Yok Don National Park. Forest Inventory and Planning Institute, Hanoi.

13 13Stibig, H.J., Achard, F. and Fritz, S. (2004) A New Forest Cover Map of Continental Southeast Asia Derived from SPOT-VEGETATION Satellite Imagery. Applied Vegetation Science, 7, 153-162.

14 Thin, N.N., Duc, N.A., Tai. V.A., Thanh, N.T.K. and Dung, N.T. (2008) Update Information of Flora and Plant's Resources of Yokdon National Park, Daclak Province.http://www.botanyvn.com/ cnt.asp?param =news &newsid=46&lg=en

15 Langner, A., Hirata, Y., Saito, H., Sokh, H., Leng, C., Pak, C. and Raši, R. (2014) Spectral Normalization of SPOT 4 Data to Adjust for Changing Leaf Phenology within Seasonal Forests in Cambodia. Remote Sensing of Environment, 143, 122-130.

16 Bhishma, P., Shiva, S.P., Ajay, P., Eak, B.R., Sanjeeb, B., Tibendra, R.B., Shambhu, C., Rijan, T., et al. (2010) Forest Carbon Stock Measurement—Guidelines for Measuring Carbon Stocks in Community-Managed Forest. Asia Network for Sustainable Agriculture and Bioresource (ANSAB), Nepal, 679 p.

17 Chaiyo, U., Garivait, S. and Wanthongchai, K. (2011) Carbon Storage in Above-Ground Biomass of Tropical Deciduous Forest in Ratchaburi Province, Thailand. World Academy of Science, Engineering and Technology, 58, 636-641.

18 Huy, B. (2008) Methodology for Research on CO_2 Sequestration in Natural Forests to Join the Program of Reducing Emission from

Deforestation and Degradation—REDD. Journal of Agriculture and Rural Development, 10, 1-10.

19 UN-REDD Vietnam Programme (2011) Technical Manual for Participatory Carbon Monitoring.

20 Trung, T.V. (1978) The Vegetation Cover in Vietnam. Chapter IV, V, 2nd Edition, Science and Technics Publishing House, Hanoi, 276 p.

21 Trung, T.V. (1998) The Tropical Forest Ecosystem in Vietnam. Chapter IV, Science and Technics Publishing House, Hanoi, 291 p.

22 UNESCO (1973) International Classification and Mapping of Vegetation. United Nations Educational, Scientific and Cultural Organization, Paris, 102 p.

23 Regulation on Criteria for Identifying and Classifying Forest (In English) (2009) No. Circular 34/TT-BNN Issued by Ministry of Agriculture and Rural Development (MARD) of Vietnamese Government. Quyđịnhtiêuchíxácđịnhvà- phânloạirừng (In Vietnamese), Tran.

24 IPCC (2006) Chapter 4: Forest Land. In: Guidelines for National Greenhouse Gas Inventories. Volume 4: Agriculture, Forestry and Other Land Use, IPCC.

25 UN-REDD Vietnam Programme (2012) Tree Allometric Equation Development for Estimation of Forest Above- Ground Biomass in Viet Nam. Part A—Introduction and Background of the Study Viet Nam.

CHAPTER 4

Estimation of Above-Ground Biomass of Wetlands

Laimdota Truus[1]

[1] Institute of Ecology at Tallinn University, Estonia

1. INTRODUCTION

Despite global importance of wetlands, estimations of their production and biomass have received little attention (Campbell et al., 2000). This chapter concentrates on analysis of the composition and above-ground biomass of floodplain grasslands and fen vegetation in the Northern forest zone. Both vegetation types were extensively used for hay and/or grazing up to the middle of the 20th century, and abandoned later.

Systematic biomass estimations were conducted in the 1970s–1980s (Estonian data from 1977–1980; most data from Canada from 1972–1978 (Campbell et al., 2000)) when they were feasible for agricultural use. Papers on vegetation production and above-ground biomass of wetlands are quite scarce nowadays. Biomass has sometimes been measured for developing community structure theories, e.g. Zobel & Liira (1997) included some wet grasslands into analysis of richness vs biomass relationship. Still, some thorough reviews can be found like an overview of biomass of rich fen types in South England and Wales by Wheeler & Shaw (1991). New interest in the subject has risen in the context of biomass use for bioenergy production (e.g. Rösch et al., 2009).

Many plant species cannot survive without special accommodation to wetland conditions. The composition of wetland vegetation is mostly controlled by the wetland water level (WL) (Bootsma & Wassen, 1996; Hájková et al., 2004; Barry et al., 2008). Wilcox & Nichols (2008) and Ilomets et al. (2010) found that the diversity and habitat value of plant communities depend on the wetland WL and the water level amplitude between dry and wet seasons (WLA). In fens with a constantly high WL rhizome-spreading graminoids and herbs dominate, while drainage and fluctuating WL support high tussock-forming graminoids.

A specific feature of both floodplain grassland and fen vegetation is high patchiness due to variations in WL and WLA caused by microtopography (Liira et al., 2009). Tussocks, formed by herbaceous plants or tree stumps, locally increase the habitat variability even more (Liira et al., 2009; Ilomets et al., 2010).

Total biomass of wetland vegetation is significantly affected by three main factors: the N:P ratio, total nutrient supply and morphological and physiological traits of plants (Güsewell, 2005). Biomass variations are higher on moister sites such as wet floodplain grasslands (Truus & Puusild, 2009) and fens (Ilomets et al., 2010). The height and coverage of tussocks increases with denser or deeper drainage. About 52% of the vascular plant species variance occurs due to four environmental variables: amplitude of WL (between spring flooding and midsummer dry period), midsummer WL, mire water pH and electrical conductivity (Ilomets et al., 2010).

Truus & Puusild (2009) found strong relation of the above-ground biomass with the management regime but not with the variations in site conditions on wet and moist floodplain grasslands. Wilson & Keddy (1986), Moore & Keddy (1989) and Garica et al. (1993) detected general hump-back relationship between species richness and biomass, but it has also been shown that a high number of factors can complicate prediction of species richness from community biomass (Gough et al., 1994).

2. FACTORS AFFECTING WETLAND PRODUCTIVITY AND SPECIES RICHNESS

2.1. Relationship Between Species Richness and Biomass

The relation between plant species richness and biomass was first discussed by Grime (1973, 1979) and Al-Mufti et al. (1977) when describing general hump-back relationship between species density and community biomass. According to these authors, maximum species richness can be found at medium values of biomass. Later, this relation has been approved (Wheeler & Giller, 1982) or denied (Gough et al., 1994). In the development of this theory Zobel & Liira (1997) attributed species richness to the plant ramet density.

Gough et al. (1994) established correlation between environmental conditions and species richness but not between biomass and environmental conditions. Therefore, the influence of environmental conditions on species richness could not be assumed strictly from biomass. Wheeler & Giller (1982),Boyer & Wheeler (1989) and Wheeler & Shaw (1991) recorded differences in biomass– species richness relation between community types (low-sedge low-productive fen, productive tall-sedge and reed fen, and fertile site communities with strong domination of *Filipendula ulmaria* or *Molinia cerulea*).

According to Gough et al. (1994), two types of processes operate in the species richness–productivity relation on wetlands:

- At low levels of productivity, species richness is primarily limited by the ability of the species to survive the abiotic conditions. In this range increase in productivity reflects a decrease in the harshness of the environment.

- At higher levels of community productivity, the decline in richness is believed to be related in some way to a greater degree of competitive exclusion with increasing productivity. For wetlands this relation was revealed by Wheeler & Giller (1982). Examining herbaceous fen vegetation, they found that species richness was negatively correlated to above-ground biomass.

Wet meadows are poorer in species than those on mineral soil. Two reasons could be pointed out:

- Hard environmental stress that excludes several plant species.

- The absence of management leading to domination of tall plants and accumulation of dead biomass on soil surface (Truus, 1998).

Strong correlation has been found in fens between the height and coverage of the tussock-forming graminoid *Molinia cerulea* in fens with fluctuating WL and midsummer WL minimum (Ilomets et al., 2010).

In general, relationship of species richness and above-ground biomass is complex and hardly predictable, especially for wetlands.

2.2. Limitations Of Productivity

2.2.1. Flood, Water Level And Water Level Amplitude

On **floodplain meadows** the duration and intensivity of flooding serve as environmental determinants of plant species selection. Riverine floodwater pulses provide water, nutrient-rich material and sediments to floodplain wetlands, but flood pulses also act as a natural disturbance by removing biomass, scouring sediments and delivering turbid waters (Bayley & Guimond, 2009). Riparian ecosystems are among the most diverse systems on the world's continents (Nilsson et al., 1997). The intensity of natural processes taking place on floodplains is variable, depending on the properties of the river and shore. Estonian rivers are usually small and floodplains narrow. Thereby most riverborn nutrients settle on the 50 m wide belt close to the river channel [1] - where productive high-growing vegetation develops. An exception is South Estonia where luxorious sandy sediments form rapidly desiccating low-productivity dry floodplain meadows.

The species composition of spring fen communities is mainly influenced by groundwater chemistry, especially pH, electrical conductivity and mineral richness (Hájek et al., 2002). It is unknown whether these factors affect species richness and the amount of above-ground biomass (Hájkova & Hájek, 2003).

2.2.2. Water And Soil Chemistry And Nutrient Availability

Water and soil chemistry and nutrient availability to plants are among the important factors controlling the diversity of wetland vegetation.

Floods bring extra nutrients to floodplain grasslands. Thus there is no N and P deficit and vegetation is luxorious. Management of grasslands removes nutrients from soil and biomass production decreases. Without management, however, annual biomass production increases.

Fens are characterized by high concentrations of cations in soil and water. The concentration of Ca, Fe, N, P and K in plants varies along the poor–rich fen vegetation gradient from poor *Sphagnum*-fens to calcareous fens, and from sedge-moss fens to forb-rich wet meadows (Rozbrojová & Hájek, 2008). The same study showed that the fertility gradient was largely independent of the poor–rich (pH/calcium) gradient. Nutrient limitations of fens are complicated: species in one community can have different limitations (Rozbrojová & Hájek, 2008). Low-productivity fen communities that support more rare species (Wassen et al., 2005) are rather P- or K-(co)limited, or limited by different environmental conditions (Rozbrojová & Hájek, 2008).

2.2.3. Management

Due to nutrient supply by floodwater, the soil of floodplain meadows is rich in nutrients and biomass productivity is high. The amounts of nutrients brought by floods is comparable to quantities taken away with the harvest or/and cattle grazing. Clipping increase species richness and shoot density but decrease above-ground biomass, thus creating more favourable conditions for more plant species. Bakker (2007) demonstrated that cutting reduces the vigour of tall competitive species, allowing smaller species coexist. Nowadays most of the floodplain meadows are left unmanaged. Hay is mown only in restricted areas for the purposes of environmental protection.

In comparison with other meadow types above-ground biomass production is lower on dry floodplain meadows and higher on floodplain marshes. Productivity is variable in all floodplain meadow community types depending on species composition (Table 1). On wet meadows the site moisture conditions are greatly responsible for plant ecological traits. On permanently wet sites both tussock-forming and mat-forming graminoids dominate while herbs dominate where soil WL drops down at least in summer (Fig. 1). Comparison of Estonian data from the period of regular management (Table 1) with the period of abandonment (Tables 2 and 3) showed that productivity had risen due to accumulation of plant nutrients on unmanaged meadow soils. Above-ground biomass varied threefold, depending on the management regime (Table 3). Liira et al. (2009) also noticed that management lowered canopy height but revealed differences in functional trait structure in more detail.

Falinska (1991, 1995) described two stages in the after-abandonment vegetation succession in *Cirsium rivularis* phytocoenosis on wet grassland. The initial stage of the succession lasted about 9 years: half of 142 plant species retreated but 12 species became dominant and a macroforb meadow community (*Lysimachio vulgaris–Filipenduletum*) meadow with mosaic structure, including species like*Filipendula ulmaria, Carex cespitosa, C. acutiformis, Lythrum salicari*a and *Lysimachia vulgaris*, was formed. During the following 15 years a specific spatial complex developed, consisting of meadow and herbaceous communities and willow shrub aggregations with the first tree species. Next the*Circaeo-Alnetum* woodland community appeared. The succession exhibits differentiation of the horizontal structure – increase in patchiness, and differentiation of the vertical structure – plant height started to increase immediately after management stopped and most of the above-ground biomass moved higher from the near-surface position.

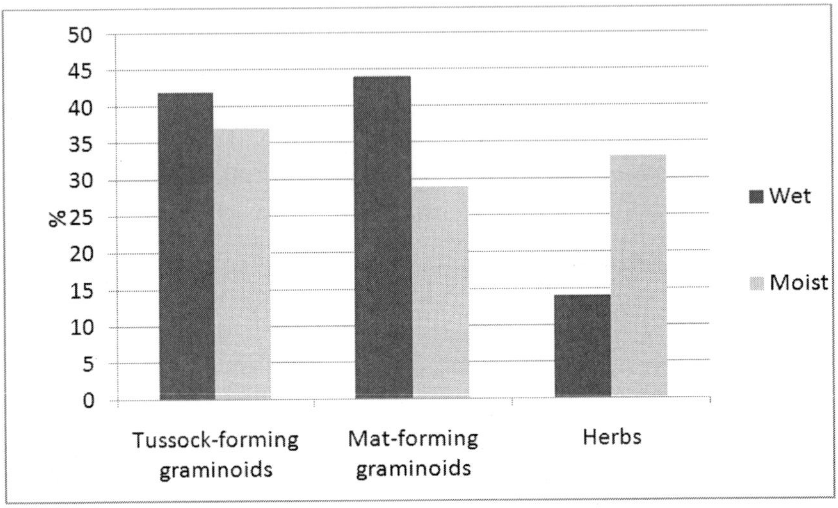

Figure 1. Life-form distribution on Soomaa (West Estonia) wet and moist floodplain meadows

The species composition and duration of this vegetation change depend on climatic and trophic conditions and hydrology, also on the ecological trait of plants and availability of diaspores. General trends, however, are: decrease in species richness, change in species composition, increase in vegetation height and above-ground biomass, and finally replacement of the herbaceous community by woodland. Re-location of most of the biomass to a higher level in the community as described byFalinska (1991, 1995) takes place if herbs dominate – on wet meadows at a drier site. No comparable data about composition and biomass change are available due to abandonment of seminatural hay lands and pastures. Just general trends in vegetation change can be followed.

Analysis of life-form distribution on Estonian floodplain meadows in periods with different management showed an increased proportion of tall herbs and graminoids instead of low herbs and graminoids in the 1960s when these areas were mostly regularly mown and the end of the 1990s when they were out of use (Fig. 2). The proportion of tall tussock-forming graminoids did not change. On floodplain grasslands these plants inhabit depressions with a higher water table and thereby were absent even in the former period.

Table 1. Mean above-ground biomass of plant communities of floodplain meadows. The analyses are means for Estonia representing seminatural hay meadows in 1978-1981[2]

Floodplain meadow type[2] English description of classification in Truus & Tõnisson, 1998	**Plant community**	**Above-ground biomass** ($g\ m^{-2}$)	**Above-ground biomass, mean for community type** ($g\ m^{-2}$)
Dry floodplain meadow	*Sesleria-Festucetum ovinaea*	150	80
	Seslerio-Nardetum	40	
	Thymo-Festucetum	30-100	
	Sieglingo-Nardetum	40-80	
	Anthoxantho-Agrostetum	40-100	
	Galio-Agrostetum tenuis	50-150	
Moderately moist floodplain meadow	*Agrostetum giganteae*	150-250	200
	Deschampsio-Festucetum rubrae	100-300	
	Alopecuretum pratensis	150-380	
Moist floodplain meadow	*Cirsio-Polygonetum bistortae*	150-300	230
	Filipendulo-Geranietum palustris	200-400	
	Deschampsieto-Caricetum caespitosae	100-250	
	Elytrigieto-Alopecuretum arundinacei	150-300	
Wet floodplain meadow with tall grasses	*Stellario-Deschampsietum*	80-200 (300)	250
	Phalaroidetum	150-500	
Wet floodplain meadow with tall sedges	*Caricetum distichae*	200-250	260
	Caricetum acutae	100-450	
	Caricetum rostrato-vesicariae	100-450	
Floodplain marshes	*Seslerio-Caricetum paniceae*	40-100	125
	Caricetum paniceo-nigrae	50-150	
	Caricetum diandro-nigrae	50-180	
	Caricetum cespitoso-appropinquatae	100-200	
	Caricetum elatae	80-300	

3. ABOVE-GROUND BIOMASS

3.1. Methods for Standing Crop Estimation

Wheeler & Shaw (1991) calculated above-ground biomass as the biomass increment between April and September. In regions with a dormant season for herbaceous plants in winter, above-ground biomass (that also represents production per year) is in its maximum in the middle of summer, but before abundant flowering. In wetlands different flowering times can be noticed: the sedges usually stop growing and flower in May and June (Leht, 1999) while common reed continues growing up to the August. In all cases, biomass samples were air-dried before measuring. Standing biomass measured in its maximum is usually equalized with production.

3.2. Above-Ground Biomass of Floodplain Meadows

In the period of regular management, mean values for above-ground biomass of Estonian floodplain meadows measured from 80 to 260 g m^{-2}, varying largely between community types and even communities[2]. On unmanaged floodplain meadows those values are more than twice higher (Tables 2and 3). Zobel & Liira (1997) presented biomass values from 300 to 600 g m^{-2} for West Estonian floodplain meadows of Sauga, Vaskjõe and Kasari (the lowest value on a dry site). High standard deviation in Tables 2 and 3 shows high variability of floodplain meadows vegetation discussed earlier. For comparison, in the Czech Republic *Molinio-Arrhenetheretea* above-ground biomass in a moist floodplain meadow was 300–350 g m^{-2} (Joyce, 2001). Values of above-ground biomass from the earlier (with regular hay cutting; Table 1) and later (without management; Tables 2 and 3) periods show an increase in standing crop that can be explained as a result of management cessation. Standing biomass also varied threefold (from 263 to 763 g m^{-2}) on floodplains in Soomaa, West Estonia (Truus & Puusild, 2009).

Table 2. Mean above-ground biomass on the Kloostri landscape transect, West Estonia. Previous hay-meadow, abandoned over 15 years

Floodplain meadow type English description in Truus & Tõnisson, 1998	**Above-ground biomass** (g m^{-2}, St.Dev in parentheses)
Dry	458 (148.6)
Moderately moist	493 (240)
Moist	350 (448.3)
Wet	(no data)
Wet with tall sedges	742 (70.3)
Floodplain marsh	376 (100.9)

Truus & Puusild (2009) studied the distribution of ecological groups (graminoids, herbs, low and tall growth-form) in relation to management cessation. The ecological group composition turned towards tussock-forming plants but the most obvious change was the increase in vegetation height (Fig. 2).

Unmanaged wetlands are dominated by powerful species (Wheeler & Giller, 1982; Truus, 1998; Truus & Puusild, 2009). On sites with a permanently high groundwater level *Deschampsia cespitosa* or*Carex cespitosa* form high tussocks while low-growing tussocks (*Nardus stricta*, *Festuca ovina*) spread on dry or moist managed grasslands. The abandonment of grasslands can lead to dominance (in some cases to almost monospecies communities) of tall herbs like *Filipendula ulmaria*. The coverage and height of tussocks of *Molinia cerulea* increase on rich fen meadows (Ilomets et al., 2010).

Table 3. Mean above-ground biomass on moist and wet floodplain meadows with different management regimes in Soomaa, West Estonia.

Floodplain meadow type English description in Truus & Tõnisson, 1998	**Above-ground biomass** (g m^{-2}, St.Dev in parentheses)
Moist, regularly mown	572 (692.3)
Moist, mown, recently abandoned	333 (167.5)
Moist, unmown but mowing reintroduced	380 (178.2)
Moist, unmown over 15 years	763 (627.5)
Wet, regularly mown	263 (108.0)
Wet, mown, recently abandoned	516 (165.9)
Wet, unmown, but mowing reintroduced	452 (398.7)
Wet, unmown over 15 years	447 (86.4)

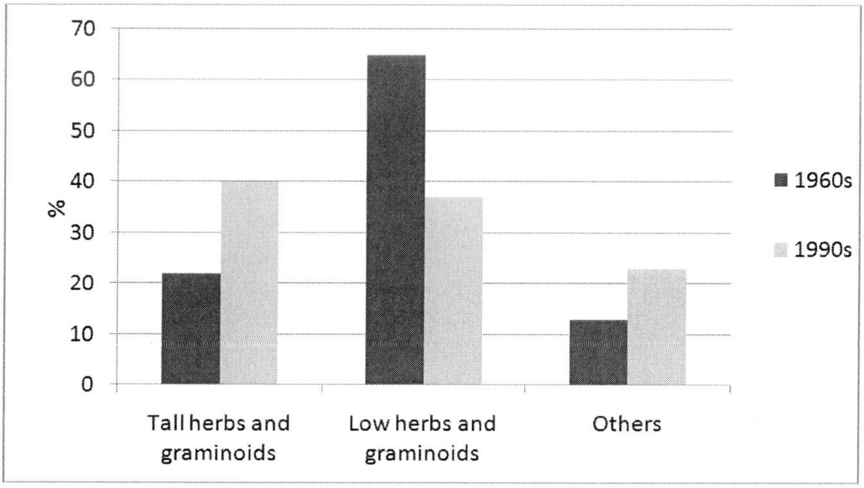

Figure 2. Proportions of the most frequent growth-forms on floodplain meadows in periods of extensive management (first half of the 20th century) and unmanagement (end of the 1990s)

3.3. Biomass of Fens

Fen vegetation presented in Table 4 is highly variable and the biomass values vary between locations. The above-ground biomass values for low-growing vegetation range from 50 to 500 g m^{-2} and from 600 to 1750 g m^{-2} for both tall graminoids and tall herbs. For comparison, in Canada and adjacent USA mean above-ground biomass was 337 ± 142 g m^{-2} for fens and bogs, and 924 ± 463 g m^{-2} for marshes and swamps (Campbell et al., 2000).

No recent data are available on biomass production on fens in Estonia. The data from 1977–1980 (Table 4) gives very low values (50 g m^{-2}) for above-ground biomass of fen meadows. The utilization of fen meadows grew in Estonia at the beginning of the 20th century. An experiment from 1922–1926 showed the yield of 140 to 450 g m^{-2} from unfertilized fen meadows.[2] -. It was also mentioned that during the experiment hay production was related to weather conditions but decreased year by year (probably because of experimental hay cutting).

4. CONCLUSIONS

Vegetation of floodplain meadows and fens varies depending on the environmental (soil, water) conditions and management regime. Both vegetation types have been in economic use but a great part of them is in the successional stage due to abandonment.

On low-productive sites plant species richness is primarily limited on abiotic conditions (WL, WLA, mineral content of soil and water, availability of plant nutrients).

The main limitation in highly productive sites is competition for light. Tall graminoids or herbs compete out low-growing plants, enabling even the development of monospecies vegetation.

The management status determines plant species richness and the above-ground biomass production. Above-ground standing biomass varied threefold due to management cessation on West Estonian floodplain grassland. Widespread cessation of management on seminatural meadows is a key for interpretation of different above-ground biomass values from different periods. Fen vegetation is probably more sensitive to above-ground biomass cutting than floodplain grassland vegetation.

It is complicated to predict species richness from community biomass, and biomass (or production) from site conditions.

Table 4. Above-ground biomass of fens with highly variable composition in different regions

Location	Vegetation community	Dry standing biomass ($g\ m^{-2}$) St.Dev. in parentheses	Reference
England and Wales	*Schoeno-Juncetum*	~ 200	Wheeler & Shaw, 1991, Fig. 1
England and Wales	*Acrocladio-Caricetum*	~ 200	
England and Wales	*Potentillo-Caricetum*	~ 200	
England and Wales	*Peucedano-Phragmitetum*	~ 300	
England and Wales	Rich-fen meadow	~ 500	
England and Wales	*Cladio-Molinietum*	~ 600	
England and Wales	*Peucedano-Phragmitetum*	~ 700	
England and Wales	*Angelico-Phragmitetum*	~ 850	
England and Wales	*Cicuto-Phragmitetum*	~ 1200	
England and Wales	*Phragmites* consociation	~ 1300	
England and Wales	*Glyceria maxima* community	~ 1500	
England and Wales	Tall herb fen	~ 1750	
England and Wales	*Phalaris arundinacea* community	900–1200	Smith et al., 1985
England and Wales	*Glyceria maxima* community	700–1200	
Siberia, Russia	*Carex*-dominating fen	200	Pjavtšenko, 1967
Switzerland	*Saxifraga hirculus* fen	152–231	Venterink & Vittouz, 2008
Netherlands	*Molinietalia* fen	~ 300–400	Van der Hoek & Sýkora, 2006
Estonia	*Drepanoclado-Schoenetum*	50	Data from 1977-1980[2]
Estonia	*Seslerio-Caricetum paniceae*	50	

Values of above-ground biomass increase from north to south but the geographical latitude (availability of photosynthetic radiation) is not as strong determinant for biomass production of wet grasslands as the local hydrological, nutritional and management status.

5. ACKNOWLEDGEMENTS

This research was financed by the Estonian Ministry of Education and Research (targeted funding project No. 0280009s07). The author is indebted to Anne Noor for linguistic help.

NOTES

[1] - Pork, K. (1984). Jõeluhtade looduslikus seisundis säilitamisest. In: Looduskaitse ja põllumajandus. Kumari, E., Randalu, I. & Hang, V. (Eds.). Academy of Sciences of the E.S.S.R, 58–70. [In Estonian]

[2] - Rinne, L. (1927). Sooheinamaa toodangu kahanemisest väetuse puudusel. Eesti Sooparanduse Seltsi teated, Vol.8&9, 3–15. [In Estonian]

REFERENCES

1. M. M. Al-Mufti, C. L. Sydes, S. B. Furness, J. P. Grime, S. R. Band, 1977 A quantitative analysis of shoot phenology and dominance in herbaceous vegetation J. Ecol., 65 759 EOF 0000-0010i313577

2. M. J. Barry, B. K. Andreas, F. A. De Szalay, 2008 Long-term plant community changes in managed fens in Ohio, USA Aquat. Conserv., 18 392 EOF 407 EOF 1099-0755

3. S. E. Bayley, J. K. Guimond, 2009 Aboveground biomass and nutrient limitation in relation to river connectivity in montane floodplain marshes Wetlands 29 4 1243 EOF 1254 EOF 0277-5212

4. M. C. Bootsma, M. J. Wassen, 1996 Environmental conditions and fen vegetation in three lowland mires Vegetatio 127 173 EOF 1385-0237

5. M. L. H. Boyer, B. D. Wheeler, 1989 Vegetation patterns in spring-fed calcareous fens: calcite precipitation and constraints on fertility J. Ecol., 77 597 EOF 0000-0010i313577

6. C. Campbell, D. H. Vitt, L. A. Halsey, I. D. Campbell, M. N. Thormann, S. E. Bayley, 2000 Net primary production and standing biomass in northern continental wetlands. Information report NOR-X-369. Canadian Forest Service, Northern Forestry Centre, 0704-7673Canada

7. K. Falinska, 1991 Plant demography and vegetation succession. Kluwer Academic Publishers, 0-79231-060-8Boston, London

8. K. Falinska, 1995Genet disintegration in Filipendula ulmaria: consequences for population dynamics and vegetation succession. J. Ecol. 83 0000-0010i313577

9. L. V. Garcia, T. Maranon, A. Moreno, L. Clemente, 1993Above-ground biomass and species richness in a Mediterranean salt marsh. J. Veg. Sci., 4 1100-9233

10. L. Gough, J. B. Grace, K. L. Taylor, 1994The relationship between species richness and community biomass: the importance of environmental variables. Oikos, 70 0030-1299

11. J. P. Grime, 1973Competitive exclusion in herbaceous vegetation. Nature, 242 0028-0836

12. J. P. Grime, 1979 Plant strategies and vegetation processes. Wiley & Sons Ltd, 04719920U.K.

13. S. Güsewell, 2005Responses of wetland graminoids to the relative supply of nitrogen and phosphorus. Plant Ecol., 176 1385-0237

14. M. Hájek, P. Hekera, P. Hájkova, 2002Spring fen vegetation and water chemistry in the West Carpathian flysh zone. Folia Geobot., 37 1211-9520

15. P. Hájkova, M. Hájek, 2003Species richness and above-ground biomass of poor and calcareous spring fens in the flysh Weat Carpathians, and their relationship to water and soil chemistry. Preslia, 75 0032-7786

16. P. Hájková, P. Wolf, M. Hájek, (2004). Environmental factors and Carpathian spring fen vegetation: the importance of scale and temporal variation, Ann. Bot. Fenn., Vol.41, 249-262, ISSN 0003-3847

17. M. Ilomets, L. Truus, R. Pajula, K. Sepp, 2010Species composition and structure of vascular plants and bryophytes on the water level gradient within a calcareous fen in North Estonia. Est. J. Ecol., 59 1 1736-7549

18. C. Joyce, 2001The sensitivity of a species-rich flood-meadow plant community to fertilizer nitrogen: the Lužnice river floodplain, Czech Republic. Plant Ecol., 155 1385-0237

19. M. . Leht, Ed., 1999 Eesti taimede määraja. EPMÜ ZBI, Eesti Loodusfoto, 998583027Tartu, Estonia (In Estonian)

20. J. Liira, M. Issak, Ü. Jõgar, M. Mändoja, M. Zobel, 2009Restoration management of a floodplain meadow and its cost-effectiveness- The results of a 6-year experiment. Ann. Bot. Fen., 46 0003-3847

21. D. R. J. Moore, P. A. Keddy, 1989The relationship between species richness and standing crop in wetlands: The importance of scale. Vegetatio, 79 1406-0914

22. D. R. J. Moore, P. A. Keddy, C. L. Gaudet, I. Wisheu, 1989Conservation of wetlands: do infertile wetlands deserve a higher priority? Biol. Conserv., 47 0006-3207

23. C. Nilsson, R. Jansson, U. Zinko, (1997, 1997Long-term responses of river-margin vegetation to water-level regulation. Science, 276 0036-8075

24. N. I. Pjavtšenko, 1967O produktivnosti bolot Zapadnoi Sibiri. Rastitelnõje Resursõ. 3 4 0033-9946In Russian)

25. Z. Rozbrojová, M. Hájek, 2008Changes in nutrient limitation of spring fen vegetation along environmental gradients in the West Carpathians. J. Veg. Sci., 19 1100-9233

26. C. Rösch, J. Skarka, K. Raab, V. Stelzer, 2009Energy production from grassland- Assessing the sustainability of different process chains under German conditions. Biomass and Bioenergy, 33 0961-9534

27. S. J. Smith, I. Ridge, R. M. Morris, 1984The biomass potential of seasonally flooded wetlands. In: Proceedings of Bioenergy' 84 World Conference, 15 21June 1984 in Goteborg, Sweden, The Bioenergy Council, 190-195, 978-0-85334-351-6Stockholm, Sweden

28. K. Zobel, J. Liira, 1997A scale-independent approach to the richness vs biomass relationship in ground-layer plant communities, Oikos. 80 0030-1299

29. L. Truus, E. Puusild, 2009Species richness, biomass production and recent vegetation changes of Estonian floodplain grassland. Pol. J. Ecol., 57 1 1505-2249

30. L. Truus, A. Tõnisson, 1998The ecology of floodplain grasslands in Estonia. In: European Wet Grasslands: Biodiversity, Management and Restoration, C.B. Joyce & P.M. Wade, (Eds.), 49 60John Wiley & Sons Ltd, 0-47197-619-9U.K.

31. L. Truus, 1998Influence of management cessation on reedbed and floodplain vegetation on the Kloostri floodplain meadow in the delta of the Kasari River, Estonia. Proc. Estonian Acad. Sci. Biol. Ecol., 47 1 1406-0914

32. D. Van der Hoek, K. V. Sýkora, 2006Fen-meadow succession in relation to spatial and temporal differences in hydrological and soil conditions, Appl. Veg. Sci., 9 1402-2001

33. M. J. Wassen, A. Barendregt, A. Palczynski, J. T. De Smidt, H. De Mars, 1990The relationship between fen vegetation gradients, groundwater flow and flooding in an undrained valley mire at Biebrza, Poland, J. Ecol., 78 0000-0010i313577

34. M. J. Wassen, H. O. Venterink, E. D. Lapshina, F. Tanneberger, 2005Endangered plants persist under phosphorus limitation, Nature, 437 22 0028-0836

35. O. H. Venterink, P. Vittoz, 2008Biomass production of the last remaining fen with saxifraga hirculus in Switzerland is controlled by nitrogen availability, Botanica Helvetica, 118 0253-1453

36. B. D. Wheeler, S. C. Shaw, 1991Above-ground crop mass and species richness of the principal types of herbaceous rich-fen vegetation of lowland England and Wales, J. Ecol., 79 0000-0010i313577

37. B. D. Wheeler, K. E. Giller, 1982Species richness of herbaceous fen vegetation in Boardland, Norfolk in relation to the quantity of above-ground plant material, J. Ecol., 70 0000-0010i313577

38. D. A. Wilcox, S. J. Nichols, 2008The effect of water-level fluctuations on vegetation in a Lake Huron wetland, Wetlands, 28 2 0277-5212

39. S. D. Wilson, P. A. Keddy, 1986Species competitive ability and position along a natural stress/disturbance gradient, Ecology, 67 0012-9658

CHAPTER 5

Landsat Imagery-Based Above Ground Biomass Estimation and Change Investigation Related to Human Activities

Chaofan Wu [1], Huanhuan Shen [1], Ke Wang [1,*], Aihua Shen [2], Jinsong Deng [1] and Muye Gan [1]

[1] College of Environmental and Resource Sciences, Zhejiang University, Hangzhou 310058, China

[2] Zhejiang Forestry Academy, Hangzhou 310023, China

ABSTRACT

Forest biomass is a significant indicator for substance accumulation and forest succession, and a spatiotemporal biomass map would provide valuable information for forest management and scientific planning. In this study, Landsat imagery and field data cooperated with a random forest regression approach were used to estimate spatiotemporal Above Ground Biomass (AGB) in Fuyang County, Zhejiang Province of East China. As a result, the AGB retrieval showed an increasing trend for the past decade, from 74.24 ton/ha in 2004 to 99.63 ton/ha in 2013. Topography and forest management were investigated to find their relationships with the spatial distribution change of biomass. In general, the simulated AGB increases with higher elevation, especially in the range of 80–200 m, wherein AGB acquires the highest increase rate. Moreover, the forest policy of ecological forest has a positive effect on the AGB increase, particularly within the national level ecological forest. The result in this study demonstrates that human activities have a great impact on biomass distribution and change tendency. Furthermore, Landsat image-based biomass estimates would provide illuminating information for forest policy-making and sustainable development.

KEYWORDS

Landsat imagery; Above Ground Biomass; Fuyang County; topography; ecological forest; human activities

1. INTRODUCTION

Being the largest terrestrial ecosystem, the forest ecosystem provides a fundamental wood supply and greatly influences global carbon stocks and carbon exchange with the atmosphere, which is relevant to the greenhouse effect [1]. Moreover, the quality of forests significantly influence human beings' daily lives [2]. Recognizing the importance of forest ecosystems, series international activities, such as reducing carbon Emissions associated with Deforestation and forest Degradation (REDD) and REDD+, have been proposed to protect global forest ecosystems and promote sustainable forest management [3]. Researchers have explored increasing numbers of studies on forest biophysical parameters, including aboveground biomass (AGB), leaf area index (LAI), and stock volume, to gain a better understanding of forest quality and productivity in recent years [4,5]. As it is an essential biophysical parameter of forest ecosystems, biomass is closely related to timber productivity and carbon cycle, and explicit spatial-temporal information on biomass could provide significant information in the understanding of the process of human–forest interactions [6].

Over the past few decades, compared to the traditional time- and labor-consuming field measurements, remote sensing provides a cost-effective and appealing way to obtain spatial and temporal forest environmental information with multiple sensors from Moderate Resolution Imaging Spectroradiometer (MODIS), Landsat, hyperspectral, Laser intensity Direction and Ranging (LiDAR) and Radio Direction and Ranging (RaDAR) springing up to promote forest research with refined spectral signals and expanding dimensions, introducing more macroscopic and valuable information for forest monitoring [7,8]. With regard to the advantages and limitations of different remote sensing images, the Landsat program is still the most prominent resource, as it possesses abundant historic spatial-temporal archives and rich spectral information for more than 30 years, since 1972, and it possesses a relatively suitable spatial resolution for forest biophysical investigation; additionally, it is a free download data, which can be obtained by the public and has an attractive large-scale availability, especially for developing countries where there is limited accessibility for high resolution images, all of the above make the data incomparable [9]. Landsat series provide an abundant data source for valuable feature extractions, from original multispectral bands to transformed spectral information, including vegetation indices that were created to improve prediction accuracy, and texture information reflecting spatial variability [10]. The newly launched Landsat 8 was further tested as the continued Landsat data record of ETM+ imagery to investigate the productivity and effectiveness of biomass estimations [11]. Furthermore, multi-temporal images and ever-increasing yearly trajectories were introduced to take advantage of phonological information, as well as disturbance and recovery variables, to improve simulation performance [12,13].

A great deal of research has been developed for remote sensing-based biomass estimation, as increasing interdependencies between remote sensing data and biomass have been increasingly discovered for empirical methods when compared to more complicated approaches based on physical mechanism models [14]. Since forests are complex ecosystems, and there are always nonlinear or more complicated relationships between their components, to overcome the weakness of traditional empirical statistic methods, which are based on the linear relation hypothesis for input variables, alternative methods in the machine learning have been introduced to establish the relationship between above ground biomass and remote sensing derived features [15,16]. Non-parametric approaches that make no assumptions about the statistical distributions of original data and relations between predictor and response variables, including K-Nearest Neighbors, Neural Networks, Support Vector Machines and Random Forest, are proliferated to probe the inconclusive relationship between remote sensing derivatives and AGB to yield more accurate predictions [12,15].

Natural environments and human activity have great influence on the biomass distributions [17]. It has been found that forest management patterns are directly instructed by forest policy [18], and biomass heterogeneity is always closely related to local topographic characteristics [19]. The main objective of this study is to (1) combine the remote sensing imagery Landsat with detailed forest inventory data to investigate the AGB estimation in Fuyang County, East China, In the past decade; and (2) analyze the AGB spatiotemporal variability across the study area corresponding to hierarchical topography and man-power management activities.

2. MATERIALS AND METHODS

2.1. Study Area

The study area, Fuyang County, is located between Latitude 29°44′45″–30°11′58.5″N and Longitude 119°25′00″–120°19′30″E in Northwest Zhejiang Province, China, with about 71% of the land covered by forest, and is approximately 38 kilometers away from the capital city, Hangzhou. The prevailing waters include the Fuchun River, with several tributaries running across the region, and the Yanshi Ridge reservoir situated in the west (Figure 1). The area is characterized as a subtropical monsoon climate with an annual average precipitation of 1441.9 mm and a mean temperature of 16.1°C. The altitude varies from 1.6 m to 1063.4 m, and the land is predominantly covered with red soil and paddy soil. Coniferous forest (*Pinus massoniana* and *Cunninghamia lanceolata*), broadleaf forest (*Lauraceae*), mixed forest, bamboo (*Phyllostachys pubescens*), and shrub are the dominant forest species, as the primeval forests have almost been exhausted as historic consumption yielded to economical development; most of current forests are secondary vegetation [20].

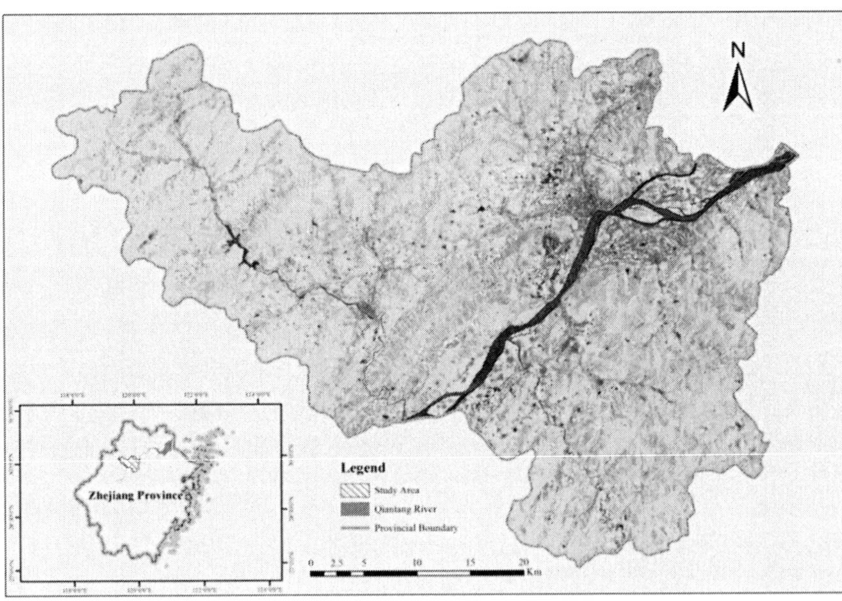

Figure 1. The location of study area with Landsat image in 2013 (RGB: 543).

2.2. Field Measurement

Field work is the foundation for remote sensing technology to extend limited stand information to large scale predictions. The two datasets used in this study are part of the field investigation data for Zhejiang Province, through a stratified random sampling approach using the same strategy in 2008 and 2013 administered by Zhejiang Forestry Academy. The allocation of hierarchical sample plots is based on a comprehensive consideration of geographical conditions and forest properties, including climate zone, tree species, age composition, and site characteristics. The theory of errors is employed to assure the quantity of typical samples, both in training and validation. The size of each inventory plot is 20 m × 20 m for trees, with three 2 m × 2 m subplots set in the diagonal line of each plot for shrubs and grasslands. Fundamental measurements are comprised of diameter at breast height (DBH), height and species recorded with Global Positioning System (GPS). The total Above Ground Biomass is the sum of tree, shrub, and herbaceous in each plot regarded and is as the final AGB with a unified unit of ton/ha. In general, six groups, including broadleaved forest, coniferous and broadleaved mixed forest, Shrub, Bamboo forest, Pine forest and Chinese fir forest, were calculated using specific allometric equations as a function of tree height and DBH, described in [21]. Main specific species included pine forest, Chinese fir, hardwood (I and II), *Phyllostachys heterocycla* cv. *Pubescens*, and so on. As the formulations developed by Yuan *et al.* have been successfully utilized to several provincial applications [22,23,24], we adopted those calculations for establishing aboveground biomass of sample plots. There are 87 and 80 sample plots for 2008 and 2013, respectively (Table 1).

Table 1. Statistics of field-based aboveground biomass.

Years	# Plots	Min AGB (ton/ha)	Max AGB (ton/ha)	Mean AGB (ton/ha)	Std.Dev.AGB (ton/ha)
2008	87	8.05291	193.2647	86.1533	40.76886446
2013	80	14.70901	219.692	98.7338	47.8469626

2.3. Remote Sensing Data Pre-Processing

As mentioned above, Landsat imagery was chosen as the main remote sensing data source for its convenient procurability and suitable spectral information. To overcome the limited availability of cloud-free images, two Landsat Thematic Mapper (TM) 5 images and one Landsat Operational Land Imager (OLI) image (path/row: 119/39), with the least clouds, were selected as the data sources from the United States Geological Survey

(USGS) website [25]. The standard level-one terrain-corrected L1T images geometrically calibrated and orthorectified to WGS-84 datum were acquired on different dates: 26 July 2004, 5 July 2008 and 19 July 2013. The images were obtained within the same month to minimize phonological influence. Visible bands and shortwave infrared bands were used as the spectral variables (except for the first blue band in 2013), and the thermal infrared channels were abandoned because of their coarser spatial resolution, both for TM and OLI. Radiometric calibration converting DN values to the top of the atmosphere radiance was conducted via the gain and offset information within the attached metadata files. Afterwards, atmospheric correction was completed by "Fast Line of sight Atmospheric Analysis of Spectral Hypercubes" (FLAASH) in ENVI software for the base image in 2008 [26], input parameters, including sensor type, flight time, atmospheric model, aerosol mode, and other parameters, were determined. Pseudo-Invariant Features (PIFs) were selected as the relative radiometric calibration method to make the 2004 and 2013 images consistent with the reference image from 2008 [27]; dark pixels located in water area and light pixels lay in roads, buildings were visually inspected and selected as invariant target pixels by referring to high resolution images and local knowledge to formulate the relationships between reference image and images to be corrected. SCS+C correction was executed to reduce topographical effect with the same resolution Digital elevation model (DEM) data [28], which would alleviate the overcorrection problem in sun-canopy-sensor (SCS) model by introducing adjustment coefficient analogous to C-correction. Here is the formulation:

$$\rho_n = \rho \times \frac{\cos\alpha \times \cos\theta + C}{\cos i + C} \tag{1}$$

where ρn is the objective reflectance, ρ is the uncorrected reflectance, α is the terrain slope, θ is the solar zenith angle, i is the incidence angle, while cosi and c are defined as follows:

$$\cos i = \cos\alpha \times \cos\beta + \sin\alpha \times \sin\theta \times \cos(\varphi - \beta) \tag{2}$$

where β is the terrain aspect and φ is the solar azimuth angle. Besides, C is calculated as the ratio of a to b, where ameans the regression slope and b refers to the intercept.

$$\rho = a + b \times \cos i \tag{3}$$

2.4. Variables Derivation

One key procedure to build and apply the relationship between remote sensing data and forest biophysical property for biomass estimation is to extract valuable candidate Landsat derivations. By referring to previous studies, apart from the original multi-spectral bands, other potentially helpful variables from the processed Landsat image were calculated. Vegetation indices were proposed as preferably important measures for forest biophysical researches. Among the vegetation indices, Normalized Difference Vegetation Index (NDVI) is the most widely used index, however, in the present study, we adopted the improved index named NDVIc as we found that it had a stronger relationship with AGB because it combined the information of shortwave infrared band, which provides valuable information to biomass retrieval [29].

The NDVIc is defined as follows:

$$NDVI_C = \frac{NIR - RED}{NIR + RED} \times \left[1 - \frac{(MIR - MIR_{min})}{(MIR_{max} - MIR_{min})}\right] \tag{4}$$

where NIR is the near-infrared band RED is the red band, MIR is the shortwave infrared band, MIR_{max} and MIR_{min} are values in the shortwave infrared band from closed canopies and open canopies. In this study, the last two values were extracted from the shortwave infrared band within the forest area for the highest value and the lowest value.

Tasseled Cap (TC) transformation was executed to reduce the primary multi-spectral information into reduced compendious features sensitive to vegetation characteristics, *viz.* brightness, greenness, and wetness [30]. Texture information was derived from the most practical method Gray Level Co-occurrence Matrix (GLCM), eight measurements including mean, variance, homogeneity, contrast, dissimilarity, entropy, second moment and correlation that were calculated from four bands (band2, band3, band4 and band5) with a window size of 3 × 3 pixels [31]. Moreover, DEM was used to generate topographical variables including slope, aspect and elevation.

In addition, the contemporaneous local Land Use and Cover maps were used as the reference to mask the non-forest area for three years to ensure that the modeling process was restricted to the forest area. Considering the positional uncertainties in GPS recordings, 3 × 3 pixels windows were used to calculate the mean values of remote sensing variables in the corresponding images.

2.5. Modeling Methods and Precision Assessment

To inspect the relationship between biomass and remote sensing variables, the field-measured AGB was considered as a dependent variable and imagery generated variables were treated as independent variables. Random forest algorithm was employed for regression as it showed significantly commendable performance than other regression techniques by previous studies and has been widely applied to environmental monitoring [32,33]. In this algorithm, numbers of decision trees are generated to the maximum extent without pruning by randomly selected two thirds of the data as training samples with bootstrapping, strengthening the flexibility by aggregating multiple classification and regression trees, and the remaining one third of data, also called out-of-bag (OOB), is used as validation samples to estimate the modeling errors. Furthermore, at each node of the decision tree, the selection of features for modeling is also stochastic, which makes the approach immune to the problem of over-fitting [34]. Therefore, there are two important parameters, respectively named *mtry*, denoted as the number of features used to split the nodes, and *ntree*, which means the number of trees to be adjusted to achieve a desirable prediction. Another advantage of the random forest algorithm is that it accomplishes excellent feature selection by automatically ranking the relative importance of variables. There are two mechanics in this algorithm to evaluate the importance of input variables, *i.e.*, mean decrease in accuracy that assesses the effect of a variable, whether it makes the mean decrease in accuracy and mean decrease in Gini Index that infer the impurity of a variable. Taking this into account, all the remote sensing generated variables were used for AGB estimation, and the mean decrease in accuracy measure was used for noting the variables' importance. The regression process was completed in the open access R statistical software [35] using the "randomForest" package [36]. The parameters *mtry* was set to the default value, one third of the total variables, and *ntree* was tested in the range of (100, 500, 800, 1000, 1500).

On account of the limited sample plots, 10-fold cross validation was employed to assess the estimated AGB performance during the modeling process. In addition, validation measures, including coefficient of determination (R^2), Root Mean Squared Error (RMSE) between simulated AGB, and field measured biomass, were calculated to assess the estimation performance.

3. RESULTS

3.1. Variable Importance for Modeling

The features adopted in the random forest regression for two years are shown in Figure 2. Non-parametric analysis Spearman's rank correlation was also performed to assess the correlations between field-based measured AGB and remote sensing variables. As a result, multi-spectral bands, including band4, band5, band7, and texture measurements, including b5_mean, b4_mean, as well as TC components wetness and brightness, were selected as the top 10 important features, both in 2008 and 2013 random forest retrievals, which was in accordance with the Spearman's rank correlation result (Table 2). Furthermore, the short wave infrared bands had a higher correlation coefficient in all strategies, which was consistent with previous studies [37]. In addition, the variable wetness presenting the moisture content was in high correlation with AGB, which may be owing to the primary water conservation forest occupying the majority in the Fuchun River watershed. However, there was some difference between the important variable selection results of random forest and Spearman's rank correlation. Although some fluctuations may appear in the RF algorithm, it should be pointed out that some variables, not selected by the Spearman analysis, still played important roles in the estimation process.

3.2. Accuracy Assessment

In the light of inevitable fluctuations in the random forest algorithm as the initial samples are randomly selected, the model processes in both years were repeated 20 times to acquire the mean values in the R statistical package, where the imputations were stabilized with the *ntree* value of 1000. Figure 3 shows the linear relationships between the estimated AGB and the field-based measured AGB, with a value of R^2 0.93 and RMSE 11.16 ton/ha in 2008, and R^2 0.90 and RMSE 16.9 ton/ha in 2013 (p value < 0.01). The results indicated that random forest, in two years, had an acceptable performance for AGB estimates. This may due to some of the following reasons: the number of plot samples used in the present study is limited with a selection of keeping homogeneous plots, while discarding the outliers using the 3 σ (standard deviation) measurement in both years; stochastic decisions in bootstrap sampling through out-of-bag error estimation, random variable selection, and taking both predictor and response variables into account, simultaneously, make the simulation effective; there are no assumptions about the population of sample plots and the relationships between Landsat image derivations and AGB for random forest regression, which is adaptive to complex forest characteristics.

Nevertheless, it should be pointed out that the phenomena that the values of highest biomass were underestimated and the values of lowest biomass were overestimated still exists, as the result in random forest for regression adopts the mean values of predictions.

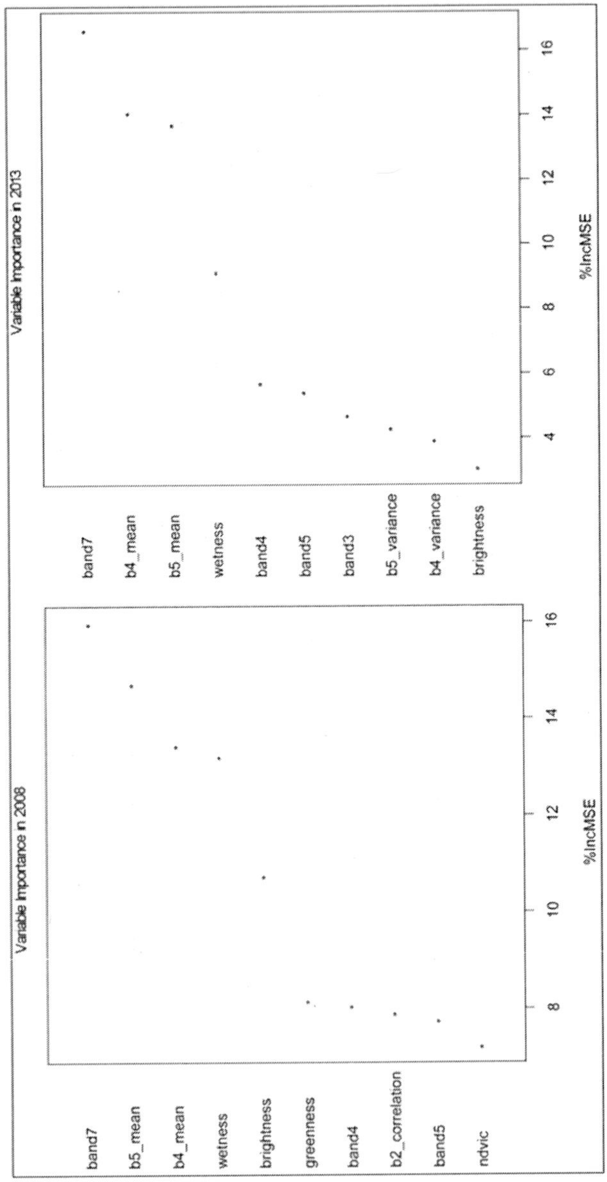

Figure 2. The top 10 variables selected in random forest in 2008 and 2013.

Table 2. Variable selection result of Spearman's rank correlation.

CorrelativeVariables in 2008		**CorrelativeVariables in 2013**	
band7	−0.514 **	band7	−0.566 **
b5_mean	−0.499 **	b5_mean	−0.539 **
wetness	0.483 **	b4_mean	−0.539 **
band5	−0.480 **	wetness	0.509 **
brightness	−0.460 **	band5	−0.493 **
b4_mean	−0.439 **	band2	−0.386 **
band4	−0.413 **	brightness	−0.376 **
ndvic	0.397 **	b2_mean	−0.369 **
greenness	−0.396 **	band3	−0.363 **
band2	−0.372 **	band4	−0.262 *
b4_contrast	−0.285 **	band1	−0.240 *
band3	−0.284 **	b2_second moment	0.235 *
b2_mean	−0.278 **	b2_entropy	−0.228 *
b4_dissimilarity	−0.248 *		
b3_mean	−0.232 *		

Note: * Significant at a 0.05 level; ** Significant at a 0.01 level.

In addition, as it is usually difficult to investigate historical biomass information in practice, previous researches recommended that the same model could be applied to time series images which lack synchronous field data but corrected using relative corrections [38], therefore the identical random forest regression model adopted in the 2008 image was employed to the relatively corrected image in 2004 to generate an estimated AGB map. In addition, the AGB map in 2013 was generated separately, based on a random forest simulation using the simultaneous field-based data.

3.3. Aboveground Biomass Estimates

3.3.1. AGB Distribution Characteristic

The estimated AGB maps of three years in Fuyang County are shown in Figure 4. The mean values of AGB were 74.24 ton/ha, 76.33 ton/ha, and 99.63 ton/ha in 2004, 2008, and 2013, respectively, showing a significant rising trend in the past decades, owning to the measures that the government has taken in order to improve forest quality, such as young forest management and forest cultivation. Similar AGB distribution patterns were observed over the three periods, from the map that high-value biomass locations were lying close to the Fuchun River, where cultivated with broadleaf and coniferous forest. While relatively lower biomass positions were primarily distributed in the northwest, which was mostly planted with shrubs and some plantations for timber production. The primary forest around the Yanshi Ridge reservoir was highwood, according to the local

Land Use and Land Cover map. Furthermore, in the southeast of the study area, as the majority of natural secondary forests were planted with *phyllostachys pubescens*, when compared to broadleaf and coniferous forest, the bamboo forest had a relatively lower biomass value. The discrepancies of AGB estimation distribution were similar to the distinct arrangement characteristic of different forest species, reflecting that the local tripartite programming had a great influence on forest allocation and development.

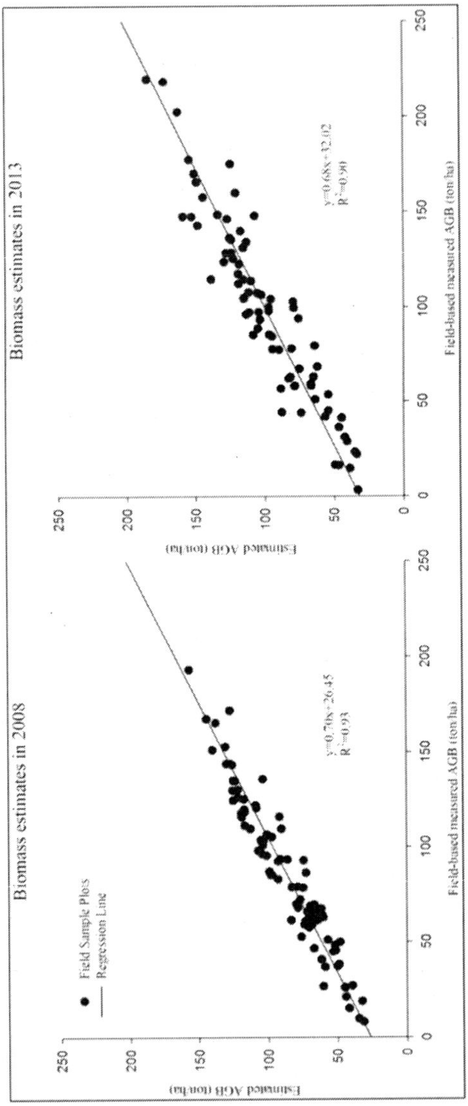

Figure 3. The relationship between estimated AGB and field-based measured AGB.

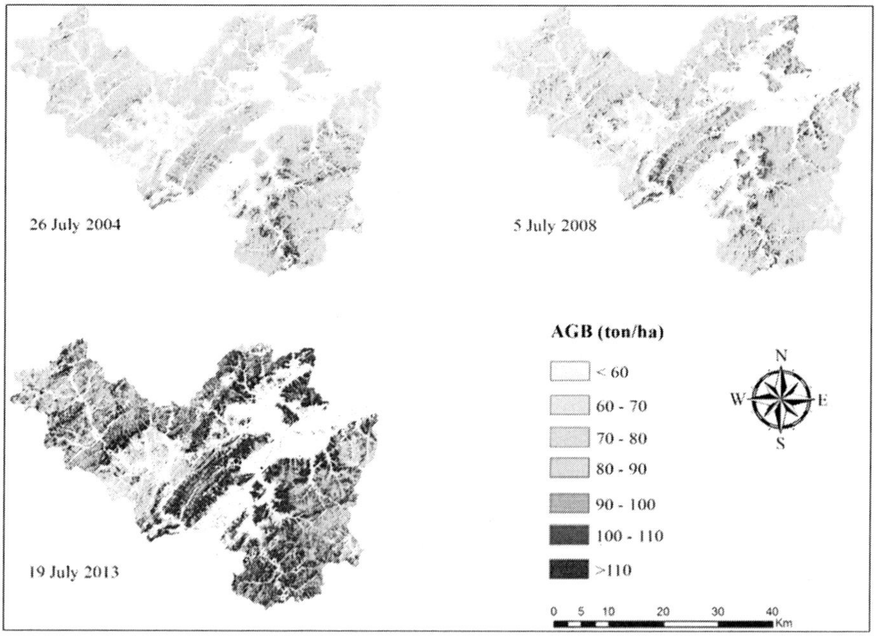

Figure 4. Estimated aboveground biomass in Fuyang County over three periods.

3.3.2. AGB Changes with Terrain

As the main soil type in the study area was red soil that mainly distributed across an elevation of 200–500 m, the terrain was divided into four stratifications (Figure 5a) to investigate the mean value of AGB change among different elevation gradients. Because temperature, precipitation and other environmental factors vary with elevation, the estimated biomass exhibits non-stationary biomass variations in terms of altitude. With the increase of elevation, the mean value of biomass was gradually increased in the three years, except in 2008, which may have been greatly influenced by the freezing rain and snow disaster at the beginning of that year, the biomass even decreased with higher elevation. Additionally, the greatest increase rate 36.46% took place in the 80–200 m gradation from 2004 to 2013, followed by the 30–80 m gradation (34.88%), when compared to the growth above 200-m elevations (30.93%).

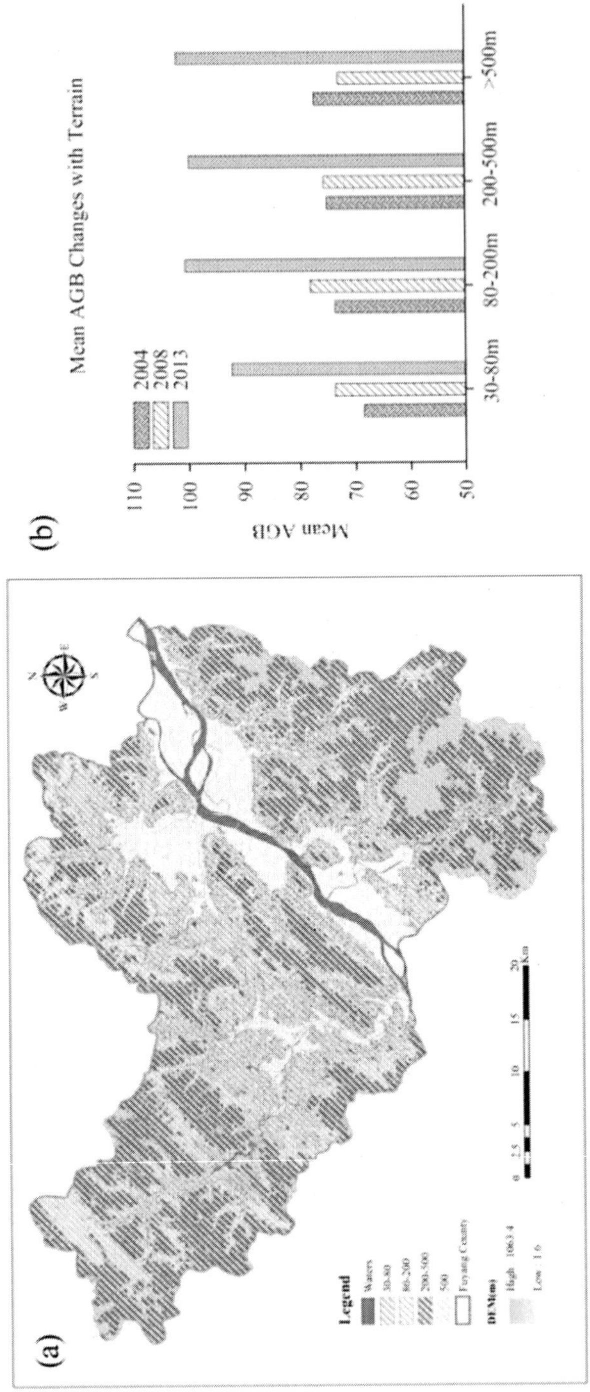

Figure 5. (**a**) Map of elevation stratification, and (**b**) change of AGB with stratified terrain.

3.3.3. AGB Change within Ecological Forest

The outcome in Figure 6 illustrates that the AGB spatial distribution exhibited different characteristics within two level ecological forests. In general, the mean value of AGB within the national ecological forest was higher than that located in the provincial ecological forest over all the periods, which conforms to the original design that national ecological forest possesses the highest susceptible location and occupied the most important geographic niches. Furthermore, AGB values in these two ecological forests were higher than that of the contemporaneous entire forest, suggesting that the established ecological forest delineation has a greater potential for local carbon sink and carbon storage. Meanwhile, the increase rate values of AGB in national ecological forest, provincial ecological forest and normal forest were 42.26%, 36.65%, and 32.19%, respectively, indicating that the policy of establishing ecological forest showed an obvious positive effect on forest ecosystem protection.

4. DISCUSSION

4.1. Reasons for AGB Changes

The reason to explain the overall increase biomass with regard to the terrain over the past decade may be due to the measurements taken by the local government. For example, in recent years, forest ecosystems along the Fuchun River banks and tributaries about 9600 hectare at low altitude were preserved with an emphasis on rebuilding zonal ecological protection forests to improve environment quality. Moreover, afforestation in the flat-land areas was promoted by changing part of cultivated land to forest along with implementing plantations to be tree-lined [20]. For mountain areas, more forest parks and nature reserves were established through enclosing the hills for natural reforestation. Figure 5b indicates the powerful restorative capability recovered from natural disasters with distinct biomass augments. Nevertheless, when the practicality is taken into consideration, geographic limitations, such as transportation convenience and water availability, areas located in higher elevations were less affected by human activities than the lower mountain areas, which may explain the phenomenon that regions located in heights below 200 m displayed larger AGB increases. However, it should be noted that effective measurements, planned to improve the forest quality, are supposed to balance natural conditions and socioeconomic development.

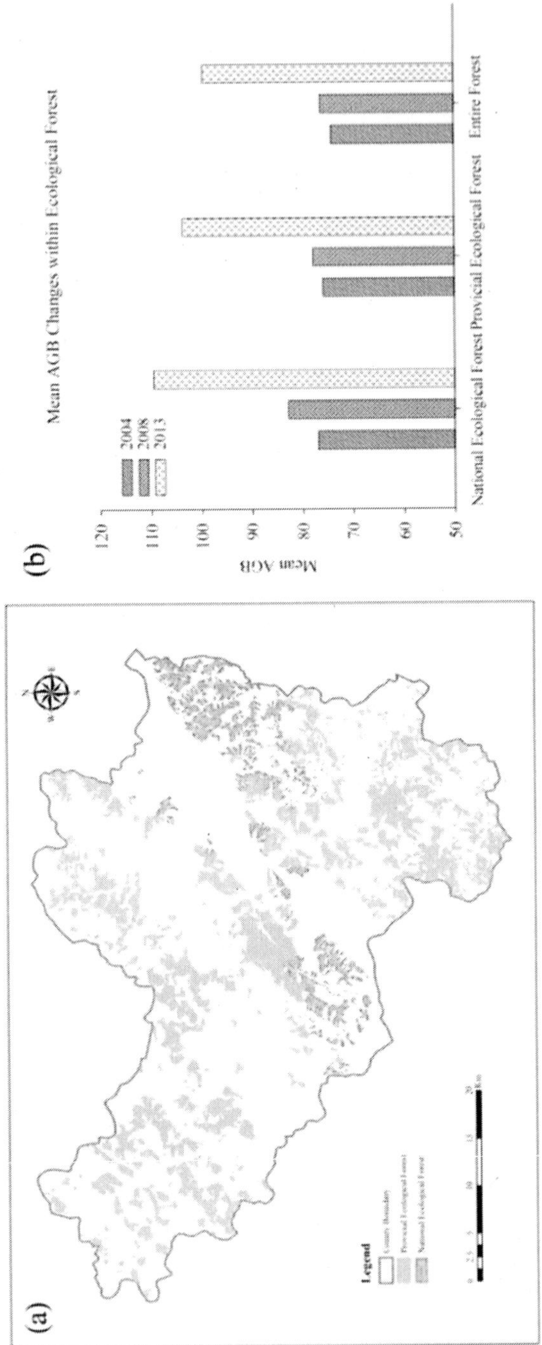

Figure 6. (**a**) Map of two-level ecological forest, and (**b**) change of AGB within ecological forest.

On the other hand, the implementation of ecological forest suggested significantly positive effects on biomass distribution and improvement. Since 2001, the government in Zhejiang Province had delimited about 197.1 × 104 hm^2 of forest (accounting for 29.43% of the forest region) as ecological forests, also named public welfare forests, which are mainly distributed in river headwaters, river banks, large reservoirs, natural reserves and famous scenery, where presents high ecological significance and low ecological vulnerability, in order to separate them from the commercial forests through different operation and management patterns. As to the implementation in Fuyang County, 423.73 km^2 area of forests were delimited as key ecological forests, of which national-level ecological forest occupied 104.27 km^2 and provincial-level took up 319.46 km^2, in total accounting for 37.83% of the entire forest. They are mainly distributed along the Fuchun River basin and national highways, reservoir, as well as scenic spots and forest parks. According to the official gazette on Fuyang key ecological forest, published in 2014, analogous to the research on riparian forests mentioned by [39], the maximal ecological benefit is for water conservation, which was evaluated to count for 56.09 billion Yuan when referring to the local Environmental Bulletin. To attract more attention of the public and to improve the awareness of ecological forest protection, the compensation funds have been gradually increased from the original 8 Yuan/mu to 30 Yuan/mu. All these measurements have promoted local forest conservation, which is reflected by the biomass increase.

4.2. Uncertainty Analysis

The reason that subspecies were not distinguished in this study, except for the limited number of sample plots, was that we wanted to accomplish recapitulative biomass estimation at the regional scale. The mean AGB for the ecological forest is 106.61 ton/ha and 99.63 ton/ha for the entire forest, compared to previous research utilizing field inventory data in Zhejiang Province. Qian *et al.* [40] predicted the mean biomass of ecological forests in the whole province would increase to 99.30 $t \cdot hm^{-2}$ in 2011, and Zhang *et al.* [22] mentioned that the mean biomass forest in Xianju County was 94.51 $t \cdot hm^{-2}$ in 2008. Other than the study conducted by Chen [41], obtaining a result of 113.33 $t \cdot hm^{-2}$ for the Liandu District ecological forest in 2008, which exhibited a higher value than our result, the others showed comparable estimates with this study.

A great deal of uncertainty still exists when estimating forest biomass [42]. Strictly speaking, complete biomass is comprised of above-ground and under-ground components, while we only focused on the above-ground biomass as the main objective. Optical imagery has obvious limitations for AGB estimates, for instance, the backgrounds, including understory vegetation and soil, can greatly influence the relationship between AGB and derived spectral bands. The spectral information is representative of tree canopy, but defective for the three-dimensional properties of the forest [43]. All this suggests that there exist gaps, but potential improvement for accuracy biomass retrieval. Since remote sensing has the advantage of macroscopic and dynamic monitoring, it provides powerful specific spectral change information and linked relationships to forest biophysical properties to investigate the interactions between environmental variables and human activities. Biomass distribution and change were simulated in the present study to quantify human activities' effects on forest ecosystems, revealing corresponding intensive biomass reactions to human interventions. Consequently, multi-source images containing more tree parameter information, associated with systematic forest administration, will be considered for further research in order to achieve more precise observations.

5. CONCLUSIONS

Remote sensing provides nondestructive and continues detection information on biomass of forest ecosystem. With the open access of Landsat imagery and rapid development of computer science, especially machine learning approaches, time-series remote sensing records could be applied to an AGB investigation, not only expanding the traditional, limited plot scale to regional or larger spatial scales, but also increasing temporal acquisitions of biomass dynamics with lower cost and higher efficiency. The economic, modern techniques, cooperating with field-based survey, helps to gain a better understanding of the interactions between human activities and forest properties in a spatially macroscopical perspective, which would present vegetation evolution processes and illuminate subsequent policy decisions.

In this study, Landsat image and field data were integrated to estimate the three period forest aboveground biomass in Fuyang County, Zhejiang Province, China, using the random forest regression with a reliable R^2 above 0.9, and RMSE below 12 ton/ha. The results showed that the estimated AGB increased distinctly from the mean value of 74.24 ton/ha in 2004 to 99.63 ton/ha in 2013, and the spatial pattern of the predicted AGB, primarily dominated by plantations, presented a close relationship with geomorphology and human behavior, dominated by local forest management. In summary, anthropological activities, including afforestation and other forest protection projects, particularly available below 200-m elevation, in conjunction with ecological forest delimitation, especially within the national level ecological forest, greatly influenced the distribution and change of forest AGB, which indicates that Landsat imagery-based

AGB estimates would provide valuable information to better understand the forest ecosystem and promote sustainable development.

ACKNOWLEDGMENTS

The authors are appreciative to the USGS and NASA for the open archives of Landsat imagery, and we are grateful to the Zhejiang Forestry Academy for their field investigations and providing of their local archives. The authors thank the Editor and two anonymous reviewers for their constructive comments, suggestions and help in enhancing the manuscript.

AUTHOR CONTRIBUTIONS

Ke Wang designed the study, Aihua Shen conducted the field investigation, Chaofan Wu created the first draft of manuscript. Chaofan Wu and Muye Gan performed data analysis. Jinsong Deng and Huanhuan Shen contributed to manuscript revision.

CONFLICTS OF INTEREST

The authors declare no conflict of interest.

REFERENCES

1 Costanza, R.; D'Arge, R.; de Groot, R.; Farber, S.; Grasso, M.; Hannon, B.; Limburg, K.; Naeem, S.; O'Neill, R.V.; Paruelo, J.; *et al*. The value of the world's ecosystem services and natural capital. *Ecol. Econ.* **1998**, *25*, 3–15.

2 Liu, J.; Dietz, T.; Carpenter, S.R.; Alberti, M.; Folke, C.; Moran, E.; Pell, A.N.; Deadman, P.; Kratz, T.; Lubchenco, J.; *et al*. Complexity of coupled human and natural systems. *Science* **2007**, *317*, 1513–1516.

3 Olander, L.P.; Gibbs, H.K.; Steininger, M.; Swenson, J.J.; Murray, B.C. Reference scenarios for deforestation and forest degradation in support of REDD: A review of data and methods. *Environ. Res. Lett.* **2008**.

4 Zhang, G.; Ganguly, S.; Nemani, R.R.; White, M.A.; Milesi, C.; Hashimoto, H.; Wang, W.; Saatchi, S.; Yu, Y.; Myneni, R.B. Estimation of forest aboveground biomass in California using canopy height and leaf area index estimated from satellite data. *Remote Sens. Environ.* **2014**, *151*, 44–56.

5 Zheng, S.; Cao, C.; Dang, Y.; Xiang, H.; Zhao, J.; Zhang, Y.; Wang, X.; Guo, H. Retrieval of forest growing stock volume by two different methods using Landsat TM images. *Int. J. Remote Sens.* **2014**, *35*, 29–43.

6 Wang, X.; Shao, G.; Chen, H.; Lewis, B.J.; Qi, G.; Yu, D.; Zhou, L.; Dai, L. An Application of Remote Sensing Data in Mapping Landscape-Level Forest Biomass for Monitoring the Effectiveness of Forest Policies in Northeastern China.*Environ. Manag.* **2013**, *52*, 612–620.

7 Lu, D.; Chen, Q.; Wang, G.; Liu, L.; Li, G.; Moran, E. A survey of remote sensing-based aboveground biomass estimation methods in forest ecosystems. *Int. J. Digit. Earth* **2014**.

8 Du, L.; Zhou, T.; Zou, Z.; Zhao, X.; Huang, K.; Wu, H. Mapping Forest Biomass Using Remote Sensing and National Forest Inventory in China. *Forests* **2014**, *5*, 1267–1283.

9 Roy, D.P.; Wulder, M.A.; Loveland, T.R.; Woodcock, C.E.; Allen, R.G.; Anderson, M.C.; Helder, D.; Irons, J.R.; Johnson, D.M.; Kennedy, R.; *et al.* Landsat-8: Science and product vision for terrestrial global change research. *Remote Sens. Environ.* **2014**, *145*, 154–172.

10 Lu, D. The potential and challenge of remote sensing-based biomass estimation. *Int. J. Remote Sens.* **2006**, *27*, 1297–1328.

11 Dube, T.; Mutanga, O. Evaluating the utility of the medium-spatial resolution Landsat 8 multispectral sensor in quantifying aboveground biomass in Mgeni catchment, South Africa. *ISPRS J. Photogramm. Remote Sens.* **2015**, *101*, 36–46.

12 Zhu, X.; Liu, D. Improving forest aboveground biomass estimation using seasonal Landsat NDVI time-series. *ISPRS J. Photogramm. Remote Sens.* **2015**, *102*, 222–231.

13 Pflugmacher, D.; Cohen, W.B.; Kennedy, R.E.; Yang, Z. Using Landsat-derived disturbance and recovery history and lidar to map forest biomass dynamics. *Remote Sens. Environ.* **2014**, *151*, 124–137.

14 Liu, Q.; Yang, L.; Liu, Q.; Li, J. Review of forest above ground biomass inversion methods based on remote sensing technology. *J. Remote Sens.* **2015**, *19*, 62–74.

15 Latifi, H.; Nothdurft, A.; Koch, B. Non-parametric prediction and mapping of standing timber volume and biomass in a temperate forest: Application of multiple optical/LiDAR-derived predictors. *Forestry* **2010**, *83*, 395–407.

16 Güneralp, İ.; Filippi, A.M.; Randall, J. Estimation of floodplain aboveground biomass using multispectral remote sensing and nonparametric modeling. *Int. J. Appl. Earth Obs. Geoinform.* **2014**, *33*, 119–126.

17 Fu, W.; Fu, Z.; Ge, H.; Ji, B.; Jiang, P.; Li, Y.; Wu, J.; Zhao, K. Spatial Variation of Biomass Carbon Density in a Subtropical Region of Southeastern China. *Forests* **2015**, *6*, 1966–1981.

18 Liu, L.; Peng, D.; Wang, Z.; Hu, Y. Improving artificial forest biomass estimates using afforestation age information from time series Landsat stacks. *Environ. Monit. Assess.* **2014**, *186*, 7293–7306.

19 Liu, C.; Zhang, L.; Li, F.; Jin, X. Spatial modeling of the carbon stock of forest trees in Heilongjiang Province, China. *J. For. Res.* **2014**, *25*, 269–280.

20 Qiu, L.; Zhu, J.; Wang, K.; Hu, W. Land Use Changes Induced County-Scale Carbon Consequences in Southeast China 1979–2020, Evidence from Fuyang, Zhejiang Province. *Sustainability* **2015**.

21 Yuan, W.; Jiang, B.; Ge, Y.; Zhu, J.; Shen, A. Study on Biomass Model of Key Ecological Forest in Zhejiang Province. *J. Zhejiang For. Sci. Technol.* **2009**, *29*, 1–5.

22 Zhang, J.; Gao, H.; Ying, B.; Wang, J.; Yuan, W.; Zhu, J.; Yi, L.; Jiang, B. The biomass dynamic analysis of public walfare forest in Xianju county of Zhejiang province. *J. Nanjing For. Univ. Nat. Sci. Ed.* **2011**, *35*, 147–150.

23 Du, Q.; Xu, J.; Wang, J.; Zhang, F.; Ji, B. Correlation between forest carbon distribution and terrain elements of altitude and slope. *J. Zhejiang AF. Univ.* **2013**, *30*, 330–335.

24 Qian, Y.; Yilita; Dou, P.; Zhu, G.; Ying, B.; Yu, S. Biomass and carbon fixation with oxygen release benefits in an ecological service forest of Jinyun County, China. *J. Zhejiang AF. Univ.* **2012**, *29*, 257–264.

25 U.S. Geological Survey. Available online: http://glovis. usgs.gov (accessed on 20 July 2015).

26 Cooley, T.; Anderson, G.P.; Felde, G.W.; Hoke, M.L.; Ratkowski, A.J.; Chetwynd, J.H.; Gardner, J.A.; Adler-Golden, S.M.; Matthew, M.W.; Berk, A.; *et al*. FLAASH, a MODTRAN4-based atmospheric correction

algorithm, its application and validation. In Proceedings of the IEEE International Symposium on Geoscience and Remote Sensing (IGARSS), Munich, Germany, 24–28 June 2002; pp. 1414–1418.

27 Myeong, S.; Nowak, D.J.; Duggin, M.J. A temporal analysis of urban forest carbon storage using remote sensing.*Remote Sens. Environ.* **2006**, *101*, 277–282.

28 Soenen, S.A.; Peddle, D.R.; Coburn, C.A. SCS+C: A modified Sun-canopy-sensor topographic correction in forested terrain. *IEEE Trans. Geosci. Remote Sens.* **2005**, *43*, 2148–2159.

29 Nemani, R.; Pierce, L.; Running, S.; Band, L. Forest ecosystem processes at the watershed scale—Sensitivity to remotely-sensed leaf-area index estimates. *Int. J. Remote Sens.* **1993**, *14*, 2519–2534.

30 Crist, E.P.; Cicone, R.C. A physically-based transformation of Thematic Mapper data—The TM Tasseled Cap. *IEEE Trans. Geosci. Remote Sens.* **1984**, *22*, 256–263.

31 Dube, T.; Mutanga, O. Investigating the robustness of the new Landsat-8 Operational Land Imager derived texture metrics in estimating plantation forest aboveground biomass in resource constrained areas. *ISPRS J. Photogramm. Remote Sens.* **2015**, *108*, 12–32.

32 Zhang, J.; Huang, S.; Hogg, E.H.; Lieffers, V.; Qin, Y.; He, F. Estimating spatial variation in Alberta forest biomass from a combination of forest inventory and remote sensing data. *Bio. Geosci.* **2014**, *11*, 2793–2808.

33 Kwon, Y.; Li, F.; Chung, N.; Bae, M.; Hwang, S.; Byoen, M.; Park, S.; Park, Y. Response of Fish Communities to Various Environmental Variables across Multiple Spatial Scales. *Int. J. Environ. Res. Public Health* **2012**, *9*, 3629–3653.

34 Breiman, L. Random forests. *Mach. Learn.* **2001**, *45*, 5–32.

35 R Core Team. R: A Language and Environment for Statistical Computing. R Foundation for Statistical Computing. Available online: http://www.R-project.org/ (accessed on 20 September 2015).

36 R Core Team. *R: A Language and Environment for Statistical Computing*; R Foundation for Statistical Computing: Vienna, Austria, 2012.

37 Baccini, A.; Laporte, N.; Goetz, S.J.; Sun, M.; Dong, H. A first map of tropical Africa's above-ground biomass derived from satellite imagery. *Environ. Res. Lett.* **2008**.

38 Lu, D.; Batistella, M. Exploring TM image texture and its relationships with biomass estimation in Rondônia, Brazilian Amazon. *Acta Amazon.* **2005**, *35*, 249–257.

39 Clipp, H.; Anderson, J. Environmental and Anthropogenic Factors Influencing Salamanders in Riparian Forests: A Review. *Forests* **2014**, *5*, 2679–2702.

40 Qian, Y.; Yi, L.; Zhang, C.; Yu, S.; Shen, L.; Peng, D.; Zheng, C. Biomass and Carbon Storage of Public Service Forests in the Central Area of Zhejiang Province. *Sci. Silvae. Sin.* **2013**, *49*, 17–23.

41 Yan-fen, C. Dynamic analysis of Vegetation Biomass and Carbon Storage of Public Welfare Forests in Liandu District.*J. Sichuan For. Sci. Technol.* **2014**, *35*, 66–69.

42 Lu, D.; Chen, Q.; Wang, G.; Moran, E.; Batistella, M.; Zhang, M.; Vaglio Laurin, G.; Saah, D. Aboveground Forest Biomass Estimation with Landsat and LiDAR Data and Uncertainty Analysis of the Estimates. *Int. J. For. Res.* **2012**.

43 Ji, L.; Wylie, B.K.; Brown, D.R.N.; Peterson, B.; Alexander, H.D.; Mack, M.C.; Rover, J.; Waldrop, M.P.; McFarland, J.W.; Chen, X.; *et al*. Spatially explicit estimation of aboveground boreal forest biomass in the Yukon River Basin, Alaska. *Int. J. Remote Sens.* **2015**, *36*, 939–953.

CHAPTER 6

Biomass Resource Assessment and Existing Biomass Use in the Madhya Pradesh, Maharashtra, and Tamil Nadu States of India

Karthikeyan Natarajan [1,*], Petri Latva-Käyrä [2], Anas Zyadin [1], Suresh Chauhan [3], Harminder Singh [3], Ari Pappinen [1] and Paavo Pelkonen [1]

[1] School of Forest Sciences, University of Eastern Finland, P.O. Box 111, Joensuu 80101, Finland

[2] Arbonaut Oy, Kaislakatu 2, Joensuu 80130, Finland

[3] The Energy and Resources Institute (TERI), IHC Complex, Lodhi Road, New Delhi 110003, India

ABSTRACT

India is experiencing energy crisis and a widening gap between energy supply and demand. The country is, however, endowed with considerable, commercially and technically available renewable resources, from which surplus agro-biomass is of great importance and a relatively untapped resource. In the policy making process, knowledge of existing biomass use, degree of social reliance, and degree of biomass availability for energy production is unequivocal and pre-conditional. Field observations, documentation, and fill-in sheet tools were used to investigate the potential of biomass resources and the existing domestic, commercial, and industrial uses of biomass in selected Indian states. To do so, a team of field observers/supervisors visited three Indian states namely: Maharashtra (MH), Madhya Pradesh (MP), and Tamil Nadu (TN). Two districts from each state were selected to collect data regarding the use of biomass and the extent of biomass availability for energy production. In total, 471 farmers were interviewed, and approximately 75 farmers with various land holdings have been interviewed in each district. The existing uses of biomass have been documented in this survey study and the results show that the majority of biomass is used as *fodder* for domestic livestock followed by in-site ploughing, leaving trivial surplus quantities for other productive uses. Biomass for cooking appeared to be insignificant due to the availability and access to Liquefied Petroleum Gas (LPG) cylinders in the surveyed districts. Opportunities exist to utilize roadside-dumped biomass, in-site burnt biomass, and a share of biomass used for ploughing. The GIS-based maps show that biomass availability varies considerably across the Taluks of the surveyed districts, and is highly dependent on a number of enviromental and socio-cultural factors. Developing competitive bioenergy market and enhancing and promoting access to more LPG fuel connections seem an appropriate socio-economic and environmental approach to reduce the use of biomass for indoor cooking and increasing the share of surplus biomass for energy production.

KEYWORDS

India; biomass resources; biomass uses; GIS applications

1. INTRODUCTION

Globally, it is estimated that approximately 2.7 billion people are heavily reliant on traditional biomass as the main fuel for cooking and heating, and approximately 1.5 billion people do not have access to electricity [1]. According to a report by the International Finance Corporation (IFC), the poor globally spend US$37 billion on low-quality energy solutions for lighting and cooking [2]. That means the poor spend three to ten times more of their disposable income on energy than the rich [3]. In India, for instance, the lowest income group spends as high as 8% of their monthly expenditure on cooking energy.

India, the world's second highest populated country after China, accounts for 17.5% of the world's population. Besides the high urbanization rate, high population growth rate, and declining opportunities in the rural areas and a low paying agriculture sector [4], the country's energy [power] sector is confronted with a plethora of impairments and challenges to the ballooning demand for energy and power, particularly in rural India. Rural India is of particular interest because it accommodates almost 70% of the Indian population. It is where the majority of socio-agricultural activities are taking place and where modern energy supply facilities and apparatuses are unequivocally needed to elevate the rural residents' living standards. Due to low household incomes, lack of adequate and reliable electricity supply, the absence of efficient energy options, and the thin markets for commercial fuels and equipment, about 64% and 26% of rural households rely on firewood, crop residues and animal wastes for cooking, respectively [5,6,7]. Due to incomplete fuel combustion in the commonly-used traditional cooking stoves, indoor air pollution has severe health implications on both mothers and their children including acute and/or chronic respiratory diseases [6,7,8,9]. Therefore, political will and determination accompanied by socially oriented public policies aiming at e.g., empowering rural areas with modern energy systems that ultimately helps in "fuel switching" or "transition" may lay the concrete foundation towards rural areas' sustainable development.

In rural areas, there exists a unique opportunity to utilize the surplus agricultural crop residues, forest residues, biomass-based industrial by-products, and the vast set-aside wastelands. If intelligently assessed and, thereafter, effectively harnessed to produce energy, it would undoubtedly improve the indoor living environment, optimize and generate other productive uses of biomass, and certainly improve the socio-economic features of rural people. In this regard, agro-biomass resource assessment and the embedded sociocultural uses must be identified and thoroughly assessed for potential energy production on mini, meso, or macro scales. In India, several studies have quantified the potentials of biomass resources available for energy production [7,10,11]. Despite slight differences in agro-biomass resources quantifications, these studies assert the potentials and availability of agro-biomass for energy production using various biomass conversion technologies mainly gasification and anaerobic digestion processes [10]. These technical studies, however, paid little attention to the existing and competing uses of biomass at e.g., household level. Furthermore, more studies are needed to investigate the nature and degree of social reliance on biomass for household use in areas where biomass-based power plants deemed projects feasible. Moreover, effective public policy in developing countries requires analysis of the factors that affect energy demand at the household level [6]. Moreover, social sustainability and corporate social responsibility are robust components of the overall energy project planning and development which, if achieved, may lead to competitive advantage, improving firm reputation, and increasing customer satisfaction [12]. Identifying the existing practices and the degree of social reliance helps quantify the biomass-based social needs thus avoid future societal conflict or grievances. In a recent study by George and Stern [6] on energy choices in two tribal villages in Maharashtra, they found that higher income is associated with the use of higher quality energy sources, which reduces the overall energy use. Additionally, they found that household size, stove ownership, and seasons influence energy choices. Fuel prices, family size, education level, and cultural factors such as religion or caste can also have pronounced influence on energy choices [6,13].

1.1. Status of Biomass-Based Industry in the Selected States

By 2013, the installed power capacity of 14 operating biomass-based power plants in Madhya Pradesh was around 59 MW_e [14]. The state aims to achieve the target of 300 MW_e biomass power by 2014. As it stands today, the registered biomass capacity in the pipeline has surpassed the target (314 MW_e), however, and due to unfavourable market conditions for biomass power production, many of the registered plants have not yet begin the construction process. Furthermore, out of 314 MWe registered capacity, about 184 MW_e of biomass power capacity had already been de-registered [14]. Maharashtra state aims to achieve 400 MW_e of biomass-based power capacity. The state has already issued all the licences to achieve the target. The licence for plant commissioning is issued under the assumption that five taluks would be able to support one 10 MW_e biomass power plant. As of 2013, the total installed biomass power capacity is around 180 MW_e (18 plants) [15]. Out of 18 power plants, 11 plants have been temporarily or permanently shut down [15]. The southernmost state of India, Tamil Nadu, is crippled by a severe shortfall of power production up to 4000 MW_e from its total demand of 13,500 MW_e. The present installed total biomass plant capacity is around 177 MW_e (19 plants—each plant capacity not greater than 15 MW_e) [16]. Most of the plants are distributed to the south of Tamil Nadu where there is an adequate supply of biomass from agriculture and wastelands. Among the existing biomass power plants, more than half of the numbers of plants (120 MWe with 80% plant load factor) have been struggling due to various reasons like unviable tariffs, restrictions on open access, rise in biomass cost, and reliable biomass supply [17,18].

This study has employed survey-based and GIS-based tools to assess the biomass resources in three different states, namely Maharashtra (MH), Madhya Pradesh (MP), and Tamil Nadu (TN). These states are selected because they produce considerable quantities of agriculture crop residues, accommodate considerable potentials of renewables, and biomass-based energy generation is one of the major focus areas of renewable energy programs in India and particularly in these states (Figure 1).

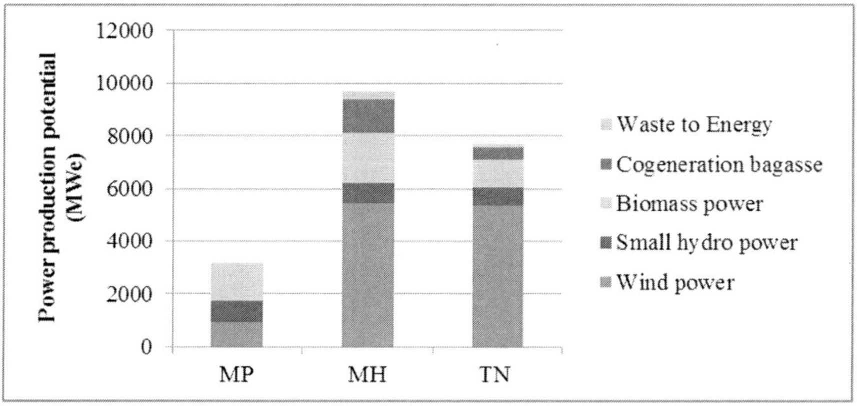

Figure 1. Source-wise renewable power production potential in the three states [19].

The main objectives of this study are to examine and document the existing biomass use practices in rural India and, based on the household biomass consumption, quantify the surplus biomass availability that can be utilized for energy production without jeopardizing the livelihood of the rural families. The implications of this study would assist in developing a new *modus operandi* and a modern biomass value-chain accompanied by technological solutions to help leapfrog the existing technical and social barriers in harnessing and utilizing surplus biomass in power sector. From a policymaking point of view, the study will assist policymakers to better understand the current social uses of biomass in the x-rayed states, thus assisting in crafting transparent and socially-friendly public policies. For investors and business makers, the study will help to identify biomass rich-zones and also poor zones where biomass utilization is socially sensitive. The study will further provide some logistical recommendations for economically reliable biomass utilization.

2. METHODOLOGY

The study area was narrowed down to three states of interest. The selected states were Madhya Pradesh (MP), Maharashtra (MH) and Tamil Nadu (TN). Both Madhya Pradesh and Maharashtra have areas of more than 300,000 km^2 and Tamil Nadu more than 130,000 km^2. The study areas cover nearly a quarter of the whole country's area and more than one fifth of the total population live in the aforementioned states. Two districts have been selected from each state (Figure 2). The selected cities were Bhopal and Indore (Maharashtra), Thane and Pune (Madhya Pradesh), and Kanchipuram and Coimbatore (Tamil Nadu). The selected cities were all the largest cities in each state. The full pilot area covered the city and the surrounding rural area. The actual border for the pilot areas were determined by the Landsat 8 image border, as each of the cities were used as the center point when looking for satellite images.

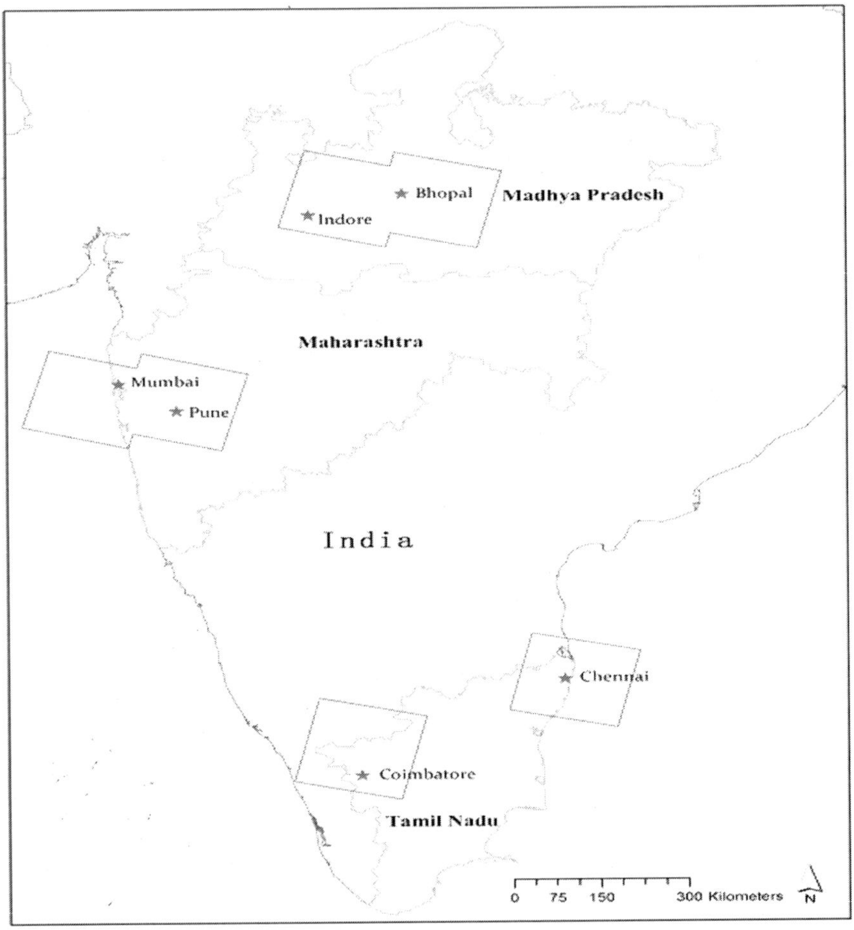

Figure 2. State-level study regions and selected pilot cities including the mapped pilot region.

For mapping the available biomass resources in pilot areas, results from field data were used. The questionnaire study was conducted in the rural parts of each pilot area. Tools were translated into Hindi, Marathi and Tamil to conduct the pen-and-paper based survey. After having consultations with various stakeholders and based on previous experience, a sample size of 75 was selected for household surveys from each selected district with approximately 150 farmers from each state. During preliminary discussions with the stakeholders, it was realized that farmers across different socioeconomic categories could have different production, use and supply patterns. Hence, farmers were divided into three categories of small (less than 5 acres), medium (5–10 acres) and large farmers (more than 10 acres). Due to limited research resources and time constraints, a sample of 25 farmers was drawn from all three categories. In addition, the sample size of 25 was considered to be representative sample size for each category, since the agricultural cropping pattern in a given area (village or taluk) does not vary greatly as most farmers would cultivate one similar crop during that season. Moreover, one can think that the biomass generated from one particular crop does not vary according to the land holding category. After this stratification, households were randomly surveyed from the villages.

The participants answered questions on their annual biomass production, yield, and residue production and the consumption of that residue biomass. To retrieve clearer insights of the biomass resource availability and distribution, literature sources and biomass databanks were also explored. For Madhya Pradesh and Maharashtra, the Biomass Resource Atlas of India was used to acquire the biomass values for agriculture and forest classes [20]. The district-wise biomass information for Tamil Nadu was acquired from a study conducted by Tamil Nadu Energy Development Agency (TEDA) and the Institute for Energy Studies (IES) [16]. Secondary data was also explored from various state reports, policy briefs from international organizations, and peer-reviewed articles. The questionnaire data was transferred from paper forms to digital format and further analyzed to calculate per hectare production and consumption of agro residue and horticulture residue biomass and eventually the total surplus biomass for agriculture land use. These surplus biomass figures were used as the amount of surplus biomass in the biomass mapping stage. To generate biomass-related maps, the GIS Arc Maps was used.

The land use mapping on the state-level was done at the National Remote Sensing Centre (NRSC). However, due to restriction on use of the data, the original land use map is not shown on this paper. The original Land Use Land Cover (LULC) map had 19 classes, and it was reclassified into five classes. It can be assumed that the reclassified map has better overall accuracy because there are fewer classes. However, the classification accuracy of the original map was not calculated. On the other hand, the overall accuracy of the reclassified map in Madhya Pradesh, Maharashtra and Tamil Nadu is 78%, 55% and 53%, respectively. The overall accuracy was relatively low, especially in Maharashtra and Tamil Nadu, at only about 50%. The corresponding kappa values were also quite low—0.55, 0.37 and 0.32, respectively. One reason why the figures are so low can be that the LULC map itself had a slight misalignment when compared to the satellite imagery. The reason for that misalignment was unclear, though, the NRSC does mention that the thematic accuracy is within one to three pixels. Because the accuracy assessment was done on a pixel-by-pixel basis; therefore, the misalignment of even one pixel can cause a specific area to have incorrect class corresponding to it.

3. RESULTS

3.1. The Existing Competing Uses of Biomass in the Selected States

Throughout the field excursions, the various uses of biomass have been documented and presented in Figure 3 below. India is a land of physical, climatic, geographic, ecological, social, cultural and linguistic diversity [4]. Therefore, the uses of biomass vary considerably across the states and are based on a plethora of socio-economic, enviromental, and cultural factors such as level of income, education level, family size, and caste and religious orientation [6,7,11,21]. Other factors such as access to LPG gas cylinders, biomass prices and availability, and availability and access to forest biomass resources are of direct influence on household demand [7,11]. In the surveyed states, the agro-biomasses are widely used for domestic cooking, livestock fodder, thatching, fodder manure, and commercial uses (*i.e.*, sold to third parties, e.g., hotels, bakeries, potteries, restaurants). In some states, field burning is traditionally practiced with respect to crop types. Apart from household and commercial use, biomass is also used in various small-scale industrial rural enterprises such as brick making, rice par-boiling, and charcoal making [21]. In the six surveyed districts, the survey of biomass uses are featured in Figure 4. In Indore and Bhopal, almost half of biomass is used as a feed for domestic livestock and a considerable share of biomass is burnt on site. In Thane and Pune, the use of biomass as a fodder for livestock accounts for almost two-thirds of the available biomass. In the Tamil Nadu state, and in the surveyed districts, the biomass resources are mainly used for animal fodder (46%) and organic fertilizer (33%), such as in Kanchipuram district where 73% is used as organic fertilizer and in Coimbatore district, where 19% is used as fodder for animals. The share of biomass being sold out to third parties varies among the surveyed districts where the highest share is being sold in Thane (30%) to zero percent share sold in Coimbatore district.

The traditional practice of field burning is common in Madhya Pradesh state in order to prepare the field for the next sowing season in a quick span of time. This is because the collection window for biomass is rather short between two seasons. Besides field burning, the soybean residuals are also dumped out on the roadside in MP. Moreover, all the selected six districts have minimal use of biomass for cooking, as the farmers have access to modern LPG cooking stoves. Overall, the results indicate that agro-biomass for fodder is the predominant use of agricultural residues in all the selected study sites except Coimbatore, where only a small share is being sold. This because in Coimbatore, the major agricultural crop residuals are from groundnut, tapioca, and cotton, where they are usually ploughed in the field to maintain and enhance the soil fertility as manure. The agricultural residuals such as sorghum stalks, paddy straws, and maize stalks are collected and used as fodder. The major buyers for agro-biomass are dairy farms and small industries like brick kilns. Furthermore, the share of surplus biomass available for other uses is rather trivial. A revisit to biomass on-site burning, roadside dumping, and ploughing is needed to explore opportunities in diverting part of such waste biomass into energy production facility.

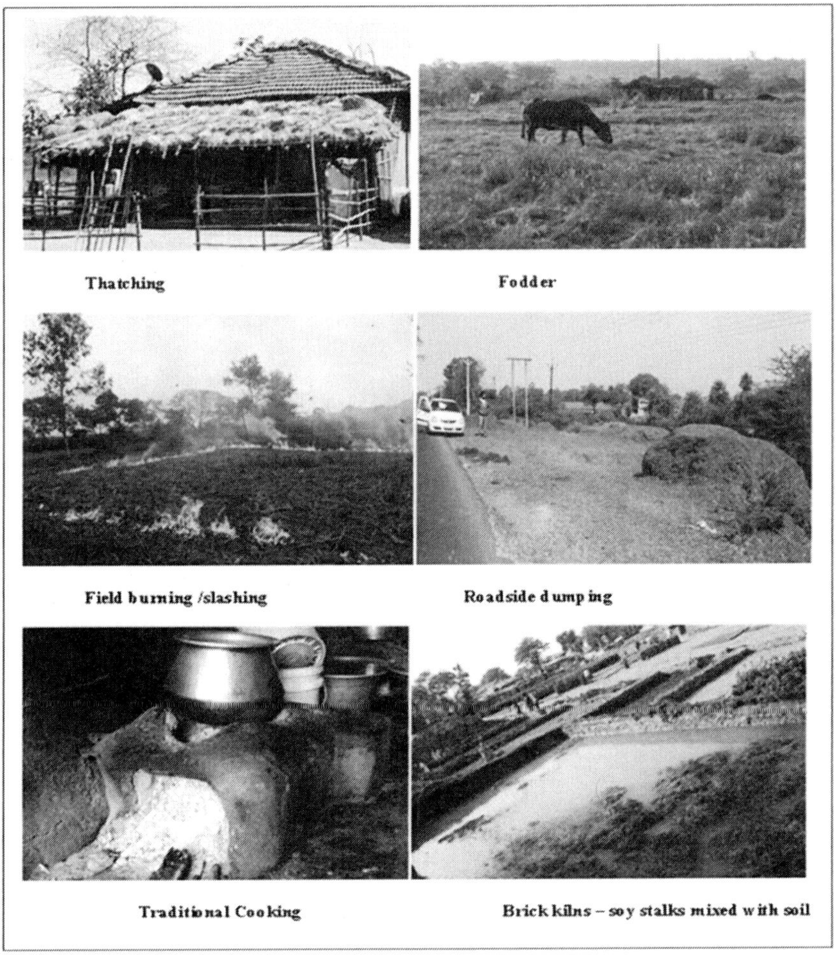

Figure 3. Field-documentation of the various biomass uses in the surveyed states.

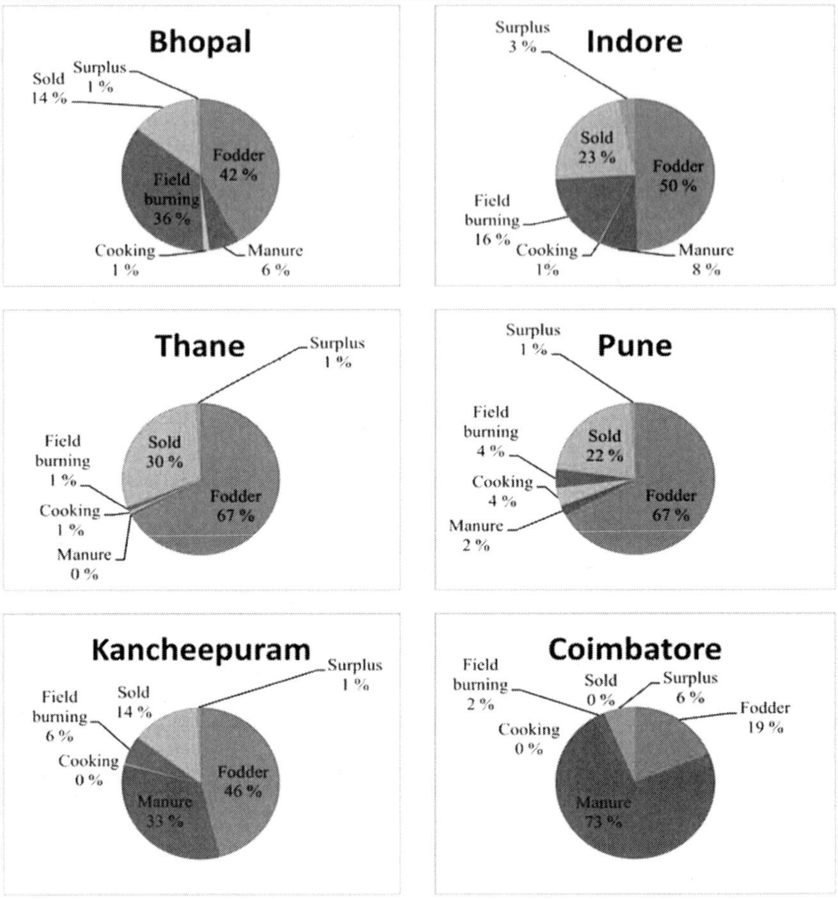

Figure 4. Share of biomass consumption and surplus availability in six pilot districts.

3.2. Mapping the Agro-Biomass and Forest Resource Potentials for Energy Production

The Biomass Resource Atlas of India (2000–2004) estimates the theoretical potential of surplus agro-biomass available for supply at 10.32 million tons in the state of Madhya Pradesh. Similarly, for Maharashtra and Tamil Nadu, the theoretical potential of surplus agro-biomass available for supply was around 14.78 million tons and 8.9 million tons, respectively [20]. For the state-level, biomass mapping (Figure 5) and for covering other land use classes than agriculture in the pilot-level mapping, literature sources were used to search the best possible biomass surplus estimates. For Madhya

Pradesh and Maharashtra, the Biomass Resource Atlas of India [20] was used to acquire the biomass values for agriculture, forest and wasteland classes. The biomass figures were for the years 2000–2004 and the biomass information was listed separately for states, districts and taluks. Biomass information for the Atlas was acquired using data from multiple sources including remote sensing data and field data. The Atlas gives area of production per specific location (state, district or taluk) and land use (Agro, forest or wasteland), and production of total biomass for all land uses as well as the crop biomass for agriculture. The surplus biomass is derived from the production and consumption of residue biomass, though consumption is not given in the table.

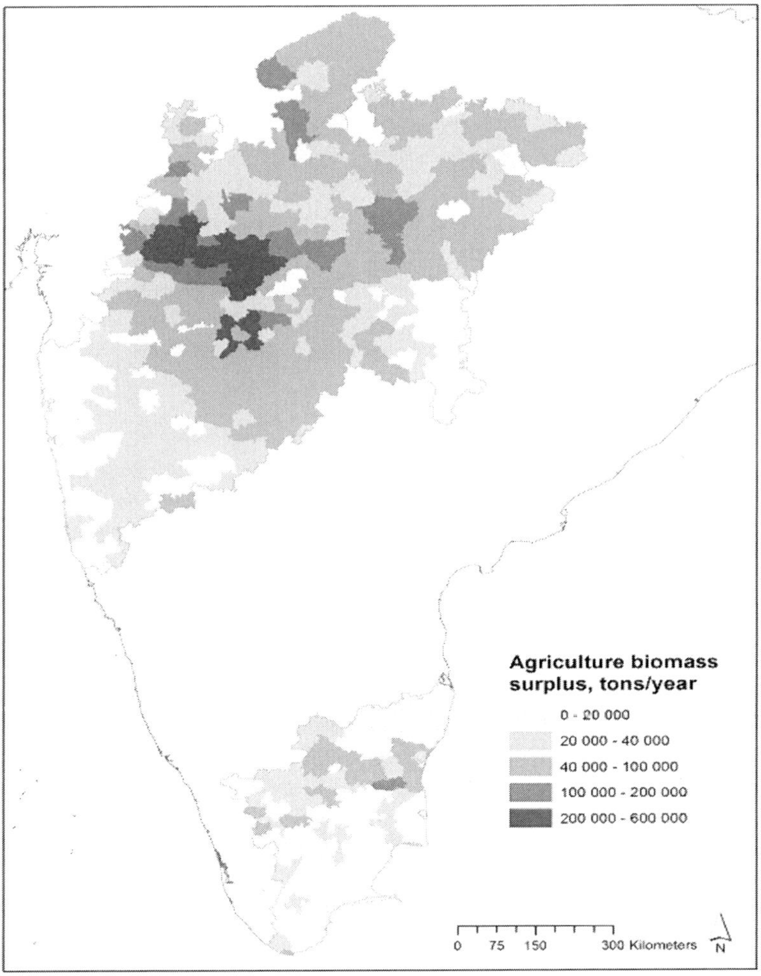

Figure 5. Surplus agro-biomass availability in MP, MH and TN.

It was decided to use the district-wise information, because it was the best combination of spatial detail and data reliability. The taluk-wise information was not used because there were many differences with the administrative taluk border layer used and the Atlas' taluk division. The district-wise biomass surplus and production figures were used for agriculture and forest land use classes. The biomass consumption was calculated based on the aforementioned figure. The values in the Atlas were given as kilotons of biomass per year. The area of specific land use within each district was used to calculate the tons of biomass per hectare figures, which were later used in map production. The district-wise biomass information for Tamil Nadu was acquired from a study conducted by the Tamil Nadu Energy Development Agency (TEDA) and the Institute for Energy Studies (IES). The District Wise Biomass Resource Assessment Study—Tamil Nadu was conducted in 2009–2010 [16].

The surplus biomass available for supply is calculated after taking into account the existing uses of biomass. In 2013, the annual biomass generation in six pilot areas were 387 thousand tonnes in Bhopal, 834 thousand in Indore, 572 thousand tonnes in Thane, 1.364 million tonnes in Pune, 160 thousand tonnes in Kanchipuram and 202 thousand tonnes in Coimbatore. The results show that the share of biomass consumption and surplus availability varied geographically which depends on many factors viz., crop production, crop types, seasonal variations, available infrastructure (e.g., access to LPG cylinders and/or forest wood resources), and socio-economic, cultural, and traditional practices. Another geographical presentation of surplus biomass availability can be found based on crop categories in Hiloidhari *et al.* [7].

The potential of utilizing forest biomass for energy generation exists; however, it is still underutilised. The degraded forest lands offer an excellent opportunity to develop energy plantations, which would also increase the livelihood opportunities for the local community through joint forest management practices. The challenges to harness the forest biomass for energy generation are manifold e.g., inaccurate data on forest land resources, encroachment, strong conservation acts and policies, wildlife, remote areas and poor infrastructure. The Biomass Resource Atlas of India (2000–2004) estimated that 59.7 million tons of surplus forest biomass can be generated annually [20]. The state-wide forest biomass generation potential was 5.4 million tonnes in MP, 5.1 million tonnes in MH, and 2.3 million tonnes in TN [20]. In our study, no field level forest inventory was conducted to study the surplus forest biomass availability; instead, the field level assumptions from [20] have been used to estimate the state-wide forest biomass distribution presented in Figure 6.

The final stage of this analysis was devoted to calculate the biomass power potentials (MW_e). In doing so, data resources from various sources such as state reports, the Biomass Atlas, peer-reviewed articles, and field data have been cross-checked to produce biomass power potentials in the three selected states. These power potential calculations took into account only surplus biomass after deducting the shares of other biomass uses. For power potential calculation, the plant parameter assumptions (average agro-biomass calorific value—3000 kcal/kg, Plant load factor—100%, specific fuel consumption—1.11 kg/kWh, station heat rate—3940 kcal/kWh) were obtained from Orient Green Power, Pollachi, Coimbatore district.

The calculated agro-biomass power potential is presented in Figure 7. The potential energy generation varies spatially explicitly as the share of biomass consumption and surplus availability varied geographically, which depends on many factors viz., crop production, crop types, seasonal variations, existing uses, and available transportation infrastructure. A study by Zyadin *et al.* [22] found that Indian farmers are very much willing to directly supply (sell) their surplus biomass quantities to a potential energy producer and that energy production is perceived to bring prosperity and wealth to their communities. However, the availability of transportation logistics, middleman reliability, and availability of seasonal workers are perceived as key obstacles to the biomass supply chain.

4. DISCUSSION AND CONCLUSIONS

The unprecedented economic growth in India has created a stampede to increase energy demand. Most Indian cities face rolling power cuts which are exacerbated by fluctuating fossil fuel costs and growing demand for more power due to rapid urbanization. The biomass-based power production holds great potential to meet India's growing energy demand, but it is not being entirely utilised. Constraints related to resource availability and seasonality, supply chain logistics and infrastructure, technological modifications, lack of strong legislative and financial measures/incentives, and policy uncertainties have resulted in the poor attraction of biomass power investments or even the shutdown of some existing biomass-powered plants.

The current traditional and cultural practices with various uses of biomass have limited the availability of biomass supply to energy generation. However, it will be unrealistic to collect the biomass for energy generation without embracing the existing particular sociocultural uses of biomass; biomass as a fodder is of critical importance in India. Therefore, it is imperative to utilise non-fodder crops (e.g., soybean husks, cotton stalks, coconut fronds) for energy generation. On the other hand, the biomass dependency for domestic purposes (cooking, thatching) could be reduced through modern cooking stoves (improved cooking stoves, subsidised LPG) and government housing programmes. Switching from traditional energy use would not only reduce the dependency on biomass but also improve the living standards of poor people. In this pretext, during Census 2010–2011, less than 50% of urban households and only 6% of rural households use LPG [23]. The remaining 80% of rural Indian households continue to use traditional fuels for cooking due to affordability, access and awareness limitations [23]. Therefore, the current LPG subsidy mechanism is heavily skewed in the favour of higher income groups and the urban areas of country [23]. Although The *Rajiv Gandhi Gramin LPG Vitaran Yojana* (RGGLVY) has increased the LPG availability in rural areas, sparsely populated and/or remote agglomerations are still underserved due to the "high cost of delivery and financial unviability of conventional distributor models" [23] (p. 10). The report [23] proposes improving LPG availability in rural areas by raising the awareness of the benefits of LPG consumption together with re-rationalizing the subsidies scheme.

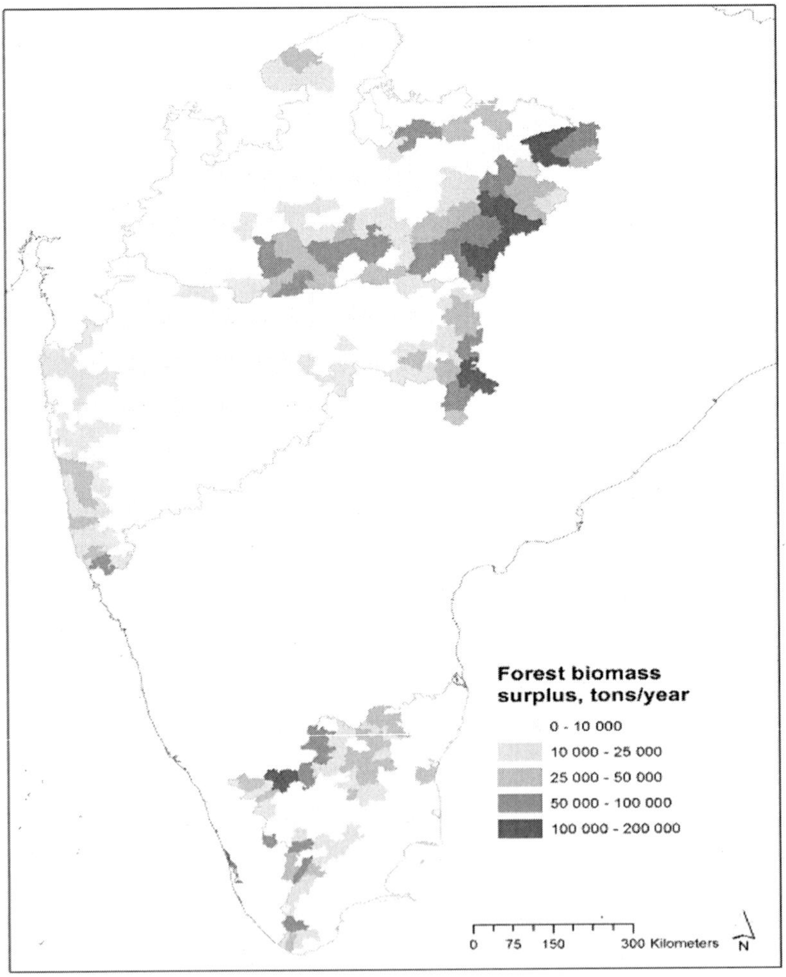

Figure 6. Surplus forest-biomass availability in MP, MH and TN.

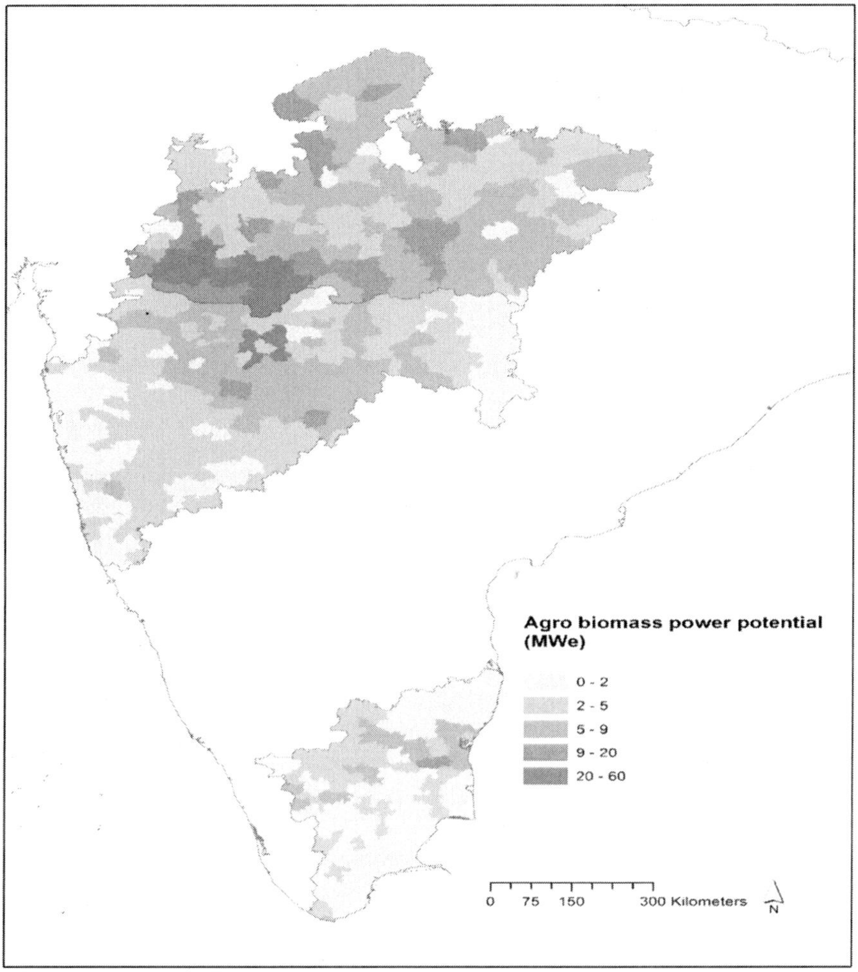

Figure 7. District wide biomass power production potential (MWe) in MP, TN and MH.

An organized biomass market is another key for successful development of the biomass industry in India. New market policies and regulations must accompany the biomass market development to avoid price fluctuations that may harm the economics of the existing or envisioned biomass-based power plants. However, paying extra attention to the sociocultural ties and uses of biomass in rural India is very crucial from a social sustainability point of view.

The present biomass industry lacks successful stakeholder models for sustainable utilisation of biomass for energy generation. For example, a biomass power plant "X" located at "Y" depends on many geographically dependent factors, e.g., continuous biomass supply, quality and mix of biomass, water resources, biomass price, power evacuation infrastructure, labour availability, public acceptance, industrial competition, and co-operation between governmental departments. The variations in any one of the factor would greatly affect the plant production. Besides these factors, commercial installations of renewable energy is very high compared to financial risks involved in other purchase options such as that of conventional non-renewable power projects. In this regard, hybrid energy systems or co-firing biomass in coal-fired power plants accompanied by green certificates-assuming biomass is carbon-neutral, would reduce emissions, and create a somewhat balanced energy production for the time being.

The organized biomass supply chain is crucial to secure and maintain reliable and stable biomass supply. The agricultural biomasses are bulky in nature and, therefore, an efficient supply chain is needed to increase the cost competiveness and energy efficiency. One could select appropriate fuel collection methods like bundling (paddy straw, sugarcane tops), chipping (e.g., eucalyptus, casuarina) with respect to fuel type, which eventually allows more biomass to be transported in a single truck. Subsequently, the biomass could be further processed using fuel processing technologies like pelleting or briquetting to increase the energy efficiency of the fuel. In addition to its increased energy value, the fuel handling becomes easier, and then the biomass can be efficiently transported to longer distances. The sustainability of biomass for energy must be evaluated in detail with respect to food security, environmental performance, and energy efficiency. Importantly, a country like India cannot afford to have pure energy plantations in agricultural lands which would eventually increase the food competition and food prices. On the other hand, agro-forestry practices (where agriculture and energy crops are cultivated together) could be adapted to meet both the agricultural and biomass needs for various food and non-food uses.

ACKNOWLEDGMENTS

The authors wish to thank the anonymous reviewers for devoting their time to comment and improve earlier versions of this article. The authors are indebted to the Indian farmers who participated in this study and provided insightful thoughts regarding biomass distribution and domestic uses. The study was supported by the School of Forest Sciences, University of Eastern Finland under BEST-SHOK project (Project: Sustainable Bioenergy Solution for Tomorrow—WP 2 Task 2.3 Case India) jointly coordinated by the Finnish Bioeconomy Cluster (FIBIC Oy) and the Cluster for Energy and

Environment (CLEEN OY) with funding from the Finnish Funding Agency for Innovation (TEKES).

AUTHOR CONTRIBUTIONS

The authors wish to thank TEKES for providing generous financial support to conduct this research project in India. Anas Zyadin and Karthikeyan Natarajan wrote the manuscript, Karthikeyan Natarajan helped in data collection, photos, and developing resources maps, Petri Latva-Käyrä developed the GIS maps, Suresh Chauhan and Singh Harminder helped in data collection and field excursions, and Paavo Pelkonen supervised the process of setting the research outline, creating survey tools, and providing assistance and commenting on earlier drafts of this manuscript. *Photos courtesy of*: Karthikeyan Natarajan.

CONFLICTS OF INTEREST

The authors declare no conflict of interest.

REFERENCES

1 Practical Action. *Poor People's Energy Outlook 2013: Energy for Community Services*; Practical Action Publishing: Rugby, UK, 2013.

2 International Finance Corporation (IFCI). *Advisory Services in Sustainable Business: 2012 Annual Review*; International Finance Corporation (IFCI): Washington, DC, USA, 2012.

3 International Labour Office (ILO), Cooperatives Unit Green, Jobs Program. *Providing Clean Energy and Energy Access through Cooperatives*; International Labour Office: Geneva, Switzerland, 2013.

4 Vij, D. Urbanization and solid waste management in India: Present practices and future challenges. *Procedia social Behav. Sci.* **2012**, *37*, 437–447.

5 Bhattacharyya, S.C. Energy access problem of the poor in India: Is rural electrification a remedy? *Energ. Policy* **2006**,*34*, 3387–3397.

6 Gregory, J.; Stern, D.I. Fuel choices in rural Maharashtra. *Biomass Bioenerg.* **2014**, *70*, 302–314.

7 Hiloidhari, M.; Das, D.; Baruah, D.C. Bioenergy potential from crop residue biomass in India. *Renew. Sustain. Energ. Rev.* **2014**, *32*, 504–512.

8 Ezzati, M.; Kammen, D.M. Household energy, indoor air pollution and health in developing countries: Knowledge base for effective interventions. *Annu. Rev. Energ. Environ.* **2002**, *27*, 233–270.

9 Bruce, N.; Perez-Padilla, R.; Albalak, R. Indoor air pollution in developing countries: A major environmental and public health challenge. *Bull. World Health Organ.* **2000**, *78*, 1078–1092.

10 Singh, J.; Gu, S. Biomass conversion to energy in India—A critique. *Renew. Sustain. Energ. Rev.* **2010**, *14*, 1367–1378.

11 Kumar, A.; Kumar, N.; Prashant Baredar, P.; Shukla, A. A review on biomass energy resources, potential, conversion and policy in India. *Renew. Sustain. Energ. Rev.* **2015**, *45*, 530–539.

12 Saeidi, S.P.; Sofian, S.; Saeidi, P.; Saeidi, S.P.; Saaeidi, S.A. How does corporate social responsibility contribute to firm financial performance? The mediating role of competitive advantage, reputation, and customer satisfaction. *J. Bus. Res.* **2015**, *68*, 341–350.

13 Masera, O.R.; Saatkamp, S.D.; Kammen, D.M. From linear fuel switching to multiple cooking strategies: A critique and alternative to the energy ladder model. *World Dev.* **2000**, *28*, 2083–2103.

14 Madhya Pradesh Urja Vikas Nigam Limited (MPREDA). Avaliable online: http://www.mprenewable.nic.in/biomass.html (accessed on 22 May 2014).

15 Maharashtra Energy Development Agency (MEDA). Power generaration from renewables: MEDA's new frontier. Avaliable online: http://www.mahaurja.com/PDF/BP_PG_Renewable.pdf (accesse d on 22 May 2014).

16 Tamil Nadu Energy Development Agency (TEDA). Bioenergy achievements. Avaliable online: http://www.teda.in/site/ index/id/ 2O8i9U4E3U (accessed on 22 May 2014).

17 A looming biomess. Avaliable online: http://www. downtoearth.org.in/ content/looming-biomess (accessed on 22 May 2014).

18 Energy Alternative India (EAI). Tamilnadu Biomass, Policy, TN Biomass Power Plants, Biomass Projects, Feedstock and Cost, Biomass Solar Hybrid Opportunities, Biomass Gassification. Avaliable online: http://www.eai.in/club/users/Shweta/blogs/1628#sthash.8wKx1C51.dpu f (accessed on 22 May 2014).

19 Ministry of Statistics and Programme Implementation (MSPI). Energy Statistics. Available online: http://mospi.nic.in/mospi_ new/upload/ Energy_stats_2014.pdf?status=1&menu_id=229 (accessed on 22 May 2014).

20 Indian Institute of Science (IISC). Biomass Resources Atlas of India 2000–2004. Available online: http://lab.cgpl.iisc.ernet.in/ atlas/Default. aspx (accessed on 22 May 2014).

21 Pachauri, S.; Jiang, L. The household energy transition in India and China. *Energ. Policy* **2008**, *36*, 4022–4035.

22 Zyadin, A.; Natarajan, K.; Chauhan, S.; Harminder, S.; Hassan, K.M.D.; Pappinen, A.; Pelkonen, P. Indian farmers' perceptions and willingness to supply surplus biomass to envisioned biomass-based power plant. *Challenges* **2015**, *6*, 42–54.

23 Abhishek, J.; Shalu, A.; Karthik, G. *Rationalizing Subsidies, Reaching the Underserved: Improving Effectiveness of Domestic LPG Subsidy and Distribution in India*; Council on Energy, Environment and Water, Thapar House: New Delhi, India, 2014.

CHAPTER 7

Introduction to Remote Sensing of Biomass

Muhammad Aqeel Ashraf[1], Mohd. Jamil Maah[1] and Ismail Yusoff[2]

[1] Department of Chemistry, University of Malaya, Malaysia

[2] Department of Geology, University of Malaya, Malaysia

1. INTRODUCTION

Planet Earth is distinguished from other Solar System planets by two major categories: Oceans and Land Vegetation. The oceans cover ~70% of the Earth's surface; land comprises 30%. On the land itself, the first order categories break down as follows: Trees = 30%; Grasses = 30%; Snow and Ice = 15%; Bare Rock = 18%; Sand and Desert Rock = 7%. Remote sensing has proven a powerful "tool" for assessing the identity, characteristics, and growth potential of most kinds of vegetative matter at several levels (from biomes to individual plants). Vegetation behaviour depends on the nature of the vegetation itself, its interactions with solar radiation and other climate factors, and the availability of chemical nutrients and water within the host medium (usually soil, or water in marine environments). A common measure of the status of a given plant, such as a crop used for human consumption, is its potential productivity (one such parameter has units of bushels/acre or tons/hectare, or similar units). Productivity is sensitive to amounts of incoming solar radiation and precipitation (both influence the regional climate), soil chemistry, water retention factors, and plant type, keeping in mind that various remote sensing systems (e.g., meteorological or earth-observing satellites) can provide inputs to productivity estimation.

Remote sensing can be broadly defined as *the collection and interpretation of information about an object, area, or event without being in physical contact with the object.* Aircraft and satellites are the common platforms for remote sensing of the earth and its natural resources. Aerial photography in the visible portion of the electromagnetic wavelength was the original form of remote sensing but technological developments has enabled the acquisition of information at other wavelengths including near infrared, thermal infrared and microwave. Collection of information over a large numbers of wavelength bands is referred to as multispectral or hyperspectral data. The development and deployment of manned and unmanned satellites has enhanced the collection of remotely sensed data and offers an inexpensive way to obtain information over large areas. The capacity of remote sensing to identify and monitor land surfaces and environmental conditions has expanded greatly over the last few years and remotely sensed data will be an essential tool in natural resource management.

1.1. Electromagnetic Energy

The electromagnetic (EM) spectrum is the continuous range of electromagnetic radiation, extending from gamma rays (highest frequency & shortest wavelength) to radio waves (lowest frequency & longest wavelength) and including visible light.

The EM spectrum can be divided into seven different regions —— gamma rays, X-rays, ultraviolet, visible light, infrared, microwaves and radio waves.

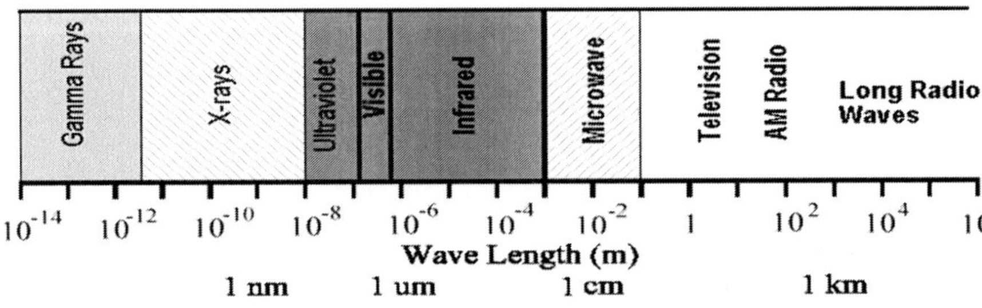

Figure 1. Electromagnetic radiation spectrum

Remote sensing involves the measurement of energy in many parts of the electromagnetic (EM) spectrum. The major regions of interest in satellite sensing are visible light, reflected and emitted infrared, and the microwave regions. The measurement of this radiation takes place in what are known as **spectral bands**. A spectral band is defined as a discrete interval of the EM spectrum. For example the wavelength range of 0.4μm to 0.5μm **(μm = micrometers or 10-6m)** is one spectral band. Satellite sensors have been designed to measure responses within particular spectral bands to enable the discrimination of the major Earth surface materials. Scientists will choose a particular spectral band for data collection depending on what they wish to examine.

The design of satellite sensors is based on the absorption characteristics of Earth surface materials across all the measurable parts in the EM spectrum.

1.2. Reflection And Absorption

When radiation from the Sun reaches the surface of the Earth, some of the energy at specific wavelengths is absorbed and the rest of the energy is reflected by the surface material. The only two exceptions to this situation are if the surface of a body is a perfect reflector or a true black body. The occurrence of these surfaces in the natural world is very rare. In the visible region of the EM spectrum, the feature we describe as the colour of the object is the visible light that is not absorbed by that object. In the case of a green leaf, for example, the blue and red wavelengths are absorbed by the leaf, while the green wavelength is reflected and detected by our eyes.

In remote sensing, a detector measures the **electromagnetic (EM) radiation** that is reflected back from the Earth's surface materials. These measurements can help to distinguish the type of land covering. Soil, water and vegetation have clearly different patterns of reflectance and absorption over different wavelengths. The reflectance of radiation from one type of surface material, such as soil, varies over the range of wavelengths in the EM spectrum. This is known as the **spectral signature** of the material.

1.3. Sensors And Platforms

A sensor is a device that measures and records electromagnetic energy. Sensors can be divided into two groups. **Passive sensors** depend on an external source of energy, usually the sun. The most common passive sensor is the photographic camera. **Active sensors** have their own source of energy; an example would be a radar gun. These sensors send out a signal and measure the amount reflected back. Active sensors are more controlled because they do not depend upon varying illumination conditions.

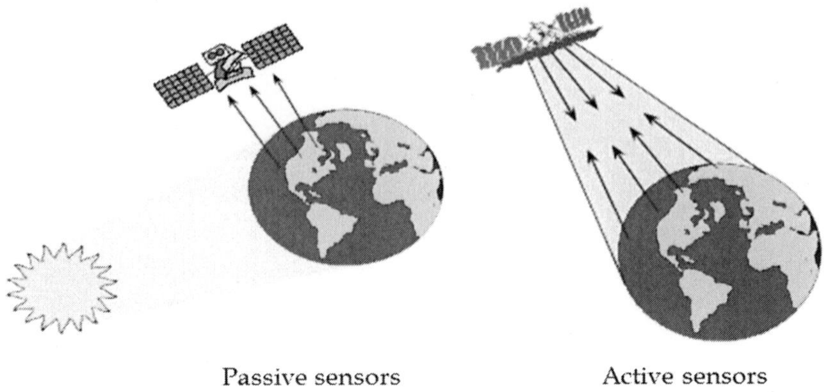

Figure 2. Active and passive sensors

1.3.1. Orbits and Swaths

The path followed by a satellite is referred to as its orbit. Satellites which view the same portion of the earth's surface at all times have geostationaryorbits. Weather and communication satellites commonly have these types of orbits. Many satellites are designed to follow a north south orbit which, in conjunction with the earth's rotation (west-east), allows them to cover most of the earth's surface over a period of time. These are Near-polar orbits. Many of these satellites orbits are also Sun-synchronous such that they cover each area of the world at a constant local time of day. Near polar orbits also means that the satellite travels northward on one side of the earth and the southward on the second half of its orbit. These are called Ascending and Descending passes. As a satellite revolves around the earth, the sensor sees a certain portion of the earth's surface. The area imaged is referred to as the Swath. The surface directly below the satellite is called the Nadir point. Steerable sensors on satellites can view an area (off nadir) before and after the orbits passes over a target.

1.3.1.1. Satellite Sensor Characteristics

The basic functions of most satellite sensors are to collect information about the reflected radiation along a pathway, also known as the field of view (FOV), as the satellite orbits the Earth. The smallest area of ground that is sampled is called the instantaneous field of view (IFOV). The IFOV is also described as the pixel size of the sensor. This sampling or measurement occurs in one or many spectral bands of the EM spectrum. The data collected by each satellite sensor can be described in terms of spatial, spectral and temporal resolution.

1.3.1.2. Spatial Resolution

The spatial resolution (also known as ground resolution) is the ground area imaged for the instantaneous field of view (IFOV) of the sensing device. Spatial resolution may also be described as the ground surface area that forms one pixel in the satellite image. The IFOV or ground resolution of the Landsat Thematic Mapper (TM) sensor, for example, is 30 m. Theground resolution of weather satellite sensors is often larger than a square kilometre. There are satellites that collect data at less than one meter ground resolution but these are classified military satellites or very expensive commercial systems.

1.3.1.3. Temporal Resolution

Temporal resolution is a measure of the repeat cycle or frequency with which a sensor revisits the same part of the Earth's surf ace. The frequency will vary from several times per day, for a typical weather satellite, to 8—20 times a year for a moderate ground resolution satellite, such as Landsat TM. The frequency characteristics will be determined by the design of the satellite sensor and its orbit pattern

1.3.1.4. Spectral Resolution

The spectral resolution of a sensor system is the number and width of spectral bands in the sensing device. The simplest form of spectral resolution is a sensor with one band only, which senses visible light. An image from this sensor would be similar in appearance to a black and white photograph from an aircraft. A sensor with three spectral bands in the visible region of the EM spectrum would collect similar information to that of the human vision system. The Landsat TM sensor has seven spectral bands located in the visible and near to mid infrared parts of the spectrum.

A **panchromatic image** consists of only one band. It is usually displayed as a grey scale image, i.e. the displayed brightness of a particular pixel is proportional to the pixel digital number which is related to the intensity of solar radiation reflected by the targets in thepixel and detected by the detector. Thus, a panchromatic image may be similarly interpreted as a black-and-white aerial photograph of the area, though at a lower resolution.

Multispectral and hyperspectral images consist of several bands of data. For visual display, each band of the image may be displayed one band at a time as a **grey scale image**, or in combination of three bands at a time as a **color composite image**. Interpretation of a multispectral color composite image will require the knowledge of the **spectral reflectancesignature** of the targets in the scene.

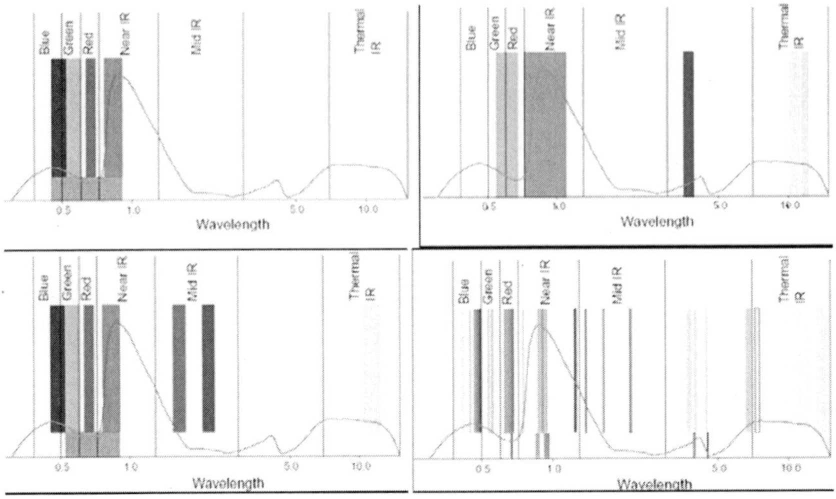

Figure 3. Electromagnetic radiation spectrum with different resolution bands

1.3.2. Platforms

Aerial photography has been used in agricultural and natural resource management for many years. These photographs can be black and white, colour, or colour infrared. Depending on the camera, lens, and flying height these images can have a variety of scales. Photographs can be used to determine spatial arrangement of fields, irrigation ditches, roads, and other features or they can be used to view individual features within a field.

Infrared images can detect stress in crops before it is visible with the naked eye. Healthy canopies reflect strongly in the infrared spectral range, whereas plants that are stressed will reflect a dull colour. These images can tell a farmer that there is a problem but does not tell him what is causing the problem. The stress might be from lack of water, insect damage, improper nutrition or soil problems, such as compaction, salinity or inefficient drainage. The farmer must assess the cause of the stress from other information. If the dull areas disappear on subsequent pictures, the stress could have been lack of water that was eased with irrigation. If the stress continues it could be a sign of insect infestation. The farmer still has to conduct in-field assessment to identify the causes of the problem. The development of cameras that measure reflectance in a wider range of wavelengths may lead to better quantify plant stress. The uses of these multi-spectral cameras are increasing and will become an important tool in precision agriculture.

Satellite remote sensing is becoming more readily available for use in precision agriculture. The**Landsat** and the **NOAA** polar-orbiting satellites carry instruments that can be used to determine crop types and conditions, and to measure crop acreage. The Advanced Very High ResolutionRadiometer (AVHRR) carried onboard NOAA polar orbiting satellites measure reflectance from the earth's surface in the visible, near infrared, and thermal infrared portions of the electromagnetic spectrum.

This spectral sensitivity makes it suitable for measuring vegetative condition and because the satellite passes overhead twice a day, it can be used to detect rapidly changing conditions.Unfortunately, its use as a precision agriculture tool is limited because the spatial resolution of the sensor is nominally 1.1km. A possible application of this scanner would be to use the thermal infrared sensor to estimate daily maximum and minimum temperatures. These temperature estimates could then be used to determine degree-days that will drive pest development models.

Degree-day models are an essential part of IPM programs and the enhanced spatial coverage provided by satellites would allow for assessment of spatial variability in predicted events that is not possible with data from sparsely spaced weather stations currently used for these models. Remotely sensed data can also be used to determine irrigation scheduling and adequacy of irrigation systems for uniformly wetting an entire field. The sensors aboard the Landsat satellite measures reflected radiation in seven spectral bands from the visible through the thermal infrared. The sensors high spatial resolution (approximately 30m) makes it useful in precision agriculture. The spectral response and higher spatial resolution make it suitable for assessing vegetative condition for individual fields but the overpass frequency is only once every 16 days. The less frequent overpass makes it difficult to use these data for assessing rapidly changing events such as insect outbreaks or water stress. New satellites with enhanced capabilities are planned and remotely sensed data will become more widely used in management support systems.

1.3.3. Common Satellites

1.3.3.1. Goes

5 spectral bands 1 - 41 km spatial resolution Geostationary

1.3.3.2. Noaa Avhrr

5 spectral bands 1.1 km spatial resolution 1 day repeat cycle

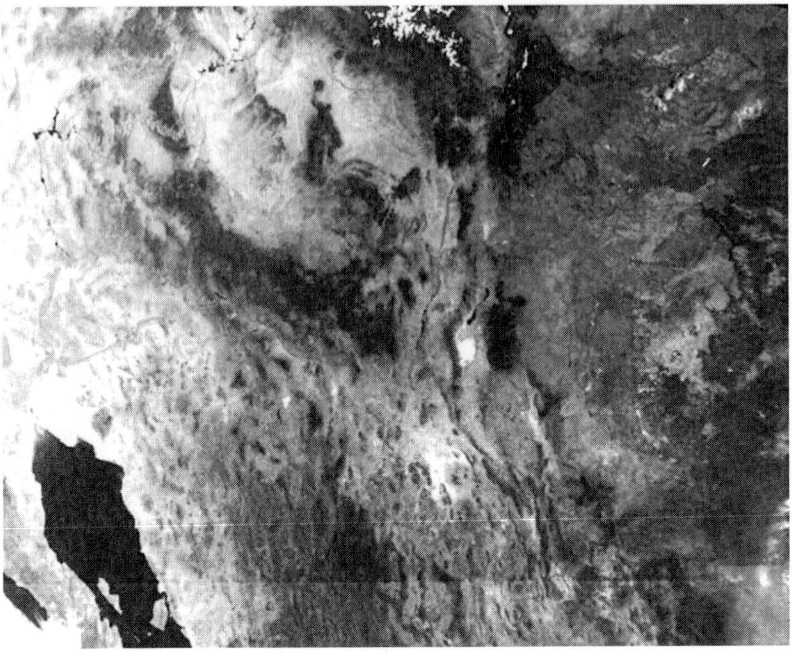

Figure 4. Figure Advanced Very High Resolution Radiometer (AVHRR) image of the southwest Untied States. Image is centred on the Las Cruces, New Mexico.

1.3.3.3. Landsat TM

7 spectral bands 30m spatial resolution 16 day repeat cycle

1.3.3.4. MODIS

Multi- spectral bands 250-1000m spatial resolution (band dependent) 1day repeat cycle

1.3.3.5. IKONOS

4 spectral Bands 4m spatial resolution 5 day repeat cycle

1.4. Spectral Signatures of Natural and Human-Made Materials

Remote sensing makes use of visible, near infrared and short-wave infrared sensors to form images of the earth's surface by detecting the solar radiation reflected from targets on the ground. Different materials reflect and absorb differently at different wavelengths. Thus, the targets can be differentiated by their spectral reflectance signatures in the remotely sensed images.

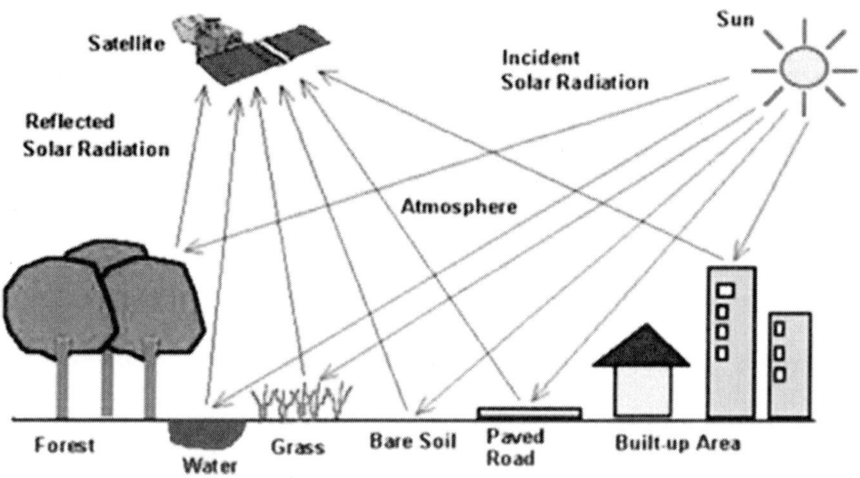

Figure 5. Refraction and diffraction of radiations by different objects

1.5. Spectral Reflectance Signature

When solar radiation hits a target surface, it may be transmitted, absorbed or reflected.Different materials reflect and absorb differently at different wavelengths. The reflectance spectrum of a material is a plot of the fraction of radiation reflected as a function of the incident wavelength and serves as a unique signature for the material. In principle, a material can be identified from its spectral reflectance signature if the sensing system has sufficient **spectralresolution** to distinguish its spectrum from those of other materials. This premise provides the basis for multispectral remote sensing. The following graph shows the typical reflectance spectra of water, bare soil and two types of vegetation.

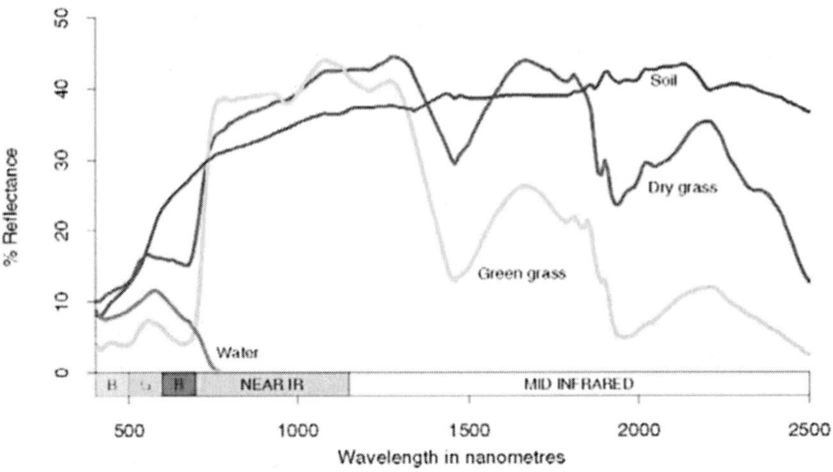

Figure 6. Spectral Resolution Of Different Materials

The reflectance of clear water is generally low. However, the reflectance is maximum at the blue end of the spectrum and decreases as wavelength increases. Hence, water appears dark bluish to the visible eye. Turbid water has some sediment suspension that increases the reflectance in the red end of the spectrum and would be brownish in appearance. The reflectance of bare soil generally depends on its composition. In the example shown, the reflectance increases monotonically with increasing wavelength. Hence, it should appear yellowish-red to the eye.

Vegetation has a unique spectral signature that enables it to be distinguished readily from other types of land cover in an optical/near-infrared image. The reflectance is low in both the blue and red regions of the spectrum, due to absorption by chlorophyll for photosynthesis. It has a peak at the green region. In the near infrared (NIR) region, the reflectance is much higher than that in the visible band due to the cellular structure in the leaves. Hence, vegetation can be identified by the high NIR but generally low visible reflectance. This property has been used in early reconnaissance missions during war times for "camouflage detection".

The shape of the reflectance spectrum can be used for identification of vegetation type. For example, the reflectance spectra of dry grass and green grass in the previous figures can be distinguished although they exhibit the generally characteristics of high NIR but low visible reflectance. Dry grass has higher reflectance in the visible region but lower reflectance in the NIR region. For the same vegetation type, the reflectance spectrum also depends on other factors such as the leaf moisture content and health of the plants. These properties enable vegetationcondition to be monitored using remotely sensed images.

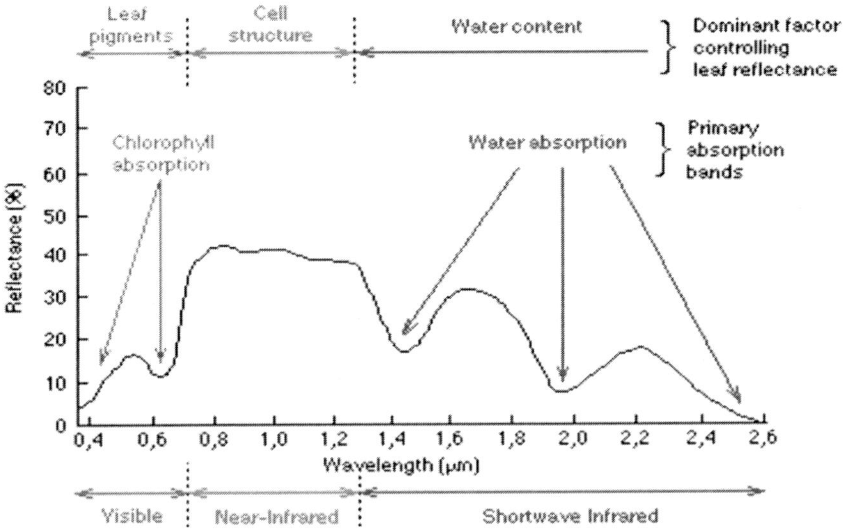

Figure 7. Reflectance spectrum of different materials

1.6. Geodesy, Geodetic Datums and Map Projections

Geodesy is the branch of science concerned with the determination of the size and shape of the Earth. Geodesy involves the processing of survey measurements on the curved surface of the Earth, as well as the analysis of gravity measurements. Knowing the exact location of a pixel on the Earth's surface (its spatial location) is an essential component of remote sensing. It requires a detailed knowledge of the size and the shape of the Earth.The Earth is not a simple sphere. Topographic features such as mountain ranges and deep oceans disturb the surface of the Earth. The ideal reference model for the Earth's shape is one that can represent these irregularities and identify the position of features through a co-ordinate system. It should also be easy to use.

1.6.1. Flat Earth Vs Curved Earth

The "flat Earth" model is not appropriate when mapping larger areas. It does not take into account the curvature of the Earth. A "curved Earth" model more closely represents the shape of the Earth. A spheroid best represents the shape of the Earth because it is significantly wider at the equator than around the poles (Unlike a simple sphere). A spheroid, (also known as an ellipsoid) represents the equator as an elliptical shape, rather than a round circle. Surveying and navigation calculations can he performed over a large area when a spheroid is used as a curved Earth reference model.

1.6.2. Sea Level and The Composition Of The Earth's Interior

The surface of the sea is not uniform. The Earth's gravitational field shapes it. The rocks that make up the Earth's interior vary in density and distribution, causing anomalies in the gravitational field. These, in turn, cause irregularities in the sea surface. A mathematical model of the sea surface can be formulated; however, it is very complex and not useful for finding geographic positions on a spheroid reference model.

1.6.3. Types Of Geodetic Datum

Based on these ideas, models can be established from which spatial position can be calculated. These models are known as geodetic datums and are normally classified into two types geocentric datum and local geodetic datum

A geocentric datum is one which best approximates the size and shape of the Earth as a whole. The center of its spheroid coincides with the Earth's center of mass. A geocentric datum does not seek to be a good approximation to any particular part of the Earth. A local geodetic datum is used to approximate the size and shape of the Earth's sea surface in a smaller area.

Datums and GIS

Having a standard accurate datum set becomes increasingly important as multiple layers of information about the same area are collected and analyzed. The layers are developed into geographic information systems (GIS), which enable the relationships between layers of data to be examined. In order to function effectively, a GIS must possess one essential attribute. It must have the ability to geographically relate data within and across layers. For example, if a dataset about vegetation is being examined against the data sets for topography and soils, the accurate spatial compatibility of the two datasets is critical.

1.6.4. Map Projection Coordinates

A map projection is a systematic representation of all or part of the Earth on a two dimensional surface, such as a flat sheet of paper. During this process some distortion of distances, directions, scale, and area is inevitable. There are several different types of map projections. No projection is free from all distortions, but each minimizes distortions in some of the above properties, at the expense of leaving errors in others. For example, the commonly used Transverse Mercator projection represents direction accurately, but distorts distance and area, especially those farthest from the equator. Greenland, for example, appears to be much larger than it really is. The Transverse Mercator projection is useful for navigation charts.

1.6.4.1. Universal Transverse Mercator (Utm)

Universal Transverse Mercator (UTM) is a global spatial system based on the Transverse Mercator projection. UTM divides the Earth into 60 equal zones, each being 6 degrees wide.Each zone is bounded by lines of longitude extending from the North Pole to the South Pole. Imagine an orange consisting of 60 segments. Each segment would be equivalent to a UTM zone. A rectangular grid coordinate system is used in most map projections. These coordinates are referred to as Eastings and Northings, being distances East and North of an origin. They are usually expressed in metres. Under the UTM system, each East and North coordinate pair could refer to one of sixty points on Earth — one point in each of the sixty zones. Because of this, the zone number needs to be quoted to ensure the correct point on Earth is being identified.

1.6.4.2. Global Positioning System

The Global Positioning System (GPS) is a satellite based system that gives real time three dimensional (3D) latitude, longitude, and height information at sub-meter accuracy. The system was developed by the United States military in the late 1970's to give troops accurate position and navigational information. A GPS receiver calculates its position on earth from radio signals broadcast by satellites orbiting the earth. There are currently twenty-four GPS satellites in this system. GPS equipment is capable of measuring a position to within centimetres but the accuracy suffers due to errors in the satellite signals. Errors in the signal can be caused by atmospheric interference, proximity of mountains, trees, or tall buildings. The government can also introduce errors in the signal for security purposes. This intentional degradation of the satellite signals is known as selective availability. The accuracy of the position information can be improved by using differential GPS. In differential GPS, one receiver is mounted in a stationary position, usually at the farm office, while the other is on the tractor or harvesting equipment. The stationary receiver calculates the error and transmits the necessary correction to the mobile receiver. GPS equipment suitable for precision agricultural cost several thousand dollars. Less expensive equipment is becoming available but the accuracy and capability is reduced.

1.6.4.3. Geographic Information System (Gis)

A Geographic Information System (GIS) is a computer-assisted system for handling spatial information. GIS software can be considered as a collection of software programs to acquire, store, analyze, and display information. The input data can be maps, charts, spreadsheets, or pictures. The GIS software can analyze these data using image processing and statistical procedures. Data can be grouped together and displayed as overlays. Overlays could be information such as soil type, topography, crop type, crop yield, pest levels, irrigation, and management information as shown.

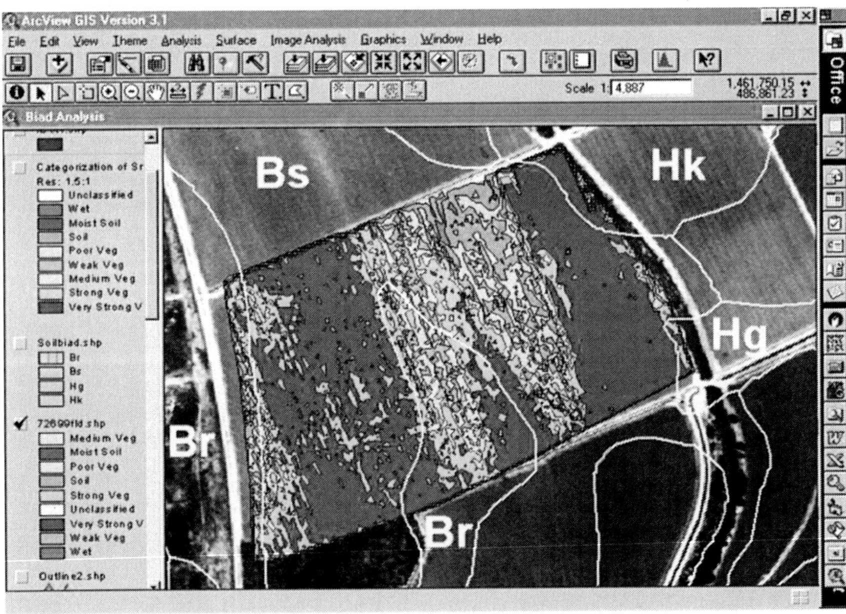

Figure 8. Topographic GIS map of the forest area

Relationships can be examined and new data sets produced by combining a number of overlays. These data sets can be combined with models and decision support systems to construct a powerful management tool. For example, we could assess how far a field was from roads or non-agricultural crops. This information could be important in pest infestation or in planning chemical application. We could also examine crop yield relationship to soil type or other factors as show in the following figure. A number of GIS software packages are now commercially available. Spatial data for the GIS is often collected using GPS equipment but another source of spatial information is aerial and satellite imagery.

1.6.4.4. Pixels, Images And Colours

1.6.4.4.1. Colour composite images

In displaying a colour composite image, three primary colors (red, green and blue) are used when these three colours are combined in various proportions, they produce different colors in the visible spectrum. Associating each spectral band (not necessarily a visible band) to a separate primary colour results in a colour composite image.

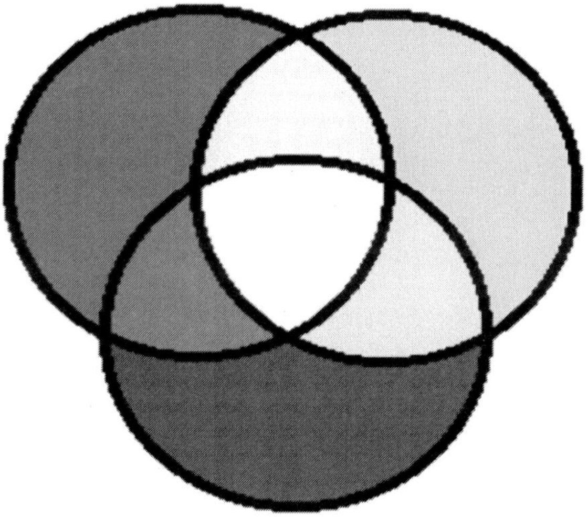

Figure 9. Primary colour composite

Many colours can be formed by combining the three primary colours **(Red, Green, Blue)** in various proportions.

1.6.4.4.2. False colour composite

The display colour assignment for any band of a **multispectral image** can be done in an entirely arbitrary manner. In this case, the colour of a target in the displayed image does not have any resemblance to its actual colour. The resulting product is known as a **false color composite** image. There are many possible schemes of producing false color composite images. However, some scheme may be more suitable for detecting certain objects in the image.

1.6.4.4.3. Natural colour composite

When displaying a natural colour composite image, the spectral bands (some of which may not be in the visible region) are combined in such a way that the appearance of the displayed image resembles a visible colour photograph, i.e. vegetation in green, water in blue, soil in brown or grey, etc. Many people refer to this composite as a "**true colour**" composite. However, this term may be misleading since in many instances the colours are only simulated to look similar to the "true" colours of the targets. For example, the bands 3 (red band), 2 (green band) and 1 (blue band) of a **AVHRR** image can be assigned respectively to the R, G, and B colours for display. In this way, the colour of the resulting colour composite image resembles closely what the human eyes would observe.

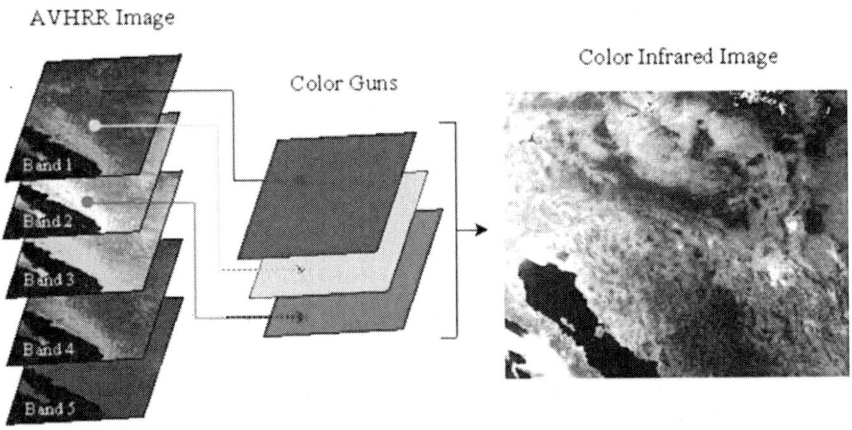

Figure 10. Development of natural colour composite

1.7. Image Processing And Analysis

Many image processing and analysis techniques have been developed to aid the interpretation of remote sensing images and to extract as much information as possible from the images. The choice of specific techniques or algorithms to use depends on the goals of each individual project. The key steps in processing remotely sensed data are **Digitizing of Images, ImageCalibration, Geo-Registration, and Spectral Analysis**. Prior to data analysis, initial processing on the raw data is usually carried out to correct for any distortion due to the characteristics of the imaging system and imaging conditions. Depending on the user's requirement, some standard correction procedures may be carried out by the ground station operators before the data is delivered to the end-user. These procedures include**radiometric correction** to correct for uneven sensor response over the whole image and **geometric correction** to correct for geometric distortion due to Earth's rotation and other imaging conditions (such as oblique viewing). The image may also be transformed to conform to a specific map projection system. Furthermore, if accurate geographical location of an area on the image needs to be known,**ground controlpoints (GCP's)** are used to register the image to a precise map (**geo-referencing**).

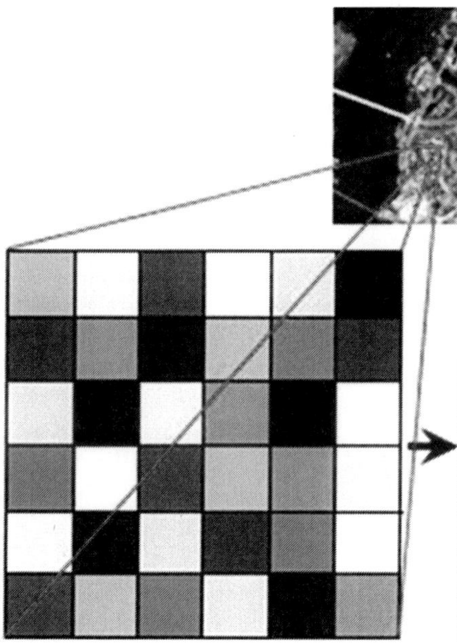

170	238	85	255	221	0
68	136	17	170	119	68
221	0	238	136	0	255
119	255	85	170	136	238
238	17	221	68	119	255
85	170	119	221	17	136

Figure 11. Georeferencing of a map

1.7.1. Digitizing Of Images

Image digitization is the conversion of an analogue image, such as a photograph, into a series of grid cells. The value of each cell is related to the brightness, colour or reflectance at that point. A scanner is a simple way to digitize images. Many modern sensors now produce raw data in digital format.

1.7.2. Image Enhancement

In order to aid visual interpretation, visual appearance of the objects in the image can be improved by**image enhancement** techniques such as grey level stretching to improve the contrast and spatial filtering for enhancing the edges. An example of an enhancement procedure is shown here.

1.7.3. Image Classification

Different land cover types in an image can be discriminated using some **image classification**algorithms using spectral features, i.e. the brightness and "colour" information contained in eachpixel. The classification procedures can be "supervised" or "unsupervised".In **supervised classification**, the spectral features of some areas of known land cover types areextracted from the image. These areas are known as the "**training areas**". Every pixel in thewhole image is then classified as belonging to one of the classes depending on how close itsspectral features are to the spectral features of the training areas.In **unsupervised classification**, the computer program automatically groups the pixels in theimage into separate clusters, depending on their spectral features. Each cluster will then beassigned a landcover type by the analyst.Each class of land cover is referred to as a "**theme**" and the product of classification is known asa "**thematic map**".The information derived from remote sensing images are often combined with other auxiliarydata to form the basis for a **Geographic Information System (GIS)**. A GIS is a database ofdifferent layers, where each layer contains information about a specific aspect of the same areawhich is used for analysis by the resource scientists.

1.8. Image Interpretation

1.8.1. Vegetation Indices

Different bands of a multispectral image may be combined to accentuate the vegetated areas.

One such combination is the ratio of the near-infrared band to the red band. This ratio is known as the Ratio Vegetation Index (RVI)

RVI = NIR/Red

Since vegetation has high NIR reflectance but low red reflectance, vegetated areas will have higher RVI values compared to non-vegetated aeras. Another commonly used vegetation index is the**Normalised Difference Vegetation Index (NDVI)** computed by

NDVI = (NIR - Red)/(NIR + Red)

Table shows equations and references for several indices that can be use in vegetation monitoring.

Table 1. Equation and references for different parameters

PARAMETER	EQUATION	REFERENCE
Normalized Difference Vegetation Index (NDVI)	(NIR-Red)/(NIR+Red)	Rouse *et al* (1974)
Water Band Index (WBI)	900/970 nm	Pefluelas *et al.* (1997)
Water Moisture Index (WMI)	1600/820 nm	Hunt and Rock (1989)
Photosynthesis Index	(531-570)/531+570)	Gamon *et al.* (1990)
Nitrogen Index (RN)	(550-600)/(800-(900)	Blackmer *et al.* (1996)
Chlorophyll based Difference Index (CI)	(850-710)/850-680)	Datt (1999)

Vegetation maps are produced by generating a normalized difference vegetation index from a infrared image and then doing a vegetation classification. Colour infrared photographs collect information in the green, red and near infrared light reflectance spectrum. Green vegetation reflects very strongly in the near infrared light range and therefore infrared images can detect stress in many crops before it is visible with the naked eye.

The Normalized Difference Vegetation Index (NDVI) is used to separate green vegetation from the background soil brightness. It is the difference between the near infrared and red reflectance normalized over the sum of these bands.

NDVI = (IR-Red)/(IR+Red)

These NDVI maps can then be classified into vegetation categories and displayed as a vegetation maps with different colours representing different levels of vegetation. In the map on the left browns and yellow represent bare soil and shades of green represent vegetation, darker greens are stronger vegetation.

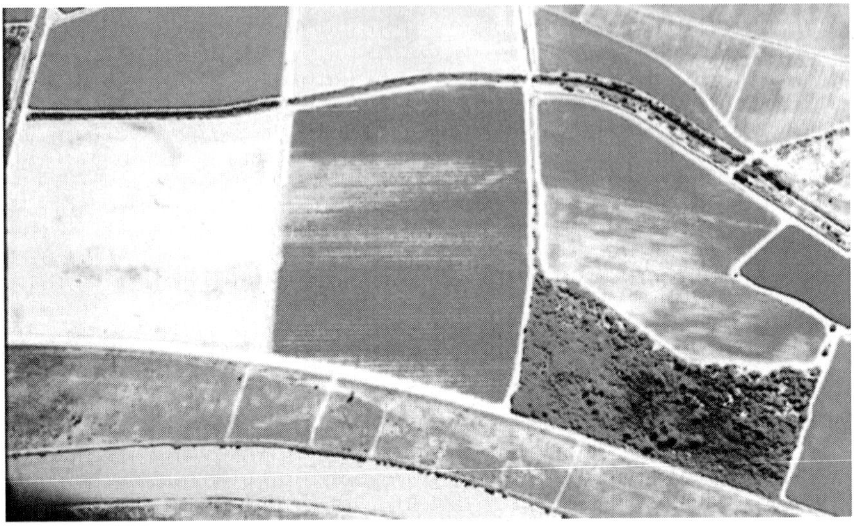

Figure 12. Example of image processing of aerial infrared photographs to produce a vegetation map for a chile field.

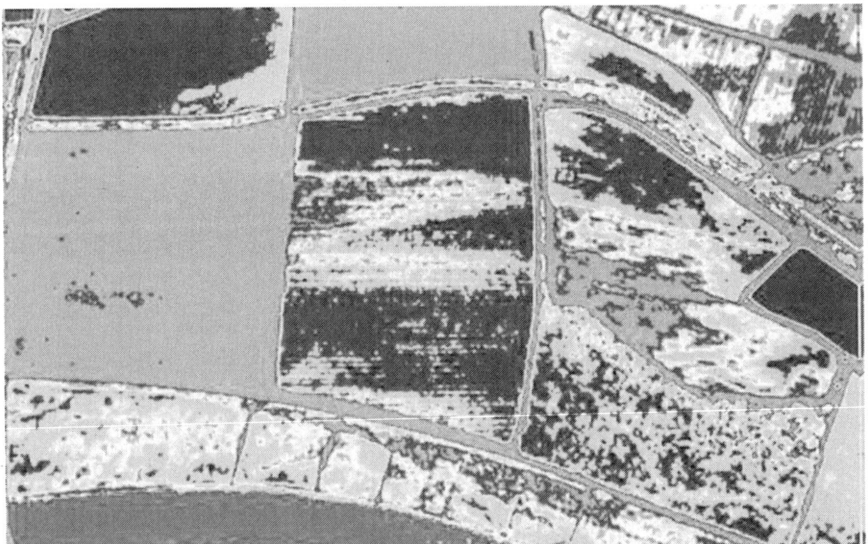

Figure 13. Example of image processing of aerial infrared photographs to produce a vegetation map for a peddy field.

1.9. Background On Remote Sensing

1.9.1. Remote Sensing

Remote sensing is the science and art of obtaining information about an object, area or phenomenon through the analysis of data acquired by a device that is not in contact with the object, area, or phenomenon under investigation. As the term indicates, it applies to any information gathering device or method where the object of observation is remote from the device.

Out of a number of devices involved in remote sensing, the most common platforms are aircraft and satellites. The sensors associated with these devices are of two types, namely passive and active sensors. In a passive system, the instrument gathers information from the radiation that happens to arrive. The main sources of radiation for such systems are either solar radiation or thermal emissions. In the active system, it is the instrument itself on board the device that is the source of radiation. It sends signals to target under investigation, and receives the return signal, having the unique characteristics of the target features. As far as satellite remote sensing is concerned, systems operating in the visible and infrared part of the electromagnetic spectrum are passive while microwave instruments are either active or passive.

Currently, satellites are the main devices in remote sensing. And the two main types of satellites are the**Polar or Near-polarOrbiting and Geostationary** satellites. The Polar or Near Polar orbiting satellites are Sun-synchronous i.e. the satellites keep a precise pace with the Sun's westward progress as the earth rotates so that they always cross the equator at precisely the same solar time. Examples can be Landsat and NOAA satellites. Geostationary satellites are satellites which travel with an angular velocity that matches the earth's rotation. As a result, they remain at the same point above the earth at all times. An example is Meteosat. These satellites are helpful in obtaining constant and persistent image of a particular area at fixed interval which is a great advantage in monitoring a location with high temporal resolution to capture the transient behavior of objects such as rain clouds.

Estimation of biomass production will provide guidance to energy development polices including:

- The impact of improved stoves on fuel wood and dung energy consumption.
- The potential of increasing the supply of fuel wood through the establishment of small scale "forest plantations"
- The potential of dung and other fuels for biomass energy supply.

1.9.2. Principles Involved

1.9.2.1. The Photon and Radiometric Quantities

Most remote sensing texts begin by giving a survey of the main principles, to build a theoretical background, mainly in the physics of radiation. While it is important to have such a framework to pursue many aspects of remote sensing, we do not delve into this complex subject in much detail at this point. Instead, we offer on this and the next several pages an outline survey of the basics of relevant electromagnetic concepts. On this page, the nature of the photon is the prime topic. Photons of different energy values are distributed through what is called the Electromagnetic Spectrum.

Hereafter in this Introduction and in the Sections that follow, we limit the discussion and scenes examined to remote sensing products obtained almost exclusively by measurements within the Electromagnetic Spectrum (force field and acoustic remote sensing are briefly covered elsewhere in the Tutorial). Our emphasis is on pictures (photos) and images (either TV-like displays on screens or "photos" made from data initially acquired as electronic signals, rather than recorded directly on film). We concentrate mainly on images produced by sensors operating in the visible and near-IR segments of the electromagnetic spectrum but also inspect a fair number of images obtained by radar and thermal sensors.

The underlying basis for most remote sensing methods and systems is simply that of measuring the varying energy levels of a single entity, the fundamental unit in the electromagnetic (which may be abbreviated "EM") force field known as the *photon*. As you will see later on this page, variations in photon energies (expressed in Joules or ergs) are tied to the parameter *wavelength* or its inverse,*frequency*. EM radiation that varies from high to low energy levels comprises the *ElectroMagnetic spectrum* (EMS). Radiation from specific parts of the EM spectrum contain photons of different wavelengths whose energy levels fall within a discrete range of values. When any target material is excited by internal processes or by interaction with incoming EM radiation, it will emit or reflect photons of varying wavelengths whose radiometric quantities differ at different wavelengths in a way diagnostic of the material. Photon energy received at detectors is commonly stated in power units such as Watts per square meter per wavelength unit. The plot of variation of power with wavelength gives rise to a specific pattern or curve that is the *spectral signature* for the substance or feature being sensed.

Now, in more detail: The photon is the physical form of a quantum, the basic particle of energy studied in quantum mechanics (which deals with the physics of the very small, that is, particles and their behavior at atomic and subatomic levels). The photon is also described as the messenger particle for

EM force or as the smallest bundle of light. This subatomic massless particle, which also does not carry an electric charge, comprises radiation *emitted* by matter when it is excited thermally, or by nuclear processes (fusion, fission), or by bombardment with other radiation (as well as by particle collisions). It also can become involved as *reflected* or *absorbed* radiation. Photons move at the speed of light: 299,792.46 km/sec (commonly rounded off to 300,000 km/sec or ~186,000 miles/sec).

Photon particles also move as waves and hence, have a "dual" nature. These waves follow a pattern that can be described in terms of a sine (trigonometric) function, as shown in two dimensions in the figure below.

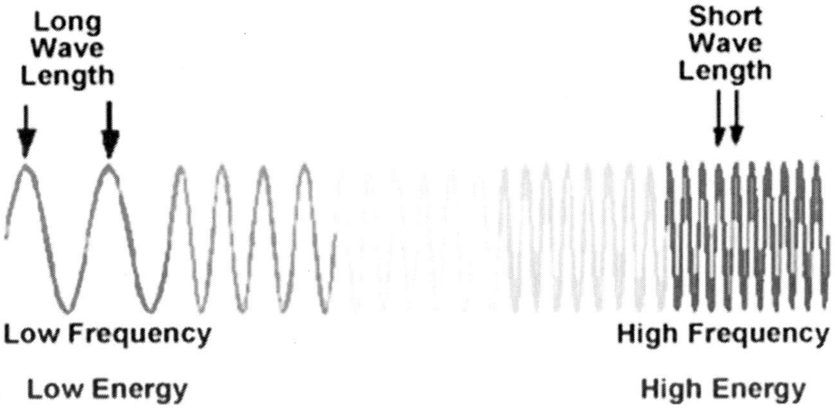

Figure 14. (NOTE: Frequency refers to number of crests of waves of same wavelength that pass by a point in one second.)Movement of photon particles as sine waves

The distance between two adjacent peaks on a wave is its wavelength. The total number of peaks (top of the individual up-down curve) that pass by a reference lookpoint in a second is that wave's frequency (in units of cycles per second, whose SI version [SI stands for System International] is known as a Hertz [1 Hertz = $1/s^{-1}$]).

A photon travels as an EM wave having two components, oscillating as sine waves mutually at right angles, one consisting of the varying electric field, the other the varying magnetic field. Both have the same amplitudes (strengths) which reach their maxima-minima at the same time. Unlike other wave types which require a carrier (e.g., water waves), photon waves can transmit through a vacuum (such as in space). When photons pass from one medium to another, e.g., air to glass, their wave pathways are bent (follow new directions) and thus experience *refraction*.

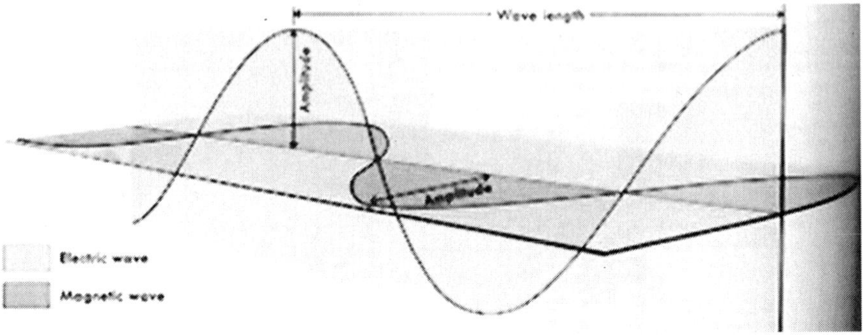

Figure 15. Dual nature (electric and magnetic field) of photon particles

A photon is said to be quantized, in that any given one possesses a certain quantity of energy. Some other photon can have a different energy value. Photons as quanta thus show a wide range of discrete energies. The amount of energy characterizing a photon is determined using Planck's general equation:

$$E = hv \tag{1}$$

where h is Planck's constant (6.6260... x 10^{-34} Joules-sec)* and v is the Greek letter, nu, representing frequency (the letter "f" is sometimes used instead of v). Photons traveling at higher frequencies are therefore more energetic. If a material under excitation experiences a change in energy level from a higher level E_2 to a lower level E_1, we restate the above formula as:

$$\Delta E = E_2 - E_1 = hv \tag{2}$$

where v has some discrete value determined by (v_2 - v_1). In other words, a particular energy change is characterized by producing emitted radiation (photons) at a specific frequency v and a corresponding wavelength at a value dependent on the magnitude of the change.

1.9.3. Sources Of Electromagnetic (Em)- Radiation

EM radiation is the energy resulting from the acceleration of electric charges and the associated electric and magnetic fields (this study is restricted to radiation emitted from the Sun and earth's surface). EM radiation is governed by the equations:

$$\Delta^2 E - \frac{\partial^2 E}{\partial t^2} = 0 \tag{3}$$

$$\Delta^2 H - \frac{\partial^2 H}{\partial t^2} = 0 \tag{4}$$

where the speed of light $c^2=1/(\mu\ \varepsilon\ )$

The energy associated with EM waves can be regarded as stream of photons travelling at speed of light, each photon having an energy hv, where h is Plank's constant and v is the frequency of the light. The EM spectrum, which is the range of wavelengths over which electromagnetic radiation extend, constitute of radio waves, micro waves, thermal infrared, infrared, visible, ultraviolet, x-ray, and gamma rays in decreasing order of wavelengths.

The ultimate source of energy for remote sensing is the Sun. Besides, all matter above absolute zero temperature emit radiation. Thus terrestrial objects are also sources of radiation, though it is considerably different in magnitude and spectral composition than that of the Sun. The emitted radiation from terrestrial objects is a function of temperature. From the principle of Black Body Radiation, the density of radiant energy U(v) emitted from a black body in the frequency range v+dv and v is:

$$U\left(v\right) d\nu = \frac{8\hbar}{C^3} \frac{v^3 dv}{\exp\left(\frac{\hbar v}{kT} - 1\right)} \tag{5}$$

which is the **Planck distribution law**. The total energy density overall frequencies is :

$$U = \int_{o}^{\infty} U(v)\, dv = \frac{8\pi^5 k^4}{15c^3h^3} T^4 = aT^4 \tag{6}$$

where a is a universal constant.

The intensity emitted from an object is therefore:

$$\mathrm{I} = \varepsilon\sigma \mathrm{T}^4 \tag{7}$$

This is the **Stefan - Boltzman** Law

The spectral distribution of emitted energy varies with temperature as shown in Figure 1. Meanwhile, the wavelength at which greatest energy density occurs varies inversely with temperature and is given by Wein's displacement law:

$$\lambda_{\max} T = \frac{hc}{4.965K} = 2.898x10^{-3} m.k \tag{8}$$

1.9.4. Energy Interaction in The Atmosphere

Atmosphere can have a profound effect on the intensity and spectral composition available to any sensing system as the radiation which reaches the sensed object passes through a certain optical path length of atmospheric air. These effects are caused principally through the mechanism of atmospheric**scattering** and **absorption**.

1.9.4.1. Scattering

As stated above, the atmosphere can have a significant effect on the incoming and outgoing radiation by scattering. There are three types of scattering depending on the size of particle involved. And these are **Rayleigh scattering, Mie scattering** and **Non-selective**scattering where Rayleigh and Non-selective scattering are the limiting cases of Mie scattering.

For Rayleigh scattering to occur, the particle size must not be larger than about $1/10^{th}$ of the wavelength of the light. In a gas with N molecules per unit volume and refractive index n, the Rayleigh extinction coefficient α for a wavelength is approximately:

$$\alpha \approx \frac{32\pi^3}{3N\dagger}(n-1)^2 \tag{9}$$

Rayleigh Sc atter $i \propto \frac{1}{\dagger}$

The extinction coefficient decreases as a wavelength increases. Specifically, the amount of scattering is inversely proportional to the fourth power of wavelength.

Mie scatter occurs for particles whose diameter is approximately equal to the wavelength. In a gas containing N spherical particles of radius R, the effective cross-section is given by:

$$\sigma = \mathbf{NAds\ R\dagger} \tag{10}$$

where Ads - is the volume in which the gas is contained, provided that no one particle lies in the shadow of another particle. If no absorption takes place, the extinction coefficient equals to scattering extinction co-efficient. Mie extinction coefficient is given by

$$\alpha = \mathbf{NK\pi R^2} \tag{11}$$

where K = the extinction factor

The ratio of scattered to incident light can be expressed as:

$$\frac{i}{I_o} = -\alpha ds \tag{12}$$

In this type of scattering, as the particles are of the order of wavelength, the light scattered from one part of the surface can be out of phase with coming from another part, unlike Rayleigh scattering were there is no phase difference between the light source and the scattered light. For Mie scattering, phase difference will be small for small scattering angle which gives rise to a large intensity in the forward direction and less in the reverse.

Non-selective scattering occurs when the diameter of the scattering particles is much larger than the wavelength. Water droplets, for example, cause such a scattering. They commonly have diameter in the range 5 to 100m and scatter all visible wavelengths, equal quantities of blue, green, and red light are scattered, making fog and clouds appear white.

1.9.4.2. Absorption

When light pass through a certain optical path in the atmosphere, it experiences absorption in addition to scattering by the existing particles. The intensity of the light diminishes according

To the equation:

$$\mathbf{I} = \mathbf{I_o exp}\left(-\alpha^1\right) \quad (13)$$

where α is the absorption coefficient

In the atmosphere, the most efficient absorbers of radiation are water vapour, carbon dioxide, and ozone.

The effect of this absorption is to leave only few regions known as atmospheric windows, in which the atmosphere transmits a substantial proportion of electromagnetic radiation. These are the only regions that can be used in remote sensing of the earth's surface.

Both scattering and absorption increase with increase in path length or with an increase in air mass.

1.9.5. Energy Interaction with The Earth's Surface

When a light wave is incident on a surface, it will be reflected, transmitted, or absorbed. Furthermore, the energy of the absorbed radiation can be re-emitted as other forms of radiation. For an incident wave of intensity I_o the intensity of the reflected wave is rI_o and the amplitude of the rest is $(1 - r)I_o$, where r is the coefficient of reflection.

When EM radiation is incident on a given surface feature, out of the three fundamental processes the reflected part is often of interest in remote sensing. (thermal emission are also often of interest). The reflected part (rI_o) will be different for different earth features depending on the type of material and the condition of the material (e.g. dry or wet). Reflectivity is also dependent on the wavelength or frequency of the incoming radiation. The function which describes the dependence of reflectivity on wavelength is called the spectral reflectance function, and is given by:

$$\rho_2 = \frac{Energy\ of\ reflected}{Energy\ of\ incident} \tag{14}$$

Different objects have very distinct spectral reflectance curves. It is the differences in spectral reflectance that allows one to distinguish different materials and objects using remotely sensed reflected radiation.

For thermal infrared wavelengths, the reflected radiation is outweighed by the emitted energy of the surface features. Hence in the thermal infrared, the radiation received from an object depends on its emissivity and temperature. Meanwhile, the temperature of an object will depend on its absorptivity (how much radiation it absorbs), its thermal conductivity (rate at which heat pass through a material), thermal capacity (ability of a material to store heat), and thermal inertia (thermal response of material to temperature change). Since our investigation focuses on non-thermal images, we will not discuss thermal remote sensing methods in detail.

1.9.6. Data Acquisition and Interpretation

Detection of EM energy can be performed either photographically or electronically. The process of photography uses chemical reactions on the surface of a light sensitive film to detect energy variation within a scene while electronic sensors generate in electrical signals that corresponds to the energy or intensity of the detected radiation. The advantage of visual (photographic) is that it is simple, it provides high good spatial detail (because of the high resolution of chemical films) and geometric integrity (geometry is not distorted). On the other hand, electronics have the advantage of broader spectral sensitivity and easier conversion of the image to digital form.

Photographic images are interpreted visually (or scanned to convert them into digital images) whereas electronic images are interpreted digitally. The electronic image constitutes an array of pixels which vary in the level of brightness in accordance with the radiation received from the surface feature they represent. Pixel brightness is converted to a binary number. In our case pixel values are 8-bit binary numbers representing integer values from 0 to 255. These are positive integers that result from quantizing of the original electrical signal from the sensor.

1.10. Remote Sensing of Biomass Production

1.10.1. Reflectance Characteristics of Green Plants

Green plants have a unique spectral reflectance curve. In the visible part of the spectrum, plants strongly absorb light in the blue (0.45μ m) and red (0.67nm) regions and reflect strongly in the green portion of the spectrum due to the presence of chlorophyll. In cases where the plant is subjected to stress or to a condition which hinders growth, the chlorophyll production will decrease. And this in turn leads to less absorption in the blue and red bands.

In the near infrared portion of the spectrum (0.7 - 1.3μm), green plant reflectance increases to 40 - 50% of incident light. Beyond 1.3μm, there are dips in the reflectance curve due to absorption by water in the leaves.

1.10.2. Principles of Detection

The differential reflection of green plants in the visible and infrared portion of the spectrum makes possible the detection of green plants from satellites. Other features on the earth surface don't have such a unique step-like character in the 0.65 - 0.75μm range of the reflectance curve. NDVI is commonly used to represent this character. It is calculated from Advanced Very High Resolution Radiometer (AVHRR) data from NOAA-8 and NOAA-9 polar orbiting satellite and is defined as:

$$NDVI = \frac{CHN2 - CHN1}{CHN2 + CHN1} \tag{15}$$

where CHN1 and CHN2 are reflectance in the visible (red) (0.58 - 0.68 μm) and near infrared channels (0.725 - 1.10 μm) respectively. NDVI is determined by the degree of absorption by chlorophyll in the red wavelengths, which is proportional to green leaf density. Therefore, NDVI correlates well with green leaf biomass, leaf area index, and other related parameters.

1.10.3. Estimation of Radiation Use Efficiency In Plants

Plants make use of specific energy wavelengths (0.4 - 0.7 μm) for the process of photosynthesis. The photo-synthetically active radiation constitutes about 50% of the energy that is emitted from the sun. Out of this phot-synthetically active radiation (PAR), about 80% of the radiation incident on a plant leaf is captured by photo-synthetically active compounds. The rest is lost by reflection and absorption by non-photosynthesizing materials. A minimum of eight photons are required to produce a glucose from a single carbon-dioxide and glucose stores 28% of the captured energy in the form of chemical energy of the molecules. And finally, as the plant produces the glucose molecule it will use about 40% of the converted energy for dark respiration. Therefore, the maximum photosynthetic efficiency is:

$$100 \times 0.50 \times 0.80 \times 0.28 \times 0.60 = 6.70 \tag{16}$$

This result applies to c_4 plants (so-called because their first product of photosynthesis is 4-carbon sugar). For c_3 plants, like wheat and rice, the efficiency is lower due to photo-respiration effects.

1.11. Remote Sensing of Radiation Intensity

1.11.1. Solar Constant

The average solar irradiance received outside the earth atmosphere is called Solar Constant. The intensity of solar radiation above the earth's atmosphere has nearly constant value unlike irradiance received at the ground. It's average value is 1367 W/m^2 though it shows some variation due to variations in solar activity. Annual fluctuations due to Earth-Sun distance give rise to a variation of ±3.4% of the extra-terrestrial irradiance and are given by

$$E_o = \langle E_0 \rangle (1 + 0.0167 \cos((2/365) * (D - 3)))^2 \tag{17}$$

where $\langle E_0 \rangle$ is the mean value of solar constant, D is the Julian days.

1.11.2. Radiation Reflected and Received By The Ground

Radiation received at the ground surface is a combination of direct radiation, which comes from the sun after passing through a path length in the transparent atmosphere, and diffuse radiation which is radiation reflected by clouds and scattered by atmosphere in general. The contribution of diffuse radiation to irradiance received by ground depends on the atmospheric thickness, moisture content, cloud frequency, turbidity of the atmosphere, and angle of zenith.

The radiation that is reflected from the ground is very small compared to that reflected from the clouds. Its value depends on the reflectance of different earth surface features. In many cases, surface albedo is taken to be uniform (0.15) across the land.

1.11.3. Atmospheric Effects

Atmosphere plays a major role at attenuation and reflection of light that pass through it. Their main effects are reflection, absorption, and scattering, depending on the wavelength and air mass ratio.

1.11.4. Air Mass Ratio

Air mass ratio is defined as the ratio of the path length of the radiation through the atmosphere at a given angle of a reference path length. The reference path length is that obtained by light traveling to a point at sea level straight through the atmosphere (vertically). The air mass ratio depends on the angle of zenith and the height above sea level of the observer. For small angles, the ratio is expressed as;

$$m = \sec \theta_z \tag{18}$$

where θ_z is the zenith angle. As the angle of zenith increases, the air mass ratio increases i.e., the attenuation increases.

1.11.5. Atmospheric Absorption and Reflection

Light passing through the atmosphere experiences absorption, scattering and reflection. Absorption causes heating and eventual re-emission of the absorbed energy as long wavelength radiation. Scattering is a wavelength dependent change in a direction. On the average 30% extra-terrestrial irradiance is reflected to outer space mainly due to cloud.

1.11.6. Irradiance Variation

Irradiance received at a given location may differ in magnitude from hour to hour, day to day, month to month, and season to season depending on air mass, turbidity, moisture content, cloud frequency, and angle of zenith. The seasonal variation give rise to a significant amount of fluctuations in the irradiance received. This fluctuation in irradiance is due to variation in the declination angle from season to season. The declination angle (δ) that the earth posses with respect to the sun varies from season to season. In the middle of march and september the declination angle, δ, is zero (0°), where as $\delta = 23.5^o$ and $\delta = -23.5^o$in the middle of June and December respectively. Analytically, the declination angle is expressed as :

$$\delta = 23.5^o \sin\left(360\frac{(284+D)}{365}\right) \tag{19}$$

where D is the Julian days.

Depending on the latitude, for a given declination angle, the irradiance increases or decreases. Moreover, irradiance varies with latitude. Irradiance variation due to seasonal variation is great at high latitudes. Variation in the earth sun distance also contributes to the variation in irradiance received although its contribution is very small.

2. APPLICATIONS

2.1. Forestry Applications

Satellite imagery is used to identify and map: -

- The species of native and exotic forest trees.
- The effects of major diseases or adverse change in environmental conditions.
- The geographic extent of forests.

This application of satellite imagery has led to the extensive use of imagery by organizations that have an interest in a range of environmental management responsibilities at a state and national level.

2.1.1. Greenhouse Gases — Sinks and Sources

Forests are often referred to as *carbon sinks.* This description is used because during photosynthesis, carbon dioxide, the major greenhouse gas, is taken from the atmosphere and converted into plant matter and oxygen.

Climate change has serious implications for Malaysia and overseas countries alike. Sustainablevland management is essential for effective greenhouse gas management; hence, it is important to acquire data on land cover in Malaysia. Remotely sensed land cover changes are used in calculations of our national emission levels, and data collected on a national scale will enable governments to develop responses to land clearing.

2.1.2. Vegetation Health

Vegetation can become stressed or less healthy because of a change in a range of environmental factors. These factors include lack of water, concentration of toxic elements/herbicides and infestation by insects/viruses. The spectral reflectance of vegetation changes according to the structure and health of a plant. In particular, the influence of chlorophyll in the leaf pigments controls the response of vegetation to radiation in the visible wavelength. As a plant becomes diseased, the cell structure of a plant alters and the spectral signature of a plant or plant community will change. The maximum reflection of electromagnetic radiation from vegetation occurs in the near infrared wavelengths. Vegetation has characteristically high near-infrared reflectance and low red reflectance. Air-borne scanners using narrow spectral bands between 0.4 urn and 0.9 urn can indicate deteriorating plant health before a change in condition is visible in the plant itself.

2.1.3. Biodiversity

Vegetation type and extent derived from satellite imagery can be combined, with biological and topographic information to provide information about biodiversity. Typically, this analysis is done with a geographic information system.

2.1.4. Change Detection

Satellite imagery is not always able to provide exact details about the species or age of vegetation. However, the imagery provides a very good means of measuring significant change in vegetation cover, whether it is through clearing, wildfire damage or environmental stress. The most common form of environmental stress is water deficiency.

2.2. Geology

Remote sensing is useful for providing information relevant to the geosciences. For example, remote sensing data are used in:

- Mineral and petroleum exploration,
- Mapping geomorphology, and
- Monitoring volcanoes.

2.3. Land Degradation

Imagery can be used to map areas of poor or no vegetation cover. A range of factors, including saline or sodic soils, and overgrazing, can cause degraded landscapes.

2.4. Oceanography

Remote sensing is applied to oceanography studies. Remote sensing is used, for example, to measure sea surface temperature and to monitor marine habitats.

2.5. Meteorology

Remote sensing is an effective method for mapping cloud type and extent, and cloud top temperature. In many of the applications identified above remotely sensed data are used with a range of other Earth science data to provide information about the natural environment. This analysis of Earth science data from a range of sources is usually done in a geographic information system (GIS).

2.6. Applications in Agriculture, Forestry, and Ecology

2.6.1.General Principles For Recognizing Vegetation

Planet Earth is distinguished from other Solar System planets by two major categories: Oceans and Land Vegetation. The oceans cover ~70% of the Earth's surface; land comprises 30%. On the land itself, the first order categories break down as follows: Trees = 30%; Grasses = 30%; Snow and Ice = 15%; Bare Rock = 18%; Sand and Desert Rock = 7%. We have already seen in previous Sections and in the Overview that in false colour imagery the remote sensing signature of vegetation is a bright red. The landscape shown in this first image could almost be on Mars except for the presence of this bright red sign of vegetation. This is the Ouargla Oasis in the Sahara Desert of southern Algeria, a concentration of trees and plants where groundwater reaches the surface:

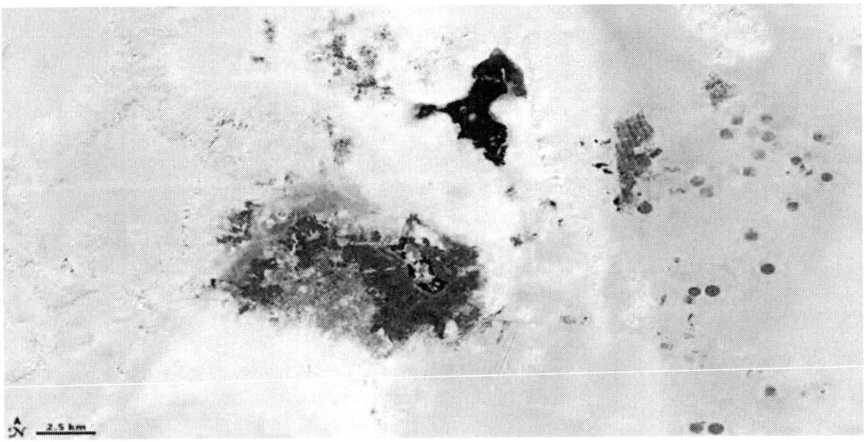

Figure 16. Image of the Ouargla Oasis in the Sahara Desert of southern Algeria

On Earth, the amount of vegetation within the seas is huge and important in the food chain. But for people the land provides most of the vegetation within the human diet. The primary categories of land vegetation (biomes) and their proportions is shown in this pie chart:

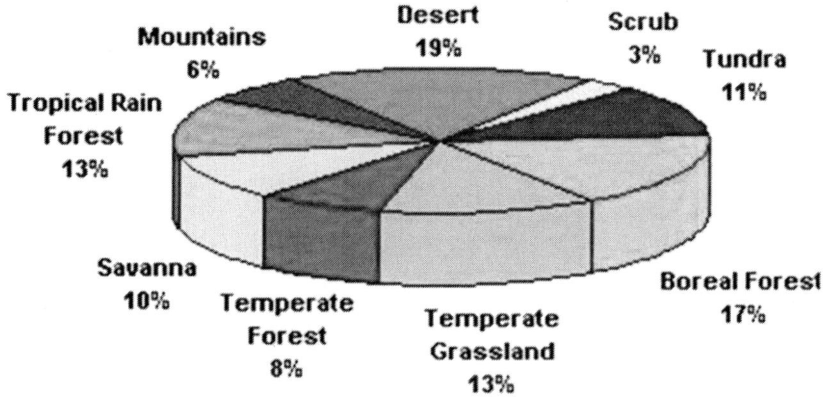

Figure 17. Pie chart for land vegetation (biomes) and their proportions

These biomes are defined in part by the temperature and precipitation controls that differentiate them:

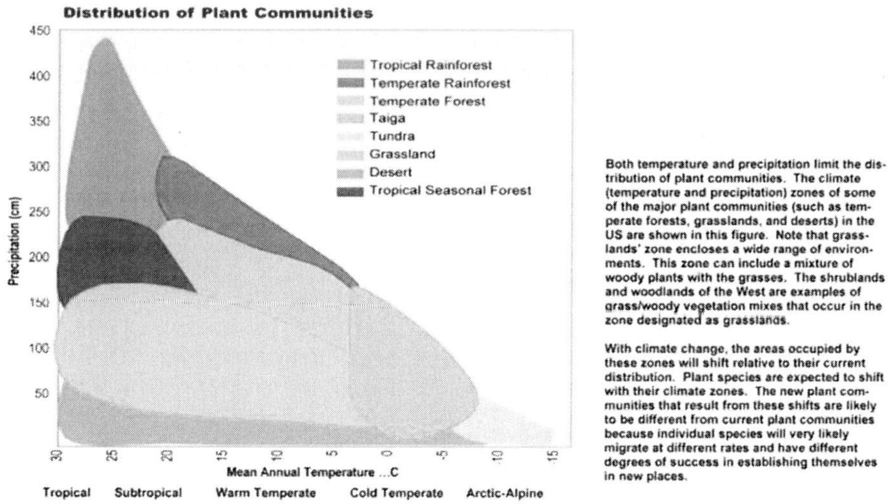

Figure 18. Distribution of land vegetation by temperature and precipitation controls

Global maps of vegetation biomes on the continents show this general distribution:

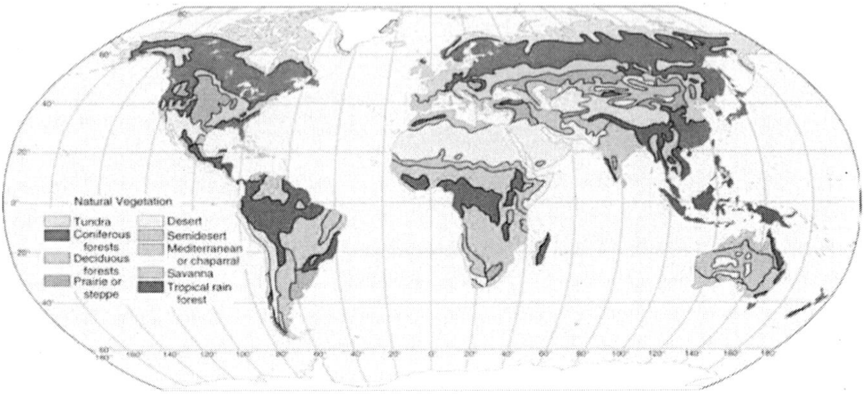

Figure 19. Global maps of land vegetation (biomes)

A fair number of global vegetation maps have been published. These usually show slight to moderate differences, depending in part with the types and numbers of classes established in the classification. There also exists a notable correlation between vegetation classes and climate. Remote sensing has proven a powerful "tool" for assessing the identity, characteristics, and growth potential of most kinds of vegetative matter at several levels (from biomes to individual plants). Vegetation behaviour depends on the nature of the vegetation itself, its interactions with solar radiation and other climate factors, and the availability of chemical nutrients and water within the host medium (usually soil, or water in marine environments). A common measure of the status of a given plant, such as a crop used for human consumption, is its potential productivity (one such parameter has units of bushels/acre or tons/hectare, or similar units). Productivity is sensitive to amounts of incoming solar radiation and precipitation (both influence the regional climate), soil chemistry, water retention factors, and plant type. Examine the diagram below to see how these interact, keeping in mind that various remote sensing systems (e.g., meteorological or earth-observing satellites) can provide inputs to productivity estimation:

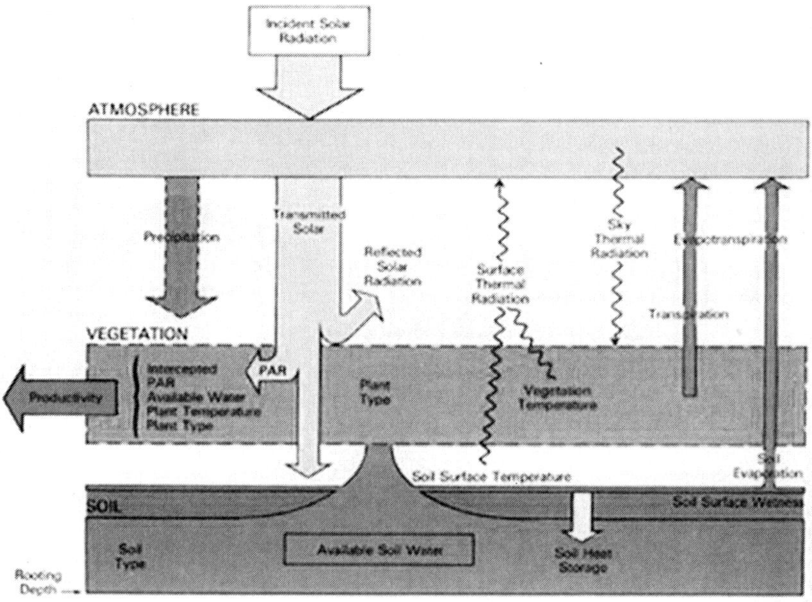

Figure 20. Interaction between productivity and solar radiations

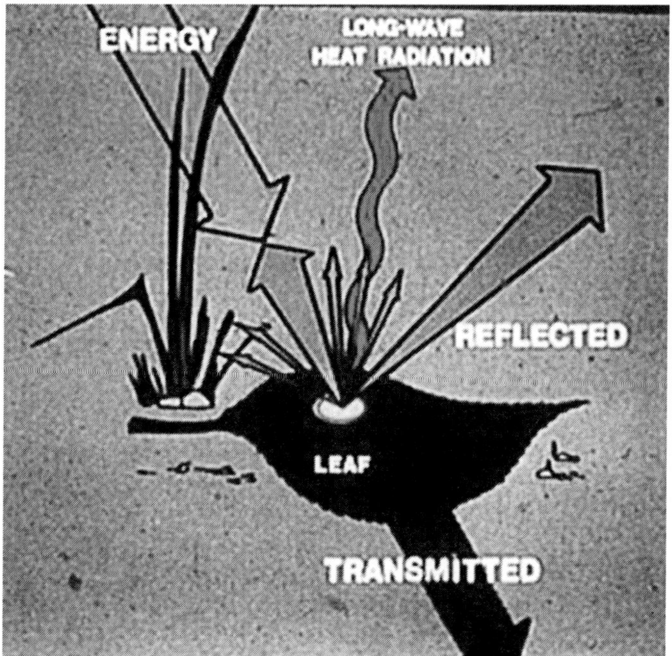

Figure 21. Reflection and absorption of radiations through biomass

Because many remote sensing devices operate in the green, red, and near infrared regions of the electromagnetic spectrum, they can discriminate radiation absorption and reflectance properties of vegetation. One special characteristic of vegetation is that leaves, a common manifestation, are partly transparent allowing some of the radiation to pass through (often reaching the ground, which reflects its own signature). The general behaviour of incoming and outgoing radiation that an act on a leaf is shown in figure 21.

Now, consider this diagram which traces the influence of green leafy material on incoming and reflected radiation.

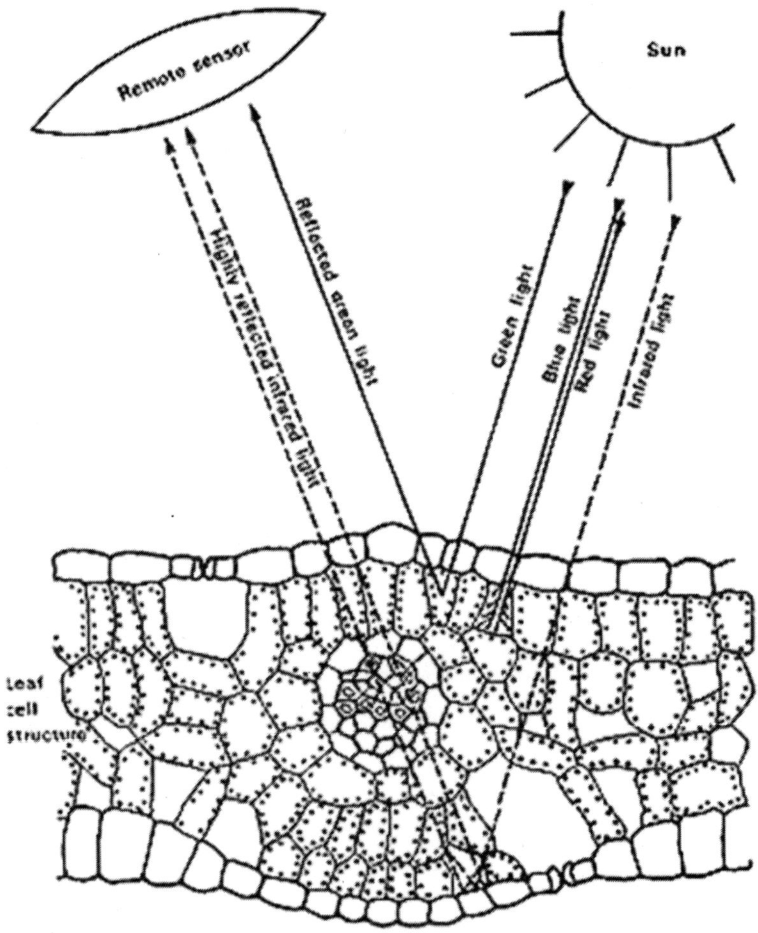

Figure 22. The influence of green leafy material on incoming and reflected radiation.

Absorption centred at about 0.65 μm (visible red) is controlled by chlorophyll pigment in green-leaf chloroplasts that reside in the outer or Palisade leaf. Absorption occurs to a similar extent in the blue. With these colours thus removed from white light, the predominant but diminished reflectance of visible wavelengths is concentrated in the green. Thus, most vegetation has a green-leafy colour. There is also strong reflectance between 0.7 and 1.0 μm (near IR) in the spongy mesophyll cells located in the interior or back of a leaf, within which light reflects mainly at cell wall/air space interfaces, much of which emerges as strong reflection rays. The intensity of this reflectance is commonly greater (higher percentage) than from most inorganic materials, so vegetation appears bright in the near-IR wavelengths (which, fortunately, is beyond the response of mammalian eyes). These properties of vegetation account for their tonal signatures on multispectral images: darker tones in the blue and, especially red, bands, somewhat lighter in the green band, and notably light in the near-IR bands (maximum in Landsat's Multispectral Scanner Bands 6 and 7 and Thematic Mapper Band 4 and SPOT's Band 3).

Identifying vegetation in remote-sensing images depends on several plant characteristics. For instance, in general, deciduous leaves tend to be more reflective than evergreen needles. Thus, in infrared colour composites, the red colours associated with those bands in the 0.7 - 1.1 μm interval are normally richer in hue and brighter from tree leaves than from pine needles.

These spectral variations facilitate fairly precise detecting, identifying and monitoring of vegetation on land surfaces and, in some instances, within the oceans and other water bodies. Thus, we can continually assess changes in forests, grasslands and range, shrub lands, crops and orchards, and marine plankton, often at quantitative levels. Because vegetation is the dominant component in most ecosystems, we can use remote sensing from air and space to routinely gather valuable information helpful in characterizing and managing of these organic systems.

This discrimination capability implies that one of the most successful applications of multispectral space imagery is monitoring the state of the world's agricultural production. This application includes identifying and differentiating most of the major crop types: wheat, barley, millet, oats, corn, soybeans, rice, and others. This capability was convincingly demonstrated by an early ERTS-1 classification of several crop types being grown in Holt County, Nebraska. This pair of image subsets, obtained just weeks after launch, indicates what crops were successfully differentiated; the lower image shows the improvement in distinguishing these types by using data from two different dates of image acquisition:

This is a good point in the discussion to introduce the appearance of large area croplands as they are seen in Landsat images. We illustrate with imagery that covers the two major crop growing areas of the United

States.The scene below is a part of the Great or Central Valley California, specifically the San Joaquin Valley. Agricultural here is primarily associated with such cash crops as barley, alfalfa, sugar beets, beans, tomatoes, cotton, grapes, and peach and walnut trees. In July of 1972 most of these fields are nearing full growth. Irrigation from the Sierra Nevada, whose foothills are in the upper right, compensates for the sparsity or rain in summer months (temperatures can be near 100° F). The eastern Coast Ranges appear at the lower left. The yellow-brown and blue areas flanking the Valley crops are grasslands and chapparal best suited for cattle grazing. The blue areas within the croplands (near the top) are the cities of Stockton and Modesto.

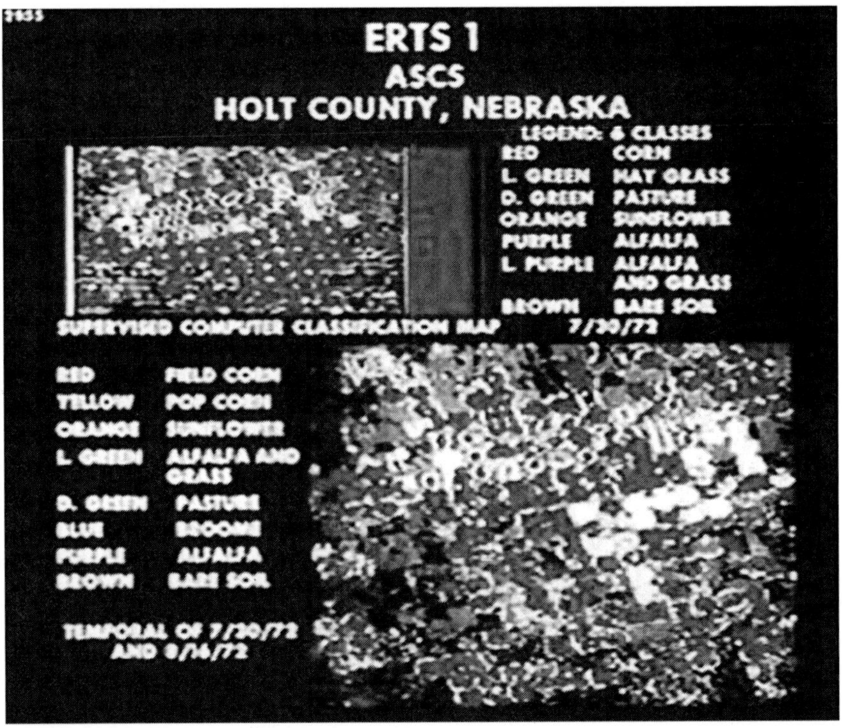

Figure 23. ERTS-1 classification of several crop types being grown in Holt County, Nebraska

Many factors combine to cause small to large differences in spectral signatures for the varieties of crops cultivated by man. Generally, we must determine the signature for each crop in a region from representative samples at specific times. However, some crop types have quite similar spectral responses at equivalent growth stages. The differences between crop (plant) types can be fairly small in the Near-Infrared, as shown in these spectral signatures (in which other variables such as soil type, ground moisture, etc. are in effect held constant).

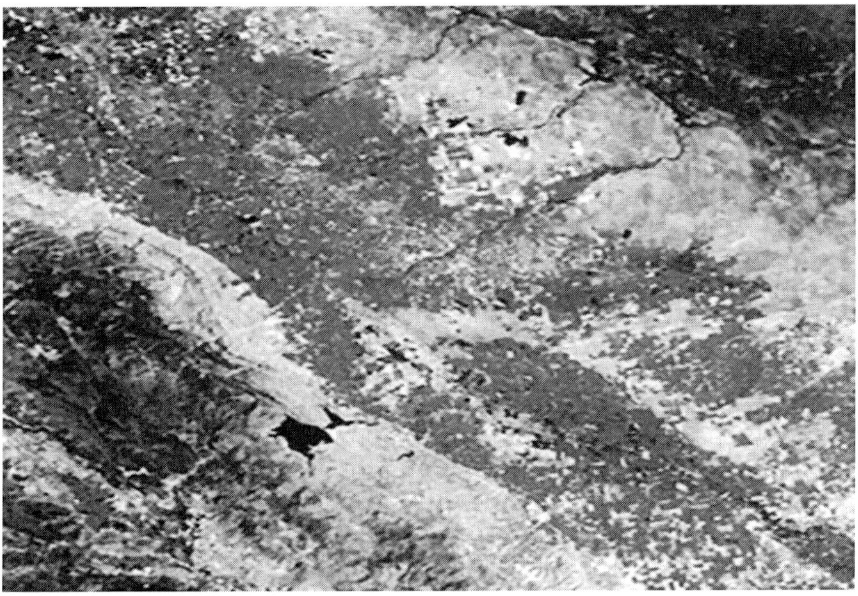

Figure 24. Landsat imagery of Great or Central Valley of California.

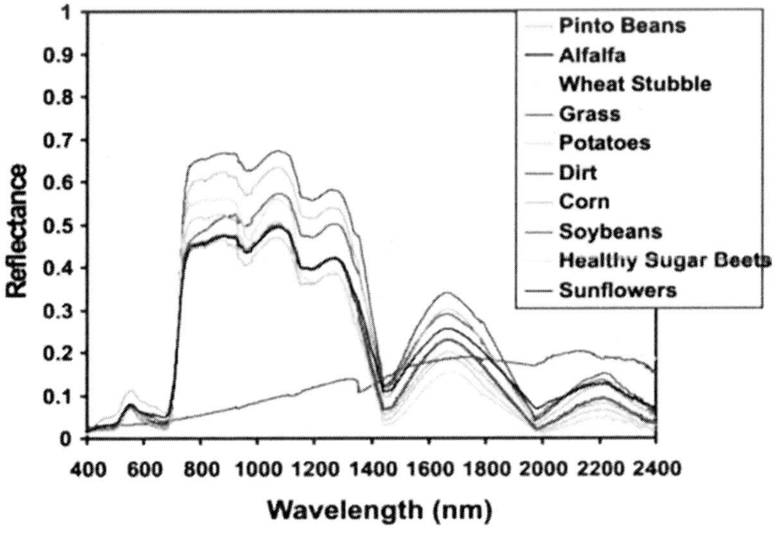

Figure 25. Spectral responses of different crops

The shape of these curves is almost identical when each crop type is compared with the others. The big difference is in the percent reflectance. The similarity in shape is explained by the fact, discussed earlier, that most vegetation matter has the same basic cell structure and similar content of chlorophyll. Yet remote sensing is reasonably effective at distinguishing and identifying different crop types.

2.6.2. Factors Affecting Spectral Signatures Of Field Crops

Read the answer to this question - it is important. The list is incomplete, but the main factors are discussed. But with so many variables involved, it is difficult to claim that each crop has a specific spectral signature. This means that, in order to identify the several crops usually present in agricultural terrain in any particular area, the most efficient course is to establish training sites, spectral characteristics are one means of identifying and classifying features in a scene. We will see how reliable this is by itself as this Section unfolds. Shape and pattern recognition are valuable inputs in determining what a feature is. The geometric shape of a field of crops sometimes is helpful in determining the actual crop itself. But field shapes tend to vary both within regions of large countries like the U.S. and in different parts of the world. This variation is evident in the illustration below

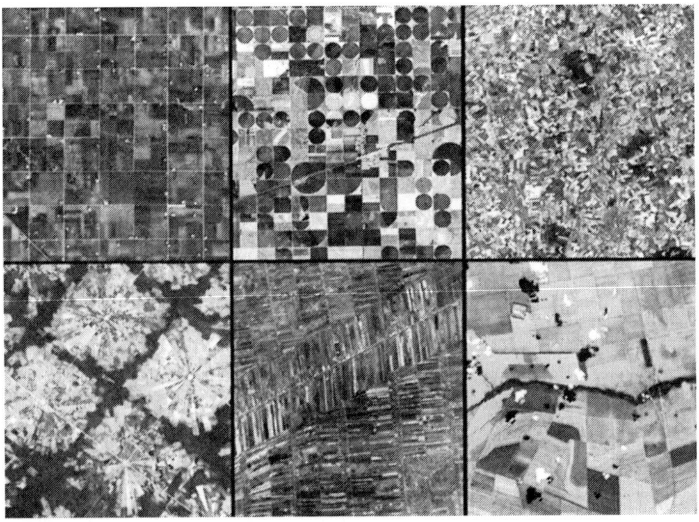

Figure 26. Landsat image showing the geometric shape of a field of different crops

Through remote sensing it is possible to quantify on a global scale the total acreage dedicated to these and other crops at any time. Of particular import is the utility of space observations to accurately estimate (goal: best case 90%) the expected yields (production in bushels or other units) of each crop, locally, regionally or globally. We can do this by first computing the areas dedicated to each crop, and then incorporating reliable yield assessments per unit area, which agronomists can measure at representative ground-truth sites. Reliability is enhanced by using the repeat coverage of the croplands afforded by the cyclical satellite orbits assuming, of course, cloud cover is sparse enough to foster several good looks during the growing season. Usually, the yield estimates obtained from satellite data are more comprehensive and earlier (often by weeks) than determined conventionally as harvesting approaches. Information about soil moisture content, often critical to good production, can be qualitatively (and under favourable conditions, quantitatively) appraised with certain satellite observations; that information can be used to warn farmers of any impending drought conditions.

Under suitable circumstances, it is feasible to detect crop stress generally from moisture deficiency or disease and pests, and sometimes suggest treatment before the farmers become aware of problems. Stress is indicated by a progressive decrease in Near-IR reflectance accompanied by a reversal in Short-Wave IR reflectance, as shown in this general diagram:

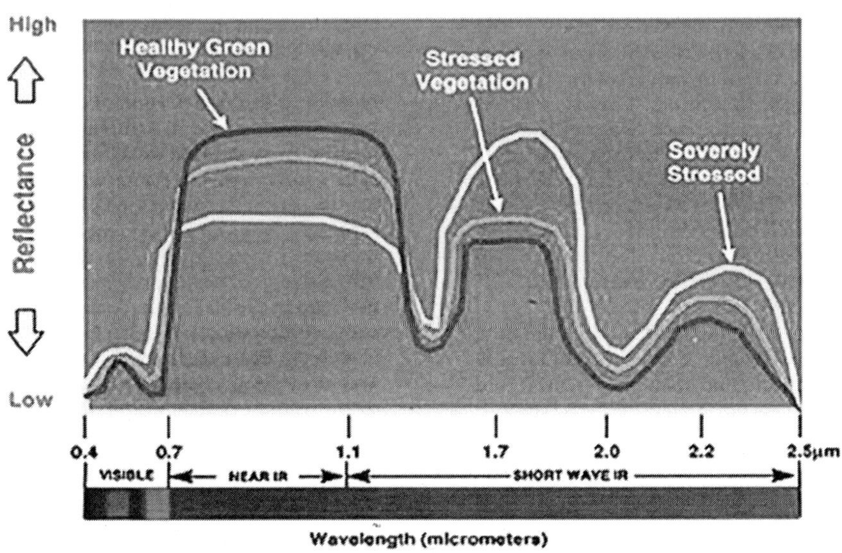

Figure 27. Crop stress by high and low reflectance

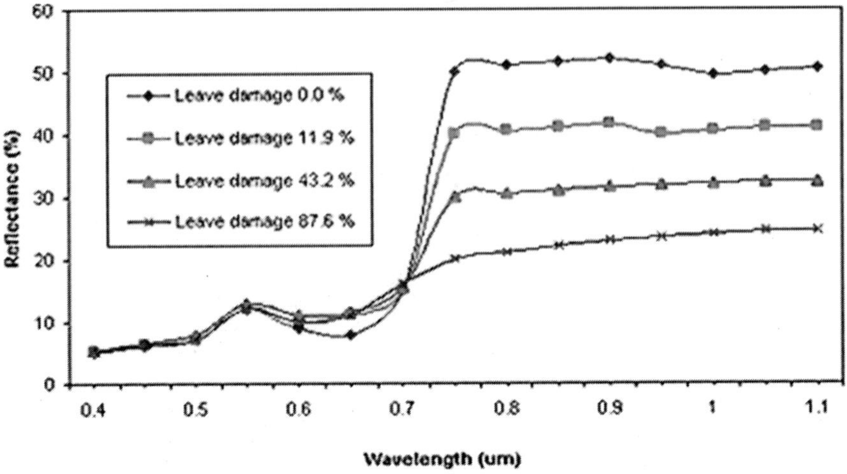

Figure 28. Soybean plant leaves indicating patterns of high and low reflectance

This effect is evidenced quantitatively in this set of field spectral measurements of leaves taken from soybean plants as these underwent increasing stress that causes loss of water and breakdown of cell walls.

For the soybeans, the major change with progressive stress is the decrease in infrared reflectances. In the visible, the change may be limited to color modification (loss of greenness), as indicated in this sugar beets example, in which the leaves have browned:

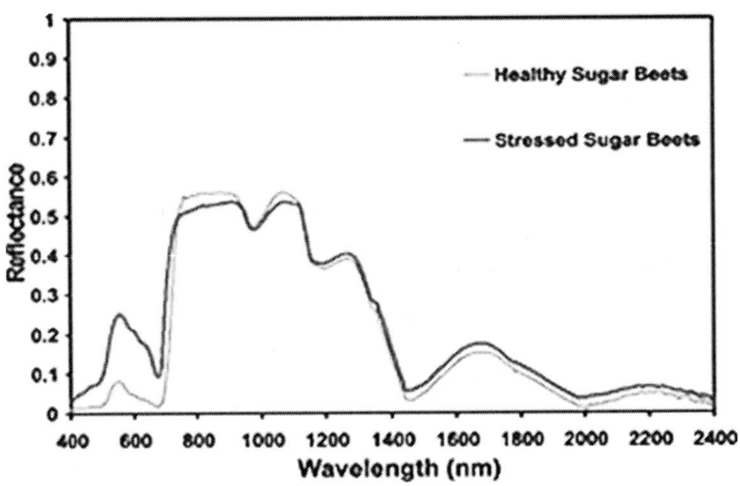

Figure 29. Sugar beets indicating patterns of high and low reflectance

Differences in vegetation vigour, resulting from variable stress, are especially evident when Near Infrared imagery or data are used. In this aerial photo made with Colour IR film shows a woodlands with healthy trees in red, and "sick" (stressed) vegetation in yellow-white (the red no longer dominates):

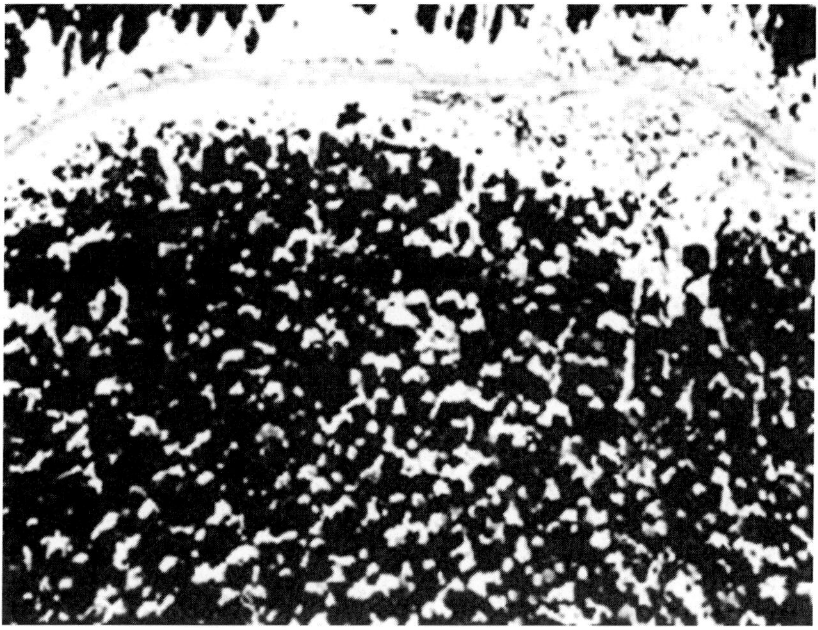

Figure 30. Colour IR film of woodland showing high and low stress

For identifying crops, two important parameters are the size and shape of the crop type. For example, soybeans have spread out leaf clumps and corn has tall stalks with long, narrow leaves and thin, tassle-topped stems. Wheat (in the cereal grass family) has long thin central stems with a few small, bent leaves on short branches, all topped by a head containing the kernels from which flour is made. Other considerations are the surface area of individual leaves, the plant height and amount of shadow it casts, and the spacing or other planting geometries of row crops (the normal arrangement of legumes, feed crops, and fruit orchards). The stage of growth (degree of crop maturity) is also a factor. For example during its development wheat passes through several distinct steps such as developing its kernel-bearing head and changing from shades of green to golden-brown.

Another related parameter is Leaf Area Index (LAI), defined as the ratio of one-half the total area of leaves (the other half is the underside) in vegetation to the total surface area containing that vegetation. If all the leaves were removed from a tree canopy and laid on the ground, their combined areas relative to the ground area projected beneath the canopy would be some number greater than 1 but usually less than 10. As a tree, for example, fully leaves, it will produce some LAI value that is dependent on leaf size and shape, the number of limbs, and other factors. The LAI is related to the the total biomass (amount of vegetative matter [live and dead] per unit area, usually measured in units of tons or kilograms per hectare [2.47 acres]) in the plant and to various measures of Vegetation Index. Estimates of biomass can be carried out with variable reliability using remote sensing inputs, provided there is good supporting field data and the quantitative (mathematical) models are efficient. Both LAI and NDVI are used in the calculations.

Satellite remote sensing is an excellent means of determining LAI on a regional or sub continental scale. In principal, actual LAI must be determined on site directly by stripping off all leaves, but in practice it can be estimated by statistical sampling or by measuring some property such as reflectance. Thus, remote sensing can determine an LAI estimate if thereflectance are matched with appropriate field truth. For remotely sensed crops, LAI is influenced by the amount of reflecting soil between plant (thus looking straight down will see both corn and soil but at maturity a cornfield seems closely spaced when viewed from the side). For the spectral signatures shown below, the Near IR reflectances will increase with LAI.

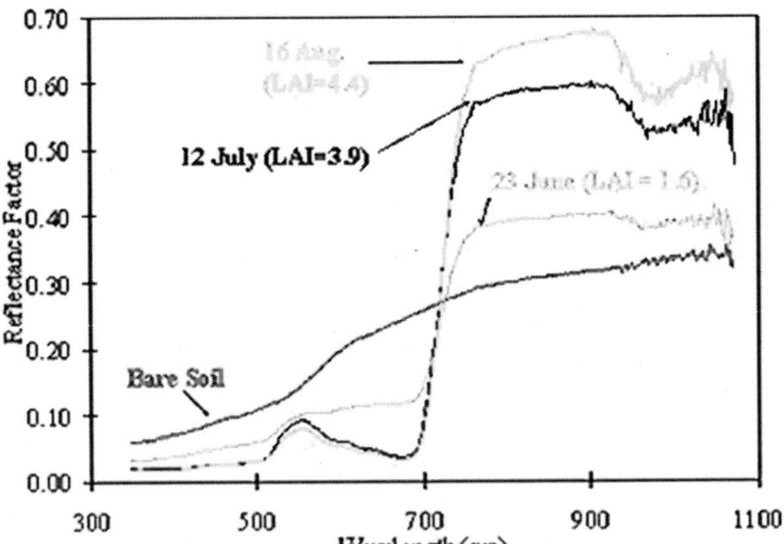

Figure 31. IR reflectance of corn and soil with LAI

This change in appearance and extent of surface area coverage over time is the hallmark of vegetation as compared with most other categories of ground features (especially those not weather-related). Crops in particular show strong changes in the course of a growing season, as illustrated here for these three stages - bare soil in field (A); full growth (B); fall senescence (C), seen in a false colour rendition:

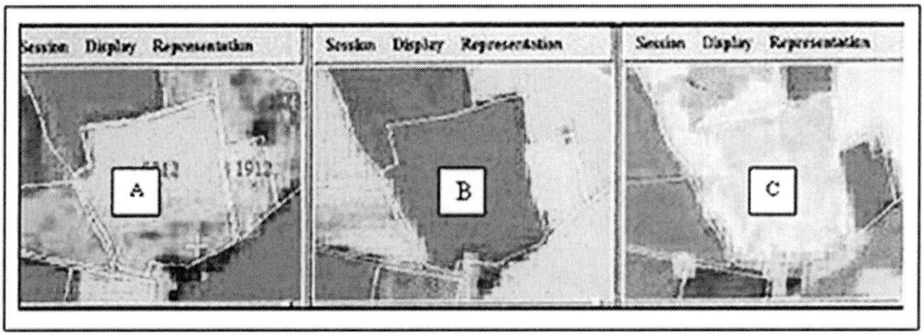

Figure 32. Land sat image of the field showing three stages - bare soil in field (A); full growth (B); fall senescence (C)

2.6.3. Detection of Dead Vegetation By Landsat

The study of vegetation dynamics in terms of climatically-driven changes that take place over a growing season is called *phenology*. A good example of how repetitive satellite observations can provide updated information on the phenological history of natural vegetation and crops during a single cycle of Spring-Summer growth is this sequence of AVHRR images of the Amu-Dar'ja Delta just south of the Aral Sea in Ujbekistan (south-central Asia).The amount of vegetation present in the delta (a major farming district for this region) is expressed as the NDVI. The Aral Sea - a large inland lake - is now rapidly drying up.

More generally, seasonal change appears each year with the "greening" that comes with the advent of Spring into Summer as both trees and grasses commence their annual growth. The leafing of trees in particular results in whole regions becoming dominated by active vegetation that is evident when rendered in a multispectral image in green tones. The MODIS sensor on Terra has several vegetation-sensitive bands used to calculate a variation of the NDVI called the Enhanced Vegetation Index (EVI).

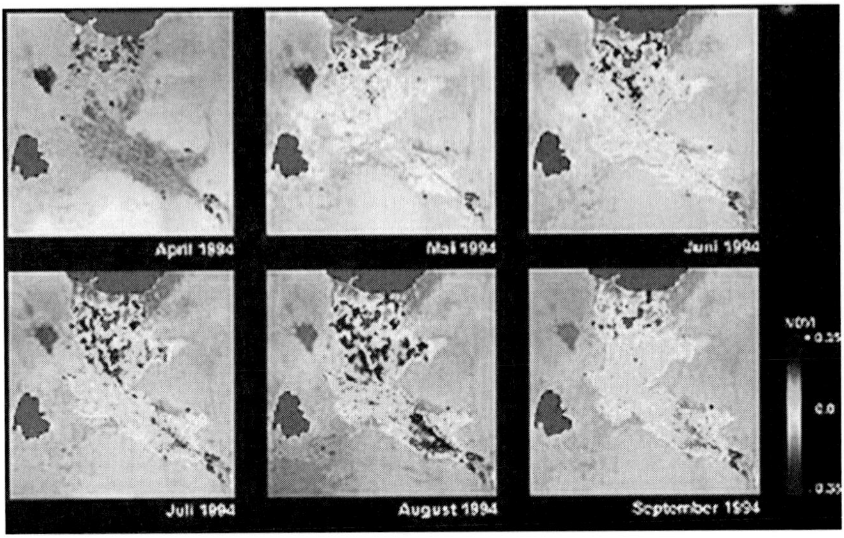

Figure 33. AVHRR images of the Amu-Dar'ja Delta, south of the Aral Sea in Ujbekistan

Now, to emphasize the variability of the spectral response of crops over time, we show these phonological stages for wheat in this sequential illustration:

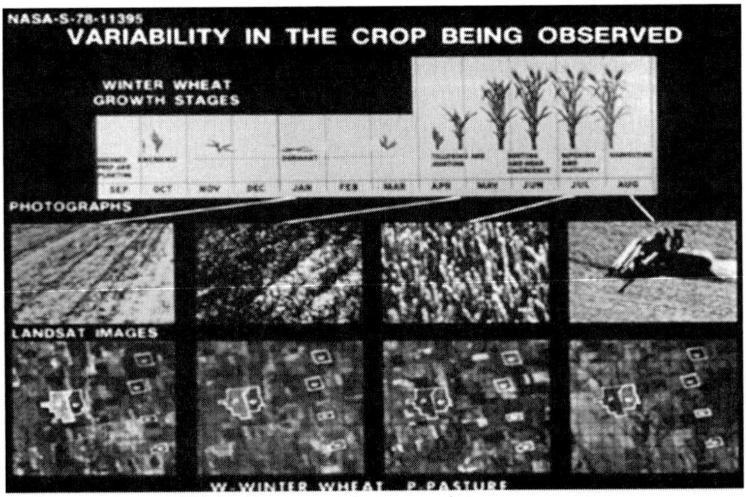

Figure 34. Enhanced Vegetation Index (EVI) showing variability of the spectral response of crops over time

Note that, in the Landsat imagery, the wheat fields (particularly the light-blue polygon in the far-left image) show their brightest response in the IR (hence red) during the emergent stage but become less responsive by the ripening stage. The grasses and alfalfa that make up pasture crops mature (redden) much later.

2.6.4. Usage Of Specific Crop Types As Training Sites Identified (Determined)?

With this survey of the role of several variables in determining crop types, let us look now at one of the most successful classifications reported to date. These are being achieved by hyper spectral sensors such as AVIRIS and Hyperion. The Hyperion hyper spectral sensor on NASA's EO-1has procured multichannel data for the Coleambally test area in Malaysia. This image, made from 3 narrow channels in the visible-Near IR, shows how the fields of corn, rice, and soybeans changed their reflectance during the (southern hemisphere) growing season: Notice the pronounced differences in crop shapes which is a big factor in producing the reflectance differences (as said above, healthy leaf vegetation generally has a spectral response that does not vary much in percent reflectance from one plant type to others, so that differences in crop shape become the distinguishing factor).

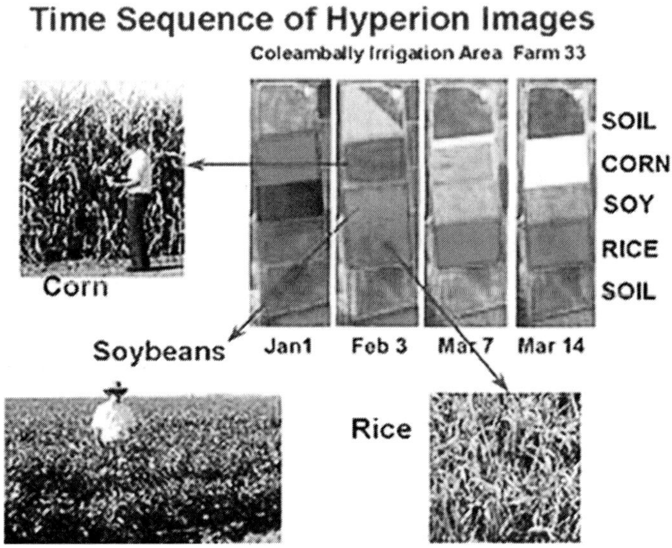

Figure 35. Visible-Near IR image showing reflectance changing in the fields of corn, rice, and soybeans during the growing season

The multichannel data from Hyperion were used to plot the observed spectral signatures for the soil and three crops, as shown here (the curves identified in the upper right [the writing is too small to be decipherable on most screens] are, from top to bottom, soil, corn, rice, and soybeans):

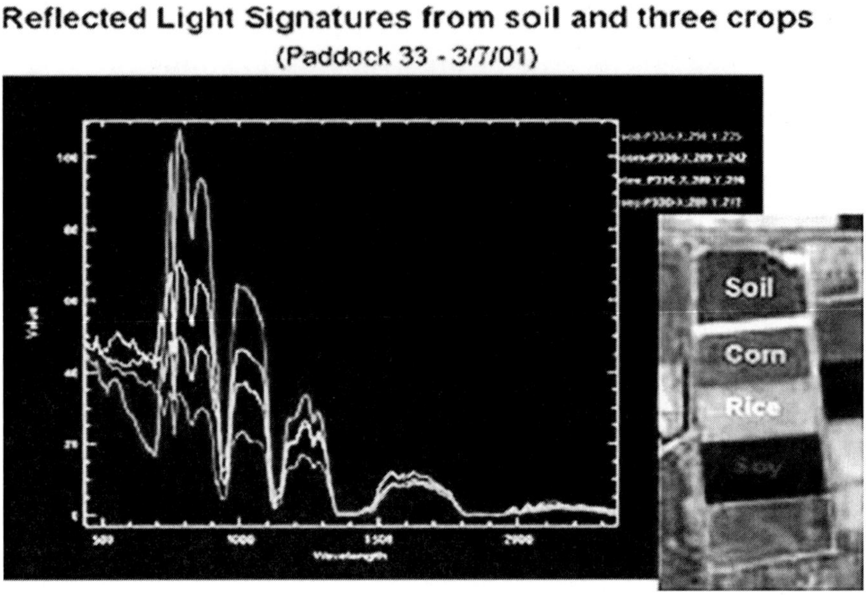

Figure 36. Reflected light signatures from soil and three crops

Using a large number of selected individual Hyperion channels, this supervised classification of the four classes in the sub scene was generated; this end result is more accurate than is normally achievable with broad band data such as obtained by Landsat:

Active microwave sensors, or radar, can use several variables to recognize crop vegetation and even develop a classification of crop types. Here is a SIR-C (Space Shuttle) image of farmland in the Netherlands, taken on April 4, 1994. The false colour composite was made with L-band in the HH polarization mode = red; L-band HV = green; and C-band HH = blue.

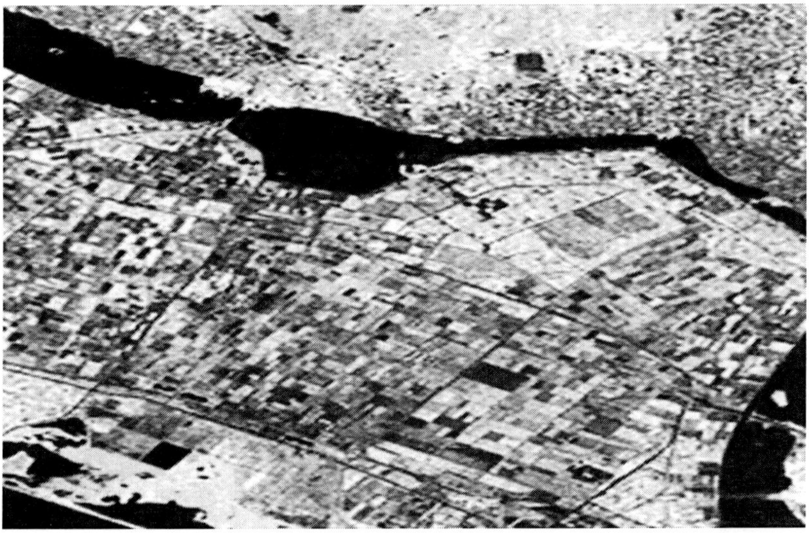

Figure 37. SIR-C (Space Shuttle) image of farmland in the Netherlands

An additional image variable is the crop's background, namely the nurturing soil, whose colour and other properties can change with the particular soil type, and whose reflectance depends on the amount of moisture it holds. Moisture tends to darken a given soil colour; this condition is readily picked up in aircraft imagery as seen in this pair of images:

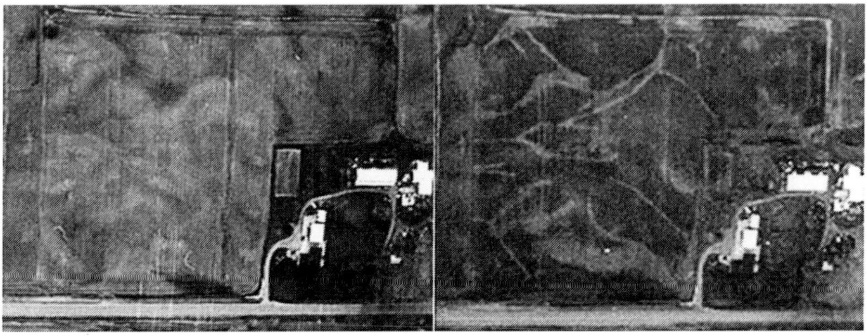

Figure 38. Aircraft imagery showing different colours due to moisture pickup

Often, the distribution of moisture, as soil dries differentially, is variable in an imaged barren field giving rise to a mottled or blotchy appearance. Thermal imagery brings out the differential soil moisture content by virtue of temperature variations. The amount of water in the crop itself also affects the sensed temperature (stressed [water deficient] or diseased crop material is generally warmer). Soil water variations are evident in this image made by an airborne thermal sensor of several fields, where high moisture correlates with blue and drier parts of the fields with reds and yellows:

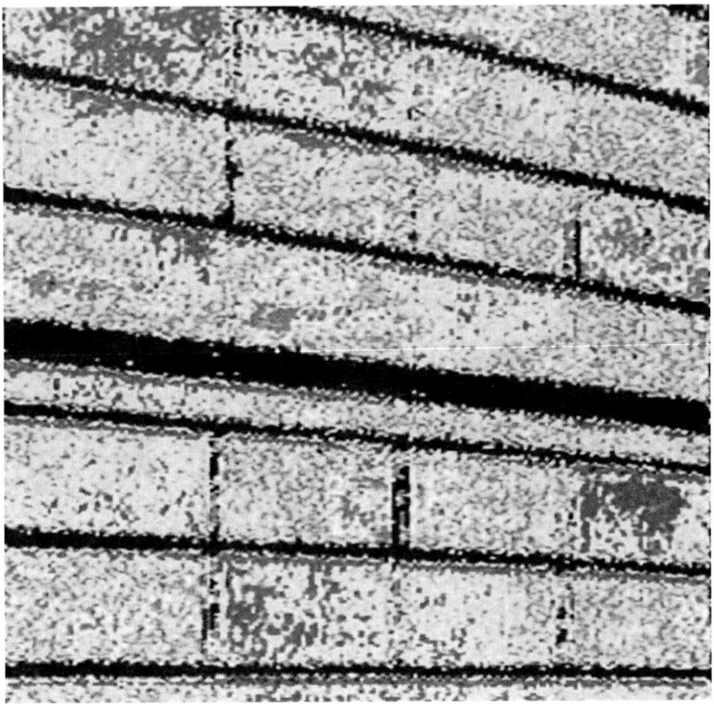

Figure 39. Image made by an airborne thermal sensor of several fields showing the soil water variations

A combination of visible, NIR, and thermal bands can pick up both water deficiency and the resulting stress on the crops in the fields. This set of three images was made by a Daedalus instrument flown on an aircraft. In the top image, yellow marks unplanted fields and those in blue and green are growing crops. The center image picks up patterns of water distribution in the crop fields. The bottom image shows levels of stress related in part to insufficient moisture.

A passive microwave sensor also picks up soil moisture. Cooler areas appear dark in images of fields over flown by a microwave sensor - although other factors, such as absence or presence of growing crops (and their types) besides moisture can account for some darker tones.

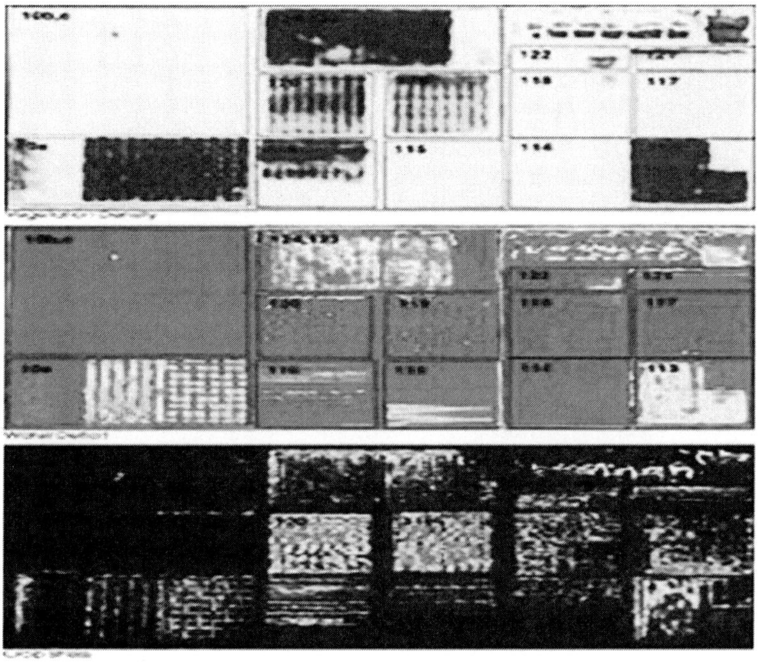

Figure 40. Image showing levels of stress related in part to insufficient moisture

REFERENCES

1. R. L. Bankert, P. M. Tag, 1998Using SSM/I Data and Computer Vision to Estimate Tropical Cyclone IntensityProceedings, 9th Conference on Satellite Meteorology and Oceanography, American Meteorological Society, Boston, MA, 226229

2. B. A. Baum, V. Tovinkere, J. Titlow, R. M. Welch, 1997Automated Cloud Classification of Global AVHRR Data Using a Fuzzy Logic ApproachJournal of Applied Meteorology3615191540

3. M. F. Baumgardner, L. F. Silva, L. L. Biehl, Stoner. E. R. And, 1985Reflectance properties ofsoils, Advances in Agronomy, 38144

4. S. Bojinski, M. Schaepman, D. Schaepfer, Itten. K. And, 2003SPECCHIO: a spectrumdatabase for remote sensing applications, Computers and Geosciences, 292738

5. F. Boochs, G. Kupper, K. Dockter, W. Kuhbauch, 1990Shape of the red edge as vitalityindicator of plants, International Journal ofRemote Sensing, 11 (10), 1741-1753.

6. J. B. Campbell, 1996An Introduction to RemoteSensing (2nd Ed), New York, The GuilfordPress.

7. R. N. Clark, T. V. V. King, C. Ager, G. A. Swayze, 1995Initial vegetation species andsenescence/stress mapping in the San LuisValley, Colorado, using imaging spectrometerdata, Proceedings: Summitville Forum 1995,

8. R. N. Clark, G. A. Swayze, A. J. Gallagher, T. V. V. King, W. M. Calvin, 1993The U. S. Geological Survey, Digital Spectral Library,Version 1: 0.2 to 3.0 microns, U.S. GeologicalSurvey Open File Report 93592pages.

9. W. Collins, 1978 Remote Sensing of Crop Typeand Maturity, Photogrammetric Engineeringand Remote Sensing, 444355

10. P. J. Curran, 1989Remote sensing of foliar chemistryRemote Sensing of Environment30271278

11. B. Curtiss, A. F. H. Goetz, 2001FielSpectrometry: techniques and instrumentation,Analytical Spectral Devices Inc,

12. B. Datt, 2000Identification of green anddry vegetation components with a crosscorrelogramspectral matching technique,International Journal of Remote Sensing, 2121332139

13. D. W. Deering, 1989Field measurements ofbidirectional reflectance: In Theory andApplications of Optical Remote Sensing, G.Asrar (Ed.), New York, Wiley and Sons, 1461

14. M. J. Duggin, W. R. Philipson, 1982FieldMeasurement of Reflectance: some majorconsiderations, Applied Optics, 21 (15), 2833-2840.

15. F. H. Goetz, L. Rowan, C., 1981 GeologicRemote Sensing. Science, 211781791

16. C. I. Grove, S. J. Hook, I. I. E. D. Paylor, 1992Laboratory Reflectance Spectra of 160 Minerals, 0.4 to 2.5 Micrometers, Jet Propulsion Laboratory Pub, 922

17. B. Hapke, 1993Theory of Reflectance and Emittance SpectroscopyUK, CambridgeUniversity Press.

18. S. B. Hooker, C. R. Mc Clain, 2000Thecalibration and validation of SeaWiFS data.Prog. Oceanogr., 45(3-4), 427-465.

19. G. R. Hunt, J. W. Salisbury, C. J. Lenhoff, 1971aVisible and Near-Infrared spectra ofminerals and rocks: III Oxides and Hydroxides, Modern Geology, 2195205

20. G. R. Hunt, 1979Near-infrared (1.3-2.4μm)spectra of alteration minerals- Potential foruse in remote sensing, Geophysics, 4419741986

21. J. R. Irons, R. A. Weismiller, G. W. Peterson, 1989Soil reflectance In Theory andApplications of Optical Remote Sensing, G. Asrar (Ed), New York, Wiley and Sons, 66106

22. T. V. V. King, R. N. Clark, C. Ager, G. A. Swayze, 1995Remote mineral mapping usingAVIRIS data at Summitville, Proceedings: Summitville Forum 1995, Posey, H. H.,Pendelton, J. A. and Van Zyl, D., (Eds.),Colorado Geological Survey Special Publication385963

23. V. M. Krasnopolsky, W. H. Gemmill, 2000Neural network multi-parameter algorithms to retrieve atmospheric and oceanic parameters from satellite data., Proceedings, Second Conference on Artificial Intelligence, AMS, Long Beach, CA, 9-14 January, 2000, 7376

24. D. A. May, J. Sandidge, R. Holyer, J. D. Hawkins, 1997SSM/I Derived Tropical Cyclone Intensities. Proceedings, 22nd Conference on Hurricanes and Tropical Meteorology, American Meteorological Society, Boston, MA, 2728

25. E. J. Milton, E. M. Rollin, D. R. Emery, 1995Advances in Field Spectroscopy, In Danson,F. M. and Plummer, S. E. (1995) Advances inEnvironmental Remote Sensing, UK: John Wileyand Sons.

26. F. Nicodemus, J. Richmond, J. Hsia, I. Ginsberg, Limperis. T. And, 1977GeometricalConsiderations and Nomenclature forReflectance, NBS Monograph 160, USDepartment of Commerce.

27. Robert. A. Pearson, D. Donald, 1999Improving Error Structure in Temperature Profile Retrievals from Satellite ObservationsBustamante th International Conference on Neural Information Processing (ICONIP'99), November 1620Perth, Australia.

28. Pfitzner, K., Bartolo, R.E., Ryan, B. and Bollhöfer,A. (2005). Issues to consider when designinga spectral library database, Spatial SciencesInstitute Conference Proceedings 2005,Melbourne, Spatial Sciences Institute, ISBN 0-9581366

29. K. Pfitzner, A. Bollhöfer, G. Carr, 2006Protocols for measuring field reflectancespectra. Supervising Scientist Report, In Press,Supervising Scientist for the Alligator RiversRegion, Canberra.

30. M. Pidwirny, 2006Introduction to Geographic Information Systems". Fundamentals of Physical Geography, 2nd Edition.

31. Posey, H. H., Pendelton, J. A., and Van Zyl,D., (Eds.), Colorado Geological Survey SpecialPublication 38, 64-69.

32. W. G. Rees, 2001Physical Principles of remotesensing, 2nd Edition, UK, Cambridge UniversityPress.

33. E. M. Rollin, D. R. Emery, E. J. Milton, 1995The design of field spectroradiometers, auser's view, In Proceedings of the 21st AnnualConference of the Remote Sensing Society,Nottingham, UK, 555562

34. J. W. Salisbury, 1998Spectral MeasurementsField Guide, Earth Satellite Corporation,April 23 1998, Published by the DefenceTechnology Information Centre as Report ADA362372

35. M. B. Satterwhite, J. P. Henley, 1990Hyperspectral Signatures (4002500nm) ofVegetation, Minerals, Soils, Rocks, and CulturalFeatures: Laboratory and Field Measurements,U.S. Army Corps of Engineers, EngineerTopographic Laboratories, Fort Belvoir, Virginia22060-5546.

36. M. E. Schaepman, 1998Calibration of aField Spectroradiometer. Calibration and Characterisation of a non-imaging fieldspectroradiometer supporting imaging spectrometer validation and hyperspectralsensor modelling, Remote Sensing Laboratories, Department of Geography, University ofZurich, 1998.

37. Silva1978Radiation and instrumentation inremote sensing, In Swain et al., (Ed.): Remotesensing- the quantitative approach, McGraw& Hill, 121135

CHAPTER 8

Evaluating Biomass of Juniper Trees (Juniperus pinchotii) from Imagery-Derived Canopy Area Using the Support Vector Machine Classifier

Mustafa Mirik*, Sriroop Chaudhuri, Brady Surber, Srinivasulu Ale, Robert James Ansley

Texas A&M AgriLife Research (TAMAR), Vernon, USA

ABSTRACT

Both temporal and spatial magnitude, structure, and distribution of rangeland aboveground biomass (AGB) are important inputs for many necessities, in particular for estimating terrestrial carbon amount, ecosystem productivity, climate change studies, and potential bioenergy uses. Much of the remote sensing research previously completed has focused on determining carbon stocks in forested ecosystems with little attention directed to estimate AGB amount in rangelands. Our objectives were to: 1) identify and delineate individual redberry juniper (Juniperus pinchotii) plants from surrounding live vegetation using the support vector machine method for classifying two-dimensional (2D) geospatial imagery with a 1-m spatial resolution at two sites; and 2) develop regression models relating imagery-derived and fieldmeasured single tree canopy area and diameter for dry AGB estimation. The regression results show that there were very close and significant relationships between field measured juniper plant AGB and canopy area derived from the image classification with $r^2 > 0.90$. These results suggest that spectral reflectance recorded on 2D high resolution imagery is capable to assess and quantify AGB as a quick, repeatable, and unbiased method over large land areas.

KEYWORDS

Remote Sensing; Geospatial Imagery; Biomass; Juniperus pinchoti; Rangeland; Bioenergy; Terrestrial Carbon Budget

1. INTRODUCTION

Aboveground vegetation biomass (biomass hereafter) distribution, structure, and amount in rangeland regions are important in estimating terrestrial carbon and energy fluxes between atmosphere and biosphere and thus are major considerations in ecosystem processes or climate change research [1-4]. Vegetation on rangelands, characterized by woodlands, shrublands, and grasslands, provides essential ecosystem services, including forage for domestic and native herbivores, but is highly variable in spatial distribution and temporal growth patterns [5-9]. A world-wide phenomenon on many rangelands has been the expansion of woody plants into grassland and savanna areas in the last 150 years [3,4,8,10]. Increases in woody-plant abundance comprise a significant but highly uncertain fraction of the carbon budget world-wide [3,6]. Projecting future states of rangeland ecosystems in response to woody invasions and changes in climateedaphic, and disturbance regimes are strongly dependent on current assessment of woody biomass and distribution and the contribution of woody plants to total terrestrial biomass amount [6].

Traditional field-based biomass estimations of woody biomass through allometric functions are accurate, but are costly, tedious, time consuming, and usually limited to small land areas. Remote sensing-based biomass prediction is the most promising method at regional and global scales [2,11-18]. Over the last decade, a large number of studies have estimated biomass using twodimensional (2D) geospatial images, synthetic aperture radar (SAR) and LIDAR [2,11,13,16,19]. Numerous studies have documented that remote sensing techniques are highly efficient to assess woody plant biomass at multiple spatial and temporal scale [11,12,20]. Although small footprint radar backscatter and LIDAR data may be more accurate than 2D geospatial imagery for characterizing woody plant attributes, these data are expensive to acquire at present, and are limited by its narrow swathcoverage on each overpass due to high spatial resolution

[4,15,21-23]. Two-dimensional high resolution geospatial imageries, such as TM, IKONOS, QuickBird, GeoEye, World View, are much more cost-effective and are now available for almost anywhere in the world [24]. Though such data have been widely used to quantify forest biomass, they have been rarely utilized for rangeland woody biomass assessment [24,25]. Research on high-resolution 2D geospatial images from satellite has evaluated algorithms to determine crown diameter, crown area, and other attributes in a wide range of forested areas [24,25]. For this reason, remote sensing studies quantifying rangeland biomass contribution to the total carbon budget are strongly needed.

Redberry juniper (Juniperus pinchotii; juniper hereafter) occupies more than 4.7 million ha of rangeland in the western half of Texas alone and extents to the neighboring states in the Southern Great Plains of the US [10]. Juniper is a native troublesome species, aggressively encroaching into rangeland due to reduced intensity and frequency of fires and livestock overgrazing. High densities of this and a closely related species in central TX, Ashe juniper (Juniperus ashei), can significantly decrease species diversity and grass production by competing for natural resources and can greatly trigger soil erosion [26].

The United States Department of Agriculture-National Agricultural Imagery Program (USDA-NAIP) imagery archive has entered public domain, providing exciting opportunities to advance rangeland research. We propose that periodically acquired NAIP images are adequate for quantifying biomass of individual juniper plants because of 1-m spatial resolution. Recently, Allometric models between field-measured redberry juniper above-ground mass (AGM) and physiognomic characteristics such as canopy area, diameter, and height were developed [10]. In addition, the potential of high-resolution QuickBird images to estimate Juniperus spp. tree volume and biomass was examined in which this type of optical imagery can be used for rapid and reliable measurements of tree volume and biomass [27,28]. The objectives of the present study were to 1) identify and delineate juniper from surrounding live vegetation using the support vector machine (SVM) classifier; 2) investigate the relationships between imagery-derived and field-measured canopy area and diameter; and 3) develop regression models relating imagery-derived and field-measured single tree attributes for estimation of total, wood, and leaf-twig biomass. Since the remote sensing biomass of juniper trees has not been well documented, we initiated this study to fill an important gap in the application of remotely assessed canopy area using the SVM method for discriminating juniper plants from background vegetation and estimating biomass components.

2. MATERIALS AND METHODS

2.1. Study Area

Data were collected from two sites near the town of Crowell about 132-km west of Wichita Falls and 241-km east of Lubbock in north central Texas (**Figure 1**). The sites were located about within 10 km of each other on similar soil types: Site 1 (Whatley Ranch), 34°4'N, 99°44'W; elev. 436-m in Foard County; Site 2 (Copper Break State Park), 34°6'N, 99°45'W; elev. 443-m in Hardeman County. Total 30 years mean annual rainfall at Crowell is 616 mm [29]. The sites were dominated by juniper and honey mesquite (Prosopis glandulosa Torr.). Herbaceous understory consists of numerous cool-season (C_3) and warm-season (C_4) grass species dominated by perennial C_4 grasses, tobosagrass (Pleuraphis mutica) and buffalograss (Bouteloua dactyloides). Other grasses are C_3mid-grass Texas wintergrass (Nassella leucotricha), C_3 annual grass Japanese brome (Bromus japonicus) and other C_4 mid-grasses such as vine mesquite (Panicum obtusum), sideoats grama (Bouteloua curtipendula), and dropseeds (Sporobolus spp.) [30]. Soils are fine-silty, mixed, thermic Typic Calciustolls of the Quanah series and fine-silty, montmorillonitic, thermic Typic Haplusterts of the Hollister series [31].

2.2. Field Sampling

A total of 54 juniper plants ranging in size from 1.53 to 73.90-m^2 canopy area were selected for the study. The trees were selected to represent the range of three diameter found at the sites, thus were not random because the objective of the study was to quantify the relationship between the tree attributes derived from the imagery and field-measured biomass through regression analysis. To randomly sample the study sites and still have the same range of canopy diameter would have required many more plots than the logistics of the study could accommodate. Selection was limited to trees that appeared healthy and undamaged and had to be at least 1-m apart from other trees. Canopy diameters along 2 directions (longest axis and perpendicular to longest) were measured on each tree followed by harvesting to the ground level during the dormant season (October-December 2010 and January-March 2011). Following harvest, leaftwig (<3-cm diameter stems) and wood (>3-cm diameter) components were manually separated and weighed. Total wet weight of each component was obtained within few hours of tree felling. Three randomly selected subsamples of each component from each tree were weighed as wet weight, oven-dried at 60°C for 60 - 70 days, and weighed after weights stabilized. Percent moisture was determined [(wet weight-dry weight)/wet weight × 100] for components and whole tree and used to determine total oven dry biomass of each tree and individual biomass components.

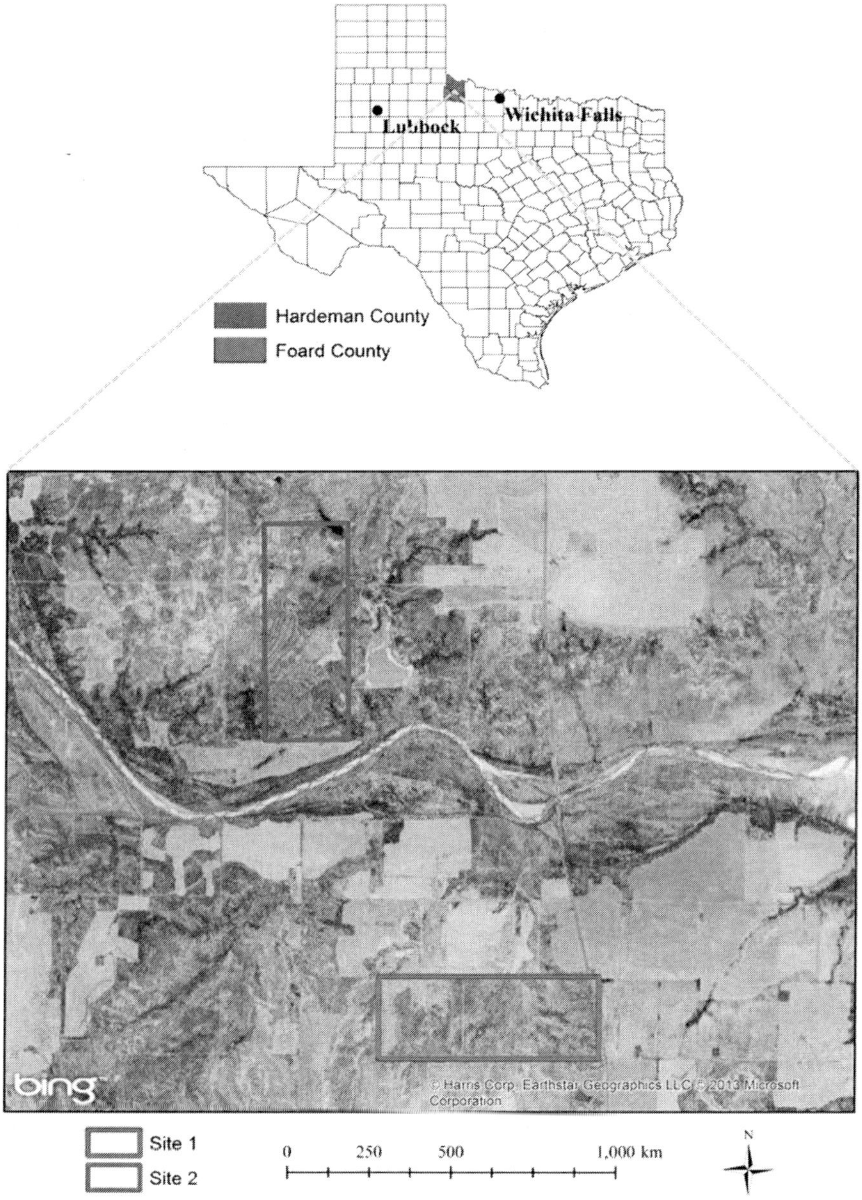

Figure 1. Location of Hardeman (top) and Foard Counties (bottom) where study sites were situated in north central Texas.

2.3. Remote Sensing Imagery and Image Classification

One county-level color infrared aerial image collected over Hardeman County, covering both sites, was obtained from the National Agricultural Imagery Program (NAIP) provided by the Natural Resources Conservation Service Geospatial Data Gateway at (http://datagateway.nrcs.usda.gov/). The NAIP imagery consisted of green, red, and near infrared bands with a spatial resolution of 1-m taken on August 12, 2010 over the sites. The image was projected to the Universal Transverse Mercator North American Datum 1983 Zone 14 North by the provider. The image was extracted for the sites using ArcGIS software suits (ESRI, Inc. Redlands, CA).

Image classifications were performed using the SVM method in Environment for Visualizing Images software (ENVI; Exelis Visual Information Solutions, Boulder, CO). The SVM is a supervised machine learning method that performs classification based on the statistical learning theory. The SVM classifies data by separating a hyperplane that provides the best separation between classes in a multidimensional feature space. This hyperplane is the decision surface on which the optimal class separation takes place. The optimal hyperplane is the one that maximizes the distance between the hyperplane and the nearest positive and negative training example called the margin. From a given set of training samples, the optimization problem is solved to find the hyperplane that leads to a sparse solution. Although the SVM is a binary classifier in its simplest form, implementation of the SVM classifier in ENVI was extended to more than two classes by splitting the problem into a series of binary class separations (ENVI User's Guide).

In order to represent more complex shapes than linear hyperplanes, a variety of kernels including the polynomial, the radial basis function, and the sigmoid can be used for performing SVM classification in ENVI. The SVM was employed using the radial basis function kernel for performing the pairwise classification. There is also a penalty parameter can be introduced to the SVM classifier to allow for misclassification during the training process. The penalty parameter was set to its maximum value, whereas a classification probability threshold of zero was used in order to classify all pixels (ENVI User's Guide). Default settings of this classifier were used for image classifications. During the classification process, only NIR band of the NAIP imagery was chosen using the spectral subset option in ENVI.

The 1-m image allowed clear and visual identification of all endmembers based on the spectral contrast among the live vegetation (juniper, mesquite, herbaceous) and senescent or non-vegetative components (road, shadow, exposed soil, water, senescent herbaceous) (**Figure 2**(a)). Previous studies found that reflectance from Ashe juniper (Juniperus ashei), mesquite, water, exposed soil, and herbaceous plants were significantly different [32,33]. In addition, reflectance variation within deciduous crown is larger than that within coniferous tree crown because of the non-conical shape, large branches, and the shade area caused by the neighboring branches [15]. Thus, juniper endmember was manually extracted from isolated trees on areas in the image [34]. Juniper endmember for each site comprised 10 polygons, each having 25 pixels, from pure juniper canopy at locations well-identified on the ground and on the image. The CEM was run for juniper endmember using covariance matrix with a 75% rule threshold and square root stretching.

2.4. Determination of Canopy Area and Development of Regression Model for Biomass Estimation

Point coordinates of the harvested trees, with sub-meter accuracy at the center of each tree following harvest, were taken with a Trimble GeoXH hand-held unit (Trimble Navigation Limited, Sunnyvale, CA) equipped with the ArcPad software (ESRI, Inc. Redlands, CA). The projection of the GPS unit was set to Universal Transverse Mercator North American Datum 1983 Zone 14 North. A unique identification number was assigned to each tree during the collection of point coordinates in the field. Spatial analyses performed for juniper canopy area determination are described below.

Following image classification using CEM, fractional abundance of juniper was converted to vector layer (polygon shapefile format) in ENVI and exported to ArcGIS for canopy area determination (**Figure 2**(b)). The point coordinates representing tree-locations were overlaid onto the vector layer (**Figure 2**(c)) and the polygons representing harvested tree were selected with the "select by location" function, where the locations were tree point coordinates. A new polygon layer including only selected polygons was created (**Figure 2**(d)). This new polygon layer and point layer, both representing harvested trees, were "joined" in order to assigned unique identification number to each polygon. Area of each polygon was determined with "calculate geometry" function and designated as canopy area. The attribute table of the circle layer was then exported to a spreadsheet in order to perform regression analysis with fieldmeasured tree attributes.

The point coordinates representing to tree-locations were overlaid onto the image where one-to-one matching with the juniper trees was verified (**Figure 2**(c)). Circles representing juniper canopy area based on point locations were blindly digitized as a polygon layer by an untrained person in ArcGIS (**Figure 2**(c)). The areas and diameters of these circles were determined by the "calculate geometry" and "field calculator" functions, respectively. The attribute table of the circle layer was then exported to a spreadsheet in order to perform regression analysis with field-measured tree attributes. Field-based canopy area (CA; m^2) determination was made using the ellipse equation: $\pi \cdot a \cdot b$, where a = radius of longest canopy axis and b = radius of perpendicular canopy axis adopted from [10].

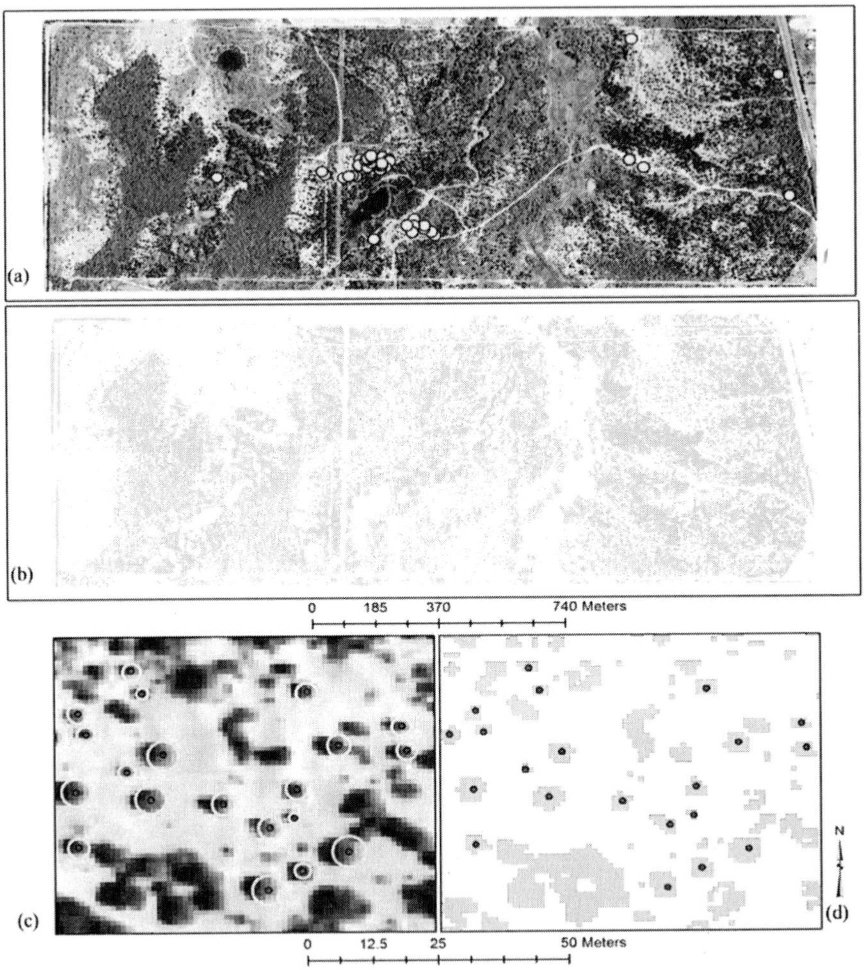

Figure 2. The false color infrared national agricultural imagery program image with 1-m spatial resolution and harvested trees represented with yellow (a); classified image with juniper: green (b); some of the harvest trees illustrated with blindly drown circles in yellow and red dots (c); classified trees shown with the red dots (d) for site 1.

Simple linear regression analyses were performed to relate image-derived tree attributes with field-measured tree variables using Statistical Analysis

Systems 9.2 (SAS Institute Inc., Cary, NC) and regression plots were created using SigmaPlot 11 (Systat Software Inc., Chicago, IL). Image-derived tree parameters were used as the independent and field-measured attributes were set as the dependent variable. Model validation was performed by randomly apportioning observations into a 70/30 split with the former fraction being used for model development, while later used to predict tree attributes. Error estimation was performed by computing the root mean squared error (RMSE) between predicted and field-measured values, as well as field-measured and imageryderived attributes.

3. RESULTS

3.1. Data Summary

Descriptive summary of variables used in regression models were presented in **Table 1**. The means and ranges confirm that a broad range of values was assessed for tree attributes. Field measured juniper plant canopy diameters ranged from 1.40 to 9.70-m with a mean and standard error ($\overline{X} \pm \varepsilon$: 5.15 ± 0.31), whereas canopy areas varied from 1.72 to 73.90-m^2 (24.73 ± 2.72). Average canopy diameters and areas derived from the imagery using both manual-extraction and classification methods were slightly higher than the field-measurements (**Table 1**).

Table 1. Summary statistics for juniper tree attributes measured in the field and extracted from the imagery with 1-m spatial resolution (n = 54).

Tree attribute	Mean	SE	Min	Max
Fmca (m^2)	24.73	2.72	1.53	73.90
Fmcd (m^2)	5.15	0.31	1.40	9.70
Fmtb [kg]	187.03	25.29	3.53	688.35
Fmwb [kg]	104.78	16.41	0.05	460.37
Fmltb [kg]	82.25	9.47	3.44	227.99
Meca (m^2)	28.21	3.27	1.72	101.92
Macd (m^2)	5.48	0.33	1.48	11.39
Cca (m^2)	27.46	3.55	0.00	105.00

Fmca: field-measured canopy area; Fmcd: field-measured canopy diameter; Fmtb: field-measured total biomass; Fmwb: field-measured wood biomass; Fmltb: field-measured leaf-twig biomass; Meca: manually-extracted canopy area; Mecd: manually-extracted canopy diameter; Cca: classified canopy area; SE: Standard Error; Min: Minimum; Max: Maximum.

Canopy diameter and area for manual extraction method ranged from 1.48 to 11.39 m (5.48 ± 0.33) and from 1.72 to 101.92-m^2 (22.84 ± 2.70), respectively. Range of canopy areas derived from classified imagery were between 0 and 105-m^2 (27.46 ± 3.55), respectively.

A juniper plant with 1.75 m diameter, and 2.3 m^2 canopy area was, however, not detected with the algorithm. Biomass varied from 3.53 to 688.85 kg (187.03 ± 24.83). Biomass was partitioned into wood biomass only with a minimum and maximum weights 0.05 and 460.37 kg (104.78 ± 16.41) and leaf-twig biomass varying from 3.44 to 227.99 kg (82.25 ± 9.47).

3.2. Biomass Estimation

Simple linear regression analysis revealed presence of robust, tight, and significant relationships between the variables of interest (Figures 3-6, **Table 2**). Predictors (classified and manually-extracted canopy area and diameter) accounted for 91% to 96% of the variation in fieldmeasured canopy area and diameter with associated RMS errors between 4.274 and 0.489, respectively, (**Figure 3**). Manually-extracted canopy area produced a slightly stronger relationship with total and wood biomass than canopy diameter (**Table 2**). Classified canopy area had equal predictive power for total and leaf-twig biomass (Figures 4(a)-(c)), while the predictive power was weaker for wood biomass (**Figure 4**(b)). The strength of the relationships between biomass components and imagery-derived canopy area or canopy diameter generally declined (r^2 = 0.88 and RMSE between 5.754 and 5.106) for leaf-twig biomass (**Figure 6**(d); **Table 2**), except for the classified canopy area (r^2 = 0.93; RMSE = 7.751; **Figure 4**(c)).

The relationships between remotely determined and field-measured tree attributes using the validation dataset confirmed robust and significant associations (Figures 5 and 6, **Table 2**). Linear regression between canopy diameter using manual extraction method and field-measured canopy diameter produced a stronger relationship (r^2 = 0.95, RMSE = 0.463) (**Figure 5**(c)) compared to canopy area calculated using both manually-extracted (r^2 = 0.94, RMSE = 4.287; **Figure 5**(a)) and classified data (r^2 = 0.94, RMSE = 4.199; **Figure 5**(b)), respectively. Total, wood, and leaf-twig biomass determined using classified canopy area accounted for 98% (RMSE = 16.644), 96% (RMSE = 15.717), and 88% (RMSE = 12.495) of the variations in field-measured counterparts (Figures 6(a)- (c)), respectively. Biomass components estimated using manually-extracted canopy area had r^2 values of 0.96, 0.96, and 0.84 for field-measured total, wood, and leaftwig biomass (**Table 2**), respectively, whereas the relationships between field-measured total, wood, and leaftwig biomass and biomass of these components determined using manually-extracted canopy diameter were 93%, 90%, and 89% (**Table 2**), respectively.

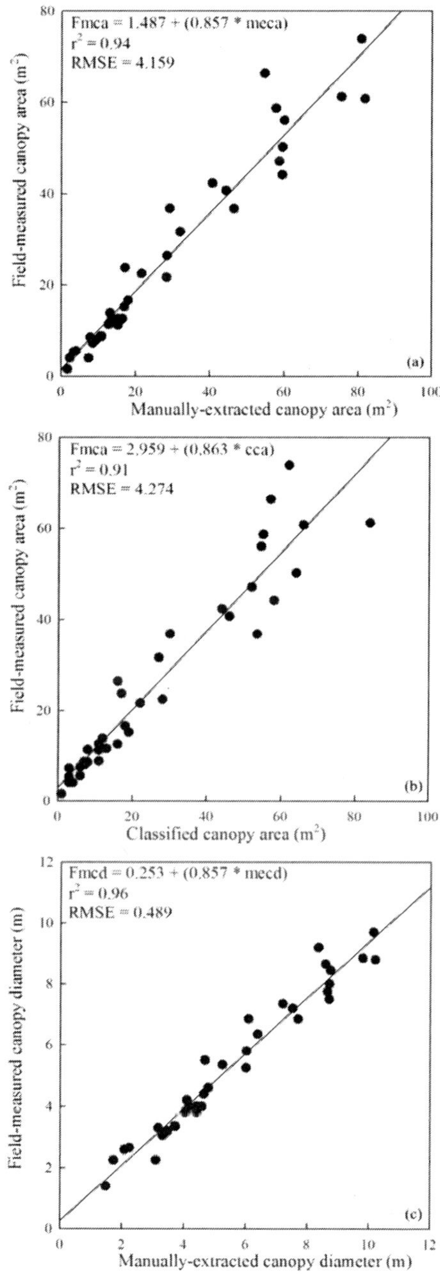

Figure 3. The relationship between manually-extracted and field-measured canopy area (a), classified and field-measured canopy area (b), and manually-extracted and fieldmeasured canopy diameter (c); n = 38, P < 0.001. Fmca: field-measured canopy area; meca: manually-extracted canopy area; cca: classified canopy area; fmcd: field-measured canopy diameter; mecd: manually-extracted canopy diameter.

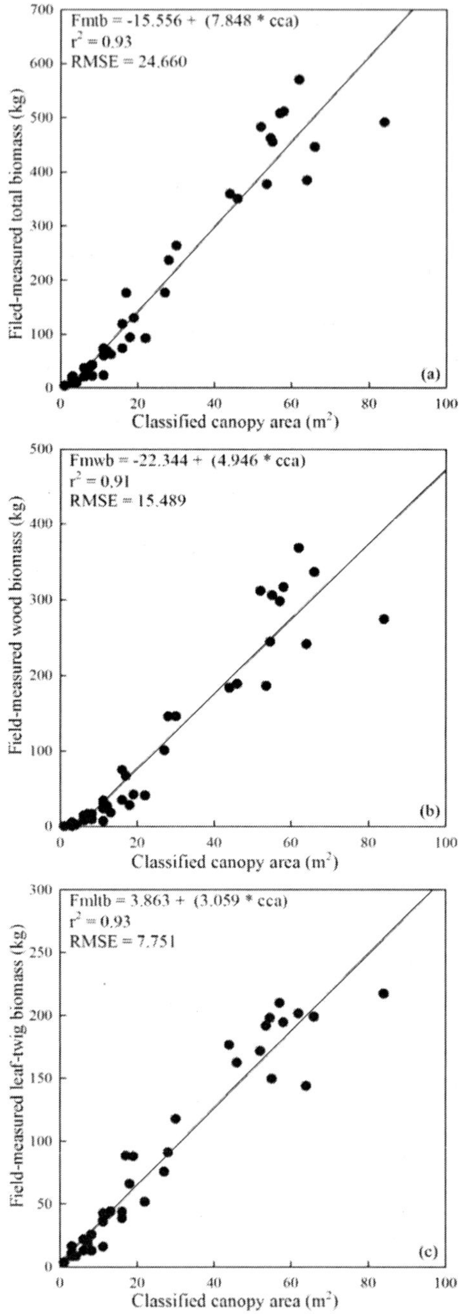

Figure 4. The relationship between classified canopy area and field-measured total (a), wood (b), and leaf-twig biomass (c); n = 38, P < 0.001. Fmtb: field-measured total biomass; cca: classified canopy area; fmwb: field-measured wood biomass; fmltb: field-measured leaf-twig biomass.

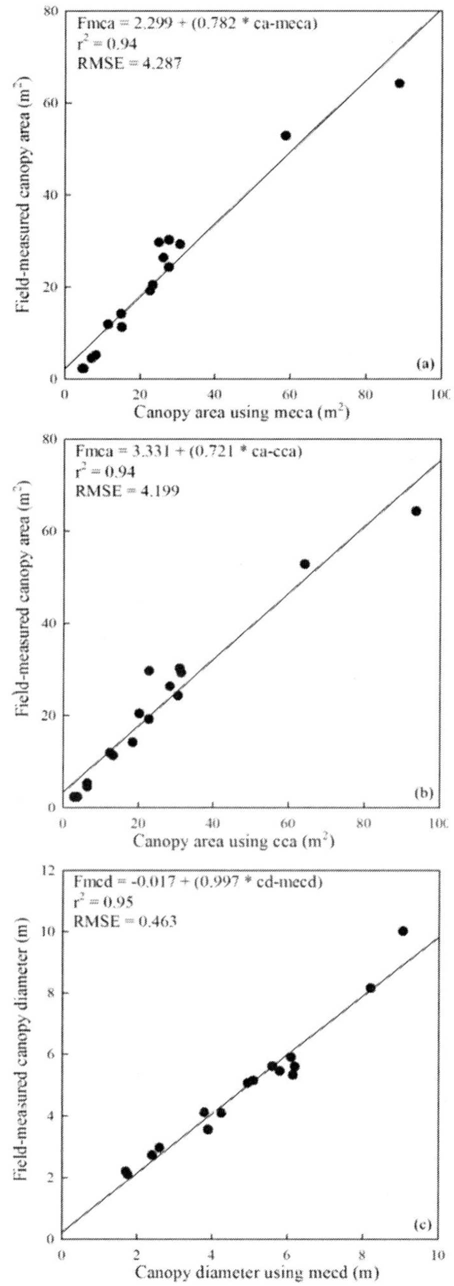

Figure 5. The relationship between canopy area using manually-extracted canopy area (meca) and field-measured canopy area (fmca) (a); canopy area using classified canopy area (cca) and fmca (b); and canopy diameter using manually-extracted canopy diameter (mecd) and field-measured canopy diameter (fmcd) (c); n = 16, $P < 0.001$.

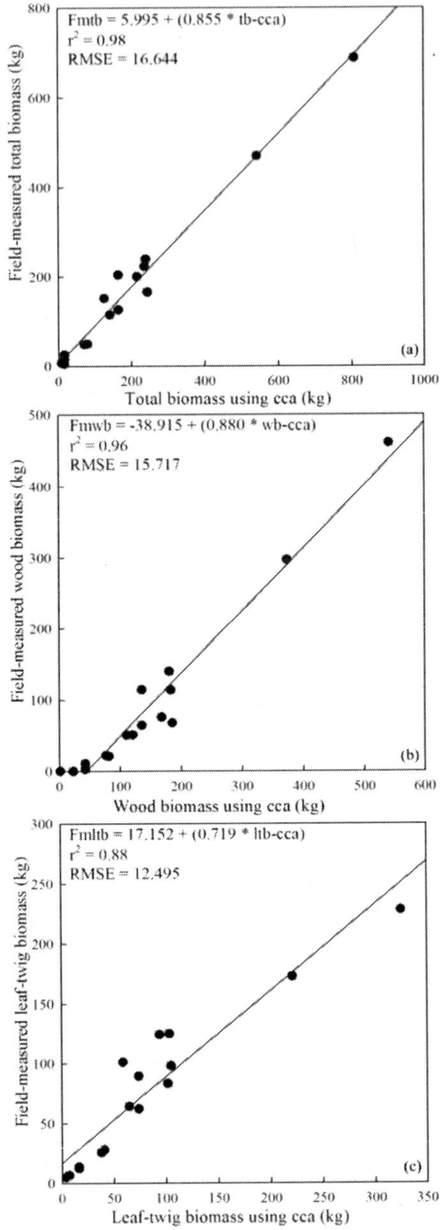

Figure 6. The relationship between total (a), wood (b), and leaf-twig biomass (c) determined from classified canopy area (cca) and field measurements; n = 16, $P < 0.001$. Fmtb: field-measured total biomass; fmwb: field-measured wood biomass; fmltb: field-measured leaf-twig biomass; tb-, wb-, ltb-cca: total, wood, and leaf-twig biomass using classified canopy area.

Table 2. The simple linear regression models with the associated statistics for manually-extracted canopy area and diameter versus predicted and field-measured total, wood, and leaf-twig biomass.

Biomass model	r^2	RMSE
Fmtb^{+} = −23.617 + (7.604*meca)	0.92	24.87
Fmwb^{+} = −30.581 + (4.903*meca)	0.93	11.58
Fmltb^{+} = 2.310 + (2.909*meca)	0.88	5.75
Fmtb^{+} = −202.34 + (71.921*mecd)	0.90	29.56
Fmtb^{+} = −142.143 + (45.704*mecd)	0.89	20.16
Fmltb^{+} = −67.776 + (27.822*mecd)	0.88	5.10
Fmtb* = 8.674 + (1.457*fmtb-meca)	0.96	16.96
Fmwb* = −11.972 + (0.992*fmwb-meca)	0.96	5.23
Fmltb* = 12.208 + (0.800*fmltb-meca)	0.84	5.65
Fmtb* = −42.420 + (1.085*fmtb-mecd)	0.93	28.21
Fmwb* =−44.061+ (1.184*fmwb-mecd)	0.90	18.48
Fmltb* =−116.266+(0.889*fmltb-mecd)	0.89	1.54

$^{+}$ and *: model development (n = 38, $P < 0.001$) and validation datasets (n = 16, $P < 0.001$), respectively; fmtb: field-measured total biomass; meca: manually-extracted canopy area; fmwb: field-measured wood biomass; fmltb: field-measured leaf-twig biomass; mecd: manually-extracted canopy diameter; ptb-meca, pwb-meca, and pltb-meca: predicted total, wood, and leaf-twig biomass using manually-extracted canopy area, respectively; ptb-mecd, pwb-mecd, pltb-mecd: predicted total, wood, and leaf-twig biomass using manually-extracted canopy diameter.

4. DISCUSSION

We evaluated and reported the usefulness of 2D geospatial aerial imagery for estimating juniper tree biomass at two rangeland sites, typical for the southern Great Plains of the US, using both automated and manual canopy area determination methods. Although accuracy assessment for classification was not conducted in this research, earlier studies found high classification accuracy for juniper species [32,33,35-38]. Overall accuracies between 80 and 92% were found for classifying Ashe juniper in central Texas using QuickBird imagery and aerial photography [32]. An airborne hyperspectral image was evaluated in order to compare classification methods for mapping Ashe juniper in central Texas [33]. The authors found that overall mapping accuracies varied from 84% to 100%. Overall classification accuracies between 80% and 92% were achieved for both Rocky Mountain juniper (Juniperus scopulorum) and Utah juniper (Juniperus osteosperma) using Landsat 5 TM imagery [38]. A mapping accuracy of 92% for western juniper (Juniperus occidentalis subsp. Occidentalis) using the NAIP imagery was reported [35].

A single juniper plant with a 2.3-m^2 canopy area (1.75-m canopy diameter) was not detected with the algorithm used to classify the imagery in this study. Visual inspection of ground-level images of this plant taken prior to harvest indicated that it was growing on 100% exposed soil without any herbaceous background cover. This suggested that 100% exposed soil background may suppress detection of smaller plants. Accurate monitoring of semi-arid vegetation using remote sensing can be hindered by the effects of bare soil [39].

Reasons for this may relate to the greater level of "brightness" associated with bare soil in arid and semiarid landscapes that saturates that portion of the image and eliminates detection of small dark objects such as a small tree canopy.

The approach developed and implemented in the current study allows accurate estimation of individual juniper tree biomass using simple linear regression for fieldmeasured biomass and automated or manual methods. The relationships observed between field-measured and image derived juniper plant variables were robust and highly significant. This indicates that remotely sensed imagery can be very useful for estimating biomass of individual juniper trees on rangeland ecosystems for both trained and untrained personnel. For example, automated canopy area determination method over large land areas can be used by trained personnel in image processing software, while manual method can be preferable by untrained rangeland managers. Remote sensing has not been used extensively for quantifying the amount and extent of woody biomass on rangelands. The bulk of the existing studies have relied on other mass quantification techniques, which usually are time-consuming measurements using field transects [9,28]. The strength of the relationships found in this study implies that these attributes can be readily obtainable from the image with a sufficient spatial resolution without a need for field measurements, especially over remote and inaccessible or large land areas. The RMSEs reported in this study were far less than that required for biomass estimation procedures in European countries, with an error not exceeding ±20% [22].

We also explored the use of 2D geospatial imagery not only for total plant biomass estimation but also for estimation of wood and leaf-twig biomass components. Estimates of woody plant components have rarely been related to remotely sensed images [40]. Our results indicated that wood and leaf-twig biomass can be estimated reasonably well with canopy area and diameter values derived from aerial images of the resolution utilized in this study. Wood biomass has the highest energy content of the plant components and would likely be the most desirable portion of woody plants from a bioenergy use perspective. Alternatively, leaf-twig biomass may be linked to estimate leaf area index (LAI), providing clues to estimate water use patterns and potential competitive effects with the herbaceous understory. Leaves also conduct photosynthesis and are the primary energy exchange medium between plant and the environment, and are thus linked to productivity and biogeochemical cycles of a site [22,40-43].

The relationships developed between image-measured canopy area and that measured on the site in this study were higher than that reported by [28]. These authors found that the QuickBird data accounted for 85% of the variation in ground-measured eastern redcedar (Juniperus virginiana) biomass. A stronger relationship ($r^2 = 0.98$) than ours between imageand ground-measured eastern redcedar canopy area was reported by [28]. An identical relationship ($r^2 = 0.92$) between LIDARand field-measured biomass to ours was reported by [44], whereas a weaker relationship ($r^2 = 0.62$) was found by [45] who related LISS-IV-estimated and field-measured biomass. A good relationship ($r^2 = 0.78$) between Aleppo pine (Pinus halepensis) biomass measured in the field and estimated from a high-quality aerial photograph [46]. Image-estimated biomass can serve as an alternative to field sampling in forest biomass research, given adequate temporal and spatial coverage of the study area [46].

Recently, there has been increasing amounts of baseline information required at large spatial scales as part of woody biomass operational management plans. Such details may include ecological diversity issues, partial harvesting (i.e., leaving old and large trees), or patch harvesting for bioenergy, wildlife or hydrological concerns. These new requirements demand a greater level of detail in remote sensing data. Higher resolution data with individual tree-scale details allows for better precision in management decisions [1,3,40,47-49]. The individual plant approach offers a better understanding of the sources of uncertainty and errors associated with remote sensing estimates when predicting biomass at a large scale [48]. With availability of high spatial and spectral resolution, multispectral and hyperspectral satellite and aerial remote sensing data in the recent times, it is now possible to estimate both individual tree and cluster or stand level biomass [28,40] at relatively low resource requirement. The equations derived and validated in this study are easy to comprehend and may be used with high confidence by managers, ecologists, scientists, and ranchers seeking rapid estimates of juniper biomass and possibly other tree species with similar growth forms for use in management and in ecological models.

Accurate estimates of biomass are also critical for monitoring carbon dynamics in rangelands that is considered essential in assessing regional or global carbon budgets. Growing interest in quantifying ecosystem carbon stocks and or potential bioenergy uses has triggered various research initiatives to explore possibilities of using non-destructive methods to estimate biomass [10, 28]. In particular, there has been a noticeable inclination towards using aerial or satellite remote sensing images to estimate biomass [3,28,50-53]. Regional companies are currently considering to use eastern redcedar in gasification facilities for the production of steam or electricity for small rural communities and in ethanol production, or to produce woody pellets for residential heating [28]. With respect to potential biomass estimation for bioenergy uses, the aerial extent of the images will have to be sufficient to cover large land areas (>50,000 ha) that is necessary for sustainable feedstock supply to a processing facility [28,54]. Such estimations may need to rely on 2D imagery such as National Agricultural Imagery Program (NAIP) of the USDA [35,53,55] or satellite images that can provide appreciable details at regional scale and can be geo-spatially integrated with other features such as road networks, waterways, etc. to facilitate harvest plans. Otherwise, if not impossible, it is too costly, labor intensive, and time consuming to estimate biomass via ground-based measurements [28].

Data reported so far worldwide have indicated that for most rangeland woody plants, the most accurate method of non-destructively estimating biomass is to measure basal stem diameter, crown diameter, plant height, and crown volume [7,56-61]. Basal stem diameter and diameter at breast height, however are not easily-measurable parameters for juniper due to its highly compacted canopy and a high density of low growing stems restricting access to the central base stem [10]. Because of spherical growth forms and dense lateral growth with very compact canopy and a high density of low growing stems, these researchers determined that canopy area, determined by measuring canopy diameter in two directions, was the best variable for predicting total tree AGM. Height was a less effective variable to predict biomass and including height to calculate canopy volume resulted in little improvement in the biomass estimation accuracy compared to canopy area alone. Since it is not possible to measure canopy height or stem diameter at breast height from 2d geospatial imagery, using canopy area and/or diameter measurements would appear to be the most suitable approach for predicting juniper tree biomass from 2D imagery. Imagery classification and converting classification to vector to obtain automated canopy area of all trees in an area are the easiest and quickest processes. The ability to remotely estimate biomass using canopy area would provide a major benefit for research and management efforts.

5. CONCLUSION

Though remote sensing data is becoming increasingly important in forest biomass estimation, little attention has been directed to rangeland woody biomass. There is an obvious need for large scale measurements to improve our understanding on the effects of ecological processes such as woody encroachment into grasslands and carbon contribution of rangeland woody plants to local or regional carbon stocks. The current study was undertaken to explore the relationship between canopy area and diameter of individual red berry juniper trees as determined via aerial images and the biomass of those trees. A major finding of this research is that the method is highly automated and repeatable, and provides the ability to estimate and map juniper biomass using image classification in addition to manual digitizing. Results suggest that 2D geospatial imagery may be a powerful tool for estimating juniper biomass and in certain situations with adequate ground-based calibration curves, could replace ground measurement in many areas. Imagery classification of woody canopies can be a relatively straightforward process when the imagery is acquired during the dormant season when there is a strong spectral contrast between evergreen juniper and leafless deciduous trees and/or dormant herbaceous plants.

6. ACKNOWLEDGEMENTS

This research was funded in part by a grant from John Deere Renewables, Inc., and the Texas AgriLife Bioenergy Initiative Fund. Copper Breaks State Park and the Whatley Ranch, Crowell, TX provided harvest sites for this project. Images used in this study were made available by the USDA-NRCS. We also thank Mimi Roy for technical discussion and Andy Bell for assisting with data collection.

REFERENCES

1 N. F. Glenn, L. P. Spaete, T. T. Sankey, D. R. Derryberry, S. P. Hardegree and J. J. Mitchell, "Errors in LiDAR-Derived Shrub Height and Crown Area on Sloped Terrain," Journal of Arid Environments, Vol. 75, No. 4, 2011, pp. 377-382.

2 J. E. Nichol and M. L. R. Sarker, "Improved Biomass Estimation Using the Texture Parameters of Two HighResolution Optical Sensors," IEEE Transactions on Geoscience And Remote Sensing, Vol. 49, No. 3, 2011, pp. 930-948.

3 E. K. Strand, L. A. Vierling, A. M. S. Smith and S. C. Bunting, "Net Changes in Aboveground Woody Carbon Stock in Western Juniper Woodlands, 1946-1998," Journal of Geophysical Research D: Atmospheres, Vol. 113, No. G01013, 2008, pp. 1-13.

4 Z. Wang, C. B. Schaaf, P. Lewis, Y. Knyazikhin, M. A. Schull, A. H. Strahler, T. Yao, R. B. Myneni, M. J. Chopping and B. J. Blair, "Retrieval of Canopy Height Using Moderate-Resolution Imaging Spectroradiometer (MODIS) Data," Remote Sensing of Environment, Vol. 115, No. 6, 2011, pp. 1595-1601.

5 K. Brinkmann, U. Dickhoefer, E. Schlecht and A. Buerkert, "Quantification of Aboveground Rangeland Productivity and Anthropogenic Degradation on the Arabian Peninsula Using Landsat Imagery and Field Inventory Data," Remote Sensing of Environment, Vol. 115, No. 2, 2011, pp. 465-474.

6 C. Huang, S. E. Marsh, M. P. McClaran and S. R. Archer, "Postfire Stand Structure in a Semiarid Savanna: CrossScale Challenges Estimating Biomass," Ecological Applications, Vol. 17, No. 7, 2007, pp. 1899-1910.

7 E. T. A. Mitchard, S. S. Saatchi, S. L. Lewis, T. R. Feldpausch, I. H. Woodhouse, B. Sonké, C. Rowland and P. Meir, "Measuring Biomass Changes Due to Woody Encroachment and Deforestation/Degradation in a ForestSavanna Boundary Region of Central Africa Using MultiTemporal L-Band Radar Backscatter," Remote Sensing of Environment, Vol. 115, No. 11, 2011, pp. 2861-2873.

8 K. P. Paudel and P. Andersen, "Assessing Rangeland Degradation Using Multi Temporal Satellite Images and Grazing Pressure Surface Model in Upper Mustang, Trans Himalaya, Nepal," Remote Sensing of Environment, Vol. 114, No. 8, 2010, pp. 1845-1855.

9 R. Sonnenschein, T. Kuemmerle, T. Udelhoven, M. Stellmes and P. Hostert, "Differences in Landsat-Based Trend Analyses in Drylands Due to the Choice of Vegetation Estimate," Remote Sensing of Environment, Vol. 115, No. 6, 2011, pp. 1408-1420.

10 R. J. Ansley, M. Mirik, B. W. Surber and S. C. Park, "Canopy Area and Aboveground Mass of Individual Redberry Juniper (Juniperus pinchotii Sudw.) Trees," Rangeland Ecology & Management, Vol. 65, No. 2, 2012, pp. 189-195.

11 M. A. Alrababah, M. N. Alhamad, A. L. Bataineh, M. M. Bataineh and A. F. Suwaileh, "Estimating East Mediterranean Forest Parameters Using Landsat ETM," International Journal of Remote Sensing, Vol. 32, No. 6, 2011, pp. 1561-1574.

12 M. L. Clark, D. A. Roberts, J. J. Ewel and D. B. Clark, "Estimation of Tropical Rain Forest Aboveground Biomass with Small-Footprint Lidar and Hyperspectral Sensors," Remote Sensing of Environment, Vol. 115, No. 11, 2011, pp. 2931-2942.

13 S. Englhart, V. Keuck and F. Siegert, "Aboveground Biomass Retrieval in Tropical Forests—The Potential of Combined Xand L-Band SAR Data Use," Remote Sensing of Environment, Vol. 115, No. 5, 2011, pp. 1260- 1271.

14 M. T. Gebreslasie, F. B. Admed, J. A. N. Van Aardt and F. Blakeway, "Individual Tree Detection Based on Variable and Fixed Window Size Local Maximum Filtering Applied to IKONOS Imagery for Even-Aged Eucalyptus Plantation Forest," International Journal of Remote Sensing, Vol. 32, No. 15, 2011, pp. 4141-4154.

15 Y. Ke and L. J. Quackenbush, "A Review of Methods for Automatic Individual Tree-Crown Detection and Delineation from Passive Remote Sensing," International Journal of Remote Sensing, Vol. 32, No. 17, 2011, pp. 4725- 4747.

16 S. C. Popescu, K. Zhao, A. Neuenschwander and C. Lin, "Satellite Lidar vs. Small Footprint Airborne Lidar: Comparing the Accuracy of Aboveground Biomass Estimates and Forest Structure Metrics at Footprint Level," Remote Sensing of Environment, Vol. 115, No. 11, 2011, pp. 2786- 2797.

17 L. R. Sarker and J. E. Nichol, "Improved Forest Biomass Estimates Using ALOS AVNIR-2 Texture Indices," Remote Sensing of Environment, Vol. 115, No. 4, 2011, pp. 968-977.

18 C. Yang, H. Huang and S. Wang, "Estimation of Tropical Forest Biomass Using Landsat TM Imagery and Permanent Plot Data in Xishuangbanna, China," International Journal of Remote Sensing, Vol. 32, No. 20, 2011, pp. 5741-5756.

19 E. Næsset, "Estimating Above Ground Biomass in Young Forests with Airborne Laser Scanning," International Journal of Remote Sensing, Vol. 32, No. 2, 2011, pp. 473-501.

20 G. Sun, K. J. Ranson, Z. Guo, Z. Zhang, P. Montesano and D. Kimes, "Forest Biomass Mapping from Lidar and Radar Synergies," Remote Sensing of Environment, Vol. 115, No. 11, 2011, pp. 2906-2916.

21 G. Chen and G. J. Hay, "An Airborne Lidar Sampling Strategy to Model Forest Canopy Height from Quickbird Imagery and GEOBIA," Remote Sensing of Environment, Vol. 115, No. 6, 2011, pp. 1532-1542.

22 T. Le Toan, S. Quegan, M. W. J. Davidson, H. Balzter, P. Paillou, K. Papathanassiou, S. Plummer, F. Rocca, S. Saatchi, H. Shugart and L. Ulander, "The BIOMASS Mission: Mapping Global Forest Biomass to Better Understand the Terrestrial Carbon Cycle," Remote Sensing of Environment, Vol. 115, No. 11, 2011, pp. 2850-2860.

23 A. Swatantran, R. Dubayah, D. Roberts, M. Hofton and J. B. Blair, "Mapping Biomass and Stress in the Sierra Nevada Using Lidar and Hyperspectral Data Fusion," Remote Sensing of Environment, Vol. 115, No. 11, 2011, pp. 2917-2930.

24 C. Song, M. B. Dickinson, L. Su, S. Zhang and D. Yaussey, "Estimating Average Tree Crown Size Using Spatial Information from Ikonos and QuickBird Images: AcrossSensor and Across-Site Comparisons," Remote Sensing of Environment, Vol. 114, No. 5, 2010, pp. 1099-1107.

25 P. Gonzalez, G. P. Asner, J. J. Battles, M. A. Lefsky, K. M. Waring and M. Palace, "Forest Carbon Densities and Uncertainties from Lidar, QuickBird, and Field Measurements in California," Remote Sensing of Environment, Vol. 114, No. 7, 2010, pp. 1561-1575.

26 R. J. Ansley, H. T. Weidemann, M. J. Castellano and J. E. Slosser, "Herbaceous Restoration of Juniper-Dominated Grasslands with Chaining and Fire," Rangeland Ecology & Management, Vol. 59, No. 2, 2006, pp. 171-178.

27 I. Ozdemir, "Estimating Stem Volume by Tree Crown Area and Tree Shadow Area Extracted from Pan-Sharpened QuickBird Imagery in Open Crimean Juniper Forests," International Journal of Remote Sensing, Vol. 29, No. 19, 2008, pp. 5643-5655.

28 P. J. Starks, B. C. Venuto, J. A. Eckroat and T. Lucas, "Measuring Eastern Redcedar (Juniperus virginiana L.) Mass with the Use of Satellite Imagery," Rangeland Ecology & Management, Vol. 64, No. 2, 2011, pp. 178-186.

29 National Oceanic and Atmospheric Administration, Climate Data Center, Asheville, 2006. http://www.ncdc.noaa.gov/ oa/ncdc.html

30 NRCS, United States Department of Agriculture, Natural Resource Conservation Service, Plants Database Website, 2011. http://plants.usda.gov

31 NRCS, United States Department of Agriculture, Natural Resource Conservation Service, Soil Series Descriptions Website, 2011. http://soils.usda.gov

32 J. H. Everitt, C. Yang and H. B. Johnson, "Canopy Spectra and Remote Sensing of Ashe Juniper and Associated Vegetation," Environmental Monitoring and Assessment, Vol. 130, No. 1-3, 2007, pp. 403-413.

33 C. Yang, J. H. Everitt and H. B. Johnson, "Applying Image Transformation and Classification Techniques to Airborne Hyperspectral Imagery for Mapping Ashe Juniper Infestations," International Journal of Remote Sensing, Vol. 30, No. 11, 2009, pp. 2741-2758.

34 B. Somers, G. P. Asner, L. Tits and P. Coppin, "Endmember Variability in Spectral Mixture Analysis: A Review," Remote Sensing of Environment, Vol. 115, No. 7, 2011, pp. 1603-1616.

35 K. W. Davies, S. L. Petersen, D. D. Johnson, D. B. Davis, M. D. Madsen, D. L. Zvirzdin and J. D. Bates, "Estimating Juniper Cover from National Agriculture Imagery Program (NAIP) Imagery and Evaluating Relationships between Potential Cover and Environmental Variables," Rangeland Ecology & Management, Vol. 63, No. 6, 2010, pp. 630-637.

36 S. L. Petersen and T. K. Stringham, "Development of GIS-Based Models to Predict Plant Community Structure in Relation to Western Juniper Establishment," Forest Ecology and Management, Vol. 256, No. 5, 2008, pp. 981-989.

37 T. T. Sankey, N. Glenn, S. Ehinger, A. Boehm and S. Hardegree, "Characterizing Western Juniper Expansion via a Fusion of Landsat 5 Thematic Mapper and Lidar data," Rangeland Ecology & Management, Vol. 63, No. 5, 2010, pp. 514-523.

38 T. T. Sankey and M. J. Germino, "Assessment of Juniper Encroachment with the Use of Satellite Imagery and Geospatial Data," Rangeland Ecology & Management, Vol. 61, No. 4, 2008, pp. 412-418.

39 K. Hufkens, J. Bogaert, Q. H. Dong, L. Lu, C. L. Huang, M. G. Ma, T. Che, X. Li, F. Veroustraete and R. Ceulemans, "Impacts and Uncertainties of Upscaling of Remote-Sensing Data Validation for a Semi-Arid Woodland," Journal of Arid Environments, Vol. 72, No. 8, 2008, pp. 1490-1505.

40 R. M. Lucas, A. C. Lee and P. J. Bunting, "Retrieving Forest Biomass through Integration of CASI and LIDAR Data," International Journal of Remote Sensing, Vol. 29, No. 5, 2008, pp. 1553-1577.

41 D. F. Levia Jr., "A Generalized Allometric Equation to Predict Foliar Dry Weight on the Basis of Trunk Diameter for Eastern White Pine (Pinus strobus L.)," Forest Ecology and Management, Vol. 255, No. 5-6, 2008, pp. 1789-1792.

42 S. D. Roberts, T. J. Dean, D. L. Evans, J. W. McCombs, R. L. Harrington and P. A. Glass, "Estimating Individual Tree Leaf Area in Loblolly Pine Plantations Using LiDAR-Derived Measurements of Height and Crown Dimensions," Forest Ecology and Management, Vol. 213, No. 1-3, 2005, pp. 54-70.

43 L. Wang, J. E. R. Hunt, J. J. Qu, X. Hao and C. S. T. Daughtry, "Towards Estimation of Canopy Foliar Biomass with Spectral Reflectance Measurements," Remote Sensing of Environment, Vol. 115, No. 3, 2011, pp. 836- 840.

44 R. M. Lucas, N. Cronin, M. Moghaddam, A. Lee, J. Armston, P. Bunting and C. Witte, "Integration of Radar and Landsat-Derived Foliage Projected Cover for Woody Regrowth Mapping, Queensland, Australia," Remote Sensing of Environment, Vol. 100, No. 3, 2006, pp. 388-406.

45 R. Madugundu, V. Nizalapur and C. C. Jha, "Estimation of LAI and Above-Ground Biomass in Deciduous Forests: Western Ghats of Karnataka, India," International Journal of Applied Earth Observation and Geoinformation, Vol. 10, No. 2, 2008, pp. 211-219.

46 A. B. Massada, Y. Carmel, G. E. Tzur, J. M. Grünzweig and D. Yakir, "Assessment of Temporal Changes in Aboveground Forest Tree Biomass Using Aerial Photographs and Allometric Equations," Canadian Journal of Forestry Research, Vol. 36, No. 10, 2006, pp. 2585-2594.

47 H. Holmström, "Estimation of Single-Tree Characteristics Using the kNN Method and Plotwise Aerial Photograph Interpretations," Forest Ecology and Management, Vol. 167, No. 1-3, 2002, pp. 303-314.

48 S. C. Popescu, "Estimating Biomass of Individual Pine Trees Using Airborne Lidar," Biomass and Bioenergy, Vol. 31, No. 9, 2007, pp. 646-655.

49 G. Whiteman and J. R. Brown, "Assessment of a Method for Mapping Woody Plant Density in a Grassland Metrix," Journal of Arid Environments, Vol. 38, No. 2, 1998, pp. 269-282.

50 G. P. Asner, S. Archer, R. F. Hughes, R. J. Ansley and C. A. Wessman, "Net Changes in Regional Woody Vegetation Cover and Carbon Storage in Texas Drylands, 1937- 1999," Global Change Biology, Vol. 9, No. 3, 2003, pp. 316-335.

51 C. Huang, G. P. Asner, R. E. Martin, N. N. Barger and J. C. Neff, "Multiscale Analysis of Tree Cover and Aboveground Carbon Stocks in

Pinyon-Juniper Woodlands," Ecological Applications, Vol. 19, No. 3, 2009, pp. 668- 681.

52 O. Masera, A. Ghilardi, R. Drigo and M. Angel Trossero, "WISDOM: A GIS-Based Supply Demand Mapping Tool for Woodfuel Management," Biomass and Bioenergy, Vol. 30, No. 7, 2006, pp. 618-637.

53 M. Mirik and R. J. Ansley, "Comparison of Groundmeasured and Image-Classified Honey Mesquite (Prosopis glandulosa) Canopy Cover in Texas," Rangeland Ecology & Management, Vol. 65, No. 1, 2012, pp. 85-95.

54 R. J. Ansley, M. Mirik and M. J. Castellano, "Structural Biomass Partitioning in Regrowth and Undisturbed Mesquite (Prosopis glandulosa): Implications for Bioenergy Uses," Global Change Biology Bioenergy, Vol. 2, No. 1, 2010, pp. 26-36.

55 E. Strand, A. Smith, S. Bunting, L. Vierling, D. Hann and P. Gessler, "Wavelet Estimation of Plant Spatial Patterns in Multitemporal Aerial Photography," International Journal of Remote Sensing, Vol. 27, No. 10, 2006, pp. 2049- 2054.

56 E. N. Chidumayo, "Above-Ground Woody Biomass Structure and Productivity in a Zambezian Woodland," Forest Ecology and Management, Vol. 36, No. 1, 1990, pp. 33-46.

57 A. Lufafa, I. Diédhiou, N. A. S. Ndiaye, M. Séné, F. Kizito, R. P. Dick and J. S. Noller, "Allometric Relationships and Peak-Season Community Biomass Stocks of Native Shrubs in Senegal's Peanut Basin," Journal of Arid Environments, Vol. 73, No. 3, 2009, pp. 260-266.

58 B. K. Northup, S. F. Zitzer, S. Archer, C. R. McMurtry and T. W. Boutton, "Above-Ground Biomass and Carbon and Nitrogen Content of Woody Species in a Subtropical Thornscrub Parkland," Journal of Arid Environments, Vol. 62, No. 1, 2005, pp. 23-43.

59 L. F. Ohmann, D. F. Grigal and R. B. Brander, "Biomass Estimation for Five Shrubs from Northeastern Minnesota," Research Paper NC-133, US Department of Agriculture, Forest Service, North Central Forest Experiment Station, St. Paul, 1976.

60 A. Rosenschein, T. Tietema and D. O. Hall, "Biomass Measurement and Monitoring of Trees and Shrubs in a Semi-Arid Region of Central Kenya," Journal of Arid Environments, Vol. 42, No. 2, 1999, pp. 97-116.

61 T. Tietema, "Biomass Determination of Fuelwood Trees and Bushes of Botswana, Southern Africa," Forest Ecol- ogy and Management, Vol. 60, No. 3-4, 1993, pp. 257- 269.

CHAPTER 9

Comparison between remote sensing and a dynamic vegetation model for estimating terrestrial primary production of Africa

Jonas Ardö

Department of Physical Geography and Ecosystem Science,
Lund University

BACKGROUND

Africa is an important part of the global carbon cycle. It is also a continent facing potential problems due to increasing resource demand in combination with climate change-induced changes in resource supply. Quantifying the pools and fluxes constituting the terrestrial African carbon cycle is a challenge, because of uncertainties in meteorological driver data, lack of validation data, and potentially uncertain representation of important processes in major ecosystems. In this paper, terrestrial primary production estimates derived from remote sensing and a dynamic vegetation model are compared and quantified for major African land cover types.

RESULTS

Continental gross primary production estimates derived from remote sensing were higher than corresponding estimates derived from a dynamic vegetation model. However, estimates of continental net primary production from remote sensing were lower than corresponding estimates from the dynamic vegetation model. Variation was found among land cover classes, and the largest differences in gross primary production were found in the evergreen broadleaf forest. Average carbon use efficiency (NPP/GPP) was 0.58 for the vegetation model and 0.46 for the remote sensing method. Validation versus in situ data of aboveground net primary production revealed significant positive relationships for both methods. A combination of the remote sensing method with the dynamic vegetation model did not strongly affect this relationship.

CONCLUSION

Observed significant differences in estimated vegetation productivity may have several causes, including model design and temperature sensitivity. Differences in carbon use efficiency reflect underlying model assumptions. Integrating the realistic process representation of dynamic vegetation models with the high resolution observational strength of remote sensing may support realistic estimation of components of the carbon cycle and enhance resource monitoring, providing suitable validation data is available.

KEYWORDS

Africa MOD17 NPP GPP LPJ-GUESS Resource assessment Carbon cycle

1. BACKGROUND

Estimates of photosynthetic assimilation and respiration of carbon (C), along with fluxes from fires and other ecosystem disturbances, form the basis for quantifying the terrestrial carbon balance. Carbon balance studies and the understanding of factors controlling carbon fluxes, as well as their spatial and temporal variation, are key features of recent research relating to climate change [1-5].

Gross primary production (GPP) is the capacity of the vegetation to capture carbon and energy during photosynthesis. Net primary production (NPP) is the net carbon stored after subtracting the autotrophic plant respiration (Ra) from GPP. Ra is commonly divided into growth respiration, often assumed to be a fixed proportion of NPP, and maintenance respiration, which is dependent on temperature [6] and nitrogen content [7]. The influence of water availability and soil moisture (in addition to temperature) on heterotrophic respiration (Rh) in drier areas is well known [8,9], but recently a drought-induced decline in Ra has been shown for trees in Amazonas [10].

While some of the annual NPP in an ecosystem may be lost by episodic events like fire, the remainder constitutes essential ecosystem services [11,12] such as fuel, food, feed, fiber and construction materials [13]. As human access to these resources and services is crucial, monitoring of primary production is important in assessing the variability of resource availability and in evaluating the potential impact of climate change on plant production [14,15] and resource availability [16].

Recent work on the carbon budget of Africa reports that the continent is a small sink of carbon (-0.61 ± 0.58 Pg C yr^{-1}) (1 Pg $= 10^{15}$ g) [17] and stresses the importance of Africa in the global carbon cycle, despite considerable uncertainty. African ecosystems contribute about 20% of global NPP, 20% of heterotrophic respiration [18] and 20% of global land use CO_2 emissions [19]. The atmospheric input from fossil fuel in Africa is low [20], but fire emissions are estimated to form about 40% of the global total, mostly from savanna burning [19,21]. Ciais *et al.* [19] used model analysis to report that GPP was more important than total ecosystem respiration (TER) in determining African net biome productivity.

Annual variability is larger for GPP than for TER and is mainly driven by rainfall [19,22], whereas TER is more dependent on temperature [23]. Jung *et al.* reported a mean GPP for Africa of 24.3 Pg ±2.9 C yr^{-1} for the period 1982–2008 [24]. Valentini *et al.*recently reported significant variability (for the period 1990–2009) in both GPP, ranging from 20.61 to 40.91 [Pg C yr^{-1}] with a mean of 28.16, and NPP, ranging from 9.25 to 20.46 [Pg C yr^{-1}] with a mean of 13.27 [17]. Much of the interannual variability of the global carbon cycle can be derived from the African continent [25], so it is important to quantify these fluxes from a carbon budget perspective as well as from a resource mapping perspective. Recent studies of potential climate change implications also stress the importance of related studies in Africa [17,19,25,26].

Remote sensing-based models, applying the concept of light use efficiency (LUE), and dynamic vegetation models (DVM) are two common approaches for assessing carbon budgets and for monitoring resources. Both methodologies can provide spatially and temporally distributed measures of GPP, NPP and Ra.

LUE-based models often assume a relatively constant assimilation rate of carbon per unit absorbed photosynthetically active radiation [27,28]. This rate is called the light use efficiency (ε) and is commonly expressed in g C MJ^{-1} APAR (absorbed photosynthetic active radiation). APAR is estimated as the product of incoming PAR and the fraction of absorbed PAR (FAPAR). FAPAR is derived from earth observation data, often with a spatial resolution of around 250–1000 m and weekly to monthly temporal resolution, from sensors such as the Advance Very High Resolution Radiometer (AVHRR), Moderate Resolution Imaging Spectrometer (MODIS) and the Satellite Pour l'Observation de la Terre (SPOT).

Vegetation indices such as the Normalized Difference Vegetation Index (NDVI) and the Enhanced Vegetation Index (EVI) are used to describe and quantify FAPAR, as they do this well [29,30]. Additional environmental constraints on assimilation, such as temperature or water availability (e.g. through soil moisture content, evaporative fraction or vapor pressure deficit), are usually estimated from meteorological data, but may also be derived directly from earth observation data [31]. This reduces dependency on data sources with comparatively low spatial resolution and potential delays in data availability through the need to process data originating from in situ measurements and meteorological reanalysis data sets. Recently suggested developments of LUE models include improved estimation of Ra, incorporation of diffuse radiation [4] and the use of variable LUE based on plant functional types or photosynthetic pathways [28]. LUE may also be determined directly using remote sensing, with a potential to provide improved estimates of the spatial variability of LUE compared to current methods [32,33].

DVMs integrate research from several disciplines, including plant geography, vegetation dynamics, biogeochemistry, plant physiology and biophysics [34]. They often present a more detailed representation of essential processes (photosynthesis, Ra, allocation of carbon, hydrology, etc.) and ecology (population dynamics, mortality, disturbances) when compared to LUE models, but are computationally more demanding. Driven by meteorology, CO_2 concentration and soil data, often with low spatial resolution, and governed by plant functional types, DVMs can be used both as a diagnostic and a prognostic tool, allowing estimates of future responses to climatic change and thereby providing valuable information on forthcoming resource availability, as well as prognoses of future carbon budgets [35]. A wide range of DVMs are available; for an overview see [34,36].

The combination of ecological process models and satellite-derived information can involve several strategies. Plummer [37] identified a remote sensing-based generation of "*spatially comprehensive and temporally repeatable global data sets for use by ecological modellers*" as one of the more central. Verstraeten *et al.* [38] integrated the C-FIX model with soil moisture data derived from an active microwave sensor, and found that soil moisture had an impact on both magnitude and spatial pattern of carbon exchange fluxes. Smith *et al.* [39] investigated the feasibility of two methods (satellite-based estimates of FPAR and stand structure descriptions) to constrain dynamic ecosystem model behavior using data from remote sensing, and concluded the combination to *"...offer a promise as a step towards the development of operational tools..."*.

This study compares and combines the LPJ-GUESS dynamic vegetation model with the earth observation-based LUE model MOD17, both described in more detail below.

The differences between DVMs and LUE models in terms of driver data and utilized concepts can result in differences in estimated vegetation productivity. This study aims to describe and quantify the differences in estimated vegetation productivity for Africa (Figure 1), and also to combine the two methodologies using a simple approach. The study is divided into three tasks:

- Comparing GPP and NPP from MOD17 and LPJ-GUESS (Null hypothesis 1: MOD17 vegetation productivity = LPJ-GUESS vegetation productivity).
- Simple integration of the two methodologies (Null hypothesis 2: NPP estimated by LPJ-GUESS = NPP estimated by the combined approach.)
- Validation versus in situ measurements of vegetation productivity (Null hypothesis 3: Model estimated vegetation productivity = in situ measured vegetation productivity).

Can knowledge that promotes reliable methods for estimation of GPP and NPP in Africa be acquired through comparison and integration of LPJ-GUESS and MOD17? Does the combination of the observational strength of high spatial and temporal resolution earth observation data with the more realistic process representation of the DVM improve estimates of net primary productivity? The central findings of this study, produced while trying to answer the questions above, included general agreement regarding estimated vegetation productivity for most land cover classes except for the evergreen broadleaf forest, a moderate relationship when comparing model-estimated vegetation productivity versus in situ data, and potential benefits through a simple integration of the two model approaches.

2. RESULTS

2.1 GPP and NPP for Africa

Mean annual GPP (2000–2010) for Africa was 22.6 ± 0.45 (± 1 standard deviation) Pg (range 21.4-23.0) for MOD17 versus 20.9 ± 0.50 Pg for LPJ-GUESS (range 20.2-21.6) (Figure 2a). Mean annual NPP (2000–2010) for Africa was 10.3 ± 0.35 Pg for MOD17 (range 9.4-10.6) versus 12.2 ± 0.31

Pg for LPJ-GUESS (range 11.7-12-6) (Figure 2a). Total $NPP_{Combined}$ was 13.3 Pg. There was a weak linear relationship ($r^2 = 0.39$) between the annual sums of GPP for MOD17 and LPJ-GUESS (Figure 2b); removing the outlier year 2005 increased r^2 to 0.55. A similar relationship was found for NPP ($r^2 = 0.43$) (Figure 2c). MOD17 GPP was systematically higher than LPJ-GUESS GPP, but the opposite applied for NPP.

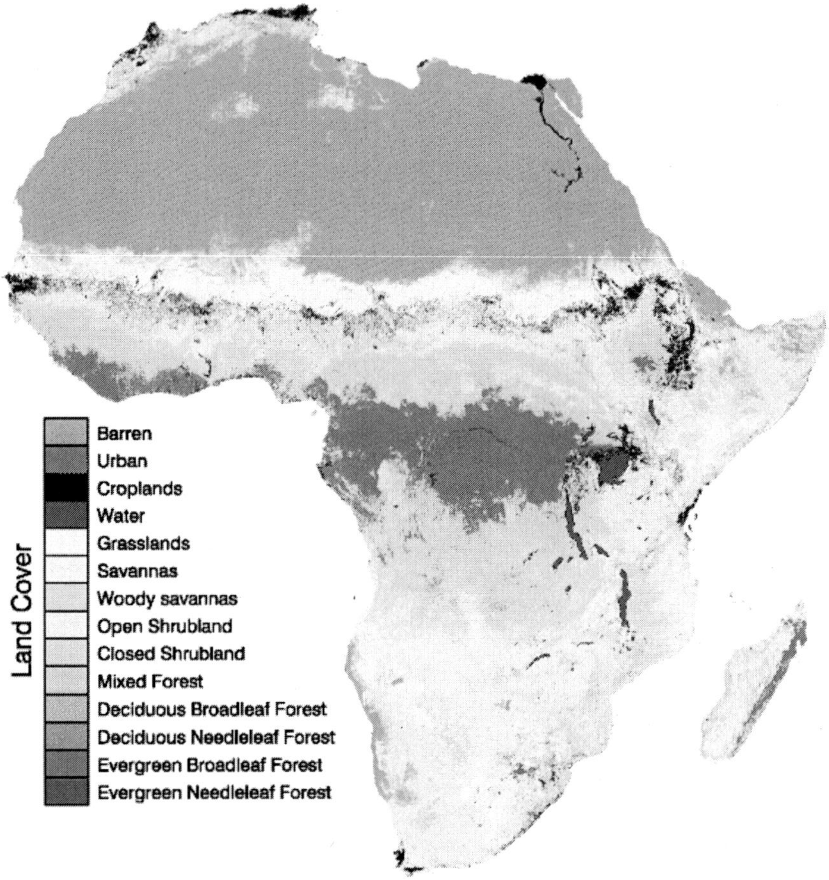

Figure 1 Study area. Land cover of Africa from MODIS (MOD12Q1). This data was used for looking up the correct biome parameters used in MOD17 from the Biome Property Look-Up Table (BPLUT), and describes the land cover classes used in analysis and their spatial distribution.

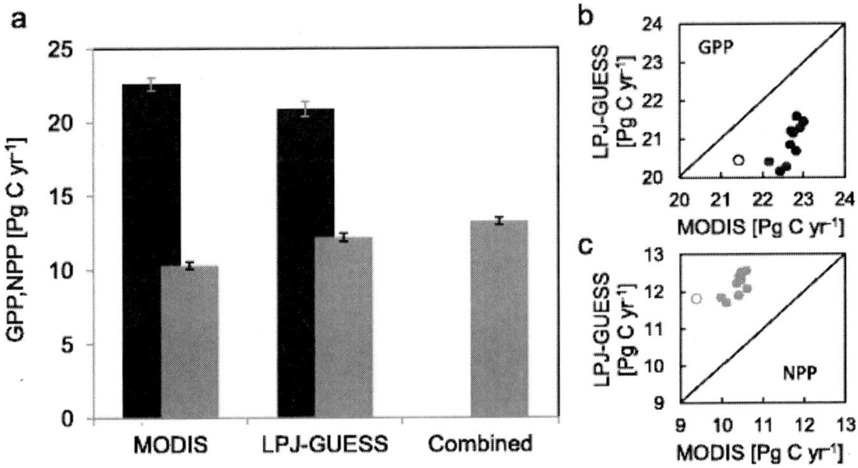

Figure 2 GPP and NPP for Africa. (a) mean GPP (black) and NPP (grey) from MOD17 and from the LPJ-GUESS model (average for the period 2000–2010), and mean $NPP_{Combined}$. Error bars illustrate ± standard deviation. GPP and NPP differ significantly (LPJ-GUESS vs MOD17, t-test, $p < 0.01$), **(b)** Annual (2000–2010) MOD17 and LPJ-GUESS GPP [Pg C] and **(c)** NPP [Pg C], the open circle in b and c denote year 2005.

The spatial pattern of NPP and GPP were similar for both methods but with some notable exceptions (Figure 3). Mean MOD17 GPP (2.41 kg C m^{-2} yr^{-1}) was, on average, 0.8 kg C m^{-2} yr^{-1} higher (t-test, $p < 0.01$) than LPJ-GUESS GPP (1.61 kg C m^{-2} yr^{-1}) for the evergreen broadleaf forest (EBF) (Figure 4a). This is equivalent to a total GPP for MOD17 exceeding LPJ-GUESS GPP by 2.4 Pg yr^{-1} for the EBF (Figure 4a). GPP of remaining forest types (DBF, DNF, ENF) differed less (<0.07 kg C m^{-2} yr^{-1}) between MOD17 and LPJ-GUESS, and ranged from 1.09 to 1.29 kg C m^{-2} yr^{-1} for MOD17 and from 1.10 to 1.21 kg C m^{-2} yr^{-1} for LPJ-GUESS (Figure 4b). These remaining forest types (DBF, DNF, EBF) have low areal extent and contribute only 2% (0.46 Pg) and 2.1% (0.44 Pg) to total GPP, for MOD17 and LPJ-GUESS, respectively (Figure 4a).

Average (2000–2010) GPP for remaining land cover classes (Wsavanna, Savanna OShrub, CShrub and Grass) differed by less than 0.2 kg C m^{-2} yr^{-1} (Figure 4b), between MOD17 and LPJ-GUESS. These land cover classes, all with large areal extent, contribute a large proportion of total continental GPP (63% for MOD17 and 71% for LPJ-GUESS). Woody savannas have the second highest GPP per area after the evergreen broadleaf forest (2.41 kg C m^{-2} yr^{-1}), averaging 1.42 kg C m^{-2} $yr^{-1}$for MOD17 and 1.32 kg C m^{-2} yr^{-1} for LPJ-GUESS.

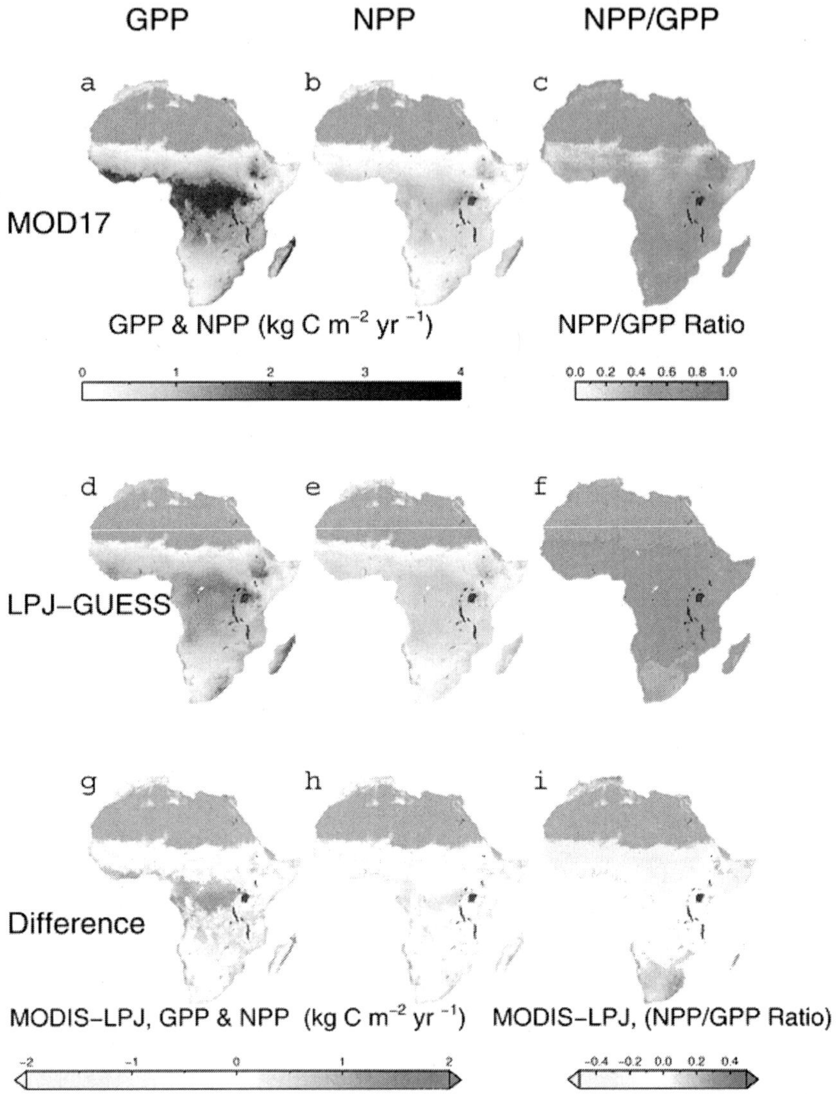

Figure 3 GPP, NPP and the NPP/GPP ratio for MOD17 and for LPJ-GUESS. Mean (2000–2010) **(a)** GPP and **(b)** NPP (both in kg C m^{-2} yr^{-1}) for MOD17 and LPJ-GUESS **(d, e)**. Mean (2000–2010) NPP/GPP ratio for MOD17 **(c)** and LPJ-GUESS **(f)**. Water is blue, urban areas are black, and barren areas are grey). Difference (MOD17-LPJ GUESS) in GPP **(g)**, NPP **(h)** and NPP/GPP ratio **(i)**.

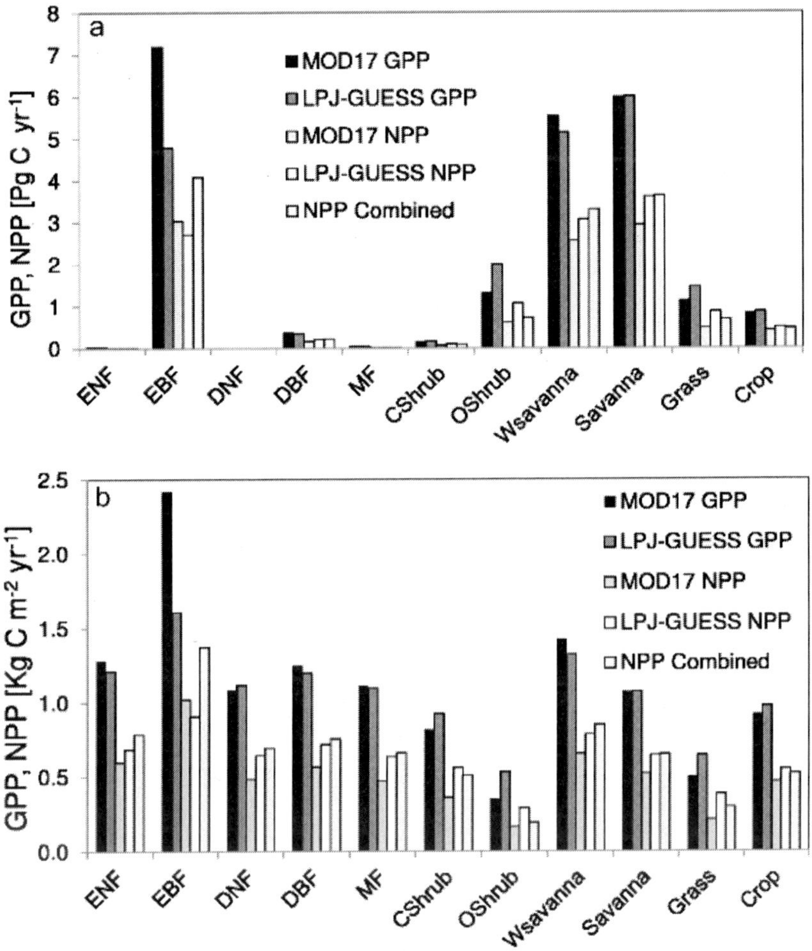

Figure 4 GPP and NPP per land cover class. (a) Totaled MOD17 and LPJ-GUESS GPP and NPP per land cover class, where GPP differs significantly (t-test $p < 0.01$) for all land cover types except for mixed forest and savannas. NPP differs significantly (t-test $p < 0.01$) for all land cover types. **(b)** Mean GPP and NPP per land cover class and unit area. Yellow bars denote $NPP_{Combined}$ (MOD17 GPP – Ra from LPJ-GUESS).

The temporal variability of each model is smaller than the differences between the models; both show a dip in 2005, but this is larger for MOD17 (Figure 5a). On average, MOD17 GPP for Africa was 1.7 Pg yr^{-1} higher than LPJ-GUESS GPP, while average MOD17 NPP was 1.9 Pg yr^{-1} lower than average LPJ-GUESS NPP. These differences were smallest for GPP (0.97 Pg) in 2005 and largest for NPP (−2.4 Pg) in 2005 (Figure 5b).

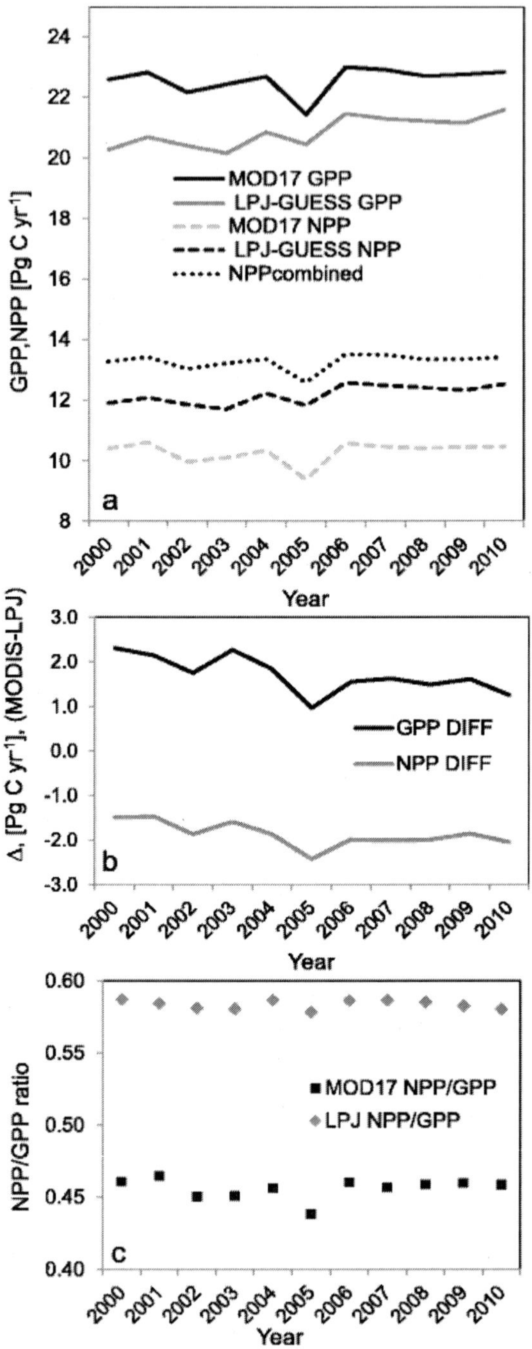

Figure 5 Time series of vegetation productivity. (a) Annual GPP and NPP for MOD17, LPJ-GUESS and the combined approach for the period 2000–2010, **(b)** differences (MOD17-LPJ-GUESS) and **(c)** the NPP/GPP ratio.

The average annual (2000–2010) NPP/GPP ratio was 0.456 (range 0.438-0.465) for MOD17 and 0.583 (range 0.578-0.587) for LPJ-GUESS (Figure 5c). For MOD17 the ratio among the land cover classes ranged from 0.35 (Grasslands) to 0.47 (Savannas), and for LPJ-GUESS from 0.55 (Woody Savanna) to 0.62 (Savannas). The NPP/GPP ratio for EBF was 0.42 for MOD17 and 0.56 for LPJ-GUESS. The temporal variability of the NPP/GPP ratio was small, especially for LPJ-GUESS and the lowest ratio for both methods occurred in 2005 (Figure 5c). Parts of southern Africa have a distinctly lower NPP/GPP ratio for LPJ-GUESS (Figure 3f). On average MOD17 assumed Ra to be about 79% (0.46/0.58) of LPJ-GUESS Ra.

2.2 MOD17 quality control (QC) data

QC values quantify the proportion of growing days (%) during the growing season that use artificially filled FPAR&LAI, so higher QC values = lower quality. High QC values are reached in the coastal areas of western Africa (QC >70%), in the Congo basin, and along a narrow band just south of the Sahara Desert (Figure 6), due to high frequency of clouds and aerosols. Southern Africa and other drier regions with less cloud have lower QC (assuming more reliable annual GPP and NPP) compared to the tropical forest areas and parts of the Ethiopian Highlands. Average QC values per land cover classes are 24% (OShrub), 32% (Crop), 33% (Savanna and Grass), 43% (Wsavanna), 36-49% (all forest types except EBF) and 65% (EBF) (Figure 6). The overall mean QC when all land cover classes are included is 39.5%.

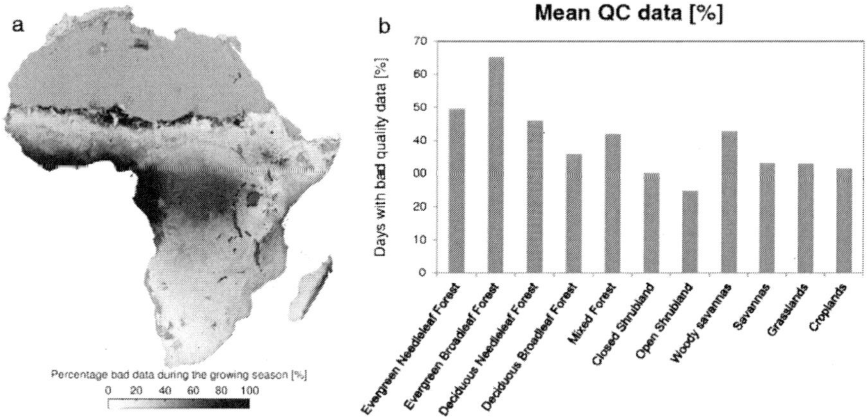

Figure 6 MODIS quality control data. (a) MOD17 QC data describing the percentage of days during the growing season with poor-quality data [%, average for 2000–2010] for Africa, **(b)** QC per land cover class.

2.3 Comparison between in situ-collected NPP and model-estimated NPP

Average MOD17 NPP (2000–2010) is strongly correlated with in situ ANPP (r = 0.80, RMSE = 153 g) (Figure 7a). Using MOD17 NPP and in situ ANPP for Sudan collected the same year reduces the linear correlation (r = 0.64, RMSE = 145 g, Figure 7b). $NPP_{Combined}$ are moderately correlated compared with in situ-collected ANPP (r = 0.64. RMSE = 176 g) for the same year. All MOD17 NPP estimates are systematically higher than the in situ data, which may partly be explained by the in situ data only representing aboveground biomass.

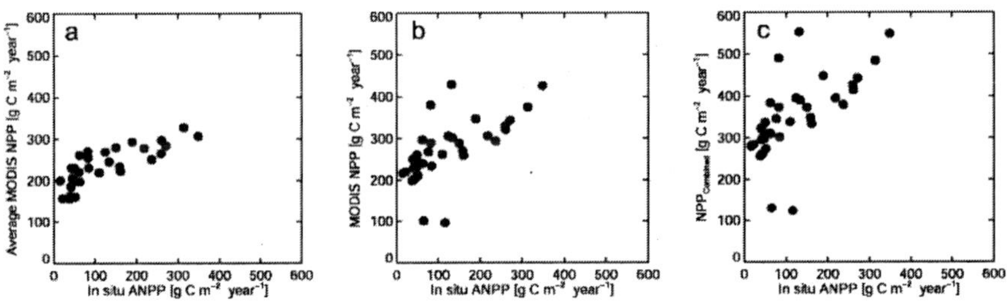

Figure 7 Validation versus in situ data from Sudan. NPP estimates versus field-based validation data of aboveground NPP (ANPP) from Sudan. **(a)** Average (2000–2010) MOD17 NPP (n = 31, r = 0.80, RMSE = 153 g), **(b)** MOD17 NPP for the same year (r = 0.64, RMSE = 145 g, n = 35), **(c)** $NPP_{Combined}$ for the same year (r = 0.64, RMSE = 176 g, n = 35).

The NPP Multi-biome data set [40] shows a strong linear relationship for LPJ-GUESS (r = 0.90, RMSE = 207 g) and a weaker linear relationship for MOD17 (r = 0.21, RMSE = 141 g) and $NPP_{Combined}$ (Figure 8), using the 2000–2010 averages. Note that Figures 7 and 8compare in situ collected aboveground NPP with total NPP (from MOD17 and LPJ-GUESS), and this influences the relationships illustrated.

NPP Combined are illustrated in Figure 9, with a more detailed comparison with LPJ-GUESS NPP for areas centered on the Ethiopian Highlands and the Congo Basin (Figure 10). The effect of the increased spatial resolution (1 × 1 km) of MOD17 is visible, but the 0.5 × 0.5 degree pattern originating from LPJ-GUESS still remains for some regions. Figure 10c and f illustrate the relationship between LPJ-GUESS NPP and $NPP_{Combined}$ for the two subareas.

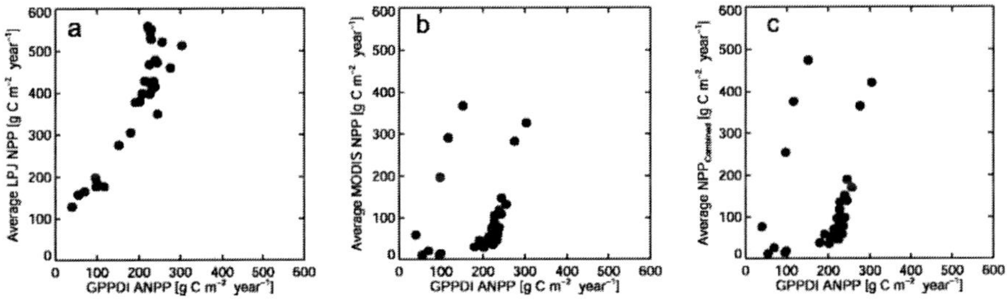

Figure 8 Validation versus NPP Multi-Biome: Global Primary Production Data Initiative (GPPDI) above ground NPP (ANPP). (a) Average (2000–2010) LPJ-GUESS NPP vs GPPDI ($r = 0.90$, RMSE $=207$ g), **(b)** Average (2000–2010) MOD17 NPP vs GPPDI ($r = 0.21$, RMSE $=141$ g) and **(c)** Average (2000–2010) $NPP_{Combined}$ vs GPPDI ($r = 0.21$, RMSE $= 142$ g), $n = 35$.

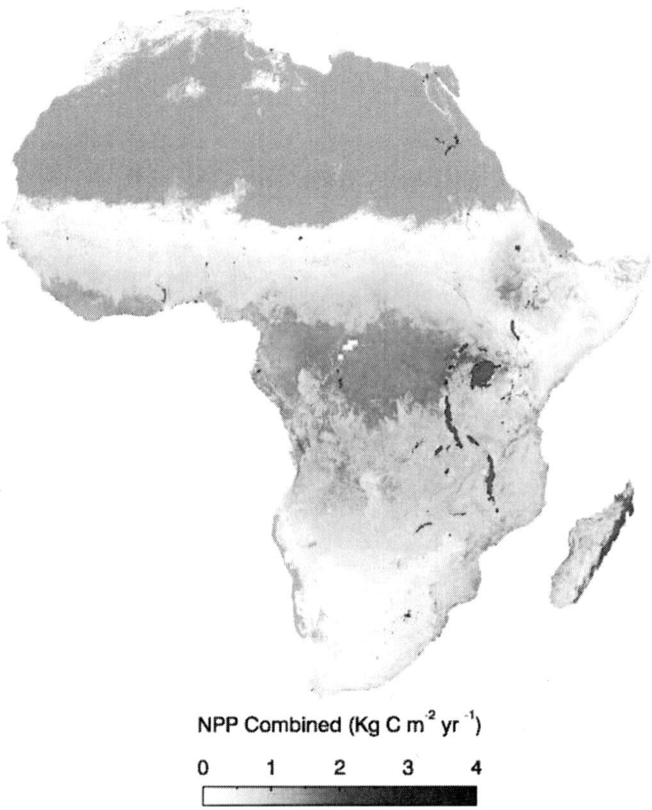

Figure 9 Integrated NPP. $NPP_{Combined}$, produced by MOD17 GPP x NPP/GPP ratio from LPJ-GUESS, average for the 2000–2010 period.

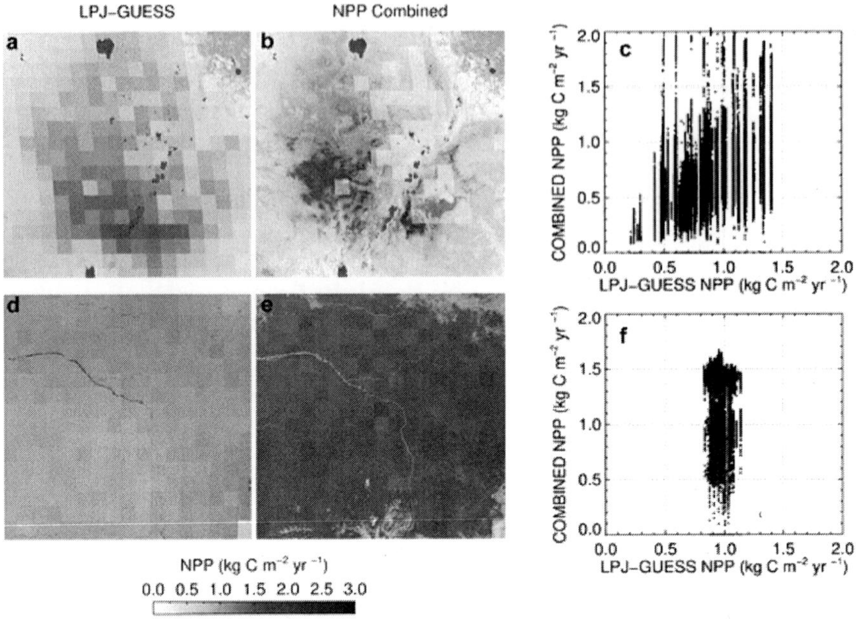

Figure 10 Dynamic vegetation model NPP vs NPP $_{\text{Combined}}$**.** NPP from **(a)** LPJ-GUESS and **(b)** $NPP_{Combined}$ for a 1000 x 1000 km area in the Ethiopian Highlands and **(c)** a scatter plot of LPJ-GUESS NPP vs $NPP_{Combined.}$ **(d-f)** show the same as **(a-c)** bur for a 1000 x 1000 km are in the Congo Basin. Urban areas are red, water is blue, and barren areas are grey. $NPP_{Combined}$ is calculated from MO17 GPP and LPJ-GUESS Ra.

3. DISCUSSION

Observed statistically significant differences in primary production between MOD17 and LPJ-GUESS support rejection of hypothesis 1 and exclude the possibility of both methods being fully correct (Figure 2). For the entire continent, MOD17 GPP exceeds LPJ-GUESS GPP by 1.7 Pg yr^{-1} on average for the study period (2000–2010). The differences are consistent over the study period (Figures 2 and 5) and can mainly be explained by the higher MOD17 GPP for the evergreen broadleaf forest (Figure 4). GPP of large land cover classes such as grasslands, savannas and woody savannas vary less. Both GPP and NPP reported here (Figure 2) are within the ranges shown in earlier results for Africa, even if the ranges are wide [17,24,41].

Average MOD17 NPP was 1.9 Pg yr^{-1} less than LPJ-GUESS NPP, which can largely be explained by a lower NPP/GPP ratio for MOD17, indicating substantially higher autotrophic respiration than LPJ-GUESS (Figures 3 and 5c). A similar result was reported from a recent study covering northern Eurasia, where a spatial correlation of 0.63 was found for mean annual GPP (2000–2009) derived from LPJG (a slightly modified version of LPJ-GUESS including methane from wetlands) versus MOD17 GPP [42]. LPJG explained about 40% of the variability found in the MOD17 product. Reported LPJG GPP was about 40% lower than MOD17 GPP, which may indicate that the LPJ-GUESS vs MOD17 GPP differences are not limited to Africa or warmer climates.

The higher proportion of GPP lost as autotrophic respiration by MOD17 has been attributed to an excessive temperature sensitivity of the MOD17 algorithm [43,44]. However, Clark *et al.* showed decreased increment in tropical trees due to high temperatures, and reported strong correlation between temperature-induced tree growth patterns and tropical CO_2 fluxes. They suggested a "*remarkable sensitivity of the net carbon balance of tropical rain forests to increasing temperature*" [45], which is also supported by other studies [46]. Mahli *et al.* reported NPP ranging from 1.0 to 1.44 kg C m^{-2} yr^{-1}, based on in situ measurements in Amazonian rainforests, close to the mean EBF NPP of MODIS (1.02 kg C m^{-2} yr^{-1}) and LPJ-GUESS (0.91 kg C m^{-2} yr^{-1}) found here (Figure 4b). Corresponding Amazonian carbon use efficiencies (NPP/GPP) ranged from 0.32 to 0.49 [47], overlapping well with the MOD17 NPP/GPP ratio of 0.42 found here for the evergreen broadleaf forest, but lower than the 0.56 of LPJ-GUESS.

For large areas of Africa, the NPP/GPP ratio for MOD17 was lower than for LPJ-GUESS (Figure 3), indicating a higher autotrophic respiration rate for MOD17. Southern Africa, Morocco & Northern Tunisia and parts of Ethiopia are exceptions to this, with lower NPP/GPP ratio for LPJ-GUESS.

In a global study, Ahlström reported that differences in meteorological forcing data used by LPJ-GUESS and MOD17 had small effects on estimated vegetation productivity [48]. However, Traore *et al.* suggested that the uncertainty in the ORCHIDEE model is strongly related to the meteorological forcing data in regions with sparse weather station data [49], something potentially affecting all models utilizing driver data derived from weather station data. From this study, no conclusions can be drawn on what determines the spatial pattern and observed differences in the NPP/GPP ratio among land cover classes, but effects of model formulation such as the temperature sensitivity and/or propertires of plant functional types (LPJ-GUESS) and biome specific parameters (MOD17) may be contributing factors.

Zhang *et al.* [50] reported a global average MOD17 NPP/GPP ratio of 0.52, higher than the results presented here for Africa (0.46). The MOD17 data used by Zhang *et al.* was driven by meteorological data from the NASA Data Assimilation Office (DAO) which is not fully comparable with later versions of MOD17 using NCEP climate driver data [50]. Amthor [51] suggested 0.35-0.80 as the 'allowable' range for the NPP/GPP ratio (with

0.45-0.60 as a more realistic alternative) and proposed that available data is not sufficient to decide how constrained the NPP/GPP ratio is across species and environments. Valentini *et al.* reported a NPP/GPP ratio ranging from 0.37 to 0.59 when comparing nine DGVMs, with a continental NPP for Africa ranging from 9.25 to 20.46 Pg C $yr^{-1}$and a GPP ranging from 20.61 to 40.91 Pg C yr^{-1}. This illustrates substantial uncertainty in vegetation productivity estimates for Africa, including both magnitudes and the carbon use efficiency (NPP/GPP) [17] in addition to the limited field data (eddy covariance measurements, long term ecological field experiments and similar) available for tropical and subtropical areas [52].

Assuming a global GPP of ~120 Pg, and applying a carbon use efficiency of 0.58 versus 0.46, yields a difference in estimated global NPP of 14.4 Pg (69.6-55.2). Even if these assumptions hardly are applicable globally, 14.4 Pg C 'lost in modelling space' is enough to encourage further investigations and additional collection of calibration & validation data and long-term ecosystem experimental data sets from tropical regions, such as Africa. Integration of different types of methods, such as remote sensing, data-oriented methods and process-oriented models, may help to produce consistent estimates of primary productivity and respired fraction, and increase knowledge about involved ecosystem processes and their drivers.

Validation of model estimates using in situ measurements provides vital information on model performance [6,53,54], even if scale differences, sampling strategies and methodological discrepancies in data collection reduce comparability. Significant positive relationships between estimated NPP versus field data were found for both models (Figures 7 and 8), indicating a general applicability of both models, as shown earlier for MOD17 [54,55] and LPJ-GUESS [56,57]. The significant positive relationships of estimated NPP versus in situ collected NPP suggest that hypothesis 3 cannot be rejected (Figures 7 and 8). A stronger linear relationship between in situ NPP data and model estimates favors LPJ-GUESS (Figure 8) whereas a lower RMSE and no systematic overestimation favor MOD17. Bias and differences arising from comparing NPP with ANPP introduce additional uncertainty, and no definite conclusion can be drawn from the current small data set available, except general significant positive relationships (Figures 7 and 8). The limited spatial distribution of the validation data (Senegal and semi-arid Sudan) limited the representativity, as major biomes such as the evergreen broadleaf forest are missing. A coordinated effort to compile continent-wide in situ data for calibration and validation of methods estimating biomass and NPP could enhance the possibilities for statistically sound and representative evaluation of methods estimating vegetation productivity for Africa.

Integrating MOD17 and LPJ-GUESS by applying the NPP/GPP ratio from the dynamic vegetation model to the observational and high spatial resolution remote sensing model GPP seems reasonable (Figure 10) if we assume a proper process representation in LPJ-GUESS. However, the validation does not support any clear improvement (Figures 7 and 8), even if estimated NPP of MOD17, LPJ-GUESS and $NPP_{Combined}$ differ on a continental scale (Figure 2) and for individual land cover classes (Figure 4). There is also a risk of violation of internal model logic due to differences in model assumptions and formulations when applying the LPJ-GUESS NPP/GPP ratio to MOD17 GPP. Consequently, there is support both for and against rejection of hypothesis 2.

The temporal variability of each method is smaller than the differences between the models. The dry year 2005 [15] yields a clear dip for MOD17 GPP but only a small dip for LPJ-GUESS GPP, whereas the lowest NPP/GPP ratio for both models occurs in 2005 (Figure 5), supporting increased respiration during dry conditions [58]. The NPP/GPP ratio in 2005 for MOD17 was 0.438 versus 0.578 for LPJ-GUESS, a deviation of 3.8% and 0.9% respectively from the 2000–2010 average NPP/GPP ratio. This indicates that MOD17 responds more strongly to the drought in 2005, potentially through higher temperature. In general, the temporal variability is similar, indicating similar forcing and similar response to precipitation and moisture availability, both important drivers of vegetation productivity in drier parts of Africa [22,59].

The evergreen broadleaf forest has the lowest satellite data reliability (Figure 6) among all land cover classes, partly due to frequent cloud cover [60]. The large proportion (QC = 65%) of FPAR data originating from MOD15 and used in MOD17 that is replaced by interpolated values may impact the GPP estimation [54] and increase the uncertainty of estimated GPP. Areas affected by frequent cloud cover, such as parts of the evergreen broadleaf forest, may then show less reliable estimates of vegetation productivity using MOD17 (or any method based on optical remote sensing). All land cover classes are affected by this, as most areas have QC values > 30%, and the overall mean is 39.5%, indicating a need for effective gap-filling methods [54,61].

Estimated global median GPP for the tropical forest, by Beer *et al.* [59] of 2.34 kg C m^{-2} yr^{-1} (median of seven different up-scaling schemes) is close to the 2.41 kg C m^{-2} yr^{-1}estimated by MOD17 (for EBF) but clearly exceeds the 1.61 kg C m^{-2} yr^{-1} estimated by LPJ-GUESS (Figures 3 and 4). Fisher *et al.* [62] estimated average GPP of the African tropical forest to range from about 1.4 to 4.0 kg C m^{-2} yr^{-1}, indicating large variability among applied global dynamic vegetation models. Without in situ validation data, the absolute magnitudes of plant productivity is difficult to evaluate, and focus is often on interannual variability related to climatic drivers [41,62].

The higher spatial resolution gained through using observational data such as MOD17 enables estimates of driver variables such as temperature, vapor pressure deficit [63] and incoming PAR [64] with high spatial and temporal resolution. This may reduce dependency on climate data sets like NCEP and CRU, facilitating high resolution estimates of vegetation productivity, especially in areas with low density of meteorological observations [62,65]. Using observational data on spatial distribution of GPP and NPP within LPJ-GUESS grid cells could increase spatial information content while keeping LPJ-GUESS within grid cell integrity (e.g. sums of GPP and NPP). From a local to regional resource monitoring perspective [16], earth observation provides additional useful spatial and temporal resolution (Figure 10), while regions with frequent cloud cover reduce the possibilities for robust continent-wide monitoring of plant productivity in Africa.

4. CONCLUSION

The results from this study suggest significant differences in (1.7 Pg C yr^{-1}) between estimated continental GPP from MOD17 and from LPJ-GUESS, mainly originating from higher MOD17 GPP for the evergreen broadleaf forest biome. The causes of this difference are not determined, but reduced availability of cloud-free earth observation data may cause uncertainties in the MOD17 estimates.

Substantial differences in carbon use efficiency (NPP/GPP ratio) result in continental NPP from LPJ-GUESS exceeding (1.9 Pg C yr^{-1}) NPP from MOD17, even if extensive land cover classes such as Savannas and Cropland show reasonable similarities in estimated GPP and NPP produced by both models.

Merging MOD17 GPP with the NPP/GPP ratio from LPJ-GUESS could help combine the high spatial resolution of the remote sensing-based MOD17 model with the more process-oriented LPJ-GUESS model. Utilization of preferred elements originating from different modelling schemes or representing different spatial & temporal regions or resolution may be beneficial in resource assessment and carbon cycle studies.

Unfortunately, as long as availability and accessibility of local meteorological data and in situ validation data (eddy covariance measurements, long-term ecological field experiments and similar) remain low, we can expect the quality and representativity of vegetation productivity estimates for Africa to remain hard to determine. Based on current available data may both methods be considered to produce plausible estimates of vegetation productivity for Africa.

5. METHODS

5.1 Study area

This study covers Africa (Figure 1) with an area of approximately 30 million km^2, including savannas (Savanna, 5.6 million km^2), woody savannas (WSavanna, 3.9 million km^2), open shrublands (OShrub, 3.7 million km^2) evergreen broadleaf forest (EBF, 3.0 million km^2), grassland (Grass, 2.2 million km^2), croplands (Crop, 0.89 million km^2), and closed shrublands (CShrub, 0.18 million km^2). Other forest types (Evergreen Needleleaf Forest (ENF), Deciduous Needleleaf Forest (DLF), Deciduous Broadleaf Forest (DBF) and Mixed Forest (MF)) cover a total of 0.37 million km^2. Other land cover classes, not considered here as MOD17 does not calculate GPP and NPP for them, include barren and sparsely vegetated areas (9.8 million km^2), water (0.25 million km^2), and urban & built up areas (53600 km^2) (Figure 1).

5.2 LPJ-GUESS

LPJ-GUESS is an "object oriented, modular framework for modelling the dynamics of ecosystem structure and functioning at scales from the patch to the globe, and at varying levels of process detail" [66]. The framework incorporates process-based representations of plant physiology and ecosystem biogeochemistry. The model is driven by atmospheric CO_2 concentration, temperature, precipitation, radiation, and soil physical properties. Photosynthesis, respiration, stomatal conductance and phenology are simulated using a daily time step. Eleven plant functional types are used to represent vegetation [48]. Model output includes GPP, NPP, respiration, carbon pools and potential vegetation among a range of other possible outputs. LPJ-GUESS performs well when compared to other vegetation models [56] and predicts present day GPP in agreement with observation-based estimates [57]. Details on the LPJ-GUESS model are available in [6,67].

Annual GPP and NPP (kg C m^{-2} year^{-1}), estimated by LPJ-GUESS and with a spatial resolution of 0.5 × 0.5 degrees (longitude, latitude), for the period 2000–2010 were used [48]. The model was forced with monthly precipitation, number of rain-days (days with >1 mm precipitation), incoming short-wave radiation and temperature from the CRU-NCEP (v2.0) dataset. Annual CO_2 concentration was set from atmospheric and ice core measurements as described in [48].

GPP and NPP were resampled to the MOD17 grid (1 km spatial resolution and an equal area Sinusoidal projection). Grid cells without valid MOD17 GPP and NPP (MOD12Q1 land cover barren, water, or urban, Figure 1) were masked out from the LPJ-GUESS data in order to make the data sets comparable (i.e. identical spatial extent, land cover classes and number of grid cells).

5.3 MOD17

MOD17 is based on the LUE concept and consists of two products, MOD17A2 and MOD17A3. MOD17A2 contains both 8-day GPP and 8-day net photosynthesis (PSNnet), whereas MOD17A3 contains annual sums of GPP, NPP and quality (QC) data [15,68].

The MOD17 algorithm calculates daily GPP as:

$$\mathrm{GPP} = \varepsilon_{\max} \times 0.45 \times SW_{rad} \times \mathrm{FAPAR} \times f(\mathrm{VPD}) \times f(T_{\min})$$

where ε_{max} is the maximal, biome-specific light use efficiency [g C MJ^{-1}], SW*rad* is incoming short-wave radiation (assuming 45% to be PAR), FAPAR is the fraction of absorbed PAR, f(VPD) and $f(T_{min})$ are linear scalars reducing GPP due to water and temperature stress.

MOD17 GPP uses National Center for Environmental Prediction-Department of Energy (NCEP-DOE) reanalysis II data for Tmin, VPD and SWrad [69,70]. The NCEP-DOE reanalysis II data is interpolated from the original resolution of approximately 1.9° latitude × 1.9° longitude to 1 × 1 km grid cells [60]. FAPAR in the MOD17 GPP algorithm is derived from the 8-day MOD15A2 1 km product, and the 1 km University of Maryland (UMD) land cover classification scheme in the MOD12Q1 product (Figure 1) is used to map biome-specific physiological parameters (ε_{max}, minimum temperature, VPD etc.) from the Biome Property Look-Up Table (BPLUT). NPP is calculated annually:

$$NPP = \sum_{i=1}^{365} PsnNet - (R_{mo} + R_g),$$

where PsnNet = GPP-R_{ml}-R_{mr}. The maintenance respiration by leaves (R_{ml}) and fine roots (R_{mr}) respectively are calculated daily. R_{mo} is the annual maintenance respiration by all other living parts except leaves and fine roots, R_g is the annual growth respiration.

A recent evaluation of MOD17 GPP for Africa, based on eddy covariance data, concluded that MOD17A2 underestimated GPP by a mean difference of 0.70 g C m^{-2} day^{-1} but seasonality was captured well [54]. The underestimation was larger for drier sites, and differences between driver data (climatology from NCEP/DOE II and FAPAR from MOD15) and field observations of the same variables were found. Several studies have pointed out problems at drier sites [71-73] and suggest that prescribed MOD17A2 ε_{max} causes underestimation of MOD17A2 GPP [54,71,73]. Plummer concluded that the global performance of the MOD17 GPP is good under unstressed conditions, but suggested adaption of ε_{max} to better account for spatial and temporal within-biome variation [74]. MOD17 PsnNet and MOD17 NPP have also been reported to underestimate NPP when compared to field-measured aboveground NPP in Senegal [75].

MOD17A3 (UM Collection 5) annual totals of GPP and NPP for the years 2000–2010 were downloaded from ftp.ntsg.umt.edu and mosaicked for Africa at a 1 × 1 km spatial resolution and an equal area sinusoidal projection. Land cover (MOD12Q1) used by the BPLUT in MOD17 (same resolution and projection as MOD17A3) were downloaded from ftp://ftp.ntsg.umt.edu/.autofs/NTSG_Products/MOD12Q1_FOR_MOD15-17 and used for land cover stratification (Figure 1).

5.4 Simple integration

The mean LPJ-GUESS NPP/GPP ratio for the 2000–2010 period was calculated (average $NPP_{(2000-2010)}$/average $GPP_{(2000-2010)}$) for each 1 × 1 km grid cell and multiplied by the 1 × 1 km MOD17 GPP, resulting in a 1 × 1 km spatial resolution NPP dataset, denoted $NPP_{Combined}$. This simple combination thereby applies the autotrophic respiration calculated from LPJ-GUESS to MOD17 GPP. The ratio of NPP to GPP is sometimes referred to as carbon use efficiency, and it is often assumed to have a constant value ~ 0.5 [76].

5.5 MOD17 QC data

A MOD17 quality control (QC) measure is used to quantify the proportion of growing days (%) during the growing season that use artificially filled FPAR/LAI (originating from the MOD15A2 FAPAR/LAI product) due to cloud cover, to calculate 8-GPP and annual GPP and NPP.

$$QC = (NUg/TOTALg) \times 100$$

where NUg is the number of days during the growing season with unreliable or missing MOD15 LAI inputs, and TOTALg is the total number of days in the growing season [60]. The growing season is defined as all days with Tmin above −8°C, also used as the minimum temperature control on photosynthesis for all biomes [60]. This temperature is only occasionally reached in Africa, and then mainly at higher elevations, so TOTALg = 365 in most cases. The QC data of MOD17A2 is inherited from the MOD15A2 FAPAR/LAI product and totaled to an annual value in MOD17A3 [60]. Average (2000–2010) QC for each land cover class was calculated.

5.6 Validation using in situ data

Scale differences and temporal sampling make evaluation of coarse to moderate spatial resolution remote sensing models and DVMs difficult using in situ measurements of NPP, as they represent distinctly smaller areas. Despite this, two field-based data sets are used for comparison with model estimates to permit validation.

Firstly, 35 sites were available in Sudan with in situ collected aboveground NPP data [77]. The sampling sites were distributed along a north to south precipitation gradient in Northern Kordofan, from approximately 200 mm yr^{-1} in the north to about 600 mm yr^{-1} in the south. Each site was an area of approximately 300 × 300 m, with homogeneous vegetation selected. The data was collected from 2008 to 2010, using nested quadrats with 10 × 10 m quadrats for tree biomass and 1 × 1 m quadrats for the field layer (herbaceous biomass). Aboveground NPP of the field layer was assumed to equal the dry weight of the green herbaceous biomass at the end of the vegetation season. Tree NPP was estimated using allometric equations [78]. On each site, 20 to 24 quadrats were sampled and on most sites only aboveground biomass data was collected; details in [77]. Biomass was assumed to contain 50% C. For each of these 35 sites, MOD17 NPP and $NPP_{Combined}$ for the corresponding grid cells and corresponding sampling year were extracted and compared to the in situ collected data. Average MOD17 NPP for the period 2000 to 2010 was also calculated for each site. Four sites without MOD17 data available for all years in the 2000–2010 period were removed when in situ NPP was compared with average MOD17 NPP. Due to differences in size, and as this in situ NPP data only overlap six different LPJ-GUESS grid cells (0.5 x 0.5 degrees), this data was not compared to LPJ-GUESS NPP.

Secondly, LPJ-GUESS NPP, MOD17 NPP and $NPP_{Combined}$ were compared to NPP data from the Global Primary Production Data Initiative [40,79]. This data was available for 32 0.5° × 0.5° cells in West Africa (Senegal) and constituted aboveground NPP (ANPP) representative of the 1987–1997 period. Even if the time period of data collection does not overlap, this data may be informative regarding the general relationship between model estimates versus in situ estimates of vegetation productivity.

ACKNOWLEDGEMENTS

This work was supported by the Swedish National Space Board. Anders Ahlström, Lund University kindly provided the LPJ-GUESS data, and the University of Montana kindly provided the MOD17 data. Abdelrahman Katir at Agricultural Research Corporation, El Obeid, Sudan, is acknowledged for providing in situ collected NPP data. Two anonymous reviewers provided valuable comments.

COMPETING INTERESTS

The author declares that he has no competing interests.

REFERENCES

1 Schimel D, House J, Hibbard K, Bousquet P, Ciais P, Peylin P, et al. Recent patterns and mechanisms of carbon exchange by terrestrial ecosystems. Nature. 2001;414:169–72.

2 Piao S, Ciais P, Friedlingstein P, Peylin P, Reichstein M, Luyssaert S, et al. Net carbon dioxide losses of northern ecosystems in response to autumn warming. Nature. 2008;451:49–52.

3 Lewis SL, Lopez-Gonzalez G, Sonke B, Affum-Baffoe K, Baker TR, Ojo LO, et al. Increasing carbon storage in intact African tropical forests. Nature. 2009;457:1003–6.

4 Mercado LM, Bellouin N, Sitch S, Boucher O, Huntingford C, Wild M, et al. Impact of changes in diffuse radiation on the global land carbon sink. Nature. 2009;458:1014–7.

5 Ballantyne AP, Alden CB, Miller JB, Tans PP, White JWC. Increase in observed net carbon dioxide uptake by land and oceans during the past 50 years. Nature. 2012;488:70–3.

6 Sitch S, Smith B, Prentice IC, Arneth A, Bondeau A, Cramer W, et al. Evaluation of ecosystem dynamics, plant geography and terrestrial carbon cycling in the LPJ dynamic global vegetation model. Global Change Biol. 2003;9:161–85.

7 Ryan MG. Effects of climate change on plant respiration. Ecol Appl. 1991;1:157–67.

8 Orchard VA, Cook FJ. Relationship between soil respiration and soil moisture. Soil Biol Biochem. 1983;15:447–53.

9 Makhado RA, Scholes RJ. Determinants of soil respiration in a semi-arid savanna ecosystem, Kruger National Park, South Africa. Koedoe [online]. 2011;53:n.1. 00-00. ISSN 0075-6458.

10 Doughty CE, Metcalfe DB, Girardin CAJ, Amezquita FF, Cabrera DG, Huasco WH, et al. Drought impact on forest carbon dynamics and fluxes in Amazonia. Nature. 2015;519:78–82.

11 Schröter D, Cramer W, Leemans R, Prentice IC, Araújo MB, Arnell NW, et al. Ecosystem service supply and vulnerability to global change in Europe. Science. 2005;310:1333–7.

12 Harfoot MBJ, Newbold T, Tittensor DP, Emmott S, Hutton J, Lyutsarev V, et al. Emergent global patterns of ecosystem structure and function from a mechanistic general ecosystem model. PLoS Biol. 2014; 12:e1001841.

13 Richmond A, Kaufmann RK, Myneni RB. Valuing ecosystem services: a shadow price for net primary production. Ecol Econ. 2007;64:454–62.

14 Schwalm CR, Williams CA, Schaefer K. Carbon consequences of global hydrologic change, 1948–2009. J Geophysical Res: Biogeosciences. 2011;116:G03042. doi:10.1029/2011JG001674.

15 Zhao M, Running SW. Drought-induced reduction in global terrestrial Net primary production from 2000 through 2009. Science. 2010;329:940–3.

16 Abdi A, Seaquist J, Eklundh L, Tenenbaum D, Ardö J. The supply and demand of net primary production in the Sahel. Environ Res Lett. 2014;9:1–11.

17 Valentini R, Arneth A, Bombelli A, Castaldi S, Gatti RC, Chevallier F, et al. A full greenhouse gases budget of Africa: synthesis, uncertainties, and vulnerabilities. Biogeosciences. 2014;11:381–407.

18 Williams CA. Integration of Remote Sensing and Modeling to Understand Carbon Fluxes and Climate Interactions in Africa. In: Ecosystem Function in Savannas. Boca Raton: CRC Press; 2010. p. 327–45.

19 Ciais P, Bombelli A, Williams M, Piao SL, Chave J, Ryan CM, et al. The carbon balance of Africa: synthesis of recent research studies. Philos T R Soc A. 2011;369:2038–57.

20 Canadell JG, Raupach MR, Houghton RA. Anthropogenic CO_2 emissions in Africa. Biogeosciences. 2009;6:463–8.

21 Roberts G, Wooster MJ, Lagoudakis E. Annual and diurnal african biomass burning temporal dynamics. Biogeosciences. 6: 849-866.

22 Hickler T, Eklundh L, Seaquist JW, Smith B, Ardö J, Olsson L, et al. Precipitation controls Sahel greening trend. Geophys Res Lett. 2005;32:L21415.

23 Mahecha MD, Reichstein M, Carvalhais N, Lasslop G, Lange H, Seneviratne SI, et al. Global convergence in the temperature sensitivity of respiration at ecosystem level. Science. 2010;329:838–40.

24 Jung M, Reichstein M, Margolis HA, Cescatti A, Richardson AD, Arain MA, et al. Global patterns of land-atmosphere fluxes of carbon dioxide, latent heat, and sensible heat derived from eddy covariance, satellite, and meteorological observations. J Geophysical Res: Biogeosciences 2011, 116:G00J07.

25 Williams CA, Hanan N, Neff J, Scholes R, Berry J, Denning AS, et al. Africa and the global carbon cycle. Carbon Bal Manag. 2007;2:3.

26 Boko M, Niang I, Nyong A, Vogel C, Githeko A, Medany M, et al. Africa. In: Parry ML, Canziani OF, Palutikof JP, Linden PJ, Hanson CE, editors. Climate Change 2007: Impacts, Adaptation and Vulnerability Contribution of Working Group II to the Fourth Assessment Report of the Intergovernmental Panel on Climate Change. Cambridge UK: Cambridge University Press; 2007. p. 433–67.

27 Monteith JL. Solar radiation and productivity in tropical ecosystems. J Appl Ecol. 1972;9:747–66.

28 McCallum I, Wagner W, Schmullius C, Shvidenko A, Obersteiner M, Fritz S, et al. Satellite-based terrestrial production efficiency modeling. Carbon Bal Manag. 2009;4:8.

29 Myneni RB, Williams DL. On the relationship between FAPAR and NDVI. Remote Sens Environ. 1994;49:200–11.

30 Zhang QY, Xiao XM, Braswell B, Linder E, Baret F, Moore B. Estimating light absorption by chlorophyll, leaf and canopy in a deciduous broadleaf forest using MODIS data and a radiative transfer model. Remote Sens Environ. 2005;99:357–71.

31 Sims DA, Rahman AF, Cordova VD, El-Masri BZ, Baldocchi DD, Bolstad PV, et al. A new model of gross primary productivity for North American ecosystems based solely on the enhanced vegetation index and land surface temperature from MODIS. Remote Sens Environ. 2008;112:1633–46.

32 Drolet GG, Middleton EM, Huemmrich KF, Hall FG, Amiro BD, Barr AG, et al. Regional mapping of gross light-use efficiency using MODIS spectral indices. Remote Sens Environ. 2008;112:3064–78.

33 Garbulsky MF, Filella I, Verger A, Peñuelas J. Photosynthetic light use efficiency from satellite sensors: from global to Mediterranean vegetation. Environ Exp Bot. 2014;103:3–11.

34 Prentice IC, Bondeau A, Cramer W, Harrison S, Hickler T, Lucht W, et al. Dynamic Global Vegetation Modeling: Quantifying Terrestrial Ecosystem Responses to Large-Scale Environmental Change. In Terrestrial Ecosystems in a Changing World. Edited by Canadell J, Pataki D, Pitelka L. Springer Berlin Heidelberg. 2007: 175–192: Global Change — The IGBP Series].

35 IPCC. Climate change 2013: The physical science basis. Contribution of working group I to the fifth assessment report of the intergovern mental panel on climate change. Cambridge, United Kingdom and New York, NY, USA: IPCC; 2013.

36 Quillet A, Peng CH, Garneau M. Toward dynamic global vegetation models for simulating vegetation-climate interactions and feedbacks: recent developments, limitations, and future challenges. Environ Rev. 2010;18:333–53.

37 Plummer SE. Perspectives on combining ecological process models and remotely sensed data. Ecol Model. 2000;129:169–86.

38 Verstraeten W, Veroustraete F, Wagner W, Van Roey T, Heyns W, Verbeiren S, et al. Remotely sensed soil moisture integration in an ecosystem carbon flux model. The spatial implication. Clim Change. 2010;103:117–36.

39 Smith B, Knorr W, Widlowski J-L, Pinty B, Gobron N. Combining remote sensing data with process modelling to monitor boreal conifer forest carbon balances. For Ecol Manage. 2008;255:3985–94.

40 Olson RJ, Scurlock JMO, Prince SD, Zheng DL, Johnson KR (eds.). NPP Multi-Biome: Global Primary Production Data Initiative Products, R2. Data set. In Book NPP Multi-Biome: Global Primary Production Data Initiative Products, R2. Data set: Available on-line [http://daac.ornl.gov] 2013.

41 Weber U, Jung M, Reichstein M, Beer C, Braakhekke MC, Lehsten V, et al. The interannual variability of Africa's ecosystem productivity: a multi-model analysis. Biogeosciences. 2009;6:285–95.

42 Rawlins MA, McGuire AD, Kimball JK, Dass P, Lawrence D, Burke E, et al. Assessment of model estimates of land–atmosphere CO_2exchange across Northern Eurasia. Biogeosciences Discuss. 2015;12:2257–305.

43 Samanta A, Costa MH, Nunes EL, Vieira SA, Xu L, Myneni RB. Comment on "drought-induced reduction in global terrestrial Net primary production from 2000 through 2009". Science. 2011;333:1093.

44 Medlyn BE. Comment on "drought-induced reduction in global terrestrial Net primary production from 2000 through 2009". Science. 2011;333:1093.

45 Clark DA, Piper SC, Keeling CD, Clark DB. Tropical rain forest tree growth and atmospheric carbon dynamics linked to interannual temperature variation during 1984–2000. Proc Natl Acad Sci U S A. 2003;100:5852–7.

46 Wang WL, Ciais P, Nemani RR, Canadell JG, Piao SL, Sitch S, et al. Variations in atmospheric CO_2 growth rates coupled with tropical temperature. Proc Natl Acad Sci U S A. 2013;110:13061–6.

47 Malhi Y, Aragao LEOC, Metcalfe DB, Paiva R, Quesada CA, Almeida S, et al. Comprehensive assessment of carbon productivity, allocation and storage in three Amazonian forests. Global Change Biol. 2009;15:1255–74.

48 Ahlström A, Miller PA, Smith B. Too early to infer a global NPP decline since 2000. Geophysical Res Lett. 2012;39:L15403. doi:10.1029/2012GL052336.

49 Traore AK, Ciais P, Vuichard N, Poulter B, Viovy N, Guimberteau M, et al. Evaluation of the ORCHIDEE ecosystem model over Africa against 25 years of satellite-based water and carbon measurements. Journal of Geophysical Research: Biogeosciences 2014:2014JG002638.

50 Zhang YJ, Xu M, Chen H, Adams J. Global pattern of NPP to GPP ratio derived from MODIS data: effects of ecosystem type, geographical location and climate. Global Ecol Biogeogr. 2009;18:280–90.

51 Amthor JS. The McCree-de Wit-penning de vries-thornley respiration paradigms: 30 years later. Ann Bot. 2000;86:1–20.

52 Piao SL, Luyssaert S, Ciais P, Janssens IA, Chen AP, Cao C, et al. Forest annual carbon cost: a global-scale analysis of autotrophic respiration. Ecology. 2010;91:652–61.

53 Sjöström M, Ardö J, Arneth A, Boulain N, Cappelaere B, Eklundh L, et al. Exploring the potential of MODIS EVI for modeling gross primary production across African ecosystems. Remote Sens Environ. 2011;115:1081–9.

54 Sjöström M, Zhao M, Archibald S, Arneth A, Cappelaere B, Falk U, et al. Evaluation of MODIS gross primary productivity for Africa using eddy covariance data. Remote Sens Environ. 2013;131:275–86.

55 Zhao M, Running SW. Response to comments on "drought-induced reduction in global terrestrial Net primary production from 2000 through 2009". Science. 2011;333:1093.

56 Ahlström A, Schurgers G, Arneth A, Smith B. Robustness and uncertainty in terrestrial ecosystem carbon response to CMIP5 climate change projections. Environ Res Lett. 2012;7:044008.

57 Piao S, Sitch S, Ciais P, Friedlingstein P, Peylin P, Wang X, et al. Evaluation of terrestrial carbon cycle models for their response to climate variability and to CO_2 trends. Global Change Biol. 2013;19:2117–32.

58 Metcalfe DB, Meir P, Aragão LEOC, Lobo-do-Vale R, Galbraith D, Fisher RA, et al. Shifts in plant respiration and carbon use efficiency at a large-scale drought experiment in the eastern Amazon. New Phytol. 2010;187:608–21.

59 Beer C, Reichstein M, Tomelleri E, Ciais P, Jung M, Carvalhais N, et al. Terrestrial gross carbon dioxide uptake: global distribution and covariation with climate. Science. 2010;329:834–8.

60 Zhao M, Heinsch FA, Nemani RR, Running SW. Improvements of the MODIS terrestrial gross and net primary production global data set. Remote Sens Environ. 2005;95:164–76.

61 Jönsson P, Eklundh L. TIMESAT - a program for analysing time-series of satellite sensor data. Comput Geosci. 2004;30:833–45.

62 Fisher JB, Sikka M, Sitch S, Ciais P, Poulter B, Galbraith D, et al. African tropical rainforest net carbon dioxide fluxes in the twentieth century. Philos Trans R Soc Lond B Biol Sci. 2013;368:20120376.

63 Hashimoto H, Dungan JL, White MA, Yang F, Michaelis AR, Running SW, et al. Satellite-based estimation of surface vapor pressure deficits using MODIS land surface temperature data. Remote Sens Environ. 2008;112:142–55.

64 EUMETSAT: Product User Manual Down-welling Surface Shortwave Flux (DSSF). EUMETSAT LSA SAF; 2011. Technical Report.

65 Ardö J, Mölder M, El-Tahir B, Elkhidir H. Seasonal variation of carbon fluxes in a sparse savanna in semi arid Sudan. Carbon Bal Manag. 2008;3:7.

66 LPJ-GUESS Ecosystem Model. http://www.nateko.lu.se/lpj-guess/index.html. Accessed October 1,2014.

67 Smith B, Prentice IC, Sykes MT. Representation of vegetation dynamics in the modelling of terrestrial ecosystems: comparing two contrasting approaches within European climate space. Global Ecol Biogeogr. 2001;10:621–37.

68 Heinsch FA, Reeves M, Votava P, Kang S, Milesi C, Zhao M, et al. User's Guide. GPP and NPP (MOD17A2/A3) Products, NASA MODIS Land Algorithm, Version 2.0. MODIS LAND TEAM; 2003. Technical Report. http://www.ntsg.umt.edu/sites/ntsg.umt.edu/files/modis/MOD17UsersGuide.pdf.

69 Kanamitsu M, Ebisuzaki W, Woollen J, Yang SK, Hnilo JJ, Fiorino M, et al. Ncep-Doe amip-Ii reanalysis (R-2). Bull Am Meteorol Soc. 2002;83:1631–43.

70 Kalnay E, Kanamitsu M, Kistler R, Collins W, Deaven D, Gandin L, et al. The NCEP/NCAR 40-year reanalysis project. Bull Am Meteorol Soc. 1996;77:437–71.

71 Coops NC, Black TA, Jassal RPS, Trofymow JAT, Morgenstern K. Comparison of MODIS, eddy covariance determined and physiologically modelled gross primary production (GPP) in a Douglas-fir forest stand. Remote Sens Environ. 2007;107:385–401.

72 Heinsch FA, Zhao MS, Running SW, Kimball JS, Nemani RR, Davis KJ, et al. Evaluation of remote sensing based terrestrial productivity from MODIS using regional tower eddy flux network observations. Ieee T Geosci Remote. 2006;44:1908–25.

73 Kanniah KD, Beringer J, Hutley LB, Tapper NJ, Zhu X. Evaluation of collections 4 and 5 of the MODIS gross primary productivity product and algorithm improvement at a tropical savanna site in northern Australia. Remote Sens Environ. 2009;113:1808–22.

74 Plummer S. On validation of the MODIS gross primary production product. Ieee T Geosci Remote. 2006;44:1936–8.

75 Fensholt R, Sandholt I, Rasmussen MS, Stisen S, Diouf A. Evaluation of satellite based primary production modelling in the semi-arid Sahel. Remote Sens Environ. 2006;105:173–88.

76 DeLucia EH, Drake JE, Thomas RB, Gonzalez-Meler M. Forest carbon use efficiency: is respiration a constant fraction of gross primary production? Global Change Biol. 2007;13:1157–67.

77 Khatir ARAI. Application of Resource Assessment and Management Support for Pastoral Systems (RAPS) Model to Analyze Pastoral Systems in North Kordofan State, Sudan. PhD-thesis. University of Kordofan, Department of Forestry and Range Sciences, Faculty of Natural Resources and Environmental Studies; 2012.

78 Sanon HA, Ledin I. Assessment of edible biomass production of *Acacia senegal*, *Guiera senegalensis* and *Pterocarpus lucens* in the Sahelian zone of West Africa. Options Mediterranéennes, A. 2009;85:117–21.

79 Zheng DL, Prince SD, Wright R. NPP Multi-Biome: Gridded Estimates for Selected Regions Worldwide, 1954–1998, R3. Data set. Available on-line [http://daac.ornl.gov] from the Oak Ridge National Laboratory Distributed Active Archive Center, Oak Ridge, Tennessee, USA 2013.

CHAPTER 10

Estimation of Biomass and Canopy Height in Bermudagrass, Alfalfa, and Wheat Using Ultrasonic, Laser, and Spectral Sensors

Jeremy Joshua Pittman [1,2,*], Daryl Brian Arnall [2], Sindy M. Interrante [1], Corey A. Moffet [1] and Twain J. Butler [1]

[1] The Samuel Roberts Noble Foundation, Ardmore, OK 73401, USA

[2] Oklahoma State University Department of Plant and Soil Sciences, Stillwater, OK 74078, USA

ABSTRACT

Non-destructive biomass estimation of vegetation has been performed via remote sensing as well as physical measurements. An effective method for estimating biomass must have accuracy comparable to the accepted standard of destructive removal. Estimation or measurement of height is commonly employed to create a relationship between height and mass. This study examined several types of ground-based mobile sensing strategies for forage biomass estimation. Forage production experiments consisting of alfalfa (*Medicago sativa* L.), bermudagrass [*Cynodon dactylon* (L.) Pers.], and wheat (*Triticum aestivum* L.) were employed to examine sensor biomass estimation (laser, ultrasonic, and spectral) as compared to physical measurements (plate meter and meter stick) and the traditional harvest method (clipping). Predictive models were constructed via partial least squares regression and modeled estimates were compared to the physically measured biomass. Least significant difference separated mean estimates were examined to evaluate differences in the physical measurements and sensor estimates for canopy height and biomass. Differences between methods were minimal (average percent error of 11.2% for difference between predicted values *versus* machine and quadrat harvested biomass values (1.64 and 4.91 t·ha^{-1}, respectively), except at the lowest measured biomass (average percent error of 89% for harvester and quad harvested biomass < 0.79 t·ha^{-1}) and greatest measured biomass (average percent error of 18% for harvester and quad harvested biomass >6.4 t·ha^{-1}). These data suggest that using mobile sensor-based biomass estimation models could be an effective alternative to the traditional clipping method for rapid, accurate in-field biomass estimation.

KEYWORDS

remote sensing; biomass estimation; mobile sensors; sensor system; data acquisition; high-throughput

1. INTRODUCTION

An effective method for in-field estimation of biomass on a dry matter (DM) basis must produce accuracy comparable to the accepted measurement standard (*i.e.*, destructive removal). Non-destructive methods for estimating dry biomass using plant or canopy measurements have been developed [1,2]. In large part, vegetative mass is considered a function of canopy or plant height [3,4]. For these methods, canopy or plant height is recorded and an empirical relationship between height and DM is developed. Devices such as the rising plate meter, capacitance meter, and meter stick are examples of devices used for physical measurements of vegetation height and biomass estimation [1,5–7]. The limitations associated with these techniques are labor and time intensiveness. Additionally, variation due to vegetation growth characteristics and spatial variability can be difficult to accurately represent by physical sample collection which limits the ability to develop a robust estimation model.

Alternatively, remote sensing strategies (ultrasonic, laser, and sensor combinations) may overcome some of the limitations encountered with physical measurement strategies. A greater number of measurements can be taken in a considerably reduced amount of time and thus a larger area can be sampled. This increased magnitude in data collection provides opportunity for development of a statistically robust estimation model as a more comprehensive representation of the area of interest (AOI) can be collected. Ultrasonic proximity sensors employ intensity differential reflectance of sound waves to approximate distances. Ultrasonic sensors have been utilized for measuring height and estimating DM in pastures [2,8,9], canopy characterization in orchards [10,11], as well as in wheat [12], cotton [13], and maize [14]. Laser proximity sensors employ time-differential reflectance of light to approximate distances. Laser sensors have been effectively used for height measurements in wheat [15,16], maize [17], rape, rye, pasture [18], standing forests [19], and miscellaneous vegetation [20]. The combination of ultrasonic and active spectral reflectance have been used to estimate biomass in white clover, red clover, alfalfa, and perennial ryegrass, with R^2 ranging from 0.90 for estimating alfalfa-perennial ryegrass mixtures to 0.99 for estimation of biomass for monoculture alfalfa [2]. Combining ultrasonic and Normalized Difference Vegetation Index (NDVI) measurements to estimate canopy height in wheat resulted in standard errors between 4.6 and 7.2 cm [12]. Similar results were found in maize using NDVI and ultrasonic sensors where an $R^2 = 0.62$ was reported for forage mass [21].

Spectral strategies seek to base biomass estimates on reflectance or absorption intensities of wavelengths from vegetation and/or soil [2,22–24]. These spectral strategies can be effective at low Leaf Area Index (LAI) and biomass, but can become less accurate as the canopy closes when a point of reflectance saturation may occur [23,25]. Some direct contribution to reflectance saturation can be attributed to increase in vegetation height, but relationships between biomass and NDVI vary logarithmically, signifying an interaction of canopy closure and height [21,26]. Normalized difference vegetation index has been employed in biomass estimation for a number of crop species. Freeman [21] employed an active spectral sensor for calculating NDVI (Greenseeker®) and recorded a positive relationship with $R^2 = 0.52$ for forage DM yield in maize. Erdle [22] reported R^2 values of up to 0.91 and 0.84 for nitrogen content and biomass, respectively, when using active spectral sensors for NDVI measurement in wheat. Additionally, Gnyp [25] observed R^2 of up to 0.69 for above-ground biomass in rice when regressed with NDVI alone, as well as a 21%–35% increase in explanation of above-ground biomass in rice when using a six-band spectral model as compared to NDVI alone.

There is limited published research on the combined use of ultrasonic, spectral, and laser sensors and their subsequent estimation models to measure forage height and DM. Therefore, the objective of this research was to evaluate the relationship between dry biomass measured via destructive removal and dry biomass estimated from a combination of sensor-measured canopy height and spectral reflectance. The evaluation was achieved by collecting both physically-measured and sensor-measured plant canopy heights as well as active and passive spectral reflectance readings via a mobile platform for vegetation at the canopy level. The intended deliverable from this research was a system containing a collection of sensors and software which would enable efficient and accurate acquisition of data by which estimation of dry biomass could be achieved.

2. MATERIALS AND METHODS

2.1. Alfalfa-Bermudagrass Mixture Experiment: Site, Design, and Management

A "600RR" alfalfa-"Midland 99" bermudagrass mixture trial was conducted at the Noble Foundation Red River Research and Demonstration Farm near Burneyville, OK, USA (33.88° N, 97.28° W; elevation 234 m. Figure 1). The soils are characterized as Slaughterville fine sandy loam (coarse-loamy, mixed, superactive, thermic Udic Haplustolls) with N-nitrate at less than 5 $g{\cdot}kg^{-1}$, soil test value of 64 $g{\cdot}P{\cdot}kg^{-1}$, 52 $g{\cdot}K{\cdot}kg^{-1}$ (amended with 0.1785 $t{\cdot}ha^{-1}$ 0-0-60), B of 0.017 $g{\cdot}kg^{-1}$(amended with 0.00745 $t{\cdot}kg^{-1}$), and pH of 6.3.

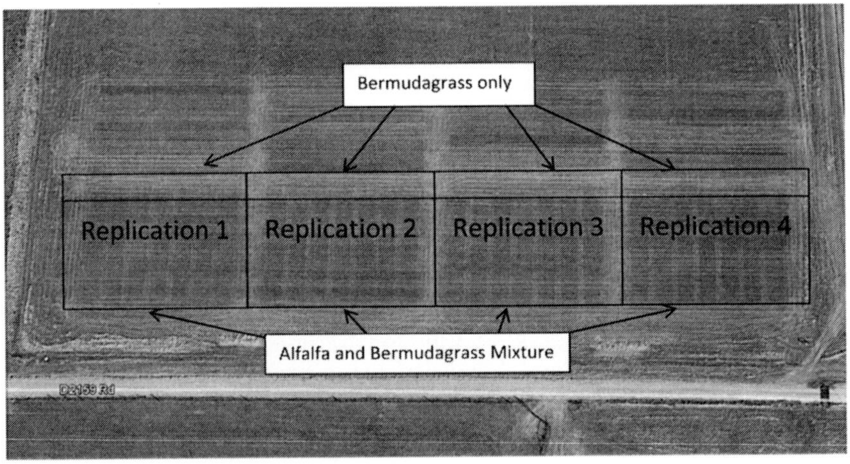

Figure 1. Aerial imagery of alfalfa and bermudagrass Trial. courtesy google earth.

A Hege 1000 cone planter no-till drill (Hege Equipment Inc., Colwich, KS, USA) was used for inter-seeding alfalfa into an established bermudagrass sward in fall 2012 and spring 2013. Data was collected the following spring and summer after establishment. Treatments were arranged in eight replications of a randomized complete block design (RCBD) with a split-split-plot arrangement. Main plots consisted of three alfalfa planting dates (September, November, and February), subplots consisted of three alfalfa seedbed preparations (mow/hay-off, mow/hay-off plus glyphosate, and tillage), and sub-subplots (1.5 m × 6 m) consisted of seven fungicide and insecticide alfalfa seed treatments. An adjacent experiment with eight replicates of 1.5 m × 6 m bermudagrass only plots treated with seven levels of N fertilizer ranging from 0 to 0.224 $t{\cdot}N{\cdot}ha^{-1}{\cdot}yr^{-1}$ was established and harvested concurrently with the alfalfa-bermudagrass mixture experiment.

2.1.1. Physical Measurements: Alfalfa-Bermuda Experiment

Data were collected from all plots four times in 2013 when alfalfa reached 10% bloom. Vegetation height measurements were taken using a meter stick and a 0.1-m^2 aluminum rising plate meter (NZ Agriworks LTD t/a Jenquip, Feilding, New Zealand) [27,28]. Species composition was estimated both visually and as hand-separated dry weights from harvested quadrats for the alfalfa and bermudagrass mixtures only [29]. Visual composition was estimated and averaged across two observers [30]. Hand-separated alfalfa and bermudagrass subsamples were dried in a forced draft oven at 50 °C for five days to a constant weight prior to weighing. Plot biomass weights were recorded on a whole plot basis by clipping plots to a 5-cm stubble height with a Cibus forage harvester (Wintersteiger Inc., Salt Lake City, UT, USA) and are reported on a DM basis.

2.1.2. Sensor Height, Spectral, and Spatial Measurements: Alfalfa-Bermuda Experiment

A ground-based mobile platform was utilized for moving sensors across the trial areas using an electric golf cart (the golf cart was selected due to minimal suspension travel Figure 2) fitted with drop spindles and oversized tires spaced at 1 m, to minimize contact with the biomass contained within the plot area (1.5 m × 6 m). The cart was custom-fitted with a mast extending from the front upon which all sensors were attached. A single deep cycle 12 V DC marine battery was added to the cart and served as the power source for all sensors. Power and/or accessory power to all sensors was routed through a system power cycle switch by which all active data acquisition could be initiated or terminated simultaneously. Additionally, a GPS with Omni Star XP GNSS positioning (repeatability <10 cm, 95% CEP) was implemented to acquire position data for all sensor readings. The

GPS was configured to output spatial data at a rate of 10 Hz such that multiple locations could be recorded within each plot. Height was measured using a single beam 660 nm time of flight laser distance sensor ("Laser"). The sensor was calibrated (calibration was performed prior to first use and verified by measurement at subsequent data collection events) to bare ground surface (0 cm) and 93 cm above ground surface as minimum and maximum heights, respectively. The laser readings were inversely related to height. The laser sensor used in this experiment differs from LIDAR laser systems which are typically aerial-based or ground-based static as opposed to mobile. Additionally, LIDAR laser systems typically scan a large area, utilize a large number of reflectance beams at numerous wavelengths, and they produce a "point cloud" [17,18]. The laser distance sensor used in these experiments emitted only one beam at one wavelength to produce a one dimensional pattern of measurements and did not have the multidimensional dynamics of a LIDAR point cloud. The laser readings characterize the height of the vegetation for a 2- to 4-mm diameter footprint which was inversely proportional to vegetation height. Two ultrasonic sensors, operating at different frequencies, were examined to observe appropriateness for use on plant material.

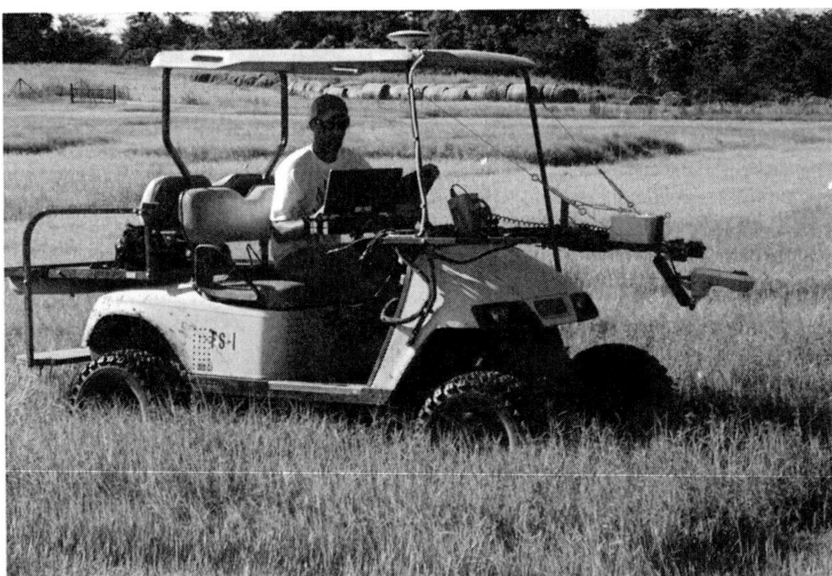

Figure 2. Electric golf cart used for transport of sensors across alfalfa-bermudagrass experiment.

Height measurements were collected using a 240 MHz ultrasonic sensor and a 120 MHz ultrasonic sensor, which were also calibrated to ground height (0 cm) and 93 cm above the ground. Ultrasonic, sensor readings were directly proportional height. Readings from the ultrasonic sensors characterized canopy height in a 7.5- to 15-cm conical footprint, which were also inversely proportional to vegetation height. As the calibration for height sensors was 0–93 cm, all were operated within effective detection limits of near 0 m to 10 m specified by the manufacturer. All height data were acquired at the default sensor output rate (50 Hz–150 Hz) and configured to collect data centered on a 0.12 m^2 area.

A Greenseeker® (Trimble, Sunnyvale, CA, USA) was employed to collect NDVI with a maximum conical footprint of 0.1 m^2 which varied inversely with forage height. Data were acquired at rate of 20 Hz from the Greenseeker® radiometer for each plot. Additionally, a CROPSCAN (CROPSCAN, Inc., Rochester, MN, USA) with a conical footprint having diameter equal to on half of height to target was also used and acquired reflectance measurements at 450, 520, 530, 570, 590, 650, 690, 710, 780 and 900 nm (8.2–13 nm band width). Sampling using the CROPSCAN was limited to two readings per plot in an east/west travel pattern as sampling time was approximately two to three seconds per acquisition. There were fewer CROPSCAN than Greenseeker® readings (two *vs.* 90 per plot, respectively) since each CROPSCAN acquisition event required a keystroke on the laptop computer compared to an automated acquisition from the Greenseeker® sensor. Prior to data acquisition for the alfalfa and bermudagrass experiment the orientation of the two instruments were adjusted such that no reflectance from the Greenseeker® radiometer influenced readings from the CROPSCAN.

2.1.3. Transport and Temporal Logistics: Alfalfa-Bermuda Experiment

Each plot was driven across at 3.2–4.8 $km \cdot hr^{-1}$ resulting in approximately five seconds of data acquisition per plot. This amount of time resulted in approximately 25–30 condensed and balanced sample values per plot per parameter (*i.e.*, laser, GPS, Greenseeker®, *etc.*). After removal superfluous data associated with the power cycling, approximately four to five averaged readings per meter were assigned to each AOI. Rate of travel was dictated by the time necessary to acquire two samples with the CROPSCAN and the more extended data output time of this sensor as compared to others used. As previously stated, each sample required two to three seconds so five seconds were necessary to acquire both samples within the plot length. Length of data acquisition time per plot varied less than one second.

The sensor array measured approximately 25 cm wide and 45 cm from front to back with the Greenseeker® radiometer located most forward and the ultrasonic proximal sensors located at the rear. The GPS was oriented approximately 75 cm to the rear of the ultrasonic sensors and approximately 45 cm right of center. This offset was accounted for in subsequent data parsing. The offset among sensors required that initiation and termination of sensor logging be timed to ensure that all vegetation measurement sensors were above the AOI while logging the data.

2.2. Wheat Experiment: Site, Design, and Management

Two wheat trials were also employed for sensor data collection. The first wheat experiment was initiated at the Noble Foundation Dupy Farm near Gene Autry, OK, USA (34.29° N, 96.99° W; elevation 220 m. Figure 3). The soils are characterized as Dale silt loam with pH of 7.3 and N-nitrate, P, and K of 14, 31 and 132 g·kg^{-1}, respectively. A Hege 500 cone planter grain drill (Hege Equipment Inc., Colwich, KS, USA) was used for planting wheat in autumn 2013, and data was collected in the spring 2014. Approximately 1200 (1.5 × 3 m) plots of 500 wheat varieties were planted as part of variety selection trials. These were arranged in completely randomized block design (CRBD) with two replications.

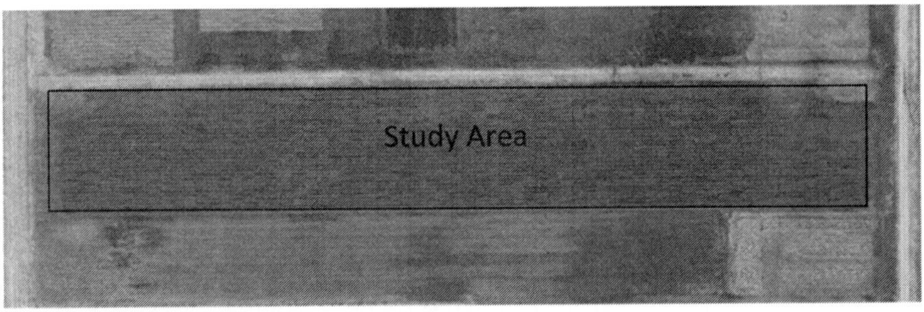

Figure 3. Aerial imagery of Dupy wheat experiment.

The second wheat experiment was initiated at the Noble Foundation Unit 3 Farm in Ardmore, OK, USA (34.17° N, 97.08° W; elevation 268 m. Figure 4). The soils are characterized as Konsil loamy fine sandy with pH of 6.8 and N-nitrate, P, and K of 28, 50 and 111 g·kg^{-1}, respectively. This trial contained 136 (1.5 × 3 m) plots comprised of 50 wheat varieties. A Hege 500 cone planter grain drill was also used for planting wheat in 2013.

Between the two wheat trials, there were seven data collection events occurring from February to April 2014.

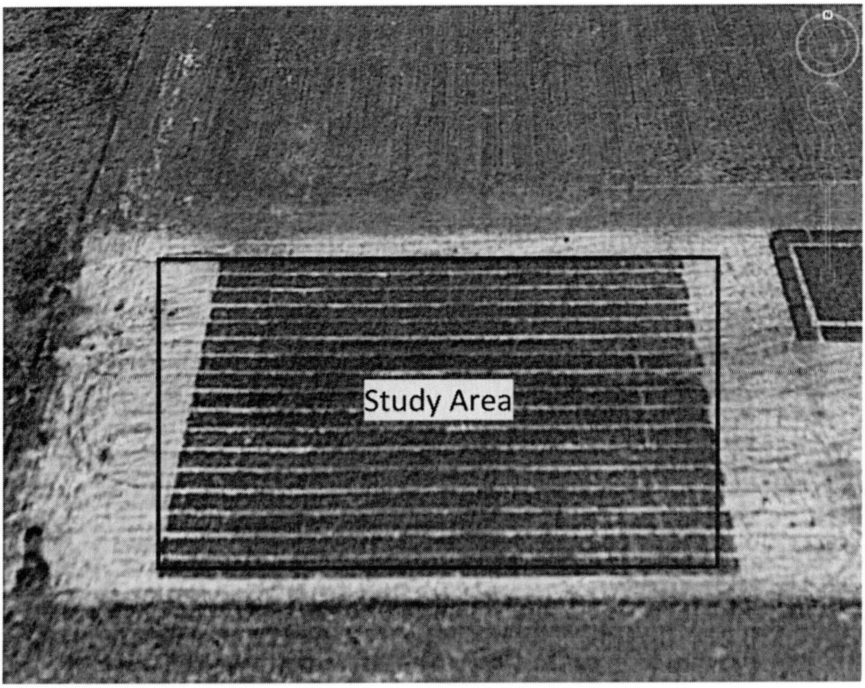

Figure 4. Aerial imagery of the unit 3 wheat experiment.

2.2.1. Physical Measurements: Wheat Experiment

Wheat biomass for both experiments was estimated by hand clipping one 0.16 m^2 quadrat per plot to a 2.5-cm stubble height. Samples were dried in a forced draft oven at 50 °C for five days prior to weighing and are reported as $kg \cdot DM \cdot ha^{-1}$.

2.2.2. Sensor Height, Spectral, and Spatial Measurements: Wheat Experiment

Sensor data was collected from the wheat trials using a gasoline-powered Spider high-clearance tractor (LeeAgra, Inc., Lubbock, TX, USA) at a ground speed of approximately 1.6–3.2 km·h^{-1} (Figure 5). The factory-installed spray mast attached to the front of the tractor was converted to a manifold configuration to accommodate the sensor array. All sensors were initially powered using the onboard, factory installed, 12 V power supply. For convenience this was later modified to use an independent 12 V power source to power sensors. Upon restarting the tractor engine a momentary power deficit would occur and required re-initializing the sensor system. The same GPS with Omni Star XP GNSS positioning as described in the alfalfa and bermudagrass trial was implemented to acquire spatial data for all sensor readings. The GPS was configured to output data at a rate of 10 Hz such that multiple locations could be recorded within each plot.

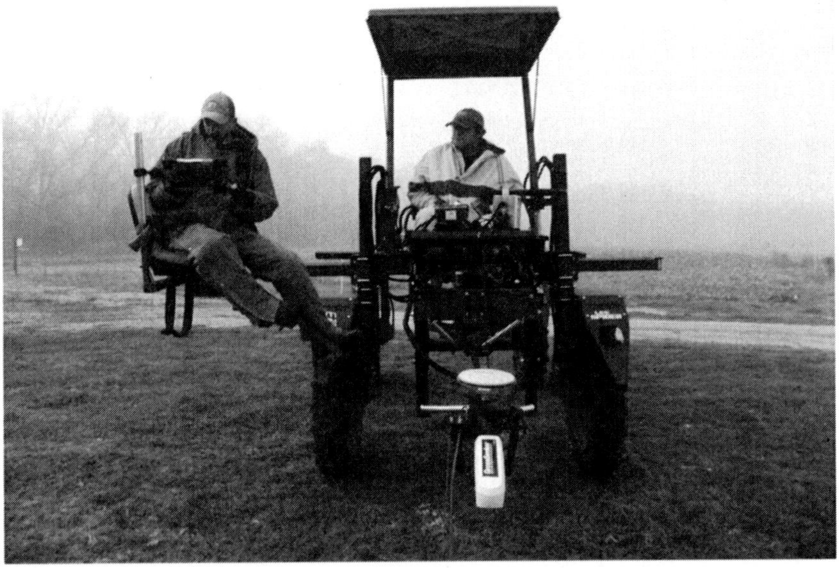

Figure 5. Spyder used for transport of sensors across wheat experiments.

Height was measured using two single 660 nm single beam time of flight laser distance sensors as well as a 120 MHz ultrasonic sensor. These sensors were the same make and model of those used in the alfalfa-bermudagrass experiment. All height sensors were calibrated at a bare ground surface and a 74 cm maximum in the same manner as those used in the alfalfa and bermudagrass experiment as well. All height data were acquired at a rate of 10 Hz and all sensors were configured to collect data centered on a 0.02-m^2 area. A Greenseeker® was employed to collect NDVI at rate of 10 Hz for each plot. The passive radiometer (CROPSCAN) was not used on the wheat experiments.

2.2.3. Transport and Temporal Logistics: Wheat Experiment

The sensor array used in the wheat trials measured approximately 20 cm long by 10 cm wide. As was previously described in the alfalfa and bermudagrass experiment, it was necessary to ensure all sensors were above the plot prior to data acquisition initiation and termination. Alley identifiers were assigned during the time spent crossing the alley areas and until all sensors were above the subsequent AOI, whereas plot identifiers were assigned to the incoming data.

Each plot was driven across at 1.6–3.2 km·hr^{-1} resulting in approximately three seconds of data acquisition per plot and due to the fact a delay buffer of approximately one second was allowed at the beginning and end of each plot. This amount of time provided approximately 25–30 readings per plot per parameter (*i.e.*, Laser, Ultrasonic, Greenseeker®). Variability in the length of data acquisition time per plot occurred but was similar to the cart configuration in the alfalfa and bermudagrass experiment and only existed on the order of less than one second.

2.3. Data Acquisition Hardware: All Experiments

For all experiments, analog data from the height measurement sensors were acquired using a data acquisition module (DAQ). Laser sensors were configured via a current loop to operate at a range of 0 to 5 V DC and were connected directly to the DAQ for voltage output. The 120 MHz ultrasonic sensor was configured to operate at a range of 0 to 5 V DC, and voltage readings were directly output to the DAQ. The 240 MHz ultrasonic sensor was operated at a range of 0 to 10 V DC and voltage readings were directly output to the DAQ. From the DAQ, all analog data were transferred as digital output to a laptop computer for the alfalfa and bermudagrass trial and ruggedized tablet computer in the wheat trials via USB connection. Data from the Greenseeker® radiometer was output directly to the tablet and laptop via serial connection as NDVI values, which were generated by the autonomous radiometer processor. CROPSCAN readings were acquired and stored in the autonomous memory contained within the radiometer hardware. It was not possible to insert plot markers into data from the CROPSCAN as it was necessary for the power source in this unit to remain autonomous and operational function could only be achieved through use of the factory provided software. However, it was possible to operate this software simultaneously on the same laptop, which was used for all other data acquisition.

2.4. Data Acquisition Software: All Experiments

For all experiments, all streams of data were captured real-time using AgriLogger and WinWedge Pro (WinWedge Pro©; TAL Technologies Inc., Philadelphia, PA, USA). These software applications were not used simultaneously for concurrent data collection. Both applications allowed for recording each stream of data with unique communication configurations. Unique configurations were necessary as retention of all data fields from all sensors was not desired and communication configurations for each stream of data or sensor were different.

Agrilogger was developed to utilize a sampling logic which resulted in only the user-specified rate of data acquisition to take place. All data was written to a single log file at the user-specified rate. In contrast, WinWedge Pro© captured all data from incoming streams at rates dictated by the transmitting hardware. When using WinWedge Pro©, it was necessary to run multiple instances of the software simultaneously, one for each data stream (*i.e.*, DAQ, GPS, and Greenseeker®). Each instance of the software produced one log file for the data stream being acquired, which resulted in multiple output files for each data collection event.

The power cycling switch used for plot delineation when acquiring data with WinWedge Pro© at no point interrupted data streams. The power was cycled on such that sensor readings were acquired and null readings were acquired when power was cycled off. These areas of null values signified non-plot areas. This strategy required combining the data from all streams post-processing. AgriLogger enabled the user to insert identifiers real-time as data were acquired. The identifiers used to delineate plot areas from non-plot areas were inserted with a mouse click or touch-screen button.

As previously stated, data acquired from the CROPSCAN were written to the autonomous storage capabilities contained within the unit. Utilization of factory included software application was necessary for post-processing reflectance data. This application produced one log file which could then be combined with data from all other sensors at post-processing based on sampling rate per plot and time stamp.

2.5. Data Post-Processing

For both WinWedge Pro© and Agrilogger, time and date fields (based on the laptop clock) were inserted into the data streams for each record received at the application level. This allowed for quality control and the ability to combine data during post-processing when using WinWedge Pro©. Combining log files produced when using WinWedge Pro© was achieved through implementation of a custom post-processing application

(DataProcessing). The primary function of the DataProcessing application was averaging data to a desired rate (*i.e.*, 5 Hz, 10 Hz, *etc.*) so as to balance the number of sensor readings across the sensors and reduce the data to a more manageable volume. The averaging was achieved by utilization of the aforementioned time stamp which had been inserted for each record. After the data were combined, it was output to a text file which contained the combined sensor data at the specified averaging interval (*i.e.*, 5 Hz, 10 Hz, *etc.*). The output file from the DataProcessing software was then manually edited by attaching range and row identifiers to plot areas. These plot areas were delineated based on the aforementioned null values. The non-plot areas were manually removed from the data, leaving only the range and row identified plot areas. These plot areas could then be assigned a unique plot identifier.

Data acquired using AgriLogger was also manually edited to remove non-plot areas. Due to the user control and plot identification features provided in this software application, the magnitude of the data contained in the single output file were of a much smaller scale than that output by WinWedge Pro©. This was due to the sampling logic data acquisition strategy implemented in AgriLogger as opposed to the constant uncontrolled streaming of data with WinWedge Pro©. A user-specified sampling rate allowed for data acquisition at rates of up to 20 Hz and output of all parameters to a single log file. No post-processing application was necessary for reduction of the data through averaging.

Post-processing data transformation was performed on laser measurements as calibrations produced readings which were inversely proportional to the height of measured vegetation. Laser readings were subtracted from the calibrated maximum reading (signifying the greatest distance from the sensor). This transformed the data to a directly varying scale which agreed with the directly varying relationships between vegetation height and readings from ultrasonic sensors. Both ultrasonic and laser readings were converted to cm values based on the minimum and maximum calibration heights at post-processing.

2.6. Data Analysis: All Experiments

Sensor readings were examined for correlation to physically-measured height and destructively-measured DM [31–33]. The combination of output from multiple sensors as constituents of a predictive model for biomass was also examined. Comparisons were examined for the accuracy in estimation of height and DM for sensor models *versus* physical measurements performed. It must be noted that destructive harvest methods differed between the alfalfa-bermudagrass and the wheat experiments. Due to the 2.5-cm difference in harvest height, data analyses for biomass were performed based on harvest method and species for model construction. Additionally, the relationship between forage harvester and quadrat measurements of forage biomass was examined by regression analysis using SAS PROC REG [34].

2.6.1. Correlation: Sensor Measurements to Physical Measurements

Physical and sensor measurement methods were examined for correlation to vegetative mass on a DM basis as well as sensor measurements to measured canopy height. These analyses were performed using SAS PROC CORR [34]. Data used for model construction were included for the examination of correlation between sensor measurements and physical measurements.

2.6.2. Model Construction

Data were split into model construction and validation sets. This division was implemented to ensure the entire range of the data would be represented in both. Two hundred-twelve samples were used to generate estimation models for alfalfa only, with a validation set containing 89 samples. Seventy-eight samples were used to construct the bermudagrass only model with 32 validation samples. Wheat biomass models were constructed from 193 samples and 97 validation samples. Since no physically-measured canopy height data was collected for wheat, no canopy height estimation models were generated. Canopy height estimation models for the alfalfa and bermudagrass trial were constructed on a vegetation composition category basis, which consisted of individual species (alfalfa, bermudagrass), mixtures of the two (MIX), and across the entirety of the alfalfa and bermudagrass experiment data (ALL). The MIX group of data from the alfalfa and bermudagrass trial was comprised of sampled verified plots having botanical compositions ranging from 80% alfalfa:20% bermudagrass to 20% alfalfa:80% bermudagrass, (n = 1002 for modeling and n = 581 for validation).

Estimation models were constructed using partial least squares (PLS) regression analyses (SAS PROC PLS) with CVTEST for selection of simplest models [34–36]. Laser and ultrasonic sensor outputs as well as NDVI from the Greenseeker® and seven spectral bands from the CROPSCAN were examined for inclusion in sensor based biomass estimation models. Laser and ultrasonic data were examined in the same manner for canopy height modeling.

Parameters included in biomass and canopy height estimation models were selected by evaluation of Variable Importance Plot (VIP) values output from SAS PROC PLS using the plots = (parmprofiles vip) option, as a filter measure [37] (Table 1). These scores represent the contribution of a variable as a predictor due to the amount of variance explained and can be viewed as a percentage in relation to one another when a number of predictor variables are simultaneously examined [37]. All components with VIP scores less than 1 were deleted from the final models for biomass and canopy height [38–40]. This strategy was adopted in order to achieve an acceptable balance in estimate accuracy and model/sensor system complexity by excluding less contributive variables and equipment from the system.

Table 1. Variable Importance Plot (VIP) scores for sensor parameters considered for model inclusion † From Greenseeker®, ‡ From CROPSCAN.

Sensor Measurement	VIP	
	DM	**Canopy Height**
Laser	1.37	1.08
120 MHz sonic	1.32	1.01
240 MHz sonic	1.11	0.95
NDVI †	1.10	
690 nm ‡	0.90	
650 nm ‡	0.83	
710 nm ‡	0.74	
590 nm ‡	0.74	
450 nm ‡	0.72	
520 nm ‡	0.71	
570 nm ‡	0.70	
530 nm ‡	0.69	
780 nm ‡	0.68	
900 nm ‡	0.66	

Upon deletion of less contributive variables, PLS models were again constructed using cross-validation (CVTEST option) with a 20-fold block training set (CV block = 20) and the SAS default of 1000 permutations [34]. Subsequently a randomly selected block of twenty observations provided cross validation analyses for model training 1000 times for construction of each model. The parameter estimates produced from these analyses were then employed in an equation for calculation of biomass and canopy height estimates (Table 2). Botanical composition based canopy height models included the laser and the 120 MHz ultrasonic (VIP scores > 1).

Table 2. Dry biomass estimation model label key for sensor and physical measures.

Model Number	Estimate	Species Specific	Number of Sensors
1	Dry biomass	Y	3
3	Dry biomass	Y	2
5	Dry biomass	Y	Meter stick
6	Dry biomass	N	Meter stick
7	Dry biomass	N	Plate meter
8	Canopy height	Y	2
9	Canopy height	N	2

2.6.3. Evaluation of Accuracy in Model Estimation for Biomass and Canopy Height

Regression analyses for canopy height and biomass estimations were performed to evaluate relationships between measured and estimated values using SAS PROC REG for samples from the validation data only [34]. Additionally, accuracy of estimation models was evaluated on a percent basis by calculating the by sample mean percent error (MPE) (Equation (1)):

$$MPE = \frac{100\%}{n}\sum_{t=1}^{n}\frac{E_t - M_t}{M_t} \tag{1}$$

where E_t is the biomass estimate for the tth plot using the method of interest, M_t is the measured biomass of the tth plot using the harvest method (*i.e.*, the accepted standard), and n is the number of plots measured.

An Error, Consistency, and Mean Agreement (ECMA) scoring system was calculated for ranking and comparison of model estimation accuracy. Calculation of this scoring system considered agreement of measured and corresponding estimated means, the by sample error estimation, and the repeatability of the error across samples in a category. The ranking calculation was compiled such that higher index scores represented more accurate estimation based on mean agreement, error, and the consistent nature of the error. The score included model error consistency (standard deviation of percent error, S_{PE}), accuracy (mean of by sample percent error, MPE), and the agreement of the mean of measured compared to mean of estimated values (R^2 of estimate to measured, as well as difference in mean of estimate "E" and measured "M") (Equation (2)):

$$ECMA = \frac{\left(\frac{r^2}{|\bar{E} - \bar{M}|}\right)}{MPE \times s_{PE}} \quad (2)$$

Least significant difference (LSD) groupings ($\alpha = 0.05$) were compared among plots grouped according to destructively-measured biomass and physically measured canopy height using the biomass and canopy height estimation models as a post-hoc analysis of accuracy (validation samples only were used in this comparison). This was done to illustrate the efficacy of using biomass or canopy height estimations calculated from sensor readings in place of destructive harvesting methods or physical height measurements for trial evaluations. Biomass comparisons groups were delineated in 1.10 $t \cdot ha^{-1}$increments from 0 to 7.72 $t \cdot ha^{-1}$. Canopy height comparisons were based on 10 physically-measured canopy height classes at ten centimeter increments. These comparisons were performed using PROC MIXED [34] in combination with the PDMIX800 macro [41,42].

3. RESULTS AND DISCUSSION

3.1. Correlation

Laser-estimated height measurements were the most correlated to physically-measured canopy height for all examinations (R = 0.88 bermudagrass to 0.78 MIX). Laser measurements were the most correlated to destructively-sampled biomass as well (R = 0.88 bermudagrass to 0.80 alfalfa). Additionally, NDVI measured using the Greenseeker® was most correlated to biomass (R = 0.75 – 0.62) for all spectral data examined (Table 3).

Additionally, regression analysis of the harvester collected to quadrat collected biomass measurements yielded results showing quadrat harvests to produce AOI DM estimates on average 5% greater than measurements acquired using the harvester.

Table 3. Pearson coefficients for sensor collected parameters correlated to physical measures. † From Greenseeker®, ‡ From CROPSCAN.

Sensor Measurement	Alfalfa	Bermudagrass	Mix	Wheat
		Destructively measured DM		
Measured height	0.83	0.83	0.82	
Plate meter	0.43	0.48	0.43	
Laser	0.80	0.88	0.86	0.86
120 MHz sonic	0.74	0.87	0.85	0.85
240 MHz sonic	0.75	0.81	0.66	
NDVI †	0.70	0.75	0.72	0.62
450 nm ‡	−0.35	−0.53	−0.41	
520 nm ‡	−0.33	−0.54	−0.36	
530 nm ‡	−0.32	−0.51	−0.32	
570 nm ‡	−0.36	−0.50	−0.37	
590 nm ‡	−0.41	−0.56	−0.38	
650 nm ‡	−0.48	−0.65	−0.51	
690 nm ‡	−0.47	−0.63	−0.54	
710 nm ‡	−0.45	−0.52	−0.27	
780 nm ‡	0.13	0.02	0.32	
900 nm ‡	0.08	0.04	0.28	
		Canopy height		
Plate meter	0.11	0.25	0.24	
Laser	0.83	0.88	0.78	
120 MHz sonic	0.76	0.82	0.73	
240 MHz sonic	0.73	0.71	0.68	

3.2. Modeling Analyses

3.2.1. Variable Inclusion Selection

All height sensor parameters were associated with VIP values greater than the exclusionary threshold of 1 [37–40] for both biomass and canopy height (Table 1). The VIP values were greater for the 120 MHz ultrasonic sensor than for the 240 MHz ultrasonic sensor. The 120 MHz ultrasonic sensor was subsequently selected for inclusion in biomass and canopy height model construction. It was apparent while post processing data from the 240 MHz ultrasonic sensor that large areas were resultant output due to loss of echo which likely diminished contribution of this device in enhancing model accuracy. It may be possible to realize more contribution from a 240 MHz ultrasonic sensor which operates in a manner that does not produce such influential quantities of superfluous data. The spectral component NDVI was selected in the biomass model based on VIP values. Data from the CROPSCAN were not employed in the construction of models due to lower VIP scores than that of NDVI from the Greenseeker®. It is likely data from the CROPSCAN were less contributive to the estimation of biomass as it was implemented from a mobile platform and data were acquired while moving across plots as opposed to a stationary orientation. The CROPSCAN was designed to be used as a stationary passive spectral radiometer but it was desired to, in this research, evaluate the potential contribution of the CROPSCAN as an element of a mobile system. It is likely additional spectral bands or indices may be contributive to modeling biomass similar to observations reported by Gnyp [25]. This would be expected whereas the sensor producing this data is an active sensor designed for high speed acquisition as opposed to a passive sensor designed for stationary use as with the CROPSCAN used in these investigations.

3.2.2. Biomass and Canopy Height Estimation Model Performance

Laser-only models explained more variation in dependent variable (VDV) for bermudagrass biomass (78%) and wheat (74%) than did ultrasonic only models for biomass and canopy height (75% and 72%, respectively). Combination models which included laser and ultrasonic improved dependent variable variation explanation in all cases except for wheat biomass (75%) and bermudagrass canopy height (77%). Inclusion of NDVI for biomass modeling improved dependent variable variation explanation by an additional 1%. Biomass models based on physically-measured canopy height were more effective than others in explanation of dependent variable variation for alfalfa only (68.5%). Plate meter-based models were less effective than others for canopy height and biomass estimation (0% to 6.1% and 18% to 23%, respectively) (Table 4). The greatest R^2 observed (0.85) for any estimated to measured biomass relationship was the dual height sensor combination for bermudagrass. Comparison of biomass model estimation based on ECMA scores showed that models which included both height sensors as well as NDVI were more accurate in all cases except for bermudagrass (Table 5). The smallest R^2 observed (0.13 to 0.25) in all cases was for the plate meter models. The meter stick measured height model was ranked second for alfalfa biomass estimation and was the only instance of a physical measurement model being ranked in the top two for biomass estimation. Regression of estimated canopy height to measured canopy height using model 9 for bermudagrass produced the greatest R^2 for all cases (0.84). Canopy height estimates in alfalfa and the legume-grass mixture produced R^2 values of 0.61 or less (Table 5).

Table 4. Explanation of variation in dependent variable (VDV) from partial least squares regression modeling for dry biomass and canopy height by sensor estimation models and model equations for height (combination ultrasonic and laser model) and biomass (two sensor model: laser and ultrasonic combination, and three sensor model: laser, ultrasonic and NDVI combination). † MIX-Mixture of alfalfa and bermudagrass; ‡ALL-All monoculture and mixed species from the alfalfa and bermudagrass experiment.

	Canopy Height	Plate Meter	120 MHz Ultrasonic	Laser
DM	VDV	VDV	VDV	VDV
Alfalfa	68.5%	18%	55%	64%
Bermudagrass	69%	23%	75%	78%
Wheat			72%	74%
MIX †	67.8%	19%	73%	73%
	3 sensor model	3 sensor equation	2 sensor model	2 sensor equation
Alfalfa	65.7%	(46.22 × Las) + 47.83(Son × NDVI)	65.5%	(46.9 × Las) + (43.13 × Son)
Bermudagrass	80.5%	(65.3 × Las) + 58.3(Son × NDVI)	81%	(65.7 × Las) + (49 × Son)
Wheat	75%	(118 × Las) + 108(Son × NDVI)	74%	231 × Las
MIX	78.9%	70.5(Las × NDVI) + 63.7(Son × NDVI)	78.5%	(61.3 × Las) + (53.9 × Son)
		Plate meter	120 MHz ultrasonic	Laser
Canopy height		VDV	VDV	VDV
Alfalfa		1.2%	57%	69%
Bermudagrass		6.1%	67%	77%
MIX		5.6%	54%	61%
ALL ‡		6.1%	55%	64%
			2 sensor model	2 sensor equation
Alfalfa			70%	(0.46 × Las) + (0.42 × Son)
Bermudagrass			77%	1.02 × Las
MIX			64%	0.017(Las × Son)
ALL			65%	(0.74 × Las) + (0.2 × Son)

Table 5. Sensor model ranking based on Error, Consistency, and Mean Agreement Score (ECMA) † MPE (0.19), Standard Deviation of MPE (0.36) and R^2 (0.87) for measured were calculated from paired bermudagrass plots. ‡ MIX-Mixture of alfalfa and bermudagrass.

Forage Type	Measure/Estimation Method	Mean	Mean-Percent Error (MPE †)	Standard Deviation MPE †	R^2-Measured to Estimated †	ECMA Score
			DM (t ha^{-1})			
Alfalfa	Measured DM	2.36				
Alfalfa	1	2.16	0.31	0.27	0.69	0.150
Alfalfa	5	3.02	0.30	0.24	0.63	0.083
Alfalfa	3	2.36	0.40	0.35	0.68	0.019
Alfalfa	7	2.16	0.53	0.67	0.13	0.005
Alfalfa	6	3.02	0.68	0.53	0.63	0.002
Bermudagrass	Measured DM †	3.33	0.19	0.36	0.87	
Bermudagrass	3	3.41	0.32	0.57	0.85	0.069
Bermudagrass	1	3.45	0.36	0.6	0.81	0.033
Bermudagrass	6	3.54	0.36	0.55	0.82	0.022
Bermudagrass	5	3.98	0.47	0.65	0.82	0.005
Bermudagrass	7	1.9	0.63	0.69	0.25	<0.000
MIX ‡	Measured DM	2.15				
MIX	1	1.83	0.30	0.26	0.79	0.035
MIX	3	2.37	0.40	0.52	0.78	0.019
MIX	6	2.76	0.68	0.79	0.55	0.002
MIX	7	1.66	0.48	0.58	0.17	0.001
MIX	5	3.1	0.85	0.91	0.55	0.001
Wheat	Measured DM	2.47				
Wheat	1	2.74	0.41	0.65	0.81	0.013
Wheat	3	3.18	0.63	0.94	0.80	0.002
			Canopy height (cm)			
Alfalfa	Measured height	30.8				
Alfalfa	9	22.5	0.30	0.17	0.61	0.04
Alfalfa	8	21.0	0.33	0.18	0.59	0.03
Bermudagrass	Measured height	36.1				
Bermudagrass	8	29.0	0.21	0.12	0.79	4.05
Bermudagrass	9	26.0	0.28	0.13	0.84	2.29
MIX	Measured height	28.2				
MIX	9	18.5	0.35	0.19	0.57	0.88
MIX	8	7.2	0.77	0.17	0.59	0.21

3.3. Post Hoc Comparisons

3.3.1. Sensor Estimation Models and Measured Biomass/Canopy Height Comparisons

Sensor models consistently overestimated small destructively measured biomass values and underestimated large values. Order of mean estimates for measured biomass and sensor-estimated biomass agreed except in the grass-legume mixture. In this case of order inconsistency, only the greatest biomass categories were inconsistent with measured values (>5.51 t·ha^{-1}).

The three sensor model (model 1) consistently produced lower biomass estimates than did the dual sensor model (model 3) for all species (Table 6).

Table 6. Mean estimates and LSD groupings for destructively measured DM and sensor modeled estimates of DM. † MIX-Mixture of alfalfa and bermudagrass.

Forage Class	DM Class	Measured DM	Sensor Estimate DM Models (t·ha^{-1})	
	(t·ha^{-1})	(t·ha^{-1})	1	3
Alfalfa	>1.1	0.85E	1.28D	1.5D
Alfalfa	1.1–2.2	1.65D	1.86C	2.09C
Alfalfa	2.2–3.3	2.72C	2.66B	2.89B
Alfalfa	3.3–4.41	3.6B	3.26A	3.45A
Alfalfa	4.41–5.51	4.88A	3.81A	4.01A
LSD		**0.22**	**0.44**	**0.44**
Bermudagrass	>1.1	0.67F	1.45E	1.58D
Bermudagrass	1.1–2.2	1.7E	1.97E	2.08D
Bermudagrass	2.2–3.3	2.96D	2.89D	2.93C
Bermudagrass	3.3–4.41	3.77C	3.8C	3.67C
Bermudagrass	4.41–5.51	4.99B	5.2B	5.02B
Bermudagrass	5.51–6.61	6.97A	6.19A	6.53A
LSD		**0.53**	**0.75**	**0.84**
MIX †	>1.1	0.83G	0.98F	1.53F
MIX	1.1–2.2	1.61F	1.26E	1.82E
MIX	2.2–3.3	2.67E	2.32D	2.84D
MIX	3.3–4.41	3.79D	3.02C	3.45C
MIX	4.41–5.51	4.92C	4.45B	5.03B
MIX	5.51–6.61	6.15B	5.06A	5.56A
MIX	6.61–7.71	7.06A	4.56B	4.94B
LSD		**0.15**	**0.28**	**0.27**
Wheat	>1.1	0.78F	1.51D	1.93D
Wheat	1.1–2.2	1.57E	1.79D	2.27D
Wheat	2.2–3.3	2.76D	2.81C	3.26C
Wheat	3.3–4.41	3.85C	4.33B	4.75B
Wheat	4.41–5.51	4.89B	4.98A	5.28B
Wheat	5.51–6.61	6.25A	5.48A	5.85A
LSD		**0.27**	**0.53**	**0.54**

Forage Class	DM Class	Measured DM	Measured height DM Estimate models (t·ha^{-1})		
			5	6	7
Alfalfa	>1.1	0.85E	1.18D	1.81D	1.7D
Alfalfa	1.1–2.2	1.65D	1.72C	2.65C	2.08C
Alfalfa	2.2–3.3	2.72C	2.39B	3.67B	2.31C
Alfalfa	3.3–4.41	3.6B	3.05A	4.68A	2.63B
Alfalfa	4.41–5.51	4.88A	3.51A	5.38A	3.07A
LSD		**0.22**	0.46	0.71	0.46
Bermudagrass	>1.1	0.67F	1.62E	1.44E	1.6B
Bermudagrass	1.1–2.2	1.7E	2.78D	2.47D	1.66B
Bermudagrass	2.2–3.3	2.96D	3.53C	3.14C	1.73B
Bermudagrass	3.3–4.41	3.77C	4.85B	4.31B	2.05B
Bermudagrass	4.41–5.51	4.99B	5.63B	5.01B	2.34A
Bermudagrass	5.51–6.61	6.97A	6.44A	5.73A	2.27B
LSD		**0.53**	0.97	0.86	0.62
MIX	>1.1	0.83G	2.23F	1.98F	1.49C
MIX	1.1–2.2	1.61F	2.88E	2.56E	1.49C
MIX	2.2–3.3	2.67E	3.26D	2.91D	1.9B
MIX	3.3–4.41	3.79D	3.56C	3.17C	1.89B
MIX	4.41–5.51	4.92C	5.46B	4.86B	2.22A
MIX	5.51–6.61	6.15B	5.95A	5.3A	2.1B
MIX	6.61–7.71	7.06A	5.38B	4.79B	2.12B
LSD		**0.15**	0.36	0.32	0.25

Sensor models consistently underestimated canopy height for taller measured values but produced estimates within 4 cm of the lowest measured height from models 8 and 9. The only exception in minimum canopy height estimation occurred in MIX model 8 estimates where the estimate was 10 cm lower than measured (Table 7).

Table 7. Mean estimates for measured canopy height (cm) and sensor model estimates of canopy height (cm). † No height data occurred in this range for bermudagrass. ‡MIX-Mixture of alfalfa and bermudagrass.

Forage Class	Height Class (cm)	Measured Canopy Height (cm)	Model 8 (cm)	Model 9 (cm)
Alfalfa	>15	12J	16CD	16DE
Alfalfa	15–20	17I	14D	15E
Alfalfa	20–25	21H	16D	18DE
Alfalfa	25–30	27G	16CD	18DE
Alfalfa	30–35	33F	22BC	22CD
Alfalfa	35–40	37E	20BCD	23CD
Alfalfa	40–45	43D	27B	28C
Alfalfa	45–50	47C	26B	29BC
Alfalfa	50–55	53B	32A	35AB
Alfalfa	55–60	57A	35A	38A
LSD		2	6	6
Bermudagrass	>15	14I	13D	11D
Bermudagrass	15–20	16I	13D	11D
Bermudagrass	20–25	21H	17CD	15CD
Bermudagrass	25–30	29G	24BCD	20BCD
Bermudagrass	30–35	31F	25BC	22BC
Bermudagrass	35–40	36E	28B	25B
Bermudagrass	40–45	42D	30B	27B
Bermudagrass	45–50†	*	*	*
Bermudagrass	50–55	54C	43A	39A
Bermudagrass	55–60	57B	47A	43A
Bermudagrass	60+	66A	51A	48A
LSD		3	12	10
MIX‡	>15	12J	2F	13E
MIX	15–20	17I	3F	14E
MIX	20–25	22H	3F	14E
MIX	25–30	27G	5E	16D
MIX	30–35	32F	7D	19C
MIX	35–40	36E	6DE	19C
MIX	40–45	42D	7DE	21C
MIX	45–50	48C	22C	34B
MIX	50–55	52B	27B	38A
MIX	55–60	57A	31A	40A
LSD		1	2	3

The LSD values for biomass and height estimation models were greater than those for the measured values. These LSD values indicated more variation within estimates for both canopy height and biomass resulting in overlapping of mean estimate groupings in some cases. Due to the fact the groupings were based on measured canopy height and measured DM, those measured groups would be expected to express the lowest variation. Additional error is also likely introduced into the modeled DM mean estimates due to the fact that the destructively measured DM does not capture in entirety the vegetation being sampled by the sensors. This error is illustrated in the stubble height remaining after destructive harvest which is embedded in and accounted for by the sensor readings and subsequently inseparable from the sensor models and sensor based estimations. This type of error could account for instances of over estimation at low biomass levels. Radial growth expansion as vegetation matured as well as under canopy fill-in may account for instances of biomass underestimation.

3.3.2. Biomass Estimation Using Physical Canopy Height Measurements

Canopy height models varied by model and species, generally overestimating at lowest biomass categories and underestimating at highest biomass categories (Table 6). Model 6 overestimated whereas model 5 underestimated alfalfa biomass. Both measured height models overestimated bermudagrass biomass except for the greatest measured biomass. Biomass estimates for the mixture for both measured height based models overestimated at lesser values (<2 $t \cdot ha^{-1}$) and underestimated at greater values (>5 $t \cdot ha^{-1}$). Plate meter biomass estimation model ordered mean estimates the same as measured for only the alfalfa and consistently overestimated low and underestimated large measured values.

3.3.3. Destructive Biomass Measurement and Model Estimate Variability

Due to the variation associated with destructively-measured biomass, it is unlikely that an estimation strategy based on this method of measure could achieve accuracy or precision in excess of the method upon which it is based. This destructively-measured variability is illustrated by the R^2 of 0.87 from paired visually identical bermudagrass plots included in Table 5. A number of factors lead to error associated with machine harvest examples of which include operator performance, height and type of vegetation, and weigh mechanism performance due to environmental variables. The use of a sensor array to estimate biomass is subject to none of the factors in the same way the machine harvest strategy would be. Subsequently, basing the estimation of biomass by sensor populated modeling when constructed from machine harvest weight data will introduce all error associated the machine harvest into the model as well as any error associated with the sensor system. This will suppress the accuracy of the modeling due to the fact the number of error terms contributing to the calculation of biomass are from both the machine harvest as well as any associated with the sensors.

4. CONCLUSIONS

Using mobile sensor systems for biomass estimation can enable a greater rate of data acquisition than manual canopy height or destructive sampling provided an appropriate software option for data acquisition is employed. Results from this study illustrate quantification of only the canopy height with ultrasonic and laser sensors can provide for biomass estimation models equivalent to and/or more effective than those which include spectral components. This is an important distinction as the cost associated with assimilation of an active spectral radiometer into such a system can greatly increase costs. An increase of approximately 1% in dependent variable variation explanation was contributed to the system at a cost in excess of US $4,000. In contrast, height sensors and a DAQ would only incur a total cost of approximately US $1,500.

Additionally, sensor estimates provide equivalent and/or superior estimates when compared to physical canopy height measurement and plate meter biomass estimation methods. It is arguable that the same is the case for collection of sensor-based canopy height data, though a maximum height threshold of accuracy is likely according to the physical limits and configuration of sensors used. Due to the commonly accepted nature of physically measured biomass estimates for research applications, sensor-based estimation strategies which utilize species differentiation in appropriate cases and ultrasonic/laser proximal sensor combinations have, in this research, been illustrated to produce comparable and/or more accurate results. Consideration should also be given to the time savings associated with using a mobile sensor system. During the course of these studies it was noted man-hours needed for physical collection of these data (30 $h \cdot rep^{-1}$) were greater by a factor of 60 than the time needed to collect data with the sensor system (0.5 h). Furthermore, processing of data acquired using AgriLogger reduced man-hour requirements by a factor of 10.

In order for the greatest level of accuracy to be obtained, it is likely necessary to implement specific models for predominant or monoculture species though a general estimation model may produce acceptable estimates for mixed species. It may also be possible to stratify implementation of models based on height measurement. This would allow adjustment of coefficients to accommodate minimum and maximum values which can be estimated imprecisely if only one model curve is applied to the entire range of canopy heights and biomass levels encountered. Further examination of spectral data as a model component may be necessary for other parameters not examined in these experiments. Future examination of additional species is also necessary to develop models for estimating DM across different environments and production systems.

Qualification of relative vegetative performance based on canopy height and/or biomass would also be possible and could contribute to variety selection for plant breeding. Difficulties in system calibration and sensor data conversion to absolute measures could be avoided in a qualitative system. It can also be asserted that results reported for research could be based on sensor-estimated biomass without the expectation of appreciable differences than would be reported from destructively sampled methods or physical measurement based estimates. Estimating biomass without vegetation removal would be useful for plant breeders needing to quantify biomass along with seed yield. In addition, forage mass could be measured prior to and post-grazing to evaluate persistence and production under grazing that currently cannot be done. Ultimately, real-world production management decisions such as stocking rate adjustments or forage harvesting intervals could be made in a much more rapid manner.

AUTHOR CONTRIBUTIONS

Jeremy Joshua Pittman—Study design, data collection and analysis, sensor system compilation/assembly/operation, manuscript composition;

Daryl Brian Arnall—Manuscript review and editing, sensor resources provision and deployment, technical equipment advisement;

Sindy M. Interrante—Data collection, manuscript review and editing, study design;

Corey A. Moffet—Manuscript review and editing, data analysis;

Twain J. Butler—Study design, data collection, manuscript review and editing.

CONFLICTS OF INTEREST

The authors declare no conflicts of interest.

REFERENCES

1 Tucker, C.J. A critical review of remote sensing and other methods for non-destructive estimation of standing crop biomass. *Grass Forage Sci.* **1980**, *35*, 177–182.

2 Fricke, T.; Wachendorf, M. Combining ultrasonic sward height and spectral signatures to assess the biomass of legume-grass swards. *Comput. Electron. Agric.* **2013**, *99*, 236–247.

3 Lati, R.N.; Manevich, A.; Filin, S. Three-dimensional image-based modelling of linear features for plant biomass estimation. *Int. J. Remote Sens.* **2013**, *34*, 6135–6151.

4 Machado, S.; Bynum, E.D.; Archer, T.L.; Lascano, R.J.; Wilson, L.T.; Bordovsky, J.; Segarra, E.; Bronson, K.; Nesmith, D.M.; Xu, W. Spatial and temporal variability of corn growth and grain yield: Implications for site-specific farming.*Crop Sci.* **2002**, *42*, 1564–1576.

5 Sanderson, M.A.; Rotz, C.A.; Fultz, S.W.; Rayburn, E.B. Estimating forage mass with a commercial capacitance meter, rising plate meter, and pasture ruler. *Agron. J.* **2001**, *93*, 1281–1286.

6 Fehmi, J.S.; Stevens, J.M. A plate meter inadequately estimated herbage mass in a semi-arid grassland. *Grass Forage Sci.* **2009**, *64*, 322–327.

7 Dougherty, M.; Burger, J.A.; Feldhake, C.M.; AbdelGadir, A.H. Calibration and use of plate meter regressions for pasture mass estimation in an Appalachian silvopasture. *Arch. Agron. Soil Sci.* **2013**, *59*, 305–315.

8 Fricke, T.; Richter, F.; Wachendorf, M. Assessment of forage mass from grassland swards by height measurement using an ultrasonic sensor. *Comput. Electron. Agric.* **2011**, *79*, 142–152.

9 Hutchings, N.J.; Phillips, A.H.; Dobson, R.C. An ultrasonic rangefinder for measuring the undisturbed surface height of continuously grazed grass swards. *Grass Forage Sci.* **1990**, *45*, 119–127.

10 Escolà, A.; Planas de Martí, S.; Rosell Polo, J.R.; Pomar Gomà, J.; Camp, F.; Solanelles Batlle, F.; Gràcia, F.; Llorens Calveras, J.; Gil Moya, E. Performance of an ultrasonic ranging sensor in apple tree canopies. *Sensors* **2011**, *11*, 2459–2477.

11 Zaman, Q.; Salyani, M. Effects of foliage density and ground speed on ultrasonic measurement of citrus tree volume.*Appl. Eng. Agric.* **2004**, *20*, 173–178.

12 Scotford, I.; Miller, P. Combination of spectral reflectance and ultrasonic sensing to monitor the growth of winter wheat. *Biosyst. Eng.* **2004**, *87*, 27–38.

13 Sui, R.; Thomasson, J. Ground-based sensing system for cotton nitrogen status determination. *Trans. ASABE* **2006**, *49*, 1983–1991.

14 Aziz, S.A.; Steward, B.L.; Birrell, S.J.; Shrestha, D.S.; Kaspar, T.C. Ultrasonic sensing for corn plant canopy characterization. Proceedings of the ASAE/CSAE Annual International Meeting, Ottawa, ON, Canada, 8 September 2004.

15 Ehlert, D.; Heisig, M.; Adamek, R. Suitability of a laser rangefinder to characterize winter wheat. *Precis. Agric.* **2010**,*11*, 650–663.

16 Fumiki, H.; Omasa, K. Estimating vertical plant area density profile and growth parameters of a wheat canopy at different growth stages using three-dimensional portable LIDAR imaging. *ISPRS J. Photogramm. Remote Sens.* **2009**, *64*, 151–158.

17 Selbeck, J.; Dworak, V.; Ehlert, D. Testing a vehicle-based scanning LIDAR sensor for crop detection. *Can. J. Remote Sens.* **2010**, *36*, 24–35.

18 Ehlert, D.; Horn, H.-J.; Adamek, R. Measuring crop biomass density by laser triangulation. *Comput. Electron. Agric.***2008**, *61*, 117–125.

19 Henning, J.G.; Radtke, P.J. Detailed stem measurements of standing trees from ground-based scanning LIDAR. *Forage Sci.* **2006**, *52*, 67–80.

20 Hopkinson, C.; Chasmer, L.; Lim, K.; Treitz, P.; Creed, I. Towards a universal LIDAR canopy height indicator. *Can. J. Remote Sens.* **2006**, *32*, 139–152.

21 Freeman, K.W.; Girma, K.; Arnall, D.B.; Mullen, R.W.; Martin, K.L.; Teal, R.K.; Raun, W.R. By-plant prediction of corn forage biomass and nitrogen uptake at various growth stages using remote sensing and plant height. *Agron. J.* **2007**,*99*, 530–536.

22 Erdle, K.; Mistele, B.; Schmidhalter, U. Comparison of active and passive spectral sensors in discriminating biomass parameters and nitrogen status in wheat cultivars. *Field Crops Res.* **2011**, *124*, 74–84.

23 Hong, S.D.; Schepers, J.; Francis, D.D.; Schlemmer, M.R. Comparison of ground-based remote sensors for evaluation of corn biomass affected by nitrogen stress. *Commun. Soil Sci. Plant Anal.* **2007**, *38*, 2209–2226.

24 Jones, C.L.; Maness, N.O.; Stone, M.L.; Jayasekara, R. Chlorophyll estimation using multispectral reflectance and height sensing. *Trans. ASABE* **2007**, *50*, 1867–1872.

25 Gnyp, M.L.; Miao, Y.; Yuan, F.; Ustin, S.L.; Yu, K.; Yao, Y.; Huang, S.; Bareth, G. Hyperspectral canopy sensing of paddy rice aboveground biomass at different growth stages. *Field Crops Res.* **2014**, *155*, 42–55.

26 Gamon, J.A.; Field, C.B.; Goulden, M.L.; Griffin, K.L.; Hartley, A.E.; Joel, G.; Penuelas, J.; Valentini, R. Relationships between NDVI, canopy structure, and photosynthesis in three Californian vegetation types. *Ecol. Appl.* **1995**, *5*, 28–41.

27 Interrante, S.M.; Biermacher, J.T.; Kering, M.K.; Butler, T.J. Production and economics of steers grazing tall fescue with annual legumes or fertilized with nitrogen. *Crop Sci.* **2012**, *52*, 1940–1948.

28 Hakl, J.; Hrevusova, Z.; Hejcman, M.; Fuksa, P. To evaluate lucerne (Medicago sativa L.) height as an important agronomic trait enabling yield estimation. *Grass Forage Sci.* **2012**, *67*, 589–596.

29 Laliberte, E.; Norton, D.A.; Tylianakis, J.M.; Scott, D. Comparison of two sampling methods for quantifying changes in vegetation composition under rangeland development. *Rangel. Ecol. Manag.* **2010**, *63*, 537–545.

30 Kercher, S.M.; Frieswyk, C.B.; Zedler, J.B. Effects of sampling teams and estimation methods on the assessment of plant cover. *J. Veg. Sci.* **2003**, *14*, 899–906.

31 Pilliod, D.S.; Arkle, R.S. Performance of quantitative vegetation sampling methods across gradients of cover in great basin plant communities. *Rangel. Ecol. Manag.* **2013**, *66*, 634–647.

32 Golodets, C.; Kigel, J.; Sapir, Y.; Sternberg, M. Quantitative vs qualitative vegetation sampling methods: A lesson from a grazing experiment in a Mediterranean grassland. *Appl. Veg. Sci.* **2013**, *16*, 502–508.

33 Brownell, D.K.; Liu, J.; Hilton, J.W.; Richard, T.L.; Cauffman, G.R.; Macafee, B.R. Evaluation of two forage harvesting systems for herbaceous biomass harvesting. *Trans. ASABE* **2012**, *55*, 1651–1658.

34 SAS Institute. *INC SAS/STAT Users' Guide Release 9.3*; STATS Publishing Inc: Cary, NC, USA, 2012.

35 Wuerschum, T.; Abel, S.; Zhao, Y. Potential of genomic selection in rapeseed (Brassica napus L.) breeding. *Plant Breed.* **2014**, *133*, 45–51.

36 Chen, P.; Zhu, Y. A new method for winter wheat critical nitrogen curve determination. *Agron. J.* **2013**, *105*, 1839–1846.

37 Wold, S.; Johansson, E.; Cocchi, M. *PLS*-Partial Least Squares Projections to Latent Structures. In *3D QSAR in Drug Design*, 1st ed.; Escom: Leiden, The Netherlands, 1993; pp. 523–550.

38 Mehmood, T.; Liland, K.H.; Snipen, L.; Saebo, S. A review of variable selection methods in partial least squares regression. *Chemom. Intell. Lab. Syst.* **2012**, *118*, 62–69.

39 Chong, G.; Jun, C.H. Performance of some variable selection methods when multicollinearity is present. *Chemom. Intel. Lab. Syst.* **2005**, *78*, 103–112.

40 Gosselin, R.; Rodrigue, D.; Duchesne, C. A bootstrap-vip approach for selecting wavelength intervals in spectral imaging applications. *Chemom. Intel. Lab. Syst.* **2010**, *100*, 12–21.

41 Saxton, A. A macro for converting mean separation output to letter groupings in proc mixed. Proceedings of the 23rd SAS Users Group International, Cary, NC, USA, 22–25 March 1998; pp. 1243–1246.

42 Lauriault, L.M.; VanLeeuwen, D.M.; Turner, J.L. Irrigation and nitrogen treatments slightly affected teff yield and quality in the southwestern USA. *Forage Grazingl.* **2013**.